Cultural Considerations

 D0348442

 Risk Factors

 Examination Step-by-Step

 Preparation for Examination

 Teaching Self Assessment

 Sample Documentation and Diagnoses

CONGRATULATIONS

You now have access to Mosby's "Get Smart" Bonus Package!

Here's what's included to help you "Get Smart":

sign on at:

http://www.harcourthealth.com/MERLIN/Barkauskas/

A website just for you as you learn health assessment with the new third edition of Health and Physical Assessment

what you will receive:

Whether you're a student, an instructor, or a clinician, you'll find information just for you, such as:
- Teaching Tips
- Content Updates
- Author Information . . .
- Frequently Asked Questions
- Links to Related Products
- and more

plus:

 WebLinks

An exciting new program that allows you to directly access hundreds of active websites keyed specifically to the content of this book. The WebLinks are continually updated, with new ones added as they develop. **Peel the top layer only from the sticker on this page and register with the listed passcode.**

Barkauskas
PASSCODE INSIDE

Lift here.

If passcode sticker is removed, this textbook cannot be returned to Mosby, Inc.

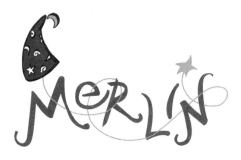

MERLIN

Mosby's Electronic Resource Links & Information Network

Mosby

A Harcourt Health Sciences Company

Health
& Physical
Assessment

Health & Physical Assessment

Third Edition

Violet H. Barkauskas, PhD, RN, FAAN
Associate Professor
School of Nursing
University of Michigan
Ann Arbor, Michigan

Linda Ciofu Baumann, PhD, RN, CS-ANP, FAAN
Professor and Associate Dean, Academic Nursing Practice
School of Nursing
University of Wisconsin-Madison
Madison, Wisconsin

Cynthia S. Darling-Fisher, PhD, RN, CS, FNP
Assistant Professor and Co-Coordinator
Family Nurse Practitioner Program
School of Nursing
University of Michigan
Ann Arbor, Michigan

Mosby

A Harcourt Health Sciences Company

St. Louis   London   Philadelphia   Sydney   Toronto

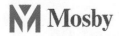

Vice President, Publishing Director: Sally Schrefer
Executive Editor: Robin Carter
Senior Developmental Editor: Kristin Geen
Editorial Assistant: Marie Thomas
Project Manager: Deborah Vogel
Project Specialist: Mary Drone
Design Manager: Bill Drone

THIRD EDITION

NOTICE

Health and physical assessment is an ever-changing field. Standard safety precautions must be followed, but as new research and clinical experience broaden our knowledge, changes in treatment and drug therapy may become necessary or appropriate. Readers are advised to check the most current product information provided by the manufacturer of each drug to be administered to verify the recommended dose, the method and duration of administration, and contraindications. It is the responsibility of the appropriately licensed health care provider, relying on experience and knowledge of the patient, to determine dosages and the best treatment for each individual patient. Neither the publisher nor the editor assumes any liability for any injury and/or damage to persons or property arising from this publication.

Mosby, Inc.
A Harcourt Health Sciences Company
11830 Westline Industrial Drive
St. Louis, Missouri 63146

Printed in the United States of America

Library of Congress Cataloging-in-Publication Data
Barkauskas, Violet.
    Health and physical assessment / Violet H. Barkauskas, Linda Ciofu Baumann, Cynthia
S. Darling-Fisher.-- 3rd ed.
      p. ; cm.
    Rev. ed. of: Health & physical assessment / Violet H. Barkauskas . . . [et al.]. 2nd ed. 1998.
    Includes bibliographical references and index.
    ISBN 0-323-01214-0
     1. Nursing assessment. 2. Medical history taking. 3. Physical diagnosis. I. Baumann,
Linda Ciofu. II. Darling-Fisher, Cynthia S. III. Health & physical assessment. IV. Title.
    [DNLM: 1. Physical Examination--Nurses' Instruction. 2. Nursing
Assessment--Nurses' Instruction. WB 200 B254h 2001]
    RT48 .H38 2001
    616.07′5--dc21
                                       2001045040

01 02 03 04 05 GW/RRDW 9 8 7 6 5 4 3 2 1

Contributors and Reviewers

CONTRIBUTORS

Mei-Wei Chang, RN, MS
University of Wisconsin-School of Nursing
Madison, Wisconsin
Chapter 6: Nutritional Assessment

Beverly Priefer, PhD, RN
Assistant Professor
Beth-El College of Nursing and Health Science
University of Colorado
Colorado Springs, Colorado
Chapter 26: Aging Clients

Gail Underbakke, MS, RD
Nutrition Coordinator
Preventive Cardiology Program, Department of Medicine
University of Wisconsin Medical School
Madison, Wisconsin
Chapter 6: Nutritional Assessment

REVIEWERS

Valerie O'Toole Baker, RN, MSN, CS
Assistant Professor of Nursing
Villa Maria School of Nursing at Gannon University
Erie, Pennsylvania

Rosa Cain, MSN, CANP
Assistant Professor, Division of Nursing
Coppin State College
Baltimore, Maryland

Rosemary Hathaway, MSN, RN
Assistant Professor, Department of Nursing
Missouri Western State College
St. Joseph, Missouri

Kerry Kokaisel, RN, MN
Instructor of Nursing
Mississippi College School of Nursing
Clinton, Mississippi

Sharon Lambert, DNS, MSN
Assistant Professor of Nursing
McKendree College
Lebanon, Illinois

Mary Ellen Lashley, RN, PhD, CRNP
Associate Professor, Department of Nursing
Towson University
Towson, Maryland

Jane A. Madden, MSN, RN
Assistant Professor of Nursing
Deaconess College of Nursing
St. Louis, Missouri

Thom J. Mansen, PhD, RN
Associate Professor, College of Nursing
University of Utah
Salt Lake City, Utah

Julie S. Snyder, MSN, RN,C
Virginia Beach, Virginia

Preface

Health and Physical Assessment reflects recent changes in the practice of health assessment by nurses. This new edition represents our beliefs in holistic health assessment as the basis for nursing intervention and practice. Health assessment is presented as the systematic collection of data that health professionals can use to make decisions about how they will intervene to promote, maintain, or restore health. Our goal for this text is to provide an innovative product that reflects and anticipates the ways in which nursing practice and health care are changing.

Health and Physical Assessment is designed for students and beginning practitioners. It contains the theory and skills necessary to collect a comprehensive health history and to perform a complete physical examination. These skills can be most effectively mastered when the text is used within a structured learning environment, which includes supervised student practice in skills laboratories or clinical settings. Because *Health and Physical Assessment* contains a great deal of substantive detail on examination techniques and findings, the student is not expected to outgrow the text but to continue to use it as a valuable reference in clinical practice.

Throughout this text, the consumer of health care is referred to as the client because the term implies the ability of a person, whether well or sick, to contract for health care as a responsible participant, along with the providers, in the health care process. Health care providers cannot expect consumers to accept assessment or intervention unless they have been actively included in the process.

ORGANIZATION

The content in *Health and Physical Assessment* is organized in four units:

Unit I: Taking the Health History, introduces the linkages from health assessment to subsequent steps of the client care process—diagnosis, care planning, and implementation. It also consists of thorough discussions of the art and science of effectively taking and recording a comprehensive health history for purposes of health or illness assessment and management. Chapter 4, which is *new to this edition,* discusses the assessment of health beliefs and behaviors.

Unit II: Holistic Assessment, with chapters on developmental, nutritional, and sleep assessment and cultural considerations in health assessment, helps the reader to understand and assess a client holistically.

Unit III: Physical Assessment, follows the traditional body-system approach and contains detailed, richly illustrated discussions of the physical examination of body systems or regions.

The chapters in Unit III are consistently organized and include the following headings and content:

Anatomy and Physiology
Examination
    Focused Health History
    Preparation for Examination: Client and
        Environment
    Technique for Examination and Expected Findings
    Screening Tests and Procedures
Variations From Health
Sample Documentation and Diagnoses
Critical Thinking Questions

Chapter 23, Integration of the Physical Assessment and Documentation, helps the reader to bring together all physical assessment components into a logical system for performing the comprehensive physical examination. Chapter 24, which is new to this edition, discusses clinical reasoning in determining health status, including an introduction to Nursing Interventions Classification (NIC), Nursing Outcomes Classification (NOC), and evidence-based practice.

This book focuses on the assessment of the healthy adult client, with a separate unit on the special assessment techniques required by clients of other age groups and with special health needs. Thus **Unit IV: Assessing Special Populations** includes chapters that present assessment techniques unique to pregnant women, children, older adults, and individuals with functional limitations. These client groups, which are frequently served by advanced practice nurses, are covered in a separate unit so the chapters can be assigned as required in a specific course of study and easily reviewed in one distinct unit.

FEATURES

- Chapter openers include the following helpful pedagogy: **Outlines** with page number references, **Learning Objectives**, and **Purpose of Examination** summaries.
- **Color photographs** of physical examination techniques are extensively used to enhance learning, and carefully crafted illustrations clarify significant aspects of the discussion, especially anatomy and physiology.
- **Preparation for Examination** boxes succinctly present needed equipment and special considerations for preparing the client and setting for an examination.
- **Helpful Hint** boxes provide tips from experienced practitioners for performing a thorough and accurate assessment.
- **Examination Step-by-Step** boxes provide a quick overview of the physical examination discussed in a chapter.
- **Risk Factors** boxes summarize the risk factors associated with common conditions and disorders for each body system.
- **Teaching Self-Assessment** is included in all applicable chapters and provides information on health promotion.
- **Cultural Considerations** boxes provide information on variations in findings that may represent cultural anomalies.
- **Sample Documentation and Diagnoses boxes** highlight the importance of documenting assessment findings and formulating nursing diagnoses and can serve as models for documentation in the clinical setting.
- **Critical Thinking Questions** help students apply what they have learned in the chapter. Answers are provided on the MERLIN website for this book.
- A **Glossary** is included as a reference at the end of the book and provides definitions of key terms that appear in the text. In this edition, glossary terms are bolded throughout the text where defined.

SUPPLEMENTS

An online **Instructor's Electronic Resource** to accompany *Health and Physical Assessment* is available. For every chapter in the text, the **Instructor's Manual** includes cognitive and psychomotor learning objectives, detailed lecture outlines, and suggested learning activities. The **Test Bank** includes more than 1000 questions in NCLEX format along with answers.

An online **Study Guide** is available that includes a variety of helpful learning exercises and answers to aid the student in obtaining a thorough understanding of the material covered in *Health and Physical Assessment*. Activities include glossary and anatomy and physiology review exercises, as well as multiple-choice, matching, short-answer questions. Laboratory and skills checklists are also included to guide the student through learning the components of physical assessment.

The new **MERLIN Website** for this book contains **WebLinks** for each chapter, **Content Updates, Teaching Tips**, and **Frequently Asked Questions** for students and instructors. It can be accessed at http://www.harcourthealth.com/MERLIN/Barkauskas/. This teaching and learning aid allows students, faculty, and clinicians to access the most current information and resources for further study and research.

ACKNOWLEDGMENTS

It is our pleasure to express gratitude to a number of individuals who helped us prepare this revision. Without their support and assistance it would not have been possible. First, we thank various editors from the Mosby and Harcourt Companies with whom we worked. During the preparation of this edition, major corporate restructuring occurred, and all of the editors and staff tried to make their organizational changes transparent to the authors. Over the revision process we worked with the following Mosby/Harcourt staff: June Thompson, Billi Carcheri Sharp, Robin Carter, Kristin Geen, Marie Thomas, Mary Drone, Deborah Vogel, and Bill Drone.

Violet H. Barkauskas
Linda Ciofu Baumann
Cynthia S. Darling-Fisher

Contents

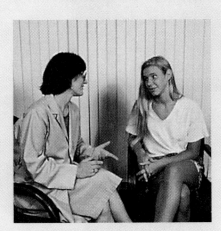

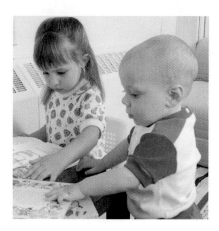

UNIT III
PHYSICAL ASSESSMENT

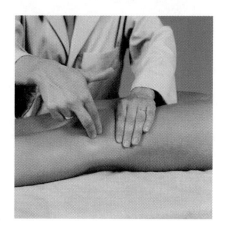

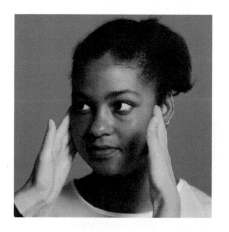

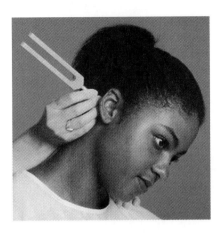

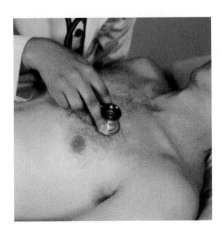

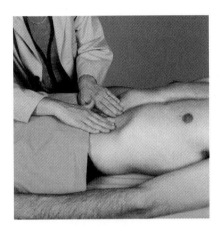

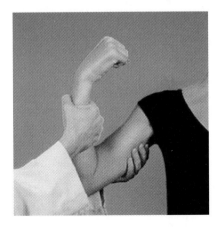

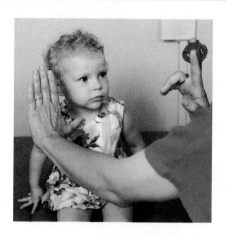

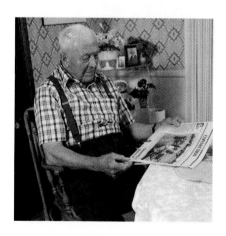

Health
& Physical
Assessment

Chapter 1

An Overview of Health Assessment

Learning Objectives

On successful study of this chapter and completion of related learning experiences, the learner will be able to:
- Describe the purposes of health assessment
- Identify the five components of the nursing process
- Explain the P-E format of nursing diagnosis
- Identify and explain how different organizing frameworks guide health assessment

Outline

PURPOSE AND SCOPE OF HEALTH ASSESSMENT

The purpose of health assessment is to collect, document, and analyze client information to determine nursing interventions that will influence the health status of a client. Health promotion expands the factors that we consider to affect a client's health. In health promotion, the practitioner assesses socioeconomic, cultural, environmental, occupational, social support, and lifestyle factors of an individual, family, or group in the community. *Healthy People 2010* is a preventive health agenda for the United States that identifies goals and priorities for health promotion, protection, and disease prevention.

The specific purpose and scope of health assessment will vary. A comprehensive, problem-focused, or emergency-focused assessment depends on a number of factors that include the setting in which assessment is taking place and the client's age, acuity level, and goals and concerns.

Comprehensive

Comprehensive assessment is usually performed when a client enters the health care system, through a visit to a primary provider or when admitted to a hospital, nursing home, or home care agency. In a primary care setting especially, a comprehensive assessment includes screening for age-specific health risks as a basis for health promotion and disease prevention services. When an ill client is admitted to a hospital, a comprehensive assessment will include data specific to the major health problem and reason for admission.

Problem-Focused

Problem-focused assessment is usually done to follow up on a previously identified problem or in response to a client's specific goals and concerns. For example, if a health care provider performs the follow-up visit for a client who was treated 2 days ago in the emergency room for a knee laceration, he or she would focus the history by asking about the degree of pain and limitation the client is experiencing and focus the physical assessment on observing for signs of wound infection.

A client might also self-initiate a problem-focused visit, such as a 35-year-old male who is concerned about his risk for skin cancer because his father was recently diagnosed with skin cancer. The focus of this assessment would be obtaining information on the history of skin problems, asking about sun-exposure and sun-protection behaviors, and performing a comprehensive skin examination.

Emergency-Focused

Emergency assessment is done to initiate lifesaving measures. Assessment is performed quickly and focuses on determining the airway, breathing, and circulation status of an individual.

THE NURSING PROCESS

The nursing process is a systematic approach used to gather client data, identify a client's response to a problem, develop expected outcomes, take action, and evaluate clinical decisions. The format of the nursing process consists of five steps: assessment, nursing diagnosis, planning, implementation, and evaluation.

Assessment

The assessment phase consists of obtaining subjective and objective data to develop a client database. Data collection includes health history and physical examination and results of laboratory and diagnostic tests. Subjective data are the client's perceptions, feelings, and memories of events that are obtained in the health history. Subjective data are difficult to measure or confirm. Objective data are observations or measurements made by the practitioner. For example, during an interview a client states that he has had an itch (a symptom) for 3 days. During the physical examination the practitioner observes a red scaly area of skin (a sign) and measures its size with a centimeter ruler. The components of the client database are shown in Box 1-1.

BOX 1-1

COMPONENTS OF A CLIENT DATABASE

Health history: subjective data, symptoms—based on what the client says
Physical examination: objective data, signs—based on what the examiner sees, hears, smells, and feels
Laboratory and diagnostic data: objective data—based on available technologies for analyzing biological, psychological, and physical functions

Once the database is collected, the practitioner may validate some of the information. This can be done through clarification with the client or by repeating any unclear or inconsistent portions of the history or physical examination. Data is then clustered into patterns based on the practitioner's knowledge and experience.

Nursing Diagnosis

The second step, diagnosing, involves interpretation or analysis of the data to determine actual or potential health problems. **Nursing diagnoses** are the basis for selecting nursing interventions. Nursing diagnoses reflect the client's response to actual or potential problems that can be prevented, resolved, or reduced through independent nursing interventions. The nursing focus is holistic and includes comfort as well as cure measures. The list of standard nursing diagnostic statements endorsed by the North American Nursing Diagnosis Association (NANDA) appears on the inside back cover of the text.

A nursing diagnosis is stated in a problem–etiology (P-E) format. Following is a sample nursing diagnosis:
   Problem (P)—Impaired physical mobility
   Etiology (E)—"related to" a fractured tibia; status after cast application
   Diagnostic statement—Impaired Physical Mobility Related to a Fractured Tibia After Cast Application
The database will include defining characteristics that support the diagnosis, such as statements by the client that she cannot walk without help and feels clumsy and observation by the practitioner that the client is wearing a short leg cast and uses crutches to ambulate.

When nursing diagnoses are recorded in this manner, any practitioner reading the diagnostic statement is able to determine how the diagnosis was reached. In addition, nursing diagnoses written in P–E format provide clues about possible nursing interventions by indicating the diagnostic label and other contributing conditions that have influenced the client's response. In this way, nursing diagnoses can also assist in the planning phase of the nursing process. For example, the diagnosis in Figure 1-1 suggests planning interventions that would allow the client to ventilate feelings regarding the loss of a leg. Another suggested intervention would be fostering the client's independence by encouraging self-care and personal decision making.

HELPFUL HINT

A nursing diagnosis is *not* a:
• Diagnostic test (schedule for mammogram)
• Nursing problem (difficulty visualizing cervix)
• Medical diagnosis (fractured tibia)
• Nursing goal (teach breast self-examination)

Whenever you develop more than one diagnosis, assign priority to each diagnosis to plan care. In your plan, first address any diagnoses that might be life threatening, such as:

Violence: risk for self-directed related to expression of suicidal thoughts and possession of a handgun.

After emergency needs are addressed, prioritize diagnoses based on what the client indicates is important to him or her. You may prioritize other needs that do not directly relate to a specific, current problem as intermediate or low priority. Some nursing diagnoses will address health promotion and protection, such as risk for injury related to not using a seatbelt when driving. An organizing framework, such as Maslow's hierarchy of needs (Box 1-2), will help you assign priorities.

Planning

In the planning step, establish goals and identify outcomes to let others know what is to be accomplished within a specific timeframe. The client's preferences and expectations must be assessed before goals are established. Short-term goals are those that can be met relatively quickly (days or weeks), and long-term goals can be met over months or years. For example, a short-term goal for a client would be,

"Increase skill in breast self-examination (BSE)." The long-term goal would be, "Client incorporates monthly BSE into lifestyle habits."

Outcomes are the specific measurable events associated with each goal, including a timeframe by which the expected outcomes should be accomplished. The *client outcome* is a statement of behavior that demonstrates an improvement in, or resolution of, the problem.

To continue with the previous example, the client outcome related to the short-term goal would be, "The client will be able to correctly perform a BSE after observing a demonstration." The outcome related to the long-term goal would be, "At 1-year follow-up the client will report performing monthly BSE." Each of these outcomes is stated in measurable terms, one verified by the practitioner observing BSE and one by client self-report (Box 1-3).

Implementation

Once you have prioritized and identified client outcomes, record a plan of action and specific nursing strategies for meeting the goals. When listing nursing interventions, include when the action should be done; who should be involved; and

---

BOX 1-2

MASLOW'S HIERARCHY OF NEEDS

1. Physiological needs—oxygen, food, elimination, temperature control, sex, movement, rest, comfort
2. Safety and security—safety from physical or psychological threat; protection, continuity, stability, lack of danger
3. Love and belonging—affiliation, affection, intimacy, support, reassurance
4. Self-esteem—sense of self-worth, self-respect, independence, dignity, privacy, self-reliance
5. Self-actualization—recognition and realization of one's potential, growth, health, autonomy

---

BOX 1-3

NURSING PROCESS OUTCOMES

- A specific health concern is identified.
- Diagnoses are prioritized based on client goals and hierarchy of needs.
- Physiological functions are addressed first.

Short-term goals	Achieved in days or weeks
Long-term goals	Achieved in months or years

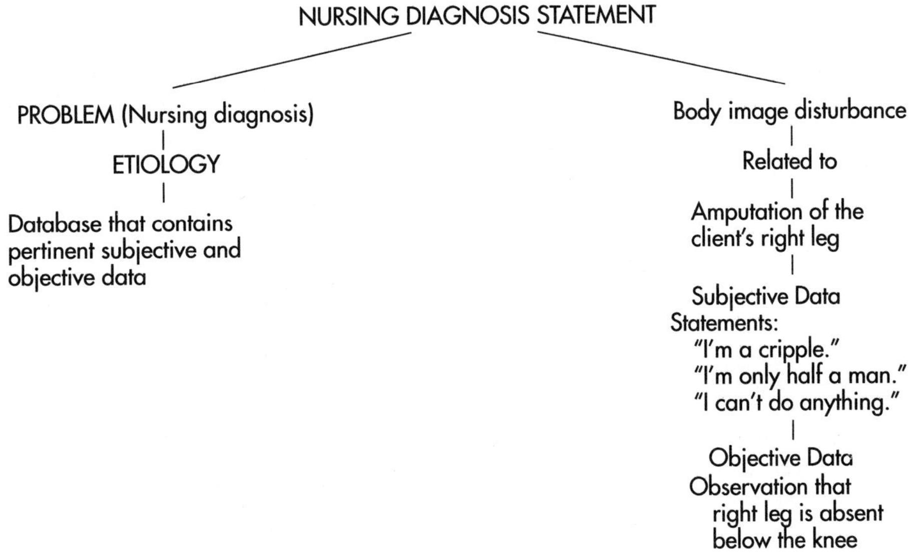

NURSING DIAGNOSIS STATEMENT

PROBLEM (Nursing diagnosis)	Body image disturbance
ETIOLOGY	Related to
Database that contains pertinent subjective and objective data	Amputation of the client's right leg
	Subjective Data Statements: "I'm a cripple." "I'm only half a man." "I can't do anything."
	Objective Data Observation that right leg is absent below the knee

Figure 1-1 Nursing diagnosis statement.

the frequency, quantity, and method to be used. For example, "The employee health practitioner will offer on-site 1-hour classes twice yearly on BSE technique to all female employees." Methods of intervention include assessing, teaching, counseling, consulting, and referring.

When implementing nursing interventions, determine the difference between nursing diagnoses and collaborative problems (Box 1-4). Nursing diagnoses relate to health problems or potential problems that health care providers can independently treat. Independent nursing interventions are within the legal scope of nursing practice and require no supervision or direction by others.

On the other hand, collaborative interventions involve direction from, or collaboration with, an appropriate and legally designated health care professional. Collaborative problems can be prevented, resolved, or reduced through collaborative or interdependent nursing interventions.

Advanced nursing practice involves a greater scope of legal authority for carrying out independent interventions. This scope of practice creates a greater overlap between medical and nursing practice. For example, advanced practice nurses who are certified through a national examination are eligible for prescriptive authority in most states.

Evaluation

The criteria for evaluation are the same as the goals or outcomes identified during planning. To evaluate goal achievement, compare the documented outcome criteria with the client's actions or behaviors. Once you have determined whether the client has achieved the outcomes, gather data you need to analyze what factors contributed to success or failure. Factors that may contribute to unsuccessful outcomes might include the following:

New problems developed
The original problem changed
The interventions were not appropriate
The goals were unrealistic
The intervention did not fit the client's needs
Incomplete information was obtained

After you have evaluated the goals and outcomes, develop a revised plan of care with new goals, outcomes, and interventions. Work with the client on all phases of this process, including how to revise the care plan. This evaluation process is ongoing as long as the practitioner has a role in caring for the client.

DOCUMENTATION

Assessment data must be recorded in an accurate and concise manner, without bias, to maximize the effectiveness of care. The written record is a legal document and a record of the client's health status. A clear record of a plan of care, expected outcomes, and evaluation criteria allow multiple providers to be involved in an informed manner in client health.

BOX 1-4

TYPES OF NURSING INTERVENTIONS

Collaborative nursing interventions—involve direction from, or collaboration with, an appropriate and legally designated health care professional
Independent nursing interventions—within the legal scope of nursing practice and require no direction by others

---

There are a number of formats used to document the nursing process. In the problem-oriented health record, a SOAP format (*s*ubjective, *o*bjective, *a*ssessment, *p*lan) is used to record problem-focused history and physical examination information, a diagnosis, and plan of care. Critical pathways are used in many managed care settings to map the outcomes or critical incidents of a client's recovery, based on a normal process of recovery from a specific medical diagnosis.

UNIQUE FOCUS OF NURSING ASSESSMENT

The specific goal of assessment varies for each type of health care professional, and each professional uses a unique organizing framework for collecting, analyzing, evaluating, and documenting the data. Although nurses and physicians seem to use the same general clinical reasoning process, these two groups of professionals reach conclusions that are different yet overlapping. The reason for this difference stems from each profession's major focus of concern.

The focus of assessment in medicine is to diagnose and treat disease. The organizing framework for medicine is the biomedical model and includes biochemical and biophysical systems. Traditionally how human psychosocial and socioeconomic factors impact health has not been a focus of medicine.

The primary focus of nursing is to diagnose human responses to actual or potential health problems. These responses may result in health problems that are not disease states, such as "risk for injury" or "caregiver role strain." Nursing assessment is holistic and focuses on the client's physical, psychological, and spiritual reactions to illness and the environment. Holistic assessment includes sociocultural factors and self-care behaviors. It goes beyond the individual to include family and community level information.

Shared Skills of Medicine and Nursing

Although assessment in both medicine and nursing is performed for different reasons, they do require the same skills for obtaining a client database. Both disciplines must be able to conduct a client interview and perform an accurate physical examination. Each professional will develop areas of expertise in assessment through acquiring knowledge, clini-

BOX 1-5

ELEMENTS OF CRITICAL THINKING

- Knowledge: past experience to build a knowledge base
- Attitudes: confidence, independence, fairness, responsibility, risk taking, discipline, perseverance, creativity, curiosity, integrity, and humility
- Intellectual: clear, precise, accurate, relevant, consistent, logical, complete, fair
- Professional: ethical standards, criteria for evaluation, professional responsibility

Modified from Kataoka-Yahiro M, Saylor C: A critical thinking model for nursing judgment, *J Nurs Educ* 33(8):351, 1994.

BOX 1-6

NINE HUMAN RESPONSE PATTERNS OF THE UNITARY PERSON FRAMEWORK

1. Exchanging: mutual giving and receiving
2. Communicating: sending messages
3. Relating: establishing bonds
4. Valuing: assigning worth
5. Choosing: selection of alternatives
6. Moving: activity
7. Perceiving: reception of information
8. Knowing: meaning associated with information
9. Feeling: subjective awareness of information

Reprinted with permission from *Nursing diagnosis reference manual,* Copyright 1991, Springhouse Corporation, Springhouse Pa.

cal experience, and exercising critical thinking for effective decision making (Box 1-5). Each professional must keep informed, through life-long learning, about new technologies for gathering objective data. Practitioners also need to be cognizant of evidence-based strategies for obtaining relevant history information to reduce the risk of health-related problems, such as obtaining a history about sexual practices to assess risk of sexually transmitted infection or screening for a woman's risk of domestic violence.

THEORETICAL FRAMEWORKS FOR HEALTH ASSESSMENT

Gordon's Functional Health Patterns

The most widely used organizing framework for nursing diagnoses is based on functional health patterns described by Marjory Gordon. The 11 health patterns allow for easy organization of basic nursing information obtained during an initial health assessment (see also Chapter 3). Gordon's functional health patterns are as follows:

1. Health perception–health-management pattern
2. Nutritional-metabolic pattern
3. Elimination pattern
4. Activity-exercise pattern
5. Sleep-rest pattern
6. Cognitive-perceptual pattern
7. Self-perception–self-concept pattern
8. Role relationship pattern
9. Sexuality-reproductive pattern
10. Coping-stress-tolerance pattern
11. Value-belief pattern

The Unitary Person Framework

Using a framework to guide assessment and decision-making is beneficial because it helps organize knowledge and provides direction for further investigation. Without the ability to systematically collect and analyze information, the nursing process is less effective in guiding care. A frame-

work also provides practitioners with specific terminology, which facilitates more effective communication between members of the same discipline.

The unitary person framework provides a model for grouping data in a holistic framework. The unitary person framework suggests that a person's health status is manifested by observable phenomena that can be classified into nine human response patterns (Box 1-6).

NANDA Taxonomy: a Nursing Classification System

The NANDA **taxonomy** is a nursing diagnosis classification system arranged in a hierarchy from the general to the specific based on the unitary person framework. The 1999-2000 NANDA taxonomy is based on the following 12 health patterns or domains:

1. Health-perception–health-management
2. Nutritional-metabolism
3. Elimination
4. Energy maintenance
5. Cognitive-perception
6. Self-perception–self-concept
7. Role relationships
8. Sexuality-reproduction
9. Coping-stress-tolerance
10. Values-beliefs
11. Safety-protection
12. Comfort

The next level of this system consists of choosing a descriptor for each pattern, such as "actual" or "at risk for." A practitioner can select the general response pattern and assess for signs and symptoms associated with that response pattern.

For example, the examiner wishing to evaluate the exchanging pattern might start by assessing the client's elimination health pattern. The examiner then decides which type of elimination to evaluate first—bowel or urinary. He or she chooses bowel elimination.

Next the examiner looks for signs and symptoms of diarrhea, constipation, or incontinence. Nursing diagnoses have been defined and determined to have certain signs and symptoms, called **defining characteristics**. These defining characteristics are cues for diagnostic reasoning.

A practitioner can also use the NANDA taxonomy to investigate a specific finding, such as an abdomen that is firm to palpation. Other cues may be associated with this finding (e.g., the client's complaint of a feeling of abdominal fullness). Based on these cues, the examiner makes a tentative diagnosis of constipation. The practitioner then tests this diagnosis by searching for the presence of its other defining characteristics (e.g., the client reports of no bowel movement for 3 days). If several of these signs and symptoms are present, the examiner can make the diagnosis of "constipation."

The predictive relationships between defining characteristics and nursing diagnoses are not perfect. These relationships are initially based on the observations of experienced clinicians who propose new nursing diagnoses. Research is currently being done to validate the defining characteristics of the diagnoses accepted by NANDA. Although the association of a cluster of signs and symptoms with a nursing diagnosis may be strong, no single group of characteristics ever absolutely indicates a particular nursing diagnosis.

Body Systems Approach

One classification system frequently used in physical assessment is the body systems approach. Using a body systems approach, an examiner might choose to evaluate the gastrointestinal system. This is a general category that consists of several organs and tissues. After choosing the system to assess, the practitioner, through history-taking and physical examination, focuses on evaluating the functioning of the various organs and tissues. With an abnormal finding, the examiner then searches for additional signs and symptoms known to be associated with this finding to make a diagnosis.

Examiners can also use the body systems approach to move from a specific complaint or finding to an evaluation of the functioning of one or more systems. For example, when investigating tachycardia, an examiner would first search for other cardiac-related signs and symptoms. However, during this search, the practitioner observes that the client has abdominal distress, has difficulty concentrating, and describes a smothering sensation. The diagnostic process might then involve assessing environmental variables for other data to confirm the tentative nursing diagnosis of anxiety related to situational crisis.

CULTURAL SENSITIVITY AND NURSING DIAGNOSES

Geissler (1991) points out that a nursing diagnosis of "impaired verbal communication related to cultural differences" directs the deficiency to the client when in reality the practitioner is equally as impaired. As the cultural diversity of the United States grows, health care providers will be challenged to develop nursing diagnoses that recognize the limitations of providers as well as clients. Cultural competence is a dynamic and conscious process of seeking skills, such as language, practices, and attitudes, to address cultural phenomena. Culture includes the values, norms, beliefs, and practices of a particular group. Culture has an effect on how an individual views the world and the meaning of events and experiences. Cultural differences and their implications for health assessment are discussed further in Chapter 7.

SUMMARY

Nursing diagnoses written in the P–E format contribute useful information to the rest of the nursing process. Nursing diagnoses are used to organize assessment data, as a basis for care planning and evaluation and as a focus for nursing documentation.

Using the NANDA taxonomy method of assessment and decision-making may be difficult at first, since practitioners traditionally have not been taught to organize their thinking in this manner. As more nursing diagnoses are developed, defined, and verified, the taxonomy will continue to be refined. This, in turn, will make the nursing diagnosis process easier.

This book introduces the practitioner to skills and techniques for obtaining and organizing data from clients. Examples in each chapter demonstrate beginning steps in clinical reasoning and documentation.

Critical Thinking Questions

1. Describe the components of the nursing process.
2. Name three frameworks used to organize health assessment data.
3. Identify whether the following information is objective or subjective:
   • A client tells you his age.
   • A client complains of insomnia.
   • You smell urine.

• You observe the client limping.
• A client states that she has diabetes.

For information that is subjective, how would the practitioner verify that the information is true or accurate?

4. A client who has had a recent below-the-knee amputation expresses concern that she will be rejected by others because of her deformity. State the nursing diagnosis using the P–E format.

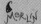 Answers are available on the MERLIN website (www.harcourthealth.com/MERLIN/Barkauskas/). And be sure to check the website regularly for additional learning activities!

Remember to check out the Online Study Guide!
www.harcourthealth.com/MERLIN/Barkauskas/

Interviewing Skills and Techniques

Learning Objectives

On successful study of this chapter and completion of related learning experiences, the learner will be able to:
- Name two types of health interviews.

- Describe techniques for conducting the interview that include types of questions, use of interpreters, validating information, and nonverbal communication.
- Identify common errors in interviewing.

Outline

PURPOSE OF THE INTERVIEW

Developing Relationships

The major purpose of interviewing a client before performing the physical examination is to obtain a **health history**. Practitioners must be skillful in communication techniques to enable a client to fully share life experiences relevant to his or her health status. In a comprehensive health interview the client has no current problem or concern. When the interview is problem focused, the practitioner also asks about the symptoms or other phenomena associated with the client's chief problems or concerns and at the same time observes for signs in the client's physical appearance or behaviors using careful observation.

Beginning with introductions, the practitioner observes and analyzes the client's reactions to the interview. The examiner must establish a climate of trust to promote interaction necessary for a **therapeutic relationship**, or an interaction that maintains a focus on the client's needs. As a practitioner, you can create a climate of trust by the way you introduce yourself, by how you conduct the interview, and through the environment you arrange for the interview. To create a respectful and warm environment, introduce yourself, including your full name and your role in the agency;

describe your understanding of the purpose of the interview; and address the client by his or her full name or surname (Figure 2-1).

Another way to promote trust and acknowledge the client as an active participant in the interview is to ask about the client's primary concerns and goals for the visit. Use communication skills that create a climate in which the client feels free to talk about his or her health condition. These strategies are necessary for obtaining the most reliable data about both the client's physical and mental status (see Chapter 19).

Adapting the Interview to the Client

The interview will be modified by the age of the client, the reason for the visit, and the existing relationship between you and the client (see Chapter 26). If a practitioner does not speak the same language as the client, an interpreter will be needed (Box 2-1). A young child will be accompanied by a parent or adult who will be the major source of information. It is important to remember that although the adult may be providing the verbal information, the child needs to feel included in the interview. Introduce yourself to the child, ask the child questions, and let the child touch equipment.

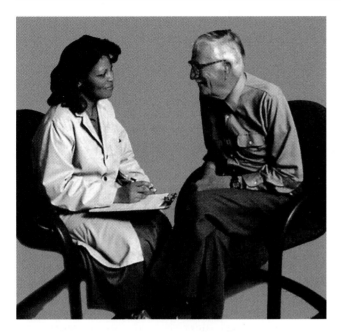

Figure 2-1 Establishing a climate that is comfortable and respectful to the client promotes communication.

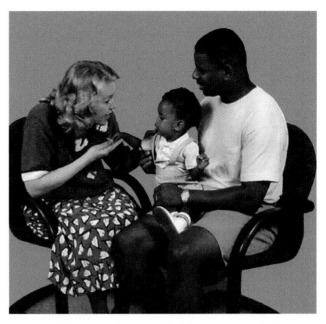

Figure 2-2 The practitioner modifies the interview by the client's age and the presence of other family members.

Adults may also prefer to have a family member or significant other with them during a health visit. Confirm that the client chooses to have another person present and acknowledge the presence and concerns of the family member or significant other (Figure 2-2).

On the first visit with a client who is being seen for a general health assessment, allow enough time to obtain baseline data and develop a relationship. When a client has an **acute** problem, spend less time on past history and put greater emphasis on understanding the immediate problem. A practitioner who has known a client or the family members for many years may be quite familiar with aspects of the client's health status and may need less time for a visit. However, a provider in this situation will need to periodically and systematically update history information.

Focusing the Physical Examination

Always ask for basic information, such as the client's reason for seeking care; his or her current health status; and information about allergies, medications taken, presence of stressors, and support available to cope with health concerns (see Chapter 3). The focus and types of questions you ask will vary according to the client's presenting problem or concerns. Chapters 10 through 28 include history questions related to specific body systems or to the health concerns of special populations, such as children, the elderly, and the functionally limited.

From information obtained in the history, you will determine what to explore in more depth during the physical examination. For example, if a client's major reason for a visit is a cough, nasal congestion, and fullness in the head, focus on examining the head, eyes, ears, nose, and throat (HEENT), as well as the lungs. A neurological or muscu-

BOX 2-1

GUIDELINES FOR THE USE OF INTERPRETERS

1. Unless you are fluent in the client's language, use an interpreter.
2. Allow extra time when using an interpreter. The interview becomes a discussion among people.
3. Avoid using family members as interpreters. They may respond to your questions based on their own knowledge without asking the client.
4. Make sure the interpreter has a basic understanding of medical terminology. Become familiar with the meaning of special words or phrases that connote practices or traditions of a particular cultural group.
5. Make sure the interpreter understands the confidential nature of the information obtained in the interview.
6. Direct questions to the client. The client may then direct responses to you directly or to the interpreter.
7. Some cultures are unfamiliar with direct questions. If necessary, adjust the type and tone of your questions to a style that is more conversational. Use short questions with minimal jargon.
8. Using repetition, validate information that you heard; summarize what you heard at the end of the interview.
9. Instructions to the client may need to be in writing in the client's language to ensure clear understanding.
10. Get feedback from the interpreter about the client's emotional state and comprehension.

loskeletal examination, for example, may not be necessary during that visit.

> **■ HELPFUL HINT**
>
> A self-administered history form helps the practitioner to focus the interview and can save time (Figure 2-3).

Therapeutic Use of Self

The use of certain personal qualities of the interviewer to support the client's perspective or feelings is called **therapeutic use of self**. For example, an interviewer might say, "As a woman I have also experienced . . ." or "As a mother I can understand how difficult this can be . . ." This technique can be especially helpful when the client's background, such as ethnicity, race, or socioeconomic status, appears to be very different from the examiner's background. It helps by establishing a common connection that can facilitate communication.

PREPARATION FOR THE INTERVIEW

A comfortable, private, and quiet environment is essential for conducting an interview. Meet the client before he or she has undressed since clothing and appearance provide valuable assessment data. In some settings, clients are asked to undress before they meet the clinician. If you are in such a situation, try to at least introduce yourself before the client undresses. Address clients using their full name or surname. Identify yourself using your full name and title. This greeting respectfully acknowledges the client and conveys your personal accountability as part of the health care team.

You and the client should both be comfortably seated and facing each other during the interview. To put the client at ease, directly state that the information you obtain will be confidential, recorded in the medical record, and shared only with those individuals directly involved in the care and treatment plan.

During the interview you will need to take some notes regarding dates, events, or short phrases related to specific aspects of the history. It is not desirable to complete the final report during the interview because doing so diverts attention from the client. You will need practice to determine what relevant information to document during the interview and what data can be later written or dictated into the permanent record. History forms that are partially completed by the client before the interview and flow sheets are useful devices for facilitating documentation of history information. Figure 2-3 is an example of a screening history form for a woman's health visit. When using a self-administered history form, know the reading level for whom the form is designed, using an assessment technique such as the SMOG. Clients who speak a language other than English should have self-administered forms available in their native language.

CONDUCTING THE INTERVIEW

Health History

Begin by finding out the client's **chief complaint**, or major reason for seeking care. It is also important to find out why the client is seeking care at this particular time. It may be that it was simply a convenient time or that an acute problem started to get worse. Other underlying concerns related to a chief complaint may exist. An individual may have had a "blue-black" mole for a number of years and now wants it evaluated "immediately." By asking what triggered the visit now, you find that a friend recently died of malignant melanoma and the client is now concerned about having cancer. Because you are aware of the concern, you can provide the appropriate evaluation, reassurance (if appropriate), and education about the warning signs of melanoma.

A client may also have a hidden agenda that is not obvious from the stated reason for a visit. By asking a question such as, "How did you hope I could help you today?" toward the end of the interview, you can identify the client's underlying concerns, as well as address the health issues obvious to a clinician (Molde, 1986).

You may also obtain data from secondary sources, such as parents, guardians, family members, significant others, written records, and interpreters. However, the client must sign a written consent for a provider to obtain information from other existing health records. The use of interpreters is discussed in more detail later in this chapter.

Client Explanatory Models

You can ask the client a series of questions to uncover his or her explanatory model (Kleinman, Eisenberg, and Good, 1978). Answers to these questions provide a meaningful explanation of the events surrounding an illness and suggest the appropriate course of action. These questions also help to uncover the client's level of understanding about a health problem and are especially useful when the client is from another culture. The following are examples of such questions.

What do you think caused your problem?
Why do you think it started when it did?
What do you think your illness does to you?
What are the symptoms?
How long do you think it will last?

Based on what you learn, you can develop a plan that will be sensitive to the client's needs and level of understanding.

INTERVIEW TECHNIQUES

Start with the concerns the client stated in the chief complaint. Be aware of the pace of your questions and the tone of your voice. You do not want to appear rushed or abrupt.

Types of Questions

Open-Ended Questions. Open the interview with a broad opening statement, such as, "Tell me what brings you here today." You can prompt the client to explain details using minimal verbal activity. For example, you might say, "Your concerns today are . . . ?"

> **■ HELPFUL HINT**
>
> To ask the clearest questions, use simple words. For example, it is better to ask, "Does Quan have pain?" than to ask, "Is Quan experiencing any discomfort?" when obtaining information from a secondary source.

UNIVERSITY HEALTH SERVICES
UNIVERSITY OF WISCONSIN-MADISON
1552 University Avenue
905 University Avenue
Madison, WI 53705

MR# _____

Name _____

BD _____ Sex _____

ID# _____

Women's Health Exam

The reason for this visit is: _____
Please list all medications you are taking: _____
Are you allergic to or ever had a reaction to:

☐ No known allergies   ☐ Sulfa   ☐ Local anesthetics   ☐ Penicillin   ☐ Aspirin   ☐ Iodine
☐ Tetracycline   ☐ Metals   ☐ Other _____

On a typical day:
1. How many cigarettes do you smoke? _____
2. How many meals do you eat? _____
3. Have you ever tried to lose or gain weight? ☐ Yes ☐ No
   Check the ways you have tried to lose weight in the past:
   ☐ none   ☐ diet pills   ☐ fasting
   ☐ laxatives   ☐ skipping meals   ☐ vomiting
   ☐ water pills   ☐ very low calorie diet   ☐ exercise
   ☐ other: _____
4. What are you doing to protect yourself against AIDS? _____
5. Do you drink alcohol or use drugs? _____
6. Do you think your use of alcohol or other drugs has ever caused problems for you? _____
7. Do you feel down hearted and blue much of the time? _____
8. Are you experiencing any mental or physical abuse in your relationships? _____

Are you currently sexually active?   ☐ yes ☐ no
   If **yes**, with: ☐ men   ☐ women   ☐ both

Do you have any specific problems related to this activity? ☐ yes ☐ no
   If **yes**, please explain _____

Has your partner(s) had more than one sex partner in the past three months?   ☐ yes ☐ no

Has your partner recently been treated for a sexually transmitted disease? (STD)   ☐ yes ☐ no

Does your partner(s) have STD symptoms?   ☐ yes ☐ no

Are you using condoms to prevent infection?   ☐ yes ☐ no

Do you have any vaginal itching or unusual discharge today?   ☐ yes ☐ no
   If **yes**, please explain _____

FAMILY HISTORY:
Birth parents, brothers or sisters ever have:

		YES	NO	
a.	Diabetes	☐	☐	_____
b.	Death from heart attack before age 50	☐	☐	_____
c.	High blood fat levels (i.e., cholesterol)	☐	☐	_____
d.	High blood pressure	☐	☐	_____
e.	Breast/uterine/ovarian cancer	☐	☐	_____

PERSONAL HISTORY: (Do you have?)

	YES	NO	
Acne	☐	☐	_____
Blood clots in veins	☐	☐	_____
Blurred, loss of or double vision	☐	☐	_____
Breast problems/lump/nipple discharge/surgery	☐	☐	_____
Cancer	☐	☐	_____
Depression	☐	☐	_____
Diabetes	☐	☐	_____
Gall Bladder Disease	☐	☐	_____
Heart problems/murmur/rheumatic fever	☐	☐	_____
High Blood Pressure	☐	☐	_____
High cholesterol	☐	☐	_____
Kidney & Bladder Problems	☐	☐	_____
Migraine Headaches	☐	☐	_____
Mom took DES to prevent miscarriage	☐	☐	_____
Mono/Hepatitis	☐	☐	_____
Neurologic disorders/seizures/numbness	☐	☐	_____
Severe pain or swelling in legs	☐	☐	_____
Severe chest pain/difficulty breathing	☐	☐	_____
Stroke	☐	☐	_____
Thyroid problems	☐	☐	_____

GYNECOLOGY HISTORY:
When did your last menstrual period begin? _____
How old were you when you first started to menstruate? _____
How long do you menstruate? _____
☐ light   ☐ moderate   ☐ heavy
Do you have cramps with your period? _____
Do you bleed or spot between periods? _____
How often do your periods come? (first day to first day) _____
Have you ever had a pelvic exam before?   YES   NO

Date of your last pap smear: _____   NORMAL ABNORMAL
Are you using contraception now?   YES   NO
   If **yes**, which method _____
Have you ever had a pelvic infection (PID)? _____
Have you ever had an ovarian cyst? _____
Have you ever been pregnant?
   If yes, check one: ☐ aborted   ☐ delivered
Were you using a birth control method? _____

PROGRESS NOTES

Figure 2-3 Self-administered history form.

The aim of an open-ended question is to elicit a response that is more than one or two words. A client will answer this type of question by describing signs or symptoms in his or her own words and at his or her own pace. Examples of open-ended questions are, "Can you tell me a little about yourself?" or "How have you been feeling since your last visit?" A risk of asking an open-ended question is that the client may be unable to focus on the topic being asked or may take an excessive amount of time to tell his or her story. In such cases you will need to focus the interview.

Closed-Ended Questions. A closed-ended question requires a response of one or two words, such as "yes" or "no," or a brief statement regarding marital status, age, or a list of medications the client may be taking. An examiner asks closed-ended questions when specific information is required, such as the client's age or the possible presence of a specific health risk (e.g., smoking), or when the client has a limited ability to respond (e.g., because of anxiety, lack of verbal skill, or physical discomfort). If a practitioner is rushed, he or she may ask more closed-ended questions to speed up the process of obtaining a history of the problem. A word of caution: Failure to allow clients to express in their own words the nature of their problem may lead to inaccurate conclusions and in the long run waste time.

Directive Questions. Directive questions lead the client to focus on one set of thoughts. This type of question is most often used in reviewing systems or in evaluating functional status. Allow the client time for reflection, at least 5 to 10 seconds, before you ask the next question. For example, you might ask, "Have you experienced any problems with urination in the past, such as infections or unusual frequency, urgency, or difficulty urinating?"

Permission-Giving Questions. Frequently you will need to ask clients questions about sensitive areas or concerns. One way to deal with such questions is to ask clients in a way that lets them know that it is all right to speak of such things to you. For example, you might tell a male client, "Many young men I see have questions or concerns about sexually transmitted infections; what questions do you have?"

Use of Silence

Periods of silence during the interview can be helpful for both you and the client. Short periods of silence allow the client to organize his or her thoughts. During silent periods, you can observe the client's emotional state and note nonverbal cues. Silence may also indicate that either you or the client need time to reflect on what was just said.

Validating Information From the Interview

Clarification

Use clarification to obtain more information about conflicting, vague, or ambiguous statements. By asking the client to elaborate on, or clarify, the thoughts and feelings he or she has expressed, you will communicate understanding. An example of clarification is, "You say you feel out of sorts. Tell me what you mean."

Restatement

Restatement involves repeating what the client has said using different words. It is a way to acknowledge that you are listening to the client and to validate your interpretation of what the client has said. An example is "I'd like to review the timing of your symptoms with you. You said that first you experienced a headache; then nausea and vomiting followed an hour later. Is that correct?"

Reflection

Reflection is repeating a phrase or sentence the client just said. This suggests to the client that you are still interested in the topic being discussed and you would like further elaboration on the facts or feelings involved. An example of reflection follows:

> Client: I love my children, but sometimes they are so
> misbehaved that I am afraid I'll hurt them.
> Interviewer: You are afraid you might hurt them?

Use reflection to describe nonverbal behavior and ask the client what it means. For example, "I notice that you haven't taken your sunglasses off. Is there a reason?" Verbalizing that you perceive what the client feels communicates empathy. For example, "I see you have tears in your eyes. You must feel quite sad about this."

Confrontation

In confrontation, you make the client aware that what you observe is not consistent with what he or she said. An example is, "You are telling me how depressed you feel, but I notice you are smiling a lot." Another example is, "You said you were so sick this morning you stayed home from work, yet you show no distress now. Can you help me understand what is going on?"

Interpretation

During **interpretation**, you share with the client the conclusion you have drawn from the information you obtained in the interview. Sharing your interpretation or the meaning of the facts provides the client with an opportunity to confirm, deny, or offer an alternative interpretation.

Summary

The use of summary is a technique that orders and condenses the information obtained during an interview to help clarify the situation being discussed. This is particularly useful when you obtain information from a client who has difficulty conveying the sequence of events.

When you terminate the interview, it may be helpful to summarize the information you obtained to highlight the main areas discussed. A summary also allows the client to assess whether information pertinent to his or her health problem was completely obtained and can help demonstrate to both the client and the examiner what was accomplished during the interview.

Focusing/Refocusing

Focusing or refocusing involves guiding the direction of the interview to ensure that specific information is obtained.

During focusing or refocusing, you attempt to help the client expand on a particular topic of concern. It is particularly useful if the client comes in for an acute complaint but has multiple health problems. It is also useful if the client begins to ramble or avoids a particular topic. When attempting to focus the interview, acknowledge the value of the information being given but redirect the discussion to the problem at hand. An example is, "I would like to hear about your past history shortly; for the moment, I need more information about your headaches."

Nonverbal Communication

Body Posture

Body language is the conveyance of messages by movements or gestures of the body or limbs, facial expressions, and eye contact. Body posture may convey anxiety, boredom, attention, or indifference. An examiner comfortably seated conveys interest in the client and readiness to listen. These nonverbal messages influence what is being verbally communicated between the examiner and the client. In a closed-body posture, one holds limbs in a defensive position, close to the body as though hugging oneself. This often conveys mistrust or anxiety. An open-body posture is one that is more relaxed, with arms extended or hanging loosely at sides. An examiner who remains standing during an interview conveys a message of time urgency. An examiner who is seated comfortably during the interview conveys to the client that he or she will take some time to conduct the interview.

Facial expressions such as frowns or smiles are indicators of emotional states such as anxiety, fear, surprise, or joy.

Eye Contact

Use eye contact and eye movement to engage or remove yourself from a situation. You may convey the message that the interview is finished by looking at a watch or clock. A client who looks around the room while answering questions or talking and avoids eye contact with the examiner may have anxiety about the situation being discussed. Prolonged direct gaze into the examiner's eyes or an excess or absence of blinking might be cues to the client's mental status.

Mirroring Activity

Mirroring involves awareness of nonverbal aspects of the client's communication to you (e.g., speed and volume of speech and body position). Imitate or mirror these characteristics in an unobtrusive way. For example, if a client is sitting forward with her arms folded across her chest, you can also fold your arms across your chest and lean forward in the client's direction. This is an action that individuals who are engrossed in a conversation frequently do without thinking. Mirroring has been shown to increase the client's comfort level and sense of rapport. It is also a nonverbal way to evaluate how comfortable the client is with the discussion. If in the course of the interview, the client suddenly changes from an open-body posture that had been similar to your own posture to a closed-body posture, the discussion may have raised a sensitive topic or the client may have lost interest in the discussion.

Interpersonal Distance

Interpersonal distance is the distance between two individuals interacting. This may vary by the nature of the relationship or cultural practices. The distance most acceptable in the dominant culture of the United States is to be close enough to be able to extend one's arm to shake hands, to hear a moderate- to low-volume voice, and to clearly observe the client. Trust is best developed from this distance.

Touch

Touch is a powerful form of communicating. It precedes speech in every person's life. Cultural traditions prescribe the ritual of touch or define the taboos. For example, in North American middle-class culture touch (when used by health care providers) conveys a message of closeness, encouragement, and caring. A warm handshake can be a familiar comfort to a client who is concerned about a health problem and who is fearful of unfamiliar surroundings.

The meaning conveyed through touch depends on personal attitudes and beliefs as well as many cultural variations on using touch in communications. Some cultural groups may express appreciation and trust in the health care provider by hugging or initiating touch, whereas other cultural groups see touch as an invasion of privacy. The practitioner must be aware of the client's reaction to touch to avoid being viewed as intrusive.

Many Asian cultures believe that the head is the most sacred part of the body. The clinician should therefore obtain permission before touching an Asian client's head. Many Asians believe that the feet are the lowest part of the body, and it is therefore disrespectful to show the bottom of your shoe to the client or point your toe toward him or her.

Cultural Variation

If you work with a particular cultural group, it is necessary to obtain some understanding of the group's health beliefs and practices, as well as some language skills to facilitate communication. The use of interpreters may be critical (see Box 2-1). A useful guide for overcoming barriers in

Cultural Considerations
Nonverbal Behavior Variations

Appropriate nonverbal behavior is subject to considerable cultural variation. In the Euro-American culture of the United States, it is important to look directly at the person with whom you are speaking. In other cultures (e.g., Asian, American-Indian, Arab, Appalachian), looking directly at another person may be a sign of disrespect or aggression. In many Asian cultures it is considered inappropriate to openly express pain or sadness to a stranger.

cross-cultural communication is the LEARN model (Berlin and Fowkes, 1983) described below:

L   Listen with sympathy and understanding to the client's perception of the problem.
E   Explain your perceptions of the problem.
A   Acknowledge and discuss the differences and similarities.
R   Recommend a course of action.
N   Negotiate an agreement.

Given current projections about the number of cultural groups who will receive health care in the United States in the next 50 years, it is unrealistic to assume that health care providers can have in-depth knowledge of the health practices and beliefs of multiple cultural groups. It is unwise to assume that because a client is a member of a particular cultural or ethnic group, he or she holds a certain belief. Beliefs within a cultural or ethnic group vary as much as they do among different groups (also see Chapters 3 and 7).

Active Listening

Listening is probably the most effective communication technique available. **Active listening** is concentrating on what the client is saying so that subtle cues may be detected. Active listening gives the client the nonverbal message that he or she is "a person of worth" whose opinions, ideas, and concerns are valued. Active listening involves blocking out environmental noise and distractions, as well as intrusive thoughts you may have about what to do next.

Providing Support

Acceptance

Never discount or judge what the person says. **Acceptance** is recognition of what is said without necessarily agreeing. An example is "You say that you fear this pain could mean you have cancer."

Openness to More Information

It is important not to appear too rushed or impatient, because the client may hesitate to share concerns that could be crucial to identifying and treating a problem. Before concluding an interview, ask, "Do you have any additional concerns you want to discuss?" This question encourages the client to bring up important issues, which may save a great deal of time in the long run.

COMMON INTERVIEWING ERRORS

Giving Advice

By giving advice you may communicate to clients that they are not capable of making their own decision about how to address the problem. You also accept responsibility for the outcomes. A health care provider should provide sufficient information about risks, side effects, and available treatment and management options so that clients can decide what is right for themselves. A client may ask your opinion about a problem. Sharing your opinion is different than giving advice. Clients may be more willing to disagree with an opin-

Cultural Considerations
Developing Cultural Sensitivity

1. Recognize that cultural diversity exists.
2. Demonstrate respect for people as unique individuals, with culture as one factor that contributes to their uniqueness.
3. Respect the unfamiliar.
4. Identify and examine your own cultural beliefs.
5. Recognize that some cultural groups have definitions of health and illness as well as practices that attempt to promote health and cure illness, which may differ from your own.
6. Be willing to modify health care delivery in keeping with the client's cultural background.
7. Do not expect all members of one cultural group to behave in exactly the same way.
8. Appreciate that each person's cultural values are ingrained and therefore very difficult to change.

From Stulc DM: The family as a bearer of culture. In Cookfair JM: *Nursing process and practice in the community*, St. Louis, 1991, Mosby.

ion of a practitioner but may be reluctant to disagree with specific advice.

Changing the Subject

Changing the subject introduces a new topic inappropriately. For example, a client may be expressing concern about the discomfort of the examination, and the practitioner asks what medication he or she is taking. Practitioners may do this unintentionally when feeling, for example, both pressured for time and anxious about ensuring that they obtain specific information.

Social Versus Therapeutic Response

A social response focuses attention on the practitioner instead of the client. An example is a client stating that she just returned from a trip to South America and the practitioner responding by talking about her own vacation. The sharing of this story by the practitioner becomes the focus of the interchange. A therapeutic response focuses attention on the client. In the previous example, after the client states that she just returned from a trip to South America, a therapeutic response by the practitioner would be, "Did you have any health problems on your trip?"

False Reassurance

In an attempt to reassure the client, statements may be made that are not true, such as, "It will be all right," "You'll be just fine," or "You'll get over it."

Overloading or Underloading the Client With Questions

Overloading is continuing to ask a client questions before he or she has a chance to answer the first one. Underloading is

Cultural Considerations
When Relating to Clients From Different Cultures

1. Assess your personal beliefs about persons from different cultures.
   - Review your personal beliefs and past experiences.
   - Set aside any values, biases, ideas, or attitudes that are judgmental and may negatively affect care.
2. Assess communication variables from a cultural perspective.
   - Determine the ethnic identity of a client, including generation in America.
   - Use the client as a source of information when possible.
   - Assess cultural factors that may affect your relationship with the client and respond appropriately.
3. Plan care based on communicated needs and cultural background.
   - Learn about the client's cultural customs and beliefs.
   - Encourage the client to reveal his or her cultural interpretation of health, illness, and health care.
   - Be sensitive to the uniqueness of the client.
   - Identify sources of discrepancy between the client's and your own conceptions of health and illness.
   - Communicate at the client's personal level of functioning.
   - Evaluate effectiveness of nursing actions, and modify the nursing care plan when necessary.
4. Modify communication approaches to meet cultural needs.
   - Be attentive to signs of fear, anxiety, and confusion in the client.
   - Respond in a reassuring manner in keeping with the client's cultural orientation.
   - Be aware that in some cultural groups, discussion concerning the client with others may be offensive and may impede the nursing process.
5. Understand that respect for the client and communicated needs are central to the therapeutic relationship.
   - Communicate respect by using a kind and attentive approach.
   - Learn how listening is communicated in the client's culture.
6. Communicate in a nonthreatening manner.
   - Conduct the interview in an unhurried manner.
   - Follow acceptable social and cultural amenities.
   - Ask general questions during the information-gathering stage.
   - Be patient with a respondent who gives information that may seem unrelated to the client's health problem.
   - Develop a trusting relationship by listening carefully, allowing time, and giving the client your full attention.
7. Use validating techniques in communication.
   - Be alert for feedback that the client is not understanding you.
   - Do not assume meaning is interpreted without distortion.
8. Be considerate of reluctance to talk when the subject involves sexual matters.
   - Be aware that in some cultures sexual matters are not discussed freely with members of the opposite sex.
9. Adopt special approaches when the client speaks a different language.
   - Use a caring tone of voice and facial expression to help alleviate the client's fears.
   - Speak slowly and distinctly, but not loudly.
   - Use gestures, pictures, and play-acting to help the client understand.
   - Repeat the message in different ways if necessary.
   - Be alert to words the client seems to understand, and use them frequently.
   - Keep messages simple, and repeat them frequently.
   - Avoid using medical terms and abbreviations that the client may not understand.
   - Use an appropriate language dictionary.
10. Use interpreters to improve communication.
    - Ask the interpreter to translate the message, not just the words.
    - Use an interpreter who is culturally sensitive.

Modified from Giger JN, Davidhizar RE: *Transcultural nursing: assessment and intervention*, ed. 3, St. Louis, 1999, Mosby.

failing to answer when a client asks a question or failing to respond to cues. An example might be:

Client: "This is going to hurt." Client is wincing, teeth clenched.

Nurse: Smiles and prepares the injection.

Jumping to Conclusions

The following is an example of jumping to conclusions, or making assumptions without verifying information: A client who is sexually active states that she does not use a birth control method and the practitioner responds, "How long have you been trying to get pregnant?" The client might lack knowledge of birth control methods or may be in a homosexual relationship in which pregnancy is not a risk.

Halo Effect

Because of the "halo effect," the practitioner may neglect to ask about potential problem areas because the client appears to be happy, prosperous, and coping well. In fact, the client may have serious financial or psychosocial problems that he or she does not feel comfortable discussing. For example, although the practitioner might say, "Oh, I never asked Mrs. Smith about her alcohol intake; she seems like such a well-adjusted person and has such a nice family," Mrs. Smith may in fact have a serious problem with alcohol.

Biased Questions

Biased questions make assumptions about the client's feelings or behavior and may lead the examiner to make false conclusions. An example is "You practice safer sex, don't you?" This question not only assumes that the client is sexually active and knows what "safer sex" means, but also conveys a certain negative judgment on the part of the practitioner toward someone who does not practice safer sex.

Box 2-2 provides examples of appropriate and inappropriate sequence of interview questions.

CONTRACTING

The initial interview is the basis for establishing a client-provider contract. **Contracting** is an agreement between the provider and client that makes explicit the expectations of each party. For example, the provider might state that for the client to receive appropriate preventive care, the client will agree to make an appointment at least yearly. The client is then encouraged to respond. It is not necessary to label this agreement a "contract," but it is important for the client and provider to agree on the plan and modify it as needed.

Sometimes contracts are written, but most often they are verbal agreements. Written contracts are often useful when using behavior modification techniques for dealing with behavior changes, such as smoking cessation or medication taking.

Timing is important when the examiner introduces discussion of a contract. Allow enough time so that you and the client have exchanged introductions and you have some awareness of the client's needs and the purpose of the visit. However, it is important not to wait until the very end of the visit to discuss a plan of care or treatment. Adequate time should be available for negotiating any modifications to the course of action or plan based on the client's response.

BOX 2-2

INTERVIEW VIGNETTES

The following is an example of an appropriate sequence of questions. Can you identify the techniques of interviewing used?

Provider: Hello, Mr. Chang, my name is Linda Jones, the nurse practitioner at the clinic. What brings you here today?

Mr. Chang: I'm worried about my heart.

Ms. Jones: Worried?

Mr. Chang: Yes. I was gardening last week and noticed that it became very hard for me to catch my breath after raking only 10 or 15 minutes. I know this is a sign of a heart problem.

Ms. Jones: Yes, shortness of breath can be a sign of a heart problem. But there can be other reasons someone becomes short of breath. I need to get more information from you before coming to any conclusions. I'm going to ask you some questions about the symptoms you experience that cause you concern . . .

The following is an example of an inappropriate sequence of questions. Can you identify the common errors discussed in the chapter?

Provider: Hello, my name is Linda. I'm a special kind of a nurse. What's your name?

Mr. Chang: George Chang.

Provider: Well, George, what's wrong with you today?

Mr. Chang: I'm not sure, but I'm worried about my heart.

Provider: Oh, at your age it's unlikely you have a heart problem. And, anyway, it's my job to diagnose the problem. I just need for you to tell me what your symptoms are. Do you have chest pain?

Mr. Chang: No.

Provider: Do you have trouble breathing?

Mr. Chang: Well, yes, as a matter of fact, that was my biggest worry.

Provider: (Interrupts.) You don't look like you're having trouble breathing to me. By the way, exactly how old are you?

? Critical Thinking Questions

1. An English-speaking practitioner is seeing a Spanish-speaking client for the first time. The client is accompanied by her granddaughter who will act as the interpreter. Discuss some of the problems with this arrangement. What would be optimal conditions for conducting this interview?

2. Role-play how you would modify the conduct of an interview for the following:
   • A client with a hearing impairment
   • An adolescent
   • A female client who is accompanied by her two children, ages 2 and 4
   • A client in acute pain
   • A client who appears to have difficulty breathing

What types of questions would be most effective?

3. A 20-year-old client identifies her chief complaint as "I may be pregnant." Develop examples of closed-ended and open-ended questions that you would use in the initial interview.

MERLIN Answers are available on the MERLIN website (www.harcourthealth.com/MERLIN/Barkauskas/). And be sure to check the website regularly for additional learning activities!

Remember to check out the Online Study Guide!
www.harcourthealth.com/MERLIN/Barkauskas/

The Health History

Outline

PURPOSE OF HEALTH HISTORY

The health history is an extremely important part of the health assessment. The history-taking interview serves as the primary vehicle by which the practitioner establishes rapport with the client. The information obtained from the history enables the practitioner to assess and diagnose the client's health needs and problems and obtain knowledge of these matters within the context of that particular client's life. The health history not only documents the client's needs and problems, but it also provides a picture of the client as a whole person, in relation to the client's social and physical environment. Thus it registers both the strengths that will support health and care interventions and the health deficits and needs.

Other important components of the history database are the client's perceptions regarding health, illness, health care interventions, and experiences with health care providers and delivery systems. Understanding these beliefs, percep-

tions, and responses is essential for providing care that is relevant and, consequently, effective.

Much of the subjective information contributing to health diagnoses is obtained through the history. The physical examination provides the objective assessment data.

The practitioner implements the health history in two phases: (1) the client interview phase, where the information is elicited, and (2) the documentation of data phase, in which the information is recorded. The sequence for obtaining and recording a history, as presented in this chapter, follows a systematic method. The client interview itself may not proceed in the same sequence because of the nature of the client's health needs or problems, the condition of the client, the purpose of the encounter, or other contextual variables. Also, the presentation in this chapter is for a comprehensive health history. In many clinical situations obtaining the complete health history on the first visit may not be feasible because of time constraints. The practitioner

needs to prioritize which components of the history are essential for a given encounter. To prioritize health history areas for a given encounter, the practitioner needs to understand fully the essential components of a health history,
develop a personal scheme for taking a health history, be
able to develop priorities for obtaining history information,
and be ready to alter the content and sequence of the interview according to the conditions and purposes of a particular encounter.

The health history is usually done in the examiner's office, in the client's home, or in the hospital room. If the interview takes place in the examiner's space, the examiner
can control the environment to facilitate privacy, comfort,
and quietness. However, if the interview is done in the
client's space, the examiner must assess the environment
and, in some instances, alter it to facilitate an adequate interview. For example, closing the curtains in a multi-bed
hospital room or requesting that the television be turned off
in the home will make the environment more conducive to
an effective interview.

Whether the examiner or the client initiates the encounter, the client will have certain ideas about its purpose
and content. Clarification of the client's purpose and expectations for the encounter and orientation of the client to the
examiner's goals and methods early in the encounter will
minimize the potential for later misunderstanding and frustration. The client's priorities may be different from those of
the examiner, or the examiner may have an inaccurate perception of the client's goals. The interviewer must clarify
any discrepancies and negotiate priorities if the encounter is
to be productive.

There are various types of health histories. These include
the following:

1. A *complete* health history, as described in this
   chapter, is taken on the initial visit to a health care
   facility, where the health care providers within that
   facility provide comprehensive and/or continuous
   care.
2. An *interval* health history is used to collect information during visits subsequent to the one in which
   the initial database was collected. Depending on
   when the history was last updated and the purpose
   of the current encounter, selected information about
   current needs and problems and updates of health
   history information are obtained. This type of
   health history is done during routine, periodic
   health assessments or as a follow-up to a visit in
   which a problem was treated. In the latter case, the
   effectiveness of the intervention is evaluated.
3. A *problem-focused* or *chief complaint–focused*
   health history is used to collect data about a specific
   problem system or region. This type of history is
   collected during episodic health care encounters
   and emergency care encounters. In these cases, the
   systems involved with the presenting health
   problem are the primary foci of the history. Examples of such health histories are included in the

systems and region examination chapters in this
book.
4. *Special* health histories are done for various screening and assessment purposes. Selected components
   of the complete health history are used depending
   on the purposes of the history. An example of such
   a history is a risk-assessment screening for health
   promotion purposes.

When eliciting the health history, the interviewer should
strive for balance between allowing clients to talk freely and
tell their story in their own way and using time efficiently.
Clients must be able to provide information that they consider relevant, especially early in the interview. However, after the client has provided an overview of the purpose of the
encounter and any information related to specific problems
or needs, the examiner must probe, clarify, and quantify
client information in structured ways. Because the examiner
is the "expert" in history taking, he or she must take the lead
in managing the interview to obtain appropriate information
as efficiently as possible. Time is not an unlimited resource.
Often other clients are waiting for services, and the examiner must control the costs of encounters.

Because it is usually not possible to record the entire
health history during the interview, the interviewer takes
notes. Forms are useful in structuring note taking and are
appropriate for many data components. The interviewer
records as much of the health history as possible during the
interview, and the remaining information is added as soon as
possible after the interview has been completed.

PREPARATION: CLIENT AND ENVIRONMENT

Organize the environment for the history in a manner that
will increase the physical and psychological comfort of the
client (Box 3-1). At the first encounter, introduce yourself to
the client with a formal greeting and use the client's full
name. In a clinic setting, seat yourself facing the client, and
allow the client to remain in street clothes until the history
portion of the assessment has been completed. In a hospital
room, seat yourself in a chair next to the bed and face the
client. In a home or other setting, organize the seating
arrangements as comfortably as possible for yourself and
the client. In all cases avoid standing during the interview or
assuming a position higher than the client, for example by
sitting on the examining table while the client sits in a chair.

Privacy may be important to the client. If others have accompanied the client to the encounter or are present, ask the
client about his or her wishes regarding others' presence
during the interview. In a home situation, others may be
asked to go to another part of the home.

Make sure that you and the client understand each
other's expectations for the encounter. Brief the client about
the purposes and structure of a health history, and ask the
client about his or her expectations and questions early in
the interaction.

BOX 3-1

PREPARATION FOR THE HEALTH HISTORY

1. Establish an environment that is conducive to effective communication—private, free of distractions and interruptions, comfortable, and quiet.
2. Introduce yourself to the client with name and title.
3. Address the client formally by his or her full name. Ask how the client wishes to be addressed throughout the history and examination.
4. If children or others are in attendance, introduce yourself, find out their relationship to the client, and determine the client's wishes about the presence of the additional person(s) during the interview and examination.
5. Allow the client to state his or her expectations for the encounter, including the problems or needs about which assistance is being sought.
6. Orient the client to the purposes, structure, and components of the health history.
7. If this is not the client's first encounter with the health system and a record exists of past data and care for the client, review the major points within the record with the client. If the most recent encounter involved treatment for a health problem, determine the effectiveness of the interventions provided on the previous encounter.
8. Make some judgment early in the interview about the priorities for the encounter, given your and the client's constraints. Communicate and negotiate priorities with the client.
9. Allow the client to remain fully dressed until you begin the physical examination.

COMPONENTS OF THE HEALTH HISTORY

The health history described in this chapter is extremely detailed and complete. In many actual client care situations, it may not be possible, or even appropriate, to obtain the complete history at the first encounter, or at all. For clients who are receiving continuous care, the history can be done in portions during several encounters. For clients who require episodic care, decisions regarding the data that are essential for immediate therapy will guide the content of the history.

The beginning health historian should practice obtaining the complete health history to develop skill in interviewing and in recording data and to establish priorities for focused interviews. During this practice process, the learner will gain an appreciation for the information obtained from each portion of the health history and skill in eliciting information logically and efficiently.

The recommended format for the complete health history is as follows (see Box 3-2 for suggested scripts for the introduction of each component):

1. Biographical information
2. Client's reason for seeking care or chief complaint

BOX 3-2

EXAMPLES OF SCRIPTS FOR INTRODUCING COMPONENTS OF THE HEALTH HISTORY

BIOGRAPHICAL INFORMATION

"I will start the history by asking you some general questions about yourself. First, could you please give me the correct spelling of your full name?"

CLIENT'S REASON FOR SEEKING CARE

"Please tell me why you came to see me today."

HEALTH HISTORY

"Because some of the health problems you had in the past may have some implications for what we do today, I will now be asking you about your health, past illnesses, health problems, and immunizations."

"Because my advice must take into account your current health habits and practices, I will now ask you various questions about your current habits and medications."

FAMILY HEALTH HISTORY

For ill client: "Because others in your family may have health problems that relate to your problems or affect your treatment, I will ask you some questions about their health."

For well client: "Because others in your family may have health problems that relate to your current health risks and future health, I will ask you some questions about their health."

REVIEW OF SYSTEMS

Physical systems and functional status: "Up to now in the interview, we have concentrated on certain parts of your body. To have a complete picture of your physical health, I will now ask you a number of questions about the other parts of your body."

Sociological systems and psychological systems: "Because I want to know more about you as a total person, I will now ask you some questions about you, your family, and your relationships with others."

Developmental data: (Usually the interview up to this point in the history will provide information for this section.)

Nutritional data: "Because nutrition is important to health, I will next ask you some questions about your diet."

3. Present health or present illness status
4. Past health history
5. Family health history
6. Review of systems
   a. Physical systems
   b. Functional status
   c. Sociological and cultural systems
   d. Psychological system
7. Developmental data
8. Nutritional data

Biographical Information

General identifying and biographical information is recorded on the first page of most health care records. Often an assistant in the health care setting records this information, or it may be on the record from a previous encounter. Obtain this information early during the client's first visit or at admission. Otherwise, the information may be omitted and unavailable when later needed in an emergency or at a time when the client is unavailable or unable to respond.

In the introductory biographical section of the history, record the information listed in Box 3-3. If the information is already recorded, be sure it is reviewed with the client on each encounter to verify that it is up-to-date.

First, record the client's name. Because persons living in an ethnically homogenous geographical area often have similar names, it is important that this key information is exact. Precise identification, including first, middle, and last names, assists in ensuring accurate information retrieval and coordination. If additional identifying information is needed in the case of names common in that health care facility, record the parents' names, including the mother's maiden name.

The practitioner must be very culturally sensitive to the conventions used to name persons in various cultures. The common convention of presenting a name in the United States (i.e., given name first followed by middle names or initials with the father's family name presented last) can not be assumed to be the convention in other cultures. Actually, substantial variability exists across cultures, and the practitioner should learn the conventions represented in the cultures seeking care in a particular situation.

Next, record the client's full mailing address and telephone numbers. Also include the name, address, and telephone num- ber of one of the client's friends or relatives. This person should be someone with whom the client is in frequent contact and who would be willing and able to relay a message to the client in an emergency or if the client cannot be located.

The birth date, sex, race, ethnicity, religion, marital status, and birthplace entries are self-explanatory. Many health problems and needs are related to age, sex, race, ethnicity, or social situation. This information provides initial insight into the client as a unique person and can be correlated with the client's needs and problems discovered later in the history.

Justifiable reasons for recording the client's Social Security number include the precise identification of each client and access to health information in other health care systems. The potential for violation of client confidentiality can be a disadvantage.

A significant difference may exist between the client's current and usual occupations. The nature of the difference may indicate the severity of the client's health problems and the level of disability resulting from them. In addition, knowledge of past occupations might provide clues to past or present environmental conditions contributing to the present illness. A factory worker with a respiratory system complaint is an example.

Knowledge of the client's birthplace provides geographical information associated with the origin of problems and cultural implications for therapy and health maintenance.

If the current health care provider is not the usual and primary source of the client's care, record the name and address of the individual or institution identified by the client. In addition, document the reason that the client is entering a new health care system. The client may be in crisis, may be dissat-

---

B O X 3 - 3

CLIENT BIOGRAPHICAL INFORMATION

Full name
Address and telephone numbers
    Client's permanent telephone number
    Contact of client (person to contact in case of emergency)
Birth date
Sex
Race
Ethnicity
Religion
Marital status
Social Security number
Occupation
    Past
    Current
Birthplace
Health insurance
Usual sources of health care
Source and reliability of information
Date of interview

Cultural Considerations
Cultural Implication of Names

Names have special cultural significance. The conventions for naming persons vary across cultures. The traditional American convention for naming people is given name first, followed by any middle names or initials, with the family name listed last (the family name is characteristically the father's family name [patrilineal]). Some other cultures use other conventions. Examples follow:
- Family name first, followed by given name (e.g., Cambodian, Chinese, and Vietnamese names)
- Given name first, followed by father's given name, adapted by adding "son" (e.g., freidriksdottir [Icelandic])
- Given name followed by the patronymic without a family name (e.g., Russian names)
- Given name followed by husband's surname (if present), father's family name, and mother's family name (e.g., names in various Hispanic cultures; in the Cuban culture, a married woman drops her mother's surname and adds her husband's surname preceded by "de" and the final part of her complete name)
- Given name followed by father's first name and the family name as the last name (e.g., Arab and Greek names)

isfied with past care, or may be "shopping." If the past source of care possesses significant data about the client's health and if the client intends to continue in the current health care system, ask the client to sign a permission for the transfer of information. Later in the health history, you will have the opportunity to record, in some detail, past patterns of health care.

The source of a client's payment for care is usually included on administrative records. However, noting this information in the health history might be useful in guiding choices of interventions.

In some health care systems the biographical information section might appropriately contain advanced directives decisions and durable power of attorney information.

Next make a statement about the source of the information to follow. In most instances the source is the client, but do not assume that this is so in subsequent encounters unless the source is specifically identified. If someone gives the information other than the client, describe the nature of the informant's contact with the client. For example, in the case of a child, a history given by a grandmother, who resides with the child, should be viewed differently from one given by a grandmother who visits the child once a week.

Along with the statement of the informant, give an evaluation of that person's reliability. For example, you could describe the informant as "inconsistent," "unclear about recent events," "evasive," or "cooperative and reliable." Such statements serve as simple criteria by which the remainder of the information in the history is judged by other health care providers. In addition, this type of information may indicate a need to retake or supplement the history at a future date or to consult with other informants to verify the data.

In some health care systems the biographical information section might appropriately contain advanced directives decisions and durable power of attorney information.

In some cases a translator will be needed to assist with the interview. The translator may be a stranger to the client or a friend or family member. If such a person has been involved, note this information on the record along with the relationship to the client (e.g., stranger, family member, friend). Note also any effect a translator may have had on the reliability of the information obtained. See Chapter 2 for guidelines regarding the use of interpreters.

■ HELPFUL HINT

For effective history-taking:
- Determine the most effective balance between allowing the client to talk in an unstructured way and the need to control the interview.
- Avoid questions that can be answered with "yes" or "no" if details are needed.
- Clarify the client's diagnostic statements and conclusions.
- Be alert to concerns that the client is having difficulty in presenting.
- Avoid the formulation of premature conclusions about the nature of the client's problem.
- Avoid judgmental statements.

It is important to date the history. In a situation in which the client's condition changes rapidly, events can be correlated only if their temporal relationships are known.

■ HELPFUL HINT

When taking a history through an interpreter:
- Ask the interpreter to translate as close to verbatim as possible.
- Advise the interpreter to clarify the meaning of a message from the practitioner if it is unclear and to avoid translating literally if the message does not seem to make sense.
- Advise the interpreter not to engage in side conversations, especially those that include the provision of advice or coaching, with the client.

Client's Reason for Seeking Care or Chief Complaint

Record the reason the client is seeking care as a short statement in the client's own words and in quotation marks. In the case of a well client, the statement of the reason for seeking care may be the client's request for a health examination for health screening or health promotion.

The statement of an ill client is sometimes called a **chief complaint** or **concern (CC)**, defined as the acute or chronic problem that is the client's priority for treatment. Whenever relevant and possible, include a notation of the duration of the problem. The duration stated by the client may not be the actual time span of the symptoms. However, it indicates the time during which the complaint was important enough to motivate the client to seek help.

Keep in mind that the reason for seeking care is not a diagnostic statement. In fact, formulating this statement in diagnostic terms can be hazardous. For example, a client who has frequent asthmatic attacks may appear for treatment with respiratory system complaints and state that he or she is having an "asthmatic attack." However, this client's diagnostic conclusion may not be accurate and could be misleading. In this early portion of the history, care must be taken to avoid client and interviewer bias. Otherwise, the interview and the problem solving may be in a potentially incorrect direction.

The following are examples of good statements of reasons for seeking care:

"Concern about change in mole."
"Chest pain for 3 days."
"Swollen ankles for 2 weeks."
"High fever and headache for 24 hours."
"Pap smear needed." (Last Papanicolaou test 9/8/99)
"Physical examination needed for camp."
In contrast, the following are examples of inadequately stated chief complaints:
Thinks she might be pregnant
"Sick"
Nausea and vomiting
Hypertension

The client's reason for seeking care may seem superfluous, especially since the next section of the history involves a description of the health need or problem in detail. However, this entry is one of the few places in the recorded histories of encounters with the health care system where clients are given the opportunity to have their needs recorded in their own words. Too often, practitioners lose sight of the clients' priorities for care. The consistent documentation of clients' reasons for seeking care assists in keeping the system responsive to clients' perceived needs.

In some instances a client presents several complaints. However, do not state more than three in this portion of the history, and note the client's priorities. Later, all the client's problems can be addressed in the present health/present illness (PH/PI) part of the health history.

Be alert to the possibility that some clients may be reluctant to state their priority for seeking health care and may provide the interviewer with a reason perceived to be more acceptable than the actual reasons, for example, abdominal pain when the actual concern is possible pregnancy. Watch for clues to any underlying and unstated concerns throughout the interview. In addition to clarifying the client's reason for seeking health care, also clarify the client's expectations about the encounter.

Present Health or History of Present Illness

The present health/present illness (PH/PI) section elaborates the information relevant to the client's reasons for seeking care. The following are the components of the present health/present illness section of the health history:

A. Introduction (for both present health and present illness interviews)
  1. Summary
  2. Usual health
B. Symptom analysis: chronological story (in cases of a present illness)
  1. Onset
    a. Date
    b. Manner (gradual or sudden)
    c. Duration
    d. Precipitating factors
  2. Course since onset
    a. Incidence (frequency)
    b. Manner
    c. Timing
    d. Duration (longest, shortest, and average times)
    e. Patterns of remissions and exacerbations
  3. Location
  4. Quality
  5. Quantity
  6. Setting
  7. Associated phenomena
  8. Alleviating and aggravating factors
  9. Client's underlying concern
C. Pertinent negative information
D. Relevant family information
E. Disability assessment

Introduction

First ask all clients to describe their present health and record it in their own words as the introduction to this section of the history. The introduction to the present illness section should be succinct. Its major purpose is to provide the reader with a general orientation to the client. Briefly summarize the client's biographical data relevant to the purpose of the encounter (usually age, race, marital status, employment status, and occupation). Describe the client's usual health; record any significant past diagnoses and past and current health problems.

State the client's previous visits or admissions, if any, to the institution or service. If the client is being hospitalized and also has been hospitalized in the past, note the client's total number of hospitalizations and the number of hospitalizations for complaints related to the present illness

For a well client, the interviewer then asks about the client's health promotion self-care practices and briefly summarizes his or her health maintenance activities and needs. For a health promotion encounter, the description of present health is usually a short summary of these self-care patterns.

When the client has a health problem, this portion of the health history challenges the practitioner's interviewing, clinical knowledge, and written communication skills. The practitioner must learn the minute details of the chief complaint and its associated phenomena. First, the information must be comprehensive. Second, it must be recorded logically and concisely. Third, it must provide the practitioner with enough information to initiate additional assessment and the intervention measures.

The interviewing and recording for the present illness portion of the health history is especially difficult for beginning practitioners because the processes involved require both skill in interviewing and history taking and clinical knowledge. Outlining the progression of the present illness before writing the narrative discussion is sometimes helpful. Although the practitioner who is learning health assessment has probably not yet studied client care management, he or she may find that the use of clinical management references for the system(s) discussed with the client will often provide valuable learning by highlighting important omissions, which can be incorporated in future interviews.

Symptom Analysis: Chronological Story

Initiate the exploration of symptoms by asking the client a question similar to the following: "Tell me about it [the problem mentioned in the chief complaint statement]," or "How did it [the problem] start, and what has happened since it started?" The client usually will respond to this inquiry with a lengthy but diagnostically incomplete discourse about the chief complaint. Exercise skill in determining when to interrupt the client—specifically, when to direct the responses by asking additional, clarifying questions and when to allow the client to continue the narration of events perceived as significant by that individual.

Create a mental or written list of the areas of symptom investigation, based on the body systems or regions affected, to be explored as an aid in attaining comprehensive information. Regardless of the nature of the problem, each of the dimensions of symptom analysis is relevant, and any health problem analysis would be incomplete without the description of all areas applicable (Box 3-4).

Onset

Determine the onset, timing, and chronological sequence of the client's problem. The client is apt to remember best the most recent episode of illness. When a prolonged illness is being discussed, the client will need direction in tracing the problem to its first symptomatic event. Once this first event has been identified, investigate it in detail and specify its date, manner of onset, duration, and precipitating factors.

Determine the usual manner of onset for the illness episodes. Note specifically any change in onset or timing. When many episodes have occurred, specify the longest, shortest, and average durations of the episodes. If there have been only several episodes, identify the length of each one.

Course Since Onset

Describe each symptom's course since onset. Determine its frequency as a specific time interval. Clients may state vaguely that they have a symptom "all the time." Such a statement may mean once a month to one client or 10 times a day to another. To obtain specific information, ask such questions as: "How many times a day (or a week or a month) does it occur?" Although suggesting answers with interview questions should be avoided, occasionally it may be necessary to pursue the issue of frequency by asking leading questions (e.g., "Does it occur more often than five times a day?").

For prolonged illnesses, describe the patterns of remission and exacerbation according to their duration and frequency. Be watchful for environmental or other clues that might be precipitating factors for illness events.

For recording the symptoms, several methods can be used to assist readers in identifying temporal relationships easily. Describe the initial event first, then the subsequent events. A chronological story can be indexed in the left-hand column of the history sheet, with prior to admission (PTA) or visit (PTV) used as a reference. For example, the chronological index can be listed as follows: "6 years PTA,"

BOX 3-4

SYMPTOM ANALYSIS

ONSET

When the symptoms started—as specific a date as possible
Manner in which the symptoms started—sudden or gradual
Duration of symptoms in the initial occurrence
Factors that seemed to precipitate or be associated with the initial event

COURSE SINCE ONSET

Frequency—in a specific time interval (e.g., per day/per month) logical to the situation
Manner of onset for subsequent events
Timing—temporal relationship of symptoms to each other or to other significant events or a daily calendar
Duration—longest, shortest, and average times
Patterns of improvement and exacerbation, including condition between episodes of the symptom(s)
Self- and professional treatment for the symptoms

LOCATION

Specific location
Radiation

QUALITY

Unique properties of the complaint (e.g., if pain—dull, aching, sharp, nagging, throbbing, stabbing, squeezing; if discharge—color, consistency, composition)

QUANTITY

Severity, size, extent, number, amount
Amount in a common measure (e.g., tablespoons)
Severity measured in estimated amount (e.g., for pain, a scale of 1 to 10) or general response (e.g., is the client able to continue what he had been doing or does he need to lie down?)
Exact size (e.g., if lesion, pinhead, dime)

SETTING

Environment—place, air quality, people, activity, etc., when symptom occurs

ASSOCIATED PHENOMENA

Occur with the chief complaint—can be precipitating, concurrent, or ensuing
Effect of chief complaint on the same or related body systems

ALLEVIATING AND AGGRAVATING FACTORS

Initial response—nature and effect
Remedies tried—nature and effect
What makes the symptom worse
What makes the symptom better
Effects of movement, position, diet, medications, and other interventions

CLIENT'S UNDERLYING CONCERN

Meaning/attribution of the symptom to the client (e.g., fear of heart attack, cancer)
Why concerned at this time (e.g., new symptom, worse episode than in the past, feeling stressed)

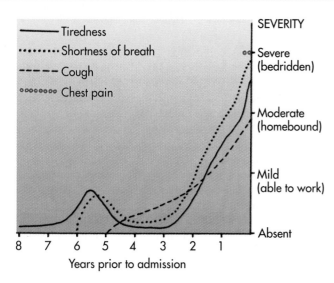

Figure 3-1 Example of a graph to illustrate symptomatic progression of an illness.

"3 years PTA," "6 months PTA," or "1 day PTA," with the corresponding narrative alongside it and continuing below the temporal index heading.

One method of demonstrating the progression of an illness is to use a diagram illustrating the disease process (see Figure 3-1 for an example). This type of diagram is especially helpful with multisymptom illnesses.

As the chronological story evolves, integrate the other areas of symptom investigation into the text of the narrative. Whenever appropriate, describe the sign's or symptom's location, quality, quantity, setting, associated phenomena, and alleviating and aggravating factors, especially when a change in pattern occurs.

Location

Determine the exact site of the sign or symptom. Subjective events, such as pain, pose certain problems. Having a client point to the exact location of pain and trace its radiation with a finger assists in determining the site. Use body hemispheres and anatomical landmarks in recording the location.

Quality

Quality refers to the unique properties or character of the complaint. Signs such as discharge are described according to their color, texture, composition, appearance, and odor. Sound and temperature may be descriptive attributes of other phenomena. Subjective events, such as pain, challenge the descriptive skills of the practitioner. The quality of pain is commonly characterized as dull, aching, sharp, nagging, throbbing, stabbing, or squeezing. Whenever appropriate, use the client's descriptions with quotation marks.

Quantity

Quantity refers to the size, extent, number, or amount (e.g., of pain, rash, discharge, or lesion). With objective events reported by the client, ask the client to refer to common mea-

surements, such as inches, cups, or tablespoons in describing approximate amounts. In describing subjective events (e.g., pain), remember that evaluations such as "a little" or "a lot" have different meanings for different persons. Describing the client's response to the symptom can sometimes more accurately convey the quality of subjective phenomena. For example, when the pain occurs, does the client stop and sit or continue with activities? Another commonly understood method of quantification is a scale of 1 to 10 to assess pain.

Setting

Whenever illness occurs, the client is in a particular environment and either with someone or alone. It is useful to ask about the setting in which certain symptoms occur because, physically or psychologically, the setting may have an effect on the client. This information can provide the practitioner with clues to the cause of the problem and implications for treatment.

Associated Phenomena

Associated phenomena are those symptoms, such as nausea and vomiting, that occur with the chief complaint. They may be related to the chief complaint or may be part of a totally different syndrome. Often the client will spontaneously identify these events. However, always ask whether anything else occurs with the chief complaint, or inquire about the presence or absence of certain specific events. Additionally, review the system or systems associated with the chief complaint. Record the client's positive responses and completely describe all reported symptoms. Document the negative responses in the negative information section.

Alleviating or Aggravating Factors

When a health problem occurs, initially the affected person often accommodates to it or attempts self-treatment. The individual may decrease activity, eat more or less, wait, or actively medicate and treat himself or herself. Often cultural responses to illness and treatment influence this self-care. The client's actions in response to the problem and the effect of these actions should be addressed in a nonjudgmental way. If professional intervention has taken place, the nature, source, and effect of each intervention need to be described. The client, through treatment or accommodation, may have discovered something that alleviates the problem. Therefore the client should be asked what makes the situation better. The client's solution may provide valuable therapeutic data and may provide insights to the individual's overall adaptation to illness. Also ask the client about what makes the chief complaint worse. Usually the client has noticed aggravating factors but may need assistance in recalling them. Inquire about the effect of movement, positioning, or eating, for example. Again, this information may offer valuable therapeutic data. Information regarding medications currently being taken is covered in the next section of the health history. At this point, ask about previous medications that may have been taken for a long time and/or those that might have an effect on the current health need or problem.

If the client has not already suggested a cause for the problem(s), ask whether the client has any thoughts about why he or she is having the problem(s) at this time.

Client's Underlying Concern

The final aspect of assessment in symptom analysis is the meaning of the symptoms to the client and any underlying concerns about them. The interviewer probes any underlying concerns and beliefs about the symptoms or needs presented and, in the case of a long-standing issue, insights into the motivation that prompted the client to seek care at this particular time.

A mnemonic device, PQRSTU, is sometimes used to recall the main components of symptom analysis. This method is presented in Box 3-5.

Pertinent Negative Information

In the analysis of a problem, negative information is as significant as positive information for determining the diagnosis. Thoroughly review each system implicated in the present illness section. Record the client's positive replies in the text of the chronological story. Document all pertinent negative information in this separate category of the present illness section. An example in the case of a chief complaint of left chest pain would be "no radiation of pain into the right chest, left arm, or lower abdomen."

Relevant Family History

Ask the client whether any problem, similar to the chief complaint, is known to exist among blood relatives. Record positive replies, specifically identifying the relative and the problem. Document negative replies in general terms (e.g., "None of the client's blood relatives has diabetes."). In the case of a client who is adopted, the family history of the biological family (if known) must be differentiated from that of the adoptive family, in which bloodlines are not shared. In the case of infectious diseases or behavioral issues, determine whether other family or household members may also be affected.

Disability Assessment

The purpose of the disability assessment is to determine the extent to which the symptoms identified in the present illness section have affected the client's total life. Note physiological effects, as well as sociological, psychological, and financial changes resultant from the problem.

Past Health History

The purpose of the past health history (PHH) section of the health history is to describe the client's current and past health and to identify all of the client's major past health problems. A recommended outline for the information is as follows:

A. General health information
 1. Usual health
 2. Allergies
    a. Environmental
    b. Food
    c. Drug
    d. Other

BOX 3-5

PQRSTU—A MNEMONIC DEVICE FOR REMEMBERING THE COMMON COMPONENTS OF SYMPTOM ANALYSIS

P: Palliative and Provocative (alleviating, aggravating, setting, and associated phenomena)
Q: Quality
R: Region and Radiation (location)
S: Severity (quantity)
T: Timing (onset and course since onset)
U: Understanding patient's perception (client's underlying concern)

 3. Habits
    a. Alcohol
    b. Tobacco
    c. Drugs
    d. Caffeine
 4. Medications taken regularly (names, dosages, frequency, intended and actual effects, and compliance)
    a. By health care provider prescription
    b. Over-the-counter medications as well as prescription medications shared by others
    c. Herbal preparation and nutritional supplements
 5. Exercise patterns
 6. Sleep patterns
 7. Immunizations
B. Past health problems
 1. Past major illnesses—resolved and chronic
 2. Childhood illnesses
 3. Accidents and disabling injuries
 4. Hospitalizations (including blood transfusions)
 5. Operations
C. Environments
 1. Community
 2. Work
 3. Recreational

Usual Health Status

Ask about the client's usual health status. Try to elicit a sense of the client's perception of, and feelings about, his or her usual health status over the past year, as well as any recent changes in that health status.

Allergies

Ask specifically about allergies to food, environmental factors, animals, and drugs. If the client reports an allergy, obtain specific information about the causative factor, reaction, diagnosis of the causative factor, therapy, and treatment outcomes. Exercise caution in assessing drug allergies. A drug reaction may not always be an allergic response. It may be an interaction with a concurrently administered drug, a misdose, a side effect, or an adverse effect.

Habits

Habits relevant to the health of an individual are excessive alcohol or caffeine ingestion, smoking, and the addictive use of legal or illegal mood-altering substances. In recording habits, note the number of cigarettes, ounces of alcohol, or tablets per day, along with the duration of the habit. Determine and record both past and current use of these substances. Obtain as specific information as possible about the types of abuse, the duration of the use or abuse in months or years, the amount of abused substance taken per day (e.g., number of tablets, ounces, bottles, injections), and the effects reflected in activities of daily living (e.g., unable to get out of bed and go to work). (Box 3-6 contains an example of a screening history for alcohol abuse.) In the case of an addiction, which is affecting health, the client has probably attempted to control the use of the unhealthy substance. Ask about previous attempts, for example, to stop smoking or control drinking, to gain insights into motivations and health promotion strategies used by the client.

Medications

If therapy is to be planned by informed practitioners, all medications currently being used by the client must be known and recorded—both those formally prescribed by health care providers as well as medications chosen by clients. For prescribed medications, clients sometimes report vague patterns, such as taking "a white pill once a day for water." This portion of the health history presents the opportunity to educate clients about the names, doses, and actions of their medications and the necessity of knowing such information. Many clients forget to mention self-prescribed or over-the-counter medications and nutritional supplements unless specifically asked about them. The practitioner should explicitly ask about such medications and supplements and record them by name and dose. The practitioner may want to ask the client to bring medications to future visits to look at self-administration and adherence pattern.

Exercise

Explore the pattern of physical and sedentary activities in the client's usual routine. Include a weekly or daily profile of the individual's usual activities. Ask the client to describe a typical day from awakening to bedtime.

Sleep

Describe the client's sleep pattern. Record the daily routine for a typical week. Determine the client's assessment of the adequacy of his or her sleep pattern and satisfaction with the pattern.

Immunizations

Record all immunizations according to type and date. Accurate immunization records are commonly kept for children but not usually for adults. For adults, obtain the exact (or at least approximate) date of the last tetanus immunization and hepatitis immunization status, as well as flu and pneumonia immunizations in the elderly and chronically ill.

Past Illnesses

Past illnesses may have some effect on the client's current health needs and problems. In addition, information about the management of and response to past problems provides some indication of the client's possible response to current and future health issues. Be sure to ask about both acute illnesses, which have been resolved or controlled, as well as chronic illnesses for which treatment or other management is continuing.

Childhood Illnesses

The recording of childhood illnesses is probably more relevant to, and more easily obtained for, a child's history than it is for an adult's. At minimum, however, ask all adults whether they have had rheumatic fever and chickenpox. Whenever a positive reply is given, determine the age of the client at occurrence, the fact or absence of a medically confirmed diagnosis, and the short- and long-term effects of the disease.

Accidents and Disabling Injuries

Ask the client to recall all accidents and disabling injuries, regardless of whether hospitalization occurred or treatment was handled on an outpatient basis. Determine and record the precipitating event, extent of injury, fact or absence of med-

BOX 3-6

SCREENING FOR PROBLEM DRINKING

The U.S. Preventive Services Task Force (1996) recommends screening to detect problem drinking for all adult and adolescent clients. The screening method endorsed is a careful history of alcohol use or the use of standard screening questionnaires. Routine measurement of biochemical markers was not recommended in asymptomatic persons. The AUDIT Structured Interview was highlighted as a useful clinical tool for screening (U.S. Preventive Services Task Force, 1996, p. 577). The tool's key questions are:

How often do you have a drink containing alcohol?

How many drinks do you have on a typical day when you are drinking?

How often do you have six or more drinks on one occasion?

How often during the last year have you found that you were unable to stop drinking once you had started?

How often during the last year have you failed to do what was normally expected of you because of drinking?

How often during the last year have you needed a first drink in the morning to get yourself going after a heavy drinking session?

How often during the last year have you had a feeling of guilt or remorse after drinking?

How often during the last year have you been unable to remember what happened the night before because you had been drinking?

Has anyone been injured as a result of your drinking?

Has a relative, doctor, or other health care worker been concerned about your drinking or suggested you cut down?

ical care, names of the practitioner and institution, and results of injury and treatment. Be alert to the possibility of patterns of injury or the presence of consistent environmental hazards. Given current concerns about blood transfusions and acquired immunodeficiency syndrome (AIDS), be sure to record information about blood transfusions in this section.

Hospitalizations

Determine whether any hospitalizations have occurred, and record descriptions of them, including all the times that the client was admitted to an inpatient unit. Include the dates of the hospitalization, the primary practitioner, name and address of the hospital, admitting complaint, discharge diagnosis, and follow-up care and treatment outcomes. Record any obstetrical hospitalizations in this section or in the review-of-systems portion of the health history (female genital system).

Operations

Record all operations together, under the specific operations category. Describe of the nature of the repair, replacement, or removal as completely as possible. Commonly, clients are unaware of the exact nature of their operations. It may be necessary to consult past records for accurate and complete information.

If the client has had major acute illnesses or chronic illnesses that have not required hospitalization, note the course of treatment, the person making the diagnosis, and the follow-up care and treatment outcomes.

Information under the categories of hospitalizations, operations, and other major illnesses may, in some instances, be redundant. Do not record detailed information more than once. Instead, state the presence of a past problem and refer the reader to the section where the full description is presented.

Environments

Ask about the client's perceptions of the health of the current and past community, work, and recreational environments. Ask about the client's general satisfaction with these environments as well as any specific safety or health risks encountered in the current situation or past situations. For the work environment, inquire about physical or chemical hazards or stressors, which might be affecting health. For recreational environments, consider exposures to allergens, chemicals, dust, or other factors that might affect health or current symptoms.

Family Health History

The purpose of the family health history (FH) section is to learn about the general health of the client's blood relatives, spouse, and children and to identify any illnesses of a genetic, familial, or environmental nature that might have implications for the client's current or future health problems and needs, or their solution or resolution. The health status of the client's family is significant for several reasons. First, the client's health status affects and is affected by health conditions in other family members. Communicable disease is an

example of this influence. Second, heredity and constitutional factors are associated with the causation of many diseases. A strong family history of certain problems might offer important clues in assessment, diagnosis, and prevention.

Genetic problems are those that are directly inherited. Familial problems are ones that have not yet been demonstrated to be genetic but appear more often in family clusters. An example of a familial problem is alcoholism. Families may also share environmental risks (e.g., exposure to toxic substances).

Inquire about the health of the client's relatives, including maternal and paternal grandparents, parents, siblings, aunts, uncles, spouse, and children. In certain situations, information regarding roommates, sexual partners, and significant others might be relevant to a family history. Information also needs to be obtained about the current health status of, presence of disease in, and current age or age at death of each family member. If a member is deceased, record the date and cause of death.

If the client has established or possible illnesses with known or suspected familial tendencies, question the client again about similar problems of family members.

Inquire about the presence of the following diseases because of their genetic, familial, or environmental tendencies: alcoholism, allergies, Alzheimer's disease, arteriosclerosis, cancer, coronary artery disease, diabetes, epilepsy, gout, hematological disorders (e.g., hemophilia, sickle cell anemia, thalassemia, hemolytic jaundice, or severe anemia), Huntington's chorea, hypertension, kidney disease, mental disorders, obesity, and tuberculosis. Often printed history forms list these diseases. Check whether the client or a family member has the diagnosis. Inquire about selected additional health problems which may be associated with the client's family history, occupation, socioeconomic status, ethnic origins, or environment.

The information in the family history section can be outlined in the record or put in the form of a family tree chart. Figure 3-2 is an example of such a chart, or **genogram**. Genograms are especially useful in situations in which genetically transmitted diseases are present or suspected or if the understanding of family composition is an important factor in management. The traditionally used symbols for genogram notations are included in Box 3-7. For an adopted individual, two genograms may be useful if the information is available. The genogram for the biological family would indicate genetic health issues and familial ones that may be genetically linked. The genogram for the adoptive family would include familial health issues and those affected by environment.

Certain health problems are linked to specific population or ethnic groups. Table 3-1 contains information about health problems that have been noted in excessively high frequencies in particular groups.

Review of Systems

The review-of-systems (ROS) portion of the history includes a collection of data about the past and present health

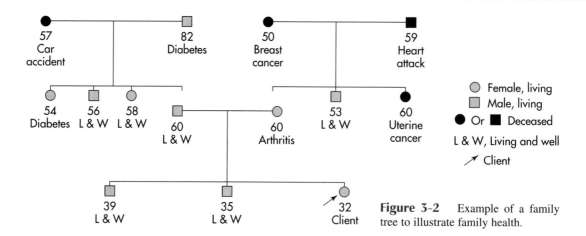

Figure 3-2 Example of a family tree to illustrate family health.

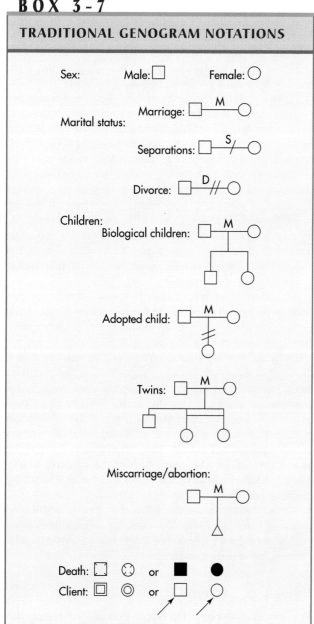

of each of the client's systems. This review of the client's physical, functional, sociological, and psychological health status may identify problems not uncovered previously in the history and provides an opportunity to indicate the client's strengths and resources.

Generally this portion of the history is organized from a head-to-toe direction and from physical to psychosocial factors. The client is told that he or she will be asked a number of questions. For both beginning and experienced interviewers, a checklist or written reminder of the ROS components is useful.

Physical Systems

In the review of physical systems, ask a question about the client's systems and related symptoms, care practices, patterns, and preventive measures; pause to let the client think and respond. If the client responds positively to symptoms, analyze the symptoms according to the characteristics of symptoms discussed in the present health/present illness section of the history. Ask questions quickly enough to be efficient, yet slowly enough to allow the client time to think. In general, emphasize the presence of past or current common anatomical or functional problems of the system as well as the health functioning and maintenance of the system.

It is important to translate the signs and symptoms into questions and terms that the client can understand. For example, questions concerning a symptom, such as intermittent claudication, need to be presented in descriptive lay terms. The following are examples of how questions related to intermittent claudication can be translated:

"Do you ever have any cramplike pains in your legs?"

"When do these cramps occur?"

"What happens to the pain if you rest your legs?"

In documenting the health history, record the presence or absence of all signs or symptoms included in the inquiry. Using the general description "negative" for a total system is meaningless. If such a broad notation is made, the reader will not know which questions were asked and consequently will not understand the context of "negative." If the reader is also the recorder, he or she probably will not, at a later time, remember which specific questions were asked. An exception might exist in a health care system where the routine review

TABLE 3-1   Distribution of Selected Genetic Traits and Disorders by Population or Ethnic Group

Ethnic or Population Group	Genetic or Multifactorial Disorder Present in Relatively High Frequency	Ethnic or Population Group	Genetic or Multifactorial Disorder Present in Relatively High Frequency
Africans	ß-Thalassemia	Jews—Ashkenazi	Bloom syndrome
	G-6-PD deficiency, African type		Factor XI (PTA) deficiency
	Hemoglobin C disease		Familial dysautonomia
	Hereditary persistence of hemoglobin F		(Riley-Day syndrome)
	Lactase deficiency, adult		Gaucher disease (adult type)
	Sickle cell disease		Niemann-Pick disease (infantile)
Amish	Ellis-van Cerveld disease		Tay-Sachs disease (infantile)
	Hemophilia B		Torsion dystonia
	Limb-girdle muscular dystrophy	Jews—Sephardi	Ataxia-telangiectasia
	Pyruvate kinase deficiency		Cystinuria
Armenians	Familial Mediterranean fever		Familial Mediterranean fever
	Familial paroxysmal polyserositis		Glycogen storage disease III
Burmese	Hemoglobin E disease	Lapps	Congenital dislocation of the hip
Chinese	Alpha thalassemia	Lebanese	Dyggve-Melchior-Clausen syndrome
	G-6-PD deficiency, Chinese type	Mediterranean peoples	ß-Thalassemia
	Lactase deficiency, adult		Familial Mediterranean fever
Costa Ricans	Malignant osteopetrosis		G-6-PD deficiency, Mediterranean type
English	Cystic fibrosis	Middle Eastern peoples	Dubin-Johnson syndrome
	Hereditary amyloidosis, type III		G-6-PD deficiency, Mediterranean type
Eskimos	Congenital adrenal hyperplasia		Ichthyosis vulgaris
	Methemoglobinemia		Metachromatic leukodystrophy
	Pseudocholinesterase deficiency		Phenylketonuria
Finns	Aspartylglycosaminuria		Werdnig-Hoffmann disease
	Congenital nephrosis	Nova Scotia Acadians	Niemann-Pick disease
	Diastrophic dwarfism		
	Generalized amyloidosis syndrome, V	Polish	Phenylketonuria
	Polycystic liver disease	Polynesians	Clubfoot
	Retinoschisis	Portuguese	Joseph disease
French Canadians	Morquio syndrome	Scandinavians	Cholestasis-lymphedema
	Tyrosinemia		Krabbe disease
Gypsies (Czech)	Congenital glaucoma		Phenylketonuria
Hopi Indians	Tyrosinase-positive albinism		Sjögren-Larsson syndrome
Icelandic peoples	Phenylketonuria	Scots	Cystic fibrosis
Indians (American Navajo)	Ear anomalies		Hereditary amyloidosis, type III
			Phenylketonuria
Irish	Phenylketonuria	Thais	Hemoglobin E disease
	Neural tube defects		Lactase deficiency, adult
Japanese	Acatalasemia	Zuni Indians	Tyrosinase-positive albinism
	Cleft lip/palate		
	Oguchi disease		

Modified from Wong DL et al.: *Whaley & Wong's nursing care of infants and children*, ed 6, St Louis, 1999, Mosby.

of physical systems section takes place and where "negative" indicates an inquiry into and a negative response to, predetermined, consistently reviewed items of exploration.

In the present health/present illness section, a body region or system may have already been reviewed, along with exploration of a health problem. In this situation, in the review of physical systems section, a notation is made that refers the reader to the present health/present illness section for information about that system.

Systems and body regions reviewed and specific areas of exploration about the health status, functional and anatomical problems, and health maintenance of those systems are pre-

sented in the following list. The purpose of the encounter, plans for care continuity, time available, and the condition of the client will affect the detail with which the review of systems is executed. The listing of areas for exploration in this chapter is very comprehensive. In actual client care situations, the practitioner would choose areas of review appropriate to the particular situation. For all systems the practitioner should, under health promotion and health maintenance exploration, ask about the usual health of the system or region. Chapters 9 through 22 contain overviews of regional health histories and analyses of common symptoms noted in those body systems or regions.

General

Usual state of health
Recent and significant gain or loss of weight (if present, amount, time interval, and possible causes are recorded)
Usual, maximum, and minimum weight
Episodes of chills
Episodes of weakness or malaise
Fatigue

Health Problem Items

Fever
Odors
Sweats

Skin

Health Promotion/Health Maintenance Items

Care habits, including use of sunscreen and skin self-examinations
History of exposure to sun, including tanning bed use and sunburns

Health Problem Items

Previously diagnosed and treated disease
Color changes
Dryness
Ecchymosis
Excessive sweating
Lesions
Masses
Odors
Petechiae
Pruritus
Rashes
Temperature changes
Texture changes

Hair

Health Promotion/Health Maintenance Item

Care patterns
Use of dyes, permanent wave solutions, or other chemicals

Health Problem Items

Alopecia, or hair loss
Excessive growth or change in distribution
Scalp lesions or itching
Texture changes

Nails

Health Promotion/Health Maintenance Items

Care patterns

Health Problem Items

Changes in appearance
Texture changes

Head and Face

Health Promotion/Health Maintenance Items

Care patterns
Use of helmets for bicycle and motorcycle riders

Health Problem Items

Dizziness
History of trauma
Injuries
Pain
Syncope
Unusual or frequent headaches

Eyes

Health Promotion/Health Maintenance Items

Date of last ophthalmological examination and glaucoma test and results
Pattern of eye examinations
Visual acuity, without and with corrective lenses, if applicable
Use of glasses or contact lenses and duration
Use of protective eyewear, if applicable

Health Problem Items

Blurred vision
Cataracts
Changes in visual fields or vision
Difficulty reading
Diplopia
Excessive tearing
Glaucoma
Infections
Pain
Photophobia
Pruritus
Redness
Swelling around the eyes
Twitching
Unusual discharge or sensations, such as "rainbows" or "halos" around lights, flashing lights, or floaters
Visual disturbances, such as "rainbows" around lights, flashing lights, or blind spots

Ears

Health Promotion/Health Maintenance Items

Care habits, especially cleaning
Hearing ability
Piercings
Use of prosthetic devices
Use of hearing protective devices in high noise areas

Health Problem Items

Changes in hearing ability
Discharge
Excess earwax
Increased sensitivity to environmental noise
Infections, including those resulting from piercings
Otalgia
Pain
Presence of excessive environmental noise
Tinnitus, buzzing, or ringing
Vertigo (subjective or objective)

Nose and Sinuses

Health Promotion/Health Maintenance Items

Olfactory ability

Health Problem Items

Change in ability to smell
Discharge (seasonal associations)
Epistaxis
Frequency of colds
Obstruction
Pain in infraorbital or sinus area
Postnasal drip
Sinus infection
Sneezing (frequent or prolonged)
Unusual snoring

Mouth and Throat

Health Promotion/Health Maintenance Items

Dental care provider
Pattern of dental care and cleaning and date of last
    examination
Pattern of dental hygiene
Use of prosthetic devices (e.g., dentures, bridges)

Health Problem Items

Abscesses
Bleeding or swelling of gums
Change in taste
Dryness
Dysphagia
Excessive salivation
Hoarseness
Lesions
Odors
Pain
Sore throats
Voice changes

Neck and Nodes

Health Problem Items

Limitation of movement
Masses
Node enlargement or tenderness
Pain with movement or palpation
Stiffness
Swelling
Tenderness

Breasts

Health Promotion/Health Maintenance Items

Mammography screening examinations
Self-examination pattern (frequency, method)

Health Problem Items

Change in appearance of breasts and nipples
Dimpling
Discharge from nipple

Masses
Pain
Surgery for enlargement or reduction
Tenderness

Respiratory and Cardiovascular Systems

Health Promotion/Health Maintenance Items

Date of last chest x-ray and electrocardiogram and results
Occupational or recreational exposure to toxins, allergens,
    fumes, and smoke (including second-hand smoke) and
    personal protection used

Health Problem Items

Past diagnosis of respiratory or cardiovascular system
    disease
Cough (add description if present)
Cyanosis
Dyspnea (if present, amount of exertion precipitating it is
    recorded)
Edema
Hemoptysis
High blood pressure
Night sweats
Orthopnea (number of pillows needed to sleep comfortably
    is recorded)
Pain (intensity [e.g., scale of 1 to 10], exact location, radia-
    tion, effect on respiration, and duration are recorded)
Palpitations
Paroxysmal nocturnal dyspnea
Smoking history
Sputum (if present, amount, color, and characteristics are
    described)
Stridor
Tuberculosis exposure
Wheezing

Gastrointestinal System

Health Promotion/Health Maintenance Items

Bowel habits
Diet (nutritional assessment can be recorded here or in a
    separate section)
Previous roentgenograms or x-ray results; endoscopic
    results (e.g., sigmoidoscopy)
Use of antacids, laxatives, and antidiarrheal medications

Health Problem Items

Abdominal pain
Appetite and changes in appetite
Ascites
Change in stool color and consistency
Constipation
Diarrhea
Dyspepsia
Dysphagia
Flatulence
Food idiosyncrasies
Hematemesis

Hemorrhoids
Hernia
Indigestion
Infections
Jaundice
Melena
Nausea
Previously diagnosed problems
Pyrosis
Recent changes in habits
Rectal bleeding
Rectal discomfort
Thirst
Vomiting

Urinary System

Health Promotion/Health Maintenance Items

Daily water intake
Usual pattern of urination

Health Problem Items

Past diagnosed problems and infections
Change in urinary stream
Dysuria
Enuresis
Flank pain
Frequency (in a 24-hour period)
Hematuria
Hesitancy of stream
Incontinence or dribbling
Nocturia
Oliguria
Pyuria
Polyuria
Retention
Stress incontinence
Suprapubic pain
Urgency
Urine color change
Urine odor change

Genital System (Male)

Health promotion/health maintenance items

Personal hygiene
Routine testicular self-examinations

Health Problem Items

Impotence
Infertility
Lesions
Masses (testicular)
Pain
Premature ejaculation
Prostate problems
Swelling
Urethral discharge

Genital System (Female)

Health promotion/health maintenance items

Personal hygiene
Frequency of Papanicolaou smear and results
Genital self-examination
Menstrual history—age at menarche, typical cycle, duration of flow, amount of flow
Date of last menstrual period (LMP)
Date of last normal menstrual period (LNMP)
History of abortions or miscarriages
Obstetrical history (for each pregnancy)
    Complications of pregnancy
    Condition, sex, and weight of baby
    Date of delivery
    Description of labor
    Duration of pregnancy
    Place of prenatal care and hospitalization
    Prenatal course
    Postpartum course
    Type of delivery (vaginal, cesarean section)

Health Problem Items

Past diagnoses
Amenorrhea
Dysmenorrhea
Dyspareunia
Fibroids
Infertility
Lesions
Menorrhagia
Metrorrhagia
Pelvic pain
Polymenorrhea
Postcoital bleeding
Pruritus
Signs and symptoms of menopause
Vaginal discharge

Sexual History (Both Sexes)

(See Box 3-8)

Extremities and Musculoskeletal System

Health Promotion/Health Maintenance Items

Repetitive motions in work or recreational activities
Risk for osteoporosis
Use of posture, exercise, and/or hose to maintain good blood circulation in legs
Past diagnosis of disease

Health Problem Items

Coldness
Crepitus
Deformities
Cramping
Discoloration
Edema

BOX 3-8

COMPONENTS OF A SEXUAL HISTORY

GENERAL SEXUAL HISTORY

Age of onset of sexual activity
Sexual preference (male, female, both)
Usual ability to perform and enjoy satisfactory sexual intercourse
Number of sexual partners
Health of sexual partners (e.g., sexually transmitted infections)
Number of sexual partners
Sexual practices
Use of condoms and other contraceptives
Sexually transmitted infections

SPECIFIC SEXUAL PROBLEMS

Changes in sex drive
Infertility
Problems with sexual function or sexuality
Sexual abuse history

Sterility
Client's perspective of the problem
Relationship of problem to time, place, and partner
Presence of loss of sex drive or dislike of sexual contact
Presence of problems in the overall relationship
Presence of stress factors in client or partner
Presence of anxiety, guilt, or anger expressed or not expressed
Presence of physical problems (e.g., pain felt by either partner)

MEDICAL HISTORY

Especially problems such as diabetes, depression, psychotic illnesses, health disease, hormone deficiencies, operations and trauma, prolactinoma, arthritis, vaginal atrophy, or phimosis

PARTNER'S VIEW OF THE PROBLEM

MEDICAL AND RECREATIONAL DRUGS

Fractures
Heat
Intermittent claudication
Joint stiffness, swelling, or redness
Limitation of movement
Pain (location, time of day, duration)
Past diagnoses and injuries
Thrombophlebitis
Weakness

Central Nervous System

Health Promotion/Health Maintenance Items

Balance
Cognitive ability
Coordination
Speech

Health Problem Items

Past diagnosis of disease
Anxiety
Aphasia
Ataxia
Changes in memory (recent and remote), attention span
Disorientation
Dizziness
Dysarthria
General behavior change
Hallucinations
Loss of consciousness
Imbalance

Mood change
Nervousness
Pain
Paralysis (partial or complete)
Paresis
Paresthesia (hyperesthesia, anesthesia)
Seizures (characteristics and treatment)
Tic
Tremor
Spasm
Sensory changes

Endocrine System

Health Promotion/Health Maintenance Items

Adult changes in size of head, hands, or feet
Hair distribution
History of physical growth and development
Hormone therapy
Presence of secondary sex characteristics

Health Problem Items

Diagnosis of diabetes or thyroid disease
Dryness of skin or hair
Exophthalmos
Goiter
Hypoglycemia
Intolerance of heat or cold
Polydipsia
Polyphagia
Polyuria

Postural hypotension
Weakness
Weight changes—sudden and unexpected

Hematopoietic System

Health Promotion/Health Maintenance Items
Iron intake

Health Problem Items
Past diagnosis of hematopoietic disease
Anemia
Bleeding tendencies
Blood transfusion
Blood type
Bruising
Exposure to radiation
History of alcoholism
History of heavy menses
Lymphadenopathy

Functional Status

If the client has functional limitations, measure the extent of abilities. Chapter 28 contains approaches and tools for the specific assessment of functional abilities. If this area of assessment is included, choose tools appropriate to the client being assessed.

Sociological and Cultural Systems

Assessment and treatment cannot be effectively managed by knowing only the client's physical status. Since the client is a unique and whole person, diagnosis and treatment must be addressed within the context of and relevant and acceptable to that person. Therefore it is necessary to gather, in some organized way, information about the client's sociological, psychological, developmental, and nutritional status.

The following is a suggested organization of sociological data:

1. Relationships with family and significant others
   a. Client's role in the family
   b. Persons with whom client lives
   c. Persons with whom client relates
   d. Recent family crises or changes
   e. Persons identified as supports
2. Environment—physical and psychological
   a. Home
      (1) Condition and physical adequacy of home
   b. Community
   c. Work
   d. Recreational
   e. Recent changes in environment
   f. Residence/travel outside of home country
3. Occupational history
   a. Jobs held
      (1) Description of jobs—physical and mental exertion
      (2) Occupational hazards (e.g., chemicals, fumes, dust, noise)
      (3) Stresses

   b. Satisfaction with present and past employment
   c. Current place of employment
4. Economic status and resources
   a. Source of income
   b. Perception of adequacy or inadequacy of income
   c. Effect of illness on economic status
5. Educational level
   a. Highest degree or grade attained
   b. Judgment of intellect relative to age
6. Daily profile
   a. Typical daily and weekend patterns
   b. Rest-activity patterns
   c. Social activities
   d. Special weekend activities
   e. Recent changes in daily activities
7. Patterns of health care
   a. Private and public primary care agencies
   b. Dental care
   c. Preventive care
   d. Emergency care
8. Relevant cultural information
   a. Where client was born—if an immigrant, length of residence in current country
   b. Ethnic affiliation and strength of ethnic affiliation
   c. Primary language and other languages spoken and read
   d. Cultural beliefs and practices as they relate to health, illness, and health care

This outline is useful for gathering the sociological and cultural data for the majority of adult clients; however, it may be necessary to make adaptations for some individuals. Many clients may be unaccustomed to extensive questioning about nonphysical matters during the taking of a health history. Therefore the use of such data may need to be explained to the client, by stating, for example, "To treat you most effectively, it is important that I know something about you as a person."

First, ask about the client's role or roles in the family and household. A member may have a socially assigned role relating to birth (e.g., that of son, father, or grandfather). In addition, the client may have a circumstantially defined role (e.g., that of provider, caregiver, or homemaker). Identify all roles.

Next, inquire about the people whom the client lives with and relates to on a regular basis. This information can be useful in hypothesizing, for example, the effect that a long illness of the care provider may have on the family. Also, identify strengths by the presence of strong family or friend relationships. Ask the client about the closeness and compatibility of these relationships. Sometimes unsatisfactory social relationships produce stress, which can be a factor in exacerbating or causing illness, and social supports can be a buffer against stress.

Ask the client whether any recent event has had a significant impact on his or her health. Resultant positive data might provide clues of causation or implications for prevention of illness.

Physical and psychological environments can have a profound effect on an individual's health status and potential.

Ask about the client's satisfaction with the appearance and general comfort of home, community, work, and recreational situations. Also, inquire whether the client considers the environment healthy or unhealthy. The pursuit of "why" when clients identify problems will provide some insight into the client's value system, possible information regarding significant health hazards, clues to the cause of the present illness, and a validation of the dissatisfaction. Again, ask about recent change or loss. Record positive responses.

Residence and travel outside of one's own country can affect health because of changes in water, food, and environmental conditions as well as response to indigenous health problems. Ask about time spent outside of the home country and recent travel.

Occupational history information can be used to specify current and past environmental hazards and sources of stress and resources; to determine the fit between personal ability and productivity; and to plan rehabilitation. Inquire about jobs held, satisfaction with those jobs, possible health and health-related hazards in those jobs, and place of current employment.

Although it is usually not always necessary to know the client's exact annual income, determine the source of that income and assessment of its adequacy in meeting current and future needs. Identify clients whose resources are insufficient to enable them to follow therapy, and make appropriate referral for financial assistance.

Determine the educational level of the client, and record the highest degree or grade completed. Also, determine literacy level and cognitive ability relative to age.

Knowing the client's daily pattern helps in understanding the client as a person who has habits that encourage or impede health. Ask the client to describe her or his typical 24-hour day and to indicate weekend differences. Specifically, identify work, activity, sleep, rest, and recreational pursuits in the recording.

Part of the client's past social interaction has been with the health care system, and past responses may predict future patterns. Ask about health agencies used for acute, preventive, and maintenance health care. Determine whether the client is a health facility "shopper" or whether his or her care has had continuity or whether care has been inaccessible because of finances or location.

Determine and record basic cultural information about the client. Basic information includes birthplace, ethnic affiliation and the strength of that affiliation, primary language spoken, and cultural beliefs and habits that may influence responses to health and illness and health care interventions. For detailed information regarding cultural assessment, see Chapter 7.

Psychological System

The following information needs to be obtained during the psychological assessment of the client:

1. Cognitive abilities
   a. Comprehension
   b. Learning patterns
   c. Memory
2. Responses to illness and health
   a. Value of health
   b. Sources of stress
   c. Stress and coping patterns
   d. Reaction to illness
3. Response to care
   a. Perceptions of caregivers
   b. Compliance with health advice and interventions
4. Cultural implications for care
   a. Patterns of illness response
   b. Acceptable and unacceptable therapeutic interventions
5. Spiritual implications for care
   a. Spiritual and religious affiliations and beliefs
   b. Spiritual beliefs affecting health practices and responses to illness

In assessing cognitive abilities, determine the client's comprehension ability. Usually, comprehension can be assessed better indirectly rather than directly. Interviewing up to this point in the history has provided the opportunity for extensive observation of the client's understanding, response, and judgment. With this experience in mind, record your judgment summary regarding the client's general comprehension ability.

Because education should be an essential component of all therapy, determine the client's health-learning patterns. Some clients need personal instructions. Others learn best through reading or group discussion. Knowing the client's preference can enable efficient use of provider effort and also involve the client in decision-making concerning the process of therapy.

Discuss the client's behavior in past illnesses and in health to help predict future responses. Ask questions such as the following: "What does health mean to you, and what do you do to keep yourself healthy?" "How do you feel, and what do you do when you become slightly ill? When you become very ill?" "Who do you go to for help if you are ill?" Most clients will be able to answer these questions easily. Record a concise summary of the client's responses. This information can indicate the client's strengths and weaknesses and possible problems in therapy.

Skill may be required in learning the client's real responses to care, since people are often placed in a position of subjugation by the health care system. Ask the client how comfortable he or she feels in asking questions of health care providers and whether he or she feels like a partner in care with them. You may record answers verbatim or summarize them.

Ask about the client's degree of adherence with past courses of therapy. If adherence has been minimal, determine the reasons for noncompliance. Problems resulting from lack of understanding and financial constraints are more easily solved than problems relating to distrust, indifference, or denial.

If the client is of a cultural group that is different from yours and that of the majority of the care providers, ask the client what he or she expects of care and therapy and whether his or her culture has particular traditions regarding persons with similar needs. If the chief complaint is an illness, ask about the feelings and responses of the client and significant others to the fact of the illness. The responses may help to guide the care provider in a more efficient direction and to avoid unacceptable routes of intervention. (For more information on the collection of culturally relevant information, see Chapter 7.)

The religion practiced by the client is usually recorded in the biographical information. In the psychological systems section, it may be useful to inquire about the client's general spiritual beliefs, which affect a person's perspectives on life, health, and death, and which may affect responses to care (Table 3-2). This data is especially useful in care systems, which respond to holistic health needs and parish ministries.

Developmental Data

A detailed description of the developmental assessment is presented in Chapter 5. At minimum, the recording of these data includes a summary of the client's development to date and a statement of current developmental functioning.

Nutritional Data

A detailed description of nutritional assessment is presented in Chapter 6. The recording of data minimally includes a description of an average day's food intake; an assessment of adequacy, inadequacy, or excess of the components of the food pyramid; and the presence of any past nutritional problems.

 ## Cultural Considerations
Selected Cultural Beliefs Related to Health and Health Care

AFRICAN-AMERICANS

Illness is either natural (due to forces of nature when not adequately protected [e.g., cold air, pollution, food and water]) or unnatural (due to evil influences [e.g., witchcraft, voodoo, hoodoo, hex, fix, rootwork]); symptoms are often associated with eating.

God sends serious illness as punishment (e.g., parents punished by illness or death of a child; can be avoided; may resist health care because illness is the "will of God").

Self-care and folk medicine are very prevalent; folk therapies are usually religious in origin; attempt home remedies first.

Poorer people do not seek help until illness occurs.

Often seek help from an "old lady" (woman with common knowledge of herbs; specializes in pediatric care); a spiritualist (received gift from God for healing incurable diseases or solving personal problems; strongly based in Christianity); a priest or priestess (most powerful leader and involved in voodoo); or a root doctor (supplies herbs, oils, candles, and ointments).

Prayer is a common means for prevention and treatment of illness.

ASIAN-AMERICANS

Filipinos

Believe God's will and supernatural forces govern the universe.

Illness, accidents, and other misfortunes are God's punishment for violations of his will.

Some use amulets as a shield from witchcraft or as a good luck piece; Catholics substitute religious medals and other items.

Chinese

A healthy body is viewed as a gift from parents and ancestors and must be cared for.

Health is one of the results of balance between the forces of yin (cold) and yang (hot)—the energy forces that rule the world; illness is caused by imbalance.

Chi is innate energy.

Blood is the source of life and is not regenerated; lack of chi and blood results in deficiency that produces fatigue, poor constitution, and long illness.

There is wide use of medicinal herbs that are applied in prescribed ways.

The goal of therapy is to restore the balance of yin and yang.

Folk healers are herbalists, spiritual healers, temple healers, or fortune healers.

Japanese

Three major belief systems are (1) Shinto (religious influence stating that humans are inherently good, evil is caused by outside spirits, and illness is caused by contact with polluting agents [e.g., blood, corpses, skin diseases]); (2) Chinese and Korean influence (health is achieved through harmony and balance between self and society, with disease caused by disharmony with society and not caring for one's body); and (3) Portuguese influence (upholds the germ theory of disease).

Believe evil is removed by purification.

Acupuncture, acupressure, massage restore energy, and moxibustion along affected meridians.

Use natural herbs.

Believe in the removal of diseased parts.

Trend is to use both Western and Eastern healing methods.

Care for disabled is viewed as the family's responsibility; take pride in their children's good health; seek preventive care and medical care for illnesses.

VIETNAMESE

Good health is a balance between yin (cold) and yang (hot).

Health results from harmony with existing universal order; attained by pleasing good spirits and avoiding evil ones.

Practice some restrictions to prevent incurring wrath of evil spirits.

Many use rituals to prevent illness.

Believe a person's life is predisposed toward certain phenomena by cosmic force.

Belief in am duc—the amount of good deeds accumulated by ancestors.

Family uses all means possible before consulting outside agencies for health care.

Fortune-tellers determine event that caused disturbance.

Modified from Wong DL et al.: *Whaley & Wong's nursing care of infants and children*, ed 6, St Louis, 1999, Mosby.

Cultural Considerations
Selected Cultural Beliefs Related to Health and Health Care —cont'd

May visit temple to procure divine instruction; use astrologer to calculate cyclical changes and forces; seek generalist health healers.

Certain illnesses, such as pustules or open wounds, are considered only temporary and should be ignored.

HAITIANS

Illness is either natural or supernatural. Supernatural illness is caused by angry voodoo spirits; enemies; or the dead, especially deceased relatives. Natural illness is due to irregularities of blood volume, flow, purity, viscosity, color, and/or temperature (hot/cold); gas; movement and consistency of mother's milk; hot/cold imbalance of the body; bone displacement; or movement of diseases. Natural illnesses are based on conceptions of natural causation.

Health is a personal responsibility.

Health is maintained by good dietary and hygienic practices.

Natural illnesses are treated by home remedies first; supernatural illness is treated by healers: voodoo priest or priestess, midwife, or herbalist or leaf doctor.

Amulets and prayer are used to protect against illness due to curses or willed by evil people.

HISPANICS
Cuban–Americans

Prevention and good nutrition are related to good health.

Diligent users of the medical model.

Have eclectic health-seeking practices, including preventive measures, extensive use of the health care system, and sometimes medicine of both religious and nonreligious origin; home remedies are used; in many instances, seek assistance from santeros (Afro-Cuban healers) and spiritualists to complement medical treatment.

Nutrition is important.

Mexican–Americans (Latinos, Chicanos, Raza-Latinos)

Health belief is strongly associated with religion; some maintain good health is a result of good luck and a reward for good behavior and that illness is punishment from God for wrongdoing or is caused by forces of nature or the supernatural.

Some believe in body imbalance causing illness, especially imbalance between caliente (hot) and frio (cold), or "wet" and "dry."

Illness is prevented by behaving properly, eating proper foods, working a proper amount of time, praying, wearing religious medals or amulets, and sleeping with relics in the home.

Seek help from curandero or curandera, especially in rural areas; this person receives his or her position by birth, apprenticeship, or a "calling" via a dream or vision; treatments involve use of herbs, rituals, and religious artifacts; for severe illnesses, make promises, visit shrines, offer medals and candles, and pray.

Puerto Ricans

Subscribe to the "hot-cold" theory of disease causation.

Some illness is caused by evil spirits and forces.

Use the health care system infrequently.

Seek a folk healer who uses herbs and rituals; consult a spiritualist medium for mental disorders. Santeria is the system, and practitioners are called santeros.

NATIVE AMERICANS

Believe health is a state of harmony with nature and the universe.

All disorders are believed to have aspects of the supernatural.

Show respect of the body through proper management.

Theology and medicine are strongly interwoven.

Seek care from medicine persons: altruistic persons who must use powers in purely positive ways; persons capable of both good and evil—perform negative acts against enemies; diviner-diagnosticians who diagnose but do not have powers or skill to implement medical treatment; specialists who use herbs as curative but nonsacred medical procedures; medicine persons who use herbs and rituals; and singers who cure by the power of their song.

TABLE 3-2	Religious Beliefs Influencing Health and Health Care
Religious Affiliation	**Beliefs**
Adventist	Some believe in divine healing and practice anointing with oil and use of prayer
	May desire communion or baptism when ill
	Believe in man's choice and God's sovereignty
	Saturday is Sabbath for many
Baptist	"Laying on of hands"
	May resist some therapies, such as abortion
	Believe God functions through physician
	Some believe in predestination; may respond passively to care

Modified from Wong DL et al.: *Whaley & Wong's nursing care of infants and children*, ed 6, St Louis, 1999, Mosby.

NOTE: Not all members of any religious affiliation believe in all formal and informal tenets across religions. The beliefs listed have been noted to be characteristic of substantial numbers of the members of the listed religions.

Continued

TABLE 3-2	Religious Beliefs Influencing Health and Health Care—cont'd
Religious Affiliation	**Beliefs**
Black Muslim	Faith healing unacceptable Maintenance of personal habits of cleanliness
Buddhist Churches of America	Illness believed to be a trial to aid development of soul; illness due to karmic causes May be reluctant to have surgery or certain treatments on holy days Cleanliness believed to be of great importance Family may request Buddhist priest for counseling Optimistic outlook; teach ways to overcome fears, anxieties, apprehension
Church of Christ Scientist	Deny existence of health crisis; see illness and sin as errors of mind that can be altered by prayer Oppose human intervention with drugs or other therapies; however, accept legally required immunizations Many adhere to belief that disease is a human mental concept that can be dispelled by "spiritual truth" to the extent that they refuse all medical treatment May desire services of practitioner or reader; will sometimes refuse even emergency treatment until a reader has been consulted Unlikely to be an organ donor
Church of Jesus Christ of Latter Day Saints (Mormons)	Devout adherents believe in divine healing through anointment with oil and "laying on of hands" by church officials (elders) Medical therapy not prohibited Financial support for the sick available through well-funded welfare system Discourage use of tobacco
Eastern Orthodox	Anointment of the sick No conflict with medical science
Episcopal (Anglican)	Some believe in spiritual healing Rite for anointing the sick available but not mandatory
Friends (Quakers)	No special rites or restrictions
Greek Orthodox	Health crisis handled by ordained priests; deacon may also serve in some cases Holy communion administered in hospital Some may desire the Sacrament of Holy Unction performed by a priest Believe every reasonable effort should be made to preserve life until termination by God
Hindu	Illness or injury believed to represent sins committed in previous life Accept most modern medical practices
Islam (Muslim/Moslem)	Faith healing not acceptable unless psychological condition of patient is deteriorating; performed for morale Ritual washing after prayer; prayer takes place 5 times daily (on rising, midday, afternoon, early evening, and before bed); during prayer, face Mecca and kneel on prayer rug Older Muslims often have a fatalistic view that may interfere with compliance with therapy
Jehovah's Witness	Adherents are generally absolutely opposed to blood transfusions, including banking of own blood; individuals can sometimes be persuaded in emergencies May be opposed to use of albumin, globulin, factor replacement, and vaccines Not opposed to giving blood sample
Judaism (Orthodox and Conservative)	May resist surgical procedures during Sabbath, which extends from sundown Friday until sundown Sunday Seriously ill and pregnant women are exempt from fasting Illness is grounds for violating dietary laws
Mennonite	Deep concern for dignity and self-determination of individual that would conflict with shock treatment or medical treatment affecting personality or will
Nazarene	Believe in divine healing, but not exclusive of medical treatment
Pentecostal (Assembly of God)	No restrictions regarding medical care Deliverance from sickness is provided for in atonement; may pray for divine intervention in health matters and seek God in prayer for themselves and others when ill Some insist illness is divine punishment; most consider it an intrusion of Satan
Orthodox Presbyterian	Blood transfusion accepted when advisable Believe science should be used for relief of suffering
Roman Catholic	Encourage anointing of sick, although this may be interpreted by older members of church as equivalent to old terminology "extreme unction" or "last rites"; they may require careful explanation if reluctance is associated with fear of imminent death Traditional church teaching does not approve of contraceptives or abortion
Russian Orthodox	Adherents believe in divine healing, but not exclusive of medical treatment
Unitarian Universalist	Most believe in the general goodness of their fellow humans and appreciate the expression of that goodness by visits from their clergy and fellow parishioners during times of illness

CONCLUDING THE HEALTH HISTORY

At the completion of the history, it is often useful to verbally summarize the key points with the client. Also, this is a good time to ask the client whether any additional pertinent information has not yet been shared.

APPLYING THE HEALTH HISTORY TO VARIOUS CLIENT GROUPS

The format and approach to the history as described in this chapter apply to general adult clients. Histories for other populations clearly need to be adapted to the characteristics and special health needs of those populations. Applications of the general history format for pregnant clients, pediatric clients, aging clients, and clients with functional limitations are presented in Chapters 25 through 28.

ORGANIZATION BY FUNCTIONAL HEALTH PATTERNS

The format for the health history presented in this chapter is based on the traditional approaches in health care delivery systems. Within nursing, alternate systems of health assessment have been developed around the organizing framework of functional health patterns (Gordon, 1994). *Functional health patterns* are defined as sequences of health behavior across time. Following is the currently used taxonomy of functional health patterns. Listed under each pattern are areas of specific assessment relevant to that health pattern.

Health Perception–Health Management Pattern

This category describes the client's perceived pattern of health and well-being and how health is managed. It includes the relevance of health perception to current activities and future planning. Also included is the individual's health risk management and general health care behavior, such as adherence to mental and physical health promotion activities, medical or nursing prescriptions, and follow-up care.

  Reason for seeking health care
  Current and usual health status
  Perception of individual's own health
  Health management and adherence behavior
  Risk factors—family history, health habits, environment
  Preventive health screening activities
  Readiness for health behavior change

Nutritional-Metabolic Pattern

This area describes the pattern of food and fluid consumption relative to metabolic need and eating patterns. It includes daily eating times, types and quantity of food and fluids consumed, particular food preferences, and use of nutrient or vitamin supplements. This area also describes breast-feeding and infant-feeding patterns. It includes reports of any skin lesions and general ability to heal; the condition of skin, hair, nails, mucous membranes, and teeth; and measurements of body temperature, height, and weight.

  General information—height, weight, appetite
  Food and fluid intake
  Weight patterns
  Activity level
  Psychosocial/cultural/personal influences
  Nutrition information
  Pertinent physiological alterations
  Drug history
  Skin and dental problems

Elimination Pattern

This category describes the patterns of excretory function (bowel, bladder, and skin). It includes the individual's perceived regularity of excretory function; use of routines or laxatives for bowel elimination; and any changes or disturbances in time pattern, mode of excretion, quality, or quantity. Also included are any devices used to control excretion.

  Bladder elimination
  Usual pattern of voiding
  Self-care practices
  Symptoms of altered bladder elimination
  Pertinent physiological alterations
  Bowel elimination
  Usual pattern of defecation
  Self-care practices
  Symptoms of altered bowel elimination
  Pertinent physiological alterations
  Skin problems

Activity-Exercise Pattern

This area describes the pattern of exercise, activity, leisure, and recreation. It includes **activities of daily living** requiring energy expenditure, such as hygiene, cooking, shopping, eating, working, and home maintenance. Also included are the type, quantity, and quality of exercise, including sports, that describe the typical pattern for the individual. Factors that interfere with the desired or expected pattern for the individual are noted (e.g., neuromuscular deficits and compensations; dyspnea, angina, or muscle cramping on exertion; and cardiac/pulmonary classification, if appropriate). Leisure patterns are also included and describe the activities that the individual undertakes as recreation either with a group or as an individual. Emphasis is on the activities of high importance or significance to the individual.

  Usual activities and exercise patterns
  Self-care activities–ADL level
  Adequacy of energy for requirements
  Symptoms related to activity and exercise
  Pertinent physiological alterations
  Functional status

Sleep-Rest Pattern

This category describes the patterns of sleep, rest, and relaxation during the 24-hour day. It includes the individual's perception of the quality and quantity of sleep and rest and perception of energy level. Also noted are aids to sleep, such as medications or nighttime routines, that the individual uses.

Usual sleep pattern
Sleep/bedtime rituals
Sleep environment
Sleep position
Psychophysiological influences
Sleep-pattern disturbance symptoms
Leisure and rest activities

Cognitive-Perceptual Pattern

This class describes the sensory-perceptual and cognitive pattern. It includes the adequacy of sensory modes, such as vision, hearing, taste, touch, and smell, and the compensation or prosthetics used for disturbances. Reports of pain perception and how pain is managed are also noted when appropriate. In addition, the **cognitive** functional abilities, such as language, memory, and decision-making, are included.

Eyes and vision
Ears and hearing
Use of hearing aids and glasses or contact lenses
Other senses
Symptoms of neurological dysfunction
Changes in memory
Pertinent physiological alterations and medications
Learning styles
Comfort

Self-Perception–Self-Concept Pattern

This area describes the self-concept pattern and the perceptions of self. It includes the individual's attitudes about himself or herself, perception of abilities (cognitive, affective, and physical), body image, identity, general sense of worth, and general emotional pattern. Patterns of body posture and movement, eye contact, voice, and speech are also noted.

Social identity
Personal identity
Physical self
Self-esteem
Self-concept threats

Role-Relationship Pattern

This class describes the pattern of role engagements and relationships. It includes the individual's perception of the major roles and responsibilities in current life situations. Satisfaction or disturbances in family, work, or social relationships, and responsibilities related to these roles are noted.

Roles
Composition of household and home environment

Family relationships
Family problems
Family functioning
Financial situation
Social functioning
Work environment
Neighborhood environment

Sexuality-Reproductive Pattern

This category describes the patterns of satisfaction or dissatisfaction with sexuality and delineates the reproductive pattern. It includes the individual's perceived satisfaction or disturbances in his or her sexuality. The female's reproductive stage, premenopausal or postmenopausal, and any perceived problems are also noted.

Sex roles and gender identification
Knowledge about sexuality and reproduction
Concerns about sexual performance and satisfaction
Reproductive history
Use of contraception

Coping–Stress Tolerance Pattern

This area describes the general coping pattern and the effectiveness of the pattern in terms of stress tolerance. It includes the individual's reserve or capacity to resist challenge to self-integrity, modes of handling stress, family or other support systems, and perceived ability to control and manage situations.

Nature of stresses
Life changes
Perception of stresses/roles
Coping strategies
Methods for resolution of stress
Sources of support

Value-Belief Pattern

This class describes the pattern of values, goals, or beliefs (including spiritual) that guide choices or decisions. It includes what is perceived as important in life; the quality of life; and any perceived conflicts in values, beliefs, or expectations that are health related.

Culture
Spirituality
Values
Perceived quality of life

COMPUTER-ASSISTED HISTORIES

Computer science is an important and permanent component of health care technology, and the computer can be an important tool in obtaining the client health history. Studies have demonstrated that the use of the computer in history taking can save the practitioner time and yield a reliable, comprehensive, and readable printout. In addition, this approach is acceptable to clients. In situations where personnel is in short supply and time allocated to history taking is routinely inadequate, the computer-assisted history can be superior to a verbal history. The computer-facilitated history may not be appropriate with client groups in which reading literacy is low.

Computer systems for history taking can be either client- or practitioner-interactive systems. The client-interactive systems are more commonly used because they can save the practitioner time. A number of client-interactive, computerized history-taking systems are available. Self-administered histories involve the client either completing a paper-and-pencil questionnaire or one on computer. With the paper-and-pencil questionnaire, the client's responses are computerized in a variety of ways, and the practitioner receives a printout of those responses. In the computerized systems, the client responds to inquiries from a computer terminal. In general, clients have viewed computer-assisted interviews favorably, and printouts from such systems have been complete, accurate, and legible.

In any client self-administered system, the practitioner's time is needed to review the client's history. Usually this review involves only a small amount of time. However, the amount of time spent by the client in the history-taking process is not shortened by the computer-assisted methods. The client's age, the number of client problems, and the time required by the client to complete the instructional portion of the computer program generally increases the overall time needed to complete a computer-assisted history. The number of the client's years of formal education decreases the overall time.

The computer-assisted history is more appropriate for the ambulatory client than for the hospitalized client. The ambulatory client can be scheduled for a computer interview or can complete a form for computerization that will yield a printout for the practitioner within several days. For hospitalized clients, information is generally needed immediately, and client access to terminals becomes problematic. Also, the hospitalized client often is too ill to complete a questionnaire or to use a computer terminal.

Practitioner-based computer systems for history taking involve either the practitioner's direct interaction with a computer, which is programmed for questions related to the history and into which answers are placed, or the practitioner's completion of a form that is computer-processed at a later time. The practitioner-interactive systems require a terminal for each practitioner—a situation that may not be cost-effective in ambulatory care situations. A more common approach is to perform computer-processing of questionnaires. The advantage of this method is that it produces a legible printout—an improvement over most handwritten documents.

The computer-assisted history can be as effective as the verbal history. In fact, it may be more effective because remembering items for review is not a problem. Any question that can be asked verbally can be programmed into a computer system, and computer technology allows for addi-

tional, branching questions if the client gives certain significant responses. Before additional assessment is done and therapy is begun, it is important for the practitioner to discuss, review, and verify the information to determine the validity of significant responses. The client may have misunderstood instructions, or mechanical errors may be reflected in the information.

As computers become more prevalent in health care systems, the use of computer-assisted histories is likely to increase. However, there will always exist situations in which the computer-assisted history is not feasible and a verbal history is necessary. Therefore skill in history taking is, and will continue to be, an important ability of the health care practitioner.

HISTORIES FOR RISK ASSESSMENT

Many health programs are providing screening services for selected potential health issues in target populations. Such programs are designed to identify individuals at higher risk for health problems and to facilitate early referral and treatment as well as health education. Often these screening services involve a short history focused on the identification of

---

BOX 3-9

COMMONLY EXPLORED AREAS IN A HISTORY FOR RISK PROFILE ASSESSMENT AND SCREENING FOR HEALTH PROMOTION INTERVENTIONS

Amount of exercise
Current work or work frequently performed in the past
Dental hygiene practices—frequency of brushing, flossing, and preventive dental care
Driving after alcohol consumption
Family history of cardiovascular disease, diabetes, or cancer
History of cardiovascular disease, diabetes, cancer, or serious infections
Immunizations
Screening tests appropriate for gender, age, and condition
Sexual intercourse patterns and numbers of partners
Smoking
24-hour dietary history recall
Typical mood
Use of alcohol
Use of car seatbelt
Use of contraceptives
Use of estrogen replacement
Use of illicit drugs
Use of prophylactic aspirin
Use of sunscreens
Use of vitamins and supplements

Data from Woolf S: The history: What to ask about it. In Woolf SH, Jonas S, Lawrence RS: *Health promotion and disease prevention in clinical practice*, Baltimore, 1996, Williams & Wilkins.

risk factors. The same principles of interviewing and history taking presented in this and the previous chapter can be applied to such histories. Because of their purpose, however, such histories are very focused and adapted to the age, gender, and other relevant characteristics of the target population. These histories are often self-administered in paper-and-pencil or computer format. The areas of assessment commonly included in such histories are listed in Box 3-9.

THE WRITTEN RECORD

The written record is the permanent, legal, and working documentation of what the practitioner sees, hears, and feels during the examination. It serves as the baseline for evaluation of subsequent changes and decisions related to therapy. This record is used health care practitioners who do not have access to the recorder and is consequently subject to interpretation.

The recorded history must be accurate, objective, clear, complete, and concise. It should also be readable by members of the health care team. Therefore, handwritten records should be legible and free of abbreviations, which are not easily decoded by health care team members. While the record does not need to contain complete sentences in all notions, take care to use proper grammar and punctuation.

The recording should be free of recorder bias. In particular, the history is not the place for the recorder to include his or her opinions of possible diagnoses. Other portions of a client's record allow for the recorder to elaborate on diagnoses and plans.

In addition, the practitioner should integrate the client's responses in an accurate but objective way. This can be accomplished in one of two ways: (1) by paraphrasing the client, using statements such as, "States he had the same symptoms 4 years ago" or "Denies chest pain," or (2) by quoting the client directly (e.g., "The pain was so severe, I fell back into the chair I had just gotten up from.").

Because most health histories are read by many health care providers over time, the clarity and organization of the presentation are important. A clear presentation is often difficult for the beginning health historian to achieve, but feedback about written histories from colleagues and instructors can assist in identifying strengths and deficits in this area. Most beginners must pay specific attention to chronology and symptom analysis.

The written record should be a complete history of the practitioner-client encounter. It should be specific enough for the reader to determine clearly what questions were asked, what areas of examination were covered, and the results of the interview and examination. An entry such as "Eyes—negative" or "Eyes—normal" does not supply information regarding what questions were asked about the eyes. The range of "normal" is wide, and any change in condition, even within the range of normal, may be significant for an individual client.

Although the written record must be complete, it should also be concise. A reader should be able to locate and read regional entries easily. A verbose and disorganized record may be even less effective than an incomplete one because its appearance may frustrate the busy reader, who simply will not read it. The record does not need to be composed of complete sentences. In fact, the use of clear phrases can save both time and space.

Two examples of documented health histories are presented in Boxes 3-10 and 3-11. One is an example of a history taken from a well client. The other is an example of a history taken from an ill client being admitted to a hospital. A sample health history form is presented in Box 3-12. An example of a recorded physical examination is included in Chapter 23.

BOX 3-10

EXAMPLE OF A RECORDED HISTORY FOR A WELL CLIENT

CLIENT: Mary Rose Doe
ADDRESS: 1056 N. East St.
   St. Louis, MO 63047
TELEPHONE: 278-9274
CONTACT: Husband, Robert Doe, at the same address,
   or Mrs. Elsa Smith (mother)
ADDRESS: 3496 Oak St.
   St. Louis, MO 63047
TELEPHONE: 926-8711
BIRTH DATE: Feb. 6, 1963   **SEX:** Female
RACE: African-American
RELIGION: Methodist (active)
MARITAL STATUS: Married
SOCIAL SECURITY NUMBER: 396-47-8911
USUAL OCCUPATION: Grade school teacher
PRESENT OCCUPATION: Same—Greenwich School
BIRTHPLACE: Greenwood, Mississippi

HEALTH INSURANCE: St. Louis Health Maintenance
   Organization, Member Number: 54983209
USUAL SOURCE OF HEALTH CARE:
   St. Louis Health Maintenance Organization,
   Primary Care Provider: Susan Crawford, FNP
   4693 C. Division St.
   St. Louis, MO 63044
SOURCE AND RELIABILITY OF INFORMATION:
   Client: cooperative, apparently reliable
DATE OF INTERVIEW: Jan. 12, 2000
REASON FOR VISIT: Annual physical examination;
   last examination, 12/98

PRESENT HEALTH STATUS
Usual Health

This is the third St. Louis HMO visit for this 37-year-old
   black, married, female school teacher who has been in good

BOX 3-10–cont'd

EXAMPLE OF A RECORDED HISTORY FOR A WELL CLIENT–cont'd

health for all of her life. Client has been hospitalized twice for the purposes of normal childbirth only. Has no major chronic disease.

Summary

Client is presently well and requests a physical examination for health maintenance and screening purposes. Is concerned about a strong family history of hypertension and believes that monitoring of her blood pressure status is important. Also requests a Pap smear and evaluation for continuance of oral contraceptives. Has been taking oral contraceptives since the birth of her last child in 1987. Client enrolled in the health plan 2 years ago.

HEALTH HISTORY

Allergies

None known. Denies allergy to penicillin, other drugs, foods, or environmental components. Has had one course of penicillin (10 days, oral) without side effects.

Immunizations

Had full DPT series when a preschooler. Had oral polio when an adolescent. No others. Has received annual flu shots for the past 3 years. Most recent tetanus 5 years ago.

Habits

Cigarettes—smoked 15 cigarettes a day for 5 years (age 20 to 25). Pack years = 3.75. No smoking since age 25.
Illicit drugs—denies past use of any.
Alcohol—drinks three to four 4-ounce glasses of red wine each weekend.
Coffee, tea—drinks approximately five 8-ounce cups of decaffeinated coffee a day. Drinks tea rarely.

Medications

Noriny/l ⅟₃₅ taken currently. Oral contraceptive used since 1987.

Aspirin (ASA) for headache—takes approximately 10 gr twice a month.
Milk of magnesia for constipation—takes 1 tablespoon about once a month.
One-A-Day multiple vitamins—takes 1 a day.

Exercise Patterns

Attends aerobics classes 2 to 3 times a week during the winter. In summer, walks 3 to 4 times a week.

Sleep Patterns

Sleeps 7 to 8 hours a night regularly with occasional naps on weekends.

Childhood Illnesses

Had rubella, chickenpox—not diagnosed by a physician. Has not had rheumatic fever.

Injuries

Broke arm in fall from bicycle when 13 years old.

Hospitalizations

See obstetrical data in Review of Physical Systems.
  1. Age 20 (1983). Childbirth.
  2. Age 24 (1987). Childbirth.

Operations

None.

Major Illnesses

None.

FAMILY HEALTH HISTORY

Strong family history for hypertension and stroke. See family tree. Denies family history of diabetes, blood disorder, gout, obesity, tuberculosis, epilepsy, kidney disease, or gastrointestinal disease.

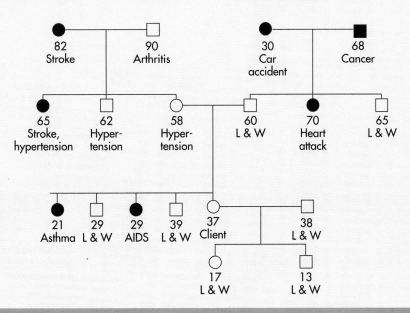

Continued

BOX 3-10–cont'd

EXAMPLE OF A RECORDED HISTORY FOR A WELL CLIENT–cont'd

REVIEW OF PHYSICAL SYSTEMS

General

Usually well. Usual-minimum-maximum weight: 140-125-160 lb. No recent increase or decrease in weight. Denies fatigue, malaise, chills, sweats, fever, seizures, or fainting. Reports height as 5 ft, 6 in.

Skin, Hair, and Nails

Denies lesions, color change, ecchymoses, masses, petechiae, texture changes, pruritus, sweating, or unusual odors. No alopecia or brittle hair. Denies brittle, cracking, or peeling nails. No birthmarks. Washes hair once a week; does not use dyes.

Head and Face

Denies pain, dizziness, vertigo, or history of injury or loss of consciousness.

Eyes

Has worn corrective lenses since age 7; currently wears contact lenses all day. Denies recent change in visual acuity, pain, infection, watery or itching eyes, diplopia, blurred vision, glaucoma, cataracts, or decreased peripheral vision. Last ophthalmoscopic examination 2 years ago. Next appointment in 2 months.

Ears

Denies hearing loss, discharge, pain, irritation, or ringing in ears. Cleans ears with cotton-tipped applicator.

Nose and Sinuses

States she has sinus pain, congestion, and subsequent nasal discharge several times each winter. Takes Sudafed prn (approximately one q 12 hours × 3 days) for each episode of rhinitis; gets relief. Denies epistaxis, soreness, excessive sneezing, obstructed breathing, or injuries. States olfaction is good.

Oral Cavity

Visits a dentist every 6 months for cleaning and examination. Brushes and flosses teeth twice a day. Denies toothache, lesions, soreness, bleeding of gums, coated tongue, disturbance of taste, hoarseness, or frequent sore throat.

Neck

Denies pain, stiffness, limitation of movement, or masses.

Nodes

Denies enlarged or tender nodes in neck, axillary, or inguinal area.

Breasts

Denies masses, pain, tenderness, or discharge. Examines breasts monthly, right after menses.

Chest and Respiratory System

Denies pain, wheezing, shortness of breath, dyspnea, hemoptysis, or cough. Denies history of asthma, pneumonia, or bronchitis. Obtains annual PPD tests—have been negative.

Cardiovascular System

Denies precordial pain, palpitations, cyanosis, edema, or intermittent claudication. Denies diagnosis of heart murmur, hypertension, coronary artery disease, or rheumatic fever.

Gastrointestinal System

Denies history of GI disease. Appetite good. Daily bowel movements; stools are always brown. Denies pain, constipation, diarrhea, flatulence, vomiting, hemorrhoids, hernias, jaundice, pyrosis, or bleeding. Has never had GI x-rays.

Genitourinary System

Denies history of bladder or kidney infections, hematuria, urgency, frequency, dysuria, incontinence, nocturia, polyuria, or VD. Menses—onset 13 years; frequency, every 26 to 30 days; duration, 5 days; flow, heavy for 3 days, light for 2 days; last menstrual period (LMP), 12/25/99. Denies dysmenorrhea, menorrhagia, discharge, or pruritus. Last Pap smear, 12/98.

Obstetrical History

1. Sept. 12, 1983. Girl, 6 lb., 8 oz. Vaginal delivery at St. Francis Hospital, St. Louis. Prenatal, intrapartum, and postpartum course normal for mother and baby.
2. Oct. 9, 1987. Boy, 7 lb, 2 oz. Vaginal delivery at St. Francis Hospital, St. Louis. Prenatal, intrapartum, and postpartum course normal for mother and baby.
3. No additional pregnancies, abortions, or miscarriages.

Sexual History

Age at first intercourse was 17 years. Enjoys intercourse with husband—no dyspareunia and able to achieve satisfactory orgasm most of the time. Using oral birth control medication. Does not want another child. Is considering a tubal ligation.

Extremities

No past problems. Denies deformities, varicose veins, thrombophlebitis, joint pain, stiffness, swelling, gout, arthritis, limitation of movement, color changes, or temperature changes.

Back

No past problems. Denies pain, stiffness, or limitation of movement; no history of disk disease.

Central Nervous System

No past problems. Denies loss of consciousness, clumsiness of movement, difficulty with balance, weakness, paralysis, tremor, neuralgia, paresthesia, history of emotional disorders, drug or alcohol dependency, disorientation, memory lapses, or seizures. Speech articulate.

Hematopoietic System

No past problems. Denies excessive bleeding and bruising, blood transfusions, or excessive exposure to x-rays or toxic agents. Blood type A, Rh positive.

BOX 3-10–cont'd

EXAMPLE OF A RECORDED HISTORY FOR A WELL CLIENT–cont'd

Endocrine System

Denies history of diabetes or thyroid disease, polyuria, polydipsia, polyphagia, intolerance to heat or cold, or hirsutism.

REVIEW OF SOCIOLOGICAL SYSTEM

Family Relationships

Lives in own home with husband and 2 children. Husband is a school teacher also; couple shares finances, childrearing, and housekeeping responsibilities. Client's parents live ½ mile away, and relationships are described as "good." Couple has several close friends; also, siblings are in frequent contact. No recent family crisis or change.

Occupational History

Has been a grade school teacher for 5 years. No other jobs. Holds bachelor's and master's degrees and feels secure that she can retain her job as long as she wants it. Enjoys children, and states job is very satisfying.

Economic Status

Client and husband achieve a combined gross income of more than $100,000 a year. Feels this is very adequate. Belongs to an HMO. Assesses coverage as "good."

Daily Profile

During the week, works 8 AM to 3 PM. Returns home around 3:30 and works until 5 PM on schoolwork. Then cooks dinner and interacts with family. Attends meetings one or two evenings a week. Weekends, client and husband usually go out one evening with friends, to movie or concert. Family attends church each Sunday. Client is involved with photography as a hobby. Frequently bicycles in summer and downhill skis in winter. Walks 2 miles a day. Tries to attend aerobics classes twice a week.

Educational Level

Highest degree attained is the master's degree. Obtains most of health knowledge by reading.

Patterns of Health Care

Has always had a primary care provider. Cared for by Dr. Richard Smith, a family practitioner until first pregnancy. Then seen regularly by Dr. Janice Lawson for obstetrical and gynecological care. Family enrolled in HMO 2 years ago. Family members see Dr. Jones and Mary Hughes, NP. Receives regular dental care.

Environmental Data

Birthplace—Greenwood, Miss. Grew up in Trenton, NJ.
Home—family lives in their own 8-room home in a residential St. Louis neighborhood. Client describes home as comfortable. Has lived there for 10 years.

Community—community is middle income, integrated, consisting primarily of young, professional families.
Work—teaches fourth grade in a community school. States that the work situation is fairly good. School is in good condition, and classes are small. A recent stress is a new assistant principal with whom client does not get along. May consider transfer to another school.

REVIEW OF PSYCHOLOGICAL SYSTEM

Cognitive Abilities

Oriented to time, place, and person (×3). Is articulate, asks questions, has a good memory. Able to understand directions.

Response to Illness

States she has never been seriously ill, so does not know what personal response would be. Feels she is "too busy" to be ill for any length of time. Uses resources of the HMO for preventive and therapeutic needs of self and family.

Response to Care

States she enjoys encounters with health care providers. States she usually follows through on the advice that is given. Feels that the services of the HMO are adequate to meet her family care needs and she has been very satisfied with the care to date.

Cultural Implications

Client states she and her family are involved in a racially integrated community. She grew up in a predominantly black northern community. Cannot identify any way in which her black culture would especially affect her response to illness or therapy in the case of illness. Active Methodist; believes that religious and spiritual beliefs would influence her responses to illness and treatment positively.

DEVELOPMENTAL DATA

Adult female: wife, mother, and career teacher.

NUTRITIONAL DATA

Diet adequate; moderately high in fats and carbohydrates. Has no food intolerances.
Usual breakfast—toast with butter, fried egg, orange juice, and coffee with cream.
Usual lunch—eats with schoolchildren; consists of meat, 1 vegetable, 1 carbohydrate, dessert, and beverage.
Dinner—meat (beef, chicken, or pork), salad, 1 vegetable, potato or bread, dessert, and coffee with cream.
Snacks—may have cheese and crackers or peanuts in the evening.

BOX 3-11

EXAMPLE OF A RECORDED HISTORY FOR AN ILL CLIENT

CLIENT: John Donald Doe
ADDRESS: 9037 N. Sheridan St.
St. Louis, MO 63125
TELEPHONE: 735-1946
CONTACT: Mrs. Clara Doe (mother)
ADDRESS: Same address as above; client will move in with mother after discharge from hospital
TELEPHONE: Same telephone number as above
BIRTH DATE: March 3, 1964
SEX: Male
RACE: White
RELIGION: Presbyterian (inactive)
MARITAL STATUS: Separated
SOCIAL SECURITY NUMBER: 097-32-7259
USUAL OCCUPATION: Offset printer
PRESENT OCCUPATION: None; on disability for 1 year
BIRTHPLACE: New York, NY
SOURCE OF REFERRAL: Self
HEALTH INSURANCE: County subsidized HMO
USUAL SOURCE OF HEALTH CARE:
Dr. Christopher Ryan
1346 W. North Ave.
St. Louis, MO 63122
SOURCE AND RELIABILITY OF INFORMATION: Client attempted to be cooperative; however, was frequently vague about the nature and time of events.
DATE OF INTERVIEW: Jan. 9, 2000
CHIEF COMPLAINT: "Pain in the left side of stomach for 2 days."

PRESENT ILLNESS
Usual Health

This is the fifth Healer's Hospital admission for this 35-year-old white, separated, unemployed male who has been drinking an average of 2 to 3 pints of hard liquor 3 to 4 times a week for the past 18 years. He states he has at least one drink of hard liquor each day. Total past admissions number 8; one of these has been for a hemorrhoidectomy. Client is presently on disability income as a result of a diagnosis of tuberculosis (11/98). Also has a history of drug abuse and gastric ulcer.

CHRONOLOGICAL STORY
18 Years PTA*

Began drinking heavily and regularly.

7 Years PTA

Diagnosed as having a gastric ulcer by Dr. Ryan. Treated by him on an outpatient basis with Maalox and Xanax prn. Had x-rays at that time. Has complained of slight to moderate gastric discomfort and food intolerance intermittently since then. Unable to relate the specific frequency or specific characteristics of episodes of illness. States that they

---
*PTA, Prior to admission.

are usually accompanied by "hangovers" and inability to remember details. Generally experiences left upper quadrant discomfort, feelings of hunger, nausea, and vomiting of mucous material 6 to 8 hours after drinking heavily. Drinks heavily 3 to 4 days a week and states symptoms occur approximately 2 times a week. Appetite generally has been fair. Meal patterns are erratic. Takes Xanax for sleep each night. Drinks two to three 8-oz bottles of Maalox per week. No pattern of follow-up care with Dr. Ryan. Symptoms relieved somewhat with Maalox. Bowel movements have been regular, formed, and brown.

1 Day PTA

Had not been drinking the night before. Awoke at approximately 7 AM and took several alcoholic drinks (amount approximately 1 cup). An hour after he attempted to drink orange juice at 9 AM, he experienced nausea and vomiting.

At 10 AM walked to his mother's home (2 blocks). On arriving, experienced a sharp, continuous, nonradiating pain in his upper left abdominal area. The intensity required him to lie down. Position changes provided no relief. A whole bottle of Maalox did not affect the pain, which built in intensity over the next 2 hours. After 2 hours the pain remained constant but was more nagging than sharp. Tried to take some soup and orange juice but immediately vomited it. At 2 PM vomited approximately 1 cup of green-colored, thick matter again, and this time there were red streaks in the vomitus. Unable to remember the exact amount of vomitus or amount of blood.

Throughout the remainder of the afternoon and early evening, took 5 mg Xanax 4 times. Obtained no relief; pain remained nagging and continuous. Was able to walk with no increase in discomfort but felt most comfortable lying down. Spent a fitful night, and the pain persisted with increased intensity. States he took his temperature at midnight and had a fever of 102° F.

Date of Admission

Rose at 9 AM and was driven to Dr. Ryan's office but found it closed. Then came directly to Healer's urgent care clinic, where he was seen and admitted.

NEGATIVE INFORMATION

Denies unusual weakness, chills, or fever before the onset of symptoms. Denies injury to the abdomen, unusual activity or exercise, pain in other locations, diarrhea, constipation, change in stools, jaundice, ascites, flatulence, hemorrhoids, rectal bleeding, or dysphagia.

RELEVANT FAMILY HISTORY

The only significant family history for a serious, persistent gastrointestinal disorder was a maternal uncle who was a heavy drinker and who died of stomach cancer at age 40. Father was an alcoholic.

BOX 3-11–cont'd

EXAMPLE OF A RECORDED HISTORY FOR AN ILL CLIENT–cont'd

DISABILITY ASSESSMENT

Client states that he has not felt really well in the past 7 years. Has not spent a great deal of time in bed but has not worked regularly and has been either drinking or "hung over" most of the time. Was diagnosed as having tuberculosis, 11/98, and was placed on a disability income plan at that time. This insurance will cover medical expenses.

PAST HEALTH HISTORY

Childhood Illnesses

Exact illnesses or dates unknown. Assumes he had all childhood illnesses (measles, mumps, chickenpox); denies history of rheumatic fever.

Injuries

Client unable to provide exact dates for any of the following:
1. Age 9 (1973). Hit in the eye by rock. States has had a permanent decrease in vision in left eye. No medical care.
2. Age 14 (1978). In an automobile accident. Was hospitalized at Lakeside Hospital, Chicago, for 1 week. Physician unknown. Discharged from hospital with no follow-up required.
3. Age 15 or 16 (1979 or 1980). Fractured right ankle while playing football. Cast applied at Johnson Hospital, Chicago, and was followed in that hospital's orthopedic clinic. Apparently healed.
4. Age 18 (1982). Head injury from blow with blunt object, which was thrown. Was unconscious for approximately 30 minutes. Head sutured in emergency room (ER) of Lakeside Hospital, Chicago. No follow-up except for removal of sutures. No complications or long-term effects.
5. Age 21 (1985). Stab wound in left shoulder; was attacked and robbed. Sutured in ER of Lakeside Hospital, Chicago. No follow-up except for removal of sutures. No complications or long-term effects.

Hospitalizations

1. Age 10 (1974). Hernia repair at Lakeside Hospital, Chicago. Dates and events of hospitalization unclear.
2. Age 14 (1978). Automobile accident. See item 2 under Injuries.
3. Age 20 (1984). Pneumonia. Under the care of Dr. Warner at St. Peter's Hospital, Chicago. Hospitalized for 2 weeks during December. No follow-up.
4. Age 23 (1987). Surgery for priapism at Lakeside Hospital. Under the care of Dr. Meyer. Follow-up for 1 year after surgery because was unable to obtain an erection. No other complications or current disability.
5. Age 24 (1988). Heroin drug overdose. Under the care of Dr. Ryan, Healer's Hospital, St. Louis. Hospitalized for 2 weeks; was to start methadone maintenance; did not. Dates of stay not known.
6. Age 26 (1990). Heroin drug overdose. Under the care of Dr. Ryan, Healer's Hospital. In the hospital for 1 week. Discharged against medical advice.
7. Age 28 (1992). Heroin drug overdose. Under the care of Dr. Ryan. Hospitalized at Healer's Hospital for 2 weeks. Discharged on methadone maintenance.
8. Age 28 (1992). Hemorrhoidectomy. Under the care of Dr. Ryan and Dr. Jones, Healer's Hospital. Hospitalized 1 week. No complications; 1 follow-up visit.

Operations

See Hospitalizations for details.
1. Age 10 (1974). Hernia repair.
2. Age 23 (1987). Correction of priapism.
3. Age 28 (1992). Hemorrhoidectomy.

Other Major Illnesses

1. Age 29 (1993). Diagnosed as having gastric ulcer by Dr. Ryan after an outpatient evaluation including x-rays. See Present Illness section for follow-up.
2. Age 34 (1998). Tuberculosis diagnosed and treated by staff of the St. Louis Health Department as an outpatient. Medications for 1 year. Off medications for the past 3 months. Followed with yearly x-rays and evaluation.

CURRENT HEALTH INFORMATION

Allergies

None known. Denies allergies to penicillin, other drugs, foods, or environmental components; has had at least 3 courses of penicillin.

Immunizations

Unknown.

Habits

Cigarettes—Has smoked an average of 1 pack a day since age 12. Pack years = 23.
Hard drugs—all types, including heroin. 1988-1992 had a "$90-a-day-habit." Was treated successfully at a methadone clinic. No recent history of drug abuse.
Alcohol—started to drink heavily at age 16. Drinking decreased during period of drug addiction. Has been drinking 2 to 3 pints of hard liquor 3-4 times a week for the past 18 years.
Coffee, tea—drinks 6 to 7 cups of caffeinated coffee a day. Does not drink tea.

Medications

Xanax 5 mg prn for gastric distress.
Maalox—for ulcer prn with varied dosage since 1993. Prescribed by Dr. Ryan. Client states he uses 2 to 3 8-oz bottles a week.
Valium—10 mg prn for ulcer and nervousness from 1983 to 1990.
Methadone—Was off and on in a treatment program during period of drug addiction. No medication taken at present.
Streptomycin—IM daily, dose? For TB, 11/98 to 9/99.
INH—tid for TB, 11/98 to 9/99.

Continued

BOX 3-11—cont'd

EXAMPLE OF A RECORDED HISTORY FOR AN ILL CLIENT—cont'd

Salve—name unknown, a nonprescription drug; topically every day for scaling skin on soles of feet; since approximately 8/93.

Magnesium citrate—for constipation approximately once a week; prescribed by self. Uses 1 tbsp prn.

Sleeping pill—1 tablet prn. Name and dose unknown. Prescribed by Dr. Ryan.

Exercise Patterns

Largely sedentary due to lifestyle and low energy. No regularly scheduled exercise.

Sleep Patterns

Sleeps about 7 to 8 hours during a 24-hour period. Often patterns are irregular because of alcohol consumption.

FAMILY HEALTH HISTORY

Maternal and paternal grandparents deceased. Ages at death and causes of death unknown. Denies family history of diabetes, blood disorders, arteriosclerosis, gout, obesity, coronary artery disease, tuberculosis, cancer, hypertension, epilepsy, kidney disease, or allergic disorders. Uncertain about health history of aunts and uncles, except for uncle with alcohol and gastrointestinal problems.

Mother—age 56; alive and well.

Father—deceased, age 50, 1979; cause unknown. Was an alcoholic.

Siblings—no maternal miscarriages.
1. ♀ Age 31; alive and well.
2. ♂ Age 20; deceased 1992; drug overdose.
3. ♀ Age 25; alive and well.
4. ♂ Age 23; alive and well.

Children
1. ♂ Age 10; alive and well.
2. ♂ Age 7; alive and well.

Wife—age 31; obese, otherwise well.

REVIEW OF PHYSICAL SYSTEMS

General

Chronically ill, white male adult; usual weight about 176 lb. Reports approximately 10 lb weight loss over the past 3- to 4-month period. Feels this is a result of not eating when drinking heavily. States he has felt a generalized fatigue and malaise for more than 1 year, since onset of TB, but denies requiring daily naps or extra sleep. States he cannot exercise because of fatigue. Denies chills (other than those associated with present illness), sweats, and seizures.

Skin, Hair, and Nails

Denies lesions, color changes, ecchymoses, petechiae, texture changes, unusual odors, or infections. Pruritus; soles of feet dry and scaling for 6 months; condition stable (using nonprescription salve, name unknown). States he has had small cracks at corners of mouth for 1 month. Denies cold sores. States hair breaks off and falls out but denies patchy alopecia. Denies brittle, cracking, or peeling nails. States bites nails. Has one birthmark on upper back but is not aware of any change in size or color.

Head and Face

Denies pain, headache, dizziness, or vertigo. History of injury with blow to forehead. Reports frequent losses of consciousness after drinking; duration unknown, probably 1 to 8 hours.

Eyes

Has worn corrective lenses since 1974, age 10. States right eye 20/20, left eye 20/50. History of one eye injury, age 9. States visual acuity decreased after injury. Denies pain, infection, watery or itching eyes, diplopia, blurred vision, glaucoma, cataracts, and decreased peripheral vision. Last ophthalmological examination 2 years ago.

Ears

Denies hearing loss. Denies discharge, pain, irritation, or ringing in ears. States he was "cut in a fight" on right auricle. Cleans ears with a toothpick.

Nose and Sinuses

Denies sinus pain, postnasal drip, discharge, epistaxis, soreness, excessive sneezing, or obstructed breathing. Denies injuries. States he has approximately two colds a year. Reports decreased sense of smell; attributes this to smoking.

Oral Cavity

Complains of frequent dryness in mouth and cracking of lips and tongue. No false teeth. Has several missing teeth. Gums bleed frequently. Denies hoarseness, pain, odor, frequent sore throats, and voice change. Dental care infrequent. Brushes teeth "occasionally."

Neck

Denies pain, stiffness, or limitation of range of motion. Denies masses.

Nodes

Denies enlarged or tender nodes in neck, axillary, or inguinal area.

Breasts

Denies surgery, pain, masses, or discharge.

Chest and Respiratory System

Denies pain, wheezing, asthma, or bronchitis. History of pneumonia, age 20 (see Hospitalizations). Denies shortness of breath or dyspnea. Sleeps on two pillows but is not dependent on them for breathing. History of TB, 1998-1999. Last chest x-ray on present admission, negative for TB. States he had one episode of hemoptysis, 1987, associated with his ulcer. Details of this unclear. States he has "smoker's cough" (dry cough in the morning) but denies sputum.

Cardiovascular System

Denies chest pain, coronary artery disease, rheumatic fever, or heart murmur. Denies hypertension, palpitations, cyanosis, or diagnosis of cardiac disorder. States he has occasional slight edema in right ankle.

BOX 3-11—cont'd

EXAMPLE OF A RECORDED HISTORY FOR AN ILL CLIENT—cont'd

Gastrointestinal System

See Present Illness. Also see Hospitalizations, re: hemor-rhoidectomy. Appetite poor. Denies melena, clay-colored stools, or diarrhea. Takes laxative, magnesium citrate, approximately once a week for constipation. Denies jaundice. Reports decreased appetite with alcohol intake but denies specific intolerance to any food.

Genitourinary System

Denies bladder or kidney infections, urgency, frequency, hesitancy, painful urination, incontinence, nocturia, polyuria, history of VD. Denies testicular pain. History of surgery for priapism with inability to have erection for 1 year after surgery. No dysfunction at present. States sex life is "fair." Alcohol decreases "urge." Heterosexual. No homosexual encounters. Has had five sexual partners in the last 5 years. Has not used condoms.

Extremities

See Past Health History. Reports swelling of ankle without pain. Denies varicose veins, thrombophlebitis, joint pain, stiffness, swelling, gout, arthritis, limitation of movement, or color changes.

Back

Denies pain, stiffness, limitation of movement, or disk disease.

Central Nervous System

Reports loss of consciousness (1982) following blow to head; duration approximately 30 minutes. Denies clumsiness of movement, weakness, paralysis, tremor, neuralgia, or paresthesia. States he is a "nervous" person but denies history of nervous breakdown. History of drug and alcohol abuse. States he will periodically (every 2 to 3 weeks) have spontaneous jerky movement of legs during rest. There are four to five movements in each episode. This has never occurred while legs were bearing weight. Denies disorientation or memory disorders. Denies seizures or epilepsy. "Passes out" frequently after heavy alcohol ingestion and sleeps for 5 to 6 hours. Wakes with headache and nausea.

Hematopoietic System

Denies bleeding, bruising, blood transfusion, or exposure to x-rays or toxic agents.

Endocrine System

Denies diabetes, thyroid disease, or intolerance to heat or cold. Growth has been within normal range.

REVIEW OF SOCIOLOGICAL SYSTEM

Family Relationships

Has been separated from wife for 6 to 7 months and is in the process of being divorced. States his marital problems do not interfere with seeing his children. Plans to move to his mother's home when discharged from hospital. States relationships with his family of origin are good. Wife and children are very concerned about alcohol abuse. Mother tolerates lifestyle.

Occupational History

Offset printer since 1986. Presently unemployed. Was advised not to work for 6 months when TB was diagnosed and has not been "able to get back to work." States he liked that occupation but expresses no urgency to return to work.

Economic Status

On disability income because of TB and need to rest. States he does not have trouble making ends meet on present income. Expresses no concern for financial status of wife and children who are on "welfare" and being assisted by wife's family.

Daily Profile

Has lived in a room since separation from wife. States he spends time during the day at home or with friends, drinking. Has no special hobbies or activities to occupy time. Has habit of heavy daily drinking. States, "I just hang around all day." Does do some spur-of-the-moment traveling. Weekdays are no different than weekends.

Educational Level

States he is "smart enough." Dropped out of college after 2 years because of disinterest. States he has no aspiration except to "get by in life."

Patterns of Health Care

Has maintained relationship with same physician for episodic care for the last 10 years. Does return for periodic examinations and follow-up when symptoms "scare him."

Environmental Data

Birthplace—New York, NY. No travel outside of USA; no armed forces duty.

Home—Plans to move to his mother's home. Will share the 5-bedroom residence with his mother and two siblings.

Neighborhood is residential; describes it as "beautiful."

REVIEW OF PSYCHOLOGICAL SYSTEM

Cognitive Abilities

Oriented to present events. Has fairly adequate vocabulary. Has a fair to poor memory. Cannot recall details of some important events. No history of psychiatric treatment.

Response to Illness

States he "quit" drinking when he entered the hospital and plans to abstain in the future. Has no specific plans for treatment. Verbalizes that his health problems are his own fault and that he will die soon if he does not resolve them. States illness does not bother him except when "it gets out of control." Definition of health entails being able to play baseball again.

Response to Care

States he has sometimes not followed medical advice because of fear or because drugs or alcohol did not allow him to think "straight." "People have been nice to me." States all care has been "OK."

Continued

BOX 3-11–cont'd

EXAMPLE OF A RECORDED HISTORY FOR AN ILL CLIENT–cont'd

Cultural Implications

Inactive Presbyterian at present but is concerned about conflict with religious beliefs and lifestyle. Fourth-generation American.

DEVELOPMENTAL DATA

Adult male who has had problems with interpersonal relationships in his marriage. Has demonstrated drug and alcohol abuse since entering adulthood. Does not express concern regarding his inability to work; has abandoned his college attendance. Immediate plans for the future involve moving in with his mother and trying to stop drinking. Speaks of his children as playmates; expresses few fathering needs or activities.

NUTRITIONAL DATA

States he does not eat or has erratic meal patterns when drinking heavily and must build his tolerance to food by taking liquids such as soup or juices after drinking. States he does eat three complete meals daily when not drinking. Includes foods from the meat and carbohydrate food groups, but does not eat fruits or green vegetables regularly.

BOX 3-12

SAMPLE HEALTH HISTORY FORM

BIOGRAPHICAL INFORMATION

Full name _____

Social Security or Clinical ID number _____

Client's permanent address _____

_____

Home telephone number _____

Work telephone number _____

Contact of client (person to contact in case of emergency)

    Name _____

    Telephone number _____

Birth date _____

Bender: male ☐   female ☐   Race _____

Ethnicity _____   Religion _____

Marital status _____

Usual occupation _____

Present occupation _____

Birthplace _____

Health insurance source and number _____

_____

Usual sources of health care _____

_____

Source and reliability of information _____

Date of interview _____

CLIENT'S REASON FOR SEEKING CARE OR CHIEF COMPLAINT

_____

_____

_____

PRESENT HEALTH OR HISTORY OF PRESENT ILLNESS

Introduction

Summary and usual health

Symptom Analysis: Chronological Story (In cases of a present illness, include information about the onset, course since onset, location, quality, quantity, setting, associated phenomena, alleviating and aggravating factors, and client's underlying concern related to each symptom.)

Pertinent Negative Information

Relevant Family Information

Disability Assessment

PAST HEALTH HISTORY

General Health Information

Usual health

Allergies

Habits (alcohol, tobacco, drugs, caffeine)

Medications taken regularly (names, dosages, frequency, intended and actual effects, and compliance)

Exercise patterns

BOX 3-12—cont'd

SAMPLE HEALTH HISTORY FORM—cont'd

Sleep patterns

Immunizations

PAST HEALTH PROBLEMS
Past major illnesses—resolved and chronic

Childhood illnesses

Accidents and disabling injuries

Hospitalizations (including blood transfusions)

Operations

ENVIRONMENTS
Community

Work

Recreational

FAMILY HEALTH HISTORY (note presence of problem and relative[s] affected)
Alcoholism

Allergies

Alzheimer's disease

Arteriosclerosis

Cancer

Coronary artery disease

Diabetes

Epilepsy

Gout

Hematological disorders (e.g., hemophilia, sickle cell anemia, thalassemia, hemolytic jaundice, or severe anemia)

Huntington's chorea

Hypertension

Kidney disease

Mental disorders

Obesity

Tuberculosis

Other: _____

REVIEW OF SYSTEMS
Physical Systems

General

Skin
Health promotion/health maintenance

Health problems

Hair
Health promotion/health maintenance

Health problems

Nails
Health promotion/health maintenance

Health problems

Head and face
Health promotion/health maintenance

Health problems

Eyes
Health promotion/health maintenance

Health problems

Continued

BOX 3-12—cont'd

SAMPLE HEALTH HISTORY FORM—cont'd

Ears
Health promotion/health maintenance

Health problems

Nose and sinuses
Health promotion/health maintenance

Health problems

Mouth and throat
Health promotion/health maintenance

Health problems

Neck and nodes
Health promotion/health maintenance

Health problems

Breasts
Health promotion/health maintenance

Health problems

Respiratory and cardiovascular systems
Health promotion/health maintenance

Health problems

Gastrointestinal system
Health promotion/health maintenance

Health problems

Urinary system
Health promotion/health maintenance

Health problems

Genital system (male)
Health promotion/health maintenance

Health problems

Genital system (female)
Health promotion/health maintenance
Menstrual history—age at menarche, typical cycle, duration
  of flow, amount of flow

Date of last menstrual period (LMP)

Date of last normal menstrual period (LNMP)

Obstetrical history

Health problems

Sexual history (both sexes)
Health promotion/health maintenance

Health problems

Extremities and musculoskeletal system
Health promotion/health maintenance

Health problems

Central nervous system
Health promotion/health maintenance

Health problems

Endocrine system
Health promotion/health maintenance

Health problems

Hematopoietic system
Health promotion/health maintenance

Health problems

FUNCTIONAL STATUS

SOCIOLOGICAL AND CULTURAL SYSTEMS
Relationships with family and significant others

Environment—physical and psychological

PSYCHOLOGICAL SYSTEM

DEVELOPMENTAL DATA

NUTRITIONAL DATA

? Critical Thinking Questions

1. How would you adapt the history to a client similar to yourself?
2. How would you adapt the history to:
   a. A 16-year-old sexually active female?
   b. A 90-year-old male who has recently lost a spouse?

3. Think about recent illnesses of yourself and family members. Describe the chief complaints using the symptom analysis criteria listed in this chapter.
4. Create a health genogram for yourself.

MERLIN Answers are available on the MERLIN website (www.harcourthealth.com/MERLIN/Barkauskas/). And be sure to check the website regularly for additional learning activities!

Remember to check out the Online Study Guide!
www.harcourthealth.com/MERLIN/Barkauskas/

Assessment of Health Behaviors

PURPOSE

Information derived from history taking provides insights into the client's overall health. When the practitioner needs to learn more about the meaning of a particular health behavior in a client's life and clues to modifying unhealthy behaviors, additional assessment areas may be pursued. *Health behaviors* are the actions persons take to maintain, promote, or improve health, well-being, and the quality of life.

This chapter provides an introduction to several of the currently used health behavior theories being applied to clinical practice and provides guidance regarding assessment of clients' thinking about particular health-related practices and factors that might influence positive health behavior change. These assessment areas are especially important in assessing clients for health promotion interventions and services. Space in this chapter permits only general introduction of the key assessment areas reflected in behavior change theories.

MAJOR HEALTH BEHAVIOR THEORIES

Transtheoretical Model

The Transtheoretical Model is commonly also termed the *Stages of Change Model*. It describes the stages through which individuals progress in the process of behavior change. This model was originally proposed by Prochaska (1979) and has been used to explain behaviors, as well as to design interventions focused on smoking cessation, contraceptive use, addictive behaviors, condom use, alcohol abuse, HIV prevention, and weight control (McKenzie and Smeltzer, 1997). The model integrates concepts and notions of behavior change from other theories. It proposes that individuals progress through various levels relating to behavior changes, from lack of awareness related to a behavior through consideration of the behavior change, testing the implementation of the change, taking focused action to make the change, and then maintaining the change. Al-

TABLE 4-1	**Stages of Change in the Transtheoretical Model**

Stages of Change	Definition of Stage	Examples of Assessing this Stage
Precontemplation	Not thinking about change in the next 6 months	Awareness of the potential impact of the focus problem
		Knowledge of methods of behavior change
Contemplation	Seriously thinking about change in the next 6 months	Perceptions about the targeted behavior
		Awareness of consequences of an unhealthy behavior
		Expected benefits of behavior change
		Awareness of the factors supporting unhealthy behavior
Preparation	Actively planning change	Establishment of a date to initiate change
		Willingness to share change decision with others
		Development of an action plan:
		• Sources of support
		• Concrete steps to effect behavior change
		• Benchmarks
		• Aids for behavior change
		• Priorities
Action	Overtly making changes	Identification of obstacles and plan to address them
		Identification of anticipated rewards for behavior change
Maintenance	Taking steps to sustain change and resist temptation	Understanding recidivism
		Plan to stay focused
		Commitment
		Incorporation of the change into lifestyle

Data from Prochaska JO, Redding CA, Evers KE: The Transtheoretical Model and stages of change. In Glanz K, Lewis FM, Rimer BK: *Health behavior and health education,* San Francisco, 1997, Jossey-Bass.

though the stage notions imply a progressive movement from a less active stage to a more active one, the progress through these levels is often nonlinear and cyclical, going through periods of relapse and restarting the process.

Research by Prochaska and colleagues (1994) has demonstrated that health promotion interventions targeted according to individuals' stages of change are much more effective than standard interventions applied equally to all clients without regard to readiness for change. Thus assessing stage of change is an important basis for tailoring interventions directed to assisting individuals to improve from one stage of change to the next. In addition to full behavior change, progress from one stage to a more action-oriented one is considered a positive outcome in itself.

The five stages of change are precontemplation, contemplation, preparation, action, and maintenance (Table 4-1). In the precontemplation stage, individuals are not thinking about changing their behavior during the next 6 months. The common timeframe for the stages in this model is 6 months. Individuals in precontemplation are generally uninformed or underinformed about the importance of the consequences of a particular unhealthy behavior to their health. They are generally unaware of the health issues that require change or for various reasons have made decisions not to initiate efforts to change their behavior. For example, in the case of a smoker, the individual adheres to a belief that smoking will cause him no harm.

In the second stage, contemplation, persons are aware that a problem exists and are considering some change regarding it, but have not yet made a commitment to action.

They are aware of the issues related to the behavior and the pros and cons of change.

In the third stage, preparation, individuals have taken some steps toward action, for example throwing away all cigarettes and buying the nicotine control patches, but have not yet fully committed to or institutionalized the behavior change.

In the fourth stage, action, individuals have actively made changes in their behaviors throughout the past 6 months to effect the behavior change in patterns of daily living or environment (e.g., the person has decreased number of cigarettes per day).

Persons who continue their actions and integrate them into their daily behavior patterns and have strategies to prevent relapse can be classified as being in the maintenance stage of change. Usually a behavior change needs to be in place for 6 months for maintenance to be established.

Sometimes a sixth stage, termination, is added to this model, especially in the case of the target area of addictions. In this stage, persons have no temptation to regress and have integrated new behaviors into daily patterns.

The model also provides guidance for analysis of factors, which influence movement from one stage to another and for the development of interventions to assist individuals to move from one stage to another. An important assessment factor is decisional balance, which reflects the individual's relative weighting of the pros and cons of changing. The knowledge of an individual's perceived pros and cons toward a particular behavior provides important insights about interventions. An example of a con related to smoking cessation is, "It helps me relax." Examples of pros toward the same behavior are, "Smoking is so expensive," or "I think smoking is affecting my health." An example of a change from a con to a pro is the following statement: "I no longer need smoking to relax me; my stress management exercises help me relax."

For a client to progress from precontemplation to contemplation, the perceived pros of change must increase, and to progress from contemplation to action, the perceived cons of changing must decrease. These pros and cons in the Transtheoretical Model are conceptually very similar to the notions of benefits and barriers observed in other health behavior theories.

Processes of change are activities that people use to progress through the stages of change. Ten so far have been tested and have received empirical support. These are listed and defined in Table 4-2.

For movement from precontemplation to contemplation, consciousness raising, dramatic relief, and environmental reevaluation processes are recommended. Self-reevaluation is recommended for movement from contemplation to preparation. Self-liberation, or giving oneself permission to change, and social liberation are strategies to assist movement from preparation to action. Action through maintenance strategies are helping relationships, counter-conditioning, contingency management, and stimulus control.

This transtheoretical theory has been used to study and design interventions directed to the following behaviors: smoking cessation, quitting cocaine, weight control, high-fat diets, adolescent delinquent behaviors, condom use, sunscreen use, radon gas exposure, exercise behaviors, mammography screening, and smoking behaviors (Prochaska et al., 1994).

Social-Cognitive Theory

The components of Bandura's (1986) Social-Cognitive Theory have served as the basis for several other health behavior theories (Figure 4-1). The theory proposes that an individual's behavior and cognitions affect future behavior. The theory's three main concepts are behavioral capacity, efficacy expectations, and outcome expectations. *Behavioral capacity* is the knowledge and skills to form a given behavior. *Efficacy expectations*, or *self-efficacy*, relate to confidence in being able to perform a particular behavior, and *outcome expectations* are beliefs that the performance of a particular behavior will produce the desired effects. These concepts connect and interact through the notion of *reciprocal determinism*, which is the dynamic interaction of the person, the behavior, and the environment in which the behavior is performed.

Self-efficacy is central to this theoretical formulation. Bandura (1977) identified four main sources of information that influence self-efficacy: past performance accomplishment, vicarious experiences (e.g., observations of the experiences of influential others), verbal persuasion (e.g., encouragement from others), and physiological arousal. These sources have implications for both assessment as well as intervention. Determining the processes by which an individual acquires self-efficacy provides substantial guidance for intervention plans related to enhancement of self-efficacy.

TABLE 4-2	**Processes of Change in the Transtheoretical Model**	
Processes of Change	**Definition**	**Stage in Which Use is Recommended**
Consciousness raising	Finding and learning new facts, ideas, and tips that support positive change	Precontemplation ➡ Contemplation
Dramatic relief	Vicarious experience of negative emotions that accompany unhealthy behaviors (e.g., through role-playing)	Precontemplation ➡ Contemplation
Environmental re-evaluation	Cognitive and affective assessment of how a particular health habit affects one's social environment	Precontemplation ➡ Contemplation
Self-re-evaluation	Cognitive and affective assessment of one's self with and without a particular unhealthy behavior Analysis of pros and cons	Contemplation ➡ Preparation
Self-liberation	Belief that one can change and the commitment and recommitment to act on that belief	Preparation ➡ Action
Social liberation	Developing appreciation that the social norms are changing in the direction of supporting the healthy behavior change	Preparation ➡ Action
Helping relationships	Seeking and using social support for the healthy behavior change	Action ➡ Maintenance
Counter-conditioning	Substituting healthier alternative behaviors and cognitions for unhealthy behaviors	Action ➡ Maintenance
Contingency management	Increasing the rewards for the positive behavior and decreasing the rewards for the unhealthy behavior	Action ➡ Maintenance
Stimulus control	Removing cues to engage in the unhealthy behavior and adding cues or reminders to engage in the healthy behavior	Action ➡ Maintenance

Data from Prochaska JO, Redding CA, Evers KE: The Transtheoretical Model and stages of change. In Glanz K, Lewis FM, Rimer BK: *Health behavior and health education,* San Francisco, 1997, Jossey-Bass.

Past performance accomplishment relates to learning through personal experience. Mastering one difficult task enhances confidence in taking on and succeeding in other difficult tasks. Vicarious experiences occur when one views others, similar to oneself, successfully performing a given behavior. Verbal persuasion is influence from a respected source toward a particular behavior. Physiological arousal can affect self-efficacy positively or negatively. For example, some negative physiological barriers (e.g., fear, hostility, and anxiety) can become barriers to change. However, these barriers can be managed by various techniques (e.g., stress management techniques or problem restructuring) if the barriers and strategies provided to manage them are identified early.

Theories of Reasoned Action and Planned Behavior

The Theories of Reasoned Action (TRA) and Planned Behavior (TPB) are a set of propositions that explain voluntary behaviors and the roles of attitudes, norms, and intentions in influencing behaviors (Fishbein and Ajzen, 1975; Ajzen, 1991) (Figure 4-2).

According to the theory of reasoned action, an individual's behavior is affected by an intention to perform a particular behavior. Intention to perform a behavior is a function of the influences of attitudes toward the behavior and normative beliefs regarding what others think about the behavior (i.e., subjective norms). Attitudes toward the behavior are a combination of behavioral beliefs and evaluation of behavior outcomes. Subjective norms are a combination of normative beliefs and motivation to comply with these normative beliefs. This theory is useful in situations in which the behavior is fully under an individual's volitional control (e.g., safe sex practices).

The Theory of Planned Behavior extends the theory of reasoned action by adding the notion of resources and constraints through the concept of perceived behavioral control. Thus a person's intention to perform a certain behavior is affected by attitude toward the behavior, normative beliefs, and perceived behavioral control. Behavior control is affected by control beliefs concerning the presence of resources for and impediments to performance and perceived

power regarding the mobilization of these resources and for overcoming impediments. The concept of perceived behavioral control is very close to the notion of self-efficacy, which is prominent in the Social-Cognitive Theory discussed in the previous section. Both theories are diagrammed in Figure 4-2.

These models have been applied to the understanding of and the designing of interventions directed toward the following behaviors: smoking cessation, condom use, participation in health screening, exercise, food choices, breast/testicular self-examination, medication compliance, weight control, and alcohol use (Connor et al., 1999).

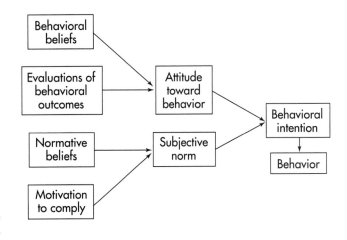

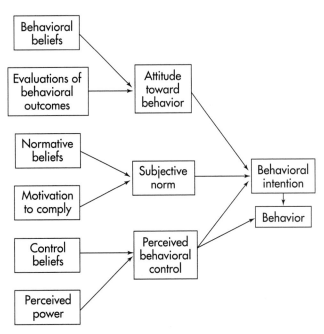

Figure 4-2 Theories of Reasoned Action and Planned Behavior. (Modified from Ajzen I: *Attitudes, personality, and behavior,* Buckingham, United Kingdom, 1988, Open University Press.)

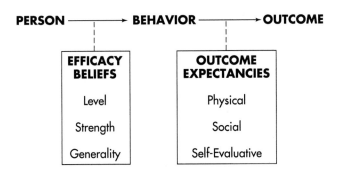

Figure 4-1 Social-Cognitive Theory. (Modified from Bandura A: *The social foundations of thought and action: a social cognitive theory,* Upper Saddle, NJ, 1985, Prentice-Hall.)

Health Belief Model

The Health Belief Model (HBM), developed by Rosenstock (1966), is one of the oldest health behavior models (Figure 4-3). This model is also based on the Social-Cognitive Theory and has been largely applied to prevention intervention programs (e.g., immunization programs). The authors of this model contend that a person's likelihood of taking recommended action is affected by several factors, including individual perceptions about the health issue, perceived benefits and barriers to the action, and behavior-specific modifying factors. Individual perceptions are the individual's perceived susceptibility to a given health problem and the perceived seriousness of disease. Modifying factors include demographic factors, knowledge, perceived threat of the health problem, and cues to action.

For a given health issue the perceived susceptibility to the particular problem and the perceived seriousness of the problem form a perception of the perceived threat of the problem. Certain demographic, psychosocial, and structural variables and cues to action mediate this perceived threat. The individual also weighs perceived benefits against perceived barriers in decisions to respond to the threat via preventive action. Thus it "is believed that individuals will take action to ward off, to screen for, or control an ill-health condition if they regard themselves as susceptible to the condition, if they believe the problem will have potentially serious consequences, if they believe that a course of action available to them would be beneficial in reducing either their susceptibility or the severity of the condition, and if they believe that the anticipated barriers to (or costs of) the action are outweighed by the benefits" (Strecher and Rosenstock, 1997, p. 44).

Health Promotion Model

The Health Promotion Model (HPM) was developed by Pender (1996) to identify the factors influencing health promotion behaviors and the relationships among those factors. The theory is built on the value expectancy notion of the Social Cognitive Theory and portrays the multidimensional aspects of persons in relationship to health behaviors (Figure 4-4). This model contains constructs similar to those seen in other models, specifically perceived benefits of action, perceived barriers to action, perceived self-efficacy, prior related behavior, interpersonal influences, situational influences, personal factors, and commitment to a plan of action. A concept unique in the model is *immediate competing demands*. However, immediate competing demands could also be considered a barrier.

In the HPM, individual characteristics and experience, prior related behavior, and personal factors influence behavior-specific cognitions and affect. These cognitions and affect include perceived benefits of action, perceived barriers to action, perceived self-efficacy, activity-related affect, interpersonal influences, and situational influences. These cognition and action variables collectively influence a commitment to a plan of action. The influence of commitment to action and immediate competing demands, along with behavior-specific cognitions and affect, combine to influence the action toward a health promotion behavior.

For example, if the health-promoting behavior is a regular sleep pattern, prior experience with sleep habits and personal emotional and physiological factors that affect sleep and rest must be assessed. Then the practitioner can work with the client to identify the perceived benefits and barriers to the improved sleep habit behavior in the context of the experience and emotional and physiological factors, the client's self-

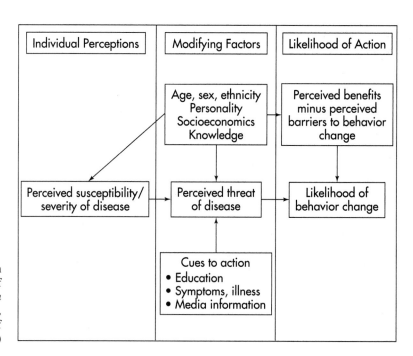

Figure 4-3   Health Belief Model. (Modified from Strecher VJ, Rosenstock IM: The Health Belief Model. In Glanz K, Lewis FM, Rimes BK: *Health behavior and health education,* San Francisco, 1997, Jossey-Bass. This material used by permission of Jossey-Bass, a subsidiary of John Wiley & Sons, Inc.)

efficacy in managing time, environments and related factors that affect sleep. Sleep is most often a pleasant experience, so attitudes toward sleep are generally positive; but the practitioner should not make that assumption and determine the client's feelings about the activity of sleep. Interpersonal influences in terms of attitudes of household members to sleep and related household patterns of activity also must be considered. Clients who share their beds with spouses or others are heavily influenced by the sleep and rest patterns of others and other situational influences related to sleep.

Once the assessment is completed and a commitment to action is made, the practitioner can help the client intervene in relevant benefit, barrier, self-efficacy, interpersonal, and environmental areas to enable changes in sleep patterns. In this example the notion of immediate competing demands will need to be carefully considered because often the reason for poor sleep habits is competing demands for the time that should be allocated to sleep.

Self-Regulation Model

Leventhal, Meyer, and Nerez (1980) developed the Self-Regulation Model (SRM), also referred to the Common-

sense Model, to explain how health beliefs influence behavioral responses to illness. The SRM is an information-processing model in which individuals are seen as motivated to construct meanings to information about their health in order to engage in self-regulating behaviors. A central feature of the model is the assumption that information processing can be explained using three sets of variables: representation, coping, and appraisal (Figure 4-5). Further, information is processed on two levels. One level of processing is done cognitively, and the other level of processing is related to emotions associated with a person's response to health information. Further information from the environment is simultaneously processed on two levels: the cognitive, or objective, level and the affective, or emotional, level. For example, a client with a headache can describe the objective characteristics of the pain but may also react with fear and anxiety about the potential seriousness of the condition.

Representation variables are dimensions that individuals use to organize and interpret information (both internal and external) and give it meaning. Information can originate from a variety of sources, including the presence of body symptoms, memories of past illness experiences, and inter-

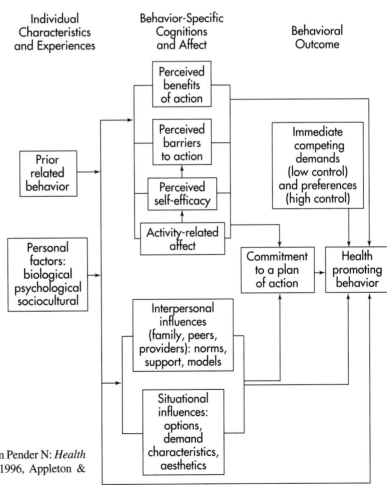

Figure 4-4 Health Promotion Model. (Modified from Pender N: *Health promotion in nursing practice*, ed 3, Norwalk, CT, 1996, Appleton & Lange.)

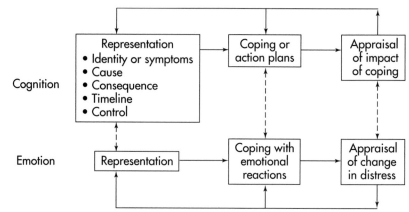

Figure 4-5 The Commonsense Model. (Modified from Leventhal H, Safer MA, Pandgis DM: The impact of communications on the self-regulation of health beliefs, decisions, and behavior, *Health Educ Q* 10(1):3-29, 1983.)

actions with others. For example, a person may feel a pounding sensation in the head and decide that this is a symptom of an illness. The individual may then search for a particular illness label to apply to the symptom. Taken together, this symptom and label comprise the identity component of the representation.

Four other components—cause, consequence, timeline, and control—are also part of the representation. Cause has to do with the individual's perceptions about the cause of illness; consequence concerns perceptions about the short- and long-term outcomes of the illness; timeline relates to ideas about the whether the illness is acute or chronic in nature; and control is one's belief that the illness can be influenced.

An example of the subjective nature of representations is found in the research done on individuals with high blood pressure. Even though hypertension is referred to the "silent killer" because it is asymptomatic, Meyer, Leventhal, and Gutmann (1985) found that more than half of newly diagnosed hypertensive clients in treatment believed that they could tell when their blood pressure was up by how they felt. The symptoms they mentioned most often were headache, dizziness, and feelings of warmth and nervousness. The authors explained how well-meaning clinicians might have reinforced the clients' belief that high blood pressure has symptoms. Taped interviews of provider-client encounters showed that practitioners would typically begin a visit by asking clients whether they had specific symptoms. The common-sense interpretation by the client was that, if the practitioner thought symptoms were so important, they must be important indicators of blood pressure control.

Representation influences *coping* and *planning* responses to information in the representation. For example, an individual who believes that a headache is a symptom of high blood pressure may cope by taking an extra dose of medication. On the other hand, someone who considers headache to be a symptom of the flu may cope by taking an aspirin and going to bed early.

The third set of variables involves appraisal or evaluation of the effectiveness of the actions taken, such as less anxiety or more physical comfort. For example, if the headache did not respond to aspirin and rest, the individual may get the idea that the headache is indicative of something more serious such as a brain tumor and seek a health care provider.

KEY VARIABLES RELATED TO HEALTH BEHAVIOR AND HEALTH BEHAVIOR CHANGE

Several health behavior models with potential for application to clinical situations have been presented. These models provide guidance for assessment areas whenever the practitioner's goal is health behavior change.

These models reflect a number of commonalties. First, the notion of perceptions is strong. These include perceptions about the actual behavior, the problem to be prevented, and the person's own ability to perform the behavior; opinions of significant others; and beliefs that the recommended behavior will achieve the desired results. Second, notions of benefits and barriers are also prominent across the theories. Benefits and barriers may be perceptual or may be real issues of available resources. Norms are prominent in the Theories of Reasoned Action and Planned Behavior and are implied in the cues to action notion in the Health Belief Model. Table 4-3 outlines approaches to the assessment of the key concepts across presented models. Definitions of the concept, assessment areas, and approaches to assessment are presented.

The student practitioner should consider the theories and various related concepts and practice obtaining related assessment information from clients to determine which concepts and theoretical formulations are most effective and functional in obtaining information to guide understanding of clients' behaviors and designing interventions to support clients' goals.

TABLE 4-3	Key Concepts of Health Behavior Theories		
Concept	Definition	Assessment Areas	Examples of Assessment Questions
Appraisal of coping (SRM)	Determination of whether coping goals were met; if not, representation is re-examined	Assessment of how well the goal of coping has been achieved	Did your actions work? Do you have less pain? Fewer symptoms? Less anxiety?
Attitudes toward health behaviors (TRA, TPB)	Beliefs that certain attributes or outcomes are associated with a particular behavior as well as the value attached to those outcomes or attributes. This idea is close to the notions of benefits and barriers but can also include the feelings about the actual behavior or behavioral outcome itself	Views of the recommended behavior. Importance of the benefits of the behavior and the specific outcome	Please tell me your opinion about the following: • Mammography detects cancer at an early stage • Mammography involves physical discomfort • Mammography exposes me to excessive radiation. How likely will using a condom decrease your sexual sensation every time you have vaginal sex during the next 3 months with your regular partner (rating: extremely likely to extremely unlikely)?
Cause (SRM)	Beliefs about the cause of problem	Causative factors	What do you think caused this problem?
Consequence (SRM)	Beliefs about the seriousness of consequences of a problem	Perceptions of the consequences	How serious do you think this is? What happens with this problem?
Control (HBM, SRM, HPM)	Beliefs about one's ability to control the problem	Perception of control over consequences	Do you think this is curable or controllable? If yes, how?
Coping or action plans (SRM)	Actions taken in response to information contained in the representation, based on beliefs about illness and prior experience	Behaviors or behavioral intentions in response to the representation	What do you plan to do about your health problem? What did you do in response to your health problem?
Identity (SRM)	The perception of body sensations attached to a verbal label	Symptom experience	What symptoms or sensations have you experienced?
Intention (HPM, TRA, TPB)	A person's perceived likelihood of performing a particular behavior	Expressions of intentions to make a change. Time period designated for the change. Evidence of preparation toward the change	How likely are you to obtain a mammogram during the next year? If you have sex during the next 2 months, how likely is that that you will always use condoms (rating: very likely to very unlikely)?
Outcome expectations (SCT, HBM)	The positive expectations resulting from the performance of a behavior; this idea is close to the notion of benefits, and the similar assessment areas apply	Beliefs about the linkage of a certain behavior and certain benefits. Positive outcomes expected as a result of a particular behavior. Value of the positive aspects of the behavior	Do you think you will be able to breathe better if you stopped smoking?
Perceived barriers/cons (HBM, HPM, SRM, TTM, SCT)	A person's opinions of the effort, resources, and costs required to achieve and maintain the recommended behavior, including giving up certain positive aspects related to the status quo	Physical costs of the behavior, including money, time, and other resources. Psychosocial costs of the behavior, including giving up familiar and habitual patterns, (e.g., smoking with friends). Perceived control over barriers	What would it take for you to lose 50 pounds? What would be the most difficult aspect of losing weight?

HBM, Health Belief Model; *HPM*, Health Promotion Model; *SCT*, Social-Cognitive Theory; *SRM*, Self-Regulation Model; *TPA*, Theory of Planned Behavior; *TRA*, Theory of Reasoned Action; *TTM*, Trans-Theoretical Model.

Continued

TABLE 4-3	**Key Concepts of Health Behavior Theories—cont'd**		
Concept	Definition	Assessment Areas	Examples of Assessment Questions
Perceived behavioral control (HPM, HBM, SCT, SRM, TPB)	A person's perceived likelihood of facilitating or constraining conditions in executing a health behavior and the personal ability to manage the performance of the behavior; this idea is close to the notion of self-efficacy, and the same assessment areas apply	Resources available to the client to make the behavior change Ability to manage the negative aspects of the behavior change	How much control do you have over your food choices and behavior patterns? How can you structure your daily patterns to achieve greater control?
Perceived benefits/pros (HBM, HPM, SCT, TTM)	A person's opinions of the positive outcomes resulting from a certain health behavior, including the efficacy of the recommended actions to achieve the result desired	Positive outcomes expected as a result of a particular behavior Value of positive aspects	What positive changes in your life would you anticipate if you lost 50 pounds?
Perceived seriousness or severity (HBM)	A person's belief regarding the seriousness of a given condition and its sequelae	Beliefs about the seriousness of a negative health outcome or its sequelae Origin of those beliefs Strength of beliefs	How do you feel about the following statement? Raising a baby alone is the same as raising a baby with a spouse (rating: strongly agree to strongly disagree).
Perceived susceptibility (HBM)	A person's opinion about the chances of getting a certain condition given certain actions or inaction	Beliefs about the probability of a negative health outcome or its sequelae Reasons for susceptibility beliefs Strength of beliefs	If you do not practice safer sex, how likely are you to get AIDS? How do you feel about the following statement? Most teenage couples who don't use contraceptives wind up pregnant (rating: strongly agree to strongly disagree).
Perceived threat (HBM)	A combination of perceived susceptibility and perceived seriousness	Overall susceptibility of the preventable problem Overall seriousness of the preventable problem	How likely are you to have health problems, given your family history, and how much of an impact would these problems have on your life?
Self-efficacy (HBM, HPM, SCT)	A person's confidence in personal ability to perform successfully a particular behavior to produce the desired outcomes	Depending on the behavior change recommended, the following assessment areas can be considered: • Concerns about performance of the behavior • Previous attempts to perform the behavior and the history and outcomes of earlier attempts • Previous attempts to perform similar or related behaviors and the history and outcomes of such attempts Resources needed to perform the behavior Overall self-confidence in establishing a goal and pursuing it to attainment	Tell me about your previous attempts to lose weight. What concerns do you have about going on a diet? What resources do you need to help you stop smoking? How confident are you that you can maintain an exercise program?
Subjective norms (HBM, TRA, TPB)	Beliefs about the opinions of persons, significant in the client's life, about the behavior, specifically approval and disapproval, and the motivation to respond to these norms	Client's perceptions of the attitudes of significant others about the behavior Importance of others' perceptions of behaviors and change	How does your boyfriend feel about using condoms? How do you feel about the following statement: "Most people who are important to me think I should take better care of myself" (rating: very true/very untrue)
Timeline (SRM)	Beliefs about duration of problem	Acute or chronic timeline	How long do you think this will last?

HBM, Health Belief Model; *HPM,* Health Promotion Model; *SCT,* Social-Cognitive Theory; *SRM,* Self-Regulation Model; *TPA,* Theory of Planned Behavior; *TRA,* Theory of Reasoned Action; *TTM,* Trans-Theoretical Model.

? Critical Thinking Questions

1. A 25-year-old woman indicated an interest in smoking cessation. She has been smoking 1½ packs of cigarettes a day for the past 9 years. She is thinking about getting pregnant and knows that smoking would be hazardous to the growing fetus and her new child. Her husband also smokes. Apply each of the health behavior models presented in this chapter to assessing this situation. Which health behavior model best fits the analysis of this situation and why? What areas of assessment would be most useful in this situation to design interventions to assist this woman to stop smoking?

2. A 55-year-old man has been recently diagnosed with several serious cardiac problems. He is 100 pounds over-weight and has a very sedentary occupation with little other exercise. His family history is positive for premature deaths of male relatives from cardiac events. Which health behavior model best fits the analysis of this situation and why? Develop an assessment for behavior change interventions for this man.

3. A 16-year-old girl has recently had her first sexual experience. She is very concerned about pregnancy and AIDS. She is seeking information and assistance regarding how to better protect herself from these problems. Which health behavior model best fits the analysis of this situation and why? What areas of health behavior change orientation would you assess?

Answers are available on the MERLIN website (www.harcourthealth.com/MERLIN/Barkauskas/). And be sure to check the website regularly for additional learning activities!

Remember to check out the Online Study Guide!
www.harcourthealth.com/MERLIN/Barkauskas/

Developmental Assessment Across the Lifespan

Learning Objectives

On successful study of this chapter and completion of related learning experiences, the learner will be able to:

- Describe the purpose of developmental assessment across the lifespan.
- Discuss selected theories of human development.

- Compare screening tools appropriate for individuals at different developmental phases.
- Describe common characteristics of physical, cognitive, and psychosocial development for each phase of the lifespan (infant, toddler, preschooler, school age, adolescent, young adulthood, middle adulthood, late adulthood).

Outline

PURPOSE OF DEVELOPMENTAL ASSESSMENT

Birth is the beginning of numerous developmental stages during the lifespan. From infancy through old age, individuals continue to develop some aspect of who they are. Each person is unique, but his or her individuality occurs within some broadly shared patterns.

The family is a powerful influence on human development. How each person develops through each phase of life and how he or she comes to view the world and interact with the people in it are largely learned within the family. While the focus of this chapter is on the individual, it is always with the acknowledgment that all individuals are part of family units, or substitutes for family units, for at least some significant portion of their lives.

Humans are dynamic, complex, changing beings. They interact continuously with the environment. Their responses to life are highly individualized. Personal growth and development patterns along with social, cultural, economic, and historical forces affect each person's responses to life.

While you are learning to obtain a health history and perform a physical examination, you are assimilating new skills, handling new tools, performing new techniques, remembering lists of questions for the health history, and performing the many components of the physical examination. However, from the onset of this learning process, you need to remember to include a perspective of the individual client as a whole person. The whole person includes the mind, body, and spirit. You cannot assess parts of the person in isolation from the other parts or from the whole. You must take into account the client's developmental processes and the phases of growth and maturation through which that person is progressing across the lifespan. Take time to assess the client as a person and to discuss and discover the client's world—in relation to his or her self-perceptions and interactions with significant others and with society at large.

Discussing issues related to current or anticipated developmental phases, stages, or crises with the client can provide greater breadth and depth of understanding about the client's life situation and its relationship to health or illness. As a health care practitioner, you are in a position to help individuals and families look at the developmental aspects of their lives. Your openness in discussing the life tasks of individuals can help them appreciate the appropriateness and normalcy of their own or their children's growth patterns, changes, behaviors, and feelings. In addition, discussion of potential challenges that individuals may face related to developmental issues may help clients and their families prepare for life changes. For example, if discussing plans for retirement with a client and his or her spouse, ask what changes they might anticipate and whether they have considered ways of adapting to meet those changes. Such anticipatory guidance may help them avoid crises that can occur when an individual who is used to a busy work life suddenly finds himself or herself with unlimited time but no idea of how to spend it. Your guidance may also assist those who are blocked in their growth to understand and deal with the problem area more effectively. Help clients review their past, compare it with the present, look at progressive phases and intervals, and plan for the future in whatever ways they feel are appropriate and necessary.

Do not expect to learn everything about a client's developmental accomplishments in one or even several interviews. This is a personal story that requires time and trust to share. Determining the presence of a developmental deficit is sometimes difficult in a busy clinical setting. You may need additional time to focus attention on assessing development, or you may need to seek the assistance of others who specialize in the field.

You can perform some developmental assessment during each encounter with a client of any age. With children, have a parent or primary caregiver present, since this person will likely be the main source of history information. With children, developmental stage expectations and concerns are more familiar to assess since there are many standardized tools and guidelines. With adults, information concerning their goals, future plans, psychosocial concerns that they are currently dealing with (e.g., school, career, parenting, relationship issues) can provide insights into their developmental status.

Record developmental assessment data in the health history.

For further information on the developmental changes of children and older adults, see Chapters 26 and 27.

STAGES OF DEVELOPMENT

Developmental stages and categories are used for purposes of organization. In life, such stages are not totally distinct or

---

BOX 5-1

SOME GENERAL CHARACTERISTICS OF GROWTH AND DEVELOPMENT

1. Growth and development are cyclical. Children tend to grow in spurts, then level off for periods. Adolescents tend to have cycles of outward activity and then inner reflection. Adults also experience periods of greater outward involvement and inner orientation.
2. Growth and development continue throughout the life cycle. From birth until death, some aspect of the complex human being is changing. This process of growth and development is both universal and unique and includes physical, emotional, psychological, social, and cognitive components. It ranges from changes that are slow, subtle, and often elusive to those that occur with astonishing rapidity.
3. All aspects of the growth and development of an individual are interrelated. The physical, mental, social, emotional, sexual, moral, and spiritual components of the self are all a part of the complex matrix that is the whole person.
4. There are periods of readiness for certain developmental tasks. During these periods a degree of maturation is necessary for the behavior to occur. If the appropriate environment or stimulus is not present, the behavior may not develop, may be delayed, or may occur in a defective way.

---

exclusive. During particular phases, certain aspects of growth may be more prominent, but many overlap. Some of the early work done on the development of children by Jean Piaget and of children and adults by Erik Erikson was based on a "stage" approach. One stage and its accomplishments was followed by another, and moving from one to the other was premised on the completion of tasks at the earlier level. Piaget asserted that biological growth combines with children's interaction with the environment to take them up a development staircase, step-by-step, with each step signaling an increase in complexity of the child's thinking. He believed that changes in memory, perceptual skills, learning ability, and other aspects of mental development all occurred in this fashion. More recently, it has been argued that more variations in children's growth can be observed and that some children develop in one area much more quickly than in others. General characteristics of growth and development are presented in Box 5-1.

SELECTED THEORIES OF HUMAN DEVELOPMENT

There are numerous theorists in the field of human development. Only a brief description of a few of them is included here. (Refer to other texts in the field for a comprehensive overview of this broad subject.) The approach in this chapter is to provide a beginning framework for assessing the personhood of each individual.

The developmental aspect of infancy and childhood has received much attention and study since the late 1800s. A considerable amount of literature has surfaced on these phases, although much still remains to be studied and understood. The focus of the more recent literature on human development is on the age span between youth and old age: middle adulthood.

This chapter organizes developmental assessment around eight major life phases based on age:

Infancy: birth to 12 months
Toddler years: 1 to 3
Preschool years: 3 to 6
School-age years: 6 to 12
Adolescence: approximately 12-19 years
Young adulthood: approximately 20 to 34 years
Middle adulthood: approximately 35 to 64 years
Late adulthood: approximately 65 to 95 + years

Characteristics of each stage are described in relation to physical, cognitive, and psychosocial issues. Note that the length of time covered in a chronological stage increases with ages, ranging from months for infants to decades for adults.

Erik Erikson: Psychosocial Development

Erikson proposed a developmental framework for the entire lifespan (Erikson, 1959, 1963, 1982). His framework is outlined here and is incorporated into the discussion at the various stages of growth used in this chapter. Erikson believed that individuals' psychosocial development or identity formation was a function of somatic, ego, and social processes. The interaction of these processes at particular times in the life cycle placed specific demands on the individual that represent psychosocial or developmental "crises" (a *crisis* is defined as a necessary turning point when development must move one way or another). Resolution of a particular crisis is the task that the individual must master in order for development to progress. Erikson (1959) described these tasks in terms of eight invariant stages. Table 5-1 summarizes the stages, the strengths and virtues resulting from their resolution, and the important external relationships that help with resolving each stage (e.g., mother, family, peers).

Each stage is characterized by the identity issue addressed (e.g., Trust and Autonomy) and the contrasting attributes that may emerge from it (Mistrust, Shame, and

TABLE 5-1   Erikson's Stages of Development

Stages	Tasks	Radius of Significant Relations	Social Modalities	Basic Strengths	Virtues
I. Infancy	Trust vs. Mistrust	Maternal person	To get To give in return	Drive	Hope
II. Early childhood	Autonomy vs. Shame/Doubt	Parental persons	To hold on To let go	Self-control	Will-power
III. Play age	Initiative vs. Guilt	Basic family	To make (going after) To make like (play)	Direction	Purpose
IV. School-age	Industry	"Neighborhood" school	To make things (complete) To make things together	Method	Competence
V. Adolescence	Identity vs. Role Diffusion	Peer groups Out groups Models of leadership	To be oneself To share being oneself	Devotion	Fidelity
VI. Young adulthood	Intimacy vs. Isolation	Partners in friendship, sex, competition, cooperation	To lose and find oneself in another	Affiliation	Love
VII. Adulthood	Generativity vs. Stagnation	Divided labor and shared household	To make be To take care of	Production	Care
VIII. Old age	Integrity vs. Despair	"Mankind" "My kind"	To be, through having been To face not being	Renunciation	Wisdom

Adapted from Erikson EH: Identity and the life cycle, *Psychol Issues* 1(1, Monograph 1), 1959; and Erickson EH: *The life cycle completed,* NY, 1982, WW Norton.

Doubt). How an individual responds will influence later attitudes and the development of personal strengths. Resolution of a particular crisis is not an either/or proposition but rather determines the relative prominence of either positive or negative attributes. If the balance is toward the positive, it will help the individual meet later crises and provide a better opportunity for unimpaired total development. However, some incidence of negative attributes, such as mistrust and self-doubt, is to be expected and even necessary for healthy development (Erikson, 1959).

Dealing with each task at a particular stage of development provides the basis for progress to the next stage. As a person faces each challenge, he or she assumes both increased vulnerability and increased potential, and new strength emerges that contributes to further development. Erikson stated that all components of the personality are present in some form even before their emergence as a "crisis" and remain systematically related to all the other components. For example, the trust developed in infancy leads to a sense of hope. In working through the tasks of adolescence, this sense of hope forms a foundation for the emerging trait of fidelity, which in adulthood is reworked into an ability to care (Erikson, 1982). Therefore optimal development depends on the proper resolution of tasks in the appropriate sequence.

Awareness of developmental issues that the client is dealing with provides insights not only into expected psychosocial concerns but also into the personal resources available to the individual to respond to stress (Erickson, Tomlin, and Swain, 1983). This awareness also can give insights into an understanding of "difficult" behaviors. An individual may be working through or reworking specific developmental tasks. Problematic behaviors may indicate progression from one stage to another rather than a static state of dysfunction.

Jean Piaget: Cognitive Development

Piaget's theory concerns cognitive, or intellectual, development. Piaget believed that cognitive acts are the act of adaptation to, and organization of, the perceived environment.

He noted certain signposts of development that indicate maturation and growth. The newborn perceives the world as a vague mass but gradually integrates the various sensory inputs from sight, sound, touch, taste, and smell. The young child does not understand that objects continue to exist even though they cannot be seen, but the child gradually learns that objects have constancy—they are in existence even when they cannot be seen. The use of symbols and language to represent reality is another developmental milestone in childhood. A young schoolchild gains the cognitive ability to focus on more than one aspect of a situation and to realize that although things may change superficially, they remain basically the same.

Piaget conceived of intellectual development as occurring through a series of four invariant stages (Table 5-2). Each stage builds on and incorporates structures from the previous stage, moving from simple to increasingly complex operations. Piaget noted that all individuals have the capability to achieve the most advanced levels of functioning. However, not all individuals will reach the final stages of development, nor will a given individual function at the same structural level for all tasks (Flavell, 1963). Piaget also noted that experiences with the environment were important in motivating development. Consequently, individuals would only show adult thought in those areas in which they had been socialized (Flavell, 1963). Social interaction in the childhood era was seen as particularly important for development.

Awareness of the type of intellectual processes the individual is using can be particularly helpful in planning interventions for clients. For example, individuals who are predominately functioning at a concrete operations level (adolescents and some adults) may not respond well to abstract instructions or future-oriented teaching. They will find specific concrete examples more helpful. It is important to remember that under stressful conditions, such as experiencing a health concern, individuals may revert to more basic levels of cognitive functioning (Erickson, Tomlin, and Swain, 1983). Designing interventions with this in mind can promote more positive outcomes.

TABLE 5-2 Piagetian Stages of Cognitive Development

Stage	Approximate Age	Ways of Understanding the World	Basic Concepts To Be Mastered
1. Sensorimotor	Birth-2 yr	Through direct sensations and motor actions	Object permanence; causality; spatial relationships; use of instruments, etc.
2. Preoperational	2-6 yr	Mental processes that are governed by the child's own perceptions and linkage of events; no separation of internal and external reality	Sense of animism; egocentrism; idiosyncratic associations; transductive reasoning
3. Concrete operational	6-11 yr	Can reason through real and mental actions on real objects; can reverse changes to the world mentally to gain understanding; can reason using a stable rule system; understands some patterns	Mass; number; volume; linear time; deductive reasoning
4. Formal operations	12 yr and older (variable)	Abstract thought; can reason about ideas, impossibilities, and probabilities; broad abstract concepts	Mastery of abstract ideas and concepts; possibilities; inductive reasoning; complex deductive reasoning

From Dixon SD, Stein MT: *Encounters with children: pediatric behavior and development*, ed. 3, St. Louis, 2000, Mosby.

Sigmund Freud: Development of Sexuality

The sex of a child is genetically determined, but the development of human sexuality is influenced by many aspects of life: physical, mental, emotional, and sociocultural. Sexuality is a large dimension of life related to many aspects of total personality functioning. It is expressed through cultural beliefs, attitudes, stereotypes, feelings, self-image, and body image.

Freud thought that sexual feelings were present from infancy, changing from one form to another into adulthood. Freud's four stages of psychosexual development center on the early years of life. At each stage, instinctual sexual energy (libido) is invested in different areas of the body. He believed that at each stage a conflict exists that must be resolved satisfactorily before the individual can progress to the next stage and that a person can become fixated at any stage. These resolutions or fixations determine how an individual interacts with others. Box 5-2 lists Freud's stages of sexual development.

Freud's theory has had a strong and lasting impact in the field of psychology. Many now feel, however, that while his focus on the sexual aspect of development was important, it was also narrow and limited and that human psychological and sexual development need to be considered in the broader context of the whole person.

Carol Gilligan: Sex Differences in Development

Recent studies focusing on men's or women's development across the lifespan have provoked controversy over the applicability of previous theories to both sexes. Many of the theories on human growth and development were developed based on research or observations of males only, or with only a small sample of females. Carol Gilligan (1982), in her study of the psychosocial processes by which women develop, takes the position that women's development does not match men's development because women's identity formation takes place in a context of an ongoing relationship with the mother rather than separation from the mother. Thus when gender identity is formed around age 3, girls tend to identify with their mothers, which fuses a sense of attachment with identity formation. For boys, this process involves separation from the mother and a firming up of boundaries. This means that for boys issues of differentiation become entwined with sexual identity.

Gilligan proposes that this differentiation continues through out the life cycle. For women themes of attachment and connectedness color all aspects of their lives. For men, themes of separation and autonomy assume primary importance. Masculine identity becomes defined through separation and may be threatened by intimacy, whereas feminine identity is defined through attachment and may be threatened by separation. This can lead to life experiences in which males may have greater difficulty with relationships, whereas females may have greater difficulty with individuation. Gilligan notes that when maturity is equated with personal autonomy, a focus on relationships is viewed as a weakness rather than a human strength, and she suggests that both forces must be in balance as the person moves toward maturity. Awareness of these potential differences may be helpful in designing interventions that are sensitive to clients' needs. For example, support groups may be more effective for women, whereas individual teaching may be more effective for men.

Comparison of Perspectives

Most providers do not subscribe to one theoretical perspective. No one theory can explain the richness of the individual's development and all the factors that contribute to it. Table 5-3 provides a comparison of three developmental approaches that are commonly used in clinical practice. The table highlights the themes and issues for each age that distinguish each stage from the next. These include familiar developmental milestones as well as developmental difficulties and frank psychopathology that may appear at various ages and which the theorists propose emerge from basic developmental processes operant at that time (Dixon, 2000). Having an understanding of these theoretical perspectives and applying knowledge of developmental perspectives in your clinical practice can enrich your encounters with clients and help you provide more holistic care.

TOOLS FOR DEVELOPMENTAL ASSESSMENT

Numerous tools are available to assess child development. Tools to assess adults tend to focus on certain aspects of adult development. Table 5-4 provides a brief overview

---

BOX 5-2

FREUD'S STAGES OF SEXUAL DEVELOPMENT

1. Oral stage—infancy through 18 months. During this period the oral region (the sensory area of the mouth, lips, and tongue) provides the greatest sensual satisfaction. Sucking and swallowing reduce tension and provide pleasure.
2. Anal stage—ages 18 months to 3 years. During this period the greatest amount of sensual pleasure is obtained from the anal and urethral areas. Toilet training is a source of tension between child and parent.
3. Phallic stage—ages 3 to 5 years. The region of greatest sensual pleasure is the genital region. The Oedipal/Electra complex occurs in the later part of the phallic stage. During this stage the child "loves" the parent of the opposite sex. The parent of the same sex is considered a rival.
4. Latency stage—ages 6 to 12 years. At the beginning of the latency stage, the child is resolving the Oedipal/Electra conflict, so this is a phase of sexual latency. During this period children form close relationships with others of their own age and sex. They direct energy to physical and intellectual quests.
5. Genital stage—puberty to adulthood. Increased hormones stimulate sexual development. Sexual urges reawaken but are now directed outside the family.

of some of the assessment tools available. Several of the more commonly used tools are described in more depth here.

Screening Tools Used With Infants and Children

Screening tools assist in determining an infant's or child's progress in accomplishing age-appropriate developmental tasks. These tools assess various components, including gross motor skills, fine motor skills, personal-social behav-

iors, and language abilities. Additional information on childhood assessment tools is presented in Chapter 26.

Denver II

The Denver II (the 1989 revision of the Denver Developmental Screening Test [DDST], Figure 5-1) is a screening tool commonly used to assess the developmental level from 1 month to 6 years of age. It is easy to administer, useful for determining developmental level, and helpful in providing guidance to parents. A series of developmental tasks are used to determine whether a child's development is within the normal

TABLE 5-3 Comparison of Developmental Perspectives of Human Behavior

| Age | Theories of Development | | | Skill Areas | | Possible Psychopathology |
	Freud	Erikson	Piaget	Language	Motor	
Birth–18 mo	Oral	Basic trust vs. mistrust	Sensorimotor	Body actions; crying; naming; pointing; shared social communication	Reflex, sitting; reaching; grasping; walking, mouthing	Autism; anaclitic depression; colic; disorders of attachment; feeding and sleeping problems
18 mo–3 yr	Anal	Autonomy vs. shame, doubt	Symbolic preoperational	Sentences; telegraph; unique utterances; sharing of events	Climbing; running; jumping; use of tools, using toilet, early self-care	Separation issues; negativism; fearfulness; constipation; shyness, withdrawal; aggressiveness
3-6 yr	Oedipal	Initiative vs. guilt	Intuition, preoperational	Connective words; can be readily understood; tells and follows stories, questions	Increased coordination; tricycle; jumping, writing	Enuresis; encopresis; anxiety; aggressive acting out; phobias
6-12 yr	Latency	Industry vs. inferiority	Concrete operational	Subordinate sentences; reading and writing; language reasoning	Increased skills; sports; recreational cooperative games	School phobias; obsessive reactions; conversion reactions; depressive equivalents; anxiety; attention deficit hyperactivity disorder
12-17 yr	Adolescence (genital)	Identity vs. role confusion	Formal operational	Reason abstract; using language; abstract mental manipulation	Refinement of skills	Delinquency; promiscuity; schizophrenia; anorexia nervosa; suicide
17-30 yr	Young adulthood	Intimacy vs. isolation	Formal operational	Reason abstract; using language; abstract mental manipulation	Refinement of specialized skills; sports skills peak	Schizophrenia; borderline personality; adjustment disorders; development of intimate relationships; difficulties with relationships
30-60 yr	Adulthood	Generativity vs. stagnation	Formal operational	Reason abstract; using language; abstract mental manipulation	Refinement of skills	Depression; self-doubts; career development issues; family, social network; neuroses
>60 yr	Old age	Ego integration vs. despair	Formal operational	Some loss of skills; decreased memory, focus	Loss of functions	Involutional depression; anxiety; anger; increased dependency

From Dixon SD, Stein MT: *Encounters with children: pediatric behavior and development,* ed. 3, St. Louis, 2000, Mosby.

TABLE 5-4	Selected Instruments to Assess Aspects of Development		
Name	**Age**	**Assessment Focus**	**Comments**
*BNBAS: Brazelton Neonatal Behavioral Assessment Scale (Brazelton, 1973; 1983)	Newborn	Neurological deficits	The most widely used neonatal behavioral assessment scale. Used with all cultural groups. Special training required to administer test. Data from the test may be used to enhance parenting skills and sensitivity to infant behaviors.
*BSID-II: Bayley Scale of Infant Development (Bayley, 1993)	1-42 months	Mental, psychomotor behavior	Used with children at risk for or suspected risk of developmental delay.
Portage Guide to Early Education (1994)	Birth-6 years	Cognitive, motor, self-help, social, communication	A home-teaching program assesses child's development, serves as an educational guide to enhance family functioning, and supports parent in child's development. Translated into 35 languages. Format: checklist.
Lollipop Test (Chew, 1992)	5 years	School readiness—visual perception, numerical ability, color recognition and visual discrimination, spatial recognition	Diagnostic screening tool.
CABS: Children's Adaptive Behavior Scale Revised (Kicklighter and Richmond, 1983)	5.0-10.11 years	Language and psychosocial	Describes language development, independent functioning, family role performance, economic-vocational activity, and socialization. Used to develop educational plans.
Carey Infant and Child Temperament Questionnaires (Carey and McDevitt, 1978; Hegvik, McDevitt, and Carey, 1982; Fullard, McDevitt and Carey, 1984)	Infants, toddlers, preschoolers	Temperament characteristics	Separate questionnaires rated by parents. Determines the patterns of temperamental attributes to determine influences on the child's relationships with parents and other caregivers.
Social Readjustment Rating Scale (Holmes and Rahe, 1967)	Adult	Stress	Measures the amount of change an individual has experienced within the last year. Based on the belief that change is stressful.
Change in Life Events Scale for Children (Coddington, 1972)	Preschool-senior high	Stress	Same as Social Readjustment Rating Scale.
Overload Index Pace of Life Index (Kemper, Giuffre, and Drabinski, 1986)	Adolescent-adult	Stress from lack of time management and pacing life	10- and 15-question indexes to help recognize sources of daily stress and teach health promotion strategies.
Personal Assessment of Intimacy Relationships (Schaefer and Olson, 1981)	Adult	Perception of intimacy and goals for the relationship	Five types of intimacy assessed: emotional, social, sexual, intellectual, and recreational.
Myers-Briggs Type Indicator (Myers, 1980)*	Adult	Personality	Used by pastors, counselors, educators. Used in premarital counseling and co-worker/manager interactions. Describes the continuum of complementary vs. opposing personality types in terms of sensing/intuitive, thinking/feeling, perceptive/judging, introvert, extrovert.
MEPSI: Modified Erickson Psychosocial Stage Inventory (Darling-Fisher and Kline Leidy, 1988)	Adolescent-adult	Adult developmental status	80-item Likert scale. Assesses the strength of psychosocial attributes arising from progression through Erickson's eight stages.
Need Satisfaction Questionnaire (Porter, 1961)	Adult	Personal needs in job	Determines how well vocation meets personal needs.
CRICHT: Chrichton Geriatric Rating Scale (Robinson, 1964)	65+	Behavior/functioning	Rates behavior and ability to perform activities of daily living.
SGSS: Stokes/Gordon Stress Scale (1986)	65+	Stress	Similar to Social Readjustment Rating Scale, using belief that change is stressful.

Modified from Wilson SF, Giddens JF: *Health assessment for nursing practice,* ed. 2, St. Louis, 2001, Mosby.
*Requires training to use.

TABLE 5-4	Selected Instruments to Assess Aspects of Development—cont'd		
Name	**Age**	**Assessment Focus**	**Comments**
Geriatric Scale of Recent Life Events (Kiyak, Liang, Kahana, 1976)	Older adult	Stress	Similar to Social Readjustment Rating Scale, using belief that change is stressful.
Modes of Adaptation Patterns Scale (Sharma, 1977; Kane and Kane, 1984)	Older adult	Coping skills	Results in four adaptive styles: high activity plus high morale (conformist), high activity plus low morale (ritualist), low activity plus high morale (passive-contented), low activity plus low morale (retreatist).
Sandor Clinical Assessment—Geriatric (SCAG) (Shader, Harmatz, and Salzman, 1974)	Older adult	Behavioral functional	Assesses behavior and ability to perform activities of daily living.
Calgary Family Assessment (Wright and Leahey, 1984)	Families	Structure, development, function	Developed for use by practitioners. Tool is easily modified to fit family being assessed.
FES: Family Environment Scale (Moos and Moos, 1976)	Families	Social environment	Compares real and ideal family social environments. Ten subscales measure relationships, personal growth, system maintenance. Results used as guide for family therapy and education.
Evaluation of Family Functioning Scale (Reidy and Thibodeau, 1984)	Families	Functioning regarding health	Developed for use by community health nurses. Dimensions evaluated include health/illness, problem solving, and coping abilities.
Parenting Satisfaction Scale (Guidubaldi and Cleminshaw, 1994, in Psychological Corporation, 1995)	Adult	Parent-child relationship	Self-report. Format: Likert scale.
FACES: Family Adaptability and Cohesion Evaluation Scales I, II, III (Olson, 1986)	Adult	Family functioning	Families are defined as enmeshed vs. disengaged and structurally rigid vs. chaotically formed.
FILE: Family Inventory of Life Events and Changes (McCubbin and Patterson, 1987)	Families	Stress	FILE and A-FILE are similar to Social Rating Scale for life stressors. Format: questionnaire.
A-FILE: Adolescent-Family Inventory of Life Events and Changes (McCubbin and Patterson, 1987)	Adolescent/ families	Stress	FILE and A-FILE are similar to Social Rating Scale for life stressors. Format: questionnaire.

range. The Denver II provides a developmental profile of the individual child in four areas: personal-social, fine motor-adaptive, language, and gross motor skills. If development in any of these four areas is questionable when compared with normal standards, refer the child for an in-depth evaluation. Children who have questionable or abnormal scores on the Denver II are at risk for developing later problems in school regardless of their intelligence. The Denver II is a screening tool; it is not a diagnostic tool, nor is it an intelligence test.

Denver Prescreening Developmental Questionnaire

The Denver Prescreening Developmental Questionnaire (PDQ) (Figure 5-2) is a brief test answered by the parent. It identifies children who will need a more thorough screening with the Denver II. It assesses the same four categories as the Denver II, and it can be administered quickly and easily. The questionnaire consists of 97 questions, divided according to

Cultural Considerations
The Denver Developmental Screening Tests

When administering the DDST, the nurse must consider cultural variations that can erroneously label the child as delayed. For example, Southeast Asian children have demonstrated delays in the areas of personal-social development because of lack of familiarity with games such as pat-a-cake and in language because of differences in word usage, such as absence of plurals (Miller, Onotera, and Deinard, 1984). The more protective parental attitude of Southeast Asians toward the young child may also prevent early learning of self-help skills (Fung and Lau, 1985). Several of these variations were noted also in native African children (Olade, 1984). Further research is needed to determine if cultural variations affect screening results with the Denver II.

From Wong DL et al.: *Whaley and Wong's Nursing care of infants and children*, ed. 6, St. Louis, 1999, Mosby.

Text continued on p. 76

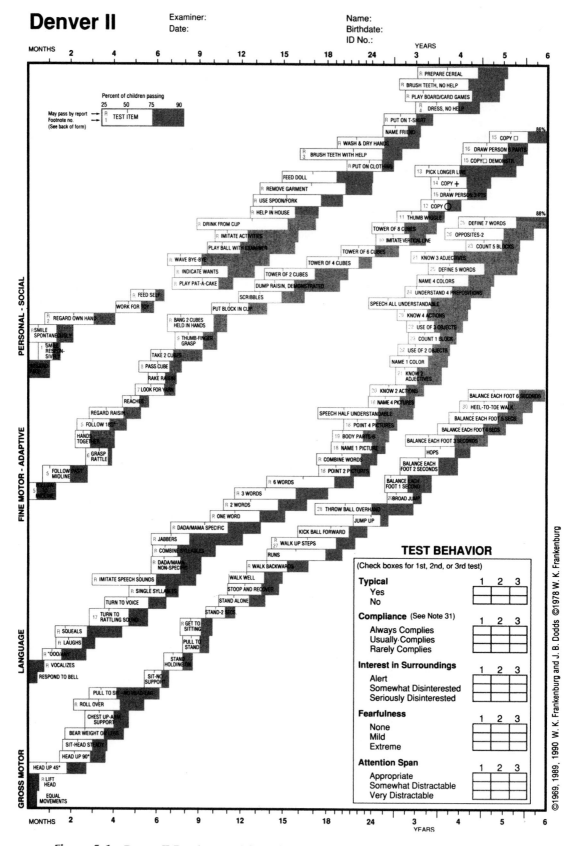

Figure 5-1   Denver II Developmental Screening Test. (From WK Frankenburg and JB Dodds, 1990.)

Continued

DIRECTIONS FOR ADMINISTRATION

1. Try to get child to smile by smiling, talking or waving. Do not touch him/her.
2. Child must stare at hand several seconds.
3. Parent may help guide toothbrush and put toothpaste on brush.
4. Child does not have to be able to tie shoes or button/zip in the back.
5. Move yarn slowly in an arc from one side to the other, about 8" above child's face.
6. Pass if child grasps rattle when it is touched to the backs or tips of fingers.
7. Pass if child tries to see where yarn went. Yarn should be dropped quickly from sight from tester's hand without arm movement.
8. Child must transfer cube from hand to hand without help of body, mouth, or table.
9. Pass if child picks up raisin with any part of thumb and finger.
10. Line can vary only 30 degrees or less from tester's line.⌐
11. Make a fist with thumb pointing upward and wiggle only the thumb. Pass if child imitates and does not move any fingers other than the thumb.

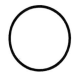   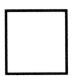

12. Pass any enclosed form. Fail continuous round motions.
13. Which line is longer? (Not bigger.) Turn paper upside down and repeat. (pass 3 of 3 or 5 of 6)
14. Pass any lines crossing near midpoint.
15. Have child copy first. If failed, demonstrate.

When giving items 12, 14, and 15, do not name the forms. Do not demonstrate 12 and 14.

16. When scoring, each pair (2 arms, 2 legs, etc.) counts as one part.
17. Place one cube in cup and shake gently near child's ear, but out of sight. Repeat for other ear.
18. Point to picture and have child name it. (No credit is given for sounds only.)
    If less than 4 pictures are named correctly, have child point to picture as each is named by tester.

    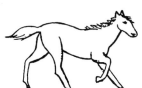   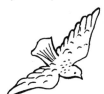   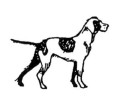   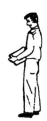

19. Using doll, tell child: Show me the nose, eyes, ears, mouth, hands, feet, tummy, hair. Pass 6 of 8.
20. Using pictures, ask child: Which one flies?... says meow?... talks?... barks?... gallops? Pass 2 of 5, 4 of 5.
21. Ask child: What do you do when you are cold?... tired?... hungry?   Pass 2 of 3, 3 of 3.
22. Ask child: What do you do with a cup? What is a chair used for? What is a pencil used for?
    Action words must be included in answers.
23. Pass if child correctly places <u>and</u> says how many blocks are on paper. (1, 5).
24. Tell child: Put block **on** table; **under** table; **in front of** me, **behind** me. Pass 4 of 4.
    (Do not help child by pointing, moving head or eyes.)
25. Ask child: What is a ball?... lake?... desk?... house?... banana?... curtain?... fence?... ceiling? Pass if defined in terms of use, shape, what it is made of, or general category (such as banana is fruit, not just yellow). Pass 5 of 8, 7 of 8.
26. Ask child: If a horse is big, a mouse is __? If fire is hot, ice is __? If the sun shines during the day, the moon shines during the __? Pass 2 of 3.
27. Child may use wall or rail only, not person. May not crawl.
28. Child must throw ball overhand 3 feet to within arm's reach of tester.
29. Child must perform standing broad jump over width of test sheet (8 1/2 inches).
30. Tell child to walk forward, ⊂⊃⊂⊃⊂⊃⊂⊃➔ heel within 1 inch of toe. Tester may demonstrate.
    Child must walk 4 consecutive steps.
31. In the second year, half of normal children are non-compliant.

OBSERVATIONS:

Figure 5-1, cont'd   For legend see opposite page.

REVISED DENVER PRESCREENING DEVELOPMENTAL QUESTIONNAIRE

(R-PDQ)
0-9 MONTHS

Child's Name _____

Person Completing R-PDQ: _____

Relation to Child: _____

CONTINUE ANSWERING UNTIL 3 "NOs" ARE CIRCLED

1. Equal Movements
When your baby is lying on his/her back, can (s)he move each of his/her arms as easily as the other and each of the legs as easily as the other? Answer **No** if your child makes jerky or uncoordinated movements with one or both of his/her arms or legs.

Yes   No   (0)   FMA

2. Stomach Lifts Head
When your baby is on his/her stomach on a flat surface, can (s)he lift his/her head off the surface?

Yes   No   (0-3)   GM

3. Regards Face
When your baby is lying on his/her back, can (s)he look at you and watch your face?

Yes   No   (1)   PS

4. Follows To Midline
When your child is on his/her back, can (s)he follow your movement by turning his/her head from one side to facing directly forward?

Yes   No   (1-1)   FMA

5. Responds To Bell
Does your child respond with eye movements, change in breathing or other change in activity to a bell or rattle sounded outside his/her line of vision?

Yes   No   (1-2)   L

6. Vocalizes Not Crying
Does your child make sounds other than crying, such as gurgling, cooing, or babbling?

Yes   No   (1-3)   L

7. Smiles Responsively
When you smile and talk to your baby, does (s)he smile back at you?

Yes   No   (1-3)   PS

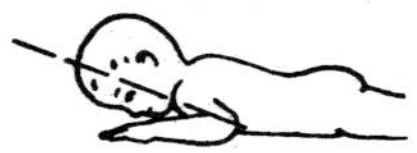

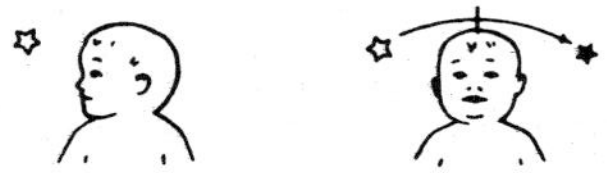

For Office Use

Today's Date: _____ yr _____ mo _____ day

Child's Birthdate: _____ yr _____ mo _____ day

Subtract to get Child's Exact Age: _____ yr _____ mo _____ day

R-PDQ Age: (_____) _____ yr _____ mo _____ completed wks)

8. Follows Past Midline
When your child is on his/her back, does (s)he follow your movement by turning his/her head from one side *almost all the way to the other side?*

Yes   No   (2-2)   FMA

9. Stomach, Head Up 45°
When your baby is on his/her stomach on a flat surface, can (s)he lift his/her head 45°?

Yes   No   (2-2)   GM

10. Stomach, Head Up 90°
When your baby is on his/her stomach on a flat surface, can (s)he lift his/her head 90°?

Yes   No   (3)   GM

11. Laughs
Does your baby laugh out loud without being tickled or touched?

Yes   No   (3-1)   L

12. Hands Together
Does your baby play with his/her hands by touching them together?

Yes   No   (3-3)   FMA

13. Follows 180°
When your child is on his/her back, does (s)he follow your movement from one side *all the way* to the other side?

Yes   No   (4)   FMA

14. Grasps Rattle
It is important that you follow instructions carefully. Do *not* place the pencil in the palm of your child's hand. When you touch the pencil to the back or tips of your baby's fingers, does your baby grasp the pencil for a few seconds?

Yes   No   (4)   FMA

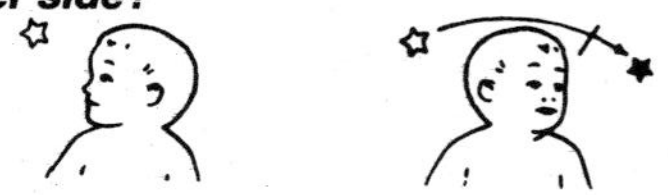

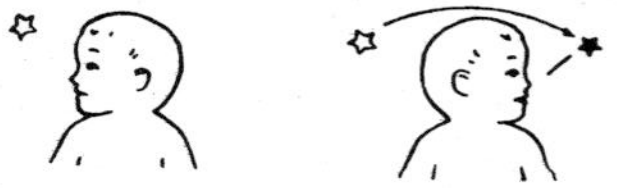

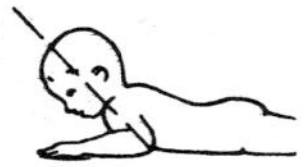

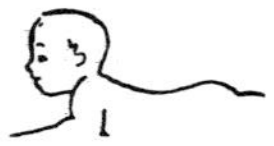

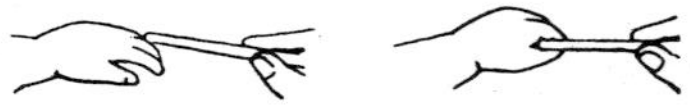

TRY THIS   NOT THIS

© Wm. K. Frankenburg, M.D., 1975, 1986

Figure 5-2 Denver Prescreening Developmental Questionnaire (PDQ). (From WK Frankenburg, 1986.)   *Continued*

0-9 MONTHS
(R-PDQ)

CONTINUE ANSWERING UNTIL 3 "NOs" ARE CIRCLED

For Office Use

15. Sits, Head Steady
When sitting, can your child hold his/her head upright and steady? Answer **No** if his/her head falls to either side or upon his/her chest. Yes No (4) GM

16. Stomach Chest Up-Arm Support
When your baby is on his/her stomach on a flat surface, can (s)he lift his/her chest using his/her arms for support? Yes No (4-1) GM

17. Squeals
Does your baby make happy high-pitched squealing sounds which are not crying? Yes No (4-2) L

18. Rolls Over
Has your baby rolled over at least 2 times, from stomach to back, or back to stomach? Yes No (4-3) GM

19. Regards Raisin
Can your child focus his/her eyes on small objects the size of a pea, a raisin, or a penny? Yes No (5) FMA

20. Reaches For Object
Can your child pick up a toy if it is placed within his/her reach? Yes No (5) FMA

21. Smiles Spontaneously
Does your child smile at crib toys, pictures, or pets when (s)he is playing by himself/herself? Yes No (5) PS

22. Pull To Sit, No Headlag
With your baby on his/her back, gently pull him/her up to a sitting position by his/her wrists. Does your baby hold his/her neck stiffly like the baby in the picture below left? Answer **No** if his/her head falls back like the baby in the picture below right. Yes No (6-1) GM

Yes   No

For Office Use

23. Sits, Looks For Yarn
Please follow directions carefully. Get your baby's attention with a scarf, handkerchief, or a tissue and then drop it *out of sight.* Did your baby try to find it? For example, did (s)he look for it under the table or continue to watch where it disappeared? Yes No (7-2) FMA

24. Passes Cube Hand To Hand
Can your baby pass something, such as a small block or a small cookie, from one hand to the other? Long objects like a spoon or rattle do not count. Yes No (7-2) FMA

25. Sits, Takes 2 Cubes
Can your baby pick up 2 things, such as toys or cookies, and hold one in each hand at the same time? Yes No (7-2) FMA

26. Bears Some Weight On Legs
When you hold your baby under his/her arms, can (s)he bear some weight on his/her legs? Answer **Yes** only if (s)he tries to stand on his/her feet and supports some of his/her own weight. Yes No (7-3) GM

27. Rakes Raisin, Attains
Can your baby pick up small objects, such as raisins or pieces of food with his/her hand using a raking or grabbing motion? Yes No (7-3) FMA

28. Sits Without Support
Without being propped by pillows, a chair, or wall, can your child sit by himself/herself for 60 seconds? Yes No (7-3) GM

29. Feed Self Crackers
Can your baby feed himself/herself a cracker or cookie? Answer **No** if (s)he has never been given one. Yes No (8) PS

30. Turns To Voice
When your child is playing and you come up *quietly* behind him/her, does (s)he sometimes turn his/her head as though (s)he heard you? *Loud sounds do not count.* Yes No (8-1) L

© Wm. K. Frankenburg, M.D., 1975, 1986

Figure 5-2, cont'd For legend see opposite page.

BOX 5-3

DENVER ARTICULATION SCREENING EXAMINATION (DASE)

DENVER ARTICULATION SCREENING EXAMINATION

(For Children 2.5 to 6 Years of Age)

Instructions: Have child repeat each word after you. Circle the underlined sounds that he or she pronounces correctly. Total number of correct sounds is the raw score. Use charts below to score results.

NAME
HOSPITAL NO.
ADDRESS

Date: _____ Child's age: _____ Examiner: _____ Raw score: _____
Percentile: _____ Intelligibility: _____ Result: _____

1. ṯable	6. zip<u>per</u>	11. <u>s</u>ock	16. <u>w</u>agon	21. <u>l</u>eaf
2. shir̲t	7. <u>gr</u>apes	12. vac<u>uu</u>m	17. <u>g</u>um	22. ca<u>rr</u>ot
3. <u>d</u>oor	8. <u>fl</u>ag	13. <u>y</u>arn	18. h<u>ou</u>se	
4. trun<u>k</u>	9. <u>th</u>umb	14. mo<u>th</u>er	19. pen<u>c</u>il	
5. jumping	10. too<u>th</u>brush	15. <u>tw</u>inkle	20. <u>f</u>ish	

Intelligibility (circle one):   1. Easy to understand   3. Not understandable
                                2. Understandable half of the time   4. Cannot evaluate

Comments:
_____

From AF Drumwright and WK Frankenburg, 1971-1973.

---

the child's age. The parent is asked to answer the questions from the appropriate age grouping.

Denver Articulation Screening Examination

The Denver Articulation Screening Examination (DASE) (Box 5-3) is used to detect articulation disorders in children ages $2\frac{1}{2}$ to 7 years. It assesses a child's ability to imitate word sounds, which provides information on a child's speech development. The child is asked to repeat 30 different sound elements; the tester listens for errors in articulation.

Draw-A-Person Test

The Draw-A-Person (DAP) test is the most current form of the Goodenough-Harris Drawing Test. It is designed to estimate the mental age of a child based on the elements present in the drawing. It is most suitable for children between 3 to 10 years old (Welch and Instone, 2000). The DAP assesses three areas of visual-motor development: visualization of the human figure, organization and interpretation (abstract conceptualization) of form, and reproduction of the visualized image through motor skills (Welch and Instone, 2000).

The child is given a blank piece of paper and a pencil and requested to draw a picture of a person. The child is told to take his or her time and draw as complete a picture as possible (without the assistance of or comments from adults). The child receives one point for each of the items present in the

drawing. One point is the equivalent of 3 months of developmental age. For each four points, add 1 year to the basal age (which is 3 years). For example, if a child scores 10 points, his or her mental age would be $5\frac{1}{2}$ years ($2\frac{6}{12} + 3$). The interpretation is based on a gradual increase in the complexity of the figures as the child becomes older. Welch and Instone (2000) describe a basic scoring scheme, which is easy to remember and apply in the clinical setting (Box 5-4).

Adult Assessment Tools

Two tools that are useful to assess life changes and their effects on adults are the Life Experiences Survey and the Hassles and Uplifts Scale. Both attempt to assess life stresses and to indicate a possible relationship between life stresses and susceptibility to physical and psychological problems or illnesses.

Life Experiences Survey

The Life Experiences Survey (Sarason, Johnson, and Siegel, 1978) is a self-report tool that allows respondents to consider events that they have experienced during the past year (Table 5-5). It includes events that occur fairly frequently and allows respondents to weigh the desirability or undesirability of events. The assumption is that negative events are more likely to be associated with stress, which in turn is related to psychological distress.

BOX 5-3—cont'd

DENVER ARTICULATION SCREENING EXAMINATION (DASE)—cont'd

To score DASE words: Note raw score for child's performance. Match raw score line (extreme left of chart) with column representing child's age (to the closest *previous* age group). Where raw score line and age column meet denotes percentile rank of child's performance when compared with other children that age. Percentiles above heavy line are *abnormal*, below heavy line are *normal*.

PERCENTILE RANK

RAW SCORE	2.5 YR	3.0 YR	3.5 YR	4.0 YR	4.5 YR	5.0 YR	5.5 YR	6 YR
2	1							
3	2							
4	5							
5	9							
6	16							
7	23							
8	31	2						
9	37	4	1					
10	42	6	2					
11	48	7	4					
12	54	9	6	1	1			
13	58	12	9	2	3	1	1	
14	62	17	11	5	4	2	2	
15	68	23	15	9	5	3	2	
16	75	31	19	12	5	4	3	
17	79	38	25	15	6	6	4	
18	83	46	31	19	8	7	4	
19	86	51	38	24	10	9	5	1
20	89	58	45	30	12	11	7	3
21	92	65	52	36	15	15	9	4
22	94	72	58	43	18	19	12	5
23	96	77	63	50	22	24	15	7
24	97	82	70	58	29	29	20	15
25	99	87	78	66	36	34	26	17
26	99	91	84	75	46	43	34	24
27		94	89	82	57	54	44	34
28		96	94	88	70	68	59	47
29		98	98	94	84	84	77	68
30		100	100	100	100	100	100	100

To score intelligibility:

	NORMAL	ABNORMAL
2.5 years	Understandable half of the time or easy to understand	Not understandable
3 years and older	Easy to understand	Understandable half of the time or not understandable

Test result: 1. Normal on DASE and intelligibility = *normal*
2. Abnormal on DASE or intelligibility = *abnormal**

*If abnormal on initial screening, rescreen within 2 weeks. If abnormal again, child should be referred for complete speech evaluation.

Ratings of events are on a seven-point scale, from extremely negative (-3) to extremely positive ($+3$). A positive change score is obtained by adding those events rated as positive, a negative change score is obtained by adding the negatively rated events, and a total change score is obtained by combining the two values. The effect of stress is also mediated by the individual's perceived control over the event, the degree of psychosocial assets, and personal characteristics (Sarason, Johnson, and Siegel, 1978).

Text continued on p. 82

BOX 5-4

SCORING CRITERIA FOR DRAW-A-PERSON TEST

1. Head present
2. Neck present
3. Neck, two dimensions
4. Eyes present
5. Eye detail: brow or lashes
6. Eye detail: pupil
7. Nose present
8. Nose, two dimensions (not round ball)
9. Mouth present
10. Lips, two dimensions
11. Both nose and lips in two dimensions
12. Both chin and forehead shown
13. Bridge of nose (straight to eyes; narrower than base)
14. Hair I (any scribble)
15. Hair II (more detail)
16. Ears present
17. Fingers present
18. Correct number of fingers
19. Opposition of thumb shown (must include fingers)
20. Hands present
21. Arms present
22. Arms at side, or engaged in activity
23. Feet: any indication
24. Attachment of arms and legs I (to trunk anywhere)
25. Attachment of arms and legs II (to trunk anywhere)
26. Trunk present
27. Trunk in proportion, two dimensions (length greater than breadth)
28. Clothing I (anything)
29. Clothing II (two articles of clothing)

From Dixon SD, Stein MT: *Encounters with children: Pediatric behavior and development,* ed. 3, St. Louis, 2000, Mosby.

TABLE 5-5   The Life Experiences Survey

Listed below are a number of events which sometimes bring about change in the lives of those who experience them and necessitate social readjustment. *Please check those events which you have experienced in the recent past and indicate the time period during which you have experienced each event.* Be sure that all check marks are directly across from the items to which they correspond to. Also, for each item checked below, *please indicate the extent to which you viewed the event as having either a positive or negative impact on your life* at the time the event occurred. That is, *indicate the type and extent of impact that the event had.* A rating of −3 would indicate an extremely negative impact. A rating of 0 suggests no impact either positive or negative. A rating of +3 would indicate an extremely positive impact.

	0 to 6 mo	7 mo to 1 yr	Extremely Negative	Moderately Negative	Somewhat Negative	No Impact	Slightly Positive	Moderately Positive	Extremely Positive
1. Marriage			−3	−2	−1	0	+1	+2	+3
2. Detention in jail or comparable institution			−3	−2	−1	0	+1	+2	+3
3. Death of spouse			−3	−2	−1	0	+1	+2	+3
4. Major change in sleeping habits (much more or much less sleep)			−3	−2	−1	0	+1	+2	+3
5. Death of close family member:			−3	−2	−1	0	+1	+2	+3
a. Mother			−3	−2	−1	0	+1	+2	+3
b. Father			−3	−2	−1	0	+1	+2	+3
c. Brother			−3	−2	−1	0	+1	+2	+3
d. Sister			−3	−2	−1	0	+1	+2	+3
e. Grandmother			−3	−2	−1	0	+1	+2	+3
f. Grandfather			−3	−2	−1	0	+1	+2	+3
g. Other (specify)			−3	−2	−1	0	+1	+2	+3
6. Major change in eating habits (much more or much less food intake)			−3	−2	−1	0	+1	+2	+3
7. Foreclosure on mortgage or loan			−3	−2	−1	0	+1	+2	+3
8. Death of close friend			−3	−2	−1	0	+1	+2	+3
9. Outstanding personal achievement			−3	−2	−1	0	+1	+2	+3

From Sarason IG, Johnson JH, Siegel JM: Assessing the impact of life changes: development of life experiences survey, *J Consult Clin Psychol* 46(5):932-946, 1978.

TABLE 5-5 **The Life Experiences Survey—cont'd**

	0 to 6 mo	7 mo to 1 yr	Extremely Negative	Moderately Negative	Somewhat Negative	No Impact	Slightly Positive	Moderately Positive	Extremely Positive
10. Minor law violations (traffic tickets, disturbing the peace, etc.)			−3	−2	−1	0	+1	+2	+3
11. *Male:* Wife/girlfriend's pregnancy			−3	−2	−1	0	+1	+2	+3
12. *Female:* Pregnancy			−3	−2	−1	0	+1	+2	+3
13. Changed work situation (e.g., different work responsibility, major change in working conditions, working hours)			−3	−2	−1	0	+1	+2	+3
14. New job			−3	−2	−1	0	+1	+2	+3
15. Serious illness or injury of close family member:			−3	−2	−1	0	+1	+2	+3
a. Father			−3	−2	−1	0	+1	+2	+3
b. Mother			−3	−2	−1	0	+1	+2	+3
c. Sister			−3	−2	−1	0	+1	+2	+3
d. Brother			−3	−2	−1	0	+1	+2	+3
e. Grandmother			−3	−2	−1	0	+1	+2	+3
f. Grandfather			−3	−2	−1	0	+1	+2	+3
g. Spouse			−3	−2	−1	0	+1	+2	+3
h. Other (specify)			−3	−2	−1	0	+1	+2	+3
16. Sexual difficulties			−3	−2	−1	0	+1	+2	+3
17. Trouble with employer (e.g., in danger of losing job, being suspended, demoted)			−3	−2	−1	0	+1	+2	+3
18. Trouble with in-laws			−3	−2	−1	0	+1	+2	+3
19. Major change in financial status (a lot better off or a lot worse off)			−3	−2	−1	0	+1	+2	+3
20. Major change in closeness of family members (increased or decreased closeness)			−3	−2	−1	0	+1	+2	+3
21. Gaining a new family member (e.g., through birth, adoption, family member moving in)			−3	−2	−1	0	+1	+2	+3
22. Change of residence			−3	−2	−1	0	+1	+2	+3
23. Marital separation from mate (due to conflict)			−3	−2	−1	0	+1	+2	+3
24. Major change in church activities (increased or decreased attendance)			−3	−2	−1	0	+1	+2	+3
25. Marital reconciliation with mate			−3	−2	−1	0	+1	+2	+3
26. Major change in number of arguments with spouse (a lot more or a lot less arguments)			−3	−2	−1	0	+1	+2	+3
27. *Married male:* Change in wife's work outside the home (e.g., beginning work, ceasing work, changing to a new job)			−3	−2	−1	0	+1	+2	+3

Continued

| TABLE 5-5 | The Life Experiences Survey—cont'd | | | | | | | | |

	0 to 6 mo	7 mo to 1 yr	Extremely Negative	Moderately Negative	Somewhat Negative	No Impact	Slightly Positive	Moderately Positive	Extremely Positive
28. *Married female:* Change in husband's work (e.g., loss of job, beginning new job, retirement)			−3	−2	−1	0	+1	+2	+3
29. Major change in usual type and/or amount of recreation			−3	−2	−1	0	+1	+2	+3
30. Borrowing more than $10,000 (e.g., buying home, business)			−3	−2	−1	0	+1	+2	+3
31. Borrowing less than $10,000 (e.g., buying car, TV, getting school loan)			−3	−2	−1	0	+1	+2	+3
32. Being fired from job			−3	−2	−1	0	+1	+2	+3
33. *Male:* Wife/girlfriend having abortion			−3	−2	−1	0	+1	+2	+3
34. *Female:* Having abortion			−3	−2	−1	0	+1	+2	+3
35. Major personal illness or injury			−3	−2	−1	0	+1	+2	+3
36. Major change in social activities, e.g., parties, movies, visiting (increased or decreased participation)			−3	−2	−1	0	+1	+2	+3
37. Major change in living conditions of family (e.g., building new home; remodeling; deterioration of home, neighborhood)			−3	−2	−1	0	+1	+2	+3
38. Divorce			−3	−2	−1	0	+1	+2	+3
39. Serious injury or illness of close friend			−3	−2	−1	0	+1	+2	+3
40. Retirement from work			−3	−2	−1	0	+1	+2	+3
41. Son or daughter leaving home (e.g., due to marriage, college)			−3	−2	−1	0	+1	+2	+3
42. Ending of formal schooling			−3	−2	−1	0	+1	+2	+3
43. Separation from spouse (e.g., due to work, travel)			−3	−2	−1	0	+1	+2	+3
44. Engagement			−3	−2	−1	0	+1	+2	+3
45. Breaking up with boyfriend/girlfriend			−3	−2	−1	0	+1	+2	+3
46. Leaving home for the first time			−3	−2	−1	0	+1	+2	+3
47. Reconciliation with boyfriend/girlfriend			−3	−2	−1	0	+1	+2	+3
Other recent experiences that have had an impact on your life. List and rate.									
48. _____			−3	−2	−1	0	+1	+2	+3
49. _____			−3	−2	−1	0	+1	+2	+3
50. _____			−3	−2	−1	0	+1	+2	+3

TABLE 5-6   The Hassles and Uplifts Scale

HASSLES are irritants—things that annoy or bother you; they can make you upset or angry. UPLIFTS are events that make you feel good; they can make you joyful, glad, or satisfied. Some hassles and uplifts occur on a fairly regular basis and others are relatively rare. Some have only a slight effect, others have a strong effect.

This questionnaire lists things that can be hassles and uplifts in day-to-day life. You will find that during the course of a day some of these things will have been only a hassle for you and some will have been only an uplift. *Others will have been both a hassle AND an uplift.*

DIRECTIONS: Please think about how much of a hassle and how much of an uplift each item was for you today. Please indicate on the left-hand side of the page (under "HASSLES") how much of a hassle the item was by circling the appropriate number. Then indicate on the right-hand side of the page (under "UPLIFTS") how much of an uplift it was for you by circling the appropriate number.

Remember, circle one number on the left-hand side of the page *and* one number on the right-hand side of the page for *each* item.

PLEASE FILL OUT THIS QUESTIONNAIRE JUST BEFORE YOU GO TO BED.

HASSLES AND UPLIFTS SCALE

HOW MUCH OF A HASSLE WAS THIS ITEM FOR YOU TODAY?	HOW MUCH OF AN UPLIFT WAS THIS ITEM FOR YOU TODAY?
HASSLES	UPLIFTS
0 = *None or not applicable*	0 = *None or not applicable*
1 = *Somewhat*	1 = *Somewhat*
2 = *Quite a bit*	2 = *Quite a bit*
3 = *A great deal*	3 = A great deal

DIRECTIONS: Please circle one number on the left-hand side *and* one number on the right-hand side for each item.

HASSLES		Item	UPLIFTS	
0 1 2 3	1.	Your child(ren)	0 1 2 3	
0 1 2 3	2.	Your parents or parents-in-law	0 1 2 3	
0 1 2 3	3.	Other relative(s)	0 1 2 3	
0 1 2 3	4.	Your spouse	0 1 2 3	
0 1 2 3	5.	Time spent with family	0 1 2 3	
0 1 2 3	6.	Health or well-being of a family member	0 1 2 3	
0 1 2 3	7.	Sex	0 1 2 3	
0 1 2 3	8.	Intimacy	0 1 2 3	
0 1 2 3	9.	Family-related obligations	0 1 2 3	
0 1 2 3	10.	Your friend(s)	0 1 2 3	
0 1 2 3	11.	Fellow workers	0 1 2 3	
0 1 2 3	12.	Clients, customers, patients, etc.	0 1 2 3	
0 1 2 3	13.	Your supervisor or employer	0 1 2 3	
0 1 2 3	14.	The nature of your work	0 1 2 3	
0 1 2 3	15.	Your work load	0 1 2 3	
0 1 2 3	16.	Your job security	0 1 2 3	
0 1 2 3	17.	Meeting deadlines or goals on the job	0 1 2 3	
0 1 2 3	18.	Enough money for necessities (e.g., food, clothing, housing, health care, taxes, insurance)	0 1 2 3	
0 1 2 3	19.	Enough money for education	0 1 2 3	
0 1 2 3	20.	Enough money for emergencies	0 1 2 3	
0 1 2 3	21.	Enough money for extras (e.g., entertainment, recreation, vacations)	0 1 2 3	
0 1 2 3	22.	Financial care for someone who doesn't live with you	0 1 2 3	
0 1 2 3	23.	Investments	0 1 2 3	
0 1 2 3	24.	Your smoking	0 1 2 3	
0 1 2 3	25.	Your drinking	0 1 2 3	
0 1 2 3	26.	Mood-altering drugs	0 1 2 3	
0 1 2 3	27.	Your physical appearance	0 1 2 3	
0 1 2 3	28.	Contraception	0 1 2 3	
0 1 2 3	29.	Exercise(s)	0 1 2 3	
0 1 2 3	30.	Your medical care	0 1 2 3	
0 1 2 3	31.	Your health	0 1 2 3	
0 1 2 3	32.	Your physical abilities	0 1 2 3	
0 1 2 3	33.	The weather	0 1 2 3	
0 1 2 3	34.	News events	0 1 2 3	
0 1 2 3	35.	Your environment (e.g., quality of air, noise level, greenery)	0 1 2 3	
0 1 2 3	36.	Political or social issues	0 1 2 3	
0 1 2 3	37.	Your neighborhood (e.g., neighbors, setting)	0 1 2 3	
0 1 2 3	38.	Conserving (gas, electricity, water, gasoline, etc.)	0 1 2 3	
0 1 2 3	39.	Pets	0 1 2 3	
0 1 2 3	40.	Cooking	0 1 2 3	
0 1 2 3	41.	Housework	0 1 2 3	
0 1 2 3	42.	Home repairs	0 1 2 3	
0 1 2 3	43.	Yardwork	0 1 2 3	
0 1 2 3	44.	Car maintenance	0 1 2 3	
0 1 2 3	45.	Taking care of paperwork (e.g., paying bills, filling out forms)	0 1 2 3	
0 1 2 3	46.	Home entertainment (e.g., TV, music, reading)	0 1 2 3	
0 1 2 3	47.	Amount of free time	0 1 2 3	
0 1 2 3	48.	Recreation and entertainment outside the home (e.g., movies, sports, eating out, walking)	0 1 2 3	
0 1 2 3	49.	Eating (at home)	0 1 2 3	
0 1 2 3	50.	Church or community organizations	0 1 2 3	
0 1 2 3	51.	Legal matters	0 1 2 3	
0 1 2 3	52.	Being organized	0 1 2 3	
0 1 2 3	53.	Social commitments	0 1 2 3	

Received March 21, 1986
Revision received July 20, 1987
Accepted August 4, 1987

From DeLongis A, Folkman S, Lazarus RS: The impact of daily stress on health and mood: psychological and social resources as mediators, *J Pers Soc Psychol* 54(3):486-495, 1988. Copyright 1988 by the American Psychological Association.

Hassles and Uplifts Scale

The Hassles and Uplifts Scale (DeLongis, Folkman, and Lazarus, 1988) (Table 5-6) assesses daily stresses. These hassles or minor-but-frequently experienced stresses have been found to correlate strongly with negative health status (Weinberger, Hiner, and Tierney, 1987). Early research found daily hassles to be a better predictor of health outcome than major life events. More recent studies found that daily hassles mediated the impact of major life events on mental health (Israel and Schurman, 1990). These results suggest that minor stresses may have both direct and indirect influences on health.

The Hassles and Uplifts scale is completed at the end of the day just before bedtime. Items are rated on a scale of 0 to 3 in relation to the degree of a hassle they are and again from 0 to 3 on how much of an uplift the same items are for the day the questionnaire is completed. The total score is obtained by summing across the ratings given to all items.

DeLongis, Folkman, and Lazarus (1988) found a significant relationship between daily stress and physical health problems, such as sore throat, back aches, headaches, and the flu. Although there were significant individual variations in response to stress, individuals with unsupportive social relationships and low self-esteem were at greater risk for both somatic and psychological health problems during and after stressful days than were individuals with positive self-esteem and supportive relationships.

Even though such questionnaires are not diagnostic tools, they can help identify areas of stress and potential risk for stress-related problems. Completion of such tools may also provide clients with some insights into areas of stress in their lives.

INFANCY: BIRTH TO 12 MONTHS

More dramatic changes occur within the brief period of infancy than during any other time of life. During the period from birth to 12 months, the child develops from a dependent, helpless newborn to a busy little person who is mobile and communicative and relates to people in terms of their importance in his or her life. Infants enter the world with all sensory systems functioning in at least a rudimentary fashion. They begin to interact with and influence their environment from the moment of birth. As the neuromuscular system becomes more integrated, they are intent on taking in everything in the environment within their reach. Soon they can display a wide range of primary, unselfconscious emotions: interest, distress, disgust, joy, anger, surprise, sadness, and fear. They are responsive to the caregiver's mood; sadness or happiness affects their behavior.

Box 5-5 summarizes child development using the categories of motor development, language development, and personal-social-adaptive development. (These categories are slightly different from, but complementary to, the categories used in the text.) Table 5-3, p. 69, identifies the individual's "skill areas" as they relate to the different developmental theories. As you design care for clients, take into account these differences, and modify your interactions and interventions to take advantage of a client's strengths and recognize his or her developmental limitations.

Physical Development

The rate of growth during the first few months and years of life is greater than at any other time. The average full-term infant weighs about 7 to 7½ pounds (3.4 kg) and is about 20 inches (50 cm) long. Birth weight is an important indicator of risk for morbidity and mortality. In the newborn period, birth weight is also used to assess the child's physiological maturity. For instance, when a newborn is preterm (born before 37 weeks gestation) or when a full-term newborn (37 to 41 weeks' gestation) is smaller than expected for gestational age, birth weight is a useful indicator of maturity. Fetal maturity reflects the ability of the infant's organ systems to adapt to extrauterine life. The New Ballard Score (Ballard et

Text continued on p. 87

BOX 5-5

CHILD DEVELOPMENT FROM 1 MONTH TO 5 YEARS

1 MONTH

Motor

1. Moro reflex present.
2. Vigorous sucking reflex present.
3. Lying prone (face down): lifts head briefly so chin is off table.
4. Lying prone: makes crawling movements with legs.
5. Held in sitting position: back is rounded, head held up momentarily only.
6. Hands tightly fisted.
7. Reflex grasp of object with palm.

Language

8. Startled by sound; quieted by voice.
9. Small throaty noises or vocalizations.

Personal-Social-Adaptive

10. Ringing bell produces decrease of activity.
11. May follow dangling object with eyes to midline.
12. Lying on back: will briefly look at examiner or change activity.
13. Reacts with generalized body movements when tissue paper is placed on face.

From Walter M. Block, MD, Child Evaluation Clinic of Cedar Rapids, Iowa, 1972.

BOX 5-5—cont'd

CHILD DEVELOPMENT FROM 1 MONTH TO 5 YEARS—cont'd

2 MONTHS

Motor

1. Kicks vigorously.
2. Energetic arm movements.
3. Vigorous head turning.
4. Held in ventral suspension (prone): no head droop.
5. Lying prone: lifts head so face makes an approximate 45° angle with table.
6. Held in sitting position: head erect but bobs.
7. Hand goes to mouth.
8. Hands often open (not clenched).

Language'

9. Is cooing.
10. Vocalizes single vowel sound, such as: ah-eh-uh.

Personal-Social-Adaptive

11. Head and eyes search for sound.
12. Listens to bell ringing.
13. Follows dangling object past midline.
14. Alert expression.
15. Follows moving person with eyes.
16. Smiles back when talked to.

3 MONTHS

Motor

1. Lying prone: lifts head to 90° angle.
2. Lifts head when lying on back (supine).
3. Moro reflex begins to disappear.
4. Grasp reflex nearly gone.
5. Rolls side to back (3-4 months).

Language

6. Chuckling, squealing, grunting, especially when talked to.
7. Listens to music.
8. Vocalizes with two different syllables, such as: a-a, la-la (not distinct), oo-oo.

Personal-Social-Adaptive

9. Reaches for but misses objects.
10. Holds toy with active grasp when put into hand.
11. Sucks and inspects fingers.
12. Pulls at clothes.
13. Follows object (toy) side to side (and 180°).
14. Looks predominately at examiner.
15. Glances at toy when put into hand.
16. Recognizes mother and bottle.
17. Smiles spontaneously.

4 MONTHS

Motor

1. Sits when well supported.
2. No head lag when pulled to sitting position.
3. Turns head at sound of voice.
4. Lifts head (in supine position) in effort to sit.
5. Lifts head and chest when prone, using hands and forearms.
6. Held erect: pushes feet against table.

Language

7. Laughs aloud (4-5 months).
8. Uses sounds, such as: m-p-b.
9. Repeats series of same sounds.

Personal-Social-Adaptive

10. Grasps rattle.
11. Plays with own fingers.
12. Reaches for object in front with both hands.
13. Transfers object from hand to hand.
14. Pulls dress over face.
15. Smiles spontaneously at people.
16. Regards raisin (or pellet).

5 MONTHS

Motor

1. Moro reflex gone.
2. Rolls side to side.
3. Rolls back to front.
4. Full head control when pulled to or held in sitting position.
5. Briefly supports most of weight on legs.
6. Scratches on tabletop.

Language

7. Squeals with high voice.
8. Recognizes familiar voices.
9. Coos or stops crying on hearing music.

Personal-Social-Adaptive

10. Grasps dangling object.
11. Reaches for toy with both hands.
12. Smiles at mirror image.
13. Turns head deliberately to bell.
14. Obviously enjoys being played with.

6 MONTHS

Motor

1. Supine: lifts head spontaneously.
2. Bounces on feet when held standing.
3. Sits briefly (tripod fashion).
4. Rolls front to back (6-7 months).
5. Grasps foot and plays with toes.
6. Grasps cube with palms.

Language

7. Vocalizes at mirror image.
8. Makes four or more different sounds.
9. Localizes source of sound (bell, voice).
10. Vague, formless babble (especially with family members).

Personal-Social-Adaptive

11. Holds one cube in each hand.
12. Puts cube into mouth.
13. Resecures dropped cube.
14. Transfers cube from hand to hand.
15. Conscious of strange sights and persons.
16. Consistent regard of object or person (6-7 months).

Continued

BOX 5-5—cont'd

CHILD DEVELOPMENT FROM 1 MONTH TO 5 YEARS—cont'd

Personal-Social-Adaptive—cont'd

17. Uses raking movement to secure raisin or pellet.
18. Resists having toy taken away.
19. Stretches out arms to be taken up (6-8 months).

8 MONTHS

Motor

1. Sits alone (6-8 months).
2. Early stepping movements.
3. Tries to crawl.
4. Stands few seconds, holding on to object.
5. Leans forward to get an object.
6. Held in sitting position: head erect but bobs.

Language

7. Two-syllable babble, such as a-la, ba-ba, oo-goo, a-ma, mama, dada (8-10 months).
8. Listens to conversation (8-10 months).
9. "Shouts" for attention (8-10 months).

Personal-Social-Adaptive

10. Works to get toy out of reach.
11. Scoops pellet.
12. Rings bell purposely (8-10 months).
13. Drinks from cup.
14. Plays peek-a-boo.
15. Looks for dropped object.
16. Bites and chews toys.
17. Pats mirror image.
18. Bangs spoon on table.
19. Manipulates paper or string.
20. Secures ring by pulling on the string.
21. Feeds self crackers.

10 MONTHS

Motor

1. Gets self into sitting position.
2. Sits steadily (long time).
3. Pulls self to standing position (on bed railing).
4. Crawls on hands and knees.
5. Walks when held or around furniture.
6. Turns around when left on floor.

Language

7. Imitates speech sounds.
8. Shakes head for "no."
9. Waves "bye-bye."
10. Responds to name.
11. Vocalizes in varied jargon-patterns (10-12 months).

Personal-Social-Adaptive

12. Plays "pat-a-cake."
13. Picks up pellet with finger and thumb.
14. Bangs toys together.

15. Extends toy to a person.
16. Holds own bottle.
17. Removes cube from cup.
18. Drops one cube to get another.
19. Uses handle to lift cup.
20. Initially shy with strangers.

1 YEAR

Motor

1. Walks with one hand held.
2. Stands alone (or with support).
3. Secures small object with good pincer grasp.
4. Pivots in sitting position.
5. Grasps two cubes in one hand.

Language

6. Uses "mama" or "dada" with specific meaning.
7. "Talks" to toys and people, using fairly long verbal patterns.
8. Has vocabulary of two words besides "mama" and "dada."
9. Babbles to self when alone.
10. Obeys simple requests, such as: "Give me the cup."
11. Reacts to music.

Personal-Social-Adaptive

12. Cooperates with dressing.
13. Plays with cup, spoon, saucer.
14. Points with index finger.
15. Pokes finger (into stethoscope) to explore.
16. Releases toy into your hand.
17. Tries to take cube out of box.
18. Upwraps a cube.
19. Holds cup to drink.
20. Holds crayon.
21. Tries to imitate scribble.
22. Imitates beating two cubes together.
23. Gives affection.

15 MONTHS

Motor

1. Stands alone.
2. Creeps upstairs.
3. Kneels on floor or chair.
4. Gets off floor and walks alone with good balance.
5. Bends over to pick up toy without holding on to furniture.

Language

6. May speak four to six words (15-18 months).
7. Uses jargon.
8. Indicates wants by vocalizing.
9. Knows own name.
10. Enjoys rhymes or jingles.

From Walter M. Block, MD, Child Evaluation Clinic of Cedar Rapids, Iowa, 1972.

BOX 5-5–cont'd

CHILD DEVELOPMENT FROM 1 MONTH TO 5 YEARS–cont'd

Personal-Social-Adaptive
11. Tilts cup to drink.
12. Uses spoon but spills.
13. Builds tower of two cubes.
14. Drops cubes into cup.
15. Helps turn page in book, pats picture.
16. Shows or offers toy.
17. Helps pull off clothes.
18. Puts pellet into bottle without demonstration.
19. Opens lid of box.
20. Likes to push wheeled toys.

18 MONTHS
Motor
1. Runs (stiffly).
2. Walks upstairs—one hand held.
3. Walks backward.
4. Climbs into chair.
5. Hurls ball.

Language
6. May say 6 to 10 words (18-21 months).
7. Points to at least one body part.
8. Can say "hello" and "thank you."
9. Carries out two directions (one at a time), for instance: "Get ball from table."—"Give ball to mother."
10. Identifies two objects by pointing (or picking up), such as: cup, spoon, dog, car, chair.

Personal-Social-Adaptive
11. Turns pages.
12. Builds tower of three to four cubes.
13. Puts 10 cubes into cup.
14. Carries or hugs a doll.
15. Takes off shoes and socks.
16. Pulls string toy.
17. Scribbles spontaneously.
18. Dumps raisin from bottle after demonstration.
19. Uses spoon with little spilling.

21 MONTHS
Motor
1. Runs well.
2. Walks downstairs—one hand held.
3. Walks upstairs alone or holding on to rail.
4. Kicks large ball (when demonstrated).

Language
5. May speak 15 to 20 words (21-24 months).
6. May combine two to three words.
7. Asks for food, drink.
8. Echoes two or more words.
9. Takes three directions (one at a time), for instance: "Take ball from table."—"Give ball to Mommy."—"Put ball on floor."
10. Points to three or more body parts.

Personal-Social-Adaptive
11. Builds tower of five to six cubes.
12. Folds paper once when shown.
13. Helps with simple household tasks (21-24 months).
14. Removes some clothing purposefully (besides hat or socks).
15. Pulls person to show something.

2 YEARS
Motor
1. Runs without falling.
2. Walks up and down stairs.
3. Kicks large ball (without demonstration).
4. Throws ball overhand.
5. Claps hands.
6. Opens door.
7. Turns pages in book, singly.

Language
8. Says simple phrases.
9. Says at least one sentence or phrase of four or more syllables.
10. Can repeat four to five syllables.
11. May reproduce about five or six consonant sounds. (Typically: m-p-b-h-w.)
12. Points to four parts of body on command.
13. Asks for things at table by name.
14. Refers to self by name.
15. May use personal pronouns, such as: I-me-you (2-2½ years).

Personal-Social-Adaptive
16. Builds five- to seven-cube tower.
17. May cut with scissors.
18. Spontaneously dumps raisin from bottle (without demonstration).
19. Throws ball into box.
20. Imitates drawing vertical line from demonstration.
21. Parallel play predominant.

2½ YEARS
Motor
1. Jumps in place with both feet.
2. Tries standing on one foot (may not be successful).
3. Holds crayon by fingers.
4. Imitates walking on tiptoe.

Language
5. Refers to self by pronoun (rather than name).
6. Names common objects when asked (key, penny, shoe, box, book).
7. Repeats two digits (one of three trials).
8. Answers simple questions, such as: "What is this?"—"What does the kitty say?"

Personal-Social-Adaptive
9. Build tower of eight cubes.
10. Pushes toy with good steering.

Continued

BOX 5-5—cont'd

CHILD DEVELOPMENT FROM 1 MONTH TO 5 YEARS—cont'd

Personal-Social-Adaptive—cont'd

11. Helps put things away.
12. Can carry breakable objects.
13. Puts on clothing.
14. Washes and dries hands.
15. Eats with fork.
16. Imitates drawing a horizontal line from demonstration.
17. May imitate drawing a circle from demonstration.

3 YEARS

Motor

1. Stands on one foot for at least 1 second.
2. Jumps from bottom stair.
3. Alternates feet going upstairs.
4. Pours from a pitcher.
5. Can undo two buttons.
6. Pedals a tricycle.

Language

7. Repeats six syllables, for instance: "I have a little dog."
8. Names three or more objects in a picture.
9. Gives sex. ("Are you a boy or a girl?")
10. Gives full name.
11. Repeats three digits (one of three trials).
12. Knows a few rhymes.
13. Gives appropriate answers to: "What: swims-flies-shoots-boils-bites-melts?"
14. Uses plurals.
15. Knows at least one color.
16. Can reply to questions in at least three-word sentences.
17. May have vocabulary of 750 to 1000 words (3-3$^1/_2$ years).

Personal-Social-Adaptive

18. Understands taking turns.
19. Copies a circle (from model, without demonstration).
20. Builds three-block pyramid.
21. Dresses with supervision.
22. Puts 10 pellets into bottle in 30 seconds.
23. Separates easily from mother.
24. Feeds self well.
25. Plays interactive games, such as "tag."

4 YEARS

Motor

1. Stands on one foot for at least 5 seconds (two of three trials).
2. Hops at least twice on one foot.
3. Can walk heel-to-toe four or more steps (with heel 1 inch or less in front of toe).
4. Can button coat or dress; may lace shoes.

Language

5. Repeats 10-word sentences without errors.
6. Counts three objects, pointing correctly.

7. Repeats three to four digits (4-5 years).
8. Comprehends: "What do you do if: you are hungry, sleepy, cold?"
9. Spontaneous sentences, four to five words long.
10. Likes to ask questions.
11. Understands prepositions, such as: on-under-behind, etc. ("Put the block *on* the table.")
12. Can point to three out of four colors (red, blue, green, yellow).
13. Speech is now an effective communication tool.

Personal-Social-Adaptive

14. Copies cross (+) without demonstration.
15. Imitates oblique cross (×).
16. Draws a man with four parts.
17. Cooperates with other children in play.
18. Dresses and undresses self (mostly without supervision).
19. Brushes teeth, washes face.
20. Compares lines: "Which is longer?"
21. Folds paper two to three times.
22. Can select heavier from lighter object.
23. Cares for self at toilet.

5 YEARS

Motor

1. Balances on one foot for 8 to 10 seconds.
2. Skips, using feet alternately.
3. May be able to tie a knot.
4. Catches bounced ball with hands (not arms) in two of three trials.

Language

5. Knows age ("How old are you?")
6. Performs three tasks (with one command), for instance: "Put pen on table—close door—bring me the ball."
7. Knows four colors.
8. Defines use for: fork-horse-key-pencil, etc.
9. Identifies by name: nickel-dime-penny.
10. Asks meaning of words.
11. Asks many "why" questions.
12. Relatively few speech errors remain—90% of consonant sounds are made correctly.
13. Counts number of fingers correctly.
14. Counts by rote to 10.
15. Comments on pictures (descriptions and interpretations).

Personal-Social-Adaptive

16. Copies a square.
17. Copies oblique cross (×) without demonstration.
18. May print a few letters (5-5$^1/_2$ years).
19. Draws man with at least six identifiable parts.
20. Builds a six-block pyramid from demonstration.
21. Transports things in a wagon.
22. Plays with coloring set, construction toys, puzzles.
23. Participates well in group play.

From Walter M. Block, MD, Child Evaluation Clinic of Cedar Rapids, Iowa, 1972.

al., 1991) is the most commonly used method of assessing gestational age (Figure 5-3, *A*). The Ballard scale is an abbreviated version of the Dubowitz scale, a standardized tool that uses the physical and neuromuscular characteristics of the infant within 48 hours of birth to determine the newborn's gestational age. The Ballard scale can be used with newborns as young as 20 weeks' gestation.

Once gestational age has been determined, it can be compared with birth weight to predict mortality risk. The newborn's birth weight, length, and head circumference are used to categorize the infant's size for gestational age in percentiles (Figure 5-3, *B*). The small-for-gestational age (SGA) infant ranks less than the 10% on the growth chart; the appropriate-for-gestational age (AGA) infant ranks be-

ESTIMATION OF GESTATIONAL AGE BY MATURITY RATING

Neuromuscular Maturity Score

	-1	0	1	2	3	4	5
Posture							
Square Window (wrist)	> 90°	90°	60°	45°	30°	0°	
Arm Recoil		180°	140° - 180°	110° 140°	90° - 110°	< 90°	
Popliteal Angle	180°	160°	140°	120°	100°	90°	< 90°
Scarf Sign							
Heel to Ear							

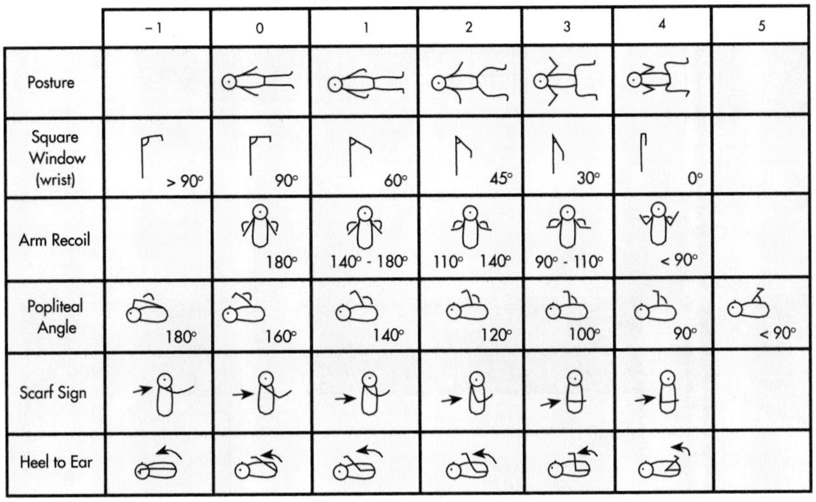

Posture. With infant quiet and in a supine position, observe degree of flexion in arms and legs. Muscle tone and degree of flexion increase with maturity. Full flexion of the arms and legs = 4.
Square window. With thumb supporting back of arm below wrist, apply gentle pressure with index and third fingers on dorsum of hand without rotating infant's wrist. Measure angle between base of thumb and forearm. Full flexion (hand lies flat on ventral surface of forearm) = 4.
Arm recoil. With infant supine, fully flex both forearms on upper arms, hold for 5 seconds; pull down on hands to fully extend and rapidly release arms. Observe rapidity and intensity of recoil to a state of flexion. A brisk return to full flexion = 4.
Popliteal angle. With infant supine and pelvis flat on a firm surface, flex lower leg on thigh and then flex thigh on abdomen. While holding knee with thumb and index finger, extend lower leg with index finger of other hand. Measure degree of angle behind knee (popliteal angle). An angle of less than 90 degrees = 5.
Scarf sign. With infant supine, support head in midline with one hand; use other hand to pull infant's arm across the shoulder so that infant's hand touches shoulder. Determine location of elbow in relation to midline. Elbow does not reach midline = 4.
Heel to ear. With infant supine and pelvis flat on a firm surface, pull foot as far as possible up toward ear on same side. Measure distance of foot from ear and degree of knee flexion (same as popliteal angle). Knees flexed with a popliteal angle of less than 10 degrees = 4.

Physical Maturity

	-1	0	1	2	3	4	5
Skin	sticky friable transparent	gelatinous red, translucent	smooth pink, visible veins	superficial peeling &/or rash, few veins	cracking pale areas rare veins	parchment deep cracking no vessels	leathery cracked wrinkled
Lanugo	none	sparse	abundant	thinning	bald areas	mostly bald	
Plantar Surface	heel-toe 40-50 mm: -1 <40 mm: -2	>50 mm no crease	faint red marks	anterior transverse crease only	creases ant. 2/3	creases over entire sole	
Breast	imperceptible	barely perceptible	flat areola no bud	stippled areola 1-2 mm bud	raised areola 3-4 mm bud	full areola 5-10 mm bud	
Eye/Ear	lids fused loosely: -1 tightly: -2	lids open pinna flat stays folded	sl. curved pinna; soft; slow recoil	well-curved pinna; soft but ready recoil	formed & firm instant recoil	thick cartilage ear stiff	
Genitals (male)	scrotum flat, smooth	scrotum empty faint rugae	testes in upper canal rare rugae	testes descending few rugae	testes down good rugae	testes pendulous deep rugae	
Genitals (female)	clitoris prominent labia flat	prominent clitoris small labia minora	prominent clitoris enlarging minora	majora & minora equally prominent	majora large minora small	majora cover clitoris & minora	

Maturity Rating

A

score	weeks
-10	20
-5	22
0	24
5	26
10	28
15	30
20	32
25	34
30	36
35	38
40	40
45	42
50	44

Figure 5-3 **A,** Ballard Scale for newborn maturity rating. The expanded scale includes extremely premature infants and has been refined to improve accuracy in more mature infants (From Wong DL et al.: *Whaley & Wong's nursing care of infants and children*, ed. 6, St. Louis, 1999, Mosby; **A,** modified from Ballard JL et al.: New Ballard Score, expanded to include extremely premature infants, *J Pediatr* 119:413, 1991.)

Continued

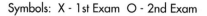

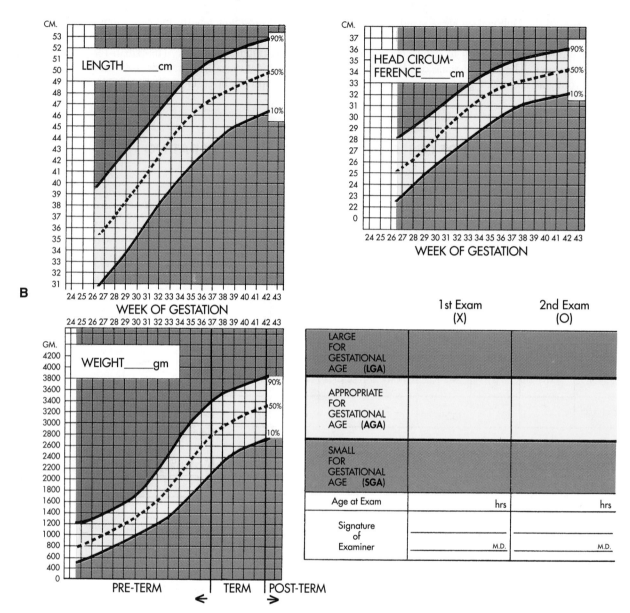

Figure 5-3, cont'd **B,** Newborn classification on maturity and intrauterine growth (From Wong DL et al: *Whaley & Wong's nursing care of infants and children,* ed. 6, St. Louis, 1999, Mosby; **B,** modified from Lubchenko LC, Hansman C, Boyd E: *J Pediatr* 37:403, 1966; and Battaglia FC, Lubchenko LC: *J Pediatr* 71:159, 1967.)

Figure 5-4 These three infants are an example of the variations in size according to gestational age. They are all 32 weeks of gestational age. They weighed 600 g (SGA), 1400 g (AGA), and 2750 g (LGA), respectively. Their associated risks of mortality are greater than 50%, 10%, and less than 4%. (From Korones SB: *High-risk newborn infants: the basis for intensive nursing care,* ed. 4, St. Louis, 1986, Mosby.)

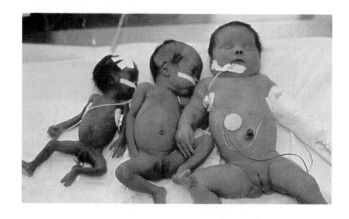

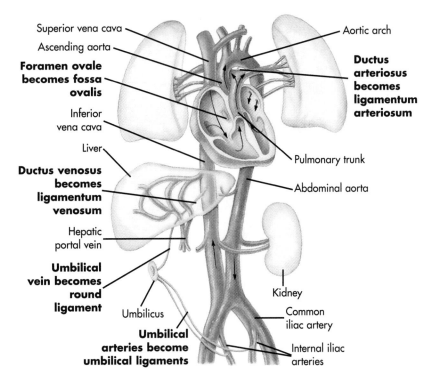

Superior vena cava

Ascending aorta

Foramen ovale becomes fossa ovalis

Inferior vena cava

Liver

Ductus venosus becomes ligamentum venosum

Hepatic portal vein

Umbilical vein becomes round ligament

Umbilicus

Umbilical arteries become umbilical ligaments

Aortic arch

Ductus arteriosus becomes ligamentum arteriosum

Pulmonary trunk

Abdominal aorta

Kidney

Common iliac artery

Internal iliac arteries

Figure 5-5   Changes in circulation after birth.   (From Thibodeau GA, Patton KT: *Anatomy & physiology*, ed. 4, St. Louis, 1999, Mosby.)

tween 10% and 90%; and the large-for-gestational age infant ranks more than 90%. Figure 5-4 illustrates the differences between infants of the same chronological age (32 weeks gestation) who fall in the different categories.

During the first few days of life, infants lose up to 10% of their birth weight but regain the lost weight within 10 days and then continue to gain steadily. In general, infants double their birth weight by 4 to 6 months and triple it by 1 year. Length increases by about 50% during the first year.

Marked changes in body contour occur during infancy. The head grows at a rapid rate during the first year, and the head circumference is greater than the chest circumference. Growth in head circumference reflects brain growth, most of which occurs during the first 2 years of life. The thickness of the subcutaneous fat increases during the first year, reaching a peak around 9 months, then decreasing during the second year. Teeth begin to erupt, and the infant advances from a liquid diet to table food.

The newborn makes many rapid adjustments necessary to sustain life outside the uterus, which are actually a continuum of the development during fetal life. At birth, respirations are initiated and changes in the circulatory system occur (Figure 5-5), the digestive system begins to assimilate the food obtained from an external source, body wastes are excreted, and maintenance of body heat depends on the infant's own resources.

Behavior includes many reflex actions that reflect the immaturity of the newborn's nervous system but also assist in adaptation with the new environment. One of the most striking physiological changes is the continuing maturation and increasing function of the nervous system. Myelination continues at a rapid rate during the first months of life but is not

completed for several years. The functional development of various body structures probably corresponds to the order of myelination and occurs in a cephalocaudal (head-to-foot) direction. The development of head control precedes sitting, standing, and walking. As the brain and central nervous system continue to develop, an increasingly sophisticated range of cognitive and behavioral skills follows.

Figures 5-6 to 5-14 provide a series of pictures of the same three children, two siblings and a friend, from infancy to early adolescence. As you read about developmental changes, note the continuities and differences that occur in these children over time.

The first 3 months of life can be called a *period of adjustment*. Reflexes become more regulated during the first month, and the infant learns how to search, suck, and let needs be known. Sleeping and feeding patterns become more regular. During the second and third months, new behaviors appear that are not reflexes. The infant begins to follow objects with the eyes, allowing exploration of the environment. There is coordination of hand-and-mouth movement, such as sucking the thumb at will. The grasp reflex gradually lessens as more purposeful movements begin. The infant begins to prolong interesting events that occur more or less by accident. The little wails that precede crying may be continued for their own sake. The squeals of the 2- to 3-month-old baby are loud, repeated, and joyful. The infant begins to smile in response to environmental stimuli and to vocalize. Most responses are generalized and commonly involve movements of the whole body. The infant during this period has developed social responses but does not discriminate; any person who can satisfy the infant's needs is accepted.

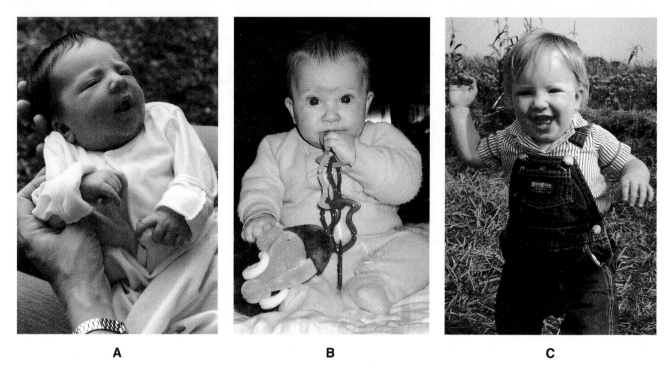

A   B   C

Figure 5-6   Infancy. Cara at **A**, 2 weeks; **B**, 6 months; **C**, 11 months

By 3 months of age, the baby becomes more discriminating and begins to differentiate his or her parents from others and produces special types of smiles and crying for parental attention. This is the beginning of attachment behavior and the development of awareness of the self as separate from the mother. Between 3 and 6 months, or even earlier, the infant repeats some actions that are interesting and prolongs those that occur accidentally, such as repeated hitting of suspended toys to produce movement. There is more imitation of facial movements and beginning imitation of sounds. The infant attempts somewhat of a search for a displaced object, but not a true search.

Infantile reflexes are replaced by purposeful movements, especially those seen in the development of eye-hand coordination. The infant begins to reach for and grasp objects with a raking motion. The tonic neck reflex and **Moro reflex** disappear during the fifth or sixth month. (The Moro reflex is a normal mass reflex in a young infant elicited by a sudden loud noise, resulting in flexion of the legs, an embracing posture of the arms, and usually a brief cry [see Table 26-20 and Figure 26-64 for more detailed descriptions]).

At 3 months the infant, while prone, can raise the head and chest from a surface with arms extended, and at 4 months the head can be held steadily while the infant is supported in the sitting position. At 6 to 7 months the infant can sit without support. Crawling typically begins at about 9 months. At about the same time, the baby will begin to pull up to a standing position while holding onto something for support. At 10 to 11 months the child starts to "cruise," walking while holding onto the furniture. Walking alone usually begins at about 12 months, though it may be several months earlier or later.

Fine motor skill development includes using the hands and fingers for grasping. The infant is born with a grasp reflex, which disappears by about 3 months. At 4 months the infant seems to discover his or her hands and inspects them. By 5 months the baby is able to grasp with two hands. By 10 months the pincer grasp, with the index finger in apposition to the thumb, is present. The child can pick up finger foods and small toys (Figure 5-6, *A* to *C).*

Cognitive Development

Piaget defined the infancy stage of cognitive development as the sensorimotor period. Mental development during this period begins with reflexes and ends with the early appearance of language and other symbolic ways of representing the world. The infant is egocentric, and sensorimotor learning is related to the self. The infant changes from responding through reflexes (e.g., crying, grasping, rooting, and sucking) to organization of sensorimotor activities in relation to the environment. Even the very young infant has the cognitive ability to perform rather sophisticated mental operations. For example, infants are more responsive to a new stimulus than to one that has been repeated several times, showing discrimination known as *habituation.* They are also able to imitate certain facial gestures, such as sticking out the tongue or opening the mouth, which are indications of early cognitive abilities and integrative function.

During the first 7 to 9 months of life, the infant's learning is focused on bodily actions. At around 8 to 9 months, the concept Piaget called "object permanence" can be observed. The infant learns that objects and people continue to exist even when he or she cannot see them. The 5-month-old infant will not reach for an object after it is hidden, but the 8-month-old infant will. Through this sequence of mental and physical actions and the gradual development of memory, the child begins to have a sense of self as separate from, and yet a part of, the environment. It is the beginning of the child's construction of reality.

The first mode of communication is crying. Although all cries may sound the same initially, by about 1 month of age, parents are usually able to differentiate the meaning of cries of varying pitch and intensity. For example, the infant has different cries for discomfort and hunger. The type of cry can also be indicative of health problems. A shrill or high-pitched cry may indicate increased intracranial pressure, and a hoarse cry may reflect hypothyroidism. Vocalization during this period changes from babbling and cooing to the use of several words that can be understood. Generally, the baby laughs at about 3 months, babbles at about 4 months, and by 9 or 10 months can imitate the sounds of others. By 12 months, several words besides "mama" and "dada" are acquired.

Psychosocial Development

During the first year of life, great strides in behavioral development occur. The infant develops social skills that bond the baby with others in the environment. Socially, the infant progresses from staring at faces and crying to smiling, demanding company, vocalizing, and actively participating in games.

The period between 6 and 12 months is dominated by the social modality of "taking and holding on" as described by Erikson. It is a period of attachment behavior. The infant at 8 to 9 months of age has a beginning concept of object permanence and becomes fearful that the mother or other primary caregiver will disappear. The infant actively initiates contact with the caregiver and seeks to maintain that contact. There is true searching for a vanished object, although the search may be in several inappropriate places. Behavior becomes more complex and aggressive. The infant coordinates earlier repetitive actions into behaviors with a purposeful aim. Now the child explores objects more fully by rubbing, banging, and chewing and by discovering the correct procedures for manipulating them. Motor development is dramatic as coordination increases. The pincer grasp, using thumb and forefinger, develops.

Erikson described this first stage of ego development as one of trust versus mistrust. During this critical period of personality development, the child develops a sense of trust based on consistent nurturing in terms of food, warmth, comfort, and the presence of the mother. Successful growth during this period means that the child comes to trust both the self and the people in the environment. The threat at this stage is mistrust of the environment and self. According to Erikson (1963), a sense of trust develops when there is a mutual regulation of the baby's pattern of accepting things and the mother's way of giving them that changes as the baby develops. The social modality of the baby's development during the first 6 months is to satisfy needs by getting, re-

ceiving, and accepting. This is not passive behavior, since the infant influences people in the environment from birth. The first reflexive behaviors of looking, rooting, sucking, and crying elicit responses in the mother or other caretaking adults that cause them to act in ways that will meet the infant's needs. Parent-child attachment is influenced by these behaviors.

The infant's social modality during the second half of the first year is taking and holding on, which begins with the eruption of teeth and the ability to sit upright and voluntarily reach out. The infant begins to be aware of being separate from the mother. The infant may become more demanding of the mother and is faced with the frustrations that result when the pleasure experienced in biting or grasping and holding on to things is met with interference. The infant displays helpless rage when strong desires are thwarted. When this behavior is understood and the infant continues to receive loving attention, trust in self and others can be maintained and strengthened. Some of the infant's early emotional expressions, such as timidity and shyness or boldness and sociability, may indicate enduring personality characteristics.

Temperament, or basic behavioral style, is inborn. Aspects of temperament include activity level; regularity in biological functioning (hunger, sleep, elimination); readiness to accept new people and situations; adaptability to change; sensitivity to noise, light, and other sensory stimuli; mood (cheerfulness or unhappiness); intensity of responses; distractibility; and persistence. Infants vary in these characteristics from birth and have a tendency to continue in one temperamental style, although parental handling and experiences may cause change.

Freud described infancy as the oral stage. The pleasure zone is the mouth; the child seeks to take in everything for sensory exploration and takes great pleasure in sucking and eating. Weaning and teething are challenges at this stage.

TODDLER: 1 TO 3 YEARS

The child enters the toddler years well-equipped to continue learning about the self and the world. Autonomy blossoms as the child begins to recognize self as separate from others. Toddlers have a sense of hope and trust and are developing intellectual and motor skills. A basic competence develops with the expansion of language, memory, and self-control. The toddler years are characterized by energetic exploration and intense inquisitiveness, and also by some obstinate and ritualistic behaviors. Ego growth is rapid during the second and third years of life as the child learns about people and objects in the environment and gradually gains increasing mastery over impulses and bodily functions (Figure 5-7, *A to C*).

Physical Development

The rate of growth in height and weight decreases during the second year of life. The toddler gains an average of 5½ pounds (2.5 kg) in weight and 4 to 5 inches (10 to 13 cm) in height. The child's adult height will be roughly twice what

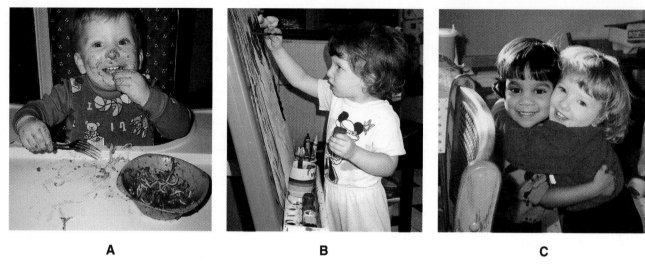

A　　　　　　　　　**B**　　　　　　　　　**C**

Figure 5-7　Toddler years. **A,** Noah, age 18 months; **B,** Cara, age 2 years; **C,** Katie and Cara, age 2½ years.

it is at age 2. As the growth rate in height and weight decreases, it becomes less consistent month by month.

The changes in the child's physical appearance are dramatic. The toddler who is beginning to walk looks top-heavy, with short legs and a potbelly. Fat pads fill the arch of the foot, and most young children appear to be flat-footed until 3 or 4 years of age. There is also a tendency for the legs to bow outward and for lordosis to be apparent. Gradually the child becomes less chubby, the abdomen becomes flatter, and the face loses its baby look. The posture and body proportions change as the chest becomes larger in proportion to the head and abdomen. After 2 years of age, the extremities continue to grow faster than the trunk, and the jaw and lower face grow more rapidly than the cranium. The subcutaneous fat decreases rapidly in thickness during the second year.

Visual acuity improves: at 2 years of age, it is about 20/40. The brain reaches 75% of its adult weight by 3 years of age. Myelination in the spinal cord is almost complete by age 2. The skin changes after the first year, becoming firmer with less water content. The primary teeth continue to erupt, and the child will have the full complement of 20 primary teeth early during the third year, when the second molars erupt.

Gross and fine motor skills increase during the toddler years as a result of the myelination of nerve fibers. Neuromuscular maturation contributes to gross motor abilities, such as sitting, crawling, standing, and walking, and to fine motor skills, such as scribbling and using a pincer grasp. The child usually walks by about 12 months, though it may be as early as 9 months or as late as 18 months. By age 2 the toddler can run and can walk up and down stairs. Toilet training, a major developmental milestone, is also dependent on neuromuscular maturation and generally occurs around age 3 (although boys may achieve this milestone later than girls).

As the toddler learns to perform self-care skills, such as drinking, eating, dressing, toothbrushing, and bathing, his or

her sense of independence and competence is enhanced. Initially, the child's efforts are clumsy and incomplete, but by about 3 years of age, the child displays a fair degree of competence in these areas. Competence increases with physical maturation and is enhanced by parents who give their child the opportunity to practice these skills.

On average, during the toddler years, girls' development tends to be a bit ahead of boys' development. Girls talk, walk, and are toilet trained a month or two earlier than boys.

Cognitive Development

During the second year of life, the child is in the sensorimotor stage as described by Piaget. The toddler, increasingly ready for independence, experiments with new ways to achieve a goal. During the last half of the second year, the child reaches a cognitive milestone: he or she becomes capable of the mental representation of external events. The toddler can think through plans to achieve a goal, rather than performing and watching what happens. The concept of object permanence is developed: the toddler searches for an object even when it is not visible.

Language skills increase dramatically during the toddler years. The use of language reflects the child's cognitive development. Speech enables the child to become more independent, as well as to better make needs known. Most children begin to use a few words at about 14 months, though some do not begin to use words until around age 2.

By age 2 most children have an effective vocabulary (words that can be spoken and/or understood) of 250 to 300 words. The first words a child learns are nouns of one syllable; subsequently the noun is connected with an action verb. During the second year, the child moves from having personal, nonverbal mental images of objects and events and the use of words and gestures invested with personal meaning, to having the capacity for thought and communicative language. A burst of vocabulary occurs toward the end of the second year. This is a period of symbolic thought, a time when the toddler can use mental symbols and words to refer to objects and people, seen and unseen, and to anticipate future events. Language develops sequentially, with adjectives and adverbs following the use of nouns and verbs. The toddler gradually learns other grammatical components of the language from 18 months on. By the third birthday the child has an effective vocabulary of about 900 words. The greater the child's vocabulary and comprehension, the more the cognitive processes can advance. As children share speech and communication with adults, they also learn ideas, attitudes, and values.

The toddler's thinking is characterized by *centering*, which means that only one aspect of an object or event is perceived by the child, and by *egocentrism*, the notion that there is only one point of view—the child's own. Toddlers are unaware of how other people think. This will be reflected in their interactions with others and in their type of play.

Psychosocial Development

Autonomy and independence are major goals for a toddler. The core task for this stage of ego development as described by Erikson is autonomy versus shame. Each child is developing a sense of individuality and separateness from other people. The toddler experiences autonomy in many ways, including the ability to gain a new level of control over motor abilities, bodily functions, and self-care skills; making and acting on decisions; coping with problems or getting the necessary help; and giving generously or holding on. Neuromuscular and cognitive development make it possible for the toddler to explore and experiment, which lead to a sense of autonomy. Failure to establish autonomy results in a sense of shame and of doubt in one's ability to function effectively.

Freud described the period from 18 months to 3 years as the anal stage of psychosexual development. The focus of this stage is on the buildup and release of tension at the orifices. The child experiences pleasure from expelling urine and feces. However, the parents begin to insist that these actions occur only at the proper time and in the proper location. Toilet training is part of socializing the child. Self-control and delayed gratification are necessary skills for socialized behavior. Freud believed that the parent's approach to toilet training and the child's response greatly influence the personality of the individual.

Socialization is an important aspect of the child's development during the toddler years. Socialization is the process by which an individual becomes a member of a social group by acquiring the group's values and behaviors. In our society, socialization during this period focuses on numerous issues, including bowel and bladder habits; cleanliness; control of anger and aggressive behaviors; acquisition of language skills; and control of excessive motor activities, egocentric behavior, and antisocial behavior.

During infancy the child had few restrictions or responsibilities. The toddler must develop new roles and relationships with the world and the people in it. The rules for acceptable behavior are changing, and the growing child must adapt. For many children, this is the time when they enter a day care or child care situation. In such situations children begin to be expected to conform to specific group behaviors. This can be a growth-producing situation or a source of conflict for the child and for the family.

Social relationships during this period continue to revolve mainly around the parents and other primary caregivers. The toddler is increasingly equipped to expand his or her social world to include siblings, other children, relatives, day care providers, and neighbors. Through social relationships the toddler learns about socially approved behaviors, such as cooperation, sharing, waiting one's turn, and respecting the feelings and possessions of others.

Socialization as a male or female begins during infancy. From 1 to 3 years of age, the child has a beginning awareness of sexual differences and sexual roles. Children begin exploring their own bodies and those of others. This is normal and is an important means for the toddler to learn about physical differences between males and females. It is important to help parents and caregivers recognize this as normal behavior and help them respond to these issues in a constructive manner.

Parents generally interact differently with boys and girls and have different expectations regarding behaviors and attitudes, such as dependence/independence, achievement, vigor, cooperation/competition, and assertiveness. The attributes that are affirmed or negated by the parents greatly influence the child's sex role development. Observation and imitation of the same-sex parent also contribute to gender identity.

The toddler is uninhibited in the pursuit of personal goals. He or she wants to explore everything in the environment. Since the toddler has not yet acquired any sense of judgment or discrimination, parents are constantly balancing the child's drive to explore and experience with the need to protect the child from situations that could be harmful or are beyond the child's ability level. This leads to conflict with the parents when the child encounters restrictions that the parent must set to protect the child or help him or her adapt to socially acceptable behaviors.

Displays of the toddler's temper are common, especially when the child is also fatigued. While temper tantrums are expressions of frustration, they may provoke fear in the child because he or she also wants to please the parent and desires the parent's love and approval. An environment that is safe for exploration and allows the child to make choices is beneficial. It is also important for the parents to maintain control of their own emotions in situations in which the toddler is not yet prepared to do so. As the toddler matures and gains greater control over self and environment, many situations become less stressful.

Play is important developmental work for the toddler. It is a process of exploration and discovery. Gradually, as the child begins to form mental images, play becomes more imaginative and imitative. The child thoroughly enjoys newly acquired abilities and manipulates objects with persistence and enthusiasm. Play provides practice for newly acquired motor skills. The toddler exhibits repetitive play and enjoys putting things in and out of containers. Children who are given the freedom to explore and make reasonable choices develop a sense of self-assurance and spontaneity. If the toddler is not allowed to play in a safe and interesting environment or if play activities are stopped by constant limit setting, the child may begin to doubt his or her ability to accomplish tasks or to meet new challenges.

Young toddlers engage in parallel play, where they play beside, but not with, each other. Initially they treat other children like objects; toddlers may push, pinch, bite, or poke others because they have no inner sense that this may hurt. Gradually the toddler moves into interactive play with peers.

The toddler gradually becomes able to play alone for longer periods, but attachment behavior continues. Periodically the toddler seeks out the parent or caregiver, particularly if there is a problem or perceived threat. When faced with a new person or situation, most toddlers have more assurance if the parent is present, and they return to the parent quickly if things become too difficult.

The toddler is sensitive to changes in the environment. If one alteration occurs in the toddler's world, it is as if everything changes and becomes strange and unmanageable. Consistent routines for daily activities are helpful. They allow the child to anticipate what will happen, learn the behaviors that are expected, and gain a sense of control. Routines, habits, or rituals may be particularly important around mealtime or at bedtime, when the child must deal with separation and darkness. If parents do everything the same way each night, the child is reassured that the world will not change while he or she sleeps.

During the toddler years the child learns to cope with separation from the parents or caregivers. Fear of separation begins at about 7 months. Between the ages of 1 and 3 years, long separations are not well-tolerated and may damage the child emotionally. Although the child is unable to express or understand the feelings he or she is experiencing, the child is able to sense loss. Learning to tolerate brief separations is an important developmental task. Developing a "good-bye" ritual when leaving the toddler with the child care provider (e.g., something brief and consistent, such as waving good-bye) is an important way to acknowledge the parent's departure. As children learn that parents will return, they become more accepting and adaptable.

Closely related to separation anxiety are the fears and fantasies commonly expressed by toddlers. The child may experience nightmares or behavioral changes, such as anxiety about taking a bath or about flushing the toilet for fear of disappearing. The toddler's feeling of power may contribute to these fears because the child believes that by wishing something, it can be made to happen. For example, the child fears that by wishing harm toward someone, it may occur. Imaginary beings and animals, some of them ferocious, are common in the imaginations of toddlers. Some of the child's own aggressive feelings may be projected onto the imaginary being. Sympathetic understanding of these fears and fantasies by the parents helps them deal with the child's concern about separation.

Emotional feelings and reactions vary in toddlers, depending on age and temperament and on how others in their environment react to them. Toddlers cannot express or explain personal emotions, so they are manifested in behaviors. These behaviors may include showing affection, shar-

ing, playing cooperatively, timidity, contrariness, selfish or aggressive behavior, temper tantrums, or dawdling. A degree of self-awareness and emotions, such as pride, sympathy, jealousy, guilt, and shame, begin to emerge during the second year. Parents need to be sensitive to the acting out of the toddler's emotions and to the need to be supportive and loving in helping the toddler as he or she learns to deal with various emotions.

The word "no" is spoken with increasing frequency during the toddler years. This is often labeled "negativism," but it is essential to the child's efforts to gain self-control and a sense of mastery over the environment. The child may say "no" and at the same time comply with the parent's request.

Children begin to develop a self-concept at a very young age. By the time a child enters the toddler years, and certainly during these years, the child has positive or negative perceptions of the self and a personal sense of worth. Adults in the child's world are very influential in determining the direction of the child's inner sense of self. Supportive reinforcement of positive feelings is essential for nurturing an emotionally healthy human being.

PRESCHOOL: 3 TO 6 YEARS

The preschool years are marked by physical, social, emotional, and intellectual development. While the child still has many dependent needs and behaviors, he or she is also beginning to exhibit more independence in actions and thoughts. The child is developing a sense of self as a social person in relation to other people and is also learning a great deal about the physical world. Preschool children are emerging from their toddler years and becoming social beings. Expanded language and gross motor skills enable them to explore further in the environment. Preschoolers are involved in increasing independence, developing basic motor and language skills, and adding to their social skills (Figure 5-8, *A to C*).

Physical Development

Physical growth continues at a slow rate. On average, the preschooler gains about 3 to 5 pounds (1.5 to 2.5 kg) in weight and 2 to 2¾ inches (5 to 7 cm) per year. The face and body become more slender as the baby fat disappears. The musculoskeletal system continues to develop, with muscles growing and cartilage changing to bone. Most of the bone growth is in the long bones. At about age 5 the child begins to lose the first set of teeth. Visual acuity reaches 20/20 between 4 and 5 years of age.

Preschoolers have an increased sense of balance and enjoy both gross and fine motor skills. Their ability to run, jump, hop, swim, skate, and ride tricycles and bicycles demonstrates their increasing gross motor abilities. Their use of building toys and art materials exhibits their increase in coordination and fine motor skills.

The preschooler is dependent on parents and other caregivers for nutritious foods and good eating habits. Family food preferences, culture, and lifestyle also influence food selections. Appetite fluctuates, and many preschoolers go

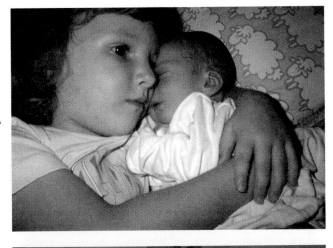

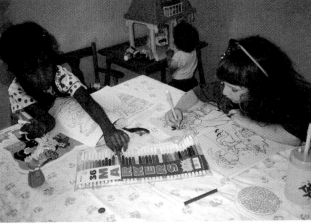

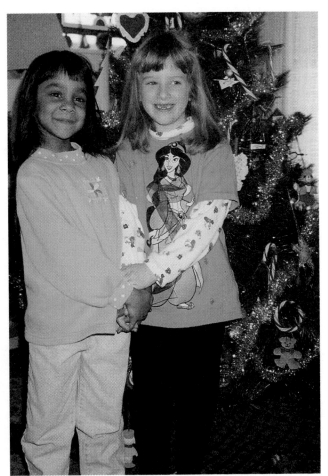

Figure 5-8   Preschool years. **A**, Cara age 4, "Big Sister" of Noah, age 2 weeks; **B**, Katie and Cara, age 5 (Noah in background, age 1); **C**, Katie and Cara, age 6.

for several months without gaining weight. However, for some preschoolers excessive eating may be a problem and is a cause for concern, since lifetime habits are beginning during these years. During the preschool years the child learns to eat with the family and to enjoy many of the foods that the family eats. The child should be able to feed himself or herself early in the preschool years and should be using eating utensils with little difficulty toward the end of the preschool years.

The preschooler shows increasing skills in dressing and other personal care skills. Toilet training is usually completed before or during the early preschool years.

Cognitive Development

Piaget described children between 2 to 7 years old as being in the preoperational stage of cognitive functioning. The child is increasingly able to use mental symbols to represent people, objects, and events. This means that the child is able to think about people, for example, without seeing or hearing them. This is liberating for the child, making it possible to act out thoughts during play. The preschooler's thinking is still limited by the inability to focus on more than one as-

pect of a situation at a time. At times, preschoolers will group unrelated characteristics of a person or event together into a confusing whole.

A major characteristic of this period is egocentric thinking: children in this stage cannot see another's point of view and assume that their own viewpoint is shared by everyone. This affects the preschooler's language, thought, and reasoning. The older preschooler begins to be able to consider more aspects of a situation, another person's viewpoint, and the intent and outcome of behavior. Cognitive growth of the preschooler includes increasing memory ability.

Language development includes use of an increasing number of words, improved articulation, use of correct grammatical structure, and a growing ability to categorize objects in the environment using words. The early preschooler uses both communicative and noncommunicative speech. When using communicative speech, the child tries to communicate a message to a listener. Noncommunicative speech consists of monologues during which the child converses out loud to himself or herself, although others may be present. The child may repeat and elaborate on statements made by parents and other adults. These monologues are often a source of great amusement to other people.

Interactions with parents, siblings, relatives, other adults, and peers all contribute to the child's educational process. In addition, many preschoolers begin structured educational programs, such as Headstart, nursery school, or preschool, when they are 3 or 4 years old. An environment at home or away from home that stimulates and affirms discovery and learning is necessary for the child to practice new skills and extend earlier experiences.

Psychosocial Development

The child identifies with the parents and is motivated to try to be what they want and to be like them. The child becomes more socially responsive and able to give love and affection. The development of initiative is characterized by the wish to "become," in which the child wants to find out what kind of person he or she can be. During the earlier years, the child broadens the sense of self as a separate person with some power to influence the environment and to control impulses and his or her own body. These accomplishments make it possible to approach new tasks with feelings of confidence and an abundance of energy. The child becomes intrusive in a desire to attack new situations. Preschool children are noisy, active, and on the move. They thrust themselves into each situation, driven by curiosity and imagination.

Erikson described this stage of ego development, particularly around 4 to 5 years of age, as one of initiative versus guilt. The child now has adequate energy, motor skills, and mental ability to attack new tasks with gusto and determination. When the parent provides encouragement and enthusiasm, while also protecting the child from harm, the child learns self-sufficiency, direction, and purpose. If the parent prevents the child from doing tasks he or she is capable of trying, or ridicules or punishes the child, the child learns guilt and shame and a sense of inadequacy. The child may then experience these negative feelings when he or she tries to do the same thing, or even when the child thinks about trying it again. This can have long-term effects on the child's psychological development.

The preschooler's social environment increasingly extends beyond the family and other primary caregivers to include other adult and peer encounters. The child learns to interact more easily with unfamiliar people. Temperament enables some children to do this with great ease; other children require more encouragement. Experiencing a variety of interactions with people of all ages is important for preschoolers to help them develop a range of personal-social behaviors.

The preschooler is able to experience many feelings, including happiness, joy, affection, excitement, wonder, anger, frustration, jealousy, sadness, loneliness, and fear—all of which are normal emotions. Emotional feelings and reactions are determined by both innate temperament (see Box 26-4) and the pattern of emotional expression of adults around the child. Children need to be able to express the range of their emotions in a supportive and loving environment and to begin to name and understand their own emotional reactions.

Death

Preschool children who experience a death, loss, separation, significant change in lifestyle, or illness require support and help in dealing with their feelings. Preschoolers may express their feelings through physical symptoms, such as headaches or stomachaches, or they may become irritable or withdrawn. The finality of death is not well understood by a child at this age. He or she may ask many questions and continue to search for the lost person. The most important aspect of dealing with a loss or death is for the parents to be gentle and honest with the child. Box 5-6 provides an overview of children's responses to death at various ages.

Negative Behaviors/Discipline

The behaviors of a preschool child are a composite of many interacting factors, including heredity, culture, the environment, and developmental level. The child continually experiments with old and new behaviors. As the child's experience moves beyond the home, he or she encounters a vast number of experiences that affect behavior. As the behavioral repertoire enlarges, the preschooler tries many new behaviors. Many of these are useful and help the child develop. However, some are negative, harmful, or dangerous and must be curtailed.

Some of the common negative behaviors of the preschooler are negative use of language, negative facial gestures, aggressive or hostile behavior, excessively dependent behavior, and noncompliance. If the parent or other caregiver does not intervene when the child displays negative behaviors, behavioral problems may develop. Some discipline is necessary, but it must be delivered within the context of love and concern for the child's present and future well-being. The preschooler is developing concepts of "good" and "bad." If a child behaves in an unacceptable manner and is told repeatedly that he or she is "bad," this affects self-image. The situation is similar with a child who is repeatedly told that he or she is "good" and then becomes limited in self-expression and self-development by aspiring to someone else's definition of "good." Adults should identify the behavior rather than labeling the child. Children become restricted by labels and may find it difficult to move beyond them to enlarge their field of experience.

Play

Play during the preschool years becomes increasingly more social, imaginative, and complex. While playing together, children develop concepts, imagination, neuromuscular coordination, and language. "Let's pretend" is a favorite phrase and activity. Through imaginative play the child tries out the roles of different people in a variety of situations. In play the child can take on any role and master fears. The child can have feelings of strength and adequacy instead of smallness and vulnerability.

Imaginary playmates are important to some preschoolers. They may include these "playmates" in dreams; fantasies; and certain daily rituals, such as eating; as well as including them in their play. Rituals continue to be a significant part of the preschooler's daily pattern.

BOX 5-6

CHILDREN'S RESPONSES TO DEATH

BIRTH TO 2 YEARS

Lacks conception of death

Can experience a sense of loss and grief

These experiences lay a foundation for developing a conception of loss and grief

2 TO 5 YEARS

Denies death as a normal process

Sees death as reversible

Has unlimited faith in his or her ability to make things happen

May react with anger or displaced anger

Gives responses that may differ little from those of his or her parents

5 TO 8 YEARS

Sees death as final; does not see it will happen to him or her

Sees death as scary

Seeks to isolate what causes death and what death means

Feels the vulnerability that accompanies death

May take on more "adultlike" caregiver roles in the family or become "self-reliant"

8 TO 12 YEARS

Views death as final and inevitable

May be unable to accept the finality of the loss

Realizes the possibilities of his or her own death; may develop fears of own mortality

Develops affective responses to death, as well as the defenses to handle his or her feelings (e.g., denial, avoidance, displacement, and reaction formation)

May create stories or jokes about death to hide fears

Experiences egocentric and magical thinking

Is aware of what this death will mean for his or her future

ADOLESCENTS

Understanding surrounding death resembles that of adulthood

Must face personal implications of death

Demonstrates risk-taking behaviors

Seriously seeks the meaning of life

More anxious about the future

Modified from Raphael B: *The anatomy of bereavement*, London, 1983, Hutchinson; Schaefer D, Lyons C: *How do we tell the children? Helping children understand and cope when someone dies*, New York, 1986, Newmarket; Wheeler SR, Pike MM. In Fawcett CS, editor: *Family psychiatric nursing*, St. Louis, 1993, Mosby; and Potter PA, Perry AG: *Fundamentals of nursing: concepts, process, and practice*, ed. 4, St. Louis, 1997, Mosby.

By internalizing the parents' standards and ideals, the child gradually develops a sense of moral responsibility and a conscience, which makes resisting temptation possible, even though the parents are not present. The child can feel guilt for misbehavior, and at about 5 years of age he or she even has some feelings of guilt for wanting to misbehave. This early conscience is modified through the years of childhood as intellectual abilities increase and the ability to identify reasons for moral action becomes more mature.

Sexuality Patterns

Love and admiration for the parents and other significant adults intensify during the preschool years. Although mixed with defiance at times, identification with the parents increases. Sexual identification began at an earlier age when the child learned that he was a boy or that she was a girl, but during the preschool years it is heightened. It becomes evident as the child begins to imitate the parent of the same sex, learns more of a sex role identity, and becomes acutely aware of sexual differences.

Interest in the parent of the opposite sex is somewhat romantic, which results in conflict when the child learns that he or she cannot replace the parent of the same sex, whom the child also loves. These feelings of intense love and the wish to be rid of one parent can cause anxiety, guilt, and fear because the child believes that wishes are as real as the actual deed. Because the child cannot compete with this larger and more powerful rival, he or she resolves the tension by identifying with the parent of the same sex. Freud called this the Oedipal complex for boys and the Electra complex for girls, named after characters in Greek mythology. Parents and other significant adults influence early sex role development.

The preschooler is very interested in his or her own body and its intactness and how it compares with that of other children. This sexual curiosity is an important developmental phase and helps the child gain an understanding of sexual identity. The child's curiosity may be manifested in direct questions to parents about sex. Such questions are an attempt to understand how the body functions and why girls and boys are different. Curiosity may also be evident in overt behaviors such as actual visual exploration of oneself or of the opposite sex.

According to Freud's psychoanalytical theory, sexual development of the preschooler also centers around resolution of the Oedipal complex for boys and the Electra complex for girls. A boy wishes to possess his mother solely and thus competes with his father to win affection from his mother. The child imitates the behaviors of the same-sex parent closely in an attempt to replace that parent, thus taking on characteristics of masculinity or femininity and resolving the complex. By the end of the preschool period, the child begins to realize that such a sexual relationship is not possible and instead expresses interest in the same-sex peer group. Nevertheless, childrearing practices and imitation of the same-sex parent influence the specific sex typing of the child.

One activity related to sexuality that tends to confuse or disturb parents is the preschooler's interest in self-stimulation of the genitals (masturbation). If this behavior is not excessive, it is both normal and healthy, since it is part of a child's bodily exploration and helps satisfy sexual curiosity. Help the parents address their own feelings about this behavior and the way they want to deal with it in their family. It is important to help parents separate their response to the behavior from their reaction to their child's developmental exploration. When assessing sex and sexuality, determine the parents' perceptions of both male and female sex roles, their understanding of sexual development in the preschooler, and any biases they may have as a result of certain attitudes or beliefs. This knowledge will help you as you design interventions for these families.

SCHOOL-AGE: 6 TO 12 YEARS

During the middle years of childhood, from ages 6 to 10, the child moves from the close ties of family and home to the larger world of peers, school, and neighborhood. The family "romance" is less intense, and the child is able to go out into the world. This is the period of latency during which the child is free from earlier concentration on sexuality and strong basic drives. The child can now direct energy toward learning the skills and competencies of the mind and body that lead to practical achievements and accomplishment in the world. Tremendous intellectual growth occurs during this lull before the "storm" of adolescence, and the child is introduced to experiences that help in learning the fundamentals of society and culture (Figure 5-9, *A* and *B*).

Physical Development

Physical growth during the middle years of childhood is relatively slow and smooth. The most pronounced period of growth usually comes toward the end of this stage, at 10 to 12 years of age. Some children begin the growth spurt as early as age 8 or 9. The increments in weight are less regular than those in the young infant and child, and weight may remain stationary for weeks at a time. The approximate annual increase in weight is about 5 to 7 pounds (2.3 to 3.2 kg). The average annual increase in height is approximately 2 to 3 inches (5 to 7.5 cm). Boys on average are taller and heavier than girls until the adolescent growth spurt, which occurs earlier in girls (see Figure 26-21 for examples of physical growth curves).

A
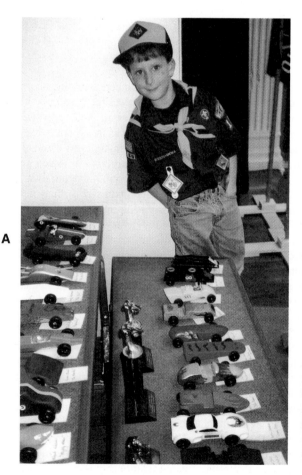

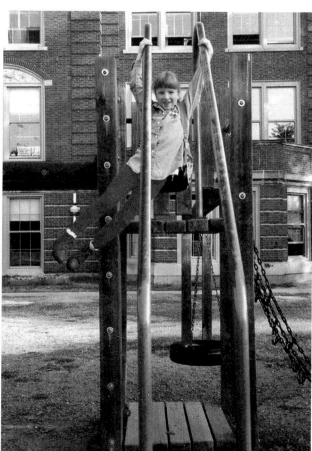
B

Figure 5-9 School-age years. **A,** Noah, age 7; **B,** Cara, age 8.

The physical changes that occur make school-age children more agile and graceful. They become slimmer, with longer legs and a lower center of gravity than the younger child. They are stronger and better coordinated and are able to fit into the adult physical environment more easily. The size of the cranium increases only slightly, because nearly 90% of the growth of the brain is accomplished by age 7. The lower parts of the face continue to grow, giving the child a more mature appearance and making room for the larger teeth to erupt. The first permanent teeth, which usually erupt at 6 to 6½ years of age, are usually the mandibular central incisors.

The eyeball continues to grow until 10 to 12 years of age. Visual acuity is usually 20/20 to 20/30 between 4 and 5 years of age, but depth perception is not very accurate until 6 to 7 years of age. Hearing is well-established at a much earlier age. Growth of lymphoid tissue increases steadily until puberty and then decreases (see Figure 26-27). This accounts for the abundance of lymphoid tissues, such as adenoids and tonsils. The skeleton continues to ossify, with cartilage being replaced by bone. The child acquires the basic neuromuscular mechanisms by age 6 or 7 and spends the school years refining physical skills, resulting in an increase in motor skills and coordination. Thus the school-age child engages in repetitive practice in all areas of neuromuscular activities from the fine motor skills of writing, drawing, and playing instruments to the large motor skills used in baseball, biking, running, and swimming, depending on individual interests.

The appetite fluctuates, and eating nutritiously may become a problem. Problems with excessive weight may also begin to occur. Although taste preferences continue to influence what the child eats, the ongoing establishment of good eating habits is important (see Chapter 6).

Cognitive Development

The cognitive development of the school-age child, according to Piaget, is characterized by the ability to begin to do mentally what the child would have had to do with real action at an earlier age. Piaget termed this the *stage of concrete operations*, meaning that the child can now use mental representations or symbols of objects and events. What had to be done physically before, the child can now experience mentally. This enables the child to use numbers, read, order objects on an increasing or decreasing scale, and classify objects by a common characteristic. The stage of concrete operations begins at about age 8.

The school-age child also begins to see the multiple characteristics of objects rather than centering on any one aspect. Piaget also found that during these years the child masters the concept of conservation. Piaget's classic test illustrating the principle of conservation is to give the child two jars of equal size containing equal amounts of liquid. The contents of one jar are then poured into two smaller containers of equal size, and the child is asked whether the amount of liquid poured into the two smaller jars is still the same as that remaining in the other container. Younger children cannot comprehend that the liquid has been conserved when placed in smaller containers. The older child comprehends that the quantity remains the same. He or she is beginning to distinguish the difference between how things seem and how they really are.

Throughout the school years, memory and language skills increase. This enhances the child's ability to share experiences and observations and to articulate questions and new understandings. Older children can think more logically because they can now make mental comparisons rather than only manipulating objects, can see the whole as well as the parts, and have mastered the concept of conservation.

As school-age children develop, thinking gradually becomes more logical. Egocentric thinking and behavior progressively diminish and are replaced by a larger view of self and others. Children begin to realize that their viewpoint is not shared by everyone and that others see things differently. This new ability to reason and to carry out mental operations in solving problems is limited in an important respect. They cannot yet differentiate clearly between their own assumptions and the facts. In other words, they treat their own hypotheses as if they were facts and reject facts that do not agree with that position.

Creativity continues to develop in the young school-age child. Frequently, however, children appear more reluctant to express creativity while they are in school, perhaps because of the responses of adults who are more interested in the "right" answers. This attitude can suppress the child's creative impulses, because adult approval is so important. The opinions of peers also assume greater importance and may also constrict creativity.

As children internalize the standards and ideals of the significant adults around them, they begin to develop a conscience and sense of moral behavior. They have greater knowledge of what is right and wrong, although they may break the rules made by adults. They begin to have feelings of guilt about misbehavior. The younger child may follow certain rules somewhat rigidly and be quick to condemn the supposed wrongs of others. This early sense of morality is expanded and modified during the years of middle childhood as intellectual skills increase and the ability to understand reasons for moral thought and action matures. Parents can enhance their child's moral growth by modeling their own values, such as honesty and fairness, at every opportunity and by helping the child understand punishment as the result of a deed and not as a judgment of the child's worth.

School is an exciting adventure, and most children anticipate it eagerly. Mixed in with the excitement are often some fears and anxieties. The child needs to separate from home and parents, adjust to new authority figures, accept restrictions on previously acceptable activities, learn new routines, and participate in large groups. These situations can create tension within the child. This may be particularly challenging for the child who has not attended a day care center or a preschool program. For children coming to school from home or from "play-based" child care programs, the increased need to focus on classroom activities may place additional demands on the child. This can also be a challenge for parents. The transition to formal schooling can be facilitated by understanding and encouragement from parents, teachers, and health care providers.

Certain characteristics are indicators of the child's readiness to enter the world of school. Some of these characteristics include the ability to communicate, ability to participate in social interactions, capacity to make friends, ongoing attainment of a basic body of knowledge, and independence in basic self-care activities.

Psychosocial Development

Erikson described the ego development stage of middle childhood as a period focused on industry versus inferiority. This is a stage when ideally the child develops a sense of industriousness and accomplishment rather than a sense of inadequacy. During this period the child leaves home for school, where the views, esteem, and approval of people outside the family become important. The child becomes a worker, one who is required to develop intellectual, physical, and social skills that contribute to a sense of adequacy. The child's attainments in cognitive, interpersonal, and social development are significant. The child is now able to see a higher organization of behavior in which to participate. The child wants to operate in socially accepted ways of thinking and behaving, can understand another person's point of view, and is able to take what he or she hears and sees and compare it with what is already known of reality. The child learns to reason and act according to rules. This promotes a positive school experience and facilitates participation in organized sports or other activities. Participation in activities that develop skills both in cooperation and competition is beneficial.

Achievement at this stage enhances feelings of competence, confidence, and industry. The child who achieves in some areas begins to feel rewarded both from outside sources, such as teachers and parents, and from within, by feelings of satisfaction. The child who does not experience some form of achievement begins to develop feelings of inferiority, low **self-esteem**, loss of confidence, and a sense of incompetence. These feelings may haunt the developing individual for many years, even when success and achievement come later.

Children experience success during this stage of industry as they participate in many productive activities. School-age children's great desire to win at games and willingness to work to achieve a variety of skills demonstrate their need to be adequate in their own eyes, as well as in the eyes of others. Parents, teachers, and other adult figures should encourage school-age children even when performance is incomplete or imperfect. Adults must realize that success comes sooner for some children than for others.

Freud described middle childhood as a period of relative sexual quiet, a time of latency. In terms of sexual development, middle childhood is a span of time between the sexual struggles and resolutions of earlier childhood and the sexual turbulence of adolescence. Awareness of sexuality is not ab-

sent; curiosity, questions, and jokes remain a part of the child's growing sexual identity.

By 6 years of age, the child's personality has become structured. Through accomplishment of earlier developmental tasks, the child has achieved a concept of the self, acquired a sense of trust, developed autonomy with some power over impulses and the environment, and incorporated standards and values of the culture as interpreted by the parents.

During these school years, the peer group becomes increasingly important, and the child needs to find a place in a group of peers. The child is ready to be involved in the private world of children where adults are not always welcome. At ages 6 and 7, peers are partners in play, with boys and girls participating together much of the time. During ages 8 and 9 the child usually selects a best friend and moves toward group activities with friends of the same sex. Feelings of group solidarity and belonging are promoted by secret languages, codes, and clubs, as well as a common culture. Together, children explore ideas and values, learn fair play, practice leadership roles, and experience cooperation and compromise. Children who show difficulty with peer relationships may have problems in developing future relationships. These children may develop into bullies or the victims of bullies. Early identification of difficulties and sensitive interventions to the child's needs can have a positive impact on later development.

As children move into the larger world of school and peers, they continue to need their parent(s). Demands for conformity are placed on them by people outside the family, such as teachers, scout leaders, and peers. The family should be children's source of strength and support. School-age children continue to need the approval of parents, teachers, and other significant adults for their uniqueness and any special talents.

As children approach adolescence, they view their parents in a more critical light. This puts a strain on the parent-child relationship and can lead to tension and arguments. Parents need to understand the changing viewpoint of the child and reassure him or her of their continuing love, even when this is difficult. Parents also need to allow greater independence and responsibility for the child in appropriate areas. This reinforces the child's sense of self and prepares the child for future developmental stages.

ADOLESCENCE: 12 TO 19 YEARS

Adolescence is the period of life beginning with puberty and extending for about 7 to 10 years to the onset of adulthood. The age boundaries of adolescence vary but range from 11-13 to 19-22, and sometimes longer. Adolescence generally extends to the time when the person is physically and psychologically mature and ready to assume adult responsibilities and be self-sufficient. Throughout the adolescent years, the individual struggles with the transition from the role of a child to the role of an adult and struggles to develop a personal identity. The adolescent moves toward greater independence and personal freedom to make decisions.

Developmental Tasks

The adolescent faces the following developmental tasks:

1. Searching for self-identity and a sense of self-worth
2. Achieving a gradual independence from parents
3. Establishing relationships with peers
4. Developing academic and vocational skills
5. Adjusting to rapid physical and sexual changes
6. Developing an internalized set of values
7. Considering choices for a career
8. Developing the ability to think logically and analytically

According to Erikson, the task of adolescence is the development of ego identity versus role confusion. The formation of a self-identity separate from others is a process that begins in infancy and continues throughout adulthood, but it has a very distinct focus during adolescence. Without the emerging understanding of self-identity as expressed through interests, preferences, and personality temperament, individuals feel confused about who they are in comparison with the group. Part of the need to identify the self as a separate person is the need to establish independence from the parents.

The word "conflict" is often associated with the words teenager and adolescent, and adolescence is truly a stage of conflict and turmoil, as well as one of high growth potential in the physical, sexual, and social areas. The adolescent must learn to cope with increasingly intense impulses, developing sexuality, and an altering body form. Spurts of growth occur, along with increased muscular energy and strength. The reproductive system matures; the individual develops secondary sexual characteristics and becomes capable of reproduction. The social world broadens in adolescence, and the individual develops a growing sensitivity to the perceived judgments of others.

Stages of Adolescence

Adolescence may be divided into four phases or stages (see Table 26-10):

1. Preadolescence
2. Early adolescence
3. Middle adolescence
4. Late adolescence

Preadolescence. Preadolescence is a stage covering the ages of 10 through 12 for girls and 10 to 11 through 13 for boys. It is characterized by increases in physical activity, energy, and restlessness. Running is more natural than walking, and sitting still even for a short time may be nearly impossible. Muscular strength, skill, and agility are very important to the individual and among peers. Adolescents may have quiet moments during which they seem to be simply staring into space. They may have fears, worries, and concerns but are generally not interested in talking about them. Signs of earlier childhood problems, such as nervous habits (e.g., nail-biting), childish antics, or bed-wetting, may reappear temporarily.

Preadolescence is a continuation of the change in primary affiliation with parents and their codes to primary affiliation with peers. These years are often trying times for parents because the parent-child bonds appear to be loosening and breaking. Although preadolescents love and feel loyalty toward their parents, they may frequently treat them with surprising suspicion, distrust, and irritability. They are easily offended and respond to seemingly minor incidents with the ready accusation that adults do not understand them and treat them unfairly. Other adults in the neighborhood may receive more admiration than the parents receive. Parental recommendations regarding use of language and matters of appearance and cleanliness are often met with indignation and conflict.

Preadolescents are increasingly sensitive about having a parent see their bodies and about public displays of affection toward parents. They are often seemingly unaware of the effect of their own inconsiderateness on the feelings of others and appear surprised when it is pointed out to them that their behavior has caused some hurt.

At this stage, boys and girls typically have little to do with each other socially. Girls may move through this phase more quickly than boys. Clique and secret club formation is a prominent characteristic. If peer codes do not meet with parental approval, they are all the more desirable. The changes of preadolescence are not easy for the parents, nor are they easy for the preadolescent. Conflicting and painful situations are common, but the preadolescent must experience these to move on in establishing an individual identity.

Early Adolescence. Early adolescence begins with puberty and lasts for several years (ages 11 to 12 through 13 to 14 for females and 12 to 14 through 15 to 16 for males) (Figure 5-10, *A* and *B*). The growth spurt focuses attention on the self and on the task of becoming comfortable with body changes and appearance. The teen tries to separate from the parents; however, the presence of parents is still important. This dependency-independency struggle is apparent by less involvement in family activities, criticism of parents, and rebellion against parental and other adult discipline and authority. Conformity to and acceptance of peer group standards and peer friendships gain importance. The peer group usually consists of same-sex friends; however, the early adolescent shows an increased interest in the opposite sex. Early adolescence usually coincides with menarche in females (see Figure 26-15) and active spermatogenesis in males (see Figure 26-16).

Middle Adolescence. Middle adolescence begins when physical growth is completed and usually extends from ages 13 to 14 through ages 16 for females and from ages 14 to 16 through ages 18 to 20 for males. The major tasks during this period are an increased sense of ego identity, attainment of greater independence, interest in the future and career possibilities, and establishment of heterosexual relationships. The individual is working to overcome feelings of insecurity and inadequacy and to move toward self-assurance and independence (Figure 5-11).

Peer group allegiance, at a peak in 15- to 16-year-olds, is manifested by clothing, food, fads, musical preference, and common jargon. Most teenagers relate increasingly with the

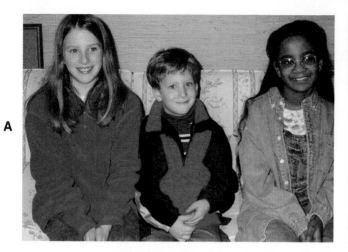
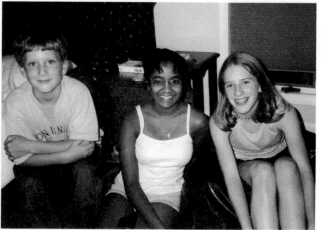

Figure 5-10 Early adolescence. **A**, Cara and Katie, age 11, with Noah, age 7; **B**, Katie and Cara, age 13, with Noah, age 9.

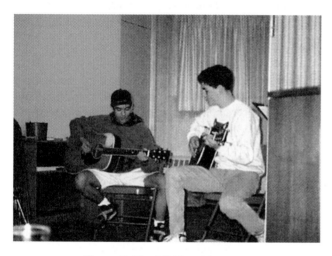

Figure 5-11 Middle adolescence.

opposite sex, whereas some begin to be aware of their homosexual orientation.

The middle adolescent gradually becomes more self-assured and able to make some independent decisions. For these reasons, the youth at this stage has particular difficulty in adjusting to controlling or confining situations. Some societal privileges and responsibilities increase during middle adolescence, such as driving a car or a first job. Experimentation with adultlike behavior and risk taking is common in an attempt to prove oneself to peers.

Sexual experimentation often begins now as a result of social exploration and physical maturation. Family relationships and communication may be disrupted as the adolescent's activity outside the home is increased. Changes in cognitive functioning may first be evident in that the adolescent moves to abstract thinking, returning to more concrete thinking during times of stress.

Late Adolescence. Late adolescence may occur from about age 17 to 18 until age 20 to 25. The person has usually finished adolescent rebellion, formed some significant views, and established a fairly stable sense of self. Many

youths are not yet committed to one occupation, and they often question relationships to existing social, vocational, and emotional roles and lifestyles.

The late adolescent may be a student or an apprentice. Lack of economic freedom may be a concern and can lead to prolonged dependence on parents. Continued dependence may lead to delayed maturity. The late adolescent is clarifying his or her value system and examining issues of philosophy, religion, life and death, and ethical decisions. The peer group has lost its primary importance, and a relationship with a particular person may become the focal point for social activity. There is more individual dating and fewer group activities with friends. Often the first emotionally intimate relationship develops at this time.

The late adolescent may take a major step in establishing independence from parents by moving away from home. Activities with family members tend to decrease, and more adultlike friendships begin between late adolescents and their parents as the earlier family turbulence subsides. At that point, the person is developmentally a young adult, having made the transition from adolescence. He or she is more realistically aware of strengths and self-limitations, as well as the limitations of others. Thought processes become more logical, and the ability to use abstract ideas increases. The end of late adolescence is marked by planning for the future in the form of higher education, occupation, and committed relationships.

Some fluctuation in this progression may continue to some degree for several years in the direction of greater maturation. The task of finding an acceptable career that is personally satisfying and potentially economically adequate assumes a more central position during the later high school years and subsequent period of college, vocational training, or apprenticeship. This is a time of becoming ready to leave the parents' home both physically and emotionally.

At age 18, people may marry without parental consent and may vote. At age 21, individuals attain most adult privileges and responsibilities conferred by society. At this time an individual is allowed to drink alcoholic beverages, sign a binding financial document, and accept full legal penalties for crimes.

The end of adolescence is more difficult to define than the beginning. Our society observes no specific ritual of passage into adulthood. The adolescent may remain dependent on the parents because of economic need or educational endeavors. In general, the adolescent moves into adulthood when he or she can prepare realistic plans for the future, including plans for education, occupation, and a shared or single lifestyle. The status of young adulthood is reached when the adolescent begins to adjust to societal responsibilities and moves toward achieving personal life goals.

Physical Development

Puberty marks the beginning of adolescence. It is characterized by dramatic physical and physiological changes, including the beginning of the ability to reproduce. There is a spurt of rapid growth in height, weight, and muscular development. Secondary sex characteristics appear, and the reproductive organs mature. In girls, puberty lasts about 3 years, from age 10 or 11 to 14. **Menarche,** the onset of menses, usually occurs at 12 to 13 years, though it may begin about 1 year earlier or several years later. It often begins just after the peak of the physical growth spurt. In boys, puberty lasts about 4 years, from ages 12 to 16.

Girls between the ages of 10 and 12 experience a spurt in height; by age 14 or 15 their growth is nearly complete. During these years, girls grow 2.5 to 5 inches (6 to 12.5 cm) and gain 8 to 10 pounds (3.5 to 4.5 kg). Boys have their rapid growth spurt between ages 12 and 14. By age 16, their growth is nearly complete. Boys grow an average of 3 to 6 inches (7.5 to 15 cm) and gain 12 to 14 pounds (5.5 to 6.5 kg). An adolescent's self-concept is continually readjusting as the body changes.

Sexual Development and Sexuality

Adolescents struggle with notions of body image and what is normal growth and development. At this stage teenagers begin to develop curiosity and interest in sexual relationships. They are very aware of the development of secondary sex characteristics and continually compare how their body looks with the appearance of their peers and to some ideal standard of attractiveness.

Frequently formerly supportive adults are confused or uncomfortable with the teenager's sexual curiosity. In addition, the changing roles of males and females leave many teenagers with little idea of what is expected from them.

Females. Menarche may occur anywhere between 10 and 16 years of age. In the United States, the average age of onset is about 12.8 years of age. Ovulation and regular menstruation usually begin 6 to 14 months after menarche. The onset of menarche varies among population groups and is influenced by heredity, nutrition, health care, and other environmental factors. Most adolescent girls view the menarche as a normal developmental milestone separating them from childhood. They may view it with curiosity or pride. Others view the onset of menstruation with fear or anxiety.

A wide variety of attitudes exist among different groups in society. The presence of physical discomfort during and/or around the time of menstruation may also lead to a negative reaction, with some females experiencing headaches, backaches, cramps, and abdominal pain. They may also experience mood changes before menstruation, such as depression, irritability, anxiety, and a sense of low self-esteem.

Secondary sex characteristics in the female begin to develop at puberty and may take 2 to 8 years for completion. Development of secondary sex characteristics occurs in a predictable sequence (described in detail in Chapter 26 [see Figures 26-6, 26-8, and 26-15]). Breast development, often the earliest sign of puberty in girls, occurs between the ages of 8 and 18. Pubic hair develops between years 11 and 14, although recent research suggests that development may occur 1 to 2 years earlier, particularly in African-American girls (Kaplowitz and Oberfield et al., 1999).

Males. **Spermatogenesis** (sperm production) and seminal emissions mark puberty and sexual maturity in the male. The first ejaculation of seminal fluid occurs about 1 year after the penis has begun its adolescent growth, and nocturnal emissions (loss of seminal fluid during sleep) occur at about age 14. Just as the onset of menstruation produces a new set of feelings in girls, nocturnal emissions may produce new feelings in boys, including pride, fear, or shame. Erotic dreams may accompany the nocturnal emissions.

Secondary sex characteristics in the male also begin before puberty and may take 2 to 5 years for completion. Changes in body shape, growth of body hair, and muscle development may continue until age 19 or 20, or even until the late 20s. Development of secondary sex characteristics occurs in a predictable sequence (described in detail in Chapter 26 [see Figures 26-7 and 26-16]). Testicular enlargement is usually the first pubescent change, starting between ages 10 and 13 and ending between ages 13 and 17. The penis and scrotum enlarge, the scrotum reddens, and scrotal skin changes texture. Hair grows at the axilla and pubic area between ages 12 and 16. The growth of facial and chest hair usually occurs somewhat later, around age 16. The voice begins to deepen at age 13 or 14.

Sexual Role Development

Maturation of an individual's sexual identity involves more than development of primary and secondary sexual characteristics and strong sexual impulses. It also involves the ability and desire to give and receive love, respect, and affection. The development of a sexual identity begins very early in life, but it is particularly strong during adolescence because of the physical changes and the search for self-identity. Conflict with parents over issues of sexual identity and behavior is common. This conflict is due in part to the changes between childhood and adolescence in what parents find acceptable, such as kissing others, and in part because of the differences between what different generations believe is acceptable.

Intellectual curiosity about sexuality and the act of sexual intercourse is a major component in adolescent sexual development. Frustration at this age results from a general lack of sufficient information about sex and mixed messages given by both the culture and the media.

Traditional attitudes and values regarding sexuality are changing. Because of the dichotomy of American values relating to sexual behavior and rules for sexual identity, present-day adolescents are left to search for their own sexual identity and moral code with very few parental or societal guidelines. Understandably, many teenagers have difficulty establishing a consistent sexual identity.

Adolescent Pregnancy

Teen pregnancies occur within all cultural and socioeconomic groups. Teenagers may find it difficult to deal with the tension between their emotional needs and their developing sexuality. During this time of sexual development and exploration of a sexual role, pregnancy may occur. Babies born to teen mothers are at risk for low birth weight and related problems. If both parents are not committed to caring for the child, this complicates the already difficult situation. Frequently the teen mother is left with little support to take on the enormous burden of rearing a child while she is still developing herself.

Educating adolescents (both males and females) about sexuality, birth control, and the realities of parenting is very important in preventing unwanted pregnancy and sexually transmitted diseases and in helping teens learn about the responsibilities of parenthood. Health care providers can have a major role both in working with adolescents and helping parents to become more comfortable with discussing sexual issues with their children.

Skin

Skin texture changes during adolescence. Sebaceous glands become more active and increase in size. Acne may develop. The sweat glands are fully developed and begin to secrete in response to emotional stimuli. Problems related to skin changes (e.g., acne) and body odor become major concerns during this period. Teaching about personal hygiene is particularly helpful at this time.

Health Risks

Physical health is generally good. Risks to the health of adolescents include poor judgment resulting in accidents, drug or alcohol abuse, unwanted pregnancy, or sexually transmitted diseases. Emotional stress due to unmet or unrealistic expectations may show up as depression, anorexia nervosa, or suicide attempts. Accidents and suicide are the leading causes of death in the adolescent population.

Helping adolescents identify healthy ways to engage in "risk taking" is a challenge to parents and health care providers. For example, trying out for an athletic team, volunteering to tutor children in need, and working to improve the environment are ways adolescents can channel their natural need to test themselves and their abilities as opposed to selecting behaviors that have more negative health outcomes.

Cognitive Development

During adolescence the mind has a great ability to acquire and use knowledge. The thought process of the adolescent becomes more logical, and the ability to use abstract ideas increases. The adolescent is working on the beginning structure of a philosophy of life. This process requires the use of abstract thinking. Piaget described this level of cognitive process as the period of formal operations. This thinking moves beyond the concrete into the area of abstract thought in which reasoning occurs and symbolic and logical processes are used.

Abstract thinking is a new and deeper level of consciousness. It allows for greater creativity and inner awareness. The individual can contemplate the past and future, as well as the present; can develop theories; and can consider scientific hypotheses. Abstract thinking liberates the person for mental processes of greater depth and breadth. This can be a period of academic and creative achievement for the adolescent.

The conscious development of a personal value system also occurs during this period. This is another component of the search for self-identity. Part of the questioning of the values of parents and institutions that occurs at this time is the process of developing a set of personal values that works for the individual. The adolescent becomes more aware of inconsistencies, hypocrisy, and injustices.

Adolescents are subject to many stresses placed on them by their families, schools, peer groups, and society at large. Adolescents are vulnerable to stress, since they have not yet developed a strong identity with sufficient coping mechanisms to deal with increasing pressures and other stressors. Problems such as teen pregnancy, drug abuse, conflict with parents, dropping out of school, or delinquency may result. As our society grows in complexity, the amount of potential stress factors which adolescents must face are likely to increase. An individual teenager's response to stress may result in growth in personal identity and self-confidence, or in vulnerability to less healthy coping patterns.

Psychosocial Development

According to Erikson, the task of adolescence is the development of ego identity versus the danger of role diffusion. Adolescents become increasingly sensitive to how they think others perceive them as compared with how they perceive themselves. Finding one's own identity is stressful and difficult work. In many ways, it is a life-long task. If the adolescent can emerge with a reasonably strong sense of his or her own identity, he or she has successfully experienced this stage. If an adolescent does not develop a personal sense of identity, an ongoing personal sense of confusion, anxiety, alienation, and incompleteness may result. The person may then look to a group outside the family for a sense of identity. The peer group becomes an important place for experimentation with various roles outside the family, and the adolescent often feels intense pressure to join one.

Adolescents may also follow or identify with popular entertainers and wear personal apparel or use speech patterns that mark them as part of a group. Because of the vulnerability of young teenagers, the pressures of peer group conformity may be harmful. Individual judgment may often be forfeited to the desires of the group as a whole, creating great stress and anxiety in some adolescents. It is the rare adolescent who has developed enough ego strength to stand alone against the crowd. Teenagers, however, perceive their behavior as highly individualistic or original because it is different from that of adults, even though it may conform to group codes.

During preadolescence, close friendships are important to identity development. During the later teen years, relationships with the opposite sex usually develop. They may take the form of group activities or couple dating. Adolescents begin to experience the possibilities for trust and intimacy with others. Some individuals become aware that they may have a homosexual orientation.

Another important characteristic is the relationship between the parent of an adolescent and his or her peer group of friends. Frequently, values and beliefs of parents are dramatically different from those of the adolescent's friends. This can result in friction between these two influential factions and can be a source of stress, especially if the teenager feels that he or she must make a choice between loved family members and friends.

The emotional life of an adolescent ranges from exhilarating peaks to depressing lows. Much energy goes into this effort to understand the meaning of this shifting complex of feelings. Outwardly these emotional expressions may be a source of tension and conflict. Gradually the emotions even out to some extent, and a sense of balance develops.

YOUNG ADULTHOOD: 20 TO 34 YEARS (Figure 5-12)

Leaving adolescence and entering young adulthood means separation from the family and its financial support as well as greater freedom to choose experiences and friends. It is also a time of taking greater responsibility for one's own life. During the first several years of early adulthood, some of the major tasks are to achieve relative independence from

parental figures; to establish an independent lifestyle; and to develop a sense of emotional, social, and economic responsibility for one's own life. The young adult faces many complex issues that affect personal and professional growth. Coping mechanisms that were developing during childhood and adolescence are challenged and expanded during the young adult years when choices and responsibilities increase. The young adult must balance the desire to explore options with the need for some stability.

During the middle years of young adulthood, there is often a period of questioning and reflection. Questions the individual reflects on may include the following: "Why am I doing this, and not something else?", "Where am I going with my life, my career?", or "What other alternatives should I consider?" This is probably the first period of conscious self-examination. Sometimes this search reaffirms the direction that a person's life is taking; sometimes change seems desirable. Depending on the set of circumstances, the person may decide to get married, change jobs, get divorced, have children, develop a career as a parent, or return to work.

This period of questioning and transition is often followed by a period of settling in with the choices that have been made. The individual can use energy to develop the chosen lifestyle and find a special place or role in a family and in society. People at this stage invest in home, career, and family.

During the later years of young adulthood the individual may establish a career commitment, form significant relationships, and even take on parenthood.

Developmental Tasks

The major developmental tasks of early adulthood include the following:
1. Becoming independent from parents
2. Establishing a household
3. Choosing and beginning to establish a career or vocation
4. Developing a personal style of living, including shared living or single living

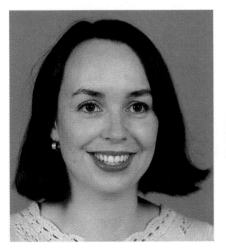 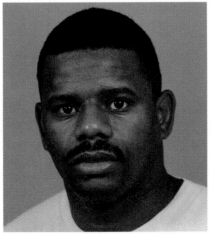 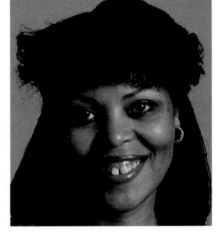

Figure 5-12 Young adulthood.

5. Establishing an intimate relationship
6. Establishing friendships and a social network
7. Choosing activities in social and community organizations
8. Developing parenting behaviors for biological offspring or in the broader framework of social parenting
9. Implementing personal values in home, employment, and community settings

Physical Development

Physical growth reaches its peak during early adulthood. The body is operating efficiently, with good muscle tone, strength, coordination, and a high energy level. The young adult has the physical strength and stamina for many activities that influence life patterns.

Sexual development is a part of this period of peak physical development. Exploration with sexuality and various sexual roles occurs at this time. During young adulthood the individual establishes a sense of identity with his or her sexual role. This is also the time for decisions on childbearing.

Nutritional needs are no longer for growth, but for maintenance and repair. Weight control becomes a problem for many adults, especially for those who continue to consume food as they did during adolescence but whose energy expenditure is less than it was during those years.

Cognitive Development

The young adult years are a time of optimal cognitive functioning. The individual is engaged in the mastery of new skills and new knowledge, and the intellect is stimulated by these exciting and challenging events. Cognitive functioning at the level of formal operations—the capacity for abstract thinking—emerged during adolescence. The young adult expands on this base by becoming less egocentric and more realistic and objective. The young adult has an excellent ability to acquire and use knowledge, and to engage in problem-solving and creative endeavors.

For many, education continues during the early years of young adulthood. College, graduate school, on-the-job training, and/or continuing education classes prepare the young adult to enter some field of work. Depending on the career path chosen, educational preparation may continue well into the 20s.

Psychosocial Development

Erikson's sixth stage, intimacy versus isolation, focuses on one of the tasks of young adulthood: forming an intimate relationship. After establishing self-identity, the individual can enter a relationship with another without losing self-identity. Because neither the development of self-identity nor readiness for an intimate relationship is clearly defined, young adults often experience some fear that they will undergo a loss of personal identity when entering a relationship. Intimacy involves more than physical contact: it is the ability to share personal identity with another without losing one's own unique identity. The desired outcome is mutual satisfaction and support.

Although Erikson focused on the heterosexual marriage relationship, intimate bonds may also be formed within a homosexual relationship. Erikson suggested that affiliation or intimacy was expressed as mutuality with a loved partner with whom one is willing and able to share the cycles of work, family life, and recreation. This bond involves the capacity to enter a committed relationship and to stand by it through difficult times.

The danger of this stage is isolation or an avoidance of those persons and settings that promote and provide intimacy. A young adult whose identity work is not well underway may settle for sets of stereotyped interpersonal relationships that lead to a deep sense of isolation. This false "intimacy" is not a love relationship; it bypasses the accomplishment of improved understanding of one's own inner resources and those of others. The person feels isolated, lonely, and withdrawn.

Another of Erikson's stages of ego development, which is important during young adulthood, but is primarily a task of middle adulthood, is the stage of generativity versus stagnation. Generativity refers to a productive life: productivity within personal relationships (family and friends), a chosen career, and in the community. Stagnation refers to self-absorption and a sense of emptiness in life.

Establishing Independence

Young adults may move out of the parental home, or they may establish a more equal role with their parents if they continue to live their parents. During difficult economic times, when jobs for high school and college graduates are hard to find, many young adults continue to live in their parents' home until they are able to establish themselves financially or return home when they find themselves in difficulty. Whether the young adult remains temporarily in the parents' home or moves out to establish an independent living situation, the young adult should work toward emotional, social, and economic independence.

Marriage or Singlehood

Marriage is increasingly viewed today in our society as a loving, sharing relationship between two people, rather than as a social institution for creating and rearing a family. While many young adults still choose marriage, singlehood is another viable option. Remaining single may meet the needs of those not ready for the complex interdependent relationship of marriage or those who by temperament are not suited to the roles of spouse and parent. Single persons may experience pressure from the family to make marriage a goal. Even people who remain single by choice may have difficulty with feelings of aloneness and lack of companionship. Singlehood, however, may increase the opportunities for career advancement, creative expression, and community service.

Divorce

The expectations for marriage as a close, loving, and sharing relationship in which both individuals benefit from the union are often unmet. Divorce is a common result in our society. Most divorces (one of two) occur during the first 3 to 5 years of married life and in individuals younger than 29 years old. Consequently, approximately 1 in 4 (25%) children lives in a single-parent home. Financial strain after divorce is a common problem, most often for the woman and children.

Divorce may be a distressing or a freeing experience depending on circumstances. Initially, it may be quite traumatic as each person deals with feelings of anger, disappointment, grief, and disillusionment. The emotions related to divorce have been compared with those experienced with death of a spouse, except that with divorce contact is often maintained, particularly when young children are involved. Divorce requires a reassessment of basic values, personal strengths and limitations, future job potential, and socioeconomic factors. After divorce, each person must move on to develop new roles. Divorced individuals often suffer emotional strain and depression. Support from family, friends, health care providers, counselors, and others may be needed to work through this process.

Parenting

Parenting tasks may be achieved by bearing children; adopting; becoming a foster parent; or reaching out in other ways, such as coaching children's teams or participating in child development organizations. The decision to rear children involves a major change in a couple's relationship. The arrival of a child is usually a happy event in the life of a couple, yet it can also bring great stress to the marriage.

The role of parent is very demanding, as well as rewarding, and requires changes in roles, relationships, and time commitments within and outside the home. Individuals struggling with infertility and the attempts to become parents also face many emotional and financial challenges related to becoming pregnant, in addition to the challenges of new parenthood. When interventions are successful, these new parents may face an even greater transition since they may have been more focused on the process of continuing a viable pregnancy than the reality of having a child.

Many individuals rear children as single parents. This may be a deliberate choice to remain single or may occur as a result of desertion, divorce, or the death of a spouse. When divorce and remarriage occur in families with children, the difficult roles of stepparent and stepchild must be worked through and established.

Support from family, friends, and health care providers is important to promote a positive family transition. Interventions need to be tailored to the needs of the mother, the father, and the child(ren).

Career, Work, and Occupation

The young adult also chooses a career or a vocation and may begin to consider how beliefs about self and society affect that choice. During these years, work is closely tied with identity. A young adult who feels satisfied with his or her work feels challenged, fulfilled, and rewarded. Frustration with work can lead to boredom and apathy. Work satisfaction is important for maturation and mental health. It can provide prestige and social recognition, a sense of self-

worth, opportunities for service, creative self-expression, varied interactions, and a means of self-support. The individual is in a position to stand on his or her own, take risks, and accept consequences for personal actions. This can produce both excitement and fear and holds great potential for personal growth. As the economy changes, it is important to be aware of its impact on employed individuals. The trend toward "right-sizing" or "down-sizing" of companies can have a major impact on the individual and the community in terms of increased stress and stress-related health problems.

Organizational Participation

During young adulthood, many individuals begin to establish connections with various organizations in the community. These affiliations may be related to commitment to a cause or belief system, development of friendship networks, physical exercise, or social purposes. Group membership serves the important purpose of providing an outlet for self-expression. However, groups may be problematic if they become a substitute for development of the individual. Maintaining a healthy balance within various group memberships and time for self-orientation is important for young adults. Self-direction, or the knowledge of one's own goals, and recognition of what membership with certain adult groups means to those goals are necessary if an individual is to achieve appropriate group affiliation.

MIDDLE ADULTHOOD: 35 TO 64 YEARS

Middle adulthood is a stage of life when growth is strongest in the areas of personal, social, and emotional development. By this time, individuals have generally chosen a lifestyle, a family or single pattern of living, and an occupation. The span of time considered to cover the middle adulthood years is variable; some consider ages 40 to 64, and others use ages 35 to 64. Stevenson (1977) uses the term **middlescence** to describe this age span. She further subdivides it into two categories: middlescence I, from 30 to 50 years, and middlescence II, from 50 to 70 years. The age boundaries of this stage of life must be considered tentative and flexible. Regardless of the parameters used, this is likely to be the longest stage of a person's life (Figure 5-13, *A*).

Developmental Tasks

The categories of early middle age and late middle age are used here to describe major developmental tasks.

The major developmental tasks for people in early middle age, between ages 35 and 50 to 55, include the following:

1. Accepting and adjusting to the physical changes of aging
2. Continuing to learn in the areas of personal and career interests
3. Reviewing, evaluating, and refining career goals (orientation) in light of a personal value system
4. Reaching the desired level of achievement in one's career

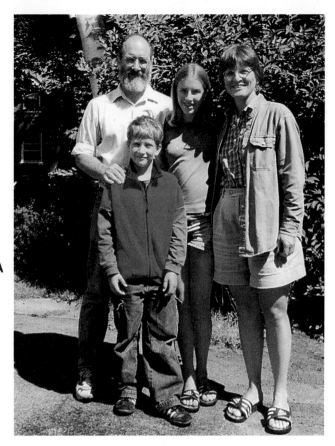
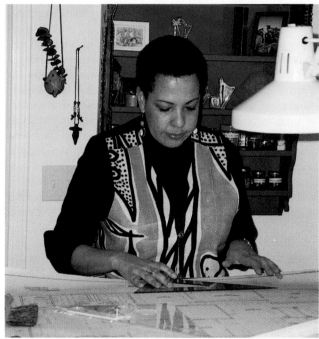

A

B

Figure 5-13, A and B Middle adulthood.

5. Working on a maturing relationship with one's spouse or significant other
6. Choosing organizational and civic activities in which to participate
7. Helping younger persons develop as they search for their own identity
8. For those without children, becoming aware of biological changes and the need to decide about possible parenthood
9. Coping with the "empty nest" as children leave home
10. Helping aging parents or planning for the time when that assistance will be necessary
11. Developing hobby and leisure activities for current enjoyment and for long-range retirement planning
12. Planning for the financial, personal, and social aspects of retirement

The major developmental tasks for persons in late middle age, between ages 50 to 55 and 65 to 70, include the following:

1. Developing supportive, interdependent relationships with grown children, their families, and other members of the younger generation
2. Enhancing the relationship with one's spouse or most significant other person
3. Adjusting to the loss of a spouse or significant other person, if necessary
4. Maintaining an affiliation with some civic, political, professional, religious, and/or social organization(s)

5. Maintaining an interest in current scientific, political, and cultural changes
6. Helping aged parents or other relatives cope with changes in their lives
7. Developing satisfying leisure time activities (Figure 5-13, *B)*
8. Preparing for or adapting to retirement, which may include another career, a move, a change in financial status, or numerous other changes
9. Adapting to changes that accompany the aging processes

Physical Changes

During the years of early middle age, physical changes are generally gradual. During the years of late middle age, they become more marked. In our society, aging changes are often the focus of humor, denial, and depression. However, many adults accept the physical changes of aging with grace.

Aging changes may begin over a wide span of time. For some people they begin in the early 30s; for others, changes do not occur until well into the 40s. The skin loses some of its elasticity: wrinkles gradually begin to form around the eyes and mouth and on the forehead. The skin sags a bit under the eyes and around the chin and jaw. The hair begins to lose pigment and turns gray or white. It may thin somewhat, and in men the hairline often recedes. Because of decreased muscular tone, the abdominal muscles are no longer as firm.

Frequently weight gain occurs, especially when the activity level decreases but caloric intake does not. Sensory function remains generally intact except for decreased accommodation for near vision (presbyopia). Internal organ function remains fairly constant in the healthy adult, although some decrease may occur in respiratory and cardiac function. If the individual actively pursues physical fitness, these changes may not occur until later.

During the late 40s or early 50s, women experience **menopause.** The menstrual cycle becomes irregular in frequency and flow pattern. Periods of heavy bleeding alternate with amenorrhea for 1 to 2 years and finally cease altogether. The decrease in the hormones estrogen and progesterone produces symptoms that may include vasomotor changes (hot flashes and sweating) and mood changes. There is an increased risk of cardiovascular problems and decrease in bone density at this time.

Men do not experience such an abrupt halt to their reproductive ability. During the late 50s or during the 60s, testosterone production decreases somewhat, leading to decreased sperm production, increased time to obtain an erection, and less intense orgasms.

During middle adulthood many individuals experience for the first time the diagnosis of a chronic health problem such as hypertension, diabetes, or arthritis. A history of smoking may lead to cardiovascular or respiratory problems, which are evident for the first time during middle age.

As the individual moves through late middle adulthood and toward late adulthood in the late 60s and into the 70s, many develop more chronic health status changes. While none of them may be life-threatening, together they do take a toll on the energy level and sense of well-being. (See also Chapter 27.)

Cognitive Development

Cognitive processes in adulthood include learning, problem solving, memory, and creativity.

Learning continues in adulthood. Much of it comes from life experiences that are integrated by thought and reflection. Adult learning is enhanced by interest, motivation, self-confidence, a sense of humor, and flexibility. The middle-aged adult is interested in how knowledge is applied to living and improving life. The growth in continuing education and outreach programs makes ongoing, life-long learning available to interested adults. These programs enable persons to update their knowledge for their profession or occupation and to develop new personal interest areas. Some adults use middle age as the opportunity to enroll in college for the first time, and others return to earn an advanced degree. Reaction time or speed of intellectual performance is individual and generally stays the same or diminishes during late middle age. Most adults experience no decrease in the ability to learn, though they may need a longer learning period.

Problem-solving abilities remain fairly constant throughout adulthood. The levels of education and intelligence and the accumulation of life experiences influence the ability to solve problems at this age, as they do at any age. People of various ages will perceive problems and situations differently. Early formative experiences differ somewhat with each generation and affect how people view problems and how they seek resolution. The older the person is, the greater the store of past experiences used to evaluate current situations. Moving through the middle adult years, individuals have the opportunity to broaden their perspectives and deepen their insights.

Memory generally remains intact during the middle adulthood years. Some decrease in recent memory may occur during the late middle years. Memory is aided by the presentation of well-organized material.

Creativity continues and may increase during middle adulthood. The insight needed for many creative thoughts, acts, and productions depends on the range of life experiences accumulated over the years.

Psychosocial Development

Erikson believed that the important task for personality development at this stage of life is resolution of generativity versus stagnation. Adults need to contribute to the next generation either by rearing children or producing something that can be passed on to subsequent generations. The latter may involve creative, socially useful work. The motivation is to create and/or nurture those who will follow and to leave a mark on the world. Generativity means sharing, giving, and contributing to the growth of others, as well as passing something on to the next generation. For some this means parenthood; for others this means generativity through creative acts of expression in the arts or through community involvement. Stagnation means experiencing boredom and a sense of emptiness in life, which leads to being inactive, self-absorbed, and self-indulgent. The individual may have difficulty accepting the changes of aging and may become overly focused on retaining aspects of youthfulness, for example, in relation to behaviors and dress.

Between the ages of 30 and 50, major life goals and activities are concentrated on the areas of self-development, career development, assistance to both the younger and older generations, and organizational endeavors. Individuals feel a need to come to terms with both their own values and society's values. Personal values undergo a major change or numerous minor changes during these years when patterns are beginning to seem set but may not feel comfortable. Individuals move into various roles in a number of settings: in the family, at work, in religious organizations, and in community and civic affairs. In Western society, much of the implementation of the goals of major institutions, such as business, industry, government, education, religion, and charitable agencies, is done by the middle-aged population.

Work/Career

Work is a major activity and motivating force during middle age. For some the work itself is rewarding and gratifying; for others the only rewards are a paycheck and fringe benefits. Success in a line of work enhances the self-image; lack of success can damage that image. As the person advances through middle age, he or she becomes more aware of the years remaining before retirement. The person reflects on whether he or she is on schedule with career goals and whether this is the desired career path for the remaining years of employment. Middle-aged individuals may realize that they have expended time and energy in doing what their family and society felt they "should" do. They may begin to feel too restricted by the career and personal choices made earlier. They may find that other aspects of themselves are struggling to surface and find expression. This reflection may involve an uprooting of the life that seemed well-grounded and striking out after a new vision. During the 40s and early 50s, individuals may be enjoying success and promotions at work or may harbor a concern that this is the last chance to "make it." Some experience tension from a fear of being passed by and are sensitive to any indications that peers or superiors are losing confidence. With so much energy going into the work setting, the home setting may suffer.

For the working woman, involvement in a career may be a source of strength, if the work brings its own rewards and sense of personal accomplishment. A mother benefits from having an identity outside her family role. However, it may also be a source of stress, since demands from both work and family may be high. Women in the work world who may already have experienced some discrimination can find promotions increasingly rare and even when they occur, they may be resented by a husband who has not been similarly recognized.

Family Roles and Relationships

New roles emerge as the middle-aged adult deals with growing children and aging parents. The adult may feel sandwiched between the concurrent needs of the older and younger generations. As the children grow through their own life stages, the parents must switch from a role of great involvement during young childhood, to lesser involvement with continued support as the offspring move through their adolescent years. When the children reach young adulthood, it is healthy for the relationship if the roles of children and parents become more equal. With aging parents, a role change for the middle-aged adult depends to a great extent on the health and dependency needs of the parents. If the parents become weak and frail, requiring more health care and a change in housing arrangements, middle-aged adults often feel as if their roles with their parents have switched; they are now increasingly in charge. When a parent dies, the middle-aged adult may feel lonely, vulnerable, and aware of the limited time to live one's life.

Caring for Children

A major family task facing the middle-aged adult with children is to help children live up to their potential and to assist them in their search for personal identity. The parent must adjust to the increasing desire of a child to be independent. As adolescence evolves, the child becomes less involved in family activities and desires increased responsibility and freedom. Some parents nurture the independence and delight in the developing individual. Others tend to be overprotective and controlling. Parents may believe they are protecting their children from the same mistakes they made as youths, but children usually resent overly protective efforts.

When the last child moves out of the family home, the middle-aged adult again needs to reconsider his or her role in the family and community. For some parents this event leaves a void; for others it presents a new opportunity for growth. A woman who has devoted years to home and family may be eager to get involved in the outside world of school, career, or community activities.

If two parents remain in the home, they need to face one another as a couple again. This opportunity can bring the positive experience of increased closeness and more time and freedom for shared activities. On the other hand, the couple may realize that their relationship was based on the children, and that apart from the children, they have little in common. A reconsideration of the marriage may occur. Changes also occur for the parent in a single-parent household. The single parent may experience loneliness, but this time may also be an opportunity for new relationships or career goals. During late middle adulthood the role of grandparent may be realized. Increasingly more middle-aged adults are experiencing situations in which grown children are moving back in with their parents due to financial constraints. This can be a very positive experience or place considerable stress on the family. Also, grandparents may find themselves rearing their grandchildren. It is important to be aware of current social trends that may place unexpected challenges on your clients.

Midlife Transition

The phrase "midlife crisis" has become popular in recent decades, but because the term crisis often has a negative connotation, the term transition is used here. Many middle-aged individuals are aware of the changes and challenges they must confront but see this more as a period of reassessment and re-evaluation than as a period of crisis. This phase may begin in the early 40s, although it may be some years earlier or later. People look at the realities of life and at the goals and dreams they have been carrying. Some of these have or can be met; others must be set aside. It is a time of taking stock, readjusting, and emerging with a new understanding. Questions frequently asked include: "What have I done with my life?", "Is this what I want out of life?", or "Have I set aside my own deepest dreams and desires for practicalities that are not satisfying?" Individuals may move their lives onto a different track, or they may accept the one they are on, adjusting to it with greater understanding.

There may be gender differences in midlife perception of the midlife transition. Men still tend to be more involved in career assessment because their traditional role has been focused on becoming established in the career world. Many women, including those who are employed, still tend to see the family as the central issue. This difference does not mean that family is not important to men or that career issues are not important to women. The occurrence of children growing in independence and leaving home differently may affect women's identity. Some may feel no longer needed in the same way; others see this as liberating, because they can now focus on their own goals with greater energy.

At about age 35, many women realize that the biological boundary of childbearing is approaching. (It must be noted, however, that with recent demographic changes, later child birth is more common, and developments in fertility technology make it increasingly possible for women to become pregnant at a later age.) Aging and biology force women to review options that were set aside and that will be closed off in the now foreseeable future. Women with or without children face this review.

Whatever the central issue, all those in midlife transition explore the meaning of their career, their family, and their personal identity. An individual who has spent some years searching for power and responsibility now may crave more inner growth and meaning. Childless couples reconsider having children, whereas those who have spent a number of years rearing young children may move toward involvement outside the home. Single people may reconsider the choice of career over marriage. The midlife transition may mean less acceptance of stereotyped roles and acknowledgment that few answers are absolute. The years 35 to 45 are a time of re-evaluating choices, purposes, and the expenditure of resources. It is a time of uncertainty and opportunity, a chance to restructure a narrower, earlier identity.

The midlife transition is variable; some may never sense a transition at all, whereas others experience profound searches and changes.

Development of Interests Outside of Work

At some point in middle age, the attitude toward work may change from one of total involvement to one of lesser involvement, with a growing interest in focusing on home and family and/or developing skill in a sport or hobby. Work may become more acceptable and be viewed more in terms of its responsibilities than in terms of power. The meaningfulness of activities is a common theme as individuals rethink daily routines at work and home and re-evaluate beliefs in religion, politics, and relationships. This situation offers the potential for psychological growth and a reintegration and stabilization of identity. During these years, aspects of the personality and talents that have been latent may begin to emerge.

Coping With Physical Changes

Part of self-knowledge and self-acceptance is an acknowledgment of the physical, emotional, and intellectual changes that accompany the aging process. Physical changes may be difficult to accept in a culture in which the signs of youthfulness are highly acclaimed. Middle-aged adults ideally find some balance between accepting the inevitable changes in appearance while striving to maintain a high level of health with positive approaches toward exercise, diet, and their socioemotional environment. On the other hand, they may also appreciate the changes of added years in terms of the emotional and intellectual benefits that accumulate.

Weight may become an eminent concern; a battle against weight gain may also be a battle against aging and the loss of physical attractiveness, and all that aging implies in our culture. Difficulties in this area may well depend on the amount of self-esteem that a person previously derived from physical attractiveness. Gray hair is yet another manifestation of a physical change accompanying aging. The adult may perceive it as a source of distress or as a sign of hard-won wisdom.

Menopause

Menopause, which normally occurs during the late 40s or early 50s, involves both physiological and psychological changes. The hormonal changes may result in episodes of rapid mood shifts, nervousness, irritability, insomnia, hot flashes, diaphoresis, and fatigue. These changes cause some women to experience confusion or depression. Other women experience relatively minor physical and psychological distress. In some cultures menopause is recognized as a time of greater wisdom, creativity, and participation in the life of the community. Menopause may be followed by increased enjoyment of sex, since concerns about pregnancy are now absent.

Loss of Peers

Many middle-aged adults are suddenly made aware of the relatively brief and fragile nature of life as a result of the death of peers. Most deaths that occur during the middle years of adulthood are due to cardiovascular disease and cancer. These events are also cause for reflection and taking stock of the meaning and direction of one's own life.

Personal Inner Growth

Individuals re-examine many issues during these years of middle adulthood—issues of personal qualities, relationships, commitments, career choices, and organizational affiliations. All of the choices and reflections concerning those issues provide an opportunity for personal growth.

Maintaining Interest in Current Affairs

People in this age group, as in any age group, are confronted with rapid changes in technology and in the social environment. However, many prefer to maintain restraint with respect to the type and rate of change. Life experiences have brought some sense of wisdom and judgment to middle-aged individuals. Although some younger people may view them as overly cautious and nonprogressive, the balance between the two views is important. At the same time, openness and flexibility continue to be important characteristics for health and well-being. Those who stay current with ideas and trends have a more positive approach to life and less need to maintain a defensive posture. They will probably also be able to communicate more effectively with younger individuals.

Retirement

Preparation for retirement is an important task, both for people who have been employed outside the home and for those who have maintained the household. For a married couple, both must readjust to more shared time. Single individuals need to adjust to more time alone. Preparation through adult education or development of new skills can pave the way for a refocusing of talents and interests. Preparation for retirement is actually life-long—both in relation to planning for financial security and in terms of personal development. People bring to retirement all that they have become during their lifetime. During the entire span of middle age, the activities an individual chooses to participate in are worthy of thoughtful consideration. A person should not delay specific planning for retirement until retirement is imminent but should integrate it throughout the adult years.

Special Characteristics of Late Middle Age

Although many of the issues and characteristics just described continue to affect the years of late middle adulthood, some changes and special characteristics may become more prominent during the 50s and 60s. Individuals in this age group have an opportunity to define and integrate the emotional and intellectual growth of the earlier adulthood years. It may be a time of changes outside the family, thus giving the individual time and energy to develop new areas of interest. In the work world, although advancement is still possible, many have attained much or most of what they can. In certain areas, such as in law, business, government, religion, and community service, this period may include the prime years of activity. People in the late middle years occupy many of the highest positions in these areas.

Within the family setting, spouses may be back to the couple stage, or fast approaching it, and must readjust to the contracted nuclear family or to life alone if a spouse should die. Grandparenting is a new role that is often acquired during this stage. Parents must reassess their relationships with their children and move from adult-child interactions to adult-adult interactions. Men may become more aware, less fearful, and more accepting of their tendencies to provide care and nurturance, whereas women may accept and develop more fully their assertiveness through an interest in business, politics, or other organizations and activities outside the home. The aging parents of 50- to 70-year-olds often require a great deal of emotional, physical, and/or financial assistance.

LATE ADULTHOOD: 65 TO 95+ YEARS

As is the case with other stages of adulthood, the parameters of late adulthood and old age are not easy to determine. Some people seem old at 40, whereas others seem young at 65. Some gerontologists have attempted to deal with this situation by setting apart the years from 60 to 75 as early old age and the years after age 75 as late old age.

Later adulthood has become a subject of increasing interest because of longer lifespans and declining death rates in Western society. The elderly are now the fastest-growing portion of the population. The larger numbers of the elderly and the changes that come with aging have created numerous challenges for individuals and for society as a whole (see Chapter 27 for a more detailed description).

Institutional forms of care (e.g., nursing homes) have been developed for care of the aged but have often proved unsatisfactory; major pieces of legislation have been passed on behalf of the elderly, but often this has not eased the financial, social, and emotional problems that develop with the passage of time. The emphasis in our society on youth and their culture, behavior, and attitudes is accompanied by a negative attitude toward those on the other end of the age continuum. This prejudice is known as "ageism," a negative attitude toward aging and discrimination based on age. This attitude characterizes the elderly as burdensome, sick, and senile and is an indication of much anxiety about aging in the American culture. This attitude, however, is changing somewhat because the ever-increasing numbers of elderly are commanding more attention to the process of aging.

In this culture it is often said that everyone wants to live long but no one wishes to grow old. This is in marked contrast to other cultures, in which old age is respected and even revered. Older adults are not a homogeneous group. Most people become more individualized as their years increase. Each individual's story, responses, and needs are unique (Figure 5-14, *A* and *B).*

Developmental Tasks

Late adulthood is similar to all other developmental stages in that individuals must be able to make certain adaptations and achieve certain developmental tasks. These tasks are different from earlier ones in that these are the final ones in life. The following are among the most significant developmental tasks in late adulthood:

1. Maintaining and developing activities that enhance self-image, contribute to a sense of worth in society, and help to retain functional capacity
2. Developing new family roles as in-laws and grandparents
3. Accepting retirement and adjusting to reduced income
4. Adapting to changes in physical status and health
5. Adjusting to changes in living arrangements
6. Adapting to losses of spouse, other family members, and friends
7. Working on a life review
8. Preparing for one's own death

Physical Changes

Individuals age at different rates. How people age depends on a number of factors. These include the following:
Personal attitude toward aging and life
Level of physical activity
Nutrition
Personal habits
Presence or absence of illness
Even in the absence of illness, some decline in physical function comes with advancing years. Usually this occurs gradually. Reaction times slow, and eyesight and hearing may diminish. In addition, older adults experience an increased incidence of chronic disease (see Box 27-1), less resistance to acute illnesses, and a slower recovery period. These physical changes produce an increase in use of the health care system (see Chapter 27 for a detailed description of physical changes and health care implications).

Some older persons adjust to these changes with an attitude of acceptance and humor. Others become preoccupied with their discomforts and ailments. Depression is a common and underdiagnosed problem in older adults and should be assessed (Table 27-1 gives an example of a short geriatric depression scale that can be used in practice).

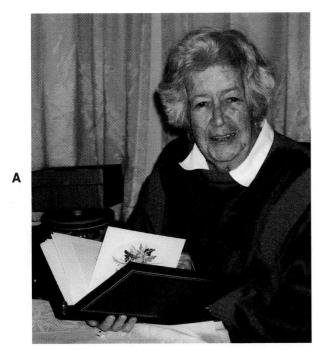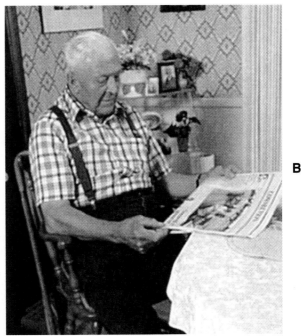

Figure 5-14, A and B Late adulthood.

Cognitive Changes

There are few predictable changes in intellectual function that accompany aging. No decrease in general knowledge occurs, and an increase in wisdom may come with advancing years. Speed in mental performance and in complex decision-making may slow. Maintenance of mental function is affected by many factors, including the following:

    Personal motivation
    Interest in the subject
    Sensory function, especially vision and hearing
    Educational accomplishments
    Recentness of learning
    Personal value of intellectual activity

Psychosocial Development

During the early part of late adulthood, the major life commitments to job and family are nearing completion. Ideally, planning for the next phase of life has been going on for many years. Most older adults have time and energy during the retirement years to further develop interests in many areas. The older adult has an opportunity to develop a new balance with others and society. It can be a time for creative endeavors.

Erikson describes the task of the last ego stage as ego integrity versus despair. Successful completion of this stage leads to the acceptance of one's life as the way it had to be, given the person, the choices, and the circumstances. The inability to come to terms with the life that one has lived can lead to negative feelings, such as despair, anger, resentment, and hopelessness.

Retirement

As both demands from work and family and living arrangements change with the onset of retirement, time becomes more available for doing other things. As mentioned previously, advance planning for retirement activities that enhance self-respect is crucial. Failure to plan can make the change come as a shock, and the hours may seem empty, heavy, or endless. If adults prepare, they can use the time to their advantage for developing new careers, hobbies, sporting skills, or community activities. This preparation will ideally enhance self-worth and promote a sense of usefulness and functional capacity. Educational opportunities for adults of all ages are increasing. For the older adult, continuing education can provide an opportunity to learn simply for the pleasure of learning or to develop another set of skills. Both physical and mental well-being depend on continuing involvement in, and contribution to, society.

When one or both elderly spouses have been employed, the marriage relationship will be affected by retirement. The couple must adjust to having more shared time and to weaving their lives together effectively. A spouse may have, at least initially, a sense of the other person being more "underfoot" and of losing privacy. Couples may develop a more equal relationship with regard to household chores and leisure activities.

How a person reacts to retirement is related to the meaning and satisfaction of his or her previous work or career. Feelings of relief and release may be present if the job lacked personal meaning and satisfaction. If the job held much meaning and gave a person satisfaction and authority, the loss is more deeply felt and may lead to depression. In addition to the loss of a job, the retiree also feels the loss of work associates and the social network and friendships they may have provided.

Retirement usually involves a financial change, typically a decrease in income. This change is difficult because it affects the person's lifestyle in the areas of daily living, home ownership and maintenance, socializing, entertainment, and travel.

New Roles

New roles emerge for older adults as their children marry and have children of their own. Acceptance of their children's spouses into the family network is instrumental in the ongoing interaction of the family. Interaction with grandchildren can be a pleasant aspect of aging if it does not become too time-consuming or burdensome. Grandparents can provide a sense of family and history. Another role that may begin in an earlier phase of late adulthood is the caring for elderly parents who may be ill or dependent. One needs to re-evaluate personal identity in light of these new roles.

Living Arrangements

The older adult may need to change living arrangements for many reasons, including physical status and finances. This may mean giving up a home of many years, with all the comfort and memories that it holds. Some individuals are able to find more suitable arrangements in single homes; others may move in with adult children or into a retirement or nursing home. In our society, the extended family is no longer expected to take care of the elders in their own homes, so a move to a facility may be seen as necessary but not desirable. Such a move usually involves giving up some or many personal belongings and some loss of privacy. These moves can, however, also involve the positive aspects of more efficient accommodations and an increase in socialization with peers.

Losses

Many of the numerous changes that occur in late adulthood are felt as losses. These include employment status, income, deaths of significant people, and changes in physical strength and sensory acuity.

The loss of a job after many years of employment may be one of the greatest developmental and situational crises in an individual's life. For many, retirement incomes are fixed, which can lead to a lowered income over time and subsequent losses. Homes, entertainment styles, and life-long travel plans may have to be given up or diminished in scope to meet the costs of food, housing, and health care.

Other losses may include the deaths of friends, a spouse, or other family members. These losses are among the most difficult aspects of later adulthood. Coping with bereavement for the person with whom one has shared life experiences, memories, and plans leaves a great personal void. Ideally, the older adult experiences the profound emotions that accompany the loss and then goes on living and fostering the development of new relationships. This process requires time and patience. Serious illnesses and deaths of people who have been close during life are also a reminder that there is an unknown but limited amount of time left to live.

Older adults may also feel physical changes as losses. Physical strength, energy, and sensory acuity of the eyes and ears typically decline gradually over the years. By age 60, most people are aware of some physical decline, and most have at least one illness or limiting condition. The occurrence of one or more chronic health conditions may affect strength, energy, and self-image. The older adult faces challenges in accepting physical changes and limitations and in using energy most effectively.

Life Review

The process of performing a life review is an important developmental task of later adulthood. The goal is to achieve a sense of integrity, acceptance, and wholeness in looking back on the life one has lived. Most older persons do spend some time reflecting on their accomplishments and failures, satisfactions, and disappointments in an effort to integrate and evaluate the diverse elements of their life so that they can reach a reasonably positive view of their life's worth. Failure to accomplish this task may lead to serious psychological problems. The life review process is far more than useless reminiscence. It allows for some gratification and also for revision in understanding and clarification of experiences that a person may have poorly understood or accepted when they occurred. It is an inventory that helps put past successes and failures into some perspective.

Encourage your clients to discuss their life with others. If considered with others, particularly with the younger generation, this review can be mutually beneficial. It gives the older person a sense of usefulness and some credit for age and wisdom and can provide the younger person with a sense of family and history. Today's older Americans have lived through more changes than any other single group in human history. (Consider events such as World Wars I and II; the Great Depression; air travel, including space exploration; and the development of antibiotics and other medical milestones, to name a few.)

Life review is one way an individual can address the tasks of this stage. Life for most people is complex, so the life review is unlikely to be entirely "good" or "bad." For most, it involves some satisfactions and some disappointments. Some hopes and dreams are realized; some remain unfulfilled. The task is to accept what happened and to accept oneself.

End of Life Issues

Preparation for one's own death, views on death and how one would like it to happen, and the possibility of an afterlife are accepted as a normal outcome of aging and part of the tasks of older adults. In fact, thoughts about these issues are likely to evolve from the life review process. For many, considering the issue of their own death is important, and they actively prepare for it in terms of finishing their business or getting their affairs in order. This preparation takes many forms, including finalizing a will, achieving some goal, resolving some or many interpersonal relationships, and saying farewell to significant family members and friends. As part of preparation, discuss with the client his or her preferences regarding advance directives specifying what medical care can be given in the event that the client becomes unable to communicate his or her decisions.

BOX 5-7

ASSESSMENT OF THE DYING PATIENT AND FAMILY

PATIENT

Age
Gender
Coping styles and abilities
Social, cultural, ethnic background
Previous experience with illness, pain, deterioration, loss, and grief
Mental health
Intelligence
Lifestyle
Fulfillment of life goals
Amount of unfinished business
The nature of the illness (death trajectory, problems particular to the illness, treatment, amount of pain)
Time passed since diagnosis
Response to illness
Knowledge about the illness/disease
Acceptance/rejection of the sick role
Amount of striving for dependence/independence
Feelings/and fears about illness
Comfort in expressing thoughts and feelings and how much is expressed
Location of the patient (home, hospital, nursing home)
Relationship with each member of the family and significant other since diagnosis

Family rules, normal, values, and past experiences that might inhibit grief or interfere with a therapeutic relationship

FAMILY

Family makeup (members of family)
Developmental stage of the family
Existing subsystems
Specific roles of each member

CHARACTERISTICS OF THE FAMILY SYSTEM

How flexible or rigid
Type of communication
Rules, norms, and expectations
Values, beliefs
Quality of emotional relationships
Dependence, interdependence, freedom of each member
How close to or disengaged from the dying member
Established extrafamilial interactions
Strengths and vulnerabilities of the family
Style of leadership and decision-making
Unusual methods of problem solving, crisis resolution
Family resources (personal, financial, community)
Current problems identified by the family
Quality of communication with the caregivers
Immediate and long-range anticipated needs

From Hess PA: Loss, grief, and dying. In Beare PG, Myers JL, editors: *Adult health nursing,* ed. 3, St. Louis, 1998, Mosby.

BOX 5-8

FACTORS INFLUENCING THE GRIEVING PROCESS

PHYSICAL

Illness involves numerous losses
Each loss must be identified
Each loss prompts and requires its own grief response
Importance of the loss varies according to meaning by individual
Sedatives—deprive experience of reality of loss that must be faced
Nutritional state—if inadequate, leads to inability to cope or meet demands of daily living numerous symptoms caused by grief
Rest—inadequate leads to mental and physical exhaustion, disease, unresolved grief
Exercise—if inadequate, limits emotional outlet, and may result in aggressive feelings, tension, anxiety, and leads to depression

PSYCHOLOGICAL

Unique nature and meaning of loss
Individual qualities of the relationship
Role body part/self-image/aspect of self was to the individual and/or family
Individual coping behavior, personality, mental health
Individual level of maturity and intelligence
Past experience with loss or death

Social, cultural, ethnic, religious/philosophic background
Sex-role conditioning
Immediate circumstances surrounding loss
Timeliness of the loss
Perception of preventability (sudden versus expected)
Number, type, quality of secondary losses
Presence of concurrent stresses/crises

SPECIFIC TO DYING/DEATH
(in addition to above)

Role decreased occupied in family or social system
Amount of unfinished business
Perception of deceased's fulfillment in life
Immediate circumstances surrounding death
Length of illness before death
Anticipatory grief and involvement with dying patient

SOCIAL

Individual support systems and the acceptance of assistance of its members
Individual sociocultural, ethnic, religious/philosophical background
Educational, economic, occupational status
Ritual

From Beare PG, Myers JL: *Adult health nursing,* ed. 3, St. Louis, 1998, Mosby.

Individuals facing death continue to feel, think, live, and respond to others around them until the moment of death. Concerns about pain and loss of control are among the dying individual's primary concerns. It is important to have an understanding of the individual's and family's spiritual and cultural beliefs related to death, dying, and bereavement in order to provide holistic care (see Chapter 7). To die in a way as close as possible to what the individual desires may be thought of as life's final developmental task.

While preparation for death is a natural component of older adult development, it is important to recognize that the individual's death will have an impact on all his or her family members, significant others, and health care providers. Addressing issues of grief and loss may be an important component of a health assessment. When assessing an individuals response to death, consider developmental differences in children and adolescents (see Box 5-6) and adjust your care accordingly. Understanding the many individual and family components that impact the response to death (Box 5-7) and attention to factors influencing the grief/loss process (Box 5-8) will help you holistically assess the needs of both the individual and family members.

Sample Documentation and Diagnoses

FOCUSED HEALTH HISTORY (SUBJECTIVE DATA)

Ms. W, age 65, has come to the clinic for a periodic blood pressure check. States she is feeling fairly well physically but is experiencing bouts of sadness and loneliness due to her recent retirement from a career in international nursing for more than 40 years. States she misses the demands of her job; the many colleagues she now sees less frequently; the travel opportunities; and, in general, the sense of meaning and purpose she had in life. Ms. W states that she was always so busy that she did not plan adequately for retirement both financially and by developing new hobbies or interests and now regrets this. Still feels capable of doing many of the things she has done before, but recognizes that certain tasks do take a bit longer. Ms. W asks whether she might be referred to a "retirement specialist." She is a single woman, never married, and has two siblings and numerous nieces and nephews, all of whom she enjoys, but she does not want to begin interfering in their lives. No recent significant weight loss or gain.

FOCUSED PHYSICAL EXAMINATION (OBJECTIVE DATA)

- Vital signs: BP 134/82 mm Hg; pulse 66, regular.
- Height 5 ft, 5 in; weight 140 lb.
- General appearance: Asian–American female who appears younger than stated age, healthy, and well-nourished; neat appearance. Handshake is warm and strong; speech is clear and articulate. Affect is somewhat sad, although she is responsive, cooperative, and eager to discuss her life situation.

DIAGNOSES

NURSING DIAGNOSES

Altered Role Performance Related to Retirement

Defining Characteristic

- Change in usual patterns of responsibilities

Social Isolation

Defining Characteristics

- Verbalization of isolation from others
- Lack of contact with significant others
- Perceived inadequacy of significant purpose in life
- Less contact with peers

Critical Thinking Questions

Review the Sample Documentation and Diagnoses Box to answer these questions.

1. What developmental stage (according to Erikson) is Ms. W facing? Describe the developmental tasks confronting Ms. W. Give specific examples of indicators of the tasks.
2. What additional information would be helpful for your developmental assessment of Ms. W?
3. What questions would you ask or tools might you use to further assess Ms. W's situation?

4. What are the key issues that Ms. W is dealing with? How might these differ (or would they differ) if she were a male?
5. How would your response to questions 1 through 4 differ if Ms. W were 35 and had just resigned from her longtime (number of years not indicated) position and was experiencing similar difficulties.

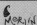

Answers are available on the MERLIN website (www.harcourthealth.com/MERLIN/Barkauskas/). And be sure to check the website regularly for additional learning activities!

Remember to check out the Online Study Guide!
www.harcourthealth.com/MERLIN/Barkauskas/

Chapter 6

Nutritional Assessment

Learning Objectives

On successful study of this chapter and completion of related learning experiences, the learner will be able to:

- Describe the recommended dietary guidelines for Americans
- Identify nutritional needs throughout the life cycle
- Outline the history pertinent to the assessment of nutritional status
- Describe the rationales for and demonstrate the anthropometrical measurements

Outline

PURPOSE OF NUTRITIONAL ASSESSMENT

The Council on Food and Nutrition of the American Medical Association defines nutrition as "the process by which an organism ingests, digests, absorbs, transports, utilizes, and excretes food substances" (Wardlaw, 1999, p. 4). Six classes of nutrients found in foods are carbohydrates, lipids (fats and oils), proteins, vitamins, minerals, and water. These nutrients provide us with energy, promote growth and development, and regulate biochemical processes. Glucose, triglycerides, and amino acids are major forms of carbohydrate, lipids, and proteins, respectively, and are energy sources for our bodies. Vitamins, either water soluble (such as vitamins B and C) or fat soluble (such as vitamins A, D, E, and K), are essential for many energy-yielding reactions. Depending on the amount we need per day, minerals can be classified as major (greater than or equal to 100 mg) or trace minerals (less than 100 mg). Major minerals include calcium, phosphorous, magnesium, sulfur, sodium, potassium, and chloride. Trace minerals are iron, zinc, iodine, copper, cobalt, selenium, molybdenum, silicon, and manganese.

Nutrition plays an important role in disease prevention, treatment, and recovery. Poor diet is a risk factor for chronic diseases such as diabetes, hypertension, obesity, heart disease, stroke, and cancer. These diseases together account for two-thirds of all deaths in the United States. On the other hand, underconsumption of nutrients is a risk factor for diseases such as osteoporosis and iron deficiency anemia.

Early detection of nutrition problems can result in health benefits and cost savings for the public. The nutrition assessment is a step-by-step process used to (a) assess the nutritional needs of an individual, (b) identify an individual at risk, (c) plan an appropriate diet for an individual client, and (d) evaluate the nutrition plan.

■ HELPFUL HINT

Energy is the capacity to do work.

A *calorie* is a measure of energy and is the amount of heat required to raise 1 g of water 1° C at atmospheric pressure.

1 kilocalorie (kcal) = 1000 calories

■ HELPFUL HINT

The 4-9-4 rule:

1 g of carbohydrate = 4 kcal of energy

1 g of fat = 9 kcal of energy

1 g of protein = 4 kcal of energy

RECOMMENDED DIETARY GUIDELINES

The Dietary Guidelines for Americans

The *Dietary Guidelines for Americans*, which emphasize both diet and physical activity, are revised by the United States Department of Agriculture (USDA) and the U.S. Department of Health and Human Services every 5 years to incorporate new scientific developments. The purpose of the guidelines is to promote health and reduce risk for chronic diseases such as diabetes, heart disease, stroke, certain cancers, and osteoporosis. The 2000 edition of *Dietary Guidelines for Americans* places new attention on food safety and reduction of saturated fat instead of total fat and carries the following three basic messages in the ABCs for good health:

Aim for fitness
Build a healthy base
Choose sensibly

The ABCs include 10 specific guidelines (Box 6-1). The Food Guide Pyramid provides a range of recommended servings to guide food choices for each of the five food groups for a nutritionally adequate diet for healthy children (ages 2 years and older) and adults (Figure 6-1 and Table 6-1).

Similar to the *Dietary Guidelines for Americans* that deemphasize the message of a low-fat diet, the American Heart Association recommends that the public consume a diet rich in whole grains, vegetables, fruits, low-fat dairy products, lean meats and poultry, fish (such as tuna and salmon), and dry beans.

Dietary Guidelines for Vegetarians

Vegetarian diets lower the risk of diet-related chronic diseases such as cardiovascular disease and cancer. A healthy vegetarian diet emphasizes a variety and abundance of five major plant food groups: (a) whole grains, (b) legumes, (c) vegetables, (d) fruits, and (e) nuts and seeds. Four optional food groups are vegetable oils, dairy, eggs, and sweets. A vegan diet excludes all animal foods such as milk, dairy products, and eggs, whereas other types of vegetarians exclude only meat and fish.

Since diet is not the only factor affecting health, the vegetarian food guide pyramid also includes physical activity, moderate sun exposure, and water intake (Figure 6-2). Table 6-2 shows food groups and serving sizes for vegetarian diets. When proper guidelines are applied, vegetarian diets can promote growth and development and meet the nutritional needs for healthy individuals.

Dietary Reference Intake

Dietary reference intake (DRI) is an umbrella term for a set of nutrient-based reference values, such as recommended dietary allowance (RDA) and tolerable upper intake levels (UL), and can be used for planning and assessing a healthy diet (Table 6-3). The RDA is the average daily dietary intake sufficient to meet the nutrient requirements of nearly all healthy men and women (97% to 98%) in a particular life stage (Table 6-4). The UL is the highest level of daily nutrient intake that is likely to pose no risk of adverse health effects to almost all individuals in the general population (Table 6-5). Megadoses of dietary or herb supplements may result in adverse health effects, such as diarrhea and gastrointestinal disturbance (vitamin C), increased tendency of hemorrhage (vitamin E), and heartburn and flatulence (garlic).

Text continued on p. 125

BOX 6-1

DIETARY GUIDELINES FOR AMERICANS FOR GOOD HEALTH

AIM FOR FITNESS
Aim for a healthy weight.
Be physically active each day.

BUILD A HEALTHY BASE
Let the Pyramid guide your food choices.
Choose a variety of grains daily, especially whole grains.
Choose a variety of fruits and vegetables daily.
Keep food safe to eat.

CHOOSE SENSIBLY
Choose a diet that is low in saturated fat and cholesterol and moderate in total fat.
Choose beverages and foods to moderate your intake of sugars.
Choose and prepare foods with less salt.
If you drink alcoholic beverages, do so in moderation.

From USDA: *Dietary Guidelines for Americans*, 2000.

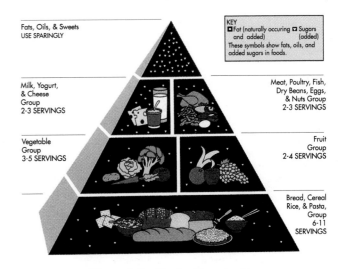

Figure 6-1 Food guide pyramid.

| TABLE 6-1 | Food Groups, Recommended Daily Servings, and Serving Size |

| Food Group | Daily Servings[a] | | | Serving Size |
	1600 calories[b]	2200 calories[c]	2800 calories[d]	
Bread, cereal, rice, and pasta (grains), especially whole grain	6	9	11	1 slice of bread About 1 cup of ready-to-eat cereal flakes ½ cup of cooked cereal, rice, or pasta
Vegetables	3	4	5	1 cup of raw leafy vegetables ½ cup of other vegetables—cooked or raw ¾ cup of vegetable juice
Fruits	2	3	4	1 medium apple, banana, orange, or pear ½ cup of chopped, cooked, or canned fruit ¾ cup of fruit juice
Milk, yogurt, and cheese (dairy)[e]—preferably fat free or low fat	2-3[f]	2-3[f]	2-3[f]	1 cup of milk[g] or yogurt[g] 1½ ounces of natural cheese[g] (such as cheddar) 2 ounces of processed cheese[g] (such as American) 1 cup of soy-based beverage with added calcium
Meat,[h] poultry,[h] fish, dry beans,[i] eggs, and nuts	2, for a total of 5 ounces	2, for a total of 6 ounces	3, for a total of 7 ounces	2-3 ounces of cooked lean meat, poultry, or fish ½ cup of cooked dry beans or ½ cup of tofu counts as 1 ounce of lean meat 2½ ounces of soyburger or 1 egg counts as 1 ounce of lean meat 2 tablespoons of peanut butter or ⅓ cup of nuts counts as 1 ounce of meat

From USDA: *Dietary Guidelines for Americans*, 2000.

[a] These are the calorie levels if you choose low-fat, lean foods from the five major food groups and if you use foods from the fats, oil, and sweets group sparingly.

[b] Children ages 2 to 6 years, women, some older adults (about 1600 calories).

[c] Older children, teen girls, active women, most men (about 2200 calories).

[d] Teen boys, active men (about 2800 calories).

[e] This includes lactose-free and lactose-reduced dairy products.

[f] Older children and teenagers (ages 9 to 18 years) and adults over the age of 50 need three servings daily. During pregnancy and lactation, the recommended number of dairy group servings is the same as for nonpregnant women.

[g] Choose fat-free or reduced fat dairy products most often.

[h] Preferably lean or low fat.

[i] Dry beans, peas, and lentils can be counted as servings in either the meat and beans group or the vegetable group. As a vegetable, ½ cup of beans counts as 1 serving. As a meat substitute, 1 cup of beans counts as 1 serving.

TABLE 6-2	Food Groups and Servings Sizes for Vegetarian Diets	
Food Group	**Daily Servings**	**Serving Size**
Bread, cereal, rice (50% whole grain)	6-11	1 slice of bread About 1 cup of ready-to-eat cereal flakes ½ cup of cooked cereal, rice, or pasta
Legumes	1-2	½ cup of cooked dry beans, lentils, peas, or limas ½ cup of tofu, soy products, or meat analogs
Vegetables, dark green and green leafy vegetables*	3-5	1 cup of raw leafy vegetables ½ cup of other vegetables—cooked or raw ¾ cup of vegetable juice
Fruits	2-4	1 medium apple, banana, orange, or pear ½ cup of chopped, cooked, or canned fruit ¾ cup of fruit juice
Nuts and seeds	1-2	About ⅓ cup of almonds, walnuts, or seeds 2 tablespoons of peanut butter, almond butter, or tahini
Milk, yogurt, and cheese—fat free or low fat	2-3	1 cup of milk† or yogurt† 1½ ounces of cheeses† 1 cup of milk fortified with calcium, vitamin D, and vitamin B_{12} alternatives
Milk alternatives (soymilk) and tofu*		1 cup of tofu
Eggs	½	3 eggs yolk/week
Fats, oils		1 teaspoon of oil, margarine, or mayonnaise 2 teaspoons of salad dressing ⅛ avocado 5 olives
Sugars		1 teaspoon of sugar, jam, jelly, honey, syrup, etc.

Modified from Haddad EH: Development of a vegetarian food guide, *Am J Clin Nutr* 59(5 suppl):1248S-1254S, 1994. (Data for table reprinted with permission by the *American Journal of Clinical Nutrition.* ©Am J Clin Nutr. American Society for Clinical Nutrition.)

*The total vegetarian meal plan must include at least two servings of calcium-rich food items daily such as 1 cup of milk alternative fortified with calcium, vitamin D, and vitamin B_{12}; 1 cup of tofu; 1 cup cooked broccoli; and 1 cup of cooked greens (e.g., collards, dandelion, kale, mustard).

†Choose fat-free or reduced fat dairy products most often.

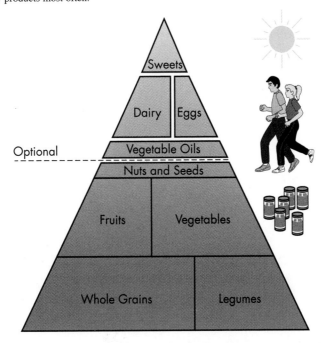

Figure 6-2 Vegetarian food guide pyramid. NOTE: A reliable source of vitamin B_{12} should be included if no dairy or eggs are consumed. (From Haddad EH, Sabate J, Whitten CG: Vegetarian food guide pyramid: a conceptual framework, *Am J Clin Nutrition* 70[3 suppl]:615S-619S, 1999. Reprinted with permission by the *American Journal of Clinical Nutrition.* ©Am J Clin Nutr. American Society for Clinical Nutrition.)

TABLE 6-3   Dietary Reference Intakes: Recommended Intakes for Individuals

Life Stage Group	Calcium (mg/d)	Phosphorus (mg/d)	Magnesium (mg/d)	Vitamin D (μg/d)a,b	Fluoride (mg/d)	Thiamine (mg/d)	Riboflavin (mg/d)	Niacin (mg/d)c	Vitamin B6 (mg/d)	Folate (μg/d)d	Vitamin B12 (μg/d)	Pantothenic Acid (mg/d)	Biotin (μg/d)	Choline (mg/d)e	Vitamin C (mg/d)	Vitamin E (mg/d)f	Selenium (μg/d)
Infants																	
0-6 mo	210*	100*	30*	5*	0.01*	0.2*	0.3*	2*	0.1*	65*	0.4*	1.7*	5*	125*	40*	4*	15*
7-12 mo	270*	275*	75*	5*	0.5*	0.3*	0.4*	4*	0.3*	80*	0.5*	1.8*	6*	150*	50*	6*	20*
Children																	
1-3 y	500*	460	80	5*	0.7*	0.5	0.5	6	0.5	150	0.9	2*	8*	200*	15	6	20
4-8 y	800*	500	130	5*	1*	0.6	0.6	8	0.6	200	1.2	3*	12*	250*	25	7	30
Males																	
9-13 y	1300*	1250	240	5*	2*	0.9	0.9	12	1.0	300	1.8	4*	20*	375*	45	11	40
14-18 y	1300*	1250	410	5*	3*	1.2	1.3	16	1.3	400	2.4	5*	25*	550*	75	15	55
19-30 y	1000*	700	400	5*	4*	1.2	1.3	16	1.3	400	2.4	5*	30*	550*	90	15	55
31-50 y	1000*	700	420	5*	4*	1.2	1.3	16	1.3	400	2.4	5*	30*	550*	90	15	55
51-70 y	1200*	700	420	10*	4*	1.2	1.3	16	1.7	400	2.4g	5*	30*	550*	90	15	55
>70 y	1200*	700	420	15*	4*	1.2	1.3	16	1.7	400	2.4g	5*	30*	550*	90	15	55
Females																	
9-13 y	1300*	1250	240	5*	2*	0.9	0.9	12	1.0	300	1.8	4*	20*	375*	45	11	40
14-18 y	1300*	1250	360	5*	3*	1.0	1.0	14	1.2	400h	2.4	5*	25*	400*	65	15	55
19-30 y	1000*	700	310	5*	3*	1.1	1.1	14	1.3	400h	2.4	5*	30*	425*	75	15	55
31-50 y	1000*	700	320	5*	3*	1.1	1.1	14	1.3	400h	2.4g	5*	30*	425*	75	15	55
51-70 y	1200*	700	320	10*	3*	1.1	1.1	14	1.5	400	2.4g	5*	30*	425*	75	15	55
>70 y	1200*	700	320	15*	3*	1.1	1.1	14	1.5	400	2.4g	5*	30*	425*	75	15	55
Pregnancy																	
≤18 y	1300*	1250	400	5*	3*	1.4	1.4	18	1.9	600i	2.6	6*	30*	450*	80	15	60
19-30 y	1000*	700	350	5*	3*	1.4	1.4	18	1.9	600i	2.6	6*	30*	450*	85	15	60
31-50 y	1000*	700	360	5*	3*	1.4	1.4	18	1.9	600i	2.6	6*	30*	450*	85	15	60
Lactation																	
≤18 y	1300*	1250	360	5*	3*	1.4	1.6	17	2.0	500j	2.8	7*	35*	550*	115	19	70
19-30 y	1000*	700	310	5*	3*	1.4	1.6	17	2.0	500j	2.8	7*	35*	550*	120	19	70
31-50 y	1000*	700	320	5*	3*	1.4	1.6	17	2.0	500j	2.8	7*	35*	550*	120	19	70

This table presents Recommended Dietary Allowances (RDAs) in bold type and Adequate Intakes (AIs) in ordinary type followed by an asterisk (*). RDAs and AIs may both be used as goals for individual intake. RDAs are set to meet the needs of almost all (97% to 98%) individuals in a group. For healthy breastfed infants, the AI is the mean intake. The AI for other life-stage and gender groups is believed to cover needs of all individuals in the group, but lack of data or uncertainty in the data prevent being able to specify with confidence the percentage of individuals covered by this intake.

Copyright 2000 by the National Academy of Sciences. Reprinted courtesy of the National Academy Press, Washington, DC.

a As cholecalciferol. 1 μg cholecalciferol = 40 IU vitamin D.
b In the absence of adequate exposure to sunlight.
c As niacin equivalents (NE). 1 mg of niacin = 60 mg of tryptophan; 0-6 months = preformed niacin (not NE).
d As dietary folate equivalents (DFE). 1 DFE = 1 μg food folate = 0.6 μg of folic acid from fortified food or as a supplement consumed with food = 0.5 μg of a supplement taken on an empty stomach.
e Although AIs have been set by choline, there are few data to assess whether a dietary supply of choline is needed at all stages of the life cycle, and it may be that the choline requirement can be met by endogenous synthesis at some of these stages.
f As α-tocopherol, α-Tocopherol includes *RRR*-α-tocopherol, the only form of α-tocopherol that occurs naturally in foods, and the 2*R*-stereoisomeric forms of α-tocopherol (*RRR*-, *RSR*-, *RRS*-, and *RSS*-α-tocopherol) that occur in fortified foods and supplements. It does not include the 2*S*-stereoisomeric forms of α-tocopherol (*SRR*-, *SSR*-, *SRS*-, and *SSS*-α-tocopherol), also found in fortified foods and supplements.
g Because 10% to 30% of older people may malabsorb food-bound vitamin B₁₂, it is advisable for those older than 50 years to meet their RDA mainly by consuming foods fortified with vitamin B₁₂ or a supplement containing vitamin B₁₂.
h In view of evidence linking folate intake with neural-tube defects in the fetus, it is recommended that all women capable of becoming pregnant consume 400 μg from supplements or fortified foods in addition to intake of food folate from a varied diet.
i It is assumed that women will continue consuming 400 μg from supplements or fortified food until their pregnancy is confirmed and they enter prenatal care, which ordinarily occurs after the end of the periconceptional period—the critical time for formation of the neural tube.

TABLE 6-4   Recommended Dietary Allowances[a] Revised 1989 (Abridged) Designed for the Maintenance of Good Nutrition of Practically All Healthy People in the United States*

Category	Age (years) or condition	Weight[b] (kg)	Weight[b] (lb)	Height[b] (cm)	Height[b] (in)	Protein (g)	Vitamin A (µg RE)[c]	Vitamin K (µg)	Iron (mg)	Zinc (mg)	Iodine (µg)
Infants	0.0-0.5	6	13	60	24	13	375	5	6	5	40
	0.5-1.0	9	20	71	28	14	375	10	10	5	50
Children	1-3	13	29	90	35	16	400	15	10	10	70
	4-6	20	44	112	44	24	500	20	10	10	90
	7-10	28	62	132	52	28	700	30	10	10	120
Males	11-14	45	99	157	62	45	1000	45	12	15	150
	15-18	66	145	176	69	59	1000	65	12	15	150
	19-24	72	160	177	70	58	1000	70	10	15	150
	25-50	79	174	176	70	63	1000	80	10	15	150
	51+	77	170	173	68	63	1000	80	10	15	150
Females	11-14	46	101	157	62	46	800	45	15	12	150
	15-18	55	120	163	64	44	800	55	15	12	150
	19-24	58	128	164	65	46	800	60	15	12	150
	25-50	63	138	163	64	50	800	65	15	12	150
	51+	65	143	160	63	50	800	65	10	12	150
Pregnant						60	800	65	30	15	175
Lactating	1st 6 months					65	1300	65	15	19	200
	2nd 6 months					62	1200	65	15	16	200

*This table does not include nutrients for which Dietary Reference Intakes have recently been established (see *Dietary reference intakes for calcium, phosphorus, magnesium, vitamin D, and fluoride* [1997], *Dietary reference intakes for thiamine, riboflavin, niacin, vitamin B₆ folate, vitamin B₁₂ pantothenic acid, biotin, and choline* [1998], and *Dietary reference intakes for vitamin E, vitamin C, selenium, and carotenoids* [2000]).

[a]The allowances, expressed as average daily intakes over time, are intended to provide for individual variations among most normal persons as they live in the United States under usual environmental stresses. Diets should be based on a variety of common foods in order to provide other nutrients for which human requirements have been less well defined.

[b]Weights and heights of Reference Adults are actual medians for the U.S. population of the designated age, as reported by NHANES II. The median weights and heights of those under 19 years of age were taken from Hamill et al. (1979). The use of these figures does not imply that the height-to-weight ratios are ideal.

[c]Retinol equivalents 1 retinol equivalent = 1 µg retinol or 6 µg β-carotene.

TABLE 6-5   Dietary Reference Intakes: Tolerable Upper Intake Levels (UL[a])

Life Stage Group	Calcium (g/d)	Phosphorus (g/d)	Magnesium (mg/d)[b]	Vitamin D (μg/d)	Fluoride (mg/d)	Niacin (mg/d)[c]	Vitamin B₆ (mg/d)	Folate (μg/d)[c]	Choline (g/d)	Vitamin C (mg/d)	Vitamin E (mg/d)[d]	Selenium (mg/d)
Infants												
0-6 mo	ND[e]	ND	ND	25	0.7	ND	ND	ND	ND	ND	ND	45
7-12 mo	ND	ND	ND	25	0.9	ND	ND	ND	ND	ND	ND	60
Children												
1-3 y	2.5	3	65	50	1.3	10	30	300	1.0	400	200	90
4-8 y	2.5	3	110	50	2.2	15	40	400	1.0	650	300	150
Males, females												
9-13 y	2.5	4	350	50	10	20	60	600	2.0	1200	600	280
14-18 y	2.5	4	350	50	10	30	80	800	3.0	1800	800	400
19-70 y	2.5	4	350	50	10	35	100	1000	3.5	2000	1000	400
>70 y	2.5	3	350	50	10	35	100	1000	3.5	2000	1000	400
Pregnancy												
≤18 y	2.5	3.5	350	50	10	30	80	800	3.0	1800	800	400
19-50 y	2.5	3.5	350	50	10	35	100	1000	3.5	2000	1000	400
Lactation												
≤18 y	2.5	4	350	50	10	30	80	800	3.0	1800	800	400
19-50 y	2.5	4	350	50	10	35	100	1000	3.5	2000	1000	400

Copyright 2000 by the National Academy of Sciences. Reprinted courtesy of the National Academy Press, Washington, DC.

[a]UL = The maximum level of daily nutrient intake that is likely to pose no risk of adverse effects. Unless otherwise specified, the UL represents total intake from food, water, and supplements. Due to lack of suitable data. ULs could not be established for thiamine, riboflavin, vitamin B₁₂, pantothenic acid, or biotin. In the absence of ULs, extra caution may be warranted in consuming levels above recommended intakes.

[b]The ULs for magnesium represent intake from a pharmacological agent only and do not include intake from food and water.

[c]The ULs for niacin and folate apply to synthetic forms obtained from supplements, fortified foods, or a combination of the two.

[d]As α-tocopherol; applies to any form of supplemental α-tocopherol.

[e]ND = Not determinable due to lack of data of adverse effects in this age group and concern with regard to lack of ability to handle excess amounts. Source of intake should be from food only to prevent high levels of intake.

NUTRITIONAL NEEDS THROUGHOUT THE LIFE CYCLE

Nutrition in Pregnant Women

The increase in the mother's basal metabolism to support the energy required for growth of the fetus and changes in her usual physical activity are factors that determine energy requirements for a pregnant woman. The estimated extra daily energy need is about 300 kcal/day throughout the pregnancy. There is a positive relationship between maternal weight gain and infant birth weight and infant health status. Therefore, it is important to monitor the amount and pattern of weight gained. Table 6-6 shows recommended total weight gain ranges for pregnant women based on prepregnancy body mass index (BMI).

Maternal iron deficiency anemia is associated with preterm delivery, low infant birth weight, and poor neonatal health. The overall iron requirement during pregnancy (30 mg/day) is significantly greater than that in the nonpregnant state (10 mg/day). As a result, iron supplements are recommended during pregnancy. Box 6-2 shows sources of iron-rich foods.

Studies have shown a relationship between periconceptional use of folic acid–containing supplements and a decrease in the occurrence of neural tube defect caused by folate deficiency. Many women of reproductive age have low dietary folate intake, and most women do not know that they are pregnant for 4 weeks, the most critical period for neural tube closure for the fetus. Therefore, for the prevention of neural tube defect, it is recommended that all women capable of becoming pregnant consume 400 μg/day from supplements or fortified foods in addition to intake of food folate from a various diet. The amount of intake needs to be sustained until after the neural tube closure is completed. Box 6-3 lists some dietary sources of folate.

Nutrition in Infancy

The energy requirement of an infant is about three to four times greater than that of an adult because of the infant's rapid growth and development and relatively high resting metabolic rate. Urine output of six to eight wet diapers per day is a good indicator of adequate amount of breast milk intake. Although breast milk has a low iron concentration, it can be absorbed well by the infant. In addition, the infant has a store of iron from birth to 4 to 6 months, after which

BOX 6-2

SOME SOURCES OF IRON*

- Shellfish like shrimp, clams, mussels, and oysters
- Lean meats (especially beef), liver† and other organ meats†
- Ready-to-eat cereals with added iron
- Turkey dark meat (remove skin to reduce fat)
- Sardines‡
- Spinach
- Cooked dry beans (such as kidney beans and pinto beans), peas (such as black-eyed peas), and lentils
- Enriched and whole grain breads

From USDA: *Dietary Guidelines for Americans,* 2000.
*Read food labels for brand-specific information.
†Very high in cholesterol.
‡High in salt.

BOX 6-3

SOME SOURCES OF FOLATE

- Organ meat such as kidney and liver
- Cooked dried beans, peas, and lentil
- Fortified ready-to-eat cereals and oatmeal
- Oranges and orange juice
- Deep green leaves such as spinach and mustard greens
- Other vegetables such as green beans, green peas, lettuce, and cabbage

Data from Institute of Medicine: *Dietary reference intakes for thiamine, riboflavin, niacin, vitamin B₆, folate, vitamin B₁₂, pantothenic acid, biotin, and choline,* Washington, DC, 1998, National Academy Press.

TABLE 6-6	**Recommended Total Weight Gain Ranges for Pregnant Women Based on Prepregnancy Body Mass Index**			
Prepregnancy Weight Classification	BMI*	% Ideal Body Weight	Recommended Total Gain† kg	lb
Underweight	<19.8	<85	12.5-18	28-40
Normal weight	19.8-26	100	11.5-16	25-35
Overweight	26-29	120	7.0-11.5	15-25
Obese	>29	>135	At least 7	At least 15

Reprinted with permission from *Nutrition during pregnancy.* Copyright 1990 by the National Academy of Sciences. Courtesy of the National Academy Press, Washington, DC.
BMI, Body mass index.
*BMI is calculated using metric units. BMI = weight (kg)/height (m²).
†Young adolescents and black women should strive for gains at the upper end of the recommended range. Short women (<157 cm or 62 in) should strive for gains at the lower end of the range.

iron supplementation needs to be considered, usually from infant iron-fortified cereal.

For a formula-fed infant, it is recommended to have no more than 32 ounces/day of iron-fortified formula. Soy-based formulas are for infants who (a) have lactose intolerance or galactosemia, (b) are fed a strict vegetarian diet, or (c) are allergic to cow's milk protein.

As the infant grows, nutrition sources change. Solids can be introduced at 4 to 6 months for both breast-fed and formula-fed babies. Earlier introduction increases the probability of development of allergies. See Chapter 26 for further discussion of nutrition for infants.

■ **HELPFUL HINT**

Progression of foods and texture beginning at 4 to 6 months of age:
Cereal ➡ vegetables and fruits ➡ meats/protein foods ➡ finger and table foods

---

Infants are susceptible to dehydration due to a greater body surface area. Conditions such as fever, diarrhea, vomiting, and illnesses increase water requirements. Fluid requirements are 125 to 150 ml/kg/day and 100 ml/kg/day for an infant whose body weight is less than 5 kg and 5 to 10 kg, respectively. Some indicators of dehydration in an infant include poor skin turgor, dry mucous membranes, and decreased urine output.

■ **HELPFUL HINT**

1 kilogram (kg) = 2.2 pounds (lb)

BOX 6-4

SOME SOURCES OF CALCIUM*

- Yougurt†
- Milk†‡
- Natural cheeses such as mozzarella, cheddar, Swiss, and parmesan†
- Soy-based beverage with added calcium
- Tofu, if made with calcium sulfate (read the ingredient list)
- Breakfast cereal with added calcium
- Canned fish with soft bones such as salmon, sardines§
- Fruit juice with added calcium
- Pudding made with milk‡
- Soup made with milk‡
- Dark-green leafy vegetables such as collards, turnip greens

From USDA: *Dietary Guidelines for Americans, 2000.*
*Read food labels for brand-specific information.
†Choose low-fat or fat-free milk products most often.
‡This includes lactose-free and lactose-reduced milk.
§High in salt.

Nutrition in Adolescents

Cognitive, psychosocial, and physiological development affect the nutritional needs of the adolescents. Common eating patterns for adolescents include skipping meals, snacking, eating meals away from home, and dieting. Before puberty, boys and girls have similar lean body mass; however, boys gain twice as much lean body mass as girls do during the growth spurt, around 13.5 to 14 years for boys and 12.5 years for girls. Due to differences in body composition between boys and girls, energy and iron requirements vary. The energy requirement for adolescents 11 to 14 years old is 2500 kcal/day for boys and 2200 kcal/day for girls. For adolescents 15 to 18 years old, 3000 kcal/day is recommended for boys and 2200 kcal/day for girls. The recommended iron intake is 12 mg/day and 15 mg/day for boys and girls, respectively. For both sexes, the recommended calcium intake is 1300 mg/day. Box 6-4 presents some sources of calcium.

Nutrition in the Elderly

The elderly are more susceptible than younger adults to be at risk for nutritional deficiency. Factors influencing nutritional status in the elderly include (a) physiological—such as loss of appetite, dental problems, and chronic disease; (b) psychological—such as depression, loneliness, and limited knowledge of nutrition; and (c) socioeconomic—such as low income, lack of access to transportation, and lack of adequate cooking facilities.

This population is at a greater risk of developing osteoporosis because of lactose intolerance, decreased calcium absorption and lean body mass, and limited physical activity. Moreover, the elderly typically have less sun exposure, which reduces metabolism of calcium and vitamin D. Thus, calcium and vitamin D fortified foods or supplements are recommended.

Since 10% to 30% of the elderly may malabsorb food-bound vitamin B_{12}, it is advisable for persons 50 years and older to meet their recommended dietary allowances through foods fortified with B_{12} or a supplement containing B_{12}. Box 6-5 shows some dietary sources of vitamin B_{12}.

BOX 6-5

SOME SOURCES OF VITAMIN B_{12}

- Beef and lamb
- Organ meats such as liver, kidney, heart, and brain
- Shellfish such as clam, oyster, mussel, crab, lobster, and scallop
- Fish such as sardines, salmon, canned tuna, catfish, pike, and whiting
- Milk and dairy products such as cheese and yogurt

Data from Institute of Medicine: *Dietary reference intakes for thiamine, riboflavin, niacin, vitamin B_6, folate, vitamin B_{12}, pantothenic acid, biotin, and choline,* 1998, Washington, DC, National Academy Press.

NUTRITIONAL ASSESSMENT

Many factors influence food intake and food utilization. Influences on food intake include (a) socioeconomic circumstances (income, location, housing, and family size); (b) food sources, accessibility, and food selection; (c) dietary patterns and eating habits; and (d) health and physical activity. The presence of disease, medications, and alcohol are other factors that influence nutrition utilization. In addition, culture, race/ethnicity, and religion affect food choice, food habits, and food-related beliefs about health. As the ethnic and racial diversity of the United States population is rapidly growing, it is important for health care providers to (a) take into consideration the variety of cultural influences affecting food choices, (b) learn more about a client's food habits, and (c) understand that no single cuisine is either completely healthful or unhealthful. Table 6-7 outlines food practices of some ethnic groups.

Cultural Considerations
"Hot" and "Cold" Foods

The concept of "hot" and "cold" foods and beliefs about their effects influence food choice during illness for Asians and Latinos. The "hot" and "cold" foods are classified differently within each cultural group. Depending on the "hot" and "cold" nature of an illness, some foods may be avoided. For example, Chinese Americans believe that diabetes is a "hot" disease so spicy, fried, or deep-fat fried "hot" foods should be avoided, and steamed and boiled foods are encouraged. In addition, postpartum women (in the first 42 days after delivery) are advised to abstain from eating fruits and vegetables ("cold" foods) since their bodies are in a "cold" state.

Religion also plays a role in food practice. Many food taboos and restrictions are related to religious beliefs. For example, black Muslims and Hindus avoid pork and beef, respectively.

TABLE 6-7 Food Practices of Some Ethnic Groups

Food Group	Common Food Practice
Mexican Americans: Diet tends to be low in vitamin A, iron, and calcium.	
Grains	Tortillas and salsa
	High in complex carbohydrates
Vegetables and fruits	High in vegetables and fruits
Milk (dairy)	Not usually consumed by adults, except cafe con leche (a blend of coffee and milk) or hot chocolate; when used, usually whole milk
	Cheese is a major part of diet
Meats, poultry, beans, and eggs	High-fat meats
	Favor beans
Food preparation	Liberal use of added fat, particularly lard
	Add sugars
Chinese Americans: Diet tends to be high in saturated fat, cholesterol, and salt.	
Grains	Rice and wheat products
Vegetables and fruits	High in vegetables and fruits
Milk (dairy)	Rarely use dairy products
Meats, poultry, beans, and eggs	Favor eggs, poultry, pork, and meats with fat
	Favor soy products
Food preparation	Rarely use butter; prefer peanut oil and corn oil
	Use oil abundantly in stir-fired meats and vegetables
American Indians: Diet tends to be high in refined sugar, fat, cholesterol, calories, and low in fiber, fruits, and nonstarch vegetables.	
Grains	Rice and bread
Vegetables and fruits	Canned and mix vegetables
	High in potatoes and squash
Milk (dairy)	Not usually consumed by adults, except milk with cereal, coffee, or tea; when used, usually whole milk
Meats, poultry, beans, and eggs	High-fat and large serving size of meats (such as bacon, hamburger, and luncheon meats)
	Green beans and peas
Food preparation	Favor frying in bacon fat, shortening, or lard
	Add butter, margarine, and mayonnaise
African-Americans: Diet tends to be high in fat and sodium.	
Grains	Rice, hot breads, and cornmeal products
Vegetables and fruits	Collards, turnip greens, dandelion greens, mustard, kale, yams, and sweet potatoes
Milk (dairy)	Not usually consumed by adults
Meats, poultry, beans, and eggs	Pork products
Food preparation	Favor frying
	Flavor black-eyed peas and greens with pork

Nutrition screening is a simple and quick process to identify a client who is at nutritional risk or is malnourished. The screening includes a nutritional health history, height, and weight and can be done by any health care provider. When a client is suspected to be at risk, a comprehensive nutrition assessment should be done. A comprehensive nutrition assessment takes time and is often done separately from a general health assessment, usually by a dietitian. There are five components of nutrition assessment: (a) nutritional health history, (b) dietary assessment, (c) anthropometric measurements, (d) biochemical and laboratory assessment, and (e) physical examination (Table 6-8).

Nutritional Health History

A nutritional health history is a comprehensive approach to assess food patterns and factors influencing the client's food habits. The method usually includes a thorough reading of the client's medical record, an extensive interview, 24-hour recall, and a food frequency questionnaire.

Focused Nutritional Health History

1. Family history
   a. Is there a history of diabetes, hypertension, obesity, osteoporosis, or anemia?
2. Self-care behaviors
   a. Who does the grocery shopping?
   b. Is income adequate for food purchases?
   c. Who prepares meals?
   d. What meal preparation facilities are available?
   e. Who do you eat with? Do you have any special traditions for meal times?

   f. Describe your activity patterns.
   g. How much exercise do you get and how often?
3. Review of systems
   a. Do any current health conditions affect your eating?
   b. Do you have difficulty chewing, tasting, or swallowing food?
   c. Do you have a loss of appetite?
   d. Do you have nausea or vomiting?
   e. Do you have problems with constipation or diarrhea?
4. Weight patterns
   a. What is your usual weight?
   b. Have you had a recent weight gain or loss?
      (1) Over what period of time did this occur?
      (2) Do you know the reason for the change in weight?
5. Eating patterns
   a. How many meals do you eat per day?
   b. What kinds and amounts of foods do you usually eat?
   c. Do you have any food preferences or dislikes?
   d. Do you have any food allergies or intolerance?
   e. Do you have religious or cultural restrictions on what you eat?
6. Use of medication and supplements
   a. Do you use any prescription or over-the-counter medications?
   b. What vitamin, mineral, or herb supplements do you take?

Dietary Assessment

The assessment of client's dietary intake is part of a comprehensive nutrition assessment. Information obtained is used to identify the presence, nature, and extent of impaired nutritional status. Methods of data collection include 24-hour recall, food record or diary, food-frequency questionnaire, and direct observation of food intake.

24-Hour Recall

The practitioner asks the client or a family member to recall the types and amounts of food eaten in the previous 24 hours or the previous day. Although it is one of the most common and easiest methods for collecting dietary intake information, it requires a skillful interviewer to ask probing questions to obtain greater accuracy. Additionally, information on 24-hour recall may not represent a typical day of food intake. Other limitations are that the client may not be telling the truth, is unable to estimate the amounts of food consumed, or cannot recall the foods eaten. Various aids such as measuring utensils, food models, pictures of foods, and utensils can be used to help with portion size estimation. It is helpful to ask questions regarding the client's sequence of activities, beginning with questions such as, "What time did you get up in the morning?" "What did you eat first?"

Food Record or Diary

Like the 24-hour recall, the food record or diary (usually includes 3 days, preferably 2 weekdays and 1 weekend) al-

TABLE 6-8	**Components of Nutrition Screening vs. Nutrition Assessment**
Nutrition Screening	**Nutrition Assessment**
Nutritional Health History	**Nutritional Health History**
	Family history
Self-care behaviors	Self-care behaviors
Review of systems	Review of systems
Weight pattern	Weight pattern
Use of medication and supplements	Use of medication and supplements
	Dietary Assessment
Anthropometric Measurements	**Anthropometric Measurements**
Height, weight, usual weight	Height, weight, usual weight, waist circumference, skinfold, and body composition
	Biochemical and Laboratory Assessment
	Physical Examination

lows for estimates of foods consumed during a specific time period. Limitations of this method are that (a) it requires literacy, (b) the client may not accurately estimate portion sizes, (c) the act of recording might alter the typical food intake, and (d) coding and analysis of the data can be costly. To minimize recording errors, the client can be instructed in advance in how to record foods eaten and how to estimate portion sizes.

Food-Frequency Questionnaire

The food-frequency questionnaire (FFQ) is usually used in combination with the 24-hour recall and is used widely for research purposes. It is a cost-effective tool for collecting dietary information but does not provide information on the quantity of food consumed. The questionnaire consists of two parts: (a) a list of foods or food groups (ranging from a brief list focusing on a specific nutrient to a list of hundreds of foods) and (b) a set of response options indicating how often foods or foods groups are consumed during a specific period, such as often, sometimes, or never. The FFQ can be self-administered or completed with a personal or telephone interview.

Direct Observation of Food Intake (Calorie Count)

Direct observation of food intake can be very useful in hospital settings. Calorie count is obtained by observing the difference between the amount of food not eaten and the amount served on the client's tray.

Analysis of Dietary Intake

Analysis of dietary intake can vary, from describing intake of foods and food groups to computations for food components, nutrients, and energy. The food scoring system based on the five major food groups from the Food Guide Pyramid (one serving size is counted as one point) is the fastest way to analyze dietary intakes. However, it may not be applica-

ble for liquid, semisolid regimens, or supplemental formula foods.

Some computer programs, tables of food composition, exchange lists, and food labels can be used to determine the nutrient content of the foods. In addition, the USDA's *Handbook #8* provides standard reference tables with code numbers to compute more detailed information on nutrients.

Anthropometrical Measurements

Anthropometrical measurements include height and weight, body mass index, waist circumference (WC), skinfold (SKF) measurement, and body composition. Standardization of equipment and methods is essential to provide accurate results.

Height

Depending on the setting, height is recorded in inches or centimeters (cm). In adults and older children, measure height by having the client stand erect and against a flat vertical measuring surface without shoes. Measurement of knee height is an alternative method used for those who are unable to stand upright because of mobility impairment or handicap. Knee height measurement is the distance from the posterior surface of the thigh, just proximal to the patella, to the sole of the foot when the knee is bent at a 90-degree angle. Table 6-9 shows recommended equations for predicting stature in African-American and Caucasian adults and children.

Weight

The platform balance scale is preferred for obtaining weight. The measurement can be recorded in kilogram or pounds. The client should wear light clothes, remove shoes and heavy jewelry, and empty pockets. A quick and easy method used to estimate an ideal weight is to assign a height of 5 feet (60 inches) to a man of 106 lb and to a woman of

---

TABLE 6-9 Recommended Knee Height* Equations for Predicting Stature in African-American and Caucasian Adults and Children

Group	Equation	Factor
African-American		
Men†	Stature = 73.42 + (1.79 × knee height)	± 7.2 cm
Women†	Stature = 68.10 + (1.86 × knee height) − (0.06 × age)	± 7.6 cm
Boys‡	Stature = 39.60 + (2.18 × knee height)	± 9.2 cm
Girls‡	Stature = 46.59 + (2.02 × knee height)	± 8.8 cm
Caucasian		
Men†	Stature = 71.85 + (1.88 × knee height)	± 7.9 cm
Women‡	Stature = 70.25 + (1.87 × knee height) − (0.06 × age)	± 7.2 cm
Boys‡	Stature = 40.54 + (2.22 × knee height)	± 8.4 cm
Girls†	Stature = 43.21 + (2.15 × knee height)	± 7.8 cm

Modified from Chumlea WC, Guo SS, Steinbaugh ML: Prediction of stature from knee height for black and white adults and children with application to mobility-impaired or handicapped persons. Reprinted by permission from *J Am Diet Assoc* 94(12):1385-1388, 1994.

*Knee height in cm.
†18 to 60 years of age.
‡6 to 18 years of age.

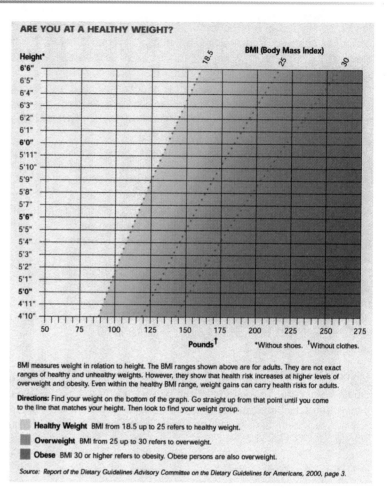

Figure 6-3   Body mass index. (From the Report of the Dietary Guidelines Advisory Committee on the Dietary Guidelines for Americans, 2000, p. 3.)

100 lb. Add an additional 6 lb for a male and 5 lb for a female for each inch over 5 feet.

Examples.   An estimated ideal weight for a man who is 6'4" (76 inches) would be:

$$106 \text{ lb} + (16 \text{ inches} \times 6 \text{ lb}) = 202 \text{ lb}$$

An estimated ideal weight for a women who is 5'5" (65 inches) would be:

$$100 \text{ lb} + (5 \text{ inches} \times 5 \text{ lb}) = 125 \text{ lb}$$

For healthy adults, body weight usually varies less than ±0.1 kg/day (0.2 lb/day). A loss of weight of greater than 0.5 kg/day (1 lb/day) indicates either negative energy, water imbalance, or a combination of both. A weight loss greater than 5% of usual body weight in the previous month or greater than 10% in the previous 6 months may indicate protein malnutrition.

◼ HELPFUL HINT

Percent of weight loss can be calculated using the following formula:

$$\% \text{ of weight loss} = \frac{(\text{Usual weight} - \text{Current weight}) \times 100}{\text{Usual weight}}$$

The measurement of height and weight and the assessment of growth for infants and very young children are discussed in Chapter 26.

Body Mass Index

The BMI, a number based on a formula for calculating weight for height (Box 6-6), is significantly associated with total body fat content and should be used to monitor changes in body weight or to assess overweight or obesity (Figure 6-3 and Table 6-10). The relationship between BMI and body fat content may vary with ethnicity, age, and sex. Clinical judgment is required when interpreting BMI in situations in which the client has edema, is highly muscular, or is very short. For example, the elderly often have less body mass but have more body fat for a given BMI than younger people.

Waist Circumference

Clients who have more abdominal fat (apple shape) are at a greater risk of type 2 diabetes, hypertension, and cardiovascular disease than clients who have more fat on extremities (pear shape) (see Figure 9-1). The WC measures abdominal fat content (Figure 6-4 and Box 6-7) and has sex-specific cutoffs for men and women (see Table 6-9). The sex-specific cutoffs may be generally applied to all adult racial and ethnic groups and should be used in conjunction with a BMI of 25 to 34.9 to identify increased disease risk. For example, a female

TABLE 6-10	Classification of Overweight and Obesity by BMI, Waist Circumference and Associated Disease Risk*			
			Disease Risk* Relative to Normal Weight and Waist Circumference	
	BMI (kg/m²)	Obesity Class	Men ≤102 cm (≤40 in) Women ≤88 cm (≤35 in)	>102 cm (>40 in) >88 cm (>35 in)
Underweight	<18.5		—	—
Normal†	18.5-24.9		—	—
Overweight	25.0-29.9		Increased	High
Obesity	30.0-34.9	I	High	Very High
	35.0-39.9	II	Very High	Very High
Extreme obesity	≥40	III	Extremely High	Extremely High

Adapted from Report of the World Health Organization Consultation of Obesity: *Preventing and managing the global epidemic of obesity,* Geneva, 1997, World Health Organization.
BMI, Body mass index
*Disease risk for type 2 diabetes, hypertension, and cardiovascular disease.
†Increased waist circumference can also be a marker for increased risk even in persons of normal weight.

BOX 6-6

CALCULATION OF BMI

$$\text{Metric conversion formula} = \frac{\text{Weight (kg)}}{\text{Height (m)}^2}$$

A person who weighs 90 kg and is 180 cm tall has a BMI of 27.8.

1 meter (m) = 100 cm $\quad \dfrac{\text{Weight (90 kg)}}{\text{Height (1.8 m)}^2} = 27.8$

$$\text{Nonmetric conversion formula} = \frac{\text{Weight (lb)} \times 704.5}{\text{Height (inches)}^2}$$

A person who weighs 150 lb and is 5 feet, 6 inches (or 66 inches) tall has a BMI of 24.3.

$$\frac{\text{Weight (150 lb)} \times 704.5}{\text{Height (66 inches)}^2} = 24.3$$

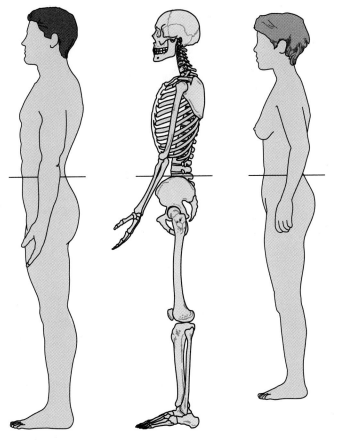

Figure 6-4   Measuring tape position for waist (abdominal) circumference. (From NHLBI Obesity Education Initiative: *Clinical guidelines on the identification, evaluation, and treatment of overweight and obesity in adults,* Bethesda, Md., 1998, Public Health Service, U.S. Department of Health and Human Services.)

client has a BMI of 28, which places her in the overweight category. If her WC is 34 inches, she would be at increased risk for type 2 diabetes, hypertension, and cardiovascular disease. However, if her WC is greater than 35 inches, she would be at a high risk for these diseases. Waist circumference may have little added predictive power of disease risk when the client has a BMI greater than or equal to 35.

Skinfold

Skinfold measurement indirectly measures the thickness of subcutaneous fat (Figure 6-5). The triceps skinfold (SKF), measured most often, and subscapular SKF measures taken together are sensitive to changes in nutritional status and reflect change in whole-body fat stores. Reliability and accuracy of the measurement depend on several factors, such as the type of SKF caliper, the technician's skill in locating and measuring SKF, and the equation used to estimate body fat. In addition, this measurement is inaccurate in very obese clients. A standardized procedure of measurement is recommended to increase accuracy and reliability of measurements (Table 6-11).

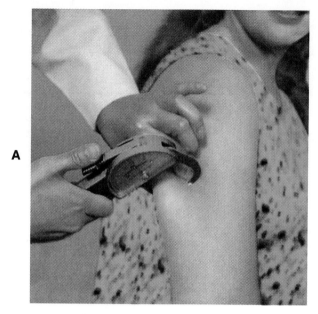

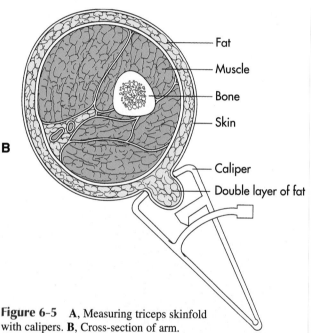

Figure 6-5 **A,** Measuring triceps skinfold with calipers. **B,** Cross-section of arm.

■ HELPFUL HINT

Take SKF measurements on the right side of the body, as recommended in the *Anthropometric Standardization Reference Manual* (Lohman et al., 1988).

Body Composition

Hydrostatic weighing is a widely used laboratory method to estimate body fat but is not a routine measurement in the clinical setting. The differences between two weights—weighing the client on a standard scale and then weighing

BOX 6-7

INSTRUCTIONS FOR MEASURING WAIST CIRCUMFERENCE, ACCORDING TO NHANES III PROTOCOL

POSITION

To define the level at which waist circumference is measured, a bony landmark is first located and marked. The subject stands, and the examiner, positioned at the right of the subject, palpates the upper hip bone to locate the right iliac crest.

LOCATION

Just above the uppermost lateral border of the right iliac crest, a horizontal line is drawn, then crossed with a vertical mark on the midaxillary line.

PLACEMENT

The measuring tape is placed in a horizontal plane around the abdomen at the level of this marked point on the right side of the trunk. The plane of the tape is parallel to the floor and is snug but does not compress the skin.

The measurement is made at a normal minimal respiration.

Modified from NHLBI Obesity Education Initiative: *Clinical guidelines on the identification, evaluation, and treatment of overweight and obesity in adults: the evidence report,* Bethesda, Md., 1998, Public Health Service, U.S. Department of Health and Human Services.

TABLE 6-11	**Standardized Sites for Skinfold Measurements**

Site	Direction of Fold	Anatomical Reference	Measurement
Triceps	Vertical (midline)	Acromial process of scapula and olecranon process of ulna	Distance between lateral projection of acromial process and inferior margin of olecranon process is measured using a tape measure on lateral aspect of arm, with elbow flexed 90 degrees. Midpoint is marked on lateral side of arm. Fold is lifted 1 cm above marked line on posterior aspect of arm. Caliper is applied at marked level.
Subscapular	Diagonal	Inferior angle of scapula	Fold is along natural cleavage line of skin just inferior to inferior angle of scapula, with caliper applied 1 cm below fingers.

Modified from Harrison GG et al.: Skinfold thicknesses and measurement technique. In Lohman TG, Roche AF, Martorell R, editors: *Anthropometric standardization reference manual,* abridged edition, Champaign, Ill, 1998, Human Kinetics, pp. 55-70.

the client again submerged in water—are used to estimate total body fat.

Bioelectrical impedance analysis (BIA) is a popular, relatively inexpensive, rapid, and noninvasive method. The method is based on differences in resistance to electrical current—lean body mass is a good conductor of electrical current, whereas fat is not. A major limitation is that it consistently underestimates and overestimates the percent of body fat in obese and very lean clients, respectively.

Biochemical and Laboratory Assessment

Lipids

Lipid protein analysis includes measurement of fasting serum levels of total cholesterol, high density lipoprotein (HDL) cholesterol, and total triglycerides. All clients 20 years and older should have serum total cholesterol and HDL cholesterol measured at least once every 5 years, and if normal, these measurements should be repeated in 5 years. For clients with total cholesterol greater than 200 mg/dl and/or HDL cholesterol less than 35 mg/dl, these measurements should be done every 1 to 2 years (Table 6-12). The results of these measurements can be inaccurate in a client with recent weight loss, a change in usual diet, acute infection, surgery, trauma, or pregnancy.

HELPFUL HINT

Fasting is defined as no caloric intake for at least 8 hours.

Carbohydrates

The fasting plasma glucose (FPG) test is a screening test for type 2 diabetes (Table 6-13). All clients 45 years and older should have FPG measured, and if normal, it should be repeated at 3-year intervals. Clients who should be tested at an earlier age or more frequently are those who (a) have a first-degree relative with diabetes; (b) are members of high-risk population such as African-Americans, Latinos, Native Americans, Asian-Americans, and Pacific Islanders; (c) deliver a baby weighing more than 9 lb; (d) are obese; (e) have HDL cholesterol less than or equal to 35 mg/dl and/or a

triglyceride level greater than or equal to 250 mg/dl; (f) have previous impaired fasting glucose (IFG) levels or impaired glucose tolerance (IGT); or (g) are hypertensive.

Protein

Blood urea nitrogen, serum creatinine, and albumin are used to measure protein catabolism and synthesis, respectively. Urea, which is formed in the liver as a by-product of the deamination of amino acid, is the end product of protein metabolism. The blood urea nitrogen (normal range is 8 to 20 mg/dl) is related to protein intake and nitrogen metabolism. Another method used to measure long-term protein in-

TABLE 6-12   Classification of Fasting Serum Lipid Levels

Fasting Serum Lipids	Classification
Total cholesterol	
<200 mg/dl (5.2 mmol/L)	Desirable blood cholesterol
200-239 mg/dl (5.2-6.2 mmol/L)	Borderline-high blood cholesterol
240 mg/dl (6.2 mmol/L)	High blood cholesterol
HDL cholesterol	
<35 mg/dl (0.9 mmol/L)	Low HDL cholesterol
Triglycerides	
<200 mg/dl (<2.26 mmol/L)	Normal blood triglycerides
200-399 mg/dl (2.26-4.51 mmol/L)	Borderline-high blood triglycerides
400-999 mg/dl (4.52-11.28 mmol/L)	High blood triglycerides
1000 (11.29 mmol/L)	Very high blood triglycerides

Modified from Expert Panel on Detection, Evaluation, and Treatment of High Blood Cholesterol in Adults: Summary of the second report of the National Cholesterol Education Program (NCEP) Expert Panel on Detection, Evaluation, and Treatment of High Blood Cholesterol in Adults (Adult Treatment Panel II), *JAMA* 269(23):3015-3023, 1993.

TABLE 6-13   Criteria for the Diagnosis of Diabetes Mellitus

Normoglycemia	IFG or IGT	DM*
FPG < 110 mg/dl 2-h PG† < 140 mg/dl	FPG ≥ 110 and <126 mg/dl (IFG) 2-h PG† ≥ 140 and <200 mg/dl (IGT)	FPG ≥ 126 mg/dl 2-h PG† ≥ 200 mg/dl Symptoms of DM and random plasma glucose concentration ≥200 mg/dl

From American Diabetes Association: Screening for type 2 diabetes, *Diabetes Care* 22[Sup]:S20-23, 1999.

IFG, Impaired fasting glucose; *IGT,* impaired glucose tolerance; *DM,* diabetes mellitus; *FPG,* fasting plasma glucose; *2-h PG,* 2-h postload glucose.
*A diagnosis of diabetes must be confirmed, on a subsequent day, by measurement of FPG, 2-h PG, or random plasma glucose (if symptoms are present). The FPG test is greatly preferred because of ease of administration, convenience, acceptability to patients, and lower cost. Fasting is defined as no caloric intake for at least 8 h.
†This test requires the use of a glucose load containing the equivalent of 75 g anhydrous glucose dissolved in water.

take is serum creatinine (normal range is 0.6 to 1.2 mg/dl). Albumin is synthesized in the liver and provides oncotic pressure that helps maintain water in circulation. Oncotic pressure or colloidal osmotic pressure is created by plasma proteins such as albumin that cannot cross the capillary membrane. Serum albumin is useful in monitoring changes in nutritional status (normal range is 3.4 to 4.7 g/dl).

Hemoglobin and Hematocrit

The hemoglobin (Hb) concentration and hematocrit (Hct) are commonly used to screen for anemia. Nutritional anemia may result from deficiency of folate, vitamin B_{12}, or iron. Iron deficiency anemia, a global nutritional problem, primarily affects infants, children, pregnant women, and women of childbearing age. The Centers for Disease Con-

---

TABLE 6-14	**Clinical Signs of Nutritional Status**	
Body Area	**Signs of Good Nutrition**	**Signs of Poor Nutrition**
General appearance	Alert, responsive	Listless, apathetic, cachectic
Weight	Normal for height, age, body build	Overweight or underweight (special concern underweight)
Posture	Erect, arms and legs straight	Sagging shoulders, sunken chest, humped back
Muscles	Well-developed, firm, good tone, some fat under skin	Flaccid, poor tone, undeveloped, tender, "wasted" appearance, cannot walk properly
Nervous control	Good attention span, not irritable or restless, normal reflexes, psychological stability	Inattentive, irritable, confused, burning and tingling of hands and feet (paresthesia), loss of position and vibratory sense, weakness and tenderness of muscles (may result in inability to walk), decrease or loss of ankle and knee reflexes
Gastrointestinal function	Good appetite and digestion, normal regular elimination, no palpable (perceptible to touch) organs or masses	Anorexia, indigestion, constipation or diarrhea, liver or spleen enlargement
Cardiovascular function	Normal heart rate and rhythm, no murmurs, normal blood pressure for age	Rapid heart rate (above 100 beats/minute, tachycardia), enlarged heart, abnormal rhythm, elevated blood pressure
General vitality	Endurance, energetic, sleeps well, vigorous	Easily fatigued, no energy, falls asleep easily, looks tired, apathetic
Hair	Shiny, lustrous, firm, not easily plucked, healthy scalp	Stringy, dull, brittle, dry, thin and sparse, depigmented, can be easily plucked
Skin (general)	Smooth, slightly moist, good color	Rough, dry, scaly, pale, pigmented, irritated, bruises, petechiae
Face and neck	Skin color uniform, smooth, healthy appearance, not swollen	Greasy, discolored, scaly, swollen, skin dark over cheeks and under eyes, lumpiness or flakiness of skin around nose and mouth
Lips	Smooth, good color, moist, not chapped or swollen	Dry, scaly, swollen, redness and swelling (chellosis), or angular lesions at corners of the mouth or fissures or scars (stomatitis)
Mouth, oral membranes	Reddish pink mucous membranes in oral cavity	Swollen, boggy oral mucous membranes
Gums	Good pink color, healthy, red, no swelling or bleeding	Spongy, bleed easily, marginal redness, inflamed gums receding
Tongue	Good pink color or deep reddish in appearance, not swollen or smooth, surface papillae present, no lesions	Swelling, scarlet and raw, magenta color, beefy (glossitis), hyperemic and hypertrophic papillae, atrophic papillae
Teeth	No cavities, no pain, bright, straight, no crowding, well-shaped jaw, clean, no discoloration	Unfilled caries, absent teeth, worn surfaces mottled (fluorosis), malpositioned
Eyes	Bright, clear, shiny, no sores at corner of eyelids, membranes moist and healthy pink color, no prominent blood vessels or mound of tissue or sclera, no fatigue circles beneath	Eye membranes pale (pale conjunctivae), redness of membrane (conjunctival injection), dryness of infection, Bitot's spots, redness and fissure of eyelid corners (angular palpebritis), dryness of eye membrane (conjunctival xerosis), dull appearance of cornea (corneal xerosis), soft cornea (keratomalacia)
Neck (glands)	No enlargement	Thyroid enlarged
Nails	Firm, pink	Spoon-shaped (koilonychia), brittle, ridged
Legs and feet	No tenderness, weakness, or swelling; good color	Edema, tender calf, tingling, weakness
Skeleton	No malformations	Bowlegs, knock-knees, chest deformity at diaphragm, beaded ribs, prominent scapulas

From Worthington-Roberts BS, Williams SR: *Nutrition in pregnancy and lactation,* ed. 6, Madison, Wisc., 1997, Brown & Benchmark.

trol and Prevention recommends periodically screening for anemia among these high-risk populations. Low Hb concentration (adult men less than 13.5 g/dl and adult women less than 11.5 g/dl) and Hct (adult men less than 39.9% and adult women less than 35.7%) are indicators of iron deficiency anemia. Hb concentration and Hct decline during the first and second trimesters among pregnant women because of an expanding blood volume. The normal values of Hb concentration and Hct in pregnant women are 11 g/dl and 33%, respectively, for the first and third trimesters and 10 g/dl (Hb) and 32% (Hct) for the second trimester.

Physical Examination

In the physical examination, the practitioner looks for signs of nutrition deficiency (Table 6-14). Clinical assessment includes general appearance of skin, eyes, tongue, rapid hair loss, sense of touch, and the ability to walk.

VARIATIONS FROM HEATH

Overweight and Obesity

Recent research shows that the prevalence of overweight (BMI 25 to 29.9 kg/m^2) and obesity (BMI greater than or equal to 30 kg/m^2) has markedly increased in the U.S. population in all age, gender, and race/ethnic groups in the past decade. Nearly 55% of American adults 20 to 74 years old are overweight or obese, which substantially increases the risk of morbidity from type 2 diabetes, hypertension, coronary heart disease, stroke, hyperlipidemia, certain cancers, and gallbladder disease. **Obesity**, the second leading cause of preventable death in the United States, is clearly related to the imbalance between calorie intake and calorie expenditure through metabolic and physical activity. A moderate reduction in calorie consumption to achieve a slow and steady weight loss is recommended (Table 6-15).

Hypercholesterolemia

An estimated 52% of American adults have **hypercholesterolemia** a total blood cholesterol level greater than or equal to 200 mg/dl. A consistent and substantial body of evidence shows an inverse relationship between low density lipoprotein (LDL) cholesterol and coronary heart disease.

To reduce elevated serum cholesterol while maintaining a nutritionally adequate eating pattern, diet therapy that progresses in two steps, Step I and Step II, is recommended

(Table 6-16). Whereas the Step I diet is recommended for the general population, the Step II diet is prescribed for the client who is already on a Step I diet at the time of detection or who cannot achieve the goals of dietary therapy on the Step I diet.

■ **HELPFUL HINT**

Saturated fats: fats are solid at room temperature.
Foods high in saturated fats tend to raise blood cholesterol.
Unsaturated fats (oils): fats are liquid at room temperature.
All kinds of unsaturated fats (oils) keep blood cholesterol low.

■ **HELPFUL HINT**

LDL can be calculated as follows*:
LDL cholesterol† = total cholesterol† − HDL cholesterol† − triglyceride/5 †

*This formula cannot be used for triglycerides greater than 400 mg/dl.
†Where all quantities are in mg/dl.

TABLE 6-15	**Low-Calorie Step I Diet**
Nutrient	**Recommended Intake**
Calories	Approximately 500 to 1000 kcal/day reduction from usual intake
Total fat	30% or less of total calories
Saturated fatty acids	8% to 10% of total calories
Monounsaturated fatty acids	Up to 15% of total calories
Polyunsaturated fatty acids	Up to 10% of total calories
Cholesterol	<300 mg/day
Protein	Approximately 15% of total calories
Carbohydrate	55% or more of total calories
Sodium chloride	No more than 100 mmol per day (approximately 2.4 g of sodium or approximately 6 g of sodium chloride)
Calcium	1000 to 1500 mg
Fiber	20 to 30 g

From NHLBI Obesity Education Initiative: *Clinical guidelines on the identification, evaluation, and treatment of overweight and obesity in adults,* Bethesda, Md., 1998, Public Health Service, U.S. Department of Health and Human Services.

TABLE 6-16	**Dietary Therapy: Step I and Step II Diets**	
	Step I Diet	**Step II Diet**
Total fat	30% or less of total calories	30% or less of total calories
Saturated fat	8%-10% of total calories	Less than 7% of total calories
Monounsaturated fat	10%-15% of total calories	10%-15% of total calories
Polyunsaturated fat	Less than 10% of total calories	Less than 10% of total calories
Cholesterol	Less than 300 mg/day	Less than 200 mg/day

Diabetes Mellitus

Diabetes mellitus is a group of metabolic diseases that is characterized by hyperglycemia resulting from defects in insulin secretion and/or insulin utilization. About 10 million American adults 20 years and older have diagnosed diabetes mellitus. The prevalence rate is higher in African-Americans (1.6 times) and Mexican Americans (1.9 times) compared with Caucasians. Type 2 diabetes, the most prevalent form, can remain undiagnosed for many years and is often asymptotic in its early stages. This chronic disease substantially increases the client's risk for coronary heart disease, stroke, and peripheral disease.

Little scientific evidence supports that simple sugars should be avoided and replaced with starches for a client with diabetes. From a clinical perspective, the total amount of carbohydrate consumed should be considered as the first priority rather than the source of the carbohydrate. Table 6-17 shows nutritional recommendations for clients with diabetes.

Hypertension

Approximately 25% of American adults have high blood pressure, and among all racial/ethnic groups, African-Americans have the highest prevalence rate. It is estimated that about 30% to 50% of clients with hypertension are sodium chloride sensitive. Results from Dietary Approaches to Stop Hypertension (DASH) recommend a diet that is low in total and saturated fat and cholesterol but rich in vegetables, fruits, and low-fat dairy foods (Table 6-18). This diet can substantially reduce blood pressure.

Cancer

Cancer is the second leading cause of death in United States. Numerous studies have reported an inverse relationship between fruits and vegetables and some types of cancers such as colon, kidney, endometrium, and breast. Even though researchers have reported that fiber, vitamin C, phytoestrogen, folic acid, and various carotenoids are the potentially protective factors against cancer, the evidence remains inconclusive.

TABLE 6-17 Nutrition Recommendations for Clients with Diabetes

Nutrient	Recommended Intake
Calories	Lose weight if overweight A moderate caloric restriction (250-500 calories less than each individual's average daily intake as calculated from a food history)
Total fat	Step I diet* Step II diet† (See Table 6-15)
Protein	10%-20% of total calories
Fiber	20-35 g/day
Alcohol	Up to 2 drinks/day for men Up to 1 drink/day for women
Sodium chloride	2.4 g of sodium or approximately 6 g of sodium chloride for general population and individuals with mild to moderate hypertension 2 g of sodium or approximately 5 g of sodium chloride for individuals with hypertension and nephropathy
Vitamin supplements	Not recommended

*Individuals who are at a healthy weight and have normal lipid levels.
†If LDL cholesterol is the primary concern, or if levels are elevated.

TABLE 6-18 The DASH Diet

Food Group	Daily Servings*	Serving Size
Bread, cereal, rice, and pasta (grains), especially whole grain	7-8	1 slice of bread About 1 cup of ready-to-eat cereal flakes ½ cup of cooked cereal, rice, or pasta
Vegetables	4-5	1 cup of raw leafy vegetables ½ cup of other vegetables—cooked or raw ¾ cup of vegetable juice
Fruits	4-5	1 medium apple, banana, orange, or pear ½ cup of chopped, cooked, or canned fruit ¾ cup of fruit juice
Milk, yogurt, and cheese (dairy)—fat free or low fat	2-3	1 cup of milk† or yogurt† 1½ ounces of cheeses†
Meats, poultry, and fish	2 or less	2-3 ounces of cooked lean meat, poultry, or fish
Nuts, seeds, and legumes	4-5 per week	About ⅓ cup of almonds, walnuts, or seeds ½ cup of cooked dry beans, lentils, peas, or limas

Modified from National High Blood Pressure Education Program: *The sixth report of the Joint National Committee on Prevention, Detection, Evaluation, and Treatment of High Blood Pressure*, Bethesda, Md., 1997, Public Health Service, U.S. Department of Health and Human Services.
*The DASH eating plan is based on 2000 calories a day. Depending on an individual's caloric needs, the number of daily servings in a food group may vary from those listed.
†Choose fat-free or reduced-fat dairy products.

Lactose Intolerance

Lactose intolerance is defined as incomplete digestion of lactose due to low levels of the enzyme, lactase. An estimated 50 million American adults are lactose intolerant. This condition occurs in more than 80% of Asian-Americans, 79% of Native Americans, 75% of African-Americans, 51% of Hispanics, and 21% of Caucasians. Lactose intolerance can result in gastrointestinal discomfort such as gas, flatulence, abdominal bloating or distention, stomach cramps, pain, diarrhea, or nausea that occurs from 30 minutes to several hours after consumption of a lactose-containing food or beverage. Most people with lactose intolerance can tolerate one serving (8 ounces) of milk and yogurt with active cultures. Additionally, encourage clients to drink milk and consume lactose-containing foods with meals to reduce the symptoms of lactose intolerance.

Nutrition Concerns in Vegetarians

Calcium can be obtained from fortified foods and beverages, supplements, foods that are naturally rich in calcium, or from a combination of these sources. Even though many leafy green vegetables (such as bok choy, broccoli, Chinese cabbage flower leaves, Chinese spinach, and kale) contain calcium, consumption of these foods may not meet the calcium needs of children, adolescents, pregnant and lactating women, and the elderly. Since vitamin B_{12} can only be found in animal foods, clients whose diets are based entirely on plants are prone to have vitamin B_{12} deficiency.

SUMMARY

Nutrition plays an important role in disease prevention, treatment, and recovery. Poor diet and underconsumption of nutrients contribute to chronic disease. To promote health and reduce risk for chronic disease, dietary guidelines with different emphasis, such as the *Dietary Guidelines for Americans*, dietary guidelines for vegetarians, and dietary reference intake, have been developed to provide guidance for meeting nutritional needs throughout the life cycle. Early detection of nutrition problems through nutrition assessment can result in health benefits and cost savings for the public. For clients with chronic diseases, following specific dietary guidelines to improve health status can delay the occurrence of disease complications.

Sample Documentation and Diagnoses

FOCUSED HEALTH HISTORY (SUBJECTIVE DATA)

Ms. Lewis is a 50-year-old African-American female who comes to clinic because she is concerned about her weight. She denies history of diabetes, hypertension, or anemia. She prepares her own meals and usually eats alone at home. Her usual daily activities include working 8 hours as a computer programmer, and in her free time she plays computer games or watches TV. She does not do any regular exercise. She denies a loss of appetite, nausea, or vomiting. She states that her usual weight is 200 lbs and reports approximately a 26-lb weight gain over the past 6 months since she moved to a new state. She has few friends here and is concerned that she eats more when she is alone. She usually eats two meals a day (lunch and dinner). Her favorite foods are fried chicken and potato chips and dip. She does not drink milk or eat cheese because of lactose intolerance. She denies any religious or cultural restrictions on what she eats and denies taking any vitamin, mineral, or herb supplements or prescription or over-the-counter medications. A 24-hour diet recall revealed that she eats high-fat content foods, few fruits and vegetables, or whole grains and drinks one cup of coffee and three cans of nondiet cola.

FOCUSED PHYSICAL EXAMINATION (OBJECTIVE DATA)

Vital signs: BP 138/86 mm Hg RAS; height 5 ft 5 in; weight 226 lbs; BMI 37.4; WC 41.8 in
Laboratory values: total cholesterol 240 mg/dl, HDL 56 mg/dl, fasting blood sugar 118 mg/dl
General appearance: Well-groomed African-American female

DIAGNOSES

HEALTH PROBLEM
Obesity; hypercholesterolemia

NURSING DIAGNOSIS

Imbalanced Nutrition: More Than Body Requirements
Defining Characteristics
- Obese
- Reported undesirable eating patterns
- Intake in excess of metabolic requirements
- Sedentary activity patterns

Critical Thinking Questions

1. Summarize the nutritional guidelines for a healthy diet for an adult. What would change if the adult were a vegetarian? A pregnant woman? A teenager? An elderly person?

2. A 35-year-old female client reports that she had her serum cholesterol measured 2 years ago. Her total serum cholesterol was 250 mg/dl, and HDL cholesterol was 32 mg/dl. She weighs 170 pounds and is 5 feet, 2 inches tall. Her WC is 34 inches. What other laboratory tests need to be done? What is her BMI? What is her ideal body weight? How would you classify her disease risk for type 2 diabetes, hypertension, and cardiovascular disease? How would you counsel her about her current weight?

3. Mr. Perez is a 45-year-old Mexican American male who has been newly diagnosed with type 2 diabetes. He needs to know how to change his diet. As the practitioner, how would you begin to assess his current nutritional status? How do you address cultural food practices? What dietary recommendations would you suggest?

 Answers are available on the MERLIN website (www.harcourthealth.com/MERLIN/Barkauskas/). And be sure to check the website regularly for additional learning activities!

Remember to check out the Online Study Guide!
www.harcourthealth.com/MERLIN/Barkauskas/

Cultural Considerations In Health Assessment

Learning Objectives

On successful study of this chapter and completion of related learning experiences, the learner will be able to:
- Describe the rationale for providing culturally competent health care.
- Discuss the impact of population trends on the current need for culturally competent health care.
- Describe the different terms associated with cultural assessment.

- Identify the major variables to be addressed in cultural assessment.
- Examine potential areas of cultural conflict between the values, beliefs, and customs of clients and those of the health care providers (yourself included) and their impact on health care.
- Conduct a comprehensive cultural assessment.

Outline

CHANGING AMERICAN DEMOGRAPHICS: THE NEED FOR CROSS-CULTURAL CARE

The American population is becoming increasingly more diverse with a rapid growth in the numbers of ethnic minorities, as well as new immigrants. Groups with a long history in this country grew at a moderate rate, but there was a major increase in the number of immigrants, in particular Hispanics and Asians, and refugees (Buchwald et al., 1994). This represents a profound shift in the demographic makeup of the United States. It is estimated that by the year 2025 the Hispanic and Asian populations will double in size. The U.S. Census Bureau estimates that by 2050 close to 50% of the United States population will consist of individuals from racial and ethnic minorities (U.S. Bureau of the Census, 1992; 1997). Table 7-1 shows racial and ethnic population projections for the early 21st Century. As our population becomes more diverse, the need for an appreciation and understanding of cultural influences on health care becomes increasingly more important.

THE HEALTH CARE CULTURE: IMPACT ON PROVIDERS AND CLIENTS AND THEIR BEHAVIOR

Cultural beliefs and personal characteristics determine health behavior in individuals and families. More than half of all health problems are the result of behavior and lifestyle. If our goal is to promote health while respecting individual value systems and lifestyles, culture-based health behavior must be understood.

TABLE 7-1	U.S. Racial and Ethnic Population Projections for the 21st Century				
	Caucasian (%)	African-American (%)	Hispanic (%)	Asian/Pacific Islander (%)	Native American (%)
1998	72.9	12.1	10.7	3.5	0.7
2005	69.9	12.4	12.6	4.4	0.8
2010	68.0	12.6	13.8	4.8	0.8
2015	66.1	12.7	15.1	5.3	0.8
2020	64.3	12.9	16.3	5.7	0.8
2030	60.5	13.1	18.9	6.6	0.8

Modified from U.S. Bureau of the Census: *Current population reports,* P25-1130, 1997, Washington, DC, U.S. Government Printing Office.

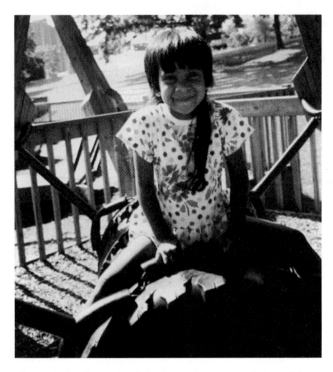

Figure 7-1 Cultural beliefs play an important role in molding a child's personality.

In North America the majority of health care providers hold values, beliefs, and attitudes that are typical of the dominant middle class. In addition, health care providers belong to a separate culture as members of the health care system. When two people of differing cultural backgrounds interact, significant communication barriers may arise unless at least one of the persons is willing and able to recognize and adapt to the other's values. To care for others, health care providers must be able to accept a wide diversity of beliefs, practices, and ideas about health and illness, including many that differ from their own.

Acceptance of alternate beliefs about health and illness can be more difficult for health care providers than might be initially assumed. As a result of being educated in and exposed to the established health care system, health care providers share certain values, attitudes, and beliefs about health and illness that they may not consciously think about. These ways of thinking have been shaped by more than 2000 years of Western thought, broadly known as *Hippocratic medicine*. Modern health care is based on rational, scientific, biomedical principles directed toward solving human health problems. As part of the dominant culture, the health care culture is interwoven with established social, religious, political, and economic systems. Certain aspects of the health care culture, such as nurse-physician relationships and provider-patient relationships, are governed by a broadly shared set of customs and protocols.

The cultural beliefs of some clients may conflict with the cultural beliefs many health care providers share. Health care providers cannot hope to plan meaningful health care for their clients without at least understanding their health beliefs. Therefore skill in performing a sensitive cultural assessment is important (see Box 7-1 for ways to develop cultural sensitivity). A thorough assessment of the cultural aspects of a client's lifestyle, health beliefs, and health practices enhances provision of comprehensive, holistic care.

TERMINOLOGY ASSOCIATED WITH CULTURAL CONSIDERATIONS

Culture is defined as a complex, integrated system that includes knowledge, beliefs, skills, art, morals, law, customs, and any other acquired habits and capabilities of a group of people. Culture is characterized by being learned, shared with others, and adapted to the environment. It is stable but subject to, and capable of, change. As a learned set of traits, culture is transmitted from one generation to the next by both formal education and imitation.

Subculture refers to a group of persons within a culture with one or more shared traits. These include age, socioeconomic status, race, ethnic origin, education, and occupation. Literally thousands of subcultures exist within a culture, and everyone is a member of several. Although subcultures have an identity uniquely their own, they are also related to the overall culture in certain ways.

Race refers to the classification of human beings on the basis of physical characteristics, such as skin pigmentation, head form, or stature, that are transmitted through genera-

BOX 7-1

WAYS TO DEVELOP CULTURAL SENSITIVITY

1. Recognize that cultural diversity exists.
2. Demonstrate respect for people as unique individuals, with culture as one factor that contributes to their uniqueness.
3. Respect the unfamiliar.
4. Identify and examine your own cultural beliefs.
5. Recognize that some cultural groups have definitions of health and illness, as well as practices that attempt to promote health and cure illness, which may differ from the nurse's own.
6. Be willing to modify health care delivery in keeping with the client's cultural background.
7. Do not expect all members of one cultural group to behave in exactly the same way.
8. Appreciate that each person's cultural values are ingrained and therefore very difficult to change.

From Stule DM: The family as a bearer of culture. In Cookfair JN, editor: *Nursing process and practice in the community,* St. Louis, 1991, Mosby.

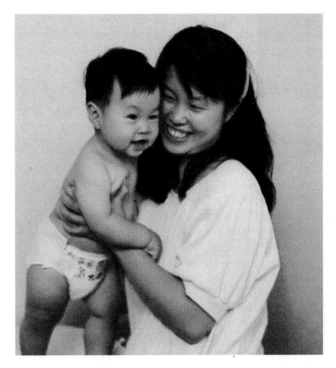

Figure 7-2 Cultural beliefs affect how mothers rear their children.

tions. Commonly recognized races are Caucasian, Negroid, and Mongoloid. However, the boundaries between races are not clearcut, and alternative systems of describing human biological variation are needed.

Ethnic groups share traits such as a common national or regional origin and linguistic, ancestral, and physical characteristics. Within the major North American subcultures, distinct ethnic groups include African, Haitian, or Dominican (Black); Mexican, Cuban, or Puerto Rican (Hispanic); Japanese, Chinese, Filipino, Korean, Vietnamese, Guamian, or Samoan (Asian); many European ethnic subcultures (German, Italian, Polish, Slavic, Scandinavian, Swiss, French, Dutch, Russian, English, Irish, Scottish); and Native American and Alaska Native subcultures. Individuals may also identify with a particular ethnic group related to their country of birth or to family genealogy that may not be obvious.

Minority group is a commonly misunderstood term. More normative than descriptive, it refers to any group that receives different and unequal treatment from others in the larger group or society and whose members see themselves as subject to discrimination. This concept is important for caregivers to understand, since many people in our society are discriminated against, and discrimination takes place in the health care system. However, an individual's membership in a minority group is not necessarily related to the individual's cultural affiliations. This distinction has an important bearing on cultural assessment.

Customs refer to the learned behaviors shared by, and associated with, a particular cultural group. They include dietary practices, communication patterns, family and kinship relations, religious practices, and health behaviors.

Rituals are highly structured patterns of behavior characteristic of cultural groups. They are prescribed ways to define basic human activities within a cultural context. Rituals may govern a group's approach to communication, traditions, taboos, religion, healing and care for the sick, trade, means of travel, sexual activities, or recreation.

Values and **norms** are judgments that cultural groups apply to behavior. Values are universal to all cultures and define the desirable or undesirable state of affairs within a culture. Norms provide direction for applying values and are the rules that govern human behavior. Cultural norms set limits. Members of a culture are rewarded or punished as they conform or deviate from them. Norms perform a number of important functions. They influence a person's perception of others. They direct a person's responses to situations and to others. They provide a basis for self-evaluation. They provide a foundation for forming opinions. They motivate behavior, and they give meaning to life and self-esteem. Values and norms exert a powerful influence over an individual's beliefs, attitudes, and practices. You must explore the client's value system to gain an appreciation for health-related behavior.

Cultural paradigms encompass abstract explanations used by groups to account for major life events. The term is synonymous with the idea of world view. The three dominant cultural paradigms are magico-religious, holistic, and scientific. This concept is crucial to health care professionals because all beliefs and values regarding health are derived from a person's basic world view. Aspects of all three world views are identifiable in most cultures, but one view usually predominates. The magico-religious paradigm offers a mystical cause-and-effect relationship between health and illness. The holistic paradigm provides the basis for a sense of balance and harmony between humans and the larger environment. The scientific view defines health as the absence of disease symptoms.

Enculturation is the process of acquiring one's cultural identity as it is transmitted by the previous generation. The degree of enculturation is important to assess before planning care, especially if you anticipate that the client will obtain health benefits by modifying some culturally based aspect of health beliefs, attitudes, or practices. You can also act as an advocate or "culture broker" for the client by educating teachers, other health care workers, or representatives of social agencies about specific cultural beliefs and practices that may influence the client's and his or her family's behaviors or response to recommendations (Tripp-Reimer, Brink, and Pinkham, 1999).

Acculturation refers to the process of adapting to a culture different from the one in which a person was enculturated. Because North America is a continent of immigrants, you will commonly encounter clients undergoing acculturation. Culture is a learned group of traits, so it is possible for an individual to acquire a new cultural identity. Again, you must assess the degree of acculturation to predict the client's inclination to comply with a desirable modification in health care beliefs, attitudes, or practices. The degree of acculturation has been shown to be related to a variety of health concerns, such as mental health (Rogler, Cortes, and Malgady, 1991), psychosocial distress (Krause and Goldenhar, 1992), and childrearing attitudes (Rauh, Wasserman, and Brunelli, 1990). When a client is undergoing acculturation, you can play a significant role in teaching the sort of acquired health behavior that the client is already attempting to learn.

Cultural determinism is simply a term for conveying the notion that a person's behavior is determined by cultural beliefs. The concept is central to cultural assessment because one must understand it to formulate client goals. A goal is something the client, not the provider, wants to achieve. A goal therefore must take into account the client's culturally determined behavior in order to be relevant and effective.

Ethnocentrism is the tendency to view people unconsciously by using one's group and one's own customs as the standard for all judgments. A practitioner with this tendency will gather data only selectively in accordance with personal standards, values, and judgments and will not be able to see what the client has to offer or the different ways in which the client views the world. This bias will limit the data a practitioner gathers and will distort interpretation.

Cultural relativity refers to the attempt to view or interpret behavior of culturally different individuals within the context of those individuals' culture. This perspective acknowledges that behavior that is appropriate in one culture may not be so defined in another culture. Providing care from a perspective of cultural relativity involves viewing behaviors within the context of the client's culture. This approach may provide meaning to behaviors that caregivers might otherwise consider negative or confusing.

Cultural competence is a complex combination of attitudes, knowledge, and skills that when integrated promote sensitive and, ideally, more effective interventions (Lipson, Dibble, and Minarik, 1996). Campinha-Bacote (1998; 1999) defines cultural competence as a process in which the health care provider continuously strives to develop the ability to effectively provide care within the client's cultural context. She

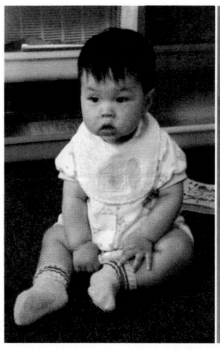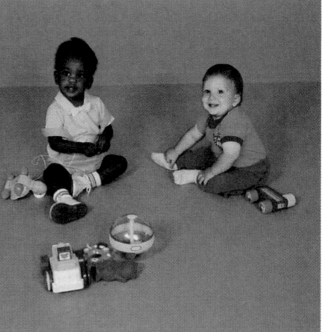

Figure 7-3   The practitioner will encounter a variety of cultural backgrounds in practice.

describes five components of cultural competence: (1) cultural awareness, (2) cultural knowledge, (3) cultural skill, (4) cultural encounters, and (5) cultural desire. Cultural awareness requires that you develop a self-awareness of your own biases and prejudices, as well as an exploration of your own cultural background. This understanding will help you become sensitive to and appreciative of the values, beliefs, practices, and problem-solving strategies of the client's culture.

Campinha-Bacote (1998, 1999) and Purnell and Paulanka (1998) describe four stages of cultural competence that are related to one's cultural awareness. These are unconscious incompetence (unawareness that one is lacking knowledge about another culture), conscious incompetence (awareness that one is lacking knowledge about another culture), conscious competence (learning about the client's culture, verifying generalizations, and providing interventions that are culturally specific), unconscious competence (the ability to automatically provide culturally congruent care to diverse clients). Purnell and Paulanka note that unconscious competence is hard to achieve. Most health care providers reach only the conscious competence stage. It is also important to be aware that the level of competence may vary according to the practitioner's experience with particular cultural groups.

Development of cultural competence occurs over time through experiences with clients from other cultures; through knowledge acquisition; through development of specific skills, such as cross-cultural communication and cultural assessment; and through the health care provider's own appreciation of, and receptiveness to, the client's values, beliefs, and customs. Cultural competence is needed to prevent mistakes such as inadvertently teaching behaviors that are inconsistent with a family's culture (e.g., encouraging a child's open expression of feelings or questioning of elders when such behavior is seen as inappropriate or disrespectful in that family's culture [Starn, 1996]).

Disease, *illness,* and *sickness* are similar terms that are commonly used and misused. The distinctions among them are important to cultural assessment. Disease is a medical term, arising from the dominant, scientifically based health care subculture. It refers to a pathological process within human structure and function. Illness is a subjective term used by both clients and clinicians to describe the symptoms of discomfort. Sickness, on the other hand, is a personal state of illness with distinct social dimensions. Depending on the norms within any given culture, role behaviors are modified when a person becomes sick. These modified role behaviors are an important aspect of cultural assessment.

MAJOR AREAS IN CULTURAL ASSESSMENT

Tripp-Reimer (1992) describes a pyramid model of the relationship between the key variables in cultural assessment. In the model, customs (or behaviors) form the top of the pyramid. They are based on beliefs (middle layer),which in turn are rooted in values (the base of the pyramid). Customs may be observed and described and therefore are the easiest to

assess. People, however, frequently learn values through an unconscious process of socialization; values are the most difficult to assess.

Values

Values provide the foundation for beliefs, attitudes, and behaviors. Often people are unaware of their values, even though they are able to describe their beliefs and customs. They acquire values through socialization early in childhood, and these values guide the individual's goals, aspirations, and behaviors. Kluckhohn (1976) describes values common to all population groups in Box 7-2. Kluckhohn proposes that variation in value orientation is one of the most important differences among people.

It is important for health care providers to recognize that the culture of the health care system has an underlying value

---

B O X 7 - 2

COMPARISON OF VALUE ORIENTATIONS

TIME ORIENTATION

Present oriented: Accepts each day as it comes; little regard for the past; future unpredictable

Past oriented: Maintains traditions that were meaningful in the past; worships ancestors

Future oriented: Anticipates "bigger and better" future; high value on change

ACTIVITY ORIENTATION

"Doing" orientation: Emphasizes accomplishments that are measurable by external standards

"Being" orientation: Spontaneous expression of self

"Being-in-becoming": Emphasizes self-development of all aspects of self as an integrated whole

HUMAN NATURE IN RELATIONS TO ORIENTATION

Human being basically evil but with perfectable nature; constant self-control and discipline necessary

Human being as neutral, neither good nor evil

HUMAN-NATURE ORIENTATION

Human being subject to environment with very little control over own destiny

Human being in harmony with nature

Human being master over nature

RELATIONAL ORIENTATION

Individualistic: Encourages individualism: impersonal relationships occur more with outsiders and less with family

Lineal: Group goals dominant over individual goals; ordered positional succession (father to son)

Collateral: Group goals dominant over individual goals: more emphasis on relationship with others on one's own level

Modified from Kluckhohn F: Dominant and variant value orientation. In Brink P, editor: *Transcultural nursing: a book of readings,* Stamford, Conn, 1976, Appleton & Lange.

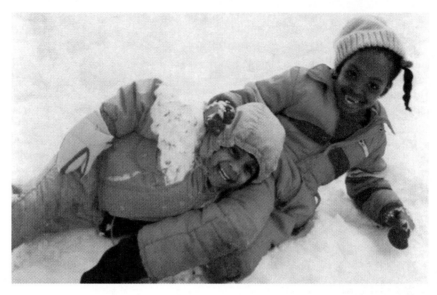

Figure 7-4   Values are acquired through socialization early in childhood, guiding the child's goals, aspirations, and behaviors.

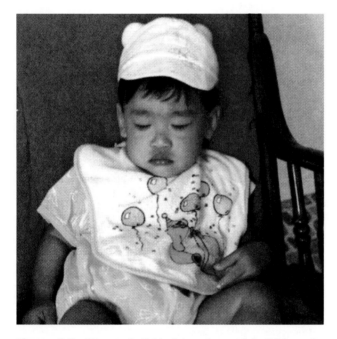

Figure 7-5   How an individual perceives a sick child can be based on cultural beliefs.

orientation that may affect providers' interactions with clients. The health care culture tends to have the following value orientations:

1. Time orientation: Has a future orientation, which means an expectation for promptness and keeping scheduled appointments.
2. Activity orientation: Values individuals for their accomplishments (a "doing" orientation), which may include getting healthy or taking medications as prescribed.

3. Human in relation to nature orientation: Views humans as having mastery over nature and values the omnipotence of technology.
4. Relational orientation: Is individualistic in its focus, emphasizing autonomy and putting the needs of the individual over the needs of the family.

It is essential to become aware of your own values in these areas. As an exercise, examine your own value orientations and compare them with the aforementioned example. When conflicts with clients arise, this self-awareness can help you understand how your expectations (based on your own value orientation) may be contributing to the difficulty.

Beliefs

Beliefs include opinions, knowledge, and faith regarding various aspects of the world. Beliefs of particular concern to health care providers are those related to illness causation, preferred method of treatment, expected outcomes, and fears about the illness. How the individual defines illness is based on his or her belief system and is largely determined by his or her culture. Tripp-Reimer (1992) notes that an individual with an obvious pathological condition may not consult the "scientific" health care professional because the condition may be ignored, undetected, or attributed to a nonscientific cause.

Chronic illnesses, such as hypertension and renal problems, may go undetected because they do not exhibit symptoms obvious to a layperson. Illnesses attributed to nonscientific causes are called "folk illnesses." A client usually seeks treatment for folk illnesses from a folk practitioner. Health professionals such as physicians and nurses are usually not seen as knowledgeable in these areas, and the client may not mention folk remedies or treatments unless specifically asked. Folk illnesses are divided into two categories:

BOX 7-3

HOT AND COLD CONDITIONS AND THEIR CORRESPONDING TREATMENT

HOT CONDITIONS	COLD FOODS	COLD MEDICINES AND HERBS
Fever	Fresh vegetables	Orange flower water
Infection	Tropical fruits	Linden
Diarrhea	Dairy products	Sage
Kidney problem	Meats such as goat, fish, chicken	Milk of magnesia
Rash	Honey	Bicarbonate of soda
Skin ailment	Cod	
Sore throat	Raisins	
Liver problem	Bottled milk	
Ulcer	Barley water	
Constipation		

COLD CONDITIONS	HOT FOODS	HOT MEDICINES AND HERBS
Cancer	Chocolate	Penicillin
Pneumonia	Cheese	Tobacco
Malaria	Temperate-zone fruits	Ginger root
Joint pain	Eggs	Garlic
Menstrual period	Peas	Cinnamon
Teething	Onions	Anise
Earache	Aromatic beverages	Vitamins
Rheumatism	Hard liquor	Iron preparations
Tuberculosis	Oils	Cod-liver oil
Cold	Meats such as beef, waterfowl, mutton	Castor oil
Headache	Goat's milk	Aspirin
Paralysis	Cereal grains	
Stomach cramps	Chili peppers	

Modified from Wilson HS, Kneisl CR: *Psychiatric nursing,* ed. 3, Upper Saddle River, NJ, 1988, Prentice-Hall.

naturalistic illness and personalistic illness (Tripp-Reimer, 1992).

Naturalistic illnesses are caused by impersonal factors that have no regard for the individual. These illnesses usually involve the concept of equilibrium. Problems develop when the balance is disturbed. One of the most common imbalances is between "hot" and "cold." These beliefs exist in Hispanic, Chinese, Filipino, and Arab cultures. In traditional Chinese health beliefs, the forces are called yin (cold) and yang (hot). Treatments usually involve restoring balance by applying opposing forces (e.g., application of the appropriate "hot" remedy to treat a "cold" illness and vice versa). Hot-cold classifications for treatments and illnesses are culturally determined and have nothing to do with actual temperature. Box 7-3 gives examples of hot-cold classifications. Understanding this belief system may help explain a client's desire for, or rejection of, a specific medical treatment. For example, the client may insist on penicillin (a "hot" medicine) or an x-ray (a "hot" treatment) for a viral respiratory infection (a "cold" condition) and may not be satisfied with his or her care without receiving what he or she believes to be an appropriate treatment.

Personalistic illnesses result from aggression directed at, or punishment of, the individual. The "evil eye" and witchcraft are two examples of personalistic folk beliefs. The "evil eye" is a concept known throughout Mediterranean (e.g., Greek and Italian) and Spanish-speaking cultures. It is usually caused unintentionally and is related to envy and admiration. Complimenting another person's child may be considered a way to "cast the evil eye," and symptoms may be interpreted as being related to this. Usually, some general methods can protect against the evil eye. Children may wear protective amulets, beads, or gold crosses, for example. Respect these cultural beliefs, and help the client determine ways to resolve the situation along with appropriate medical interventions, if they are required.

Belief in witchcraft as a cause of illness is prevalent in many cultures in the United States and around the world (Giger and Davidhizar, 1999). Snow (1981) noted evidence of this belief in Puerto Ricans, Haitians, and African-Americans. He estimated that one third of African-American clients treated in psychiatric centers in the southern United States believed that they were victims of witchcraft. The common theme Snow noted was that someone had done something to cause another person's injury, illness, or death.

Clients usually seek out a folk healer for treatment of these conditions. For many clients, the practitioner can be most helpful by working in a collaborative and cooperative manner with the folk healer to provide holistic care to the

TABLE 7-2 Folk Healing Practices

Practice Name	Ethnicity	Practice Procedure	Purpose
Acupuncture	Asian (Chinese)	Needles in meridians (energy lines), herbs	Pain, sinus problems, injuries, stress, stroke, deafness, epilepsy, and so on
Cao Gio	Vietnamese, Cambodian	Coining produces ecchymosis, petechiae	Coughing, congestion, fever
Curanderismo	Hispanic	Bleeding, herbs, emetics, diuretics, prayers, penance, miracles	Physiological or psychological problems, social maladjustment
Folk practitioners	Haitian	Poltices, voodoo	Evil eye lifted
Hilot	Filipino	Faith healing through prayer, herbal medicine, massage, manipulation of bones and tissues	Most illness
Medicine men	Native American	Meditation, sweat lodges, herbal medicine, ritual	Any disease caused by an imbalance with nature
Moxa	Chinese	Burning of a plant on the skin	Mumps, convulsions, epistaxis
Root doctor	African-American	Herbs, laying on of hands	Any illness
Spiritual healer	White	Laying on of hands	Physiological, psychological, or social problems

From Starn J: Family culture and chronic conditions. In Jackson PL, Vessey JA, editors: *Primary care of the child with a chronic condition,* ed. 2, St. Louis, 1996, Mosby.

TABLE 7-3 Healers and Their Scope of Practice

Culture/Folk Practitioner	Preparation	Scope of Practice
Hispanic		
Family member	Possesses knowledge of folk medicine.	Common illnesses of a mild nature that may or may not be recognized by modern medicine.
Curandero	May receive training in an apprenticeship. May receive a "gift from God" that enables her/him to cure. Knowledgeable in use of herbs, diet, massage, and rituals.	Treats almost all of the traditional illnesses. Some may not treat illness caused by witchcraft for fear of being accused of possessing evil powers. Usually admired by members of the community.
Espiritualista or spiritualist	Born with the special gifts of being able to analyze dreams and foretell future events. May serve apprenticeship with an older practitioner.	Emphasis on prevention of illness or bewitchment through use of medals, prayers, amulets. May also be sought for cure of existing illness.
Yerbero	No formal training. Knowledgeable in growing and prescribing herbs.	Consulted for preventive and curative use of herbs for both traditional and Western illnesses.
Sabador (may refer to a chiropractor by this title)	Knowledgeable in massage and manipulation of bones and muscles.*	Treats many traditional illnesses, particularly those affecting the musculoskeletal system. May also treat nontraditional illnesses.
Black		
"Old lady"	Usually an older woman who has successfully raised her own family. Knowledgeable in child care and folk remedies.	Consulted about common ailments and for advice on child care. Found in rural and urban communities.
Spiritualist	Called by God to help others. No formal training. Usually associated with a fundamentalist Christian church.	Assists with problems that are financial, personal, spiritual, or physical. Predominantly found in urban communities.
Voodoo priest(ess) or hougan	May be trained by other priest(esses). In the United States the eldest son of a priest becomes a priest. A daughter of a priest(ess) becomes a priestess if she is born with a veil (amniotic sac) over her face.	Knowledgeable about properties of herbs; interpretation of signs and omens. Able to cure illness caused by voodoo. Uses communication techniques to establish a therapeutic milieu like a psychiatrist. Treats blacks, Mexican-Americans, and Native Americans.
Chinese		
Herbalist	Knowledgeable in diagnosis of illness and herbal remedies.	Both diagnostic and therapeutic. Diagnostic techniques include interviewing, inspection, auscultation, and assessment of pulses.

From Hautman MA: Folk health and illness beliefs, *Nurse Pract* 4(4):23-31, 1979.
*Preparation is for *sabador,* not chiropractor.

client. An example of this approach is the effort of the Indian Health Service to involve traditional healers in the client's care and make the services of traditional healers accessible to clients even when they are hospitalized (Giger and Davidhizar, 1999). Table 7-2 describes different folk healing practices. Table 7-3 describes different types of folk healers, their preparation, and practice.

Assessment of Beliefs

Understanding the client's beliefs related to health problems is particularly important for the development of an effective plan of care. Kleinman, Eisenberg, and Good (1978) suggest the following set of questions to elicit the client's explanatory model:

1. What do you think caused your problem?
2. Why do you think it started when it did?
3. What does your sickness do to you? How does it work?
4. How severe is your sickness? Will it have a long or a short duration?
5. What kind of treatment do you think you should receive?
6. What are the most important results you hope to receive from this treatment?
7. What are the chief problems your sickness has caused you?
8. What do you fear most about your sickness?

Customs

Customs are learned behaviors that you can easily assess through observation and direct questioning. However, problems and misunderstandings can arise if you do not assess customs or if you do not validate the meaning of observed behaviors. Customs include dietary practices, communication patterns, family and kinship relations, religious practices, and health behaviors. Tables 7-4 and 7-5 describe examples of behaviors relevant to the health care of different cultural groups, and the implications for health care.

Diet and Nutrition

Anthropologists have shown that cultural groups differ in their dietary beliefs and practices, but this is obvious to anyone who associates particular foods with specific ethnic

TABLE 7-4   Cultural Behaviors Relevant to Health Assessment

Cultural Group	Cultural Variations (Common Belief/Practice)	Nursing Implications
African-Americans	Dialect and slang terms require careful communication to prevent error (e.g., "bad" may mean "good").	Question the client's meaning or intent.
Mexican-Americans	Eye behavior is important. An individual who looks at and admires a child without touching the child has given the child the "evil eye."	Always touch the child you are examining or admiring.
Native Americans	Eye contact is considered a sign of disrespect and is thus avoided.	Recognize that the client may be attentive and interested even though eye contact is avoided.
Appalachians	Eye contact is considered impolite or a sign of hostility. Verbal patter may be confusing.	Avoid excessive eye contact. Clarify statements.
American Eskimos	Body language is very important. The individual seldom disagrees publicly with others. Client may nod yes to be polite, even if not in agreement.	Monitor own body language closely as well as client's to detect meaning.
Jewish-Americans	Orthodox Jews consider excess touching, particularly from members of the opposite sex, offensive.	Establish whether client is an Orthodox Jew and avoid excessive touch.
Chinese-Americans	Individual may nod head to indicate yes or shake head to indicate no. Excessive eye contact indicates rudeness. Excessive touch is offensive.	Ask questions carefully and clarify responses. Avoid excessive eye contact and touch.
Filipino-Americans	Offending people is to be avoided at all cost. Nonverbal behavior is very important.	Monitor nonverbal behaviors of self and client, being sensitive to physical and emotional discomfort or concerns of the client.
Haitian-Americans	Touch is used in conversation. Direct eye contact is used to gain attention and respect during communication.	Use direct eye contact when communicating.
East Indian Hindu–Americans	Women avoid eye contact as a sign of respect.	Be aware that men may view eye contact by women as offensive. Avoid eye contact.
Vietnamese-Americans	Avoidance of eye contact is a sign of respect. The head is considered sacred; it is not polite to pat the head. An upturned palm is offensive in communication.	Limit eye contact. Touch the head only when mandated and explain clearly before proceeding to do so. Avoid hand gesturing.

Modified from Giger JN, Davidhizar RE: *Transcultural nursing: assessment and intervention,* ed. 2, St. Louis, 1995, Mosby.

TABLE 7-5   Cross-Cultural Examples of Cultural Phenomena Impacting on Nursing Care

Nations of Origin	Communication	Space	Time Orientation	Social Organization	Environmental Control	Biological Variations
Asian China Hawaii Philippines Korea Japan Southeast Asia (Laos, Cambodia, Vietnam)	National language preference Dialects, written characters Use of silence Nonverbal and contextual cuing	Noncontact people	Present	Family: hierarchial structure, loyalty Devotion to tradition Many religions, including Taoism, Buddhism, Islam, and Christianity Community social organizations	Traditional health and illness beliefs Use of traditional medicines Traditional practitioners: Chinese doctors and herbalists	Liver cancer Stomach cancer Coccidioidomycosis Hypertension Lactose intolerance
African West Coast (as slaves) Many African countries West Indian Islands Dominican Republic Haiti Jamaica	National languages Dialect: pidgin, creole, Spanish, and French	Close personal space	Present over future	Family: many female, single parent Large, extended family networks Strong church affiliation within community Community social organizations	Traditional health and illness beliefs Folk medicine tradition Traditional healer: root-worker	Sickle cell anemia Hypertension Cancer of the esophagus Stomach cancer Coccidioidomycosis Lactose intolerance
Europe Germany England Italy Ireland Other European countries	National languages Many learn English immediately	Noncontact people Aloof Distant Southern countries: closer contact and touch	Future over present	Nuclear families Extended families Judeo-Christian religions Community social organizations	Primary reliance on modern health care system Traditional health and illness beliefs Some remaining folk medicine traditions	Breast cancer Heart disease Diabetes mellitus Thalassemia
Native American 500 Native American tribes Aleuts Eskimos	Tribal languages Use of silence and body language	Space very important and has no boundaries	Present	Extremely family oriented Biological and extended families Children taught to respect traditions Community social organizations	Traditional health and illness beliefs Folk medicine tradition Traditional healer: medicine man	Accidents Heart disease Cirrhosis of the liver Diabetes mellitus
Hispanic countries Spain Cuba Mexico Central and South America	Spanish or Portuguese primary language	Tactile relationships Touch Handshakes Embracing Value physical presence	Present	Nuclear family Extended families *Compadrazzo:* godparents Community social organizations	Traditional health and illness beliefs Folk medicine tradition Traditional healers: *curandero, espiritista, partera, señora*	Diabetes mellitus Parasites Coccidioidomycosis Lactose intolerance

From Potter PA, Perry AG: *Fundamentals of nursing*, ed. 5, St. Louis, 2001, Mosby. Compiled by Rachel Spector, RN, PhD.

groups. The development of a national cuisine is a complex process related to the availability of certain kinds of food, the price, the efficiency of its distribution, the subjective preferences of taste and spices, and patterns of trade and commerce. Hotter, spicier food is preferred by groups living relatively closer to the equator, where the climate is warmer. Groups living in higher latitudes in more temperate climates prefer relatively less spicy food. The variety of foods available in industrialized countries is greater than that in developing countries.

Apart from its nutritional value, food carries a range of symbolical meanings. Food that is popular in one society may be rigorously forbidden in another. Food and the social aspects of eating food play a central role in daily life. Consequently, the practitioner should appreciate that dietary beliefs and practices are notoriously difficult to change, even if they interfere with adequate nutrition.

Before attempting to change nutrition practices, try to understand the ways in which various cultures view their food and the ways food is classified. Food is usually classified into (1) definitions of what is edible and what is not, (2) what is sacred and what is profane, (3) the ways food is grouped, (4) food as medicine, and (5) social food. For example, rancid butter is not normally considered edible in North American culture, yet it is a standard condiment in tea in many central Asian regions. By the same token, food commonly eaten in North America, such as pork rinds, would be considered repulsive in some other cultures. Snails and eels are considered delicacies by some cultures but inedible by others.

In the United States and Canada, industrialized countries with many immigrants, few foods are generally considered profane. But among specific religious groups, some examples of sacred and profane foods are familiar. Many Jews will not eat pork, and strict Catholics will not eat meat on Fridays (although this has become a less common practice). In addition to religious-based sanctions, many people are vegetarians and other groups avoid highly processed foods.

Medicinal qualities are ascribed to various foods (rightly or wrongly) across the world. North Americans have their own widely shared beliefs associating food with medicine. "Apples keep doctors away." "Honey and lemon help reduce congestion." "Fish is brain food." "Citrus fruits provide protection from colds." "Oats unclog arteries."

Finally, all cultures tend to associate foods with social occasions unique to their cultures. Some occasions seem to demand wine, and others seem to demand hot chocolate. Certain foods are consumed at baseball games, whereas other foods are eaten as family traditions on various holidays.

Other cultures are no different from the dominant culture in these broad aspects of food. Only the foods that carry strong cultural preferences or taboos vary from one culture to another.

Communication Patterns

Communication patterns are closely intertwined with culture and may be the source of misunderstandings between you and your client. Communication patterns include both

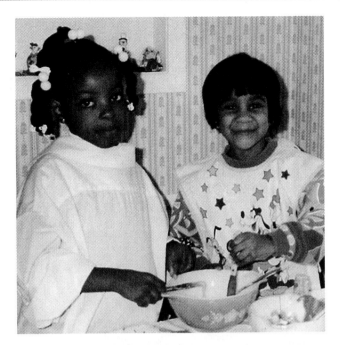

Figure 7-6 Cultural groups may differ in their dietary beliefs and practices.

verbal and nonverbal behaviors. Verbal behaviors include language, vocabulary, grammatical structure, voice qualities, intonation, speed, pronunciation, and silence. Nonverbal behaviors include touch, facial expression, eye movement, posture, personal space, and distance.

Determining what language is spoken at the client's home is an important part of a cultural assessment. Find out how well the client understands written and spoken English, since this is important for both verbal interactions and for giving the client written information, such as health education pamphlets. Even when the client speaks English, colloquialisms may be confusing. For example, "bad" may have a negative connotation for one group and a more positive connotation for another group. Certain groups may use lay terms such as "high blood" for hypertension and "low blood" for anemia. These may vary among different ethnic groups, so confirm your understanding of the term with the client.

Also, be aware of cultural norms related to the way you address clients (e.g., whether you address them by their first name or use a more formal title). Proper forms of address may vary according to ethnic or regional groups.

Nonverbal communication may also have different meanings in different cultures. In North American middle-class culture, looking directly at the person with whom you are speaking is important. However, in many cultures (Asian, Native American, Indochinese, Arab, Appalachian), looking directly at another person may be a sign of disrespect or aggression. Touch also has many different interpretations by different cultural groups. Some groups, such as those of Mediterranean descent, use touch to communicate feelings, whereas other groups see touch as an invasion of privacy. Many Asian groups believe that the head is the most sacred part of the body (see Chapter 2); therefore obtain permission before touching the client's head. The feet are the lowest part of the body, so showing the bottom of your shoe or pointing your toe at the client is seen as being disrespectful.

Family Relationships

Attitudes toward family structure and family roles and relationships have been traditionally mediated by cultural considerations. However, cultural differences related to families, once a defining characteristic of different cultural groups, have been rapidly changing. Our society has become highly mobile and more integrated, tearing down barriers

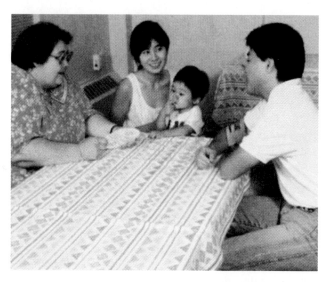

Figure 7-7 Making assumptions about the relationship between family and culture should be avoided, since cultural differences related to families are rapidly changing in today's society.

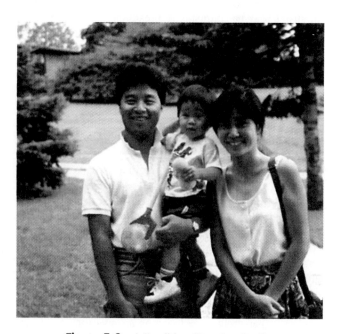

Figure 7-8 A "traditional" nuclear family.

that previously kept family norms intact within subcultures. The media has focused attention on alternative family arrangements and practices, making them more familiar and thus acceptable.

In the past, the concept of the nuclear family was predominant. Typically, married couples tended to share the same race, religion, and socioeconomic status. They had children, and the mother provided child care while the father earned the income. They tended to stay married for life. With the advent of mass communication, easy access to cheap and fast transportation, and economic changes promoting urbanization, today's young people often move far away from their parents. More young people attend college and use this opportunity to migrate elsewhere. Far from the daily influences of their families, new group affiliations develop based on common interests, education, and jobs. There has been an increased incidence and acceptance of divorce, dual-income families, single-parent families, same-sex families, teenage parents, and involvement of fathers in child care. According to the U.S. Bureau of Labor Statistics (1999), only 13% of all families fit the traditional model of husband as wage-earner and wife as homemaker. Of families with children, dual-earning working couples represent the majority (42%), followed by single-parent families (22%). Culturally mediated family practices that used to distinguish one cultural group from another are also now less distinct.

This is not to say that cultural differences in attitudes toward family structure and roles no longer exist. Rather, they cannot be taken for granted. Therefore, avoid making any assumptions about the relationship between family and culture. Take a value-free approach to assessing family dimensions, which can be so important to health and well-being.

To assess the client's family, first determine the family structure. Use a simple family tree or family diagram (called a **genogram**) to establish who the members of the family are and how the client fits in (Figure 7-9, *A*). Constructing a genogram entails gathering three levels of information: (1) mapping family structure, (2) recording family demographic information, and (3) delineating family relationships. To further examine the family's relationships within the community, it is helpful to construct an ecomap. The ecomap diagrams the client's relationships with individuals/groups in his or her social network. This includes the client's significant others, friends, neighbors, peers, and associates, as well as significant community groups such as school, church, and health care providers. Figure 7-9, *B,* shows an example of an ecomap; note that the genogram forms the center of the ecomap.

Constructing both a genogram and an ecomap allows you to get a clear picture of family structure and to explore roles and relationships both within and outside the family. This helps determine to whom the client is attached (or in conflict with) and how the dynamics of various relationships work. Relationships, both within families and in broader associations, can be close or distant, dependent or hostile. In each relationship the sharing of power and decision making, as well as approaches to problem solving, can vary widely.

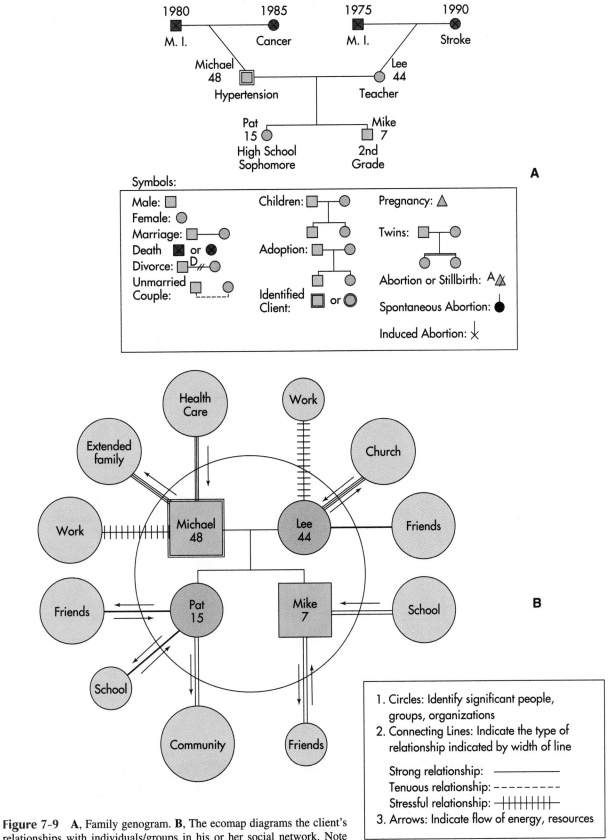

Figure 7-9 A, Family genogram. **B**, The ecomap diagrams the client's relationships with individuals/groups in his or her social network. Note that the genogram forms the center of the ecomap. (From Bomar PJ: *Nurses and family health promotion: concepts, assessment, and interventions,* ed. 2, Philadelphia, 1996, WB Saunders.)

It is important to determine who is the family's key decision maker related to health issues, as well as who is the primary provider of care. For example, the grandmother may be the decision maker about health issues or a daughter-in-law may be expected to provide primary care for her husband's elderly mother. Inclusion of these important individuals in your plan of care will have a significant impact on its effectiveness.

Assess family function in areas such as communication patterns and attitudes toward expressing feelings and offering support. Many tools exist that provide a systematic assessment of family roles and functions. A familiar one that assesses the person's satisfaction with relationships in the immediate family (and is reliable, valid, and clinically useful) is the family APGAR (Box 7-4).

Keep in mind that despite the rapid change in family structure and function associated with distinct cultural groups, cultural considerations remain very important for many individuals.

Religious Practices and Spirituality

Religion and spirituality have an influence on the lifestyles of people in most cultures and may affect nutrition and health care practices. Religion and spirituality are terms often used interchangeably; however, understanding the distinction between these terms is important for conducting a holistic assessment. *Religion* refers to an organized system of beliefs, knowledge, and practices centered around the worship of a higher being and which lends purpose and meaning to life (O'Neil and Kenny, 1998). *Spirituality* is a broader concept that reflects a sense of connectedness within oneself, with others, and with a higher being. *Spiritual well-being* is defined as a sense of inner peace, reverence for life, compassion for others, and appreciation of both diversity and unity. It also includes a relationship with a higher being, a conviction that there is a purpose and meaning in life, and a realistic sense of adversity and loss (Hanson and Boyd, 1996). Although the impact of religion on health and health behavior is important to assess, the

---

BOX 7-4

FAMILY APGAR

DEFINITION	FUNCTIONS MEASURED BY THE FAMILY APGAR	RELEVANT OPEN-ENDED QUESTIONS
Adaptation is the use of intrafamilial and extrafamilial resources for problem solving when family equilibrium is stressed during a crisis.	How resources are shared, or the degree to which a member is satisfied with the assistance received when family resources are needed.	How have family members aided each other in time of need? In what way have family members received help or assistance from friends and community agencies?
Partnership is the sharing of decision making and nurturing responsibilities by family members.	How decisions are shared, or the member's satisfaction with mutuality in family communication and problem solving.	How do family members communicate with each other about such matters as vacations, finances, medical care, large purchases, and personal problems?
Growth is the physical and emotional maturation and self-fulfillment that is achieved by family members through mutual support and guidance.	How nurturing is shared, or the member's satisfaction with the freedom available within the family to change roles and attain physical and emotional growth or maturation.	How have family members changed during the past years? How has this change been accepted by family members? In what ways have family members aided each other in growing or developing independent lifestyles?
Affection is the caring or loving relationship that exists among family members.	How emotional experiences are shared, or the member's satisfaction with the intimacy and emotional interaction that exists in the family.	How have family members reacted to your desires for change? How have members of your family responded to emotional expressions such as affection, love, sorrow, or anger?
Resolve is the commitment to devote time to other members of the family for physical and emotional nurturing. It also usually involves a decision to share wealth and space.	How time (and space and money) is shared, or the member's satisfaction with the time commitment that has been made to the family by its members.	How do members of your family share time, space, and money?

Data from Smilkstein G: The Family APGAR: a proposal for a family function test and its use by physicians, *J Fam Pract* 6:1231-1239, 1978.

client's spirituality or spiritual well-being also needs to be considered.

Most religions have rituals or ceremonies that mark life cycle stages such as birth, entrance into adulthood, marriage, and death. Religions may have certain dietary restrictions, such as prohibitions against eating pork (Jewish and Muslim religions) or abstaining from specific foods on certain days (Roman Catholic). Religions may prohibit certain types of health care interventions, such as the administration of blood (Jehovah's Witnesses) or use of medications containing caffeine or made from pork products. Table 3-2 describes a variety of religious beliefs that may affect nursing care. Remember that the strictness of adherence to these rules varies among individuals and subgroups within the religion.

Religious beliefs may influence a client's perception of the cause of an illness, its severity, and the type of healer required. The religion and religiosity of the individual determine the role that religious faith plays in the recovery process. In many instances religiosity also affects the response to a specific treatment and the process of healing. Although cultural heritage and religion may be interrelated, do not assume that membership in a particular ethnic or cultural group is equated with membership in a specific religion. For example, although many Mexican-Americans are Catholic, do not assume that your Mexican-American client is Catholic and in a time of crisis offer to contact a priest for support. This approach, although well-intentioned, may add to the client's stress and sense of frustration. Gathering initial information about the client's religious affiliation and the role that religious beliefs and practices play in health and illness helps avoid mistaken assumptions and provides information that is important to the client's care.

Spiritual Assessment.   In assessing the client's spiritual needs, several areas need to be considered. Purnell and Paulanka (1998) propose that the nurse assess three areas: (1) the client's religious practices and use of prayer; (2) what the client feels gives meaning to life and his or her sources of strength; and (3) the relationship between the client's spiritual beliefs and health care practices. Shelly and Fish (1988) suggests four areas to explore (environmental, behavioral, verbal, and interpersonal relationship information) in order to better understand the spiritual needs of culturally diverse clients.

Specifically, the practitioner should observe whether the client:

1. Has religious objects (e.g., Bible, Koran, prayer book, religious medals, sculptures, photographs of religious leaders) in the environment
2. Wears clothing, jewelry, or undergarments that have religious significance
3. Receives greeting cards that are religious in nature or from a religious representative
4. Appears to pray at certain times of the day or before meals
5. Subscribes to a specific diet (e.g., kosher; vegetarian; or a diet free from pork, caffeine, shellfish, or other specific food items) for religious reasons
6. Reads religious books, pamphlets, or magazines

7. Mentions God (Allah, Yahweh, Buddha, or another supreme being), prayer, faith, church, or other religious topics
8. Requests a visit by a clergy member or other religious representative
9. Expresses fear or anxiety about suffering, pain, or death
10. Has visitors, including a rabbi, priest, church elder, or other religious representative
11. Prefers to remain alone or interact with others. What is the quality of his or her interactions with visitors, staff, roommate(s)?

An understanding of the client's spiritual needs can provide important information that may have a significant impact on the client's response to care.

Health and Illness Behaviors

Culture also influences the client's attitudes toward health; response to illness; and even experience of symptoms, such as pain. Individuals learn about health behaviors through socialization in their families. Beliefs about illness and alternative types of health care providers are discussed earlier in the section on beliefs. Specific illness behaviors also are culturally determined. Zola (1966) examined the differences in symptoms that caused clients to seek health care by a physician. In his comparison of diagnostically matched clients from different ethnic groups, he found that the definition of an illness and the pattern of response to symptoms varied according to ethnic group. The experience of pain is another symptom that is strongly influenced by culture.

Pain.   Pain is among the most common symptoms in clinical practice, yet it is not purely a neurophysiological response. Pain is influenced by social, psychological, and cultural factors. Culture influences both pain intensity and pain tolerance. Culture determines a person's attitudes toward pain and beliefs about it. Emotions associated with the context in which pain is experienced can have a powerful effect on how pain is felt. Sometimes soldiers are wounded in battle and do not realize it until afterward. In some cultures meditation or religious trances dissipate the sensation of pain, as in the firewalkers of Sri Lanka, who are apparently oblivious to the expected intensity of the pain they experience. Other cultures value the ability to withstand pain without complaint or physical manifestations, as in the case of certain Native Indian and African tribes, who demonstrate their adulthood by withstanding painful stimuli.

It is difficult to separate culturally determined pain from pain that is mediated by neurological mechanisms. Health care providers often encounter the so-called "placebo effect," in which an inactive drug relieves suffering. A simple belief in the effectiveness of the placebo can release endorphins in the brain, actually providing physiological pain relief.

Culture also determines when pain is abnormal, requiring medical attention and treatment. The extent to which pain is considered a normal part of life also affects a person's willingness to withstand it. Studies show, for instance, that Polish women are far more able to accept the pain associated with childbirth than their Polish American counterparts, who have greater access to anesthesia during labor.

Each culture has its own language of distress, which includes facial expressions, changes in activity, sounds, and words describing feeling. These norms determine acceptable ways clients express pain to others. For example, Zborowski (1952) in a classic study found that Italian-Americans tended to dramatize their pain as a means of allaying anxiety and dissipating the pain. Irish-Americans, by contrast, were more reticent about their bodily complaints. Villarruel and Ortiz de Montellano (1992) identified themes related to the cultural meanings of pain and pain-related behaviors in Mesoamerican cultures (with particular reference to Mexican-Americans).

Pain is a subjective sensation that has physiological, cultural, and emotional components. The actual cause or intensity of pain is difficult to assess. In treating pain, remember that it is the client's experience of pain, as the client feels it, that determines how you treat it. Carefully assess cultural considerations that may affect a client's ability or willingness to report pain as a sign of illness as well as an inclination to seek treatment.

Other Variables to Consider

Heredity

Information concerning ethnic, cultural, or racial heritage is also important for assessing the client's susceptibility to specific genetic disorders. Because of intermarriage within a relatively narrow range of ethnic, geographical, or religious groups, certain traits are passed on that place members of those groups at risk for genetic disorders. (See Table 3-1 for an overview of disorders and genetic traits for a variety of population or ethnic groups.) Knowledge of these susceptibilities is important for screening clients for problems, providing interventions to prevent complications related to problems, and counseling clients who are considering having children and are concerned about the risks of passing on such traits.

Biological Variation

The significance of specific biological, physical, and physiological variations among individuals in various racial groups has gained greater recognition in the nursing literature (Giger and Davidhizar [1999]; Purnell and Paulanka [1999]). Giger and Davidhizar (1999) note that most studies of biological baseline data in growth, development, nutrition, and other biological phenomena were conducted on Caucasian subjects, therefore, the subsequent "norms" developed may not be appropriate when applied to individuals from other racial groups. Significant differences have been noted in terms of skin color, body structure, body weight, disease risks and health conditions, and variations in drug metabolism (Purnell and Paulanka, 1998). For example, skin color changes, such as pallor or erythema, are manifested differently in persons of light and dark colored skin. Table 10-2 provides more in-depth descriptions of such differences. Differences in normal growth patterns have been noted between Caucasian and Asian infants. Vietnamese infants were found small by American standards. However, when weight for stature graphs were plotted, these infants fell in the normal range

(Felice, 1986). This indicates a need for growth parameters that reflect differences in specific racial and ethnic groups.

In relation to disease conditions, there is an increased genetic susceptibility to specific diseases and conditions in some ethnic groups. For example, the prevalence of diabetes among African-Americans is about 70% higher than among Caucasian Americans, and the prevalence among Hispanics is nearly double that for Caucasian Americans. The prevalence of diabetes among Native Indians and Alaska Natives is more than twice that for the total population (CDC, 1995). Recent research has also noted variation in drug metabolism among diverse racial and ethnic groups. For example, increased sensitivity to alcohol has been noted in both Chinese and Native American groups. Psychotropic drugs and specific classes of antihypertensive medications are also metabolized differently depending on race (Campinha-Bacote [1998]; Giger and Davidhizar [1999]; Purnell and Paulanka [1998]). Awareness that biocultural variations exist is essential as you consider both physical findings and interventions for your clients.

Socioeconomic Status

Socioeconomic status (SES) is related to education, income, and occupation. A client's SES may have a stronger influence on health and access to health care than ethnicity or racial status (Lipson, Dibble, and Minarik, 1996). Public health research shows that people in lower socioeconomic groups have the highest rates of death and disease resulting from virtually every health problem. Thus, although speaking of "a culture of poverty" is incorrect, socioeconomic status is an important predictor of health and disease. People in poverty make less use of the health care system. They also have greater difficulty accessing the health care system. Their choice of providers, as well as their criterion for seeking health care, is different from the frequency and criterion associated with more affluent individuals. Therefore an awareness of a client's economic status has implications for care.

CLINICAL APPLICATIONS OF CULTURAL ASSESSMENT

Health care providers often want detailed descriptions of characteristics of different cultural groups to help guide their care. There are several excellent texts that present such information (e.g., Giger and Davidhizar, 1999; Lipson, Dibble, and Minarik, 1996; and Purnell and Paulanka, 1998, as well as others listed in the Bibliography). It is important to keep in mind that these descriptions are generalizations meant to be used as guidelines only.

Cultural traits are not uniform and static. How important cultural influences are to health care concerns varies according to the degree of enculturation and acculturation, the type of problem, and the congruence with the health care culture. Knowledge of cultural factors provides a context for understanding behaviors and designing care to meet the client's (or family's) needs. A cultural assessment does not require exhaustive information on every element of the culture. Make sure to identify major values, beliefs, and behaviors related to particular health concerns. (Figure 7-10 summarizes Giger and Davidhizar's model and the components that need to be

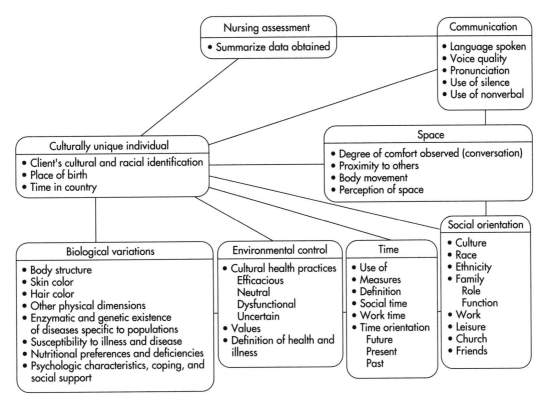

Figure 7-10 Giger and Davidhizar's transcultural assessment model. (From Giger JN, Davidhizar RE: *Transcultural nursing: assessment and intervention*, ed. 3, St. Louis, 1999, Mosby.)

considered in a cultural assessment). Tailor actual assessments and interventions to the individual client and family. Also avoid making assumptions about cultural beliefs and behaviors without receiving validation from the client. Cultural assessment involves a shared negotiation between you and the client in which each person is equal in bringing important and relevant information to the interview.

Cultural affiliation cannot be determined by an individual's appearance or surname. Therefore it is important that every client have a cultural assessment. Lipson, Dibble, and Minarik (1996) recommend that at a minimum the following content be included in the cultural assessment of any client:

1. Where was the client born. If an immigrant, how long has the client lived in this country?
2. What is the client's ethnic affiliation, and how strong is the client's ethnic identity?
3. Who are the client's major support people: family members, friends? Does the client live in an ethnic community?
4. What are the primary and secondary languages? What is the client's speaking and reading ability in these languages?
5. How would you characterize the client's nonverbal communication style?
6. What is the client's religion? What is its importance in daily life and current practices?
7. What are the client's food preferences and prohibitions?
8. What is the client's economic situation, and is the income adequate to meet the needs of the client and family?

9. What are the health and illness beliefs and practices?
10. What are the customs and beliefs around transitions such as birth, illness, and death?

Table 7-6 provides an example of a more detailed cultural assessment of a family with a chronically ill member. This could be easily modified for an acutely ill client or one with health promotion needs.

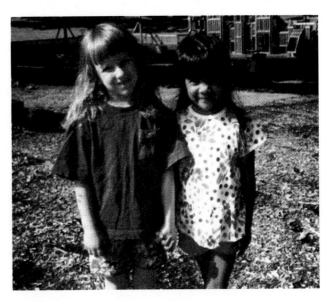

Figure 7-11 Knowledge of cultural factors provides a context for understanding behaviors and designing care to meet the client's needs.

TABLE 7-6	Sample Format for a Cross-Cultural Assessment of a Family With a Member With a Chronic Condition

Area of Concern	Sample Questions
Family demographics	Who lives in your family (i.e., members, ages, sexes)?
	What kind of work do members of the household do?
	What is your family's socioeconomic status?
	What kind of health insurance coverage do you have?
	Which family members are covered?
	What chronic conditions or symptoms do you have?
	How would you describe the problems that have brought you here today?
	Who is the primary care taker in your family?
Orientation	Where were the members of the family born?
	What is the ethnic background of the family members?
	How many years have family members lived in the United States? (NOTE: Only ask if appropriate.)
	In your family is it important to be on time for an appointment or to get to an appointment when possible based on everyone's schedule for that day?
	Why do you think you have (the above-named) chronic condition (e.g., punishment for a parent's past behavior, such as conceiving a child out of wedlock; the result of a genetic problem; or a gift given because of the family's patience and love)?
Communication	What language(s) and dialect(s) are spoken at home?
	Who reads English in the family? If no one reads English, in what language would you prefer printed materials?
	Do parents and children look when spoken to or do they look down? To whom should questions be addressed? (NOTE: Avoid using a child as a translator, if at all possible, because of the strain this task imposes.)
Family relationships	Besides the immediate household, who else makes up the members of this family?
	Who makes the decisions in this family (e.g., mother-in-law, father, both partners, other family or friends, group decision)?
	Who cares for the client and the client's medical needs?
	What are the housing arrangements (e.g., space, number of rooms, members living in the home)?
	What is the family's usual daily routine like?
	To whom do you turn when you need help with, or have questions about, your condition?
Beliefs about health	What is the present health status of family members?
	What illnesses or conditions are present in the current family members?
	What illnesses or conditions were present in deceased family members?
	How often and for what reasons have family members used Western medicine in the past?
	What complementary therapies are used by your family routinely and specifically for the client (e.g., acupuncture, healers, prayer, massage)?
	What do you do when you are in pain?
	Is it important to keep the client at home or to use institutional placement?
	What do you think will help clear up the problem?
	Are there things that help you get better that the health care providers should know?
	What problems has your illness caused your family?
Education	How much schooling have family members completed?
	What ways are best for you to learn about your condition (e.g., pamphlets, videos, direct patient teaching, home visits, return demonstrations)?
	From whom are you most comfortable learning about your condition (e.g., doctor, nurse, social worker, home health aide, other family members)?
Religion	What religion(s) are practiced in your family?
	What religious practices do you do to help yourself or your family (e.g., pray, meditate, attend a support group, practice the laying on of hands)?
	What practices does your religion say you should *not* do (e.g., have blood transfusions, allow strangers or dangerous circumstances to affect you or your family)?
Nutrition	When are usual mealtimes for your family?
	With whom do you eat?
	What foods do you usually eat?
	What special foods do you eat when you are sick?
	What foods do you *not* eat and when?

Modified from Starn J: Family culture and chronic conditions. In Jackson PL, Vessey JA: *Primary care of the child with a chronic condition,* ed. 2, St. Louis, 1996, Mosby.

Health care providers need to consider ways to modify care to meet both the provider's professional standards of practice and the client's cultural beliefs and practices. Tripp-Reimer, Brink, and Pinkham (1999) propose a model for negotiation when cultural discrepancies or conflicts arise between clients and health care providers. The goal of negotiation is to reduce cultural conflict in a way that promotes cooperation and allows clients and providers to achieve an outcome satisfactory to both parties. Their recommended model is presented in Box 7-5.

Health care providers need to consider ways that the health care system in which they function can be more responsive to the needs of culturally diverse populations. Box 7-6 provides an excellent summary of the ways providers can promote culturally sensitive health care services. Analyze your health care agency to see whether these activities are a routine part of it functioning, and consider ways that individual providers as well as the agency as a whole can promote culturally competent care. This will become increasingly important given the demographic changes predicted for the future.

BOX 7-5

STEPS FOR NEGOTIATION WHEN CONFLICTS ARISE BETWEEN CLIENTS AND PROVIDERS

1. The health professional asks questions to find out how the client explains the illness or health problem.
2. The health professional then clearly and fully presents (in lay terms) an explanation of the disorder, including the recommended treatment, and invites questions from client and family, to which full explanations are given. The point here is to work within the client's frame of reference and level of understanding.
3. A working alliance is possible when the client's explanation of the illness either agrees with or shifts to the health professional's model, or if the recommendations of the health professional shift more toward the client's expectations of treatment.
4. At times, discrepancies remain. When this occurs, the health professional can openly acknowledge and clarify conflict. The health professional is ethically entitled to provide references and data to support his or her position but should also allow the client and the client's family to provide references and data to argue their position. The

health professional continues to elicit the client's explanatory model until understanding is reached.
5. At this juncture, either the professional or the client will change sides to arrive at a mutually desired treatment.
6. When a conflict cannot be resolved, the health professional should attempt to arrive at an acceptable compromise of treatment based on biomedical knowledge, knowledge of the client's point of view, and ethical standards.
7. When all else fails, the health professional needs to recognize that the role is to provide expert advice and rationale for the treatment recommendations but that it is the client (or client's family) who is the final decision-maker in the situation. If a complete stalemate is reached, the health professional is responsible for offering a referral to another person. Finally, the client may seek advice from another health provider without fear of reprisal by the system.
8. Throughout this process, each negotiation involves an ongoing monitoring of the agreement and of each party's participation in the agreement (Katon and Kleinman, 1981).

From Tripp-Reimer T, Brink P, Pinkham C: Culture brokerage. In Bulechek GM, McCloskey JC, editors: *Nursing interventions: effective treatments,* ed. 3, Philadelphia, 1999, WB Saunders.

BOX 7-6

HALLMARKS OF CULTURALLY SENSITIVE CAREGIVING SYSTEMS

1. The asset model is based on recognizing cultural differences in childrearing, family strengths, and culturally based coping methods.

   The provider gathers data based on reviewing previous health care records, reading about the specific culture to learn about basic beliefs and values, and asking family members questions. This model asks what the family's strengths are (e.g., family members present, ways the family cares for their child, types of complementary therapies the family has used, ways family members find support or coping techniques, shared caregiving by all family members). These strengths are then built on by the primary care provider to foster care.
2. Providers seek community participation in all stages of program design, development, implementation,

outreach, policy making, problem solving, and evaluation.

   Informal and formal community leaders need to be involved in and approve of assessment and intervention approaches. This means talking to church leaders, various traditional healers, and elders who are respected in each ethnic community to learn what they think is culturally appropriate and sensitive care. Primary care providers may also seek out leaders of support groups for clients with special needs.
3. Community outreach to families is ongoing and culturally appropriate.

   Providers and support staff who either speak the language of the clients or are from the same ethnic group are sought. Interpreters are hired when necessary to provide outreach at

Modified from Starn JR: Family culture and chronic conditions. In Jackson PL, Vessey JA, editors: *Primary care of the child with a chronic condition,* ed. 2, St. Louis, 1996, Mosby.

Continued

BOX 7-6–cont'd

HALLMARKS OF CULTURALLY SENSITIVE CAREGIVING SYSTEMS—cont'd

schools, churches, or ethnic gathering places. Practitioners must explain concepts of confidentiality and privacy to interpreters. Health care providers should also look at the client/parent when the interpreter is translating, unless direct eye contact is contraindicated in the culture (e.g., Native American or Filipino cultures).

4. Intake systems are sensitive to family and cultural values. Providers should ask the family appropriate questions about the family's culture. However, intake may take several visits if privacy and mistrust of outsiders are issues that must be resolved before effective service can begin. Limit the number of professional care providers present. Encourage the family to have those family members who are important to them and the interpreter present. Conduct the meeting in either an informal or a formal manner based on the family's values.

5. Families are involved directly in the family treatment and service plan.

   Families help prioritize the goals. The family decision-makers are consulted in determining the plan. The family's orientation to primary care providers as authority figures or joint decision-makers is determined before attempting to develop the service plan. Family caregivers and decision-makers are involved in the ways that the family deem acceptable when developing the individualized service plan.

6. Family goals permit intracultural variation on a case-by-case basis.

   Standard care plans are altered based on family needs to include alternative modes of therapy, such as healers, acupuncture, or other practices of importance to the family.

7. Emphasis is placed on maintaining and improving the self-esteem, cultural identification, and goal-setting ability of each family to foster self-sufficiency.

   Family decision-makers and the caregivers are acknowledged. Family strengths are praised.

8. The teaching of parent-child interaction patterns must fit ideal family cultural values.

   For example, a Filipino or Native American child is not pushed to look at authority figures or to speak up in a disagreement; deference and avoidance of eye contact are culturally appropriate.

9. Team members have ongoing, culturally appropriate training.

   Team members are either of the same cultural background and speak the same language as the family or they have taken workshops given by ethnic leaders or others with expertise in the cultural group receiving care.

10. Educational materials, media, evaluation, and monitoring instruments are field-tested for cultural appropriateness and congruency in language content and emotional meaning.

11. Typical cultural and familial celebrations and symbolism are incorporated within services. Special holidays may be acknowledged by families sharing native foods and holiday traditions with care providers and other families.

12. Continuous evaluation is mandated to ensure cultural appropriateness and program effectiveness. The client's progress is monitored internally and by external evaluators. Assess the family's perceptions of the intervention. Determine whether the family is meeting goals and prioritizing these goals.

? Critical Thinking Questions

1. List four ways in which you might enhance your personal cultural sensitivity.
2. Conduct a cultural self-assessment. Describe (verbally to a friend or write it out for yourself) your own:
   • Ethnic affiliation
   • Religious affiliation/religious or spiritual practices
   • Family traditions
   • Family attitudes/values about education, sex/marriage, work, illness, death, and dying; roles of extended family members
   • Dietary patterns/traditions
   • Health practices used to both keep healthy and treat illnesses

3. Consider how your cultural belief (as evidenced by your responses to question 2) might influence your experience as a client in the current U.S. health care system.
4. Consider how your cultural beliefs (based on your responses to question 2) might influence your assessment of and care for a client from another country. How would you modify an interview or care for a client who is, for example, Muslim or Hispanic?
5. List eight questions used to assess a client's beliefs related to health problems. Answer your questions, using a situation when you had a health problem. Ask a friend, family member, or colleague to respond to these questions. Consider their implications for your (or your interviewee's) health care.

Answers are available on the MERLIN website (www.harcourthealth.com/MERLIN/Barkauskas/). And be sure to check the website regularly for additional learning activities!

Assessment Techniques

Learning Objectives

On successful study of this chapter and completion of related learning experiences, the learner will be able to:
- Discuss seven basic principles used in conducting an examination.

- Name four examination techniques.
- Identify equipment used for examination.
- Describe how to modify the examination for special populations.

Outline

Purpose Of Examination

The overall goals of the physical examination are to (1) obtain baseline data on the individual client, (2) identify variations from the normal state, and (3) validate information obtained in the health history. The health assessment database consists of both subjective and objective information. Subjective information is the client's verbalized perceptions and interpretations. In the interview, the history and review of systems provide subjective information. This information alerts the practitioner to areas to focus on during the examination. The practitioner obtains objective information through the physical examination by observation and measurement of data using all of the senses. This information is used to support the subjective information given by the client during the interview.

CONDUCTING THE EXAMINATION
Basic Principles

The examiner's goal is to conduct an efficient and complete examination that involves as little trauma and fatigue to the client as possible. Accomplishing this goal requires a consistent, systematic pattern of performing the examination. Following such a pattern will prevent omitting a step and possibly vital information. The practitioner must be thorough and exact in the examination routine. With experience, he or she will develop an individual examination technique and sequence. However, the following general principles will help to ensure that the examiner conducts a comprehensive examination in a logical order:

1. Explain the procedures to clients at the beginning of the evaluation, and restate them as the examination proceeds. Assist clients in appropriate positioning, and warn them of any uncomfortable maneuvers. Instruct clients as to how to cooperate with any special maneuvers.
2. Use a head-to-toe approach. The head and face are examined before the genitals or feet because this sequence is generally more acceptable to the adult client.
3. Move from external to internal. Begin with observation, and then use instruments or perform digital examinations. Initial observations are general impressions, such as the client's appearance. Later observations might involve using an instrument such as an otoscope to identify anatomical landmarks of the eardrum, or tympanic membrane. Any intrusive procedure is done last.
4. Examine normal or unaffected areas before observing abnormal areas or parts of the body where the client describes symptoms. The regions that are to be examined must be exposed completely to ensure an accurate finding. Be sensitive to the client's anxiety and possible embarrassment when certain areas of the body are exposed.
5. Observe for body **symmetry,** comparing one side with the other. Although minor asymmetry may be a normal finding, right-to-left differences in leg circumference or joint movement may be the first clue to other problems.
6. Perform the physical examination while standing on the client's right side. This consistency of examiner position will help to locate anatomical landmarks as the examination is performed.
7. The examination environment should have adequate lighting, quiet, privacy, and all necessary equipment readily available.

Safety

Health care providers must be aware of the need to protect themselves and their clients from the risk of infection. Whenever a health care provider comes in close physical contact with a client, infection can be transmitted. Hand

BOX 8-1

SAFETY FIRST

The goal of Standard Precautions is that the health care provider will avoid contact with all of the client's body fluids. This approach involves wearing latex gloves whenever examining an area of the client's body (e.g., mouth, genitals) or obtaining a specimen (e.g., blood, sputum) when there is potential for contact with body fluids. Protective eyewear should be worn when dealing with secretions that can be passed through the air and might come in contact with the examiner's eye (e.g., during suctioning). Protective clothing, such as a fully buttoned laboratory coat, a disposable gown, or a uniform, should be worn to reduce the risk of transmission of infectious organisms.

Risk of transmission of infection to the practitioner and to housekeeping and maintenance personnel can be reduced by proper disposal of any equipment that has come in contact with the client's body fluids. Needles should not be recapped. Needles and other sharp objects should be disposed of in a "sharps" container to avoid accidental puncture or laceration wounds.

washing is one of the most effective methods of reducing the transmission of infection and must be done before and after any physical contact with a client during an examination (Box 8-1).

Simple hand washing is an effective method for preventing transmission of microorganisms. Hand washing consists of cleansing the fingers, nails, palms, backs of hands, and wrists for 10 to 30 seconds. Use running warm water, clean soap or cleanser, and friction to remove debris and microorganisms. Dry hands thoroughly with a clean towel, and then turn off the water without contaminating clean hands.

EQUIPMENT PREPARATION

Equipment needed in a comprehensive health assessment is shown in Figure 8-1. The examiner should keep all equipment within easy reach and place it on a table before beginning the examination. In addition to the equipment shown in the figure, the examiner may use a thermometer and a visual acuity chart during a screening examination. The purpose of each piece of equipment is discussed in detail in the various assessment chapters.

EXAMINATION TECHNIQUES

The four assessment techniques used in the physical examination are inspection, palpation, percussion, and auscultation. Positioning of the client is sometimes used as a fifth assessment technique. The examiner uses these techniques as an organizing framework for bringing the senses of sight, hearing, touch, and smell into focus. These techniques are

TABLE 8-1	Discriminating Areas of the Hands Used in Palpation	

Discriminating Sense	Sensitive Regions
Pulses	Fingertips
Fine tactile discrimination	
Skin texture	General differences: fingertips
	Fine discrimination: back of the hands and fingers
Position, shape, and consistency of a structure or mass	Fingertips using the grasping action of fingers and thumb
Vibration	Palmar aspects of the metacarpophalangeal joints (ball of the hand)
	Alternatively: ulnar side of the hand
Temperature	Dorsa of the hands or fingers (back of the hand)

From Talbot LA, Meyers-Marquardt M: *Pocket guide to critical care assessment*, ed. 3, St. Louis, 1997, Mosby.

explained further in the chapters that deal with their application to specific organs and systems.

Inspection

During **inspection** the examiner concentrates attention on a thorough and unhurried visualization of the client. Inspection also involves listening to any sounds coming from the client and being aware of any odors that may be present. The inexperienced examiner often moves too quickly to a "hands on" technique and may miss information that can be obtained only through careful observation. Up to 80% of diagnoses are based on data obtained from a history and inspection. Observing for body symmetry is one of the first steps in examining a body system (see Figures 14-8 and 19-14).

Lighting must be adequate for inspection. Either daylight or artificial light is suitable. Tangential lighting is a method of directing light from an adjustable lamp at a right angle to the area being observed. This technique produces shadows that are useful in assessing movements, such as abdominal pulsations, jugular vein distention, or precordial movement.

Palpation

In performing **palpation**, the skilled examiner uses the most sensitive parts of the hand for each type of palpation (Table 8-1). For example, pulses are best assessed using the third and fourth fingers, and vibrations are best felt with the palmar or ulnar surfaces of the hand. The examiner's hands should be warm, and the nails should be well-trimmed. Gloves should be worn for any examination of mucous membranes or any area where contact with body fluids or drainage is likely. Touch is used to examine the skin and

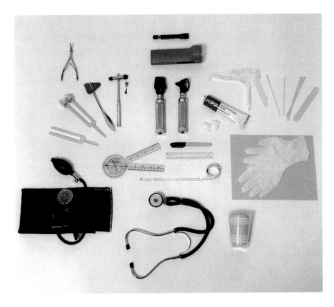

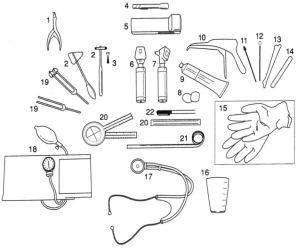

Figure 8-1 Equipment used during the physical examination. *1,* Nasal speculum; *2,* reflex hammer (two types shown); *3,* dull-end object for sensory examination; *4,* penlight; *5,* flashlight; *6,* ophthalmoscope; *7,* otoscope; *8,* cotton balls; *9,* lubricant; *10,* disposable vaginal speculum; *11,* cervical brush; *12,* cotton-tip applicator; *13,* cervical spatula; *14,* tongue depressor; *15,* disposable gloves; *16,* specimen cup; *17,* stethoscope; *18,* sphygmomanometer and blood pressure cuff; *19,* tuning fork (two types shown); *20,* centimeter ruler and goniometer; *21,* tape measure; *22,* marking pen.

hair for moisture and texture, to determine the extent of tenderness, and to note any tremor or spasm of muscle tissues. It is also used to elicit **crepitus**, or crackling, in bones and joints.

The examiner may palpate individual structures within body cavities, particularly the abdomen, for position, size,

■ HELPFUL HINT

Always palpate areas of tenderness last.

shape, consistency, and mobility. The examining hand can be used to detect masses. Palpation may also serve as a means of evaluating abnormal collections of fluid. Both light and deep palpation are used in the examination. Light palpation involves applying slight pressure to the area being examined to assess skin, tenderness, or pulsations. Deep pal-

pation is done to assess the size or contour of organs, such as the liver or kidney (see Figure 17-26). Light palpation should always be performed first because it is less likely to create discomfort for the client.

Percussion

Percussion involves tapping on the surface of the skin. This tapping creates a vibration of underlying organs and tissues that produce sound. For example, solids, liquids, and gases that are sufficiently elastic to convert energy to motion can transmit sound. Direct, or immediate, percussion is the striking of a finger or hand directly against the body. Indirect, or mediate, percussion is using the middle finger of the dominant hand (plexor) to strike against the middle finger (pleximeter) of the other hand immediately distal to the distal interphalangeal joint. Only the distal portion of the finger of the pleximeter hand is placed firmly against the skin. A crisp and sharp blow is delivered with the plexor at a 90-degree angle to the pleximeter. In Figure 8-2 the examiner is bracing the middle plexor finger with her index finger to provide more control when striking the pleximeter.

Wrist action of the plexor controls the speed and force of a blow. The wrist is flexed and then brought forward with a quick, snapping motion to deliver a fast strike and rapid removal of the plexor to avoiding dampening the vibration. The fingernails of the plexor finger must be kept short to avoid cutting the skin of the pleximeter. The vibration produced through percussion involves only the tissue adjacent (3 to 5 cm) to the pleximeter. Other examples of mediate percussion are shown in Figures 15-17, 17-13, and 17-16.

Fist percussion involves striking with the hand in a fisted position. The blow is delivered with the lateral aspect of the hand. The purpose of this type of percussion is to elicit sensation by the vibration of the tissue, which stimulates pain or tenderness of organs (e.g., liver, kidneys). Fist percussion may be direct or indirect. When indirect fist percussion is used, the blow is delivered to the dorsal surface of the opposite hand (see Figures 17-17 and 17-36).

The examiner evaluates the following characteristics of percussion sounds: intensity, pitch, and quality (Table 8-2).

Intensity

Intensity refers to the loudness of sound. As a sound wave travels, air molecules are compressed and then expanded in the wake of the compression wave. The difference between

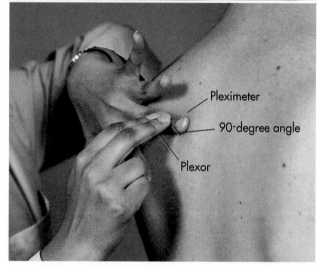

Figure 8-2 Indirect percussion. **A,** Positioning of the hands. **B,** Hand movement. The plexor blow to the pleximeter hand is delivered with a crisp, sharp wrist action.

TABLE 8-2 **Sounds Produced by Percussion**

Record of Finding	Intensity	Pitch	Quality	Example of Where Sounds May Be Heard
Tympany	Loud	High	Drumlike	Gastric air bubble
Hyperresonance	Very loud	Very low	Booming	Air-filled lungs (e.g., in emphysema)
Resonance	Loud	Low	Hollow	Normal lung
Dullness	Moderate	Moderate	Thudlike	Liver
Flatness	Soft	High	Flat	Muscle, bone

maximum pressure and minimum pressure is the amplitude of the sound wave. The greater the amplitude, the more movement will occur during vibration of the tympanic membrane, and the louder the perception of sound will be. Loudness is a subjective quality. The perception of loudness is affected by the attentiveness of the individual or competing sounds in the environment.

Pitch

Pitch is related to the frequency of sound. It is the number of vibrations of sound per second. The waveform of a sound of single frequency is sinusoidal,

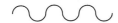

with perfectly matched peaks and valleys. The distance from one peak to the next is one cycle. The recording of frequency is done in cycles per second (cps) or hertz (Hz). The human ear can detect sounds in the frequency range of 20 to 20,000 Hz. With advancing age, the human ear becomes progressively less sensitive to the higher sound frequencies. The loss of the sounds of speech and music (300 to 3000 Hz) is most common in elderly persons.

Quality

The term *harmonic* refers to the physical property of sound that causes the effect called quality or *timbre*. The examiner records the quality in descriptive terms, such as humming, buzzing, or musical.

The more air that the tissue contains (i.e., the less dense the tissue), the deeper and louder the sound will be. The denser the tissue, the higher and fainter the sound will be. The examiner records sounds elicited in percussion in relation to the density of the tissue being vibrated. The least dense tissues produce **tympany**. Successively denser tissue results in hyperresonance, **resonance, dullness**, and flatness.

The change from resonance (less density) to dullness (greater density) is more easily perceived than the change from dullness to resonance. Thus percussion should be done from more resonant to less resonant areas.

Auscultation

Auscultation is the process of listening for the sounds that the human body produces. The particularly important sounds are those produced by (1) the thoracic and abdominal viscera and (2) the movement of blood in the cardiovascular system. Direct auscultation involves listening with the unassisted ear (i.e., without any amplifying device). However, auscultation is routinely done with a stethoscope, an instrument developed by René Laënnec in 1816. The purpose of the stethoscope is to exclude environmental sound and to augment internal sound.

The acoustic stethoscope is the type currently used (Figure 8-3). It is a closed cylinder that captures sound waves produced by the sound source. The diaphragm of the stethoscope is most effective in assessing high-frequency sounds, such as breath and bowel sounds. The diaphragm is applied

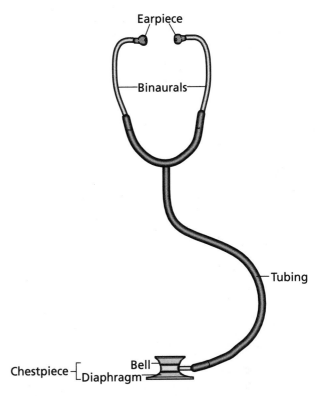

Figure 8-3 Parts of a stethoscope. (From Potter PA, Perry AG: *Basic nursing: a critical thinking approach*, ed. 4, St. Louis, 1999, Mosby.)

firmly to the skin so that it creates a seal between the skin surface and the diaphragm (see Figure 16-25).

The bell-type head of the stethoscope is most effective in detecting low-frequency sounds, such as vascular sounds or blood pressure (see Figures 16-26 and 16-28). It is important to avoid pressing the bell too firmly on the skin surface because stretching the skin inhibits vibration by actually converting the tissue to a diaphragm. The bell chestpiece should be wide enough to span an intercostal space in an adult and deep enough so that it will not fill with tissue.

Several sizes of earpieces are supplied with better stethoscopes. The examiner should determine which size fits his or her ear most snugly. The earpiece should occlude the external meatus, thus blocking extraneous sound. However, the earpiece should not cause the examiner pain. The binaurals (metal tubing) are angled slightly toward the nose of the wearer to project the sound onto the tympanic membrane. The direction of the angle may be adjusted by the tension spring. The tubing should not be longer than 30 to 35 cm to minimize sound distortion. Longer tubing increases the chance of diminishing the sound.

> ### ■ HELPFUL HINT
> Don't wear a stethoscope backwards. Make sure the earpieces, when held in front of you, angle forward.

TABLE 8-3   Positions for Examination

Position	Areas Assessed	Rationale	Limitations
Sitting	Head and neck, back, posterior thorax and lungs, anterior thorax and lungs, breasts, axillae, heart, vital signs, and upper extremities	Sitting upright provides full expansion of lungs and provides better visualization of symmetry of upper body parts.	Physically weakened client may be unable to sit. Examiner should use supine position with head of bed elevated instead.
Supine	Head and neck, anterior thorax and lungs, breasts, axillae, heart, abdomen, extremities, pulses	This is most normally relaxed position. It provides easy access to pulse sites.	If client becomes short of breath easily, examiner may need to raise head of bed.
Dorsal recumbent	Head and neck, anterior thorax and lungs, breasts, axillae, heart, abdomen	Position is used for abdominal assessment because it promotes relaxation of abdominal muscles.	Clients with painful disorders are more comfortable with knees flexed.
Lithotomy*	Female genitalia and genital tract	This position provides maximal exposure of genitalia and facilitates insertion of vaginal speculum.	Lithotomy position is embarrassing and uncomfortable, so examiner minimizes time that client spends in it. Client is kept well draped.
Sims'	Rectum and vagina	Flexion of hip and knee improves exposure of rectal area.	Joint deformities may hinder client's ability to bend hip and knee.
Prone	Musculoskeletal system	This position is used only to assess extension of hip joint.	This position is poorly tolerated in clients with respiratory difficulties.
Lateral recumbent	Heart	This position aids in detecting murmurs.	This position is poorly tolerated in clients with respiratory difficulties.
Knee-chest*	Rectum	This position provides maximal exposure of rectal area.	This position is embarrassing and uncomfortable.

From Potter PA, Perry AG: *Basic nursing: theory and practice*, ed. 3, St. Louis, 1995, Mosby.
*Clients with arthritis or other joint deformities may be unable to assume this position.

Auscultation can also be done using a Doppler monitor. A Doppler monitor is a battery-operated instrument that is placed on the body surface to amplify quiet sounds. A seal is created between the skin and the instrument with a water-soluble gel. A Doppler monitor is commonly used to listen to fetal heart tones and peripheral pulses not easily detected by palpation (Figure 8-4).

Special Maneuvers—Positioning

Positioning the client can help in using the four modalities described here. For example, positioning the client in a right side-lying position will aid in palpating the spleen. Positioning also makes certain body areas more accessible to the examiner. Table 8-3 summarizes the positions used for assessing different body parts. The inability of a client to as-

Examination Step-by-Step

The techniques of examination to assess the lungs include the following steps:
1. Inspection
2. Palpation
3. Percussion
4. Auscultation
5. Positioning the client to maximally expose an area for examination

sume a position may be an important objective finding. For example, the inability to lie flat may be a sign of a cardiovascular or pulmonary problem.

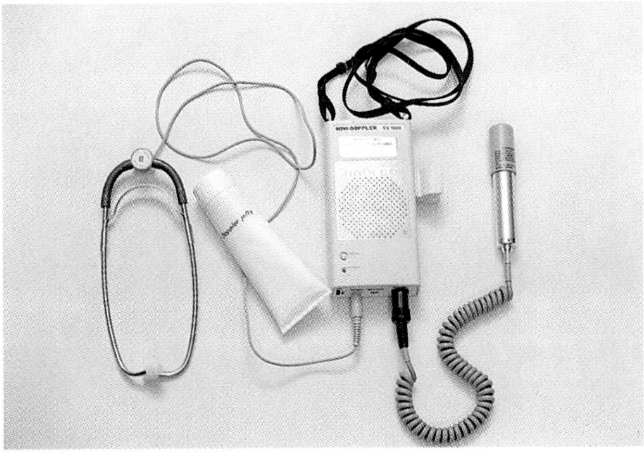

Special Populations

The examiner needs to adapt his or her approach to the physical examination for special populations. For a client with a cognitive deficit, the presence of a familiar person may help to ensure cooperation during the examination. For a client who is wheelchair bound, most of the physical examination can be performed with the client sitting. Assistance may be needed for the client to assume a standing or supine position. The physical examination will need to be modified for

Figure 8-4 Doppler. (From Seidel HM et al.: *Mosby's guide to physical examination,* ed. 4, St. Louis, 1999, Mosby.)

an unconscious client who will not be able to follow instructions. For a bed-ridden client, most of the examination can be performed in supine and side-lying positions. The length of the examination needs to correlate with the client's mental and physical levels of tolerance. For example, recovery from brain damage is often associated with fatigue. A client in acute pain may not be able to cooperate with the examiner's instructions (see also Chapter 28).

? Critical Thinking Questions

1. Name three purposes of the physical examination.
2. Demonstrate direct and indirect percussion. Give an example of when would you use each technique. How would you describe the findings of percussion over puffed-out cheeks? Lungs? The anterior surface of the thigh?

3. What are the uses for the bell and the diaphragm of a stethoscope? Describe the specific techniques for using each of these stethoscope heads.
4. A client who is in the office for a general physical examination tells you that he has a sore right knee. How will you apply the basic principles of conducting a physical examination to determine the sequence of the examination?

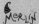 Answers are available on the MERLIN website (www.harcourthealth.com/MERLIN/Barkauskas/). And be sure to check the website regularly for additional learning activities!

Remember to check out the Online Study Guide!
www.harcourthealth.com/MERLIN/Barkauskas/

General Assessment, Including Vital Signs

Learning Objectives

On successful study of this chapter and completion of related learning experiences, the learner will be able to:

- Identify components of the assessment for general appearance.

- Describe the steps in accurate assessment of temperature, respiration, pulses, and blood pressure.
- Name three conditions related to variations in blood pressure.

Outline

Purpose of Examination

A physical examination should be tailored for the client's individual needs. A complete physical examination is done for (1) health promotion and disease prevention purposes, (2) a preoperative evaluation, and (3) when a more complete database is needed for diagnosing or planning treatment. After interviewing the client and obtaining subjective data from the health history, the examiner proceeds to the physical examination. Physical examination will provide the objective measurements of health assessment.

The examiner's observations and measurements are essential in verifying the client's description of symptoms and in identifying signs or objective findings. The tools of physical assessment also allow the examiner to explore facets not usually available to the client. Conclusions about an individual's health status are drawn from synthesizing information from the client's description and the examiner's assessment.

GENERAL INSPECTION

General inspection is the first step in performing an initial screening examination. The steps for performing an initial screening examination are listed in Box 9-1. Begin by observing the client entering the room, during introductions, and as he or she follows instructions before the interview begins. *General observation* is the overall impression given by the client's general state of health and outstanding characteristics.

Inspect the client from head to toe. Inspection is a more detailed observation that includes smell, hearing, and touch, as well as visual inspection. Make observations only in good light, particularly when assessing skin color.

Make every attempt to concentrate on the person being examined. With practice and by carefully guarding against distractions, either from the environment or unrelated thoughts, you will learn to become completely absorbed with the client. Total and focused concentration on the client allows the examiner to process information using all sensory modalities.

■ HELPFUL HINT

Give the client total attention. Do not allow yourself to be interrupted to take phone calls or to be distracted by other responsibilities. Consider the time with the client as precious.

The general observations continue throughout the interview. In some cases, the initial impression sets the focus of the interview and the physical examination. For instance, some feature of the client's appearance may point immediately to the problem. Slow speech and a hoarse voice, for example, may indicate the need to look further for the dry skin and sluggish movements of hypothyroidism.

Although the initial inspection is a scanning procedure, the astute practitioner gathers information that may be used as the basis for planning portions of the examination that deserve special attention.

ASSESSMENT OF BODY MORPHOLOGY AND GAIT

Body Types

Although body **morphology**, or the size and physical shape of a person, is to some degree genetically determined, the environment (e.g., exercise and diet) plays a significant role in altering body type. Variations in body shape and content are shown in Figure 9-1.

Mesomorphic Type

The **mesomorphic** body type is characterized by average height, well-developed musculature, wide shoulders with a subcostal angle that is approximately a right angle, and a flat abdomen.

Ectomorphic Type

The **ectomorphic** body build is often described as tall and willowy. The musculature and subcutaneous fat are poorly developed. The extremity bones are long and thin. The clavicles, ribs, and spinous processes protrude because of the deficient subcutaneous fat. The chest is long and narrow. Because abdominal muscles are not as well-developed, the abdominal wall may sag outward. The neck is long.

Endomorphic Type

The **endomorphic** body build is short, stocky, and the most likely of the body types to be obese. The neck is short and thick. The extremities are large and sturdy. Compared with the mesomorphic and ectomorphic types, the chest is shorter and broader and the costal margin is a wider angle (obtuse). Fat distribution in the endomorphic body type can be described as "apple shape" if the fattest area is the waistline; "pear shape" refers to fat distribution that is greatest in the hips, thighs, and buttocks. An apple shape is associated with a greater risk of heart disease.

Symmetry

The arrangement of most structures of the human body is symmetrical; that is, the size and shape of right and left structures correspond. If inspection reveals areas that obviously lack symmetry, note this and investigate it later.

Posture

Posture is a part of body image. Good body alignment is a sign of good health. Correct posture is the position in which minimum stress is applied to each joint. Minimum muscular effort is required to maintain an upright posture, which is achieved when the line of the center of gravity bisects the principal weight-bearing joints and is the same distance from each foot. Frequent changes of posture are necessary for comfort. Good posture depends on a normal sense of bal-

---

B O X 9 - 1

SCREENING EXAMINATION

Steps for performing an initial screening:
1. Working from head to toe, perform a general inspection for an overall impression of the client's apparent state of health, outstanding characteristics, and signs of distress.
2. Note the apparent age, sex, race, body type, stature and symmetry, weight and nutritional status, posture and motor activity, and general skin condition.
3. When establishing verbal exchange, note the client's apparent mental status and characteristics of speech.
4. Assess the vital signs. Take the temperature, pulse, respiratory rate, and blood pressure, using the techniques of inspection, palpation, and auscultation, and percussion.

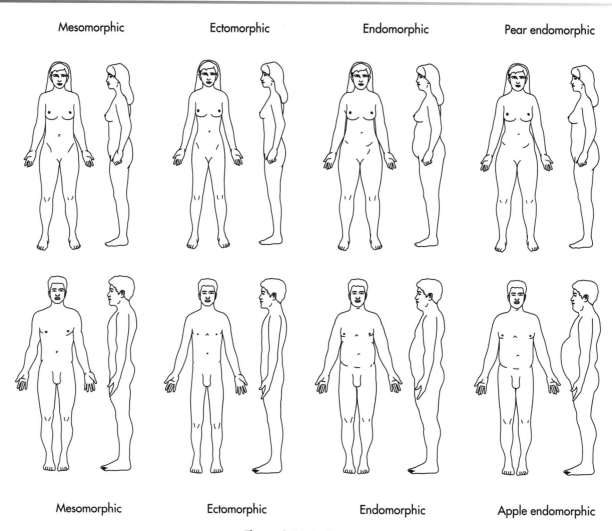

Figure 9-1   Body types.

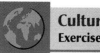

Cultural Considerations
Exercise Influences

Some evidence points to appropriate exercise as an aid to maintaining erect posture. Chinese shadowboxing exercises are purported to maintain body awareness and erect posture despite advancing years.

ance and muscular coordination. Faulty posture is any position that increases stress to joints (Figure 9-2). Posture can be altered by pain, injury, or psychological state.

Aging and Posture

Bone and joint changes contribute to the bent posture often seen in the elderly. Joint degeneration and osteoporosis occur with aging. Aging changes, such as widening and flattening of the third cervical vertebrae and drying of the intervertebral disks, may result in a decrease from baseline adult height of as much as 2 to 3 cm (1 to 1.5 inches).

Although all muscles decline in girth and strength with aging, the muscles of the trunk are particularly affected. Weakness of the abdominal muscles also contributes to the slumped posture of the elderly.

Gait

The phases of normal **gait** are stance and swing (Figure 9-3). The stance phase occurs when the foot is on the ground and bearing weight. The lower leg supports the body weight, and the body advances over the supporting limb. The five components of stance are (1) initial contact, (2) loading response, (3) midstance, (4) terminal stance, and (5) preswing.

The normal heel strike is quiet and smoothly coordinated with the knee extended. The loading response, the movement to full contact of the foot with the floor, should be complete and proceed smoothly. The midstance of the foot is the shift of weight onto the foot. The weight should be supported evenly by all aspects of the foot, and the knee is slightly flexed. In the terminal stance, the metatarsal pushoff is a smoothly coordinated lift off the floor. The swing phase

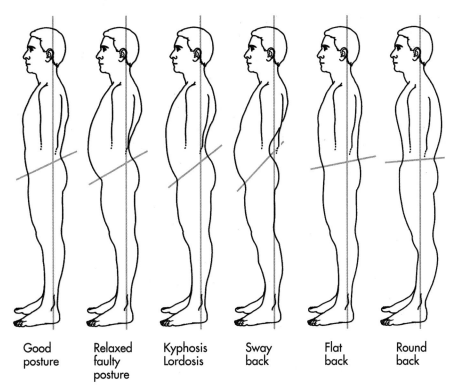

Good posture | Relaxed faulty posture | Kyphosis Lordosis | Sway back | Flat back | Round back

Figure 9-2 Good posture and types of faulty posture.

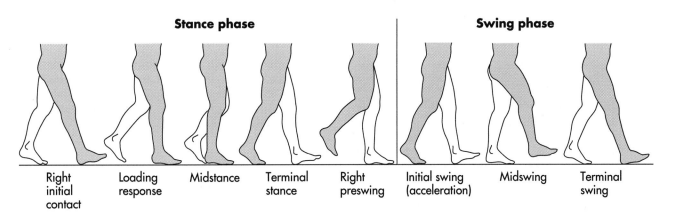

Stance phase   **Swing phase**

Right initial contact | Loading response | Midstance | Terminal stance | Right preswing | Initial swing (acceleration) | Midswing | Terminal swing

Figure 9-3 Stance and swing phase of gait. (Modified from Magee DJ: *Orthopedic physical assessment*, ed. 3, Philadelphia, 1997, WB Saunders.)

occurs when the foot is non–weight bearing and moving forward. The swing phase allows the toes to clear the floor and the swing leg to advance forward.

Technique for Assessment of Posture and Gait

Develop a protocol for observing the main postures of the body in all its common acts. Watch the client come into the room and sit down, and observe while the client lies on the examining table. It is important to note whether the client sits tensely or slumps in the chair.

The characteristics of the client's walk provide clues to the client's problems. Ask the client to walk a straight line

for a short distance both toward and away from you. Note the speed of the client's step, as well as the smoothness and style of movement.

ASSESSMENT OF GENERAL APPEARANCE

Weight

Weight is sometimes considered a vital sign because unexplained weight loss is an early sign of illness. Aging and a sedentary lifestyle contribute to weight gain. Body fat distribution changes with age; abdominal and truncal fat increases, and the extremities thin.

Adipose deposition varies by gender. Women have fat deposits over the shoulders, breasts, buttocks or lateral aspect of the thighs, and pubic symphysis. The fat deposits in men are more evenly dispersed throughout the body.

An essential part of the assessment of children or anyone who has not completed the growth cycle is the accurate, serial measurement of height and weight. Growth charts (see Figure 26-21), which are assembled from data gathered from large populations, allow the examiner to compare an individual client's pattern of growth with national standards. Body mass index (BMI) is a measure based on height and weight that places an adult into underweight, normal, overweight, or obese weight categories (see Chapter 6).

Hair Growth Patterns

Hair growth is influenced by hereditary and racial factors. Excessive hairiness is thought to be a dominant hereditary trait related to the presence of androgens, whereas thinning or absent hair is a recessive trait.

Hair grows at various rates. The most rapid rate of growth is that of the beard, followed by that of the scalp, axillae, thighs, and eyebrows. The rate of hair growth is affected by environmental temperature and by the general state of health. Exposure to extremely cold temperatures impedes hair growth.

A heavier distribution of hair is correlated with darker hair pigmentation (i.e., the brunette individual is more likely to have more hair than the blonde person).

Cultural Considerations
Hair Growth Variations

Caucasian persons have more abundant and coarser body hair than Asians. Facial hirsutism, or excessive hair growth, occurs in more than 40% of Caucasian women. Asian women, on the other hand, do not develop excessive facial hair growth, and Asian men have sparser beards than Caucasian men. African-Americans have kinky hair, whereas Caucasians have straight or wavy-to-curly hair. Native Americans have straight hair.

Some male hair growth characteristics may be normal for women of certain ethnic or familial groups and could include sideburns; hair growth on the upper lip, abdomen, and lower limbs; and hair growth around the areola of the breasts (see also Chapter 10).

Alopecia (balding) is more frequently noted in individuals with abundant coarse-hair growth on the body. Alopecia is thought to be related to androgen production. Male pattern baldness is recession of the hairline and baldness of the crown (see Figure 10-8). As a rule, women do not bald unless androgens are present in relatively increased amounts or the baldness occurs as a result of disease or chemotherapy.

Technique for Assessment of General Appearance

Weight

Weigh the client and measure his or her height to calculate the BMI (see Chapter 6). Record weight in kilograms or pounds and height in centimeters or inches, depending on the requirements of the particular setting.

■ HELPFUL HINT

Weigh the client with or without clothes; however, record whether the client was clothed. The client should not wear shoes when height is measured.

Hair

Inspect for hair growth on the following body regions: scalp, face, ears, thoracic area, lower limbs, genital area, lumbosacral area, upper back, midphalangeal area, pubis, and axillae. Observe hair for growth characteristics, distribution, density of growth, appearance, and hygiene.

Nails

The nails may indicate the level of concern and care the client has for appearance. Inspect the nails for length, cleanliness, neatness of filing, and the presence of polish. Inspection of the nail is obscured in women who use artificial nails

TABLE 9-1	Association of Breath Odors to Disease		
	Breath Odor	**Description**	**Associated Condition**
	Halitosis, foul	Odor of necrotic tissue	Pyorrhea
			Poor dental hygiene
			Tonsillitis
			Sinusitis
			Lung abscess
			Bronchiectasis
	Feculent	Odor of feces	Bowel obstruction
	Fetor hepaticus	"Fishy" odor	Hepatic failure
	Acid	Odor of acid	Peptic disease
	Ammonia	Odor of urine	Renal failure
	Acetone	Odor of acetone ("fruity")	Diabetic ketoacidosis
	Bitter almonds	Odor of almonds	Cyanide poisoning

that are glued to the nailbed. Note the texture, thickness, and contour.

Personal Hygiene

General cleanliness of the body is an important indication of the individual's self-esteem and access to necessary supplies to maintain good body care. Standards of cleanliness are a sociocultural value. Deodorants are not used in all cultures. Although shaving the legs is a common practice in some groups of women in the United States, it is not practiced by all women. However, although norms may vary, poor personal hygiene can indicate serious mental or physical illness.

Odors

Note odor of the body and breath. The smell of alcohol on the client's breath should alert one to look for other effects of alcohol, a central nervous system (CNS) depressant. Foul breath points to the possibility of an oral or pulmonary infection or may simply be the result of poor oral hygiene. The odor of ammonia may be detectable in the patient with uremia. Body odor may be related to the activities of the sweat and sebaceous glands and to the general cleanliness of the body.

The odors emanating from the client may provide clues helpful in defining the client's condition. Some diseases are characterized by particular mouth odors. The odors known to have diagnostic importance are listed in Table 9-1.

Manner of Dress

Note the fit of clothing, as well as its appropriateness to the season or room temperature. General grooming may provide clues to the client's socioeconomic condition, as well as ego strength and self-image. If a client is unshaven or unwashed, this may be a sign of self-neglect or neglect by relatives or others on whom the client is dependent. Carefully note such signs of neglect.

ASSESSMENT OF VITAL SIGNS

The most common clinical measurements made by the health practitioner are temperature, pulse, respiratory rate, and blood pressure. Because these measures provide such valuable data about the client's state of health, they have been termed the **vital** or **cardinal signs**. Obtain vital signs at the beginning of any examination.

Variations from the client's baseline values or from the previous measurement are clinically significant. The client's baseline measures are important because there is considerable variability among individuals. The examiner assesses vital signs to establish a database; data obtained on future occasions may then be compared with baseline values.

Bear in mind that your manner of approach to the client may alter the client's vital signs, especially if the client reacts emotionally to your actions. For instance, a curt, impatient, rude interaction or awkward handling of the instruments may upset the client, increasing the pulse rate, respiration rate, blood pressure, and even temperature if the interaction is prolonged.

Temperature

For most individuals the optimum temperature for metabolic function of all cells of the human body is 37° C (98.6° F). The core temperature of the body is maintained within very narrow limits. The normal ranges for temperature are 36.4° to 37.2° C (97.5° to 99° F). Factors that influence temperature are described in Box 9-2.

Temperature Regulation

Body temperature is an excellent example of both **homeostasis** and biological rhythms (Figure 9-4). The hypothalamus serves as the body's thermostat. Two hypothalamic centers trigger heat-dissipating or heat-conserving mechanisms.

BOX 9-2

FACTORS INFLUENCING TEMPERATURE

Biological rhythms are reflected in temperature assessment (Figure 9-4). Diurnal variations of up to 1° C are observed; the trough, or low point, occurs in the hours before waking; the peak occurs in the late afternoon or early evening.

Hormones can increase temperature. Increased secretion of thyroid hormone increases body temperature. Progesterone secretion at the time of ovulation correlates with temperature increases of 0.5° C, which continue until the menses.

Environment affects temperature. Body temperature is altered little by seasonal changes in temperature. Hot and cold baths produce temporary changes in temperature.

Exercise increases body temperature because of the physiological changes incurred.

Eating food is associated with a rise in temperature as a result of the specific dynamic action (SDA) of the food.

Age is a factor in temperature assessment. Because heat control mechanisms are not as well-established in the child as in the adult, considerable variation in a child's temperature may occur. Normal body temperature declines with age, from 37.2° C (99.0° F) in young children, to 37° C (98.6° F) in adults, to 36° C (96.8° F) in older adults.

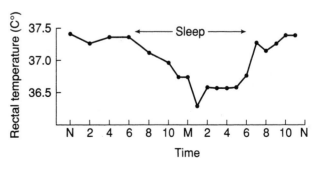

Figure 9-4 Biological rhythms for temperature in a 24-hour cycle. (From Mountcastle VB: *Medical physiology*, vol. 2, ed. 14, St. Louis, 1980, Mosby.)

The delivery of overwarmed blood to thermoreceptors in the anterior hypothalamus results in sweating and redistribution of blood, which dilates surface capillaries and causes flushing. Temperature loss from the skin occurs when blood flow to the skin increases and sweat evaporates. This heat loss is related to the temperature difference between the skin and external environment.

Conduction, convection, radiation, and evaporation are the physical phenomena involved in temperature regulation. **Conduction** is heat loss from the object of higher temperature to the object of lower temperature, such as when a client is bathed in cool water. **Convection** is the loss of heat to the molecules of air, especially to moving air from a fan or breeze. Conduction and convection occur only when the ambient temperature is lower than the body temperature.

Radiation is the loss of heat by electromagnetic infrared waves. The radiation does not heat the air through which it passes. Heat radiates from the skin to a cooler environment, such as skin in contact with an ice bag. **Evaporation** is the conversion of liquid (sweat) to gaseous form. Vaporization of perspiration depends on ambient humidity and does not occur when air is very humid.

Heat-conserving mechanisms are activated when overcooled blood is delivered to thermoreceptors in the posterior hypothalamus. These mechanisms include reducing blood flow to the distal extremities and constricting peripheral capillary beds (blanching). Compensatory heat production is enhanced both at the metabolic level (nonshivering thermogenesis) and through voluntary muscle contraction and shivering. Shivering occurs when vasoconstriction is ineffective in preventing heat loss.

Temperature Acclimatization

Clients who have spent a good deal of time in very cold climates show an increased ability to tolerate cold. These individuals show (1) an increased metabolic rate with increased rates of secretion of thyroid hormones, (2) reduction in shivering, and (3) an increased rate of hair growth.

Adaptation to heat changes the secretion of sweat. The amount of sweat produced declines from the profuse, dripping, early response to a quantity that will evaporate on reaching the air.

Temperature Recording

Record body temperature in degrees Celsius (°C) or in degrees Fahrenheit (°F) according to the protocol of the practice setting. The metric system is generally the preferred system in health care.

To convert Celsius to Fahrenheit, subtract 32 and divide by 1.8. To convert Fahrenheit to Celsius, multiply by 1.8 and add 32.

Figure 9-5 equates Fahrenheit and Celsius temperatures in the compatible range for human survival.

Technique for Temperature Measurement and Normal Findings

For accurate temperature measurement, insert the glass or electronic thermometer properly, and leave it in place for the recommended length of time. Explain to the client what is

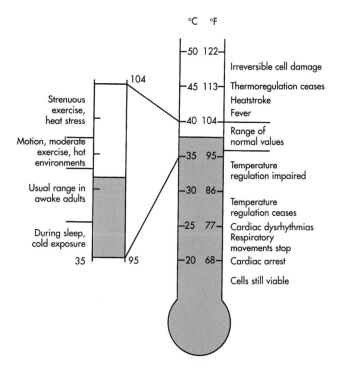

Figure 9-5   Body temperature. Diagram, modeled after a thermometer, shows some physiological consequences of an abnormal body temperature. The normal range of body temperature under various conditions is shown in the inset. (From Thibodeau GA, Patton KT: *Anatomy and physiology*, ed. 4, St. Louis, 1999, Mosby.)

BOX 9-3

PROPER PLACEMENT OF A THERMOMETER

ORAL TEMPERATURE

1. Ask the client to open his or her mouth and to place the tip of the tongue against the upper teeth.
2. Insert the thermometer tip gently under the tongue between the frenulum and the lower gum.
3. Leave in place at least 3 minutes.

RECTAL TEMPERATURE

1. Assist the client to a lateral position with the upper leg flexed.
2. Separate the buttocks to view the anus while instructing the client to breathe deeply.
3. Insert the lubricated thermometer 3 to 4 cm for an adult and 1 to 2 cm for an infant.
4. Leave in place at least 2 minutes.

AXILLARY TEMPERATURE

1. Insert the thermometer into the center of the axilla, and lower the client's arm over the thermometer.
2. Fold the client's arm over his or her chest to keep the thermometer in place.
3. Leave in place at least 5 minutes in children and longer in adults.

being done. Three types of glass thermometers are oral thermometers with a slender tip, stubby thermometers with a short tip used for axillary temperatures, and rectal thermometers with a blunt end to prevent trauma when inserted. Box 9-3 describes the proper placement of a thermometer.

Oral Temperature.   The oral temperature is the most convenient method for registering body temperature in the alert, adult client. Normal oral temperature in adults is 37° C (98.6° F). Wait 15 minutes before taking a temperature if the client has smoked or ingested hot or iced liquids. Place an oral glass mercury thermometer in the mouth for 3 to 5 minutes, although the oral thermometer may take as long as 7 minutes to reach maximum temperature. An electronic thermometer has the advantages of registering temperature within 30 seconds and reducing risk of mercury spills.

Rectal Temperature.   The rectal site for registering temperature is preferable for the client who is confused or comatose, is unable to close his or her mouth, or is receiving oxygen. The normal rectal temperature in adults is 37.5° C (99.5° F). The lubricated thermometer placed in the rectum will register within 2 minutes.

Axillary Temperature.   The axillary method is safe and accurate for infants and small children but is not often used with adult clients unless oral and rectal routes are not accessible. The normal axillary temperature in adults is 36.5° C (97.7° F). It can take up to 10 minutes for the full registration of axillary temperature in adults and about 5 minutes in children.

Tympanic Temperature.   Tympanic thermography is a noninvasive technique for assessment of body temperature. It uses an infrared sensor to detect the temperature of blood flowing through the eardrum. The probe tip is shaped like the end of an otoscope, the instrument used to examine the ear. The tympanic thermometer registers an electronic display within 2 seconds (Figure 9-6).

Respiration

Use inspection to assess the rate and effort of respirations. Observe for chest or abdominal movement to assess the rate. Count respirations that occur at regular intervals for 15 seconds and multiply by 4. In most adults the resting respiratory rate is 12 to 20 breaths per minute. For irregular respiratory patterns, the rate may need to be assessed for a longer time—30 seconds to 1 minute. For clients whose respirations are difficult to observe, lightly place your hand on the client's upper chest to assess the rate. (see also Figure 15-12).

Pulses

General assessment usually includes assessment of the peripheral (radial) or apical **pulse** for rate, rhythm, and volume. The nature of the peripheral pulse gives an indication of cardiac function and perfusion of the peripheral tissues. Use pads of the second and third fingers to assess pulses. Never use the thumb for palpation since it may be less sensitive.

Pulse Rate

The adult heart rate is between 50 and 100 beats per minute. Table 9-2 shows normal variations in pulse rate by age. The pulse rate is lowest in the early morning and most rapid in the late afternoon and evening. When obtaining baseline data, count the pulse rate for 1 full minute to accurately evaluate the rate, rhythm, and volume. Normal rhythm is an even tempo. For subsequent measurements, count 15 to 30 seconds and multiply by 4 and 2 respectively, if pulses are regular. Auscultate the apical pulse for 1 minute if irregularities are felt. Place the diaphragm of the stethoscope over the chest area palpated to have the strongest impulse and count each pair of "lub dub" sounds as one pulse (see also Figure 16-25).

Pulse Volume

Pulse volume represents the strength of left ventricular contraction, or stroke volume. Estimate pulse volume from the feel of the vessel as blood flows through it with each heartbeat. **Bounding** is the descriptive term used to describe the full pulse that is difficult to depress with the fingertips. The normal pulse is easily palpable, does not fade in and out, and

TABLE 9-2	Age Variations in Pulse Rate
Age	**Pulse Rate (beats/min)**
Infants	120-160
Toddlers	90-140
Preschoolers	80-140
School agers	80-130
Adolescent	60-90
Adult	60-100
Conditioned athlete	50

Modified from Hazinski MF: Children are different. In Hazinski MF, editor: *Nursing care of the critically ill child*, St. Louis, 1984, Mosby; and Kinney MR et al.: *AACN's clinical reference for critical care nursing*, ed. 3, St. Louis, 1993, Mosby. In Potter PA, Perry AG: *Basic nursing: a critical thinking approach*, ed. 4, St. Louis, 1999, Mosby.

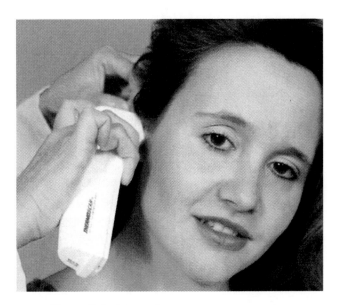

Figure 9-6 Tympanic temperature measurement.

is not easily obliterated. "Weak," "feeble," and "thready" are descriptive words for the pulse of a vessel with low volume. The artery with low volume is readily compressed.

Pulse volume can also be graded on force or amplitude using the following four-point scale:

4+	bounding
3+	increased
2+	normal
1+	weak
0	absent

Technique for Assessment of Vital Signs

The modalities used to assess vital signs include inspection, palpation, auscultation, and the use of instruments to obtain specific measures of physiological functioning.

Inspection

Inspect for changes in color, such as the flush of fever, the pallor in response to cold, or the dusky blueness of cyanosis.

Palpation

Palpation to Assess Body Temperature.   Palpate to determine temperature using the dorsal aspect of your hand or fingers, which are more sensitive to temperature variation. Palpation may reveal moisture and texture variations, as well as the vibration of shivering.

Palpation to Assess Arterial Pulses.   The pulse is best palpated over arteries that are close to the surface of the body and that lie over a bony surface. Feel bilateral pulses simultaneously to assess symmetry.

Radial Pulse.   Clinicians most frequently use the radial pulse to initially assess the rate and rhythm of pulsation, the pattern of pulsation, and the shape (consistency) of the arterial wall. The examiner has easy access to this pulse. Other pulses in the upper extremity that are easy to evaluate are the ulnar and brachial pulses (Figure 9-7).

Evaluate the radial pulse by placing the pads of your first and second fingers on the palmar surface of the client's relaxed and slightly flexed wrist medial to the radius bone (Figure 9-8). (Occasionally the arteries run in a deeper and

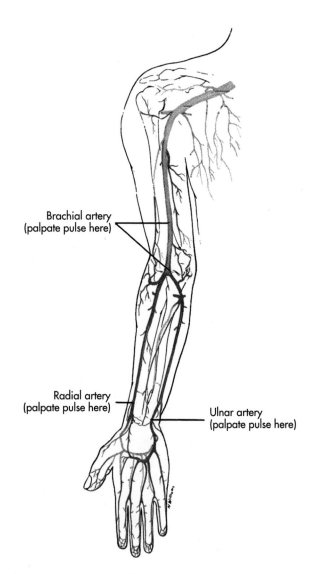

Brachial artery (palpate pulse here)

Radial artery (palpate pulse here)

Ulnar artery (palpate pulse here)

Figure 9-7   Arteries of the upper extremity. (Modified from Francis CC, Martin AH: *Introduction to human anatomy*, ed. 7, St. Louis, 1975, Mosby.)

BOX 9-4

NORMAL VARIATIONS IN BLOOD PRESSURE

Blood pressure varies continually with respiration, autonomic state, emotional levels, and biological rhythms. Furthermore, successive readings of indirect measures of blood pressure by the same or different observers may differ by as much as 10 mm Hg.

The change from a supine to an erect position causes a slight decrease in systolic blood pressure (less than 15 mm Hg) and a slight rise in diastolic pressure (less than 5 mm Hg).

The blood pressure also shows a circadian pattern; it is higher in the afternoon and evening hours and lower in the late hours of sleep.

Because blood pressure is readily altered by stressful events, an effort should be made to relax the client as much as possible before taking the blood pressure.

The blood pressure in the arm increases when the arm is lower than the level of the heart; conversely, raising the arm above the level of the heart lowers the blood pressure. If you are measuring a standing blood pressure, rest the elbow of the client's arm in your hand, with the weight of his or her forearm on your arm.

more lateral course.) Exert sufficient pressure to occlude the artery during diastole yet allow the vessel to return to normal contour during systole.

Brachial Pulse.   The brachial pulse is palpated and auscultated as part of the blood pressure evaluation. Palpate the pulse over the antecubital fossa (anterior surface of the elbow joint). The brachial artery is medial to the biceps tendon.

The major pulses of the lower extremities are palpated over the femoral, popliteal, dorsalis pedis, and posterior tibial arteries (Figure 9-9). Palpate the femoral pulse midway between the anterosuperior iliac crest and the symphysis pubis, below and medial to the inguinal ligament. Palpate the popliteal pulse by pressing deeply into the dorsal aspect of the knee while the knee is slightly bent. Palpate the dorsalis pedis pulse by applying light touch about midway between the ankle and toes on the dorsum of the foot. Palpate the posterior tibial pulse slightly below and posterior to the medial malleolus of the ankle (Figure 9-10).

Blood Pressure

Anatomy and Physiology

Blood pressure is the result of the interaction of cardiac output and peripheral resistance and is dependent on the velocity of the arterial blood, the intravascular volume, and the elasticity of the arterial walls (see Box 9-4 for normal variations in blood pressure). Arterial pressure is the force exerted

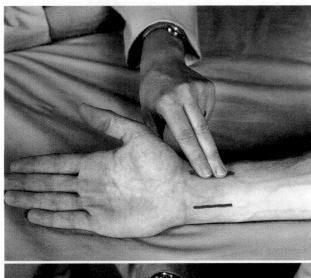

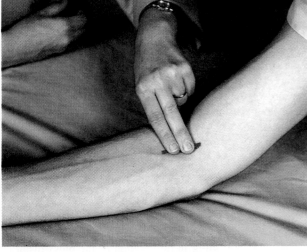

Figure 9-8   A, Palpation of the radial pulse. The site for palpation of the ulnar artery is also marked. **B,** Palpation of the brachial pulse.

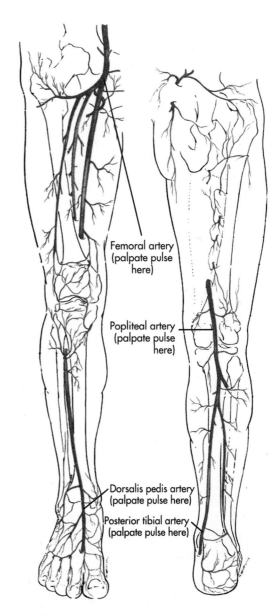

Figure 9-9 Location of pulses for palpation. (From Francis CC, Martin AH: *Introduction to human anatomy,* ed. 7, St. Louis, 1975, Mosby.)

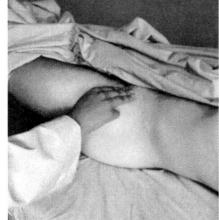

A

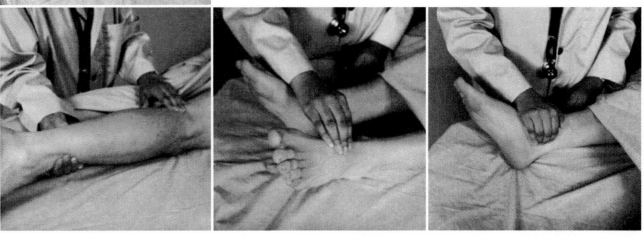

Figure 9-10 Palpation of various pulses. **A**, Femoral pulse. **B**, Popliteal pulse. **C**, Dorsal pedal pulse. **D**, Posterior tibial pulse.

B   C   D

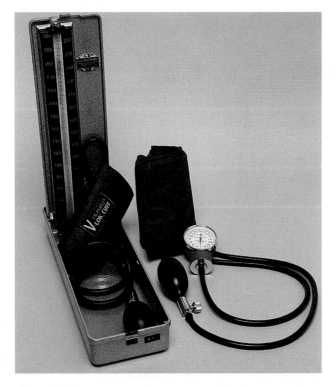

Figure 9-11 Mercury column and aneroid sphygmomanometers. (From Potter PA, Perry AG: *Basic nursing: a critical thinking approach*, ed. 4, St. Louis, 1999, Mosby.)

by the blood against the wall of the artery as the heart contracts and relaxes. **Systolic (systole)** blood pressure is the force exerted against the wall of the artery when the ventricles are contracting, and **diastolic (diastole)** blood pressure is the force of the blood when the heart is in the filling phase and the ventricles are relaxed. **Pulse pressure** is the difference between the systolic and diastolic blood pressures. The usual pulse pressure is between 30 and 40 mm Hg.

The examiner may assess the systemic arterial blood pressure by direct or indirect methods. The direct method requires the insertion of a small tube called a *cannula* directly into the artery. The cannula is then attached to a manometer to obtain a blood pressure reading. The direct technique is used in critical care settings. Indirect blood pressure measurement can be made without opening the artery.

Indirect Measurement of Blood Pressure

Indirect measurement of blood pressure takes into account the following: (1) the arterial wall may be occluded by direct pressure, resulting in obliteration of the pulse distal to the compression, and (2) oscillations that vary directly with the amount of applied pressure may be measured from the compressed artery.

The most commonly used method of indirect assessment of blood pressure is the auscultatory technique. The proper

BOX 9-5

BLOOD PRESSURE EQUIPMENT

A *stethoscope* is used to listen to sounds produced by each type of the blood pressure measurement devices described in the following paragraphs.

The *mercury column manometer* is a straight glass tube connected to a reservoir of mercury. The reservoir in turn is connected to the pressure bulb so that pressure created on the bulb causes the mercury to rise in the tube. Because the weight of mercury depends on gravity, a given amount of pressure will always support a column of mercury of the same height if the tube is straight and of uniform diameter. The mercury manometer does not need further calibration after the initial setting.

The *aneroid sphygmomanometer* is made up of a metal bellows connected to the compression cuff. The movement of the bellows rotates a gear that moves a pointer across the calibrated dial. The aneroid sphygmomanometer is calibrated against a mercury manometer because the more complex mechanisms have been shown to need routine and frequent adjustment. This is simply done by using a connecting Y tube between the manometers.

Electronic devices are available for blood pressure measurement and are used for continuous blood pressure monitoring, as well as for self-monitoring of the client's blood pressure at home. The electronic units determine blood pressure by analyzing the sounds of blood flow or measuring oscillations. A cuff is automatically inflated to occlude the artery. Battery-operated units produce a digital readout of the systolic and diastolic measures after the cuff is manually inflated.

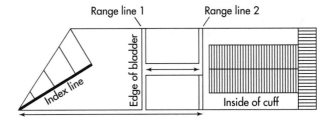

Figure 9-12 Selection of proper cuff size. The index line should reach halfway around the arm diameter. The range lines define the minimum and maximum arm sizes on which the cuff can be used. The end of the cuff must fall between range lines 1 and 2 when the cuff is applied. (From American Heart Association of Wisconsin: *Blood pressure measurement education program instructor's manual*, Milwaukee, 1996, The Association.)

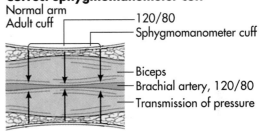

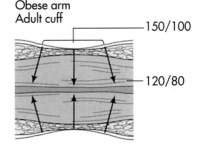

Figure 9-13 Longitudinal sections of arms of different diameters to which sphygmomanometer cuffs have been applied. **A**, Normal arm with correct cuff size. **B**, Obese arm, cuff size too small.

application of the auscultatory method yields values that are within 4 to 5 mm Hg of the results of the direct method of measurement.

The two types of sphygmomanometers that clinicians commonly use to assess arterial blood pressure are the mercury column and the aneroid instruments (Figure 9-11 and Box 9-5). Each instrument includes a pressure manometer, an inflatable rubber bladder encased in a cloth cuff that is used for occluding an artery, and a rubber hand bulb with a pressure control valve. The mercury column sphygmomanometer is considered to be the most accurate and reliable measure when properly used.

Cuff Size. The size of the cuff must always be checked in relation to the size of the arm on which it will be used. The width of the bladder should reach halfway around the arm. The length of the bladder should reach 80% around the arm. To determine the correct cuff size, many manufacturers premark the cuffs with three lines: the index line and range lines 1 and 2 (Figure 9-12). The index line and range line 1 mark the ends of the rubber bladder. A proper-sized cuff edge should fall between range lines 1 and 2 when the cuff is applied.

If the cuff is too narrow or applied too loosely, the blood pressure reading will be erroneously high because more pressure is required to occlude the brachial artery. Using a cuff that is too small is a common error in blood pressure

measurement (Figure 9-13). Cuffs may be obtained in several sizes, as shown in Figure 9-14.

Technique for Blood Pressure Measurement and Normal Findings

Auscultatory Method of Blood Pressure Assessment. When the cuff is properly placed on the client's limb, the arterial blood can flow past the cuff only when arterial pressure exceeds that in the cuff. Partial obstruction of arterial blood flow disturbs the laminar flow pattern, creating turbulence. This turbulence produces sounds called **Korotkoff sounds**, which can be heard over arteries distal to the cuff through a stethoscope (Figure 9-15). See Box 9-6 for steps in taking a blood pressure.

Record the systolic blood pressure at the point when you initially hear Korotkoff sounds. This is also the beginning of phase I, which starts with faint, clear, and rhythmic tapping

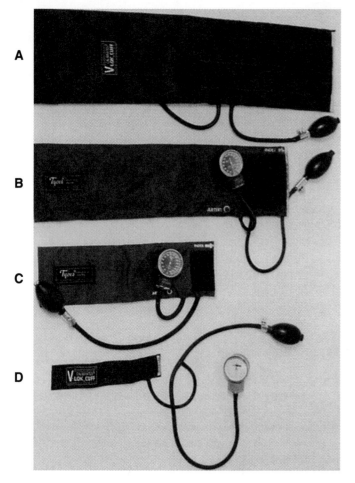

Figure 9-14   Blood pressure cuff sizes. **A**, Thigh. **B**, Large adult. **C**, Adult. **D**, Neonate.

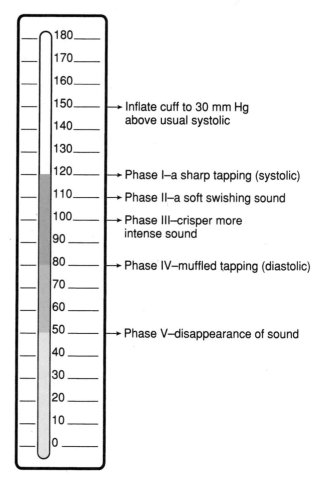

Figure 9-15   Phases of Korotkoff sounds that would be recorded as a blood pressure of 120/80/50 mm Hg.

BOX 9-6

TAKING A BLOOD PRESSURE STEP-BY-STEP

1. Situate the client in a comfortable sitting position, with the arm resting on a flat surface at heart level and the palm turned upward. Expose the upper arm fully. Have the person rest 5 minutes before taking the blood pressure. Wait 30 minutes if the client has smoked or ingested caffeine.
2. Palpate the brachial artery. Center the bladder of the cuff over the brachial artery with the bottom edge of the cuff 2.5 cm (1 inch) above the antecubital space. Do not rely on cuff markings; find the center by folding the bladder in half.
3. If you do not know the client's usual blood pressure, estimate the systolic pressure first by applying the cuff, palpating the radial pulse, and inflating the cuff until the pulse disappears. The point when the pulse disappears is the estimated systolic pressure. Deflate the cuff completely and wait 30 seconds before measuring the blood pressure.
4. Be sure the cuff is fully deflated. Wrap the cuff evenly and snugly around the upper arm. Place the manometer at eye level.

5. Place the stethoscope over the brachial artery. Apply light pressure to ensure good skin contact. Heavy pressure may distort sounds.
6. Close the valve of the pressure bulb clockwise until tight.
7. Rapidly and steadily inflate the cuff to 30 mm Hg above the client's normal or estimated systolic level.
8. Slowly release the valve, allowing the mercury to fall at a rate of 2 to 3 mm Hg per second.
9. Note the point on the manometer at which the first clear sound is heard (phase I). This is the systolic pressure. Continue to deflate the cuff, noting the point at which sound is muffled (phase IV) and when sound disappears (phase V). In children, record phase IV and phase V for the diastolic pressure. In adults, record phase V.
10. Listen 10 to 20 mm Hg below the last sound, then deflate the cuff rapidly and remove it from the client's arm. If repeating the procedure, wait 1 to 2 minutes.

When initially evaluating a client, take blood pressure measures in both sitting and lying positions on each arm. There may be a decrease in blood pressure, less than 10 mm Hg, from supine to sitting.

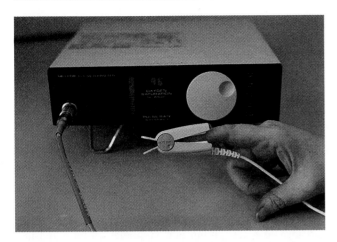

Figure 9-16 Pulse oximeter. (From Potter PA, Perry AG: *Basic nursing: a critical thinking approach*, ed. 4, St. Louis, 1999, Mosby.)

noises that gradually increase in intensity. At this point the intraluminal pressure is the same as the cuff pressure, but it is not great enough to produce a radial pulse.

Phase II is characterized by a murmur, or swishing sound, that is heard as the vessel distends with blood. Phase III is the period when the sounds are crisper and more intense. In phase III the vessel remains open in systole but obliterated in diastole.

Phase IV is when the sounds become muffled and low pitched. The pressure at this point is the closest to the diastolic arterial pressure measured by a direct method.

Cessation of sound is phase V. During the entire phase V the vessel remains open.

In children the muffling of sound (phase IV) is regarded as the true diastolic pressure, since sounds may be heard until 0 on the manometer. In adults, diastolic pressure is the disappearance of sound (phase V).

Normal Systolic and Diastolic Pressure. In adults a normal systolic blood pressure is less than 130 mm Hg. Normal diastolic pressure is less than 85 mm Hg. A client with a systolic blood pressure less than 55 mm Hg, for example, may be considered hypotensive, although there is no numerical guideline to label blood pressure hypotensive. Hypotension in the absence of other signs and symptoms is generally innocent, although the blood pressure must be high enough to perfuse blood to the kidneys, brain, and other tissues.

Blood pressure gradually increases until late adolescence, when adult blood pressure levels are reached (see also Chapter 26). To get the best estimate of a person's usual blood pressure, take two or three readings and average them with the client in a sitting position. A single blood pressure reading is not a reliable measure.

Measurement of Blood Pressure in the Leg. Measure blood pressure in the leg when the arms are not available. With the client lying prone, if possible, apply a large cuff (thigh) to the lower third of the thigh. Center the bladder of the cuff over the popliteal artery. Auscultate in the popliteal fossa. The systolic blood pressure is normally 20 to 30 mm Hg higher in the leg than in the arm.

Auscultatory Gap. Occasionally, as the cuff is deflating, the Korotkoff sounds disappear and then are heard 10 to 15 mm Hg later. This is called an *auscultatory gap.* When this happens, the examiner may seriously underestimate the systolic pressure or overestimate the diastolic pressure. An auscultatory gap occurs in about 5% of adults and is prevalent in individuals with hypertension. The auscultatory gap can be avoided if the examiner palpates the pulse for disappearance while the cuff is inflated to 30 mm Hg above the point at which the artery is occluded.

> ### ■ HELPFUL HINT
> Place the bell lightly over the skin. The bell of the stethoscope transmits low-frequency sounds better than the diaphragm.

> ### ■ HELPFUL HINT
> If you have not inflated the cuff 30 mm Hg above the systolic pressure (obliteration of the pulse) and begin to listen during phase II, the sounds may be too soft to hear.

Absent Phase V. In some individuals the Korotkoff sounds do not disappear but are heard until the manometer falls to 0 mm Hg. This is especially common in children. In this situation, phase IV, or the change in Korotkoff sounds, is a more reliable estimate of the diastolic pressure than phase V. The blood pressure would be recorded as 110/70/0.

Blood Pressure in Children

Obtain a blood pressure measurement during well-child visits beginning at age 3. Blood pressure measurement in children should be obtained on the right arm for two reasons. Initial studies to determine "normal" blood pressure in children were done using the right arm. Also, if a child has a narrowing of the aorta or subclavian artery, the effect on the left-arm blood pressure reading will be greater.

The screening examination may yield an incidence of hypertension in fewer than 3% of children 4 to 15 years old. However, early detection of hypertensive children may mean that early diagnosis and treatment may prevent the sequelae of the underlying disease process (see also Chapter 26).

Pulse Oximetry

A pulse oximeter is a probe with a light-emitting device (LED) and photodetector connected by a cable to an oximeter (Figure 9-16). This device is used to assess the amount of oxygen concentration in blood. Light emitted by the LED is absorbed differently by oxygenated and deoxygenated hemoglobin. To use the device, attach the photosensor to clean skin at the finger or ear. The photodetector calculates pulse oxygen saturation (SpO_2). Normal SpO_2 ranges between 90% to 100%. Less than 85% is abnormal, indicating impaired oxygenation of peripheral blood.

Pulse oximetry is used in emergency settings for clients who have respiratory symptoms and to evaluate initial and ongoing tissue oxygenation to assist in decision making about therapies.

VARIATIONS FROM HEALTH

General Inspection

Observe for signs of distress in the client. Some of the signs that may indicate a need for immediate intervention are (1) anxiety, indicated by a clenched jaw, fidgety movements, and an apparent inability to process questions; (2) pain, indicated by moaning, writhing, facial grimacing, or guarding

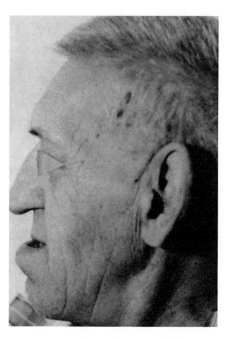

Figure 9-17 Acromegaly. Note the prominent jaw and forehead, the large zygomatic arches and supraorbital ridges, enlarged nose, and coarse and oily skin. (From Mazzaferri EL: *Endocrinology case studies*, ed. 2, Flushing, NY, 1975, Medical Examination Publishing. Modified from the American Heart Association Biostatistical Fact Sheet, 1998.)

of the painful part; (3) cardiopulmonary distress, signaled by labored breathing, coughing, cyanosis, and/or pallor; (4) alteration in consciousness; or (5) observable injury. If you detect distress, you may need to deal with the underlying problem immediately and postpone the full interview and physical examination to a later time.

Facial Expression

Individuals with Parkinson's disease tend to have motionless faces because of limited movement of the musculature. In addition, their blinking rate is slowed so that these clients appears to stare.

The facial changes that occur with acromegaly, caused by excessive growth hormone production, include a prominent supraorbital ridge, jutting jaw, and enlarged nose and lips (Figure 9-17).

In myxedema (hypothyroidism) the facial features are flattened because they are swollen from fluid retention that is caused by the accumulation of mucopolysaccharides. The face appears heavy and coarse.

Posture

Faulty posture is most likely to result from postural or structural problems. Postural problems result from poor posture habits, muscle imbalance, or pain. Examples are the deviation of the spine toward the affected side in sciatica (irritation to the sciatic nerve) and the maintenance of a position that elevates the clavicles, such as leaning forward on extended arms, by the client with chronic obstructive lung disease. Children may have poor postural habits such as a slouch because they do not want to appear taller than their peers.

Occupations that require positions that deviate from normal alignment may result in chronic pain or deformity. Examples include bent shoulders in mine workers and painful shoulders in sewing machine operators.

Structural factors, especially spinal deformities, can also cause faulty posture (see Figure 9-2). Disordered body alignment may lead to changes of the surrounding soft tissue. An example of this is the change in lung volume and ventilation, as well as in circulation, that occurs with scoliosis or lateral curvature of the spine (Figure 9-18).

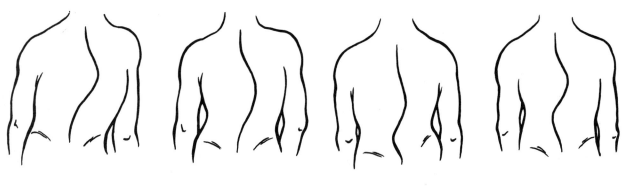

Right thoracic curve

Right thoracic lumbar curve

Left lumbar curve

Right thoracic and left lumbar curve (double major curve)

Figure 9-18 Examples of scoliosis curve patterns.

Weight

Anorexia nervosa is a psychological disorder in which the person has a distorted body image and perceives that he or she needs to lose weight. To lose weight, the person with anorexia nervosa severely restricts his or her food intake. Bulimia nervosa includes cycles of bingeing and purging by vomiting or using laxatives. Anorexia nervosa and bulimia occur mostly in adolescent females and is associated with amenorrhea. Anorexia nervosa is present if the client is at or below 85% of his or her expected weight (Figure 9-19). Even though more than 40% of clients recover from anorexia nervosa, it is associated with a fivefold increase in mortality when compared with the general population of the same age and sex.

Obesity is a body weight that is 20% greater than the ideal weight for height. Obesity is also defined as a BMI greater than 30. The prevalence of overweight varies by race, ethnicity, and gender. (For ideal body weight values, see Chapter 6.)

Alterations in Appearance From Endocrine Disorders

When hypothyroidism begins in infancy, it is called **cretinism** and is characterized by retarded bone maturation and multiple abnormal areas of epiphyseal ossification. Juvenile myxedema is also a cause of retarded growth.

In adults hypothyroidism is identified by the presence of generalized signs and symptoms such as fatigue, modest weight gain, dry skin, cold intolerance, constipation, slowed pulse, and periorbital swelling.

Gigantism is caused by excess growth hormone (GH) before puberty and before the ossification of the epiphyseal plates. The excess results in the overgrowth of the long bones.

Acromegaly is a disease caused by hypersecretion of GH secondary to pituitary tumor; it is usually detected in the fourth or fifth decade of life. In most instances growth of the acral (small) parts proceeds so slowly that it is not noticed until the changes are well-advanced. Bony changes in the skull are most apparent. The mandible is increased in length and width. There is little increase in height because the epi-

physeal plates have closed. The features are exaggerated as a result of the expansion of the facial, molar, and frontal bones. The skull itself, as well as the sinuses, may be markedly enlarged. Arthralgia and arthritis are commonly present in acromegaly.

Cushing's syndrome is a disease caused by an excess of endogenous cortisol or exogenous glucocorticoids. The fat distribution that is characteristic of Cushing's syndrome (hyperadrenalism) or administration of the glucocorticoid hormone is in the facial, nuchal (neck), truncal, and girdle areas. Cushing's syndrome (Figure 9-20) is characterized by thin skin, purplish striae, plethora (red cheeks), muscle weakness, evidence of osteoporosis, redistribution of fat deposits, truncal obesity, "buffalo hump" (cervicodorsal fat), "moon facies" (fat cheeks), and thin extremities.

Hair

In starvation general protein production is inhibited, which leads to reduced hair growth, dullness in appearance, and loss of color. In some ethnic groups, especially those with black or dark brown hair, this loss of hair pigment results in a reddish brown hair color.

Chemotherapeutic drugs inhibit cell division and thereby inhibit hair growth.

Increased hair growth in normal sites has been associated with adrenal tumors.

Hirsutism, the appearance of excessive hair in normal and abnormal sites caused by increased androgens, has been observed in the following pathophysiological conditions: polycystic ovary, Cushing's syndrome, and ovarian tumor. Hirsutism can be most disturbing to the female client. The degree of overgrowth need not be marked to pose a threat to the client's feelings of femininity. When the examiner notes hirsutism in a female client, he or she should also be alerted to the presence of other virilizing signs, which include a deepening of the voice, clitoral enlargement, and changes in fat distribu-

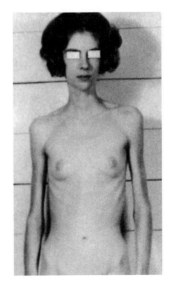

Figure 9-19 Young female with anorexia nervosa. (From Ezrin C, Godden JO, Volpe R: *Systematic endocrinology*, ed. 2, New York, 1979, Harper & Row.)

Cultural Considerations
Overweight Variations

Race	Gender	% Overweight
Caucasion	M	39.6
	F	23.0
African-American	M	36.2
	F	29.2
Hispanic	M	44.0
	F	33.4

Data from 1988-1991 (NHANES III) and HHANES 1982-1984. In American Heart Association: *Heart and stroke facts 1996*, supplement, Dallas, 1996, The Association.

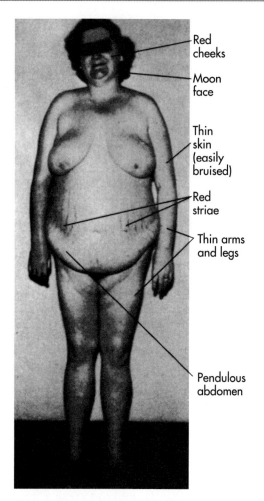

Figure 9-20 Physical characteristics of Cushing's syndrome. Prominent features include moon facies, red cheeks, thin skin, bruisability, red striae, and poor wound healing. Fat distribution is in the trunk with thin arms and legs. (Modified from Prior JA, Silberstein JS, Stang JM: *Physical diagnosis: the history and examination of the patient,* ed. 6, St. Louis, 1981, Mosby.)

tion. Because of the identity confusion that may exist in the presence of hirsutism, approach the problem with sensitivity.

Fungal infections (tinea capitis) may cause hair loss. The fungal contamination is commonly acquired from pets and contaminated cosmetics.

Chemical and thermal treatment of the hair can cause damage to the surface, characterized by breaking and splitting.

Structural Variations

Defects of the thoracic cage might change the nature of respiration. Some defects are pectus carinatum, in which the sternum is markedly protuberant (as in a bird); funnel chest, or pectus excavatum, in which the sternum is retracted; and barrel chest (Figure 9-21).

Fever

Fever, or **pyrexia**, is the elevation of body temperature above normal limits compared with a given individual's basal data. For example, a temperature of 37° C (98.6° F) in a client whose normal temperature is 36.1° C (97° F) would

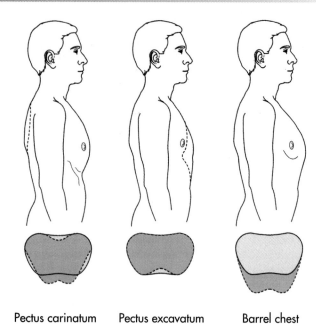

Pectus carinatum   Pectus excavatum   Barrel chest

Figure 9-21 Chest deformities. Lower vertical views show change in chest wall contours with deformity. (Modified from Magee DJ: *Orthopedic physical assessment,* ed. 3, Philadelphia, 1999, WB Saunders.)

be considered a fever. Fever is described in three stages: cold; hot; and defervescence, or decline.

Cold Stage

The cold stage is the period of a developing increase in core temperature and is characterized by heat conservation reactions. Cutaneous circulation is decreased, and the skin looks blanched and feels cold. Heat production produces shivering and piloerection ("goose pimples"). Chills and rigor are the extremes of shivering and produce rapid increases in temperature.

Hot Stage

The hot stage is the period after the fever has peaked. During this stage, blood flow to the periphery is increased. The body radiates excess heat, feels hot, and is flushed.

Defervescence

The stage of **defervescence** is the period of fever abatement and is characterized by heat-loss mechanisms, particularly vasodilation and sweating. Diaphoresis is diffuse perspiration, which may accompany fever abatement.

Variations in Pulse

Table 9-3 shows the variations in arterial pulse volume, rate, and rhythm.

Tachycardia

Rates that are persistently more than 100 beats per minute (**tachycardia**) suggest some abnormality. Heart rates are increased during fever, anemia, hypoxia, and low-volume states (shock). However, tachycardia can also be a result of exercise, anger, anxiety, or fear.

TABLE 9-3 Arterial Pulse Abnormalities

Type	Description	Possible Causes
Diminished, weak, thready	Pulse is difficult to feel, easily obliterated by the fingers, and may fade out Pulse is slow to rise, has a sustained summit, and falls slowly	Hypovolemia Aortic stenosis Decreased cardiac output
Full, strong, bounding	Pulse is readily palpable, not easily obliterated by fingers Pulse is felt as a brisk impact; can occur with or without increased pulse pressure	Anemia Exercise Fever Hyperthyroidism
Water-hammer, collapsing	Pulse has greater-than-normal amplitude Pulse is marked by rapid rise, followed by a sudden descent	Chronic aortic regurgitation Patent ductus arteriosus
Pulsus bisferiens (double peaked)	Best felt by palpating carotid artery Two systolic peaks can occur in disorders that cause rapid left ventricular ejection of large stroke volume with wide pulse pressure	Aortic regurgitation Patent ductus arteriosus
Pulsus alternans	Pulses have large-amplitude beats followed by pulses of small amplitude Rhythm remains normal	Left-sided congestive heart failure
Bigeminal pulse	Normal pulses are followed by premature contractions Amplitude of premature contraction is less than that of normal pulse Rhythm is irregular	Premature ventricular or atrial contraction
Pulsus paradoxus	Pattern is exaggerated (>10 mm Hg) during inspiration, and amplitude is increased during expiration Heart rate and rhythm are unchanged	Cardiac tamponade Constrictive pericarditis Pulmonary emphysema (noncardiac)

Inspiration   Expiration   Inspiration

Modified from Canobbio MM: *Cardiovascular disorders*, St. Louis, 1990, Mosby.

Bradycardia

Bradycardia is a slow heart rate of less than 50 beats per minute. A slow rate may indicate stimulation of the parasympathetic system or failure in the electrical conduction system of the heart. Bradycardia may be caused by overdoses of digitalis. Bradycardia occurs normally in the well-trained athlete. This is due to heart muscle increasing in strength with development of skeletal muscle. This increased strength results in greater stroke volume, which in turn requires fewer beats per minute to maintain cardiac output.

Palpitations

When the client describes feeling his or her heartbeat, this feeling is referred to as a **palpitation**. Common terms used by clients to describe this phenomenon are "pounding," "thudding," "fluttering," "flopping," and "skipping." Palpitations are more common just before falling asleep or during sleep.

Palpitations may be experienced by an individual after strenuous exercise or when that person is aroused emotionally or sexually. In this case the cardiac contraction is of a greater rate and amplitude. A common feature of the anxiety

TABLE 9-4	Classification of Blood Pressure for Adults Ages 18 Years and Older*		
Category	Systolic (mm Hg)		Diastolic (mm Hg)
Optimal†	<120	and	<80
Normal	<130	and	<85
High normal	130–139	or	85–89
	Hypertension‡		
Stage 1	140–159	or	90–99
Stage 2	160–179	or	100–109
Stage 3	≥180	or	≥110

From Joint National Committee on Prevention, Detection, Evaluation, and Treatment of High Blood Pressure: *The sixth report of the Joint National Committee on Detection, Evaluation, and Treatment of High Blood Pressure*, NIH Publication No. 98-4080, Bethesda, Md., 1997, National Institutes of Health.

*Not taking antihypertensive drugs and not acutely ill. When systolic and diastolic pressures fall into different categories, the higher category should be selected to classify the individual's blood pressure status. For instance, 160/92 mm Hg should be classified as stage 2, and 174/120 mm Hg should be classified as stage 3. Isolated systolic hypertension (ISH) is defined as systolic blood pressure (SBP) ≥140 mm Hg and diastolic blood pressure (DBP) <90 mm Hg and staged appropriately (e.g., 170/82 mm Hg is defined as stage 2 ISH). In addition to classifying stages of hypertension on the basis of average blood pressure levels, clinicians should specify presence or absence of target organ disease and additional risk factors. This specificity is important for risk classification and treatment.

†Optimal blood pressure with respect to cardiovascular risk is less than 120/80 mm Hg. However, unusually low readings should be evaluated for clinical significance.

‡Based on the average of two or more readings taken at each of two or more visits following an initial screening.

state (arousal) is palpitations caused by the increased adrenergic activity. The relationship between anxiety and palpitations creates some problem for the examiner; because the presence of palpitations commonly creates anxiety, ask questions carefully so as not to cause further anxiety.

Palpitations are also associated with anemia, fever, hypoglycemia, and thyrotoxicosis.

Variations in Blood Pressure

Differences in Blood Pressure Indicating Disease

On initial examination, measure blood pressures in both arms. Differences in blood pressure between the two arms may be caused by congenital aortic obstruction (**coarctation**), acquired conditions such as aortic dissection, or obstruction of the arteries of the upper arm.

Sudden changes in blood pressure may produce changes in body function, and sudden drops in blood pressure may result in fainting. Fainting is observed in **orthostatic hypotension**, defined as a systolic blood pressure decrease of 30 mm Hg and an increase in pulse of 10 to 20 beats per minute when moving from a lying to a standing position. In orthostatic hypotension, the blood pressure may be normal when an individual is reclining but drops when he or she rises to a sitting or standing position, particularly when the position change is rapid. Faintness and dizziness from orthostatic hypotension is common in individuals taking antihypertensive medications or in individuals who are elderly, volume depleted, or confined to bed.

Hypertension

The screening examination is especially important for recognizing the client who has **hypertension** (persistently ele-

vated blood pressure). Because hypertension may be present without symptoms, it is known as the *silent disease*. A client who does not feel ill does not usually come to a clinic or hospital for health care. Thus the screening examination may be instrumental in prompting the hypertensive client to begin early treatment to prevent some of the complications of untreated hypertension.

The sixth Joint National Committee on Prevention, Detection, Evaluation, and Treatment of High Blood Pressure (1997) defines hypertension as being at least two blood pressure readings that average more than 140/90 mm Hg (Table 9-4) or as requiring antihypertensive medication to maintain a blood pressure less than 140/90. Hypertension should be diagnosed not on the basis of a single blood pressure reading but on the basis of several readings. The timing of subsequent readings should be based on the initial blood pressure level. Table 9-5 presents follow-up criteria for ranges of systolic and diastolic readings.

One in four American adults has high blood pressure. Ninety percent of adults who have high blood pressure have essential or idiopathic hypertension. In essential hypertension, no physiological cause is identified for the elevated blood pressure level. Hypertension prevalence is highest in African-Americans, at 34.6%, compared with other racial/ethnic groups.

HELPFUL HINT

An adult is advised to engage in at least 30 minutes of moderate intensity activity most days of the week for good health.

| TABLE 9-5 | Recommendations for Follow-Up Based on Initial Blood Pressure Measurements for Adults (Initial Screening Blood Pressure [mm Hg])* |||

Systolic	Diastolic	Follow-up recommended†
<130	<85	Recheck in 2 years
130–139	85–89	Recheck in 1 year‡
140–159	90–99	Confirm within 2 months‡
160–179	100–109	Evaluate or refer to source of care within 1 month
≥180	≥110	Evaluate or refer to source of care immediately or within 1 week depending on clinical situation

From Joint National Committee on Prevention, Detection, Evaluation, and Treatment of High Blood Pressure: *The sixth report of the Joint National Committee on Detection, Evaluation, and Treatment of High Blood Pressure*, NIH Publication No. 98-4080, Bethesda, Md., 1997, National Institutes of Health.
*If the systolic and diastolic categories are different, follow recommendation for the shorter-time follow-up (e.g., 160/86 mm Hg should be evaluated or referred to source of care within 1 month).
†Modify the scheduling of follow-up according to reliable information about past blood pressure measurements, other cardiovascular risk factors, or target-organ disease.
‡Provide advice about lifestyle modifications.

Teaching Self Assessment

WEIGHT CONTROL

Maintaining a normal weight reduces the risk of hypertension. Weight loss often results in a substantial decrease in blood pressure, even when ideal weight is not achieved. Restriction of daily dietary sodium to 2 g is also recommended. Alcohol consumption should not exceed 8 ounces of wine or 24 ounces of beer (see also Chapter 6). Other risk-reducing behaviors include avoiding tobacco use, following a regular program of exercise, and using behavior modification therapies such as relaxation and biofeedback.

Exercise.   Instruct clients to measure their maximal heart rate to assess the amount of exertion in physical exercise. To do this, subtract one's age from 220. To exercise aerobically, the pulse must reach 80% of an individual's maximal heart rate. The client should obtain a radial or carotid baseline pulse before exercising by feeling the pulse, counting for 10 seconds, and then multiplying that count by 6. The count should be repeated immediately after exercise to obtain the maximal heart rate and 2 minutes later to assess recovery to baseline. If after 2 minutes the pulse has not returned to near baseline, the exercise involved too much exertion.

Sample Documentation and Diagnoses

FOCUSED HEALTH HISTORY (SUBJECTIVE DATA)

Mrs. H, a 78-year-old Caucasian female, was brought into the emergency room by her daughter, who found her confused and slumped in a chair in an extremely hot apartment. Mrs. H states she has black spots in front of her eyes, a very bad headache, and nausea.

FOCUSED PHYSICAL EXAMINATION (OBJECTIVE DATA)

Vital signs: BP 100/50 mm Hg right arm, lying down; pulse 120, weak, regular; respirations 32, labored and shallow; Temperature 40° C (104° F) (rectal).

General appearance: Elderly woman who appears weak, unable to stand or sit. Skin is flushed. Client is oriented to person, time, and place. Daughter is present during the examination at request of the client.

Physical examination: Skin is flushed, cool to touch on extremities, warm and dry to touch on trunk. Oral mucosa dry. Peripheral pulses barely palpable.

DIAGNOSES

HEALTH PROBLEM

Hyperthermia

NURSING DIAGNOSES

Hyperthermia Related to Exposure to Hot Environment

Defining Characteristics

- Fever
- Flushed skin, warm to touch
- Increased respiratory rate
- Tachycardia

Activity Intolerance Related to Generalized Weakness

Defining Characteristics

- Weakness
- Shallow, labored breathing
- Confusion

Altered Tissue Perfusion Related to Hyperthermia

Defining Characteristics

- Decreased peripheral pulses
- Cool peripheral skin

? Critical Thinking Questions

Review the Sample Documentation and Diagnoses box to answer questions 1 and 2.

1. What pulses would you monitor in the case of Mrs. H? Based on the information provided, how would you grade the pulses measured?
2. In the case of Mrs. H, what factors contributed to her hyperthermia? Using the principles of temperature regulation, what measures could be started to accelerate heat loss?
3. A 32-year-old African-American male who smokes comes to a blood pressure screening clinic and has a blood pressure of 130/86 mm Hg based on the average of two readings. How would you classify his blood pressure? What follow-up would you recommend? What lifestyle modifications should be discussed?

Answers are available on the MERLIN website (www.harcourthealth.com/MERLIN/Barkauskas/). And be sure to check the website regularly for additional learning activities!

Remember to check out the Online Study Guide!
www.harcourthealth.com/MERLIN/Barkauskas/

Chapter 10

MERLIN www.harcourthealth.com/MERLIN/Barkauskas/

Skin, Hair, and Nails

Learning Objectives

On successful study of this chapter and completion of related learning experiences, the learner will be able to:

- Describe the anatomy and physiology of the skin and its appendages.
- Identify the history questions needed to conduct a thorough assessment of the skin, hair, and nails.
- Explain the process of describing and classifying skin lesions.
- Describe common patterns and lesions seen in individuals of different ages and races.
- Describe methods to assess skin, hair, and nail changes in light and dark-skinned individuals.
- Recognize variations from health in the assessment of the skin, hair, and nails.
- Describe information necessary to help clients reduce their risk for skin cancers.

Outline

Purpose of Examination

The skin, or integumentary system, is an organ system readily accessible to examination. It provides a membrane barrier between the individual and the external environment. The skin responds to changes in the external environment. It also reflects changes in the internal environment. A careful examination of the skin may yield valuable information about the client's general health. It can provide specific information needed to identify a systemic disease or a skin problem. A description of the skin of the healthy client, as well as a description of the client with a skin problem, is important. The examiner should pay special attention to any deviation from normal.

Examination of the skin requires understanding of the structure and function of the system and familiarity with the appearance of the skin, hair, nails, and mucous membranes in health and disease. This chapter includes a brief discussion of the anatomy and function of the skin, hair, and nails; methods for conducting a health history; and the systematic examination of the skin, hair, and nails. (The examination of the sclera and conjunctiva is discussed in Chapter 12, and the examination of the oral mucosa is discussed in Chapter 13.)

ANATOMY AND PHYSIOLOGY

The skin, combined with its appendages (the hair, nails, sebaceous glands, and eccrine and apocrine sweat glands), is the largest organ of the body. It has many important functions:

- Provides a barrier to loss of water and electrolytes
- Provides protection from external agents injurious to the internal structures
- Regulates body temperature and blood pressure
- Acts as a sense organ for touch, pressure, temperature, and pain
- Maintains body surface integrity by ongoing cell replacement and increased regeneration for wound repair
- Maintains a buffered protective skin film by eccrine and sebaceous glands to protect against microbial and fungal agents
- Participates in production of vitamin D
- Delays hypersensitivity reactions to foreign substances
- Indicates emotion through color change

Skin

The skin is composed of three distinct layers: the epidermis, the dermis, and the subcutaneous tissue (Figure 10-1).

Epidermis

The epidermis is the outermost layer of the skin. It acts as a barrier to external penetration and also retains substances inside. It varies in thickness from about 0.3 to 1.5 mm, depending on the individual's age and the body region. The epidermis is an avascular, cornified cellular structure that depends on the underlying dermis for its nutrition. It is continuous with the mucous membranes and the lining of the ear canals. It is composed chiefly of keratinocytes, cells that produce keratin. The epidermis is divided into several layers. The outermost, or horny, layer is the stratum corneum. Keratin is its principle structural element. Stratified layers of dead keratinized cells form the stratum corneum and are constantly shed and replenished as new skin cells are pushed up from the lower layers. There is almost a complete cell turnover every 3 to 4 weeks. The stratum corneum is an important barrier to water loss and to environmental threats. The innermost layer of the epidermis, the stratum germinativum, or basal cell layer, contains the **melanocytes**, which produce melanin, the pigment that gives color to the skin and hair. Melanocytes also filter ultraviolet light.

Dermis

The dermis underlies the epidermis and constitutes the bulk of the skin. It is often referred to as the "true skin." The der-

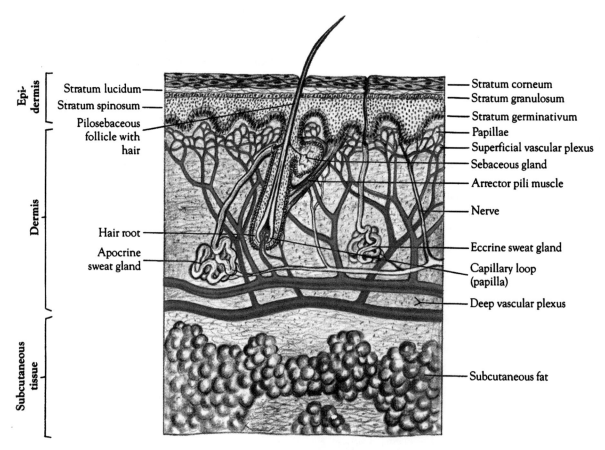

Figure 10-1   Structures of the skin. (From Thompson JM et al: *Mosby's clinical nursing*, ed. 4, St. Louis, 1997, Mosby.)

mis is about 20 times thicker than the epidermis in certain areas of the body. It is a tough connective tissue that contains lymphatics and nerves and is highly vascular. The dermis contains collagen fibers and elastic fibers, which provide resilience, strength, and support. The dermis nourishes and supports the epidermis. Nerve fibers in the dermis provide sensations of temperature, touch, and pain and also include autonomical nerves that innervate the glands, blood vessels, and arrector pili muscles.

Subcutaneous Tissue

The subcutaneous layer, or superficial fascia, lies immediately under the dermis. It is composed of adipose tissue. It stores fat for energy, generates heat, and provides temperature insulation.

Epidermal Appendages

The **sebaceous** glands, eccrine sweat glands, apocrine sweat glands, hair, and nails are considered appendages of the epidermis. They are formed by invagination of the epidermis into the underlying dermis. Keratin is the principal constituent of the nails and hair.

Sebaceous Glands

The sebaceous glands usually arise from the hair follicles and produce sebum, which has a lubricating effect on the horny outer layer of the epidermis. Sebaceous glands are on all parts of the body except the palms and soles. Secretory activity of the glands is stimulated by sex hormones and varies throughout the lifespan in response to hormonal levels. Sebaceous glands are most abundant on the forehead, face, chin, and scalp. Excessive production of sebum is called *seborrhea*.

Sweat Glands

There are two types of sweat glands: eccrine and apocrine. The eccrine sweat glands open onto the surface of the skin and produce a dilute saline solution, or sweat. They are distributed throughout the body and in great density on the palms and other parts of the hands. They have an important function in regulating body temperature. Body heat is dissipated as sweat is produced and evaporates. The apocrine sweat glands are found in the axillary and genital areas. They are larger and deeper than the eccrine glands and usually open into the hair follicles. They produce a milky, viscid fluid or sweat. The sweat produced by the apocrine glands decomposes when it is contaminated by bacteria, resulting in its characteristic body odor. The apocrine glands do not function until a person reaches puberty. Secretion occurs during emotional stress and sexual stimulation.

Hair

Hair is formed by invagination of epidermal cells into the dermal layers. Hair consists of a root, shaft, and hair follicle. Hair follicles are formed *in utero* and continue functioning through old age. No new follicles are formed after birth. Hair follicles produce the keratin of mature hair. Melano-cytes in the shaft provide hair color. Adults have two types of hairs: vellus hairs (which are short, fine, and nonpigmented) and terminal hairs (which are thick, coarse, and pigmented). Terminal hairs are found most extensively on the scalp, brows, and extremities.

Each hair goes through cyclic growth phases: a growing (anagen) phase, a transition (catogen) phase lasting only a few days, and a resting (telogen) phase. Ninety percent of normal scalp hairs are in the growing phase, and 10% are in the resting stage. Hairs in the resting stage are subsequently expelled by the regenerating new hair. Hair on the head, on average, grows about 12 mm ($\frac{1}{2}$ inch) per month or about 11 cm (5 inches) a year. Hair growth is different depending on its location. Axillary, pubic, beard, and body hair is influenced by hormones. Hair on the scalp, eyelashes, and extremities does not require hormonal stimulus. Hair loss may be related to factors such as destruction of the hair matrix, slowing of hair growth due to medications or metabolic disorders, and genetic characteristics. With aging, hair color and texture changes. Color changes are related to a decrease in the number of functioning melanocytes. Onset and number of graying hairs will also be genetically determined. Texture changes may be related to hormonal changes that occur with age. Nutrition changes will also have an impact on texture and, in some instances, color. With inadequate nutrition, hair becomes brittle, dry, and lusterless.

Nails

The nails are keratinized appendages of the epidermis. The nails consist of (1) the nail matrix (root), where the nailplate is developed; (2) the nailplate; (3) the nailbed, which is attached to the nailplate; and (4) the periungual tissue, including the eponychium and the perionychium (Figure 10-2).

The nail matrix, the site of nail growth, is not visible. The lunula, located at the base of the visible nail, has the shape of a half-moon and marks the end of the nail matrix. A bluish hue is visible in the nails of more darkly pigmented individuals. The size of the lunula is variable; it may not be visible in older individuals. The nailplate is a horny, semitransparent structure with a dorsal convexity. The nailplate rests on and adheres to the nailbed. The nailbed has a rich capillary network, which shows through the nailplate as a pink surface. Normal thickness of the nail is 0.3 to 0.65 mm (0.012 to 0.025 inch); it is somewhat thicker in men. The free edge of the nailfold is continuous with the cuticle, which is an extension of the stratum corneum of the dorsum of the finger. The eponychium lies below this and is the anterior extension of the roof of the nailfold on the nailplate. The hyponychium is the portion of the fingertip underlying the free portion of the nail. The perionychium is the epidermis bordering the nail.

The nailplate is formed continuously and uniformly at all points in the matrix. Fingernail growth rates in the normal adult vary from 0.1 to 1 mm per day. The rate varies with nutrition, age, activity level, and seasonal rhythms. Nail growth is greater in warm seasons than in cold, and accelerated growth has been observed in warm climates. The growth rate slows with aging. The total time required for the nail to grow from the lunula to the free margin of the nail is

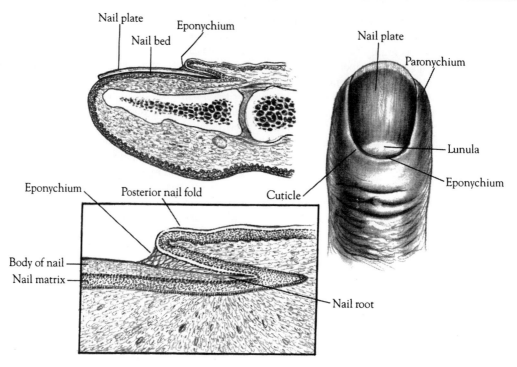

Figure 10-2 Structures of the nail. (From Thompson JM et al.: *Mosby's clinical nursing*, ed. 4, St. Louis, 1997, Mosby.)

called the *migration time* and is normally 130 days. The time required for complete renewal of the fingernail *(regeneration time)* is 170 days. Regeneration of the toenail takes 1 to 1½ years.

EXAMINATION

Focused Health History

Present Health/Illness Status

1. Chief complaint or concern
2. Usual condition of skin, hair, and nails, including usual skin tone and hair color
3. Allergies: medications, foods, pollens, seasonal allergies
4. Exposures: travel, environmental or occupational hazards or irritants, frequent sun exposure, use of tanning salons, frequent hand washing or immersion in water, family members or close contacts with skin problems, seasonal changes, heat, cold
5. Medications: prescribed or over-the-counter, topical or systemic, new or previously taken
6. Skin care habits: cleansing patterns, skin care products used (e.g., soaps, oils, astringents, alcohol, facials), use of sunscreens, recent changes in skin care habits or products
7. Nail care habits: difficulty cutting or clipping toenails and/or fingernails, types of instruments used, nail biting, use of adhesives for false fingernails
8. Hair care habits: cleansing routines; recent changes in routine or products used; use of dyes, hair straighteners, permanents, or other chemical treatments; hair styles that put tension on the hair

9. Diet: any recent dietary changes, nutritional supplements, new foods
10. Recent life changes, losses, or psychological or physiological stress

Past Health History

1. Previous occurrences of the problem and its resolution
2. Skin problems: history of allergies, eczema, lesions, and their response to treatment
3. Hair problems: loss; unusual growth or distribution; thinning, breakage; response to treatment
4. Nail problems: injury, infections, allergic reactions (to nail care products), response to treatment
5. Systemic health problems: cardiac, endocrine, respiratory, liver, hematological, or other systemic diseases
6. Tolerance to sunlight, history of sunburns

Family Health History

1. History of allergic diseases such as asthma, hay fever, or other sensitivities
2. Dermatological disorders: skin cancer; melanoma; psoriasis; eczema; infestations (e.g., lice, scabies); infections
3. Familial patterns of hair loss, coloration, or distribution

Personal and Social History

1. Significant others: who is in the home, current support system
2. Usual activities: work, school, day care; hobbies
3. Recent life changes: (positive and negative), stresses, losses, anniversaries of losses
4. Cultural practices: related to skin, hair, and nail care; adornments; braiding; body piercing; tattoos; shaving;

folk remedies (e.g., coining, cupping, application of ointments, plasters, herbs)

Specific Problems/Symptom Analysis

Skin

Changes in usual state of health: rashes or lesions; excessive bruising; lumps; pruritus; pigmentation changes; texture; dryness, oiliness; odor; changes in or new presentation of wart or mole; lesion that is repeatedly irritated or that is slow to heal

1. **Onset:** sudden or gradual; specific date of onset
2. **Course since onset:**
   Frequency: previous occurrence or progressive problem; give specific time interval
   Timing: relationship of symptoms to specific events or other symptoms; with rashes, determine activities, signs, or symptoms that preceded the rash (e.g., hiking, fever, ingestions)
   Duration: how long has problem persisted (days, weeks, years)
3. **Location:** where did the lesion start, has it spread, is it on extensor or flexor surfaces, skinfolds, is it generalized or localized, any progression of rash or pattern?
4. **Quality:**
   Color: generalized (pallor, jaundice, cyanosis) or localized (hypopigmentation or hyperpigmentation, erythema)
   Itching: (pruritus), mild or intense; any pattern of occurrence (e.g., increases at night), pain, or paresthesia
5. **Quantity:** exact size and number of lesion(s)
6. **Setting:** travel; other family members or close contacts at home, school, or work with a similar problem; recreational activities (e.g., camping, hiking, working with chemicals, paints, dyes); tanning salon; sun bathing
7. **Associated phenomena:** recent viral illness, high fever, headaches, chills, systemic diseases, immunizations, relationship to leisure activities or stress
8. **Alleviating and aggravating factors:** medications; relaxation; not using certain products or avoiding contact with allergens; over-the-counter (OTC) or prescription medications or home remedies; response to treatment; change in skin care products; use of different perfumes, detergents, or other products that come in contact with the skin; diet changes; new pet; stress-related reactions; heat, cold
9. **Underlying concern:** fear of melanoma, cancer, disfigurement, social isolation

Hair

Changes in usual state of health; thinning or hair loss; excess hair; distribution of hair; color change

1. **Onset:** sudden or gradual; specific date of onset; asymmetrical or symmetrical pattern
2. **Course since onset:**
   Frequency: previous occurrence or progressive problem; give specific time interval
   Timing: relationship of symptoms to specific events or other symptoms
   Duration: how long has problem persisted
3. **Location:** body part affected, generalized or localized
4. **Quality:**
   Color change: generalized or localized
   Texture: any changes
5. **Quantity:** hair loss or unusual growth
6. **Setting:** home, school, work, exposure to environmental or occupational hazards
7. **Associated phenomena:** any other health problems, fever, skin disorders, hormonal changes (medications or menarche, pregnancy, menopause), thyroid disease
8. **Alleviating and aggravating factors:** discontinuance of particular products, dietary changes, dieting (particularly liquid protein diet), malnutrition, hair care products/chemicals, medications or home remedies, response to treatment
9. **Underlying concern:** fear of systemic disease; concern about aging, rejection by peers

Nails

Changes in usual state of health: splitting, breaking, biting, thickening, discoloration; separation from nailbed; inflammation

1. **Onset:** sudden or gradual; specific date of onset; related to illness or trauma
2. **Course since onset:**
   Frequency: recurrent or intermittent; how often
   Timing: relationship of symptoms to specific events or other symptoms
   Duration: how long has problem persisted
3. **Location:** where did the lesion start; generalized or localized
4. **Quality:** change in color, shape; pain
5. **Quantity:** number of nails affected, amount of pain/tenderness
6. **Setting:** home, school, or work
7. **Associated phenomena:** other health problems, such as cardiac or respiratory disease, psoriasis, hypothyroidism
8. **Alleviating and aggravating factors:** diet; cessation of specific behaviors; exposure to drugs, chemicals; immersion in water; nail care products; medications or home remedies; response to treatment
9. **Underlying concern:** cosmetic issues; systemic disease

Preparation for Examination: Client and Environment

The examination of the skin is important in the assessment of the client's overall health and as a screening for skin cancer. A complete examination of the skin needs to be a part of every complete physical examination. This requires that you take a brief but careful view of the entire body and then examine specific areas in more detail. Provide a warm examining room with sufficient privacy. Have the client remove clothing so that you can fully view each section of the body. Protect client modesty by draping areas you are not examining.

Technique for Examination and Expected Findings

The examination of the skin and appendages needs to include a general inspection of the entire body, followed by a detailed regional examination. A good source of illumination is necessary; indirect natural daylight is preferred. Consider using a small magnifying glass to aid in examining individual lesions of the skin. Use a clear, flexible centimeter ruler to assess the size of the lesions. Always wear gloves when examining lesions.

When doing a complete physical examination, begin the skin examination with the exposed areas (hair, face, hands, and arms). This technique may be less threatening to the client. Then inspect and palpate the skin, mucous membranes, and epidermal appendages of each body part as you examine it. Examine the entire body (with the client disrobed) at the end of the examination when the client is standing. For example, when examining the spine, assess the skin on the back, buttocks, and legs before or after the spine examination.

Research indicates that detailed full-body examinations reveal several times as many melanomas than less-detailed examinations. This thoroughness is particularly important for clients at risk for melanoma.

If the client's main reason for being examined is to evaluate a skin problem, first note the client's general appearance since that may give clues as to whether the problem is related to an acute illness syndrome, a chronic illness syndrome, or a generalized or localized problem. Next do a full-

Preparation for Examination

EQUIPMENT

Item	Purpose
Metric ruler	To measure lesions
Flashlight	To illuminate lesions
Magnifying glass (optional)	To aid in evaluation of lesions
Disposable latex gloves	To protect examiner when examining lesions
For special procedures:	
Wood's lamp (filtered ultraviolet light)	To assess for tinea capitis
Glass slides and 20% KOH solution	To assess for fungal infection, tinea versicolor

CLIENT AND ENVIRONMENT

1. Provide a warm room with adequate lighting.
2. Protect the client's modesty while exposing areas to be examined as fully as possible.
3. Explain examination before beginning.
4. Use short, clear instructions.

Risk Factors
Malignant Melanoma

Malignant melanoma is the most rapidly increasing form of cancer in the United States. Surgical treatment of early stages is usually curative, whereas treatment of later stages results in a poor prognosis. Those at high risk for melanoma have one or more of the following:
1. Large number of typical moles
2. Presence of atypical moles
3. Family history of melanoma
4. Prior melanoma
5. History of repeated severe sunburns, ease of burning, freckling, or inability to tan

The NIH Consensus Development Panel on Melanoma (1992) recommends that individuals be taught self-examination of the skin, know the warning signs of melanoma, and contact their health care provider if such signs appear. Warning signs include these *ABCDEs* of melanoma (Figure 10-3):

Asymmetry: Early melanoma is asymmetrical. Most typical or common moles are symmetrical.

Border: Melanomas may have notching, scalloping, or poorly defined borders. Most common moles have very clear-cut borders.

Color: Melanomas are usually variegated. They may have shades of brown, tan, red, white, blue/black, or combinations thereof. Common moles tend to be uniform in color.

Diameter: Melanomas are commonly larger than 6 mm in diameter, although they may be diagnosed at a smaller size. Most common moles are less than 6 mm in diameter (about the size of a pencil eraser).

Elevation: Melanomas are almost always elevated; surface distortion can be assessed by side lighting. (Melanoma *in situ* and acral letiginous lesions may be flat.)

Enlargement: A history of increasing size of the lesion is perhaps one of the most important signs of malignant melanoma.

Risk Factors
Skin Cancer

- Older than 50
- Male
- Family history of skin cancer, especially melanomas
- Fair skin and light-colored hair or eyes
- Precancerous skin lesions (dysplastic nevi, certain congenital nevi)
- Extended periods of exposure to sunlight (occupational or recreational)
- Tendency to burn easily
- Geographical location—high altitudes or near equator
- Exposure to radium, isotopes, x-rays, ultraviolet light
- Exposure to coal, tar, arsenic, creosote, and/or petroleum products
- Repeated skin trauma or irritation
- History of childhood sunburns and sunlight exposure

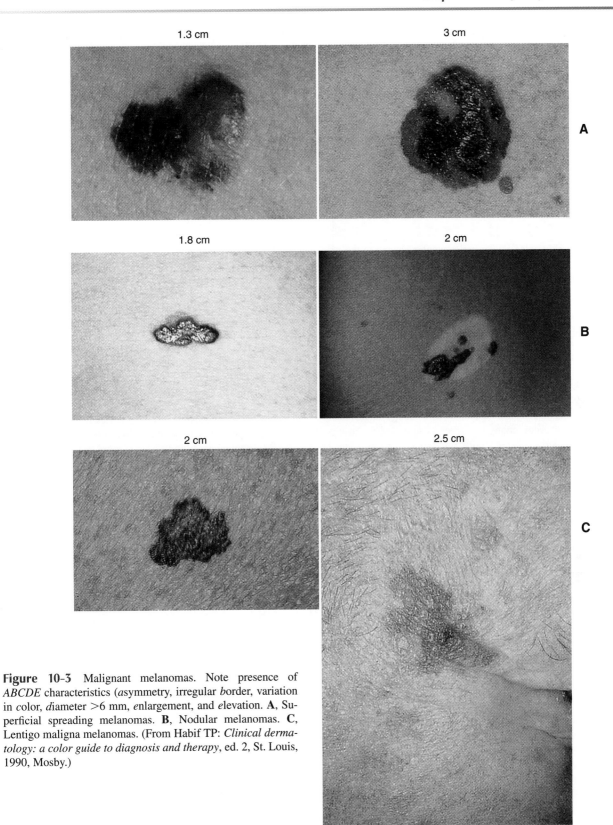

Figure 10-3 Malignant melanomas. Note presence of *ABCDE* characteristics (*a*symmetry, irregular *b*order, variation in *c*olor, *d*iameter >6 mm, *e*nlargement, and *e*levation. **A,** Superficial spreading melanomas. **B,** Nodular melanomas. **C,** Lentigo maligna melanomas. (From Habif TP: *Clinical dermatology: a color guide to diagnosis and therapy*, ed. 2, St. Louis, 1990, Mosby.)

body inspection to get an idea of the distribution pattern and extent of any lesions. Follow this with a detailed examination of the specific areas affected.

Ask the client whether his or her skin is its usual color to establish the baseline reference point. Compare symmetrical anatomical areas throughout the examination. Also compare sun-exposed areas with areas not exposed to the sun. Examine intertriginous areas (those with skinfolds), which are dark, warm, and moist, such as large breasts, the groin, or an obese abdomen, for signs of irritation and/or infection. Make sure to have the client remove the socks, and examine the feet, including the toenails and the areas between the toes.

Skin

Inspection. Inspect the skin for color and vascularity and for evidence of perspiration, edema, injuries, or skin lesions. During the examination, think about the underlying structures and the particular kind of exposure of a body part. Note changes in the skin that indicate past injuries and habits, such as calluses, stains, scars, needle marks, or insect bites. Also note the grooming of hair and nails.

> **■ HELPFUL HINT**
>
> In evaluating skin color, if you notice a color change in the client's skin, consider:
> * The lighting in the examination room
> * The position of the client or the client's extremity
> * The room temperature
> * The client's emotional condition
> * The cleanliness of the skin
> * The presence of edema

Color. Skin color varies from person to person. It is important to ask the client about his or her usual skin coloring before the examination. This baseline knowledge is important in assessing color change. Expected skin color varies from light tan to dark brown with pinkish or yellow overtones, depending on race. Skin color also varies from one part of the body to another. The exposed areas of the body, including the face, ears, back of the neck, and backs of the hands and arms, are noticeably different from the unexposed areas. Exposed areas may be more damaged after long exposure to the sun and weather.

The vascular flush areas (cheeks, bridge of the nose, neck, upper chest, flexor surfaces of the extremities, and genital area) may appear pink or red with anxiety, excitement, or temperature elevation. Compare them with areas of less vascularity. The pigment-labile areas are the face, backs of the hands, flexors of the wrists, axillae, mammary areolae, midline of the abdomen, and genital area. These areas may show normal systemic pigmentary changes, such as during pregnancy.

Changes in skin color may also provide evidence of systemic disease. These changes include the following:

1. **Cyanosis,** a dusky blue color, may be visible in the nailbeds and in the lips and the oral mucosa. It results from decreased oxyhemoglobin binding, or decreased oxygenation of the blood, and can be caused by pulmonary or heart disease, by abnormalities of hemoglobin, or by cold.
2. **Jaundice,** a yellow or green hue, occurs when tissue bilirubin is increased and may be visible first in the sclerae and then in the mucous membranes and the skin.
3. **Pallor,** or decreased color in the skin, results from decreased blood flow to the superficial vessels or from decreased amounts of hemoglobin in the blood. Pallor is most evident in the face, the palpebral conjunctiva, the mouth, and the nailbeds.

> **■ HELPFUL HINT**
>
> In assessing dark skin, consider the following:
> 1. Skin color should be observed in the sclera, conjunctiva, buccal mucosa, tongue, lips, nailbeds, palms, and soles.
> 2. Inspection should be accompanied by palpation, especially if inflammation or edema is suspected.
> 3. Findings should always be correlated with the client's history to arrive at a nursing diagnosis.
> 4. *Pallor* in brown-skinned patients may present as a yellowish brown tinge to the skin. In a black-skinned patient the skin will appear "ashen gray." It can be difficult to determine. Pallor in dark-skinned individuals is characterized by absence of the underlying red tones in the skin.
> 5. *Jaundice* may be observed in the sclera but should not be confused with the normal yellow pigmentation of the dark-skinned patient. The best place to inspect is in that portion of the sclera that is observable when the eye is open. If jaundice is suspected, the posterior portion of the hard palate should also be observed for a yellowish cast. This is most effective when done in bright daylight.
> 6. The *oral mucosa* of dark-skinned individuals may have a normal freckling of pigmentation that may also be evident in the gums, the borders of the tongue, and the lining of the cheeks.
> 7. The *gingiva* normally may have a dark blue color that may appear blotchy or be evenly distributed.
> 8. *Petechiae* are best observed over areas of lighter pigmentation: the abdomen, gluteal areas, and volar aspect of the forearm. They may also be seen in the palpebral conjunctiva and buccal mucosa.
> 9. To differentiate petechiae and ecchymosis from erythema, remember that pressure over the area will cause erythema to blanch but will not affect either petechiae or ecchymosis.
> 10. *Erythema* usually is associated with increased skin temperature, so palpation should also be used if an inflammatory condition is suspected.
> 11. *Edema* may reduce the intensity of the color of an area of skin because of the increased distance between the external epithelium and the pigmented layers. Therefore, darker skin would appear lighter. On palpation the skin may feel "tight."
> 12. *Cyanosis* can often be difficult to determine in dark-skinned individuals. Familiarity with the precyanotic color is often helpful. However, if this is not possible, close inspection of the nailbeds, lips, palpebral conjunctiva, palms, and soles should show evidence of cyanosis.
> 13. *Skin rashes* may be assessed by palpating for changes in skin texture.

Used with permission from *Nursing 77* 7(1):48-52, January 1977. © Springhouse Corporation, www.springnet.com.

4. **Erythema,** or an intense redness of the skin, may be generalized or localized. Generalized redness of the skin may be caused by fever, whereas defined areas of redness may be the result of a localized infection or sunburn.
5. **Pigmentation changes** or alterations in the normal pattern of pigmentation result from changes in the

TABLE 10-1	**Conditions Causing Variation in Pigmentation**	
Condition	**Characteristic Color**	**Location**
Diffuse Hyperpigmentation		
Addison's disease, ACTH-producing tumors	Tan to brown, "bronzing"	Generalized, more marked on exposed areas, flexures, mucous membrane of mouth
Arsenic toxicity	Dusky, diffuse, paler spots	Trunk, extremities
Chloasma (mask of pregnancy), phenytoin ingestion	Tan to brown	Forehead—adjacent to hairline, malar prominence, upper lip, chin
Hemochromatosis	Bronze to grayish brown, deposits of hemosiderin	Generalized
Ichthyosis	Tan, fine to coarse scales	Generalized
Malabsorption syndrome (sprue)	Tan to brown patches	Any area of body
Scleroderma	Yellow to tan (may also have depigmentation)	Generalized
Uremia (chronic renal failure)	Yellow-brown, retention of urinary chromogens	Generalized
Lack of Pigmentation		
Vitiligo	Circumscribed lack of pigmentation	Face, eyelids, neck, axillae, hands, wrists, groin
Albinism—hereditary	Complete or partial lack of melanin	Generalized (universal albinism), skin, hair, eyes

ACTH, Adrenocorticotropic hormone.

distribution of melanin or in the function of the melanocytes in the epidermis. Either hyperpigmentation or depigmentation can occur. A **nevus**, or birthmark, is an example of a defined area of hyperpigmentation that may be an innocent manifestation, such as the Mongolian spots found on infants, or it may be a more serious finding, such as the numerous café-au-lait spots of neurofibromatosis. Depigmentation of the skin, which occurs in vitiligo, may involve only one or a few areas or may be more generalized. Common sites of vitiligo are the face, neck, axillae, groin, anogenital area, eyelids, hands, and wrists. Table 10-1 lists other conditions causing variations in pigmentation.

Pigmentation differences related to skin tone and racial characteristics will impact the manifestation of the aforementioned color changes. It is important to be knowledgeable of the ways these problems present in clients of different skin tones in order to make an accurate assessment. Table 10-2 compares the differences in assessment of color changes in light-skinned and dark-skinned individuals.

Palpation

Palpate the skin to augment your findings on inspection. In general, perform palpation simultaneously as you examine each body part. Note changes in temperature, moisture, texture, and turgor.

Temperature. Skin temperature increases when blood flow through the dermis increases. Localized elevations in skin temperature occur with a burn or a localized infection. A generalized increase in skin temperature may occur with a fever, which may be due to a localized infection or systemic disease. The temperature of the skin is reduced when blood flow through the dermis decreases. Generalized skin coolness occurs when the client is in shock. Localized hypothermia occurs in conditions such as arteriosclerosis. Always check for bilateral symmetry. Inequality in temperature may indicate circulatory problems or infection.

Moisture. Moisture on the skin varies from one body area to another. The soles of the feet, palms of the hands, and intertriginous areas (i.e., where two surfaces are close together) contain more moisture than other parts. The amount of moisture found over the entire integument also varies with changes in the environmental temperature, muscular activity, and body temperature. The skin regulates body temperature by producing perspiration when the temperature increases. Evaporation of the sweat then lowers the body temperature. The skin is normally drier as the individual ages and during the winter months when environmental temperatures and humidity are lower. Abnormal dryness of the skin occurs with dehydration. In this instance, the skin feels dry even when the temperature increases. In addition, the normally smooth and moist oral mucous membranes become dry, and the lips are dry and cracked. Dryness of the skin also occurs in conditions such as myxedema and chronic nephritis.

Texture. Texture refers to the fineness or coarseness of the skin. Changes in skin texture may indicate local irritation or trauma to defined skin areas or may be associated with problems of other systems. The skin becomes soft and smooth in hyperthyroidism and rough and dry in hypothyroidism.

Turgor. Turgor refers to the elasticity of the skin. You can most easily determine turgor by picking up a fold of skin over the abdomen and observing how quickly it returns to its normal shape (Figure 10-4). A loss of turgor is associated with dehydration. The skin demonstrates a laxness and a loss of normal mobility, returning to place slowly. Loss of turgor is also associated with aging; the skin becomes wrinkled and lax from loss of elasticity. Increased turgor is associated with

TABLE 10-2 Differences in Color Changes in Light and Dark Skin

Etiology	Light Skin	Dark Skin
Pallor		
Anemia—decreased hematocrit Shock—decreased perfusion, vasoconstriction	Generalized pallor, loss of rosy glow in skin, especially in face; skin with natural yellow tones appears more yellow, may be mistaken for mild jaundice	Brown skin appears yellow-brown, dull; black skin loses its red undertones and appears ashen gray; skin loses its healthy glow—check areas with pigmentation, such as conjunctivae, mucous membranes
Local arterial insufficiency	Marked localized pallor (e.g., lower extremities), especially when elevated	Ashen gray, dull; cool to palpation
Albinism—total absence of pigment melanin throughout integument	Whitish pink skin; white or pale blond(e) hair; pink irises	Tan, cream, or white skin; white or pale blond(e) hair; pink irises
Vitiligo—patchy depigmentation from destruction of melanocytes	Patchy milky white spots, often symmetrical, bilaterally, especially around mouth	Patchy milky white spots, often symmetrical bilaterally
Cyanosis		
Increased amount of unoxygenated hemoglobin Central—chronic heart and lung disease cause arterial desaturation	Skin, lips, and mucous membranes look blue tinged; nailbeds, and conjunctivae are blue	Skin dark but dull, lifeless; natural skin tone will influence color of cyanotic skin*
Peripheral—exposure to cold, anxiety	Nailbeds dusky	Nailbeds dusky
Erythema		
Hyperemia—increased blood flow through engorged arterioles, such as in inflammation, fever, alcohol intake, blushing	Red, bright pink; easily seen anywhere on body; inflammation accompanied by higher temperature at site	Redness may be difficult to detect; localized inflamed areas may appear purple; rely on palpation for increased temperature, hardness, swelling, or edema
Polycythemia—increased red blood cells, capillary stasis	Ruddy blue in face, oral mucosa, conjunctiva, hands and feet	Difficult to detect; check lips for redness
Carbon monoxide poisoning	Bright cherry red in face and upper torso	Cherry red color in nailbeds, lips, and oral mucosa
Venous stasis—decreased blood flow from area, engorged venules	Dusky rubor of dependent extremities; a prelude to necrosis with pressure sore	Easily masked; use palpation for warmth or edema

In the Cyanosis / Dark Skin cell:

Natural		Cyanotic
black	→	gray
brown	→	dark blue
red	→	purple
tan	→	blue
yellow	→	green
white	→	blue

Cyanosis may be undetectable except for ashen gray lips, tongue, oral mucous membranes, nailbeds; conjunctivae may appear pale or blue tinged

*As described by Gaskin (1986).

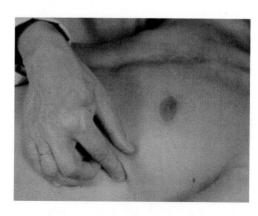

Figure 10-4 Testing skin turgor.

TABLE 10-2 Differences in Color Changes in Light and Dark Skin—cont'd

Etiology	Light Skin	Dark Skin
Purpuras		
Ecchymosis (bruise) Large patch of capillary bleeding into tissue secondary to trauma	Color goes from: 1. Red-blue or purple within 24 hours of trauma 2. Blue to purple (1–5 days) 3. Green (5–7 days) 4. Yellow (7–10 days) 5. Brown to disappearing (10–14 days)	Deeper dark purple, bluish, or black tone; difficult to see unless it occurs in an area of light pigmentation
Petechiae Due to bleeding from superficial capillaries; infection	Lesions appear as small, reddish purple pinpoints; may be seen in mouth, buccal mucosa, and conjunctiva; on skin especially noticeable on abdomen, buttocks, and inner surfaces of arms or legs	Difficult to see; may be evident in buccal mucosa, sclera, and conjunctiva; also look in areas of lighter melanization such as abdomen, buttocks, and inner surface of forearm
Jaundice		
Increased serum bilirubin, over 2 to 3 mg/dl, due to liver inflammation or hemolytic disease, such as after severe burns and some infections	Generalized; also see yellow in sclera, hard palate, oral mucosa, fingernails, palms of hands, and soles of feet	Check sclera for yellow near limbus; do not mistake normal yellowish fatty deposits in periphery under eyelids for jaundice—jaundice best noted in junction of hands and soft palate and also on palms of hand and soles of feet
Carotenemia—increased serum carotene from ingestion of large amounts of carotene-rich foods	Yellow-orange in forehead, palms and soles, and nasolabial folds, but no yellowing in sclera or mucous membranes	Yellow-orange tinge on palms of hands and soles of feet; no yellowing of sclera or mucous membranes
Uremia—renal failure causes retained urochrome pigments in blood	Generalized pallor and yellow or orange-green or gray overlying pallor of anemia; may also have ecchymoses and purpura; does not affect conjunctiva or mucous membranes	Difficult to discern and easily masked; rely on laboratory and clinical findings; does not affect conjunctiva or mucous membranes
Brown-Tan		
Addison's disease—cortisol deficiency stimulates increased melanin production	Bronzed appearance, an "eternal tan"; most apparent around nipples, perineum, genitalia, and pressure points (inner thighs, buttocks, elbow, axillae)	General deepening of skin tone, but is easily masked; rely on laboratory and clinical findings
Rash		
Various causes	May be visualized, as well as felt with light palpation	Not easily visualized but may be felt with light palpation
Scar		
Multiple causes	Generally heals, showing narrow scar line	Frequently has keloid development, resulting in a thickened, raised scar

an increase in tension, which causes the skin to return to place quickly when pinched. Increased turgor occurs in progressive systemic sclerosis (PSS), a connective tissue disorder.

Lesions

Perform the initial examination of any skin lesion at a distance of 3 feet or more to determine the general characteristics of the eruption. This first observation provides the opportunity to determine the location, distribution, and configuration of the lesions. Next, carry out a closer examination to determine the type of lesion(s): its color, size, shape, texture, firmness, and morphological characteristics.

Type of Lesion. The morphological classification of skin lesions is based on the size, shape, and elevation or depression of the lesions. Determining the morphological structure of the individual lesion (macule, papule, vesicle, etc.) helps identify the specific problem. Table 10-3 provides detailed parameters for classification of skin lesions.

Classify lesions as primary, secondary, or vascular. Primary lesions are those that appear initially in response to some change in the external or internal environment of the skin. Secondary lesions do not appear initially but result from modifications such as trauma, chronicity, or infection in the primary lesion. For instance, the primary lesion may be a vesicle, which is a small, circumscribed, elevated lesion containing clear fluid. The vesicle will rupture, leaving a small moist area, which is classified as a secondary lesion called an erosion. Tables 10-4 and 10-5 illustrate some of the primary and secondary lesions. Table 10-6 describes types

of skin lesions that characterize acute, subacute, and chronic stages of dermatitis. Primary and secondary lesions may occur at the same time.

Vascular lesions usually appear as red pigmented lesions. They may be indicative of problems such as bleeding (petechiae and ecchymoses) or liver disease (spider angioma), or they may be due to benign conditions such as telangiectasia. Determining whether the lesion blanches (diascopy) will help differentiate purpuric lesions. Place a glass slide over the lesion and apply pressure. This expresses blood from the capillaries and superficial venules, and the lesion fades. Petechial or purpuric lesions, which are caused by extravasation of blood into the dermis, will not blanch. Erythematous lesions (hives), which are caused by increased blood in dilated blood vessels in the skin, and vascular lesions with intact vessel walls (telangiectasia), do blanch. Vascular lesions are described in Figure 10-5.

Measure the lesion with a small, clear, and flexible ruler. Report sizes in centimeters (inches may also be used but are less desirable). Measure all the dimensions possible (length, width, height/depth). If possible, draw a diagram with location and dimensions included. This will help you monitor the progression or resolution of the lesion. The term used to

Text continued on p. 204

■ HELPFUL HINT

When assessing skin lesions, if a lesion is present, consider the following:
• Are there any associated symptoms (e.g., pruritus)?
• What is the chronology of the appearance of these lesions?
• Are they changing in morphology? Are they disappearing?
• Are there associated variables or precipitants, such as the following:
  Environmental exposures
  Injury
  Infection
  Use of medications (prescribed or self-treatment)
  Diet
  Clothing
  Emotional factors
  Personal care items, such as soaps and cosmetics

TABLE 10-3   Identification of Skin Lesions

	Name of Lesion	Description	<1 cm	>1 cm
Type:				
Primary lesion	Macule—patch	Flat, circumscribed discoloration	Macule	Patch
	Papule—plaque	Solid, elevated lesion	Papule	Plaque
	Nodule—tumor	Solid, elevated lesion; also has depth	Nodule	Tumor
	Vesicle—bulla	Fluid, filled, superficial, elevated	Vesicle	Bulla
Primary lesions of varying sizes	Pustule	Vesicle or bulla containing pus		
	Wheal	Lesion caused by cutaneous edema; irregular in shape; elevated; transient		
	Telangiectasia	Dilated capillary; fine red line(s)		
	Cyst	Elevated, circumscribed, encapsulated lesion		
Secondary lesion	Scale	Accumulation of loose surface epithelium		
	Crust	Dried surface fluids: serum or pus		
	Excoriation	Scratch mark		
	Erosion	Superficial denuded lesion		
	Scar	First red, then pale, smooth hyaline wound repair; may be flat, depressed, elevated		
	Keloid	Hypertrophic scar		
	Ulcer	Loss of tissue from a surface caused by destruction of a superficial lesion		
	Atrophy	Thinning of skin; loss of hair and sweat glands		
	Fissure	Linear crack in skin that extends to dermis		
	Lichenification	Thickening of skin caused by chronic scratching		

Number: ☐ Single   ☐ Numerous   ☐ Actual count
Size: (Measure [cm])
Shape: ☐ Round   ☐ Oval   ☐ Umbilicated   ☐ Irregular
Color: ☐ Red   ☐ Brown   ☐ Black   ☐ Gray-blue   ☐ White   ☐ Purple
              ☐ Orange   ☐ Yellow   ☐ Circumscribed?   ☐ Diffuse?   ☐ Change with diascopy?*
Configuration   ☐ Single   ☐ Grouped   ☐ Herpetiform   ☐ Linear   ☐ Annular   ☐ Archiform
(see Figure 10-6):   ☐ Reticular   ☐ Scattered
Distribution   ☐ Localized   ☐ Generalized   ☐ Symmetrical
(see Figure 10-7):
   Site of predilection _____

*Diascopy consists of the application of firm pressure against a microscopic slide or clear plastic placed over a skin lesion, allowing identification of capillary dilation and thus differentiating telangiectasia from purpura. The technique also makes lymphoma, sarcoidosis, and tuberculosis of the skin appear yellow-brown.

TABLE 10-4	**Primary Skin Lesions**

Description	Examples		
Macule A flat, circumscribed area that is a change in the color of the skin; less than 1 cm in diameter	Freckles, flat moles (nevi), petechiae, measles, scarlet fever	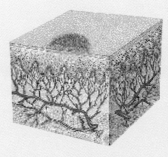	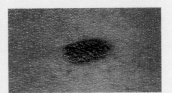 Flat nevi. (From Habif TP: *Clinical dermatology: a color guide to diagnosis and therapy,* ed. 2, St. Louis, 1990, Mosby.)
Papule An elevated, firm, circumscribed area less than 1 cm in diameter	Wart (verruca), elevated moles, lichen planus	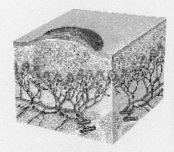	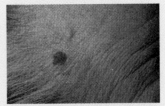 Cherry angioma. (From Baran R, Dawber RPR, Levene GM: *Color atlas of the hair, scalp, and nails,* London, 1991, Wolfe.)
Patch A flat, nonpalpable, irregular-shaped macule more than 1 cm in diameter	Vitiligo, portwine stains, mongolian spots, café au lait spot	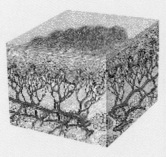	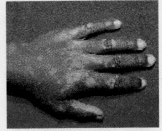 Vitiligo. (From Weston WL, Lane AT: *Color textbook of pediatric dermatology,* St. Louis, 1991, Mosby.)
Plaque Elevated, firm, and rough lesion with flat top surface greater than 1 cm in diameter	Psoriasis, seborrheic and actinic keratoses	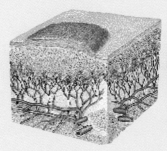	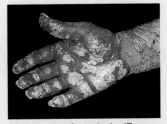 Plaque type of psoriasis. (From Goldstein BG, Goldstein AO: *Practical dermatology,* ed. 2, St. Louis, 1997, Mosby.)

From Wilson SF, Giddens JF: *Health assessment for nursing practice,* ed. 2, St. Louis, 2001, Mosby.

Continued

TABLE 10-4	**Primary Skin Lesions—cont'd**

Description	Examples		

Wheal

Elevated irregular-shaped area of cutaneous edema; solid, transient; variable diameter

Insect bites, urticaria, allergic reaction

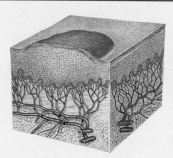 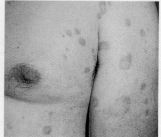

Wheals of urticaria. (From Goldstein BG, Goldstein AO: *Practical dermatology,* ed. 2, St. Louis, 1997, Mosby.)

Nodule

Elevated, firm, circumscribed lesion; deeper in dermis than a papule; 1 to 2 cm in diameter

Erythema nodosum, lipomas

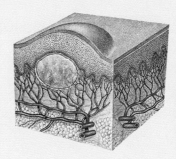 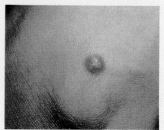

Dermatofibroma. (From Goldstein BG, Goldstein AO: *Practical dermatology,* ed. 2, St. Louis, 1997, Mosby.)

Tumor

Elevated and solid lesion; may or may not be clearly demarcated; deeper in dermis; greater than 2 cm in diameter

Neoplasms, benign tumor, lipoma, hemangioma

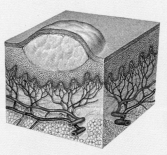 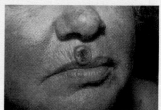

Tumor of upper lip. (From Goldstein BG, Goldstein AO: *Practical dermatology,* ed. 2, St. Louis, 1997, Mosby.)

Vesicle

Elevated, circumscribed, superficial, not into dermis; filled with serous fluid; less than 1 cm in diameter

Varicella (chickenpox), herpes zoster (shingles)

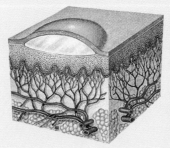 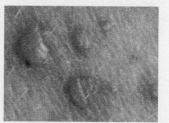

Vesicles. (From Farrar WE et al.: *Infectious diseases,* ed. 2, London, 1992, Gower.)

TABLE 10-4	**Primary Skin Lesions—cont'd**		
Description	**Examples**		

Bulla

Vesicle greater than 1 cm in diameter

Blister, pemphigus vulgaris

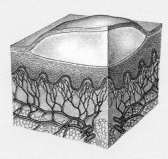 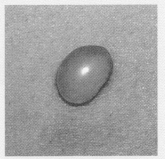

Blister. (From White GM: *Color atlas of regional dermatology,* St. Louis, 1994, Mosby.)

Pustule

Elevated, superficial lesion; similar to a vesicle but filled with purulent fluid

Impetigo, acne

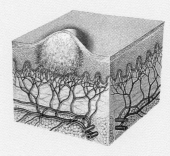 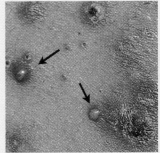

Acne. (From Weston WL, Lane AT: *Color textbook of pediatric dermatology,* ed. 2, St. Louis, 1996, Mosby.)

Cyst

Elevated, circumscribed, encapsulated lesion; in dermis or subcutaneous layer; filled with liquid or semisolid material

Sebaceous cyst, cystic acne

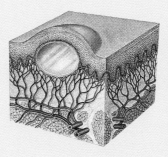 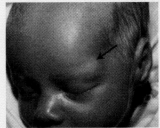

Sebaceous cyst. (From Weston WL, Lane AT: *Color textbook of pediatric dermatology,* ed. 2, St. Louis, 1996, Mosby.)

Telangiectasia

Fine, irregular red lines produced by capillary dilation

Telangiectasia in rosacea

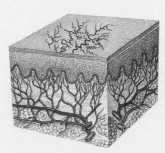 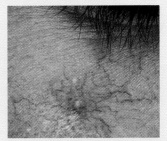

Vascular spider. (From Habif TP: *Clinical dermatology: a color guide to diagnosis and therapy,* ed. 3, St. Louis, 1996, Mosby.)

From Wilson SF, Giddens JF: *Health assessment for nursing practice,* ed. 2, St. Louis, 2001, Mosby.

TABLE 10-5	**Secondary Skin Lesions**

Description	Examples		
Scale Heaped-up keratinized cells; flaky skin; irregular; thick or thin; dry or oily; variation in size	Flaking of skin with seborrheic dermatitis following scarlet fever, or flaking of skin following a drug reaction; dry skin	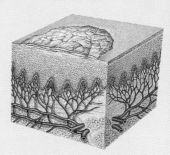	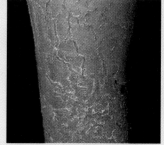 Scaling. (From Habif TP: *Clinical dermatology: a color guide to diagnosis and therapy,* ed. 3, St. Louis, 1996, Mosby.)
Lichenification Rough, thickened epidermis secondary to persistent rubbing, itching, or skin irritation; often involves flexor surface of extremity	Chronic dermatitis	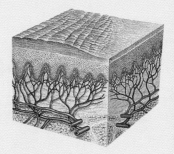	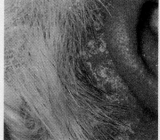 Stasis dermatitis in an early stage. (From Marks Jr JG, DeLeo VA: *Contact and occupational dermatology,* St. Louis, 1992, Mosby.)
Keloid Irregular-shaped, elevated, progressively enlarging scar; grows beyond the boundaries of the wound; caused by excessive collagen formation during healing	Keloid formation following surgery	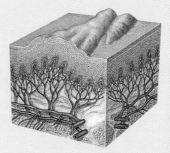	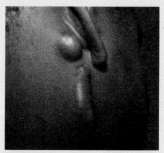 Keloid. (From Weston WL, Lane AT: *Color textbook of pediatric dermatology,* ed. 2, St. Louis, 1996, Mosby.)
Scar Thin to thick fibrous tissue that replaces normal skin following injury or laceration to the dermis	Healed wound or surgical incision	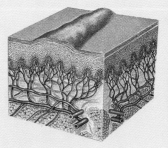	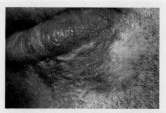 Hypertrophic scar. (From Goldman MP, Fitzpatrick RE: *Cutaneous laser surgery: the art and science of selective photothermolysis,* St. Louis, 1994, Mosby.)

From Wilson SF, Giddens JF: *Health assessment for nursing practice,* ed. 2, St. Louis, 2001, Mosby.

TABLE 10-5	**Secondary Skin Lesions—cont'd**

Description	Examples		
Excoriation Loss of the epidermis; linear hollowed-out crusted area	Abrasion or scratch, scabies	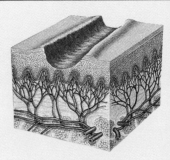	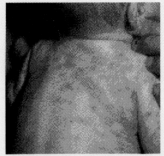Scabies. (From Weston WL, Lane AT: *Color textbook of pediatric dermatology,* ed. 2, St. Louis, 1996, Mosby.)
Fissure Linear crack or break from the epidermis to the dermis; may be moist or dry	Athlete's foot, cracks at the corner of the mouth	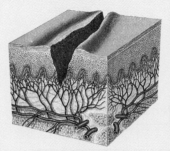	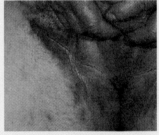Fissure. (From Habif TP: *Clinical dermatology: a color guide to diagnosis and therapy,* ed. 3, St. Louis, 1996, Mosby.)
Erosion Loss of part of the epidermis; depressed, moist, glistening; follows rupture of a vesicle or bulla	Varicella, variola after rupture	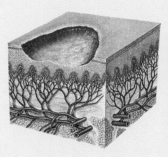	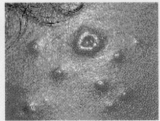Erosion. (From Cohen BA: *Atlas of pediatric dermatology,* St. Louis, 1993, Mosby.)
Ulcer Loss of epidermis and dermis; concave; varies in size	Decubiti, stasis ulcers	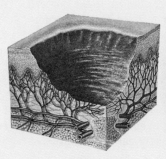	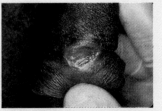Ulcer caused by syphilis. (From Goldstein BG, Goldstein AO: *Practical dermatology,* ed. 2, St. Louis, 1997, Mosby.)

Continued

TABLE 10-5	**Secondary Skin Lesions—cont'd**

Description	Examples	
Atrophy		
Thinning of skin surface and loss of skin markings; skin translucent and paperlike	Striae; aged skin	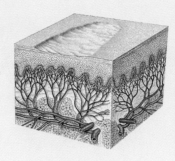 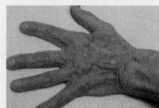 Aged skin. (From Seidel HM et al.: *Mosby's guide to physical examination,* ed. 4, St. Louis, 1999, Mosby.)

From Wilson SF, Giddens JF: *Health assessment for nursing practice,* ed. 2, St. Louis, 2001, Mosby.

TABLE 10-6	**Stages of Dermatitis**

Stage	Lesions
Acute	Erythema, edema, vesicles, exudate, crusting
Subacute	Erythema, residual crusting, scaling
Chronic	Scaling, hyperpigmentation, lichenification, fissuring

describe a lesion will vary with its size. For example, a vesicle is a fluid-filled lesion and is less than 1 centimeter in diameter. If it is greater than 1 centimeter, it is called a bulla.

Always wear gloves when palpating a skin lesion. Gently palpate lesions to determine their texture, firmness, and tenderness and in some instances to determine the actual shape of the lesions.

Color. Describe the color of the individual lesion. There may be no discoloration, or you may see many colors. For example, with ecchymosis the initial dark red and dark blue colors fade and a yellow color appears. Lesions may be well-defined, with the color changes limited to the borders of the lesion. These lesions are referred to as "circumscribed." Lesions may have "diffuse" borders that are undefined, with the color changes spread over a large area.

Distribution. Describe the distribution of skin lesions according to the location or body region affected and the symmetry or asymmetry of findings in comparable body parts. Keep in mind that there are characteristic patterns for many skin disorders. These may provide a major clue in the diagnosis of a specific skin problem. Figure 10-6 illustrates distribution patterns observed in selected problems. Table 10-7 lists the regional distribution of common skin growths and rashes.

Configuration. Note the configuration, or arrangement, of skin lesions, which is equally important in defining the problem. Configuration refers to the arrangement or position of several lesions in relation to each other. For example, the skin lesions of tinea corporis, which is ringworm of the body, have an annular configuration that is circular. Figure 10-7, within Table 10-8, illustrates some configurations, and Table 10-8 describes their characteristics and provides example dermatoses.

Sebaceous Glands

The sebaceous glands, which are more numerous over the face and scalp areas, normally become more active during adolescence. This increased activity results in more oil in the skin. A sudden increase in the oil of the skin at other ages is not normal and may suggest an endocrine problem.

Hair

Inspection and Palpation. Examine the hair and scalp for any lesions. Separate the head hair into sections to fully inspect the scalp. Examine the hair over the entire body to determine the color, distribution, quantity, and quality.

Distribution. Hair may be present on the scalp, lower face, nares, ears, neck, axillae, anterior chest, back and shoulders, arms, legs, buttocks and pubic area, and around the nipples. Coarse terminal hair occurs on the scalp, on the pubic and axillary areas, and in the male's beard. The body is covered with fine vellus hair. A normal male or female hair pattern evolves after puberty. The pattern of hair distribution in the male genital area is diamond shaped, whereas the pattern of hair distribution in the female genital area is an inverted triangle. A deviation may indicate an endocrine problem.

Text continued on p. 209

Purpura—red-purple nonblanchable discoloration greater than 0.5 cm diameter.
Cause: Intravascular defects, infection

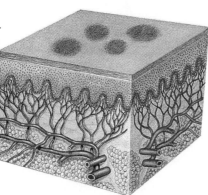

Petechiae—red-purple nonblanchable discoloration less than 0.5 cm diameter
Cause: Intravascular defects, infection

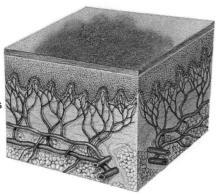

Ecchymoses—red-purple non-blanchable discoloration of variable size
Cause: Vascular wall destruction, trauma, vasculitis

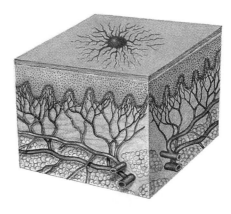

Spider angioma—red central body with radiating spiderlike legs that blanch with pressure to the central body
Cause: Liver disease, vitamin B deficiency, idiopathic

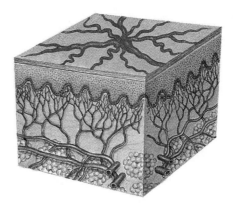

Venous star—bluish spider, linear or irregularly shaped; does not blanch with pressure
Cause: Increased pressure in superficial veins

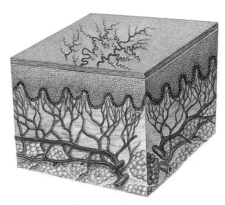

Telangiectasia—fine, irregular red line
Cause: Dilation of capillaries

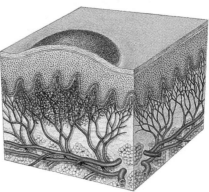

Capillary hemangioma (nevus flammeus)—red irregular macular patches
Cause: Dilation of dermal capillaries

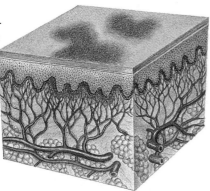

Figure 10-5 Characteristics and causes of vascular lesions. (Modified from Seidel HM et al: *Mosby's guide to physical examination*, ed. 4, St. Louis, 1999, Mosby.)

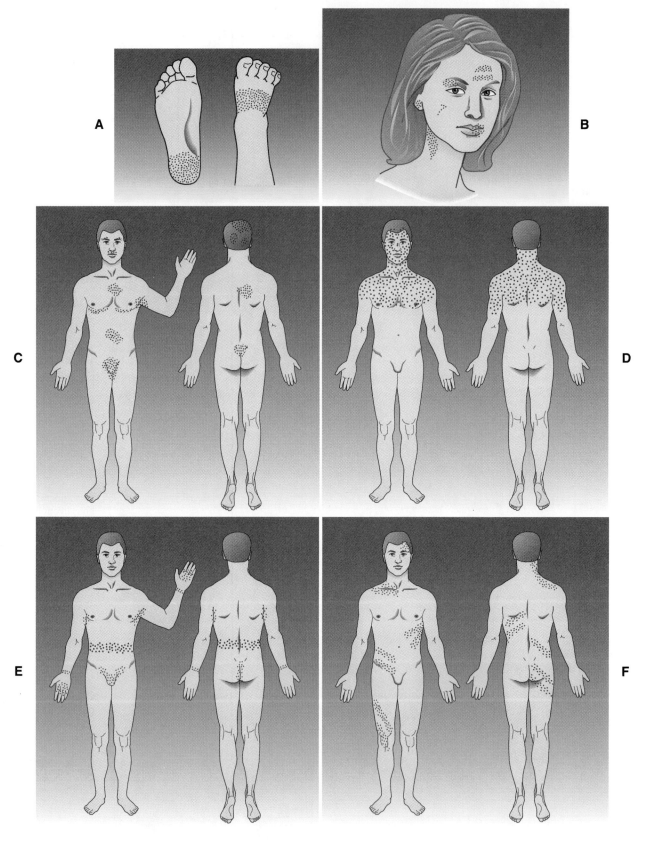

Figure 10-6   Distribution of lesions in selected problems of the skin. **A,** Contact dermatitis (shoes). **B,** Contact dermatitis (cosmetics, perfumes, earrings). **C,** Seborrheic dermatitis. **D,** Acne. **E,** Scabies. **F,** Herpes zoster.

TABLE 10-7   Regional Distribution of Skin Lesions

Growths	Rashes	Growths	Rashes
Scalp		**Extremities**	
Nevus	Seborrheic dermatitis (dandruff)	Nevus	Atopic dermatitis
Seborrheic keratosis	Psoriasis	Dermatofibroma	Contact dermatitis (from plants)
Pilar cyst	Tinea capitis	Wart	Psoriasis
	Folliculitis	Xanthoma	Insect bites
		Seborrheic keratosis	Erythema multiforme
Face		Actinic keratosis	Lichen planus (wrists and ankles)
Nevus	Acne		Actinic purpura (arms)
Lentigo	Acne rosacea		Stasis dermatitis (legs)
Actinic keratosis	Seborrheic dermatitis		Vasculitis (legs)
Seborrheic keratosis	Contact dermatitis (cosmetics)		Erythema nodosum (legs)
Sebaceous hyperplasia	Herpes simplex		
Basal cell carcinoma	Impetigo	**Hands (Dorsa)**	
Squamous cell carcinoma	Pityriasis alba	Wart	Contact dermatitis (occupational)
Flat wart	Atopic dermatitis	Actinic keratosis	Scabies (interdigital)
Nevus flammeus	Lupus erythematosus	Actinic lentigo	
		Squamous cell cancer	
Trunk		Keratoacanthoma	
Nevus	Acne	**Hands (Palmar)**	
Skin tag	Tinea vesicolor	Wart	Nonspecific eczematous dermatitis
Cherry hemangioma	Psoriasis		Atopic dermatitis
Seborrheic keratosis	Pityriasis rosea		Psoriasis
Epidermal inclusion cyst	Scabies		Tinea manuum
Lipoma	Drug eruption		Erythema multiforme
Basal cell carcinoma	Varicella		Secondary syphilis
Keloid	Mycosis fungoides		
Neurofibroma	Secondary syphilis	**Feet (Dorsa)**	
		Wart	Contact dermatitis (shoe)
Genitalia		**Feet (Plantar)**	
Wart (condyloma acuminatum)	Herpes simplex	Wart (plantar)	Tinea pedis
Molluscum contagiosum	Scabies	Corn	Nonspecific eczematous dermatitis
	Psoriasis	Nevus	Psoriasis
	Lichen planus		Atopic dermatitis
	Syphilis (chancre)		
Groin (Inguinal)			
Skin tag	Intertrigo		
Wart	Tinea cruris		
Molluscum contagiosum	Candidiasis		
	Pediculosis pubis		
	Hidradenitis suppurativa		
	Psoriasis		
	Seborrheic dermatitis		

Modified from Lookingbill D, Marks J: *Principles of dermatology,* ed. 2, Philadelphia, 1993, WB Saunders.

TABLE 10-8   Descriptive Dermatologic Terms

Lesion*		Characteristics	Examples
Annular		Ring shaped	Ringworm
Arcuate		Partial rings	Syphilis

*Examples of different configurations of skin lesions and their descriptions are contained within Table 10-8 as Figure 10-7. (From Swartz MH: *Textbook of physical diagnosis: history and examination,* ed. 3, Philadelphia, 1998, WB Saunders.)
Continued

TABLE 10-8	Descriptive Dermatologic Terms—cont'd	
Lesion	**Characteristics**	**Examples**
Bizarre	Irregular or geographic pattern *not* related to any underlying anatomic structure	Factitial dermatitis
Circinate	Circular	
Confluent	Lesions run together	Childhood exanthems
Discoid	Disc shaped without central clearing	Lupus erythematosus
Discrete	Lesions remain separate	
Eczematoid	An inflammation with a tendency to vesiculate and crust	Eczema
Generalized	Widespread	
Grouped	Lesions clustered together	Herpes simplex
Iris	Circle within a circle; a bull's-eye lesion	Erythema multiforme (iris)
Keratotic	Horny thickening	Psoriasis
Linear	In lines	Poison ivy dermatitis
Multiform	More than one type of shape or lesion	Erythema multiforme
Papulosquamous	Papules or plaques associated with scaling	Psoriasis
Reticulated	Lace-like network	Oral lichen planus
Serpiginous	Snake-like, creeping	Cutaneous larva migrans
Telangiectatic	Relatively permanent dilation of the superficial blood vessels	Osler-Weber-Rendu disease
Universal	Entire body involved	Alopecia universalis
Zosteriform†	Linear arrangement along a nerve distribution	Herpes zoster

†Also known as dermatomal.

Quantity. Changes in the quantity of the hair are also important. **Hirsutism**, increased hair growth, occurs in conditions such as Cushing's syndrome, polycystic ovary disease, and acromegaly. Decreased hair growth or loss of hair may be associated with hypopituitarism or a pyogenic infection. Patterns of hair loss may also be hormonally regulated, as with male-pattern baldness (Figure 10-8). Table 10-9 lists types of alopecia, or hair loss.

Texture. Hair in the pubic and axillary areas is coarse. Scalp hair may be thick or thin, coarse or fine, straight, curly, or kinky. It should be shiny, smooth, and resilient. These characteristics may be affected by the use of beauty products, such as rinses, hair straighteners, dyes, or permanents. Texture may also change with systemic illnesses. For example, changes in the texture of hair associated with hypothyroidism include dryness and coarseness, and changes associated with hyperthyroidism include increased silkiness and fineness. Texture and color determine the quality of the hair. Palpate the hair for texture and the scalp for dryness, flakiness, or lesions.

Color. Hair color may vary from light blond(e) to black. Changes in color such as graying occur normally with aging. Premature graying may be indicative of underlying disease such as pernicious anemia. Patchy gray hair may develop after nerve injuries. Hair color also may change as a result of malnutrition. Use of dyes, rinses, or permanents also influence hair color.

Nails

Inspection and Palpation. The assessment of the nails is important to determine not only their condition, but also possible evidence of systemic diseases. Examine the nails for shape, normal dorsal curvature, adhesion to the nailbed, regularity of the nail surface, color, cleanliness, and thickness. Examine the skinfolds around the nails for any color changes, swelling, increased temperature, or tenderness (see Figure 10-2). Complete absence of the nail, or anonychia, is usually congenital.

Curvature. The nail surface is usually flat or slightly curved. The nail edges should be rounded and smooth. The normal angle of the nail base is 160 degrees. **Clubbing**, which is associated with respiratory and cardiovascular problems, cirrhosis, colitis, and thyroid disease, occurs when the angle of the nail base exceeds 180 degrees (Figure 10-9). With clubbing, the nail becomes thickened, hard, shiny, and curved at the free end. In advanced cases the entire nail is

TABLE 10-9	Alopecia—Hair Loss
Type of Alopecia	**Description**
Androgen (in female)	Thinning of scalp hair, male pattern; hirsutism on body
Areata	Circumscribed bald areas; sudden onset, usually reversible
Chemical	Hair brittle, breaks off
Cicatricial	Permanent localized loss of hair associated with scarring
Drug or radiation	Generalized loss of hair caused by antineoplastic agents, such as gold, thallium, and arsenic, or by radiation
Male pattern	Receding of anterior hairline, temples, and vertex; hereditary
Mucinosis	Erythmatous papules or plaques without hair
Syphilitic	Generalized thinning of hair or baldness; mucous patches without hair

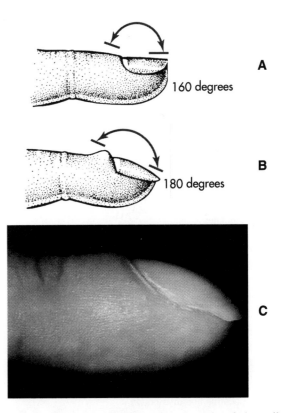

Figure 10-9 Finger clubbing. **A,** Normal angle of the nail. **B,** Abnormal angle of the nail seen in late clubbing. **C,** The distal phalanges are enlarged to a rounded bulbous shape. The nail enlarges and becomes curved, hard, and thickened. (**C** from Habif TP: *Clinical dermatology: a color guide to diagnosis and therapy,* ed. 3, St. Louis, 1996, Mosby.)

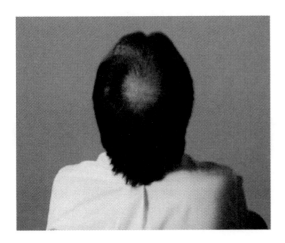

Figure 10-8 Male-pattern baldness.

pushed away from the base at an angle greater than 180 degrees and feels "spongy."

Nail Ahesion.   The nail should be firmly adherent to the nailbed, and the nail base should be firm to palpation. To test for adherence, gently squeeze the nail between your thumb and the pad of your finger (Figure 10-10). Examine the nailfolds for swelling, redness, pus, warts, or tumors. **Paronychia** is an inflammation of the folds of tissue surrounding the nails, leading to erythema, with inflammation, swelling, and induration of the nailfold accompanied by pain and tenderness (Figure 10-11). It is the most common complaint related to the nails.

Nail Surface.   The nail surface should be smooth and flat. Inspect for grooves, depressions, pitting, and ridging. Longitudinal ridging may be a normal variant (Figure 10-12) or may occur with **lichen planus** (Figure 10-13). The client may have transverse grooves related to repeated injury to the nail, as with picking at the nail.

Nail Color.   Nail color should be pink, although pigment bands may normally be present in the nailbeds of dark-skinned individuals (Figure 10-14). Sudden appearance of a pigment band in white individuals may indicate melanoma.

Nail Thickness.   Thickening, or hypertrophy of the nail, is generally caused by trauma. The nail of the small toe is often the only one affected; it takes on a clawlike shape. Thickening of the nails has been associated with psoriasis, fungal infection, a defective vascular supply, and trauma. Thinning of the nail has been linked to defective peripheral circulation and nutritional anemias. Brittleness of the nails is a common finding and may be related to prolonged exposure to water and alkaline substances. Systemic diseases commonly associated with brittle nails are nutritional anemias and impaired peripheral circulation.

Screening Tests and Procedures

Fungal Examination

To confirm the presence of a fungal infection, take fungal scrapings from scaling and vesicular lesions. Using a scalpel, collect scales from the edge of the lesion. Place them on a glass slide. Place one or two drops of 10% to 20% KOH (potassium hydroxide) solution on the scrapings and cover them with a coverslip. Gently heat the slide for 20 to 30 seconds and then cool it for 10 minutes. Examine the slide with a microscope, using both high and low power. If a fungal infection exists, hyphae and spores will be visible as refractile tubules and oval bodies.

Tinea capitis (ringworm of the scalp) has commonly been assessed with a Wood's lamp. However, this is useful for only certain fungal forms of tinea (Habif, 1996). Darken the room and then shine the light on the suspected area. Tinea capitis will fluoresce a characteristic bright blue-green if the infecting organism is *Microsporum canis*. However, the majority of current tinea cases in North America are due to *Trichophyton tonsurans*, which does not fluoresce. Tinea versicolor fluoresces a golden yellow.

Examination Step-by-Step

SKIN

1. Perform an overall inspection of the entire body.
2. Inspect each area of the body for the following:
   a. Color
   b. Symmetry
   c. Uniformity
   d. Thickness
   e. Pigmentation
   f. Lesions
3. Palpate the skin in each area of the body for the following:
   a. Moisture (dry, sweaty, oily, scaly)
   b. Temperature
   c. Thickness
   d. Mobility/turgor
4. Inspect and palpate lesions for the following:
   a. Size
   b. Color
   c. Surface texture (flat, raised, indurated)
   d. Pattern
   e. Location and distribution
   f. Exudates

HAIR

1. Inspect the hair for the following:
   a. Quantity
   b. Distribution
   c. Pattern of loss
   d. Color
   e. Scalp lesions

NAILS

1. Inspect the nails for the following:
   a. Angle
   b. Contour
   c. Color
   d. Ridges
   e. Symmetry
   f. Cleanliness
2. Palpate the nailplate for the following:
   a. Texture
   b. Consistency
   c. Thickness
   d. Adherence to the nailbed

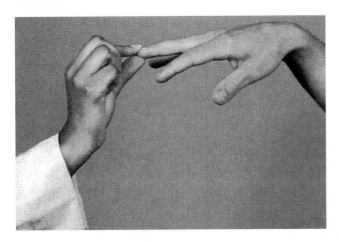

Figure 10-10 Palpate the nail to test for adherence.

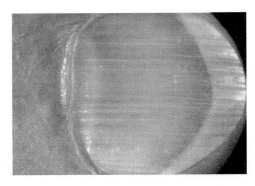

Figure 10-12 Longitudinal ridging. Parallel elevated nail ridges are a common aging change and do not indicate any deficiency. (From Habif TP: *Clinical dermatology: a color guide to diagnosis and therapy*, ed. 3, St. Louis, 1996, Mosby.)

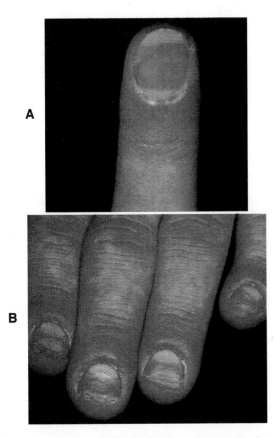

A

B

Figure 10-11 Paronychia. **A,** Acute paronychia. Erythema and purulent material occur at the proximal nailfold. **B,** Chronic paronychia. Erythema and swelling of the nailfolds. The cuticle is absent. Chronic inflammation has caused horizontal ridging of the nails. (From Habif TP: *Clinical dermatology: a color guide to diagnosis and therapy*, ed. 3, St. Louis, 1996, Mosby.)

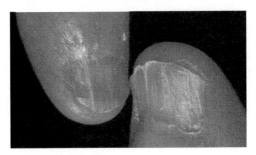

Figure 10-13 Lichen planus. Inflammation of the matrix results in adherence of the proximal nailfold to the scarred matrix. (From Habif TP: *Clinical dermatology: a color guide to diagnosis and therapy*, ed. 2, St. Louis, 1990, Mosby.)

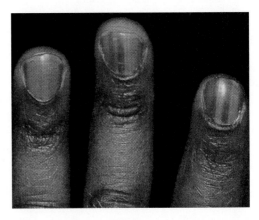

Figure 10-14 Pigmented bands occur as a normal finding in more than 90% of African-Americans. (From Habif TP: *Clinical dermatology: a color guide to diagnosis and the*rapy, ed. 3, St. Louis, 1996, Mosby.)

VARIATIONS FROM HEALTH

The particular manifestations of the many skin problems that you will see in practice are too numerous to discuss here. This section presents a few examples of skin problems commonly seen in practice. For more specific details, consult a textbook on dermatology.

Tables 10-10 and 10-11 provide an overview of common skin lesions. Figures 10-15 through 10-41 illustrate common skin lesions and common problems of the hair and nails.

Teaching Self Assessment

Several professional organizations recommend teaching the client to do regular monthly (ideally) self-examination of the skin for abnormal lesions, in addition to annual complete skin examinations by a health care provider. The U.S. Preventive Services Task Force finds no evidence for or against skin self-examination. However, there is agreement that individuals at high risk for melanoma (see Risk Factors box on malignant melanoma, p. 192) can benefit from close monitoring and self-examination. In addition, organizations such as the American Academy of Dermatology and the U.S. Preventive Services Task Force (1996) recommend that individuals limit their exposure to sunlight, use sunscreen preparations (rated at least 15 SPF), and wear protective clothing when exposed to the sunlight.

Suggestions from the National Cancer Institute for individuals for performing self-examination include the following:

1. Use a good light: adjust position to avoid glare.
2. Use a full-length mirror and hand-held mirrors to examine your back and other hard-to-see areas. If possible, ask a relative or close friend to help inspect areas you are unable to see.
3. Begin with your face and scalp and work your way down your body.
4. Concentrate on areas where dysplastic nevi are most common—the shoulders and back—and least common—scalp, breasts, and buttocks. Make sure to check between your toes and the soles of your feet.
5. Keep a record, or take pictures, of moles, birthmarks, and other lesions. Note their location, size, and appearance.
6. Compare photographs or your information about your moles to see whether there is any change in appearance.
7. Consult your health care provider promptly if you notice any of the following:
   a. Any of the *ABCDEs* of melanomas (see Risk Factors box on malignant melanoma, p. 192)
   b. Existing moles that have changed in other ways, such as bleeding, or development of an ulcer or nodule
   c. New moles
   d. Sores that do not heal
   e. Persistent swelling or lumps

TABLE 10-10 Common Lesions of the Skin

Condition	Lesion	Location
Actinic keratosis	Macule; scaling; red	Areas exposed to sunlight; scalp; ears
Atopic dermatitis	Dry, scaling inflammation; pruritus; excoriated lichenification; abnormally sensitive to environmental irritants	Forehead; cheeks; flexure regions; may be generalized
Contact dermatitis	Erythema; pruritus resulting from environmental irritant	Area of contact
Discoid lupus erythematosus	Discrete with hyperkeratotic plugs; scaling; central atrophy; scarring, red	Paranasal area; eyebrows; upper midback
Eczema		
Allergic	Erythema to exudate	Scalp; nose; forehead; eyelids; neck (from shampoo or hair dye); feet (from shoes); ears (from hearing aids or glasses); hands (from rubber gloves)
Chronic hereditary	Laminated silvery scales, tiny bleeding spots if scale pulled off	Points of trauma; genitalia
Nummular	Round lesions; moist surface; crusting; excoriation	Extensor surfaces of arms and legs
Intertrigo	Moist patches or erosions; borders well demarcated; red; associated with friction; macerated	Skinfolds (warm and moist); breasts; axilla; inguinal regions; between toes; marked in obesity
Pityriasis rosea (unknown cause)	Macules; scaling, oval shape; long axis follows lines of cleavage; red	Herald patch; then generalized
Psoriasis	Early lesion discrete; deep red patches; scaling; later discrete or confluent patches; plaques; gray-white thick scale; scale may appear shiny (disorder of keratin synthesis, hereditary)	May arise in one skin area or may appear as generalized skin involvement
Rosacea	Papules; pustules; oiliness; erythema; telangiectasia may be present	Face

TABLE 10-10 Common Lesions of the Skin—cont'd

Condition	Lesion	Location
Seborrhea	Noninflammatory dryness and scaling "dandruff" or oiliness	Scalp; face
Seborrheic dermatitis	Inflammation; dryness; scaling (loose, flaky); oiliness; pruritus; may be crushed; eczematous	Scalp; ears; face (nasolabial fold, temples, eyelids); shoulders; navel; perianal region
Seborrheic keratosis	Early lesion—tan macule; progresses to papules, plaques; surface brown, rough	Any area; common on trunk
Scleroderma	Indurated; atrophic, shiny; skin appears tight, fastened down; hyperpigmentation or depigmentation	Generalized; tight facies; claw fingers
Systemic lupus erythematosus	Purpuric lesions; erythema; telangiectasia	Malar prominence; over joints
Vascular		
Nevus flammeus (port wine stain)	Plaque; plexus of capillaries may have rough surface; red or purple	Present at birth; 50% on nuchal area
Nevus vasculosus	Capillary hemangioma; single tumor; rough surface; bright or dark red	75% in head region; appear in first or second month; most disappear by age 7
Spider nevus (arteriolar spider or spider angioma)	Small branching arteriole; red; blanches on pressure	Any area; most common on face, neck, arms, and upper trunk
Telangiectasia	Capillary dilatation; red; blanches on pressure	Lips, tongue, nose, palms, and fingers
Extravasation of Blood		
Senile purpura	Ecchymoses; large areas blue-black, then green-yellow, then yellow; lesions do not blanch	Usually occurs on dorsum of hand or forearm
Neoplasia		
Paget's disease	Crusted dermatitis; moist verrucous surface; pruritus	Nipple and areola (manifestation of deeper intraductal malignancy)
Kaposi's sarcoma (associated with AIDS)	Reddish brown plaques and nodules often associated with lymphedema	Most commonly seen on lower extremities
Scar		
Striae	Linear; depressed; red-blue first, then silvery white	Abdomen, buttocks, or breasts; less often on thighs, upper arms, and back
Bacterial Infection		
Erysipelas	Acute; edematous; red; tender	Face; limbs; abdomen
Impetigo	Yellow crusts; erythematous base; rapid spreading	Facial area; may be localized or may spread
Leprosy	Macules—tan to pink; nodules—yellowish; may ulcerate; incubation about 3 years	
Scarlet fever	Confluent, diffuse, blanching dermatitis; erythematous 1–7 days after—sore throat, fever	Generalized
Syphilis (secondary)	Macules; papules; lymphadenopathy; malaise, myalgia; low-grade fever	Mucous membranes; palms; soles
Syphilitic chancre	Small, round, red macule; erodes to indurated ulcer (1–2 cm); regional lymphadenopathy)	Breast, vulva; penis
Trichomonal Infection		
Trichomoniasis	Granular vaginal mucosa; bright red; petechiae may be present; discharge "foamy"	Vagina, labia
***Candida* Infection**		
Candida	Patch borders well demarcated; flaccid pustules; patches creamy white; erythematous base; curdlike white discharge, pruritus patches; erythema	Inguinal region, vagina; glans penis

AIDS, Acquired immunodeficiency syndrome.

Continued

TABLE 10-10	Common Lesions of the Skin—cont'd	
Condition	**Lesion**	**Location**
Viral Infection		
Rubella, rubeola, roseola	Macules; discrete; erythematous; fever; lymphadenopathy (rubella); Koplik's spots (rubeola); 2- to 3-week incubation (rubella); then malaise, fever	Appear on trunk first; spread peripherally
Varicella (chickenpox)	Papule; vesicle; erythematous base; first clear fluid, then turbid; crusting on fourth day; 2-week incubation; 24-hour fever; malaise	First on chest and back; then face, arms, and legs
Variola (smallpox)	Macules; erythematous; progress to umbilicated lesions; then pustules, firm, round, then crusting; 2- to 3-week incubation; 5-day prodromal; toxic myalgia; fever	More lesions on face, extremities
HIV Infection	Variety of dermatoses (macules, papules, nodules, plaques): bacterial, fungal, parasitic, viral; worsening of psoriasis, seborrheic dermatitis; herpes simplex, herpes zoster, oral candidiasis	Anywhere on body, including all mucosal surfaces
Fungal Infection		
Tinea corporis (ringworm)	Scaling; red with pale center; vesicular border; pruritic	Face; neck; extremities
Tinea cruris	Scaling; crescentic; red-brown	Axilla; inguinal region
Tinea pedis (fungal infection of foot)	Scaling; circular; vesicular border; red; chronic hyperkeratotic	Feet
Infestations		
Pediculosis capitis	Pruritus; white concretions on hair—nits	Hair of scalp
Variation in Pigmentation		
Café au lait spots	Patches; light tan (six or more larger than 1.5 cm indicative of neurofibromatosis)	Anywhere on skin
Freckle (ephelis)	Discrete; macule; tan to brown	Pigmenting increased in areas exposed to sun
Lentigo		
Juvenile	Discrete macule; brown	Not affected by sun exposure
Senile	Single macule; scaling; yellow-brown; may be dark brown	Exposed surfaces, forehead, cheeks, extensor surfaces of limbs
Malignant	Mottled; irregular macule; enlarging: tan-brown, black-white; may ulcerate—then red	Face; also eyelids, conjunctiva, lips, penis, axilla
Mongolian spots	Patch; irregular, dark blue or purple (chromophobe-like cell in skin)	Sacrum; present at birth; more common with darker-pigmented individuals; disappear spontaneously by age 4
Nevus	Macule; pigmented or nonpigmented; may be present at birth or arise later	
Peutz-Jeghers syndrome	Brown spots; abdominal pain	Lips; fingers; toes
Depigmentation		

Vitiligo
  Addison's disease
  Pernicious anemia
  Thyrotoxicosis
	Circumscribed patch(es) of depigmentation	Face, neck, axillae, groins, anogenital area, eyelids, hands, and wrist

HIV, Human immunodeficiency virus.

TABLE 10-11	**Common Raised Lesions**	
Condition	**Lesion**	**Location**
Acne vulgaris	Comedones; papules; pustules; cysts; scars	Face; back; shoulders; upper arms
Dermatitis herpetiformis (chronic)	Macules; papules; vesicles; excoriated vesicles; pruritus (intense); residual hyperpigmentation; hereditary	Scalp; interscapular, sacral
Leukoplakia	Plaque; thick; indurated; white	Mucous membrane; mouth; labia; vagina
Lichen planus (unknown cause)	Maculopapular lesion; deep red to purple; pruritus; hyperkeratotic	Flexor surfaces of wrists; palms; soles; ankles; abdomen; sacrum
Lichen simplex (chronic)	Plaque; dry; lichenification; hyperpigmentation	Scalp; labia
Seborrheic keratosis	Single plaque; soft lesion with rough surface; brown	Back; chest; scalp; face; back of hands; and external surfaces of forearms
Lipid Disorder		
Xanthelasma	Papules or plaques; yellow; lipid deposits	Eyelids
Cysts		
Epidermoid and sebaceous cysts	Fluctuant, globular lesions	Scalp; face; back; or scrotum
Milia	Pinhead (1–2 mm) white, sebaceous cyst	Infraorbital skin; nose; chin; common in newborn
Neoplasia		
Acrochordon (skin tag)	Pedunculated skin tag; skin color	Neck; axilla; groin
Basal cell carcinoma	Nodular—rolled edge; tendency to ulcerate in center	Face; scalp; ears; or neck
Basal cell epithelioma	May follow actinic keratosis; papule or nodule—rolled edge; ulcer—nonhealing	Face; scalp; upper back
Squamous cell carcinoma	Nodule; indurated; ulcer—nonhealing; history of overexposure to sun, x-ray films; often opaque	Often on head (75%); hands (15%)
Dermatofibroma	Tumor; discrete, dome shaped; brown; smaller than 1 cm	Usually legs
Lipoma	Fatty tumor; soft	Trunk; nuchal area; arms; and thighs
Malignant melanoma	Arises from pigmented nevus; indurated; may be flat or elevated, eroded, or ulcerated	Any area of skin or mucous membrane
Neurofibroma	Pedunculated; soft; flaccid lesion; skin color black, brown, rose, white	Anywhere on skin, including palms and soles
Pigmented nevus	Single or multiple dome-shaped lesions; may be hairy; brown to black; present at birth	Anywhere on skin
Vascular		
Angioma (sometimes called senile angioma)	Papule; vascular; cherry red; pinhead (1–3 mm); most adults after climacteric	Usually on trunk
Hyperkeratosis		
Clavus (corn)	Hyperkeratosis; hard; tender; shape—inverted cone	Dorsum of toes; most common on fifth toe
Cutaneous horn	Horn projection of hyperkeratotic lesion	Face; arms; scalp; and dorsum of hand
Wheals		
Dermographism	Wheal in response to scratch or pressure; (histamine easily released)	Anywhere on skin

Continued

TABLE 10-11	**Common Lesions of the Skin—cont'd**

Condition	Lesion	Location
Wheals—cont'd		
Erythema multiforme (varied causes)	Wheal-like; round, darker, depressed center (target appearance)	Arms and legs first; then on body
Urticaria	Wheal; pale on erythematous base; pruritus; transient	Usually trunk but may appear anywhere on body
Bullae		
Pemphigus	Bullae; flaccid, moist, fluid-filled rupture easily bleeds; erythematous base; from lack of mucopolysaccharide protein for intercellular cement	Skin and mucous membranes
From Bacterial Infection		
Chancroid	Vesicopustule; ulcer; ragged, undermined edges; shallow; may be multiple; red; lymphadenopathy	Genitalia—male and female
Folliculitis	Discrete perifollicular papules and pustules; erythematous	Any hairy area
Furuncle	Swelling becomes pustular; red; tender; painful	Any hair site but most common on neck, buttocks, wrists, and ankles
From Viral Infection		
Herpes simplex	Vesicles; grouped; may be recurrent	Lips; anywhere on face
Herpes zoster	Tenderness, burning; pruritus; vesicles later crusting; erythematous base; hypersensitivity; localized lymphadenopathy	Pathway of a peripheral nerve; may have postherpetic neuralgia
Molluscum contagiosum	Multiple, discrete globules; waxy depression in center	Trunk
Verruca acuminata	Papillary (cauliflower-like); red; soft	Penis; vulva; perianal area
Verruca plantaris (plantar wart)	Circumscribed callus; surrounded by hyperkeratosis; black dots; tender	Plantar surface of foot or toes
Verruca vulgaris (wart)	Single or multiple; tan	Hands
From Infestation		
Pediculosis corporis (body lice)	Wheal; central hemorrhagic spot; linear excoriations; later dry, scaly pigmentation	Trunk; can be generalized
Pediculosis pubis (pubic lice)	Papules; discrete; excoriated; gray-white dots at base of hair—nits; lice may be seen at base of hairs	Genital region; lower abdomen; chest; axillae; eyebrows; eyelashes
	Gray-blue macules	May be present on abdomen; chest; axillae; eyebrows; eyelashes
Scabies	Vesicles; papules; pruritus	Skinfolds

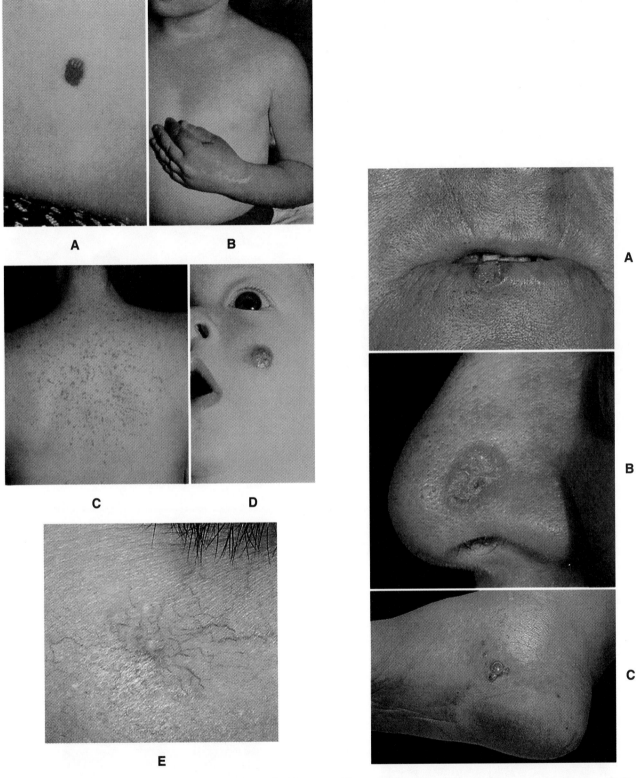

Figure 10-15 Vascular lesions. **A**, Cherry angioma. **B**, Nevus flammeus. **C**, Telangiectasias. **D**, Strawberry hemangioma. **E**, Spider angioma. (Courtesy American Academy of Dermatology and Institute for Dermatologic Communication, Schaumburg, Ill.)

Figure 10-16 Neoplasias. **A**, Squamous cell carcinoma. **B**, Basal cell carcinoma. **C**, Kaposi's sarcoma. (From Habif TP: *Clinical dermatology: a color guide to diagnosis and therapy*, ed. 3, St. Louis, 1996, Mosby.)

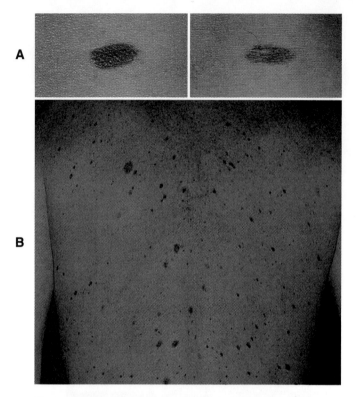

Figure 10-17   Melanocytic growths. **A,** Common typical moles: junction nevus—flat, black, and uniform; compound nevus—center is elevated. **B,** Dysplastic nevi—numerous large nevi are present. (From Habif TP: *Clinical dermatology: a color guide to diagnosis and therapy,* ed. 3, St. Louis, 1996, Mosby.)

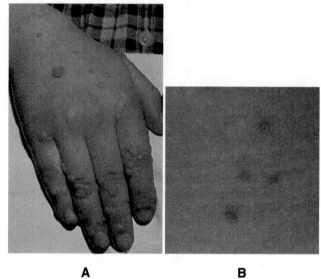

A   B

Figure 10-18   Warts. **A,** Verruca vulgaris. **B,** Molluscum contagiosum. (Courtesy American Academy of Dermatology and Institute for Dermatologic Communication and Education, Schaumburg, Ill.)

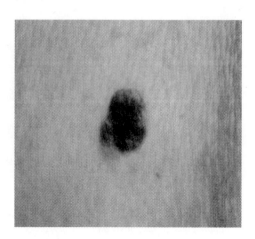

Figure 10-19   Seborrheic keratosis.

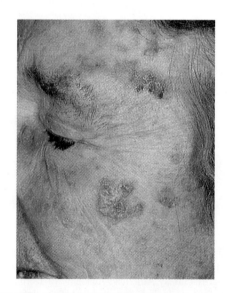

Figure 10-20   Actinic keratosis. Early lesions are present on the forehead. A more advanced lesion with yellow scale is on the cheek. (From Habif TP: *Clinical dermatology: a color guide to diagnosis and therapy,* ed. 3, St. Louis, 1996, Mosby.)

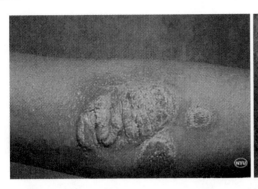
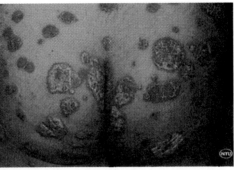

Figure 10-21 Psoriasis. (Courtesy American Academy of Dermatology and Institute for Dermatologic Communication and Education, Schaumburg, Ill.)

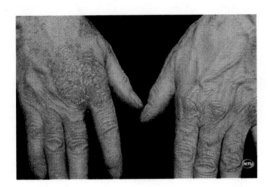

Figure 10-22 Nummular eczema. (Courtesy American Academy of Dermatology and Institute for Dermatologic Communication and Education, Schaumburg, Ill.)

A

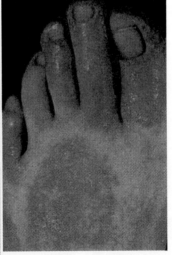

B

C

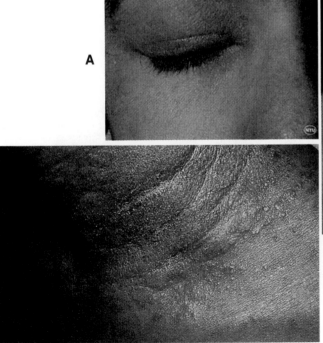

Figure 10-23 Contact dermatitis. **A,** From shampoo. **B,** From shoes. **C,** From application of Lanacaine. (**A** and **B** courtesy American Academy of Dermatology and Institute for Dermatologic Communication and Education, Schaumburg, Ill.; **C** from Cohen BA: *Atlas of pediatric dermatology*, London, 1993, Mosby-Wolfe.)

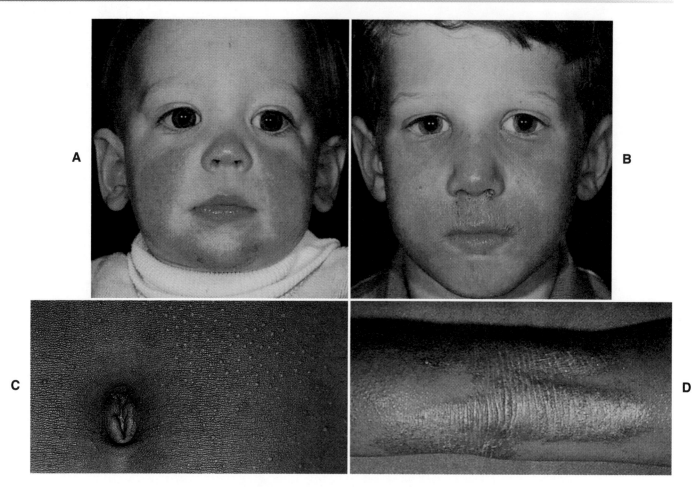

Figure 10-24   Atopic dermatitis. **A** and **B**, In light-skinned children. **C**, Follicular hyperkeratosis on the abdomen in a dark-skinned client. **D**, Lichenification of the popliteal fossa from chronic rubbing of the skin in a dark-skinned client. (**A** and **B** from Habif TP: *Clinical dermatology: a color guide to diagnosis and therapy*, ed. 3, St. Louis, 1996, Mosby; **C** and **D** from Weston WL, Lane AT, Morelli JG: *Color textbook of pediatric dermatology*, ed. 2, St. Louis, 1996, Mosby.)

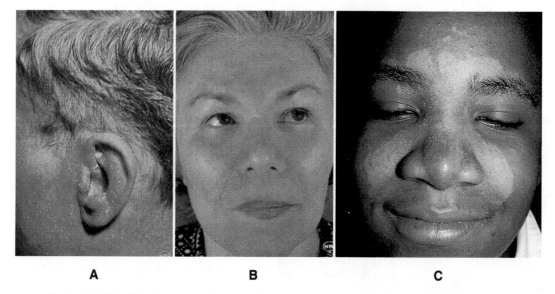

Figure 10-25   Seborrheic dermatitis. **A** and **B**, In light-skinned clients. **C**, In a dark-skinned client. (**A** and **B** courtesy American Academy of Dermatology and Institute for Dermatologic Communication and Education, Schaumburg, Ill.; **C** from Cohen BA: *Atlas of pediatric dermatology*, London, 1993, Mosby-Wolfe.)

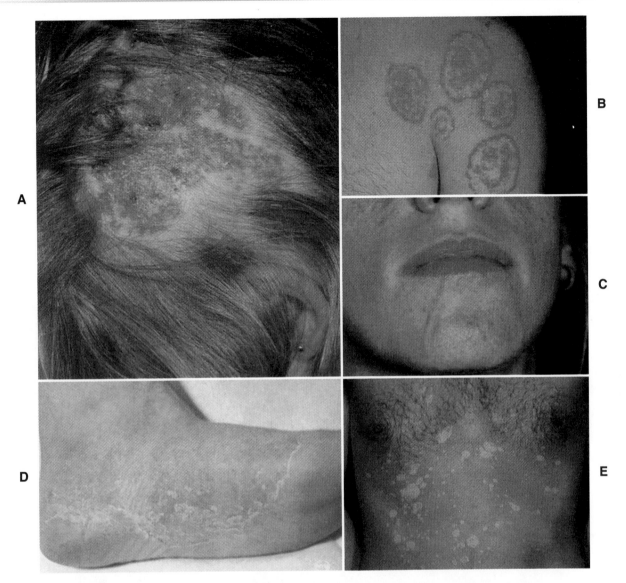

Figure 10-26   Tinea infections. **A**, Tinea capitis. **B**, Tinea corporis. **C**, Tinea of the face. **D**, Tinea pedis. **E**, Tinea versicolor. (**A** to **C** and **E** from Habif TP: *Clinical dermatology: a color guide to diagnosis and therapy*, ed. 3, St. Louis, 1996, Mosby; **D** courtesy American Academy of Dermatology and Institute for Dermatologic Communication and Education, Schaumburg, Ill.)

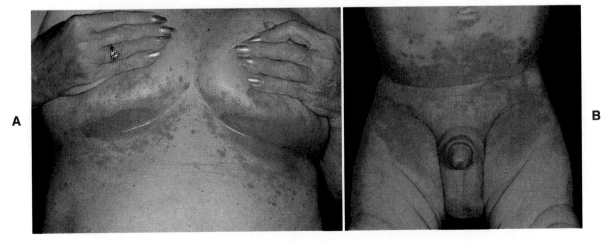

Figure 10-27   Candidiasis. **A**, Candida intertrigo. **B**, Diaper candidiasis. (From Habif TP: *Clinical dermatology: a color guide to diagnosis and therapy*, ed. 3, St. Louis, 1996, Mosby.)

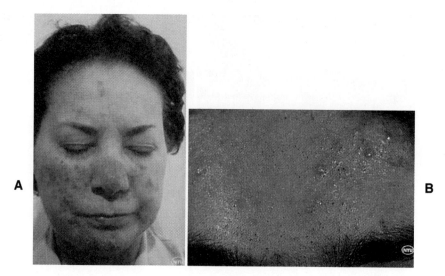

Figure 10-28   Acne. **A**, Acne rosacea. **B**, Acne vulgaris. (Courtesy American Academy of Dermatology and Institute for Dermatologic Communication and Education, Schaumburg, Ill.)

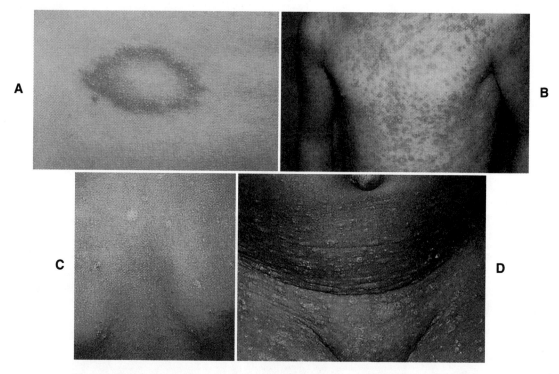

Figure 10-29   Pityriasis rosea. **A**, Large herald patch on the chest shows central clearing, mimicking tinea corporis. **B**, Oval lesions on the chest. **C**, Back of an African-American client; note the Christmas tree pattern. **D**, Small papular lesions, as well as larger scaly patches, are prominent on the abdomen and thighs. (From Cohen BA: *Atlas of pediatric dermatology*, London, 1993, Mosby-Wolfe.)

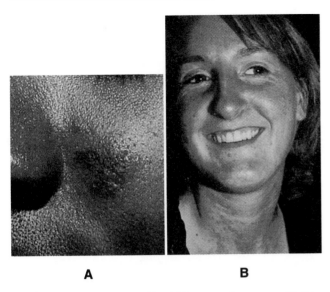
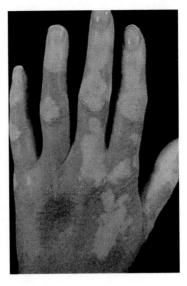

A   **B**

Figure 10-30   Lupus. **A**, Discoid lupus erythematosus. **B**, Systemic lupus erythematosus. (Courtesy American Academy of Dermatology and Institute for Dermatologic Communication and Education, Schaumburg, Ill.)

Figure 10-31   Vitiligo. (Courtesy American Academy of Dermatology and Institute for Dermatologic Communication and Education, Schaumburg, Ill.)

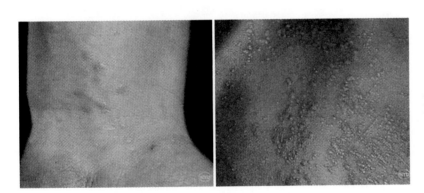

Figure 10-32   Lichen planus. (Courtesy American Academy of Dermatology and Institute for Dermatologic Communication and Education, Schaumburg, Ill.)

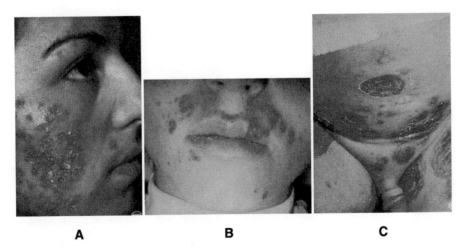

A   **B**   **C**

Figure 10-33   Impetigo. **A**, Impetigo contagiosa. **B** and **C**, Impetigo (bullous). (Courtesy American Academy of Dermatology and Institute for Dermatologic Communication and Education, Schaumburg, Ill.)

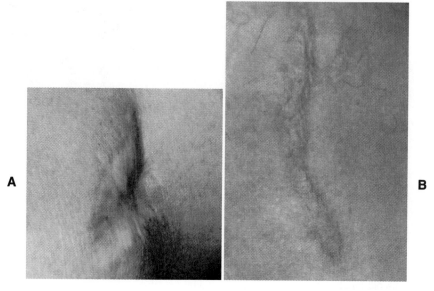

Figure 10-34   Scars. **A,** Scar on the knee. **B,** Scar from a second-degree burn on the leg.

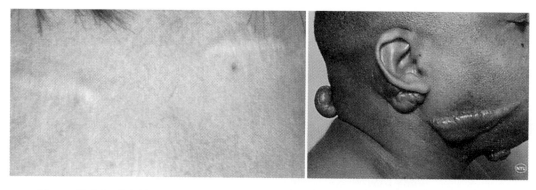

Figure 10-35   Keloids. (Courtesy American Academy of Dermatology and Institute for Dermatologic Communication and Education, Schaumburg, Ill.)

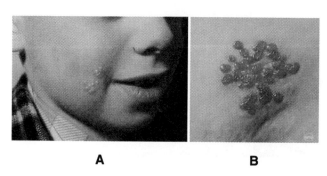

Figure 10-36   Herpes. **A,** Herpes simplex. **B,** Herpes zoster. (Courtesy American Academy of Dermatology and Institute for Dermatologic Communication and Education, Schaumburg, Ill.)

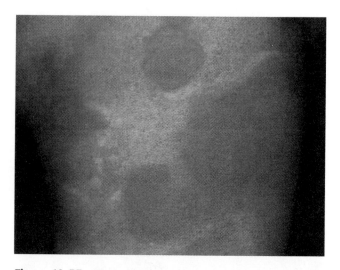

Figure 10-37   Hives. The most characteristic presentation is uniformly red, edematous plaques surrounded by a white halo. (From Habif TP: *Clinical dermatology: a color guide to diagnosis and therapy*, ed. 3, St. Louis, 1996, Mosby.)

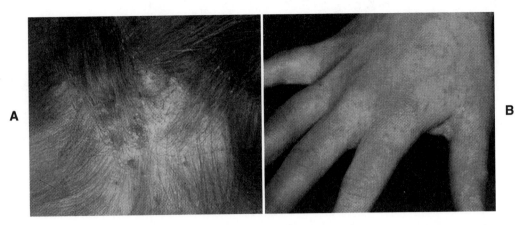

Figure 10-38   Infestations. **A**, Lice. **B**, Scabies. (From Habif TP: *Clinical dermatology: a color guide to diagnosis and therapy*, ed. 3, St. Louis, 1996, Mosby.)

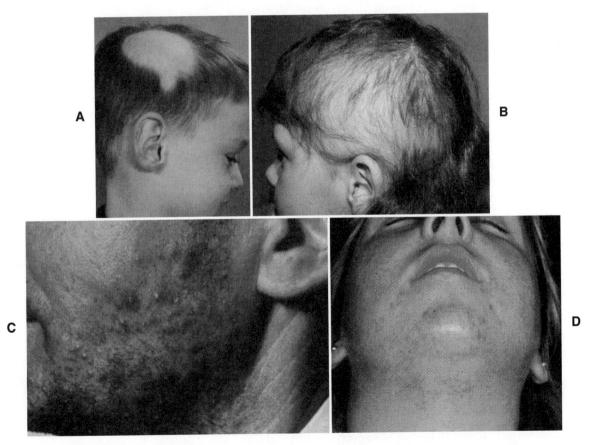

Figure 10-39   Hair disorders. **A**, Alopecia areata. **B**, Trichotillomania. **C**, Folliculitis. **D**, Hirsutism. (**A** and **C** courtesy American Academy of Dermatology and Institute for Dermatologic Communication and Education, Schaumburg, Ill.; **B** and **D** from Habif TP: *Clinical dermatology: a color guide to diagnosis and therapy*, ed. 3, St. Louis, 1996, Mosby.)

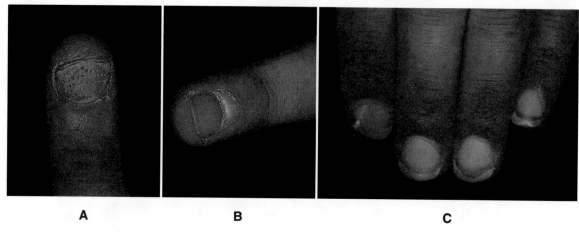

A   **B**   **C**

Figure 10-40 Nail changes associated with systemic disease. **A,** Psoriasis. Pitting is the most common change found in psoriasis. **B,** Beau's nails. A transverse depression of the nails occurs several weeks after certain illnesses. **C,** Terry's nails. The nailbed is white with only a narrow area of pink at the distal end. Findings are associated with cirrhosis, congestive heart failure, diabetes mellitus, and aging. (From Habif TP: *Clinical dermatology: a color guide to diagnosis and therapy,* ed. 3, St. Louis, 1996, Mosby.)

Sample Documentation and Diagnoses

FOCUSED HEALTH HISTORY (SUBJECTIVE DATA)

Mr. J, a 50-year-old white male, states that 2 days ago he noticed that a mole at his back waistline had changed color (from brown to blue-black) and bled slightly yesterday. States that his waistband aggravates the mole. He is concerned about skin cancer and has monitored the mole for the past few years. Measurement of the mole approximately 2 months ago was 5 mm in diameter; at that time it was round, flat, and brown. Denies any skin reactions or other lesions, as well as any pain or pruritus, any change in scalp/body hair, or excessive sun exposure. Denies previous history of atypical moles or skin cancer and family history of melanoma or skin cancer. States that he has been in good health, with no other problems.

FOCUSED PHYSICAL EXAMINATION (OBJECTIVE DATA)

General appearance: Appears quite anxious about change in mole.
Skin: Fair/pink, cool, smooth; elastic turgor. Hyperpigmented macules across shoulders; 5-mm round, raised nevus at waistline—blue-black in color; excoriation, with some crusting noted at edges.
Hair: Male distribution, thinning at hairline.
Nails: No clubbing, deformities, or change in color. Nailbeds pink; brisk capillary refill.

DIAGNOSES

HEALTH PROBLEM

Recent change in mole; rule out skin cancer

NURSING DIAGNOSES

Impaired Skin Integrity Related to Mechanical Irritation of Mole
Defining Characteristics
- Color change in mole
- Elevation change in mole
- Bleeding noted from mole
- Waistband rubs against mole, causing irritation

Anxiety Related to Potential Diagnosis of Cancer
Defining Characteristic
Apprehensive with reassurance-seeking behavior

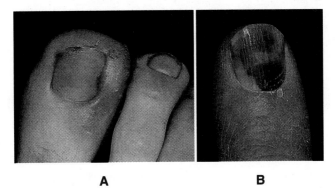

A   **B**

Figure 10-41 Nail changes associated with injury or infection.
A, Ingrown toenail. **B**, Subungual hematoma.

? Critical Thinking Questions

Review the Sample Documentation and Diagnoses section to answer these questions.
1. What additional history information would be helpful in determining Mr. J's risk for melanoma? What other information might you seek if he were younger, older, or female?

2. How would Mr. J's risk status change if he were of a different race (e.g., African-American, Asian-American)?
3. What additional information would be helpful to address Mr. J's anxiety?
4. What information would you give Mr. J to help him reduce his risk for skin cancers?

Remember to check out the Online Study Guide!
www.harcourthealth.com/MERLIN/Barkauskas/

Face, Head, Neck, and Regional Lymphatics

Learning Objectives

On successful study of this chapter and completion of related learning experiences, the learner will be able to:
- Describe the anatomy and physiology of the face, head, and neck region and the regional lympathic system.
- Identify history questions pertinent to a focused assessment of this region.

- Describe techniques used to assess the face, head, neck, and regional lymphatic system.
- Recognize variations from health in the assessment of this region.

Outline

Purpose of Examination

Facial expression and appearance are likely to be the first observations that a practitioner will make about a client. The regional part of the physical examination routinely begins with the face, head, and neck. The head and neck provide the protective casing for the special sense organs, brain, and upper spinal column. Many structures and portions of body systems are located in this region, including structures for sensation and expression; skin and hair; and components of the musculoskeletal, vascular, lymphatic, and glandular systems.

This chapter focuses on the elements and factors to be considered in assessment, including the face—appearance, expression, and landmarks; the head—bony structures, position, and scalp; and the neck—muscles, trachea, thyroid gland, and cervical vertebrae. The beginning practitioner will gradually learn to incorporate all of these components into the examination.

For assessment of other structures of the face, head, and neck, see Chapters 10, 12, 13, and 19.

ANATOMY AND PHYSIOLOGY

Face

As an individual grows and develops from infancy throughout mature adulthood, the facial appearance changes. The distribution of underlying fat undergoes modification, nasal cartilage enlarges, and the features become more pronounced.

The external portions of the special sense organs of the face and head are generally symmetrical. These include the eyes, nose, mouth, and ears. The palpebral fissures and the nasolabial folds are also symmetrical. The palpebral fissures are the openings between the margins of the upper and lower eyelids. The nasolabial folds are the creases in the skin extending from the angle of the nose to the corner of the mouth (Figure 11-1).

Two cranial nerves mediate the sensation and motion of the face: the trigeminal nerve and the facial nerve. The **trigeminal nerve,** cranial nerve (CN) V, carries sensation of the face (Figure 11-2). The trigeminal nerve has three sensory branches: ophthalmic, maxillary, and mandibular. The **facial nerve,** CN VII, innervates the muscles of facial expression.

The artery accessible to examination on the face is the **temporal artery,** which runs anterior to the ear over the temporal bone and onto the forehead (Figure 11-3).

Head

The skull protects the sensitive structures of the brain. In infancy the cranial bones that compose the skull are soft and separated along suture lines, but by adulthood they have become fused along these suture lines (Figure 11-4). The following cranial bones make up the skull:

Frontal
Parietal
Temporal
Occipital

The facial bones give the face its contours, allow jaw mobility, and offer protection for the special sense organs. The fused bones of the face include the following:

Frontal
Nasal
Zygomatic
Lacrimal
Sphenoid
Maxilla

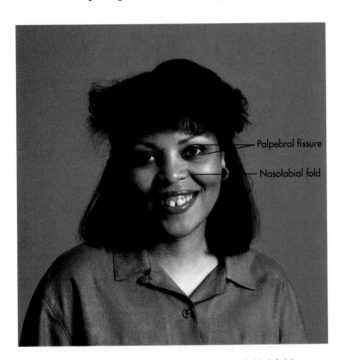

Figure 11-1   Palpebral fissures and nasolabial folds.

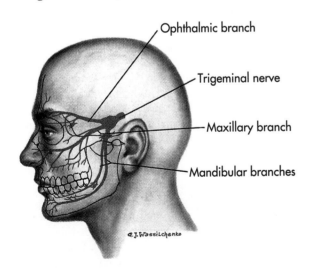

Figure 11-2   Trigeminal nerve with innervation to the face by ophthalmic, maxillary, and mandibular branches. (From Rudy EB: *Advanced neurological and neurosurgical nursing*, St. Louis, 1984, Mosby.)

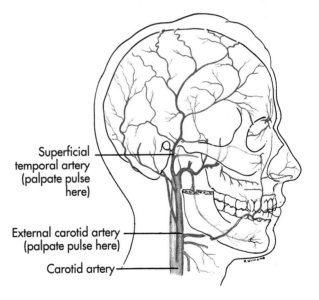

Figure 11-3   Temporal artery. (Modified from Francis CC, Martin AH: *Introduction to human anatomy*, ed. 7, St. Louis, 1975, Mosby.)

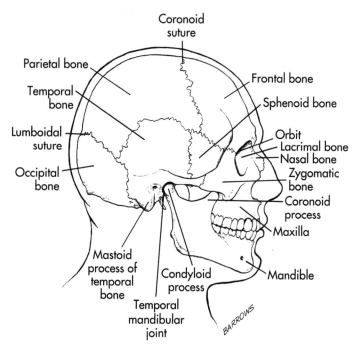

Figure 11-4 Bones of the skull.

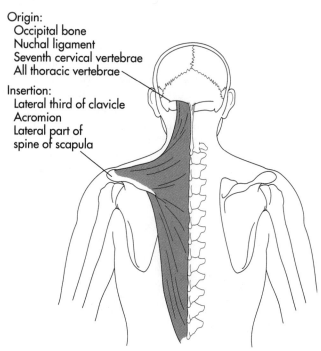

Figure 11-6 Trapezius muscle.

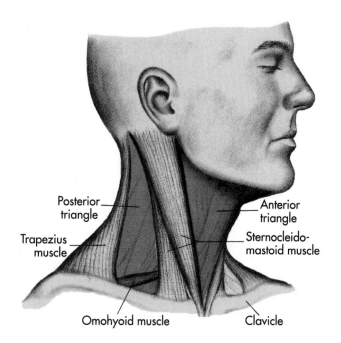

Figure 11-5 Sternocleidomastoid and trapezius muscles. Anterior and posterior triangles. (From Seidel HM et al: *Mosby's guide to physical examination*, ed. 3, St. Louis, 1995, Mosby.)

The mandible, or lower jaw bone, is not fused. It is connected to the temporal bone of the skull at the temporomandibular joint.

When you examine the head and face, use the bones as landmarks to identify the regions of the head and their overlying structures.

Neck

The following components are the major structures of the neck:

Sternocleidomastoid and trapezius muscles
Trachea
Thyroid gland
Carotid arteries and jugular veins (see Chapter 16)
Cervical lymph nodes
Cervical vertebrae

Neck Muscles

The two major muscles of the neck are the sternocleidomastoid muscle and the trapezius muscle (Figures 11-5 and 11-6). These symmetrical muscles provide support and allow movement of the neck, enabling it to flex, extend, and rotate. They are innervated by the spinal accessory nerve, CN XI. Both sets of muscles and their position in relation to adjacent bones form triangles that are used to describe anatomical landmarks and physical findings. Each **sternocleidomastoid muscle** extends from the upper sternum and the proximal portion of the clavicle to the mastoid process of the temporal bone behind the ear. This pair of muscles provides for turning and lateral flexion of the head.

For the purpose of describing findings, each side of the neck can be divided into two triangles called the **anterior** and **posterior triangles** (see Figure 11-5). Forming the anterior triangle are the edge of the mandible (superiorly), the sternocleidomastoid muscle (laterally), and the midline of the trachea (medially). Composing the posterior triangle are the sternocleidomastoid muscle (laterally), the trapezius muscle (posteriorly), and the clavicle (inferiorly).

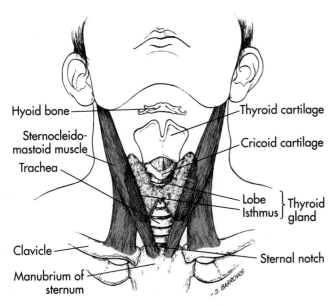

Figure 11-7 Anterior midline neck structures.

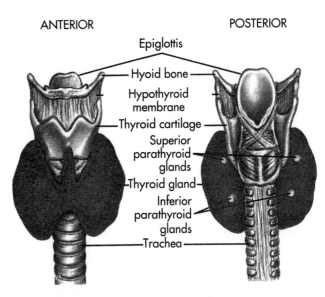

Figure 11-8 Thyroid gland. (From Thompson JM et al.: *Mosby's clinical nursing*, ed. 4, St. Louis, 1997, Mosby.)

Within the anterior triangle are the anterior cervical lymph nodes, the carotid artery, and the internal jugular vein. Several groups of lymph nodes lie within the posterior triangle.

The **trapezius muscles** (see Figure 11-6) are large, flat, and triangular. Each one extends from the cervical and thoracic vertebrae and from the spine of the scapula to the occipital bone of the skull. The trapezius muscles are involved in the movements of shrugging the shoulders, pulling the scapulae downward and toward the vertebral column, rotating the head to the side, and extending the head backward.

Midline Neck Structures

As shown in Figure 11-7, the anterior midline neck structures include the following:

Hyoid bone
Thyroid cartilage
Cricoid cartilage
Tracheal rings
Isthmus of the thyroid gland

The hyoid bone lies just below the mandible at the angle of the floor of the mouth. The thyroid cartilage is shaped like a shield, with a notch at the upper edge that marks the level of bifurcation, or division, of the common carotid artery into the internal and external carotid arteries. The thyroid is the largest of the cartilaginous structures of the neck. The cricoid cartilage, the uppermost ring of the trachea, lies just below the thyroid cartilage. The isthmus of the thyroid gland is found across the trachea and below the cricoid cartilage. The cartilaginous trachea is located below the cricoid cartilage and continues to the lungs, where it divides into two bronchi.

Thyroid Gland

The **thyroid gland** (Figures 11-7 and 11-8) is the largest endocrine gland in the body and the only one that is accessible to direct physical examination. It is butterfly shaped with a lobe on each side of the trachea. A connecting isthmus joins the lower part of the lobes just below the cricoid cartilage. The lobes curve posteriorly and are largely covered by the sternocleidomastoid muscles. Each lobe is somewhat irregular and cone shaped. The normal consistency of the thyroid can be described as "meaty" or "rubbery." The thyroid arteries supply the highly vascular thyroid tissue.

The thyroid gland produces two hormones: thyroxine (T_4) and triiodothyronine (T_3). The functions of these hormones are essential for normal physical growth and development in infancy and childhood and for the maintenance of metabolic stability throughout life. These hormones influence the concentration and activity of numerous enzymes and the metabolism of substrates, vitamins, and minerals. They also affect the secretion and degradation rates of all other hormones and their target tissue responses. Thus thyroid hormones affect virtually all the tissues and organ systems of the body. It is important to note that changes due to altered thyroid function can occur in other body systems even when there is no change in the thyroid gland that is detectable on physical examination. Thyroid tissue may enlarge retrosternally or in areas that are not accessible to palpation. If a thyroid disorder is suspected, clinical assessment must include other body systems, such as the cardiovascular, gastrointestinal, integumentary, and neurological systems.

Lymph Nodes

In this text, examination of the lymphatic system is described by body region; therefore the system is described in this chapter and also in the chapters on assessment of the ears, nose, and throat (Chapter 13); breasts (Chapter 14); and genitalia (Chapters 20 and 21). Since this text follows a head-to-foot examination format, the first lymph nodes to be examined are those in the head and neck. General material about the lymphatic system is included in this chapter.

The lymphatic system consists of a network throughout the body, including lymph fluid; collecting ducts; lymph nodes; the spleen; the thymus; the tonsils; the adenoids; and small amounts of lymph tissue found in other places in the body, such as the bone marrow, the appendix, and Peyer's patches in the intestinal wall. The lymphatic system is a complete circulatory system distinct from, but closely linked to, the blood circulatory system.

The fluid and proteins that compose the lymphatic fluid move from the vascular system into the interstitial spaces. Here they are collected by microscopic lymphatic tubules that return the fluid to the cardiovascular system. Lymphatic vessels originate as microscopic, open-ended tubules that merge to form large collecting ducts. Lymph nodes are small oval clumps of lymphatic tissue occurring in groups along the lymph vessels. Superficial lymph nodes lie in the subcutaneous connective tissues; the deeper nodes are beneath the muscular fascia or in various body cavities. Some nodes have a diameter of 0.5 cm (0.25 inch), but most are smaller. The lymphatic ducts merge into two main trunks that drain into the venous system at the subclavian veins. The right lymphatic duct receives the lymphatic fluid from the right side of the head and neck, the right arm, and the right side of the chest wall. It drains into the right subclavian vein. The lymphatic duct drains the rest of the body and empties into the left subclavian vein (Figure 11-9)

The lymphatic system has no pumping device of its own. Its movement is much slower than that of the blood circulatory system. Factors affecting the movement of lymph include arterial pulsation; compression of lymphatic vessels by contracting skeletal muscles; and contraction of the smooth muscles in the walls of the lymphatic vessels, lymph nodes, and collecting ducts. Mechanical obstruction slows or stops the movement of lymph, causing the nodes to dilate.

A primary purpose of the lymphatic system is to protect the body from infection by providing immunity against foreign substances. The lymphatic system functions to do the following:

1. Filter and engulf bacteria, certain other cells, foreign particles, or toxins in the lymph nodes, thus providing defensive immunity against microorganisms and abnormal cells
2. Return fluid, proteins, and electrolytes from tissue space to the blood
3. Absorb fat and fat-soluble substances from the intestinal tract
4. Produce lymphocytes in the lymph nodes, tonsils, adenoids, spleen, and bone marrow
5. Produce antibodies

The lymphatic system is also a pathway for the spread of malignancy.

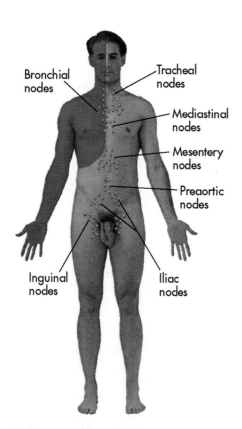

Figure 11-9 Lymphatic drainage pathways. Shaded area of the body is drained via the right lymphatic duct, which is formed by the union of three vessels: right jugular trunk, right subclavian trunk, and right bronchomediastinal trunk. Lymph from the remainder of the body enters the venous system by way of the thoracic duct. (From Seidel HM et al.: *Mosby's guide to physical examination*, ed. 4, St. Louis, 1999, Mosby.)

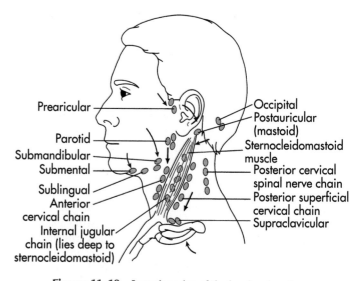

Figure 11-10 Lymph nodes of the head and neck.

Lymph Nodes of the Head and Neck

The head and neck are richly supplied with lymph node groups (Figure 11-10). Some of the groups are known by several names. The following is one commonly used system of terms:

Lymph nodes of the head

Occipital—at the base of the skull

Postauricular (mastoid)—behind the ear, slightly anterior to the mastoid process

Preauricular—in front of the ear

Parotid—near the angle of the jaw

Submandibular (submaxillary)—midway between the angle of the jaw and the tip of the mandible

Sublingual—near the midline, beneath the tongue

Submental—in the midline posterior to the tip of the mandible

Lymph nodes of the neck (these lie in the anterior or posterior triangle or under the sternocleidomastoid muscle)

Anterior cervical chain—over and anterior to the sternocleidomastoid muscle, in the anterior triangle

Internal jugular chain—behind and largely covered by the sternocleidomastoid muscle

Posterior cervical spinal nerve chain—near the cervical vertebrae (located in the posterior area of the neck)

Posterior superficial cervical chain—along the anterior edge of the trapezius, in the posterior triangle

Supraclavicular—just above the clavicle in the angle formed by the clavicle and sternocleidomastoid muscle

EXAMINATION

Focused Health History

Present Health/Illness Status

1. Usual state of health: exercise and sleep patterns; presence of stress, tension; demands at home, work, or school
2. Environmental exposure to injury: use of handrails; presence of electrical cords, loose rugs; use of helmet, protective eye shields; exposure to toxins; participation in activities with potential for risk of injury, such as active sports; recent travel to areas of infectious outbreaks; exposure to infection (including human immunodeficiency virus [HIV])
3. Nutrition: eating habits, food intolerance, recent weight gain or loss
4. Use of tobacco, alcohol, intravenous drugs, medications: analgesics, anticonvulsants, cardiac preparations, thyroid preparations, oral contraceptives, antibiotics, chemotherapy

Past Health History

1. History of head or facial trauma, injury, blood transfusions
2. History of surgery; tumor; seizure disorder; radiation exposure to the head, neck, thyroid, or upper chest
3. Unusual or frequent headaches

4. Systemic health problems: chronic illness, Hodgkin's or other lymphoma, cancer, HIV infection, mononucleosis
5. Recurrent infections, including sexually transmitted infections

Family Health History

1. Malignancy
2. Blood disorders: anemia, hemophilia, agammaglobulinemia
3. Recent infections
4. Tuberculosis
5. History of headaches, thyroid disorders

Specific Problems/Symptom Analysis

Headache

1. **Onset:** time of day or night; gradual or sudden
2. **Course since onset:** frequency and timing (e.g., occasional, clustering, headache-free periods), duration (e.g., minutes, hours, days, weeks)
3. **Location:** entire head, unilateral, one spot, sinus region, behind the eyes, "hatband" distribution, frontal, temporal, occipital, neck pain
4. **Quality of pain:** throbbing, pounding, boring, shock-like, dull, sharp, nagging, constant, intermittent; effect of motion; change in level of consciousness as pain increases
5. **Quantity or severity of pain:** same or different with each event; ask the client to grade the pain using a scale of 1 to 10
6. **Setting:** description of headache over course of day—worse or better as day progresses; occurrence during sleep, home, work
7. **Associated phenomena:** visual prodrome such as scotoma (a defect of vision in a defined area); hemianopia (vision loss in half of a visual field); distortion of size, shape, or location of object; nausea, vomiting, diarrhea; visual disturbances, such as photophobia (abnormal sensitivity to light); increased tearing; difficulty falling asleep; nasal discharge; tinnitus; paresthesias; impaired mobility; fever
8. **Alleviating and aggravating factors:** fatigue, stress, food or food additives, alcohol, seasonal allergies, pattern with menstrual cycle, intercourse, oral contraceptives, feelings of anxiety or depression; activities during 24 hours preceding onset; ask about client's efforts to treat with analgesics, vasodilators, bron-

Risk Factors
Headache

Anxiety or tension
Substance use or withdrawal (e.g., alcohol, tobacco, caffeine)
Poor dental hygiene
Sinus congestion or inflammation
Trigger foods, especially those with tyramine (aged cheese), sulfites (red wine), and nitrites (smoked meats)

chodilators, and stimulants such as caffeine; sleep; meditation; other approaches

9. **Underlying concern:** high stress level

A sample headache record, such as the one shown in Table 11-1, is useful in helping the client record the pattern of headaches for a certain amount of time. The record helps to assess the type of headaches that the client is experiencing.

Head Injury

1. **Onset of traumatic event:** nature of the event, any loss of consciousness, duration of unconsciousness, behaviors after event; (it may be useful to have an observer's description of the event in addition to the client's account)
2. **Course since onset:** changes since onset, light-headedness, fainting, seizures
3. **Location:** local tenderness, location of injury
4. **Quality:** characteristic of pain as sharp, stabbing, burning
5. **Quantity:** frequency of sensations, 1 to 10 pain severity rating
6. **Setting:** relationship of injury to activities
7. **Associated phenomena:** visual changes, blurred or double vision, change in level of consciousness, nausea and vomiting, change in breathing pattern, discharge from nose or ears, head or neck pain, laceration
8. **Alleviating and aggravating factors:** effects of movement, swallowing, use of home remedies
9. **Underlying concern:** limitations in function

Neck Pain

1. **Onset:** sudden or gradual, history of trauma
2. **Course since onset:** frequency, timing, and duration of pain
3. **Location:** describe point of origin; point of maximum pain; areas of radiation patterns to shoulders, arms, and back
4. **Quality of pain:** burning, cramping, throbbing, dull, sharp
5. **Quantity or severity:** rate pain severity using 1 to 10 rating scale
6. **Setting:** relationship to activities
7. **Associated phenomena:** limited movement; difficulty swallowing; bacterial or viral infection; swelling; neurological symptoms such as clumsiness, numbness, weakness, emotional stress, headache
8. **Alleviating and aggravating factors:** what makes the pain better; what makes it worse; efforts to treat; and effectiveness of treatment, heat, cold, medication, movement, positioning
9. **Underlying concern:** neck injury or strain

Thyroid Function

1. **Onset:** sudden or gradual, of irritability, nervousness, lethargy, disinterest, altered sensitivity to heat or cold, change in menstrual pattern, weight gain or loss
2. **Course since onset:** frequency, timing, and duration of symptoms
3. **Location:** general or local symptoms

Risk Factors
Head Injury

Substance abuse
Failure to use seatbelts
Failure to wear protective headgear for activities such as biking, motorcycling, or skateboarding
Participation in contact sports

Risk Factors
Thyroid Disease

History of radiation of the head or neck
Family history of thyroid cancer
Male gender has higher incidence of thyroid disease
Obesity

TABLE 11-1   **Sample Headache Record**

Date	Time of Onset	Duration	Location	Severity 1 = mild 10 = severe	Efforts to Relieve	Results	Possible Precipitating Factors

4. **Quality:** characteristic of a neck mass as mobile, non-mobile, smooth, irregular
5. **Quantity:** severity of symptoms
6. **Setting:** change in usual energy level at home, work, recreation
7. **Associated phenomena:** swelling; redness in the neck; change in texture of hair, skin, or nails; increased pigmentation of skin at pressure points; increased prominence of eyes; puffiness in periorbital area; blurred or double vision; dyspnea on exertion; tachycardia; palpitations; cardiac irregularity
8. **Alleviating and aggravating factors:** effects of swallowing, eating, talking, medication
9. **Underlying concern:** thyroid dysfunction

Enlarged Lymph Nodes

1. **Onset:** sudden or gradual, of infection, surgery, trauma, swelling or enlarged nodes that client may describe as lumps, bumps, kernels, or swollen glands
2. **Course since onset:** frequency, timing (intermittent or constant), duration
3. **Location:** unilateral or bilateral
4. **Quality:** tenderness, pitting, fixed or mobile
5. **Quantity:** number of nodes, size in centimeters
6. **Setting:** variations during the day, changes in environment
7. **Associated phenomena:** pain, fever, redness, warmth, itching, ulceration, bleeding (note site and character), fatigue, weakness, weight gain or loss
8. **Alleviating and aggravating factors:** effect of medications, treatment efforts and effect (e.g., support stockings, elevation)
9. **Underlying concern:** infection, serious illness

Risk Factors
Lymphatic Enlargement

Inadequate primary defenses, such as broken skin or stasis of body fluids
Inadequate secondary defenses, such as suppressed inflammatory response
Immunosuppression
Chronic disease
Malnutrition
Risk factors for cancers that involve the lymph nodes, such as lymphomas, breast cancer, lung cancer, and prostatic cancer

Preparation for Examination

EQUIPMENT

Item	Purpose
Gloves	For palpation of head and hair
Stethoscope	For auscultation of temporal artery and thyroid
Glass of water	For observation and palpation of thyroid
Ruler	To measure enlarged lymph nodes

Preparation for Examination: Client and Environment

The examination room should provide privacy and a comfortable temperature for the client. The room should be well lighted and quiet.

Technique for Examination and Expected Findings

Face

The techniques of inspection and palpation are used to perform a complete examination of the face.

Inspection. To begin, observe the client's facial expression and appearance. Facial expression is frequently a guide to a person's feelings. However, it is important to remember that cultures vary in the degree and style of facial expression. Persons from certain cultures use pronounced facial expressions along with hand gestures and words. Those from other cultures are less expressive, particularly with strangers.

Inspect the color and condition of the facial skin and the shape and symmetry of the facial features, including the eyebrows, eyes, palpebral fissures, mouth, and nasolabial folds. The head is normally upright and still. The facial features should be symmetrical at rest and with a change of expression, although a slight degree of asymmetry is common.

Test facial muscular and neurological function by asking the client to elevate and lower the eyebrows, frown, close the eyes tightly so that the practitioner cannot open them, puff the cheeks, show the teeth, and smile. This test is used to evaluate the function of the facial nerve, CN VII (see Chapter 19).

Palpation. Palpate the temporal arteries bilaterally just anterior to and slightly above the tragus of the ear (Figure 11-11). Note any thickening, hardness, or tenderness of the vessel. Use the bell of the stethoscope to auscultate the temporal artery for a bruit, which is a soft blow-

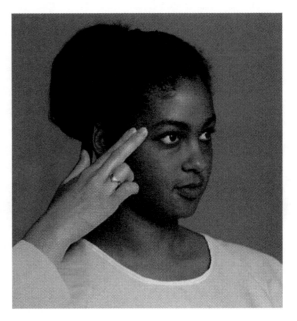

Figure 11-11 Palpation of the temporal artery.

ing sound of blood flowing through a stenosed (narrowed) vessel. A bruit is not normally present.

Palpate the temporomandibular joint. To locate this joint, place your fingertips just anterior to the tragus of the ear (Figure 11-12). Rest your fingertips over this area, and ask the client to open and close the mouth and move the joint from side to side. The temporomandibular joint should move smoothly up and down and to the right and left. Check for swelling or crepitus.

Head

The techniques of inspection and palpation are used for examination of the head.

Inspection.   Observe the head for size, shape, symmetry, position, and any unusual movements. To inspect the scalp, part the hair in several areas. Check behind the ears

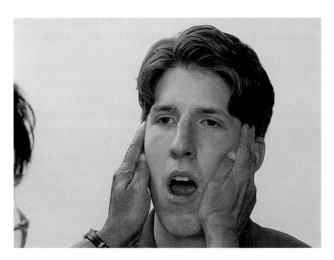

Figure 11-12   Position fingers in front of each ear to examine the temporomandibular.

and along the hairline. Hair condition and styling may be useful indicators of the client's social group identification, emotional status, and personal hygiene.

Palpation.   If the client wears a wig or other hairpiece, ask him or her to remove it. Using the pads of the second, third, and fourth fingers, palpate the scalp in several areas with a gentle rotary motion. The scalp should move freely over the skull. Normally, there are no depressions, swelling, or tenderness. Inspect the distribution and texture of the hair, and note the use of coloring or lubricating agents.

Neck

In a case involving traumatic neck injury, do not manipulate or examine the cervical spine. Stabilize the spine until further studies can be performed.

The techniques of inspection, palpation, and auscultation are used for examination of the structures of the neck.

Inspection.   Inspect the neck for symmetry of the muscles and trachea and for stability in normal position. The neck muscles should be symmetrical, with no masses or swelling noted. To assess muscular function, ask the client to perform range of motion by flexing the chin to the chest (Figure 11-13, *A*), turning the head in lateral rotation (Figure 11-13, *B*), and slightly hyperextending the neck backward (Figure 11-13, *C*). These motions should be smooth and should not cause pain or dizziness. Inspect the midline cartilages, including the thyroid and cricoid cartilages, and the tracheal rings, assessing for symmetry. The trachea should be centered and equidistant from each sternocleidomastoid muscle. Look for fullness at the base of the neck. Inspect the posterior aspect of the neck. The cervical vertebrae should be in alignment. The neck should be symmetrical, and no masses or swelling should be present.

Palpation.   Test the sternocleidomastoid muscle by having the client turn the head to one side and then to the other against the resistance of your hand (see Figure 19-16). Test

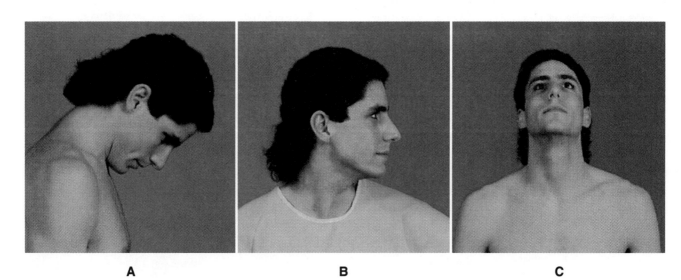

A   B   C

Figure 11-13   **A**, Flexion of the neck. **B**, Lateral rotation of the neck. **C**, Extension of the neck.

for trapezius muscle strength by asking the client to shrug the shoulders against the resistance of your hands (see Figure 19-7). If the client has pain, palpate the sternocleidomastoid for tenderness, spasm, swelling, and trigger points. When you test the strength of the neck muscles, you are also assessing CN XI, the spinal accessory nerve. (The neurological examination of these muscles and their innervation are discussed in Chapter 19.) Gently palpate the midline cartilages. They should be smooth and nontender. Palpate the occipital area, the mastoid process, and the spinous processes of the cervical vertebrae. These should be symmetrical, without tenderness, pain, or swelling.

Thyroid Gland

The techniques used to examine the thyroid gland include inspection, palpation, and auscultation. The thyroid is assessed for enlargement, tenderness, nodules, and bruits. The normal thyroid gland is not visible or palpable, or only slightly so. Examining the thyroid is easy if the neck is long and slender. If the neck is short or thick or if the client has had neck surgery, examination may be difficult. Note that determination of thyroid function includes more than assessment of the neck. Since effects of thyroid activity are widespread, observations of behavior, appearance, skin, eyes, hair, and cardiovascular status are also important.

Inspection. To inspect the thyroid gland, stand in front of the client and observe the lower half of the neck—first in normal position, next in slight extension, and then while the client swallows a sip of water (Figure 11-14). The movements of the cartilages are fairly easy to observe. Note any unusual bulging of thyroid tissue in the midline, at the base of the neck, or of the lobes behind the sternocleidomastoid muscles. Normally, none is seen.

Palpation. After inspection, palpate the neck for the presence of an enlarged thyroid, for consistency of the gland, and for any nodules. The lobes of the thyroid gland

are generally not palpable. In a thin neck the isthmus is occasionally palpable. The thyroid is also sometimes palpable during pregnancy. In a short, stocky neck, even an enlarged gland may be difficult to palpate. Palpation may be done with the examiner standing either in front of or behind the client. Although several techniques can be used for palpation of the thyroid, the underlying principles for each technique include the following:

1. Movement of the gland while the client swallows
2. Adequate exposure of the gland by tilting the head to one side to relax the muscles
3. Manual displacement of surrounding structures to better expose the gland
4. Comparison of one side with the other

Since the sternocleidomastoid muscles are strong and large, it is important to relax them. The thyroid gland is fixed to the trachea and rises during swallowing. This feature distinguishes the thyroid from other neck structures. Palpate the area where the isthmus and lobes are located to determine the gland's size, consistency, degree of enlargement, presence of nodules, and surface characteristics.

Posterior Approach. The posterior approach is easier and less awkward for the practitioner than the anterior approach. Stand behind the client, who is seated on a chair or examining table. Ask the client to lower the chin to relax the sternocleidomastoid muscles. Curve your fingers anteriorly so that your fingertips rest on the lower half of the neck over the trachea below the cricoid cartilage (Figure 11-15). Ask the client to swallow a sip of water while you palpate for any enlargement of the thyroid isthmus. Next, to examine each lobe separately, ask the client to lower the chin and turn the head slightly to the right. With the fingers of your left hand, gently displace the thyroid cartilage slightly to the right while you use the fingers of your right hand to palpate the area next to the midline cartilage where the thyroid lobe lies (Figure 11-16). This procedure is then repeated with the

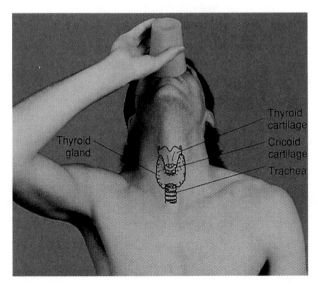

Figure 11-14 Inspection of the neck for enlargement of the thyroid gland.

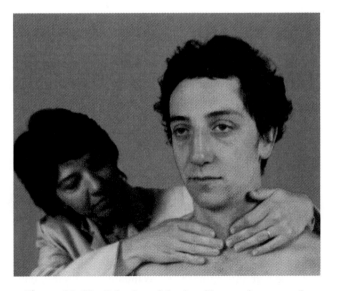

Figure 11-15 Palpation of the thyroid: posterior approach.

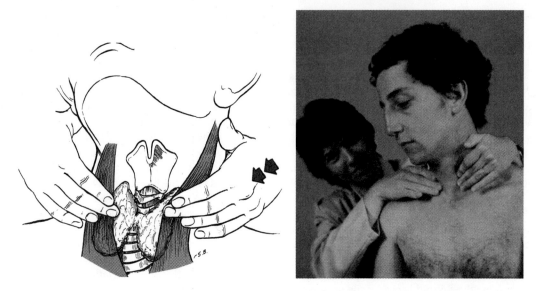

Figure 11-16 Posterior approach to thyroid examination. To examine the right lobe of the thyroid gland, the examiner displaces the trachea slightly to the right with the fingers of the left hand and palpates for the right thyroid lobe with the fingers of the right hand.

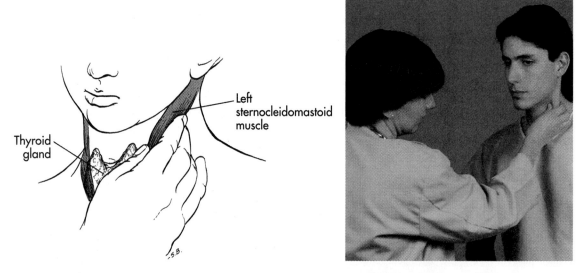

Figure 11-17 Anterior approach to thyroid examination. The examiner grasps around the left sternocleidomastoid muscle with the right hand to palpate for an enlarged left thyroid lobe.

client turning the chin to the left while you palpate with the fingers of your left hand. Having the client swallow a sip of water during this procedure may be helpful.

Anterior Approach. Stand in front of the seated client. Using the fingertips of your index and middle fingers, palpate below the cricoid cartilage for the thyroid isthmus as the client swallows a sip of water. As in the procedure used for the posterior approach, ask the client to flex the head and turn it slightly to one side and then to the other. Palpate the left lobe by displacing the thyroid cartilage slightly toward that lobe with the left hand and examining the thyroid with the right hand. This area can be more deeply palpated by hooking the thumb and fingers around the sternocleidomas-

toid muscle (Figure 11-17). Estimate the size of palpable masses or nodules, and describe their location, tenderness, shape, consistency, surface characteristics, and fixation to surrounding tissue.

Auscultation. If enlargement of the gland is detected or suspected, perform auscultation over the lobes of the thyroid by using the bell of the stethoscope (Figure 11-18). Increased blood flow to the thyroid gland produces vibrations that may be heard as a soft rushing sound or bruit.

Lymph Nodes

The lymphatic system is not generally accessible to examination in healthy people. When infection or malignancy is

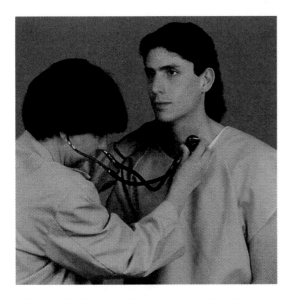

Figure 11-18 Auscultation over the thyroid gland.

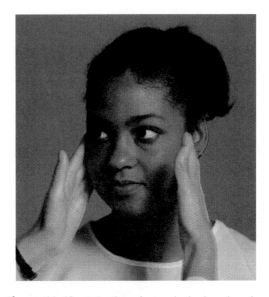

Figure 11-19 Palpation of preauricular lymph nodes.

present, the nodes typically enlarge. Those nodes lying near the surface of the body can be palpated. Some healthy people have a few discrete (separate or distinct), movable, small, nontender nodes present. These are typically less than 1 cm in diameter. They are sometimes referred to as "shotty" nodes.

The techniques of inspection and palpation are used to examine the lymph nodes.

Inspection.   In the healthy client, lymph nodes are not visible. With infection or neoplasm, the areas where the nodes are located may appear swollen. Inspect the areas where the superficial lymph nodes are located, and observe any swelling, edema, skin lesions, erythema, or red streaks on the skin. Often the enlargement is subtle, so observation is based on a careful history and is carefully integrated with palpation. Observe the areas of the head and neck where lymph nodes are grouped.

Palpation.   Palpate groups of lymph nodes in the head and neck using the pads of the second, third, and fourth fingers. Use a gentle, circular motion. Move the skin lightly over the underlying tissues rather than moving the examining fingers over the skin. Press lightly at first, increasing the pressure gradually, if needed. Heavy pressure can push the nodes into the deeper soft tissues so that their presence may be missed. You may palpate the nodes on each side of the head simultaneously. When you palpate the nodes in the neck that lie near the carotid sinus, palpate one side at a time because pressure over the carotid sinus can result in a drop in blood pressure and lead to syncope.

To examine the lymph nodes of the head, begin node palpation at the base of the skull (occipital nodes) and move toward the areas posterior and anterior to the ear (postauricular and preauricular nodes) (Figure 11-19), along the angle of the jaw (parotid nodes), then along and under the mandible (submandibular, sublingual, and submental nodes).

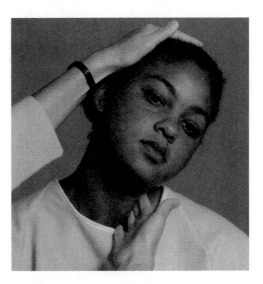

Figure 11-20 Palpation of anterior cervical lymph nodes.

<table>
<tr><td>■ **HELPFUL HINT**</td></tr>
</table>

The groups of lymph nodes are not always as distinctive as the drawings indicate. If you are not certain which group you are palpating, describe them by location as precisely as possible. (See Box 11-1 for terms commonly used to describe some of the characteristics of enlarged nodes.)

When examining the neck nodes, ask the client to bend his or her head slightly downward (Figure 11-20). This position reduces muscle tension and enhances accurate palpation. Palpate the node chains superficially and then more deeply in the soft tissues of the anterior triangle (anterior cervical chain, Figure 11-20) and posterior triangle (posterior superficial cervical chain). The internal jugular chain is difficult to examine, particularly if pressed too heavily. Probe gently, with your thumb and fingers around the sternocleidomastoid muscle (Figure 11-21).

■ **HELPFUL HINT**

Whenever a lesion is present, look for involvement of the regional lymph nodes that drain it. Whenever a node is enlarged or tender, look for a source of infection or neoplastic growth in the area that it drains.

To examine the supraclavicular nodes, palpate into the soft tissue just above the clavicle (Figure 11-22, *A*). As with the other neck nodes, it is helpful to ask the client to bend his or her head slightly downward (Figure 11-22, *B*).

If any nodes are detected, describe them according to the following:

1. Location
2. Size
3. Shape
4. Number of nodes
5. Surface characteristics
6. Consistency
7. Tenderness

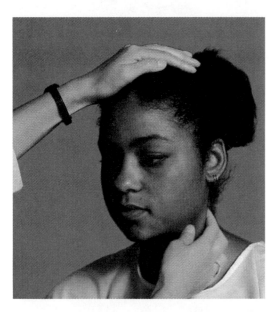

Figure 11-21   Palpation of deep cervical lymph nodes.

BOX 11-1

TERMS USED TO DESCRIBE THE CHARACTERISTICS OF ENLARGED LYMPH NODES

Location: use imaginary body lines, such as the midclavicular line; bony prominences, such as the mandible; or muscles, such as the sternocleidomastoid, to describe specific location.

Size: measure in centimeters.

Shape: usually oval.

Surface characteristics: smooth, nodular, irregular, singular or matted (in groups).

Consistency: soft, firm, hard, rubbery, spongy, cystic.

Mobility/fixation: describe whether node moves freely or is attached to adjacent structure or underlying tissue.

Tenderness: describe whether node is painful without palpation and/or tender with palpation.

Signs of inflammation: erythema, increased warmth.

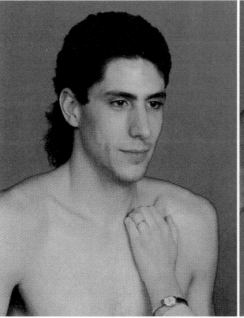

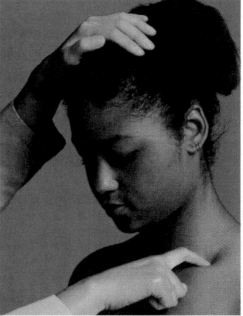

Figure 11-22   Palpation of the supraclavicular lymph nodes.

8. Mobility or fixation to surrounding tissues
9. Discreteness or matting—whether the nodes are palpated as separate from or connected to each other
10. Signs of inflammation

Nodes enlarged because of infection are likely to be tender and matted (Box 11-1). Nodes enlarged because of a malignancy are likely to be hard, discrete, asymmetrical, and not tender. When you find enlarged lymph nodes, explore the areas drained by those nodes for signs of infection or malignancy.

Screening Tests and Procedures

A common laboratory test for clients with head and neck symptoms is a test of thyroid function. Listed in Table 11-2 are common laboratory tests used to help evaluate the client who has signs and symptoms of thyroid dysfunction. Since

Examination Step-by-Step

Make sure that the examination room has good lighting, a comfortable temperature, and privacy for the client. Have the necessary equipment—a stethoscope, glass of water, ruler, and gloves—ready.

INSPECTION
1. Face: appearance, expression, symmetry of structure and features, skin color, movements
2. Head: size; shape; symmetry; condition of skin, hair (distribution, texture, quantity), and scalp (deformities, lesions); unusual movements
3. Neck: symmetry, mobility, range of motion, neck vessels

PALPATION
1. Head: scalp (tenderness, deformities, lesions), hair (if indicated), temporal artery pulses, temporomandibular joint, lymph nodes
2. Neck: anterior midline neck structures, thyroid gland, carotid artery pulses, lymph nodes, muscle strength, cervical vertebrae

AUSCULTATION
1. Neck: carotid arteries and thyroid gland for bruits

TABLE 11-2	Some Tests Used To Determine Altered Thyroid Function
Test	Comments
TSH—thyroid stimulating hormone	Elevated with hypothyroidism Lowered with hyperthyroidism
Total serum T$_4$	Elevated with hyperthyroidism Lowered with hypothyroidism
Thyroid scan	Evaluates functional status of nodular goiter
Ultrasonography	Evaluates status of single nodules

values may differ among laboratories, the normal value range for the specific laboratory that provides the results must be determined.

VARIATIONS FROM HEALTH

Face

Changes in Coloration
1. Cyanosis: occurs with poor circulation to local structures or when the amount of unsaturated hemoglobin in the body tissues is increased, as may occur with cardiac or pulmonary disease; lips, nose, cheeks, ears, and oral mucosa may become bluish.
2. Pallor: results from decreased vascular supply, as in shock.
3. Jaundice: results from decreased liver function or obstruction and increased bilirubin deposits in the skin; before the yellow color of jaundice is evident in the skin, it may be observed in the sclera of the eyes and mucous membranes of the mouth.
4. Lupus erythematosus: an erythematous discoloration in a butterfly pattern bridges the cheeks and nose.
5. Other: localized color changes from acne, moles, or scar tissue.

Changes in Shape
1. Edema: excess accumulation of fluid in the tissues may result from cardiovascular or renal disease; often initially evident in the eyelids, where it is called *periorbital edema*, this condition can involve the entire face.
2. Protrusion of eyeballs (exophthalmos) and elevation of upper lids; result of hyperthyroidism; gives face a staring or startled expression.
3. Puffiness with dry skin and coarse features: result of hypothyroidism; called *myxedema facies* (Figure 11-23).

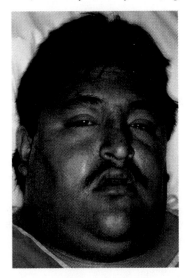

Figure 11-23 Myxedema facies. Note dull, puffy, yellowed skin; coarse, sparse hair; temporal loss of eyebrows; periorbital edema; prominent tongue. (From Lemmi FO, Lemmi CA: *Physical assessment findings CD-ROM,* Philadelphia, 2000, WB Saunders.)

4. Face rounded, cheeks red: result of increased adrenal hormone production (Cushing's syndrome) or secondary to intake of synthetic adrenal hormones; called *moon facies* (see Figure 9-20).
5. Face sunken, skin rough and dry: prolonged illness, dehydration, or starvation may produce this cachectic face; eyes, cheeks, and temples appear sunken, and nose appears sharp.

Changes in Symmetry

1. Asymmetry, abnormal movements, or both may result from facial nerve lesions or from central nervous system lesion, such as results from a cardiovascular accident.
2. Paralysis of CN VII, or Bell's palsy, causes changes on affected side; eyelid does not close completely, lower eyelid and corner of mouth droop, and nasolabial fold disappears.

Changes in Hair Distribution

1. For women in some ethnic groups, increased facial hair, often above the upper lip, is a normal finding.
2. Excessive hair growth in mustache, sideburn, and chin areas results from elevated production of adrenal hormones.
3. Thinning of scalp hair and eyebrows is a result of increased thyroid activity.

Pain

1. Trigeminal neuralgia (tic douloureux): this neurological abnormality is caused by degeneration of or pressure on one or all of the three divisions of the trigeminal nerve, CN V (see Figure 11-2 for distribution pattern of this nerve):
   a. Ophthalmic (first division)—pain around eyes and over forehead
   b. Maxillary (second division)—pain in nose, cheek, and upper lip
   c. Mandibular (third division)—pain in lower lip and side of tongue
   The pain is aching, burning, flashing, or stablike, and attacks cause the person to wince with facial contractions. Pain attacks may occur spontaneously or may be evoked by pressure on a trigger zone, cold air, a light touch, biting, swallowing, chewing, laughing, talking, yawning, or sneezing. The pain may last from a few seconds to a few minutes. Cycles of pain and abatement may continue for hours. Trigeminal neuralgia affects persons in middle to late adulthood.
2. Herpes zoster may affect any sensory nerve, but the virus typically tends to invade the posterior root ganglia associated with the thoracic and trigeminal nerves. The pain may be constant or intermittent, superficial or deep.
3. Sinus tenderness results from inflammation of one or more of the paranasal sinuses. The client may experience pressure and pain in the area of the sinuses, headache, fever, and local tenderness to palpation.

4. Temporomandibular joint pain dysfunction syndrome is an abnormal condition marked by painful jaw movement and mandibular dysfunction. The joint may snap, lock, or "pop." The pain may be referred to other points on the face and neck.

Head

Changes in Size

1. Abnormally large head in children: caused by accumulation of fluid in the ventricles of the brain (hydrocephalus).
2. Large head in adults: results from osteitis deformans (Paget's disease) or acromegaly (see Chapter 9).

Changes in Shape

1. Sebaceous cysts on scalp: result from occlusion of sebaceous gland ducts; palpable as smooth, rounded nodules attached to the scalp.
2. Trauma or surgical removal of a portion of the skull alters shape.

Changes in Hair

1. Coarse, dry, brittle: results from hypothyroidism.
2. Fine, silky, soft: results from hyperthyroidism.
3. Thinning or hair loss (alopecia): may be hereditary (especially in men), a side effect of chemotherapy, or a result of prolonged illness or emotional stress.
4. Hair and scalp should be checked for dandruff and parasites.

Pain

Headaches are one of the most common symptoms experienced, resulting more often from tension or emotional distress than from organic disease. They also may be the presenting symptom of an injury or severe illness, such as cerebral hemorrhage, brain tumor, or meningitis. Whatever their cause, headaches can be associated with intense and debilitating pain. In addition, individuals may suffer from more than one type of headache at a time.

Headaches can be classified in numerous ways. One approach is to divide them into primary headaches with three main groups: (1) muscle contraction, or tension, headaches; (2) migraine headaches; and (3) cluster headaches (Table 11-3). These headaches are classified as primary because they are not directly related to a specific underlying cause.

Secondary headaches are due to structural or physiological problems. They include traction and inflammatory headaches, which are caused by disease or injury, such as sinus inflammation, cranial hemorrhage, or brain tumor, to some structure of the head or neck (e.g., brain, meninges, arteries, veins, eyes, ears, teeth, nose, paranasal sinuses, jaw, neck joints). Secondary headaches may also be due to a systemic cause, such as allergies, hormones, toxins, infection, or exertion. The nature of the headache depends on the underlying disorder. Secondary headaches occur less frequently than primary headaches. However, it is very important to rule out the underlying, possibly life-threatening,

TABLE 11-3	Characteristics of Primary Headaches		
	Muscle Contraction or Tension Headaches	Migraine Headaches	Cluster Headaches
Age at onset	Adolescence through adulthood	Childhood, adolescence, or young adulthood	Young to middle adulthood
Sex distribution	Occur more frequent in females	Occur more frequently in females	Occur more frequently in males
Typical onset	Gradual, often following stress	Begins as dull ache, progresses to intense pain; occurs anytime during day; may have aura of warning symptoms	Sudden; reaches peak intensity in several minutes; often occurs during evening or night; may awaken client
Location	"Hatband" distribution; may radiate to occipital area and around eyes	Generally unilateral; may be frontal around eye or cheek, may alternate from side to side with subsequent attacks, or may be bilateral	Unilateral, involving facial area from neck to temple; may be around eye
Character of pain	Dull, bandlike, constricting, persistent, with occasional episodes of severe pain	Intense, pulsating, throbbing, one-sided	Sharp, intense, deep, burning, boring, stabbing, excruciating, steady
Duration	Hours to days or months	Several hours to several days	Several minutes to several hours
Frequency	Varies	Varying intervals from several times per month to several times per year; may have a pattern, as with menstrual cycle	May be daily for several weeks in repetitive clusters several times per year
Associated symptoms	Neck stiffness, shoulder ache, nausea	Photophobia, nausea, vomiting, dizziness, tremors, sensitivity to sound	Tearing of eye and stuffiness of nostril on affected side; facial flushing; modified Horner's syndrome with mild ptosis (drooping of upper eyelid) and miosis (constriction of pupil) on affected side
Precipitating factors	Fatigue, stress, anxiety, depression, or no obvious precipitant	Fatigue, prolonged hunger, menstruation, birth control pills, stress, bright sunlight, foods or drugs containing vasoactive chemicals	Alcohol, vasodilators, cigarette smoke, caffeine
Other factors	Most common type of head pain; may result from depression or anxiety or from organic problems, such as cervical arthritis	Familial	
Prodromal events		Complex of neurological events that may precede the migraine include paresthesias, aura, visual changes such as flashing lights, scotomata (blind spots), hemianopia (loss of vision on one side), distorted perception of size and shape of objects	

cause(s) of the headache before deciding on a diagnosis of a primary headache.

Sinus headaches are the most common type of secondary headaches. They are caused by inflammation of one or more of the paranasal sinuses. These headaches may be a complication of a respiratory infection, dental infection, allergy, or change in atmospheric pressure (e.g., air travel, swimming), or they may result from a structural defect. Swelling of the nasal mucous membranes obstructs the openings from the sinuses to the nose, resulting in an accumulation of secretions; this situation may cause tenderness, pressure, and headache.

Temporal Arteritis

Arteritis is an inflammatory condition of one or more layers of an arterial wall. Temporal arteritis usually affects individuals older than 50 years and is characterized by flulike symptoms, polymyalgia, ocular symptoms, and headache.

The skin over the temporal artery becomes red, swollen, and tender. The temporal pulse may be strong, weak, or absent. Temporal arteritis is considered an emergency condition since the major danger is sudden and irreversible blindness.

Neck

If traumatic neck injury has occurred, the neck should not be moved.

Neck Muscles

Common variations from health of the neck muscles include stiffness and pain caused by tension, cervical arthritis, or meningitis.

Temporomandibular Joint Disease

Pain in the area of the **temporomandibular joint** results from dislocation of the condyle, osteoarthritis, rheumatoid arthritis, or a myofascial pain syndrome. Pain is often localized to the neck and ear in the area adjacent to the joint. The client has limited motion of the jaw; muscle tenderness; and, occasionally, joint crepitus.

Polymyalgia Rheumatica

This syndrome is characterized by an aching pain, tenderness, and stiffness in the neck and shoulders, which may extend to the upper arms, forearms, hips, and legs. Aching is increased with motion.

Hypothyroidism and Hyperthyroidism

In general, with hypothyroidism there is a slowing of body functions; with hyperthyroidism there is an acceleration of body functions. Signs and symptoms of either are initially often subtle. The thyroid gland may have diffuse or local enlargement. Symmetrical enlargement may occur with dietary iodine deficiency. Localized or nodular enlargement consists of one or more nodules and may be found in the lobes or the isthmus. Solitary nodules are suggestive of carcinoma, particularly in young adults. Thyroid dysfunction, either hypothyroidism or hyperthyroidism, cannot be determined by the size of the gland alone. If thyroid dysfunction is suspected, thyroid function studies are necessary. The effects of excessive or inadequate amounts of thyroid hormones on body structures and systems are shown in Table 11-4.

TABLE 11-4   **Effects of Hyperthyroidism and Hypothyroidism on Body Systems and Structures**

Body System or Structure	Hyperthyroidism	Hypothyroidism
General		
Weight	Loss	Gain
Temperature intolerance	Heat	Cold
Energy level	Sense of increased energy and alertness	Fatigue, exercise intolerance
Sleep	Insomnia	Drowsiness, difficulty sleeping, obstructive sleep apnea
Skin	Warm, moist; increased sweating; smooth texture; diffuse pigmentation; erythema; brittle nails	Cool, pale, dry, rough, scaly, itchy, facial edema, decreased sweating
Hair	Fine texture, loss, inability to hold a permanent	Thin, dry, poor growth, loss
Cardiovascular/pulmonary	Increased cardiac output, increased blood pressure, wide pulse pressure, tachycardia, atrial dysrhythmias, systolic murmur, palpitations, angina, dyspnea, edema, increase in rate or depth of respirations, bruit over thyroid	Congestive heart failure, angina, bradycardia, cardiomegaly, pericardial or pulmonary effusions, slow and shallow respirations, upper airway obstruction, dyspnea on exertion
Gastrointestinal	Indigestion, anorexia, polyphagia, diarrhea, increased appetite	Thickened tongue, decreased appetite, constipation, abdominal distention
Renal	Polydipsia, polyuria, urgency	Decreased output
Nervous	Restlessness, irritability, anxiety, memory loss, easy distractibility, decreased ability to concentrate, emotional liability, panic attacks, hyperreflexia, tremor	Reduced concentration and memory, irritability, slowed thought processes and speech, inability to concentrate, apathy, depression, slowed motor functions, delayed relaxation of deep tendon reflexes, coma
Muscular	Weakness, tremulousness	Stiffness, aching, pain, weakness, muscle cramps, arthralgias
Eyes	Lid lag and lid retraction (startled look), tearing, conjunctival irritation	Periorbital puffiness
Voice		Deep, hoarse
Hearing		Acuity may diminish
Reproductive		
Women	Hypomenorrhea, amenorrhea	Menorrhagia, amenorrhea, infertility, anovulatory cycles
Men	Decreased libido and potency	Decreased libido and potency

Lymph Nodes

Lymph Node Enlargement

Enlarged lymph nodes may be due to acute or chronic infections. Examples of acute conditions are infectious mononucleosis, tonsillitis, or streptococcal meningitis. Acute infections may cause lymph nodes to be firm, tender, matted, or discrete. Sharply localized tender nodes suggest infection at a distal focus. More serious illnesses related to the immune system, such as cancer and acquired immunodeficiency syndrome (AIDS), may also present clinically in the lymph nodes. For example, the first clinical sign of metastatic disease is the involvement of lymph nodes in the region draining the site of neoplastic growth. The lymph nodes may be hard, fixed to surrounding tissue, and nontender. In a person infected with HIV, nodes of any chain may be enlarged, but those of the head and neck are most commonly involved.

Acute Infections

Streptococcal Pharyngitis. Symptoms of streptococcal pharyngitis usually include a sore throat and runny nose and may include headache, fatigue, myalgias, and abdominal discomfort. Anterior cervical nodes are commonly palpable and tend to be firm, discrete, mobile, and tender.

Epstein-Barr Virus Mononucleosis. Epstein-Barr virus mononucleosis (infectious mononucleosis) is most common in adolescents and young adults. Lymph node enlargement may be generalized but is most common in the anterior and posterior cervical chains. Nodes vary in firmness, are generally discrete, and may be tender. Early symptoms include pharyngitis, fever, fatigue, and malaise. Splenomegaly, hepatomegaly, and a rash may develop.

Lymphadenitis. Lymphadenitis is an inflammatory condition of the lymph nodes resulting from bacterial infection, neoplastic disease, or other inflammatory conditions. The nodes may be enlarged, hard, tender, smooth, or irregular.

The overlying skin may become edematous, red, and warm. The site of the affected node indicates the site of the origin of the disease.

Metastatic Disease. Malignant lymphomas, including Hodgkin's disease, cause nodes to be large, discrete, nontender, and firm to rubbery in consistency. Such nodes may be localized to any area but are occasionally generalized. **Lymphadenopathy**, an inflammatory condition of the lymph nodes, may be due to chronic lymphocytic leukemia. Lymph nodes due to metastatic cancer are nontender, have a firm to hard consistency, may be discrete or matted, and tend to be localized initially. The various lymphomas differ in degree of cellular differentiation and content, but the manifestations are similar in all types. Characteristically the appearance of a painless, enlarged lymph node or nodes in the neck is followed by weakness, fever, weight loss, and anemia.

Hodgkin's disease is a malignant disorder characterized by painless, progressive enlargement of lymphoid tissue, which is usually first evident in cervical lymph nodes. Symptoms include anorexia, weight loss, generalized pruritus, low-grade fever, and night sweats.

Acquired Immunodeficiency Syndrome. Acquired immunodeficiency syndrome (AIDS) is a disease involving a defect in cell-mediated immunity. This syndrome is caused by human immunodeficiency virus infection. It is characterized by the loss of T_4 lymphocyte cells, which leads to progressive loss of immune system competency, with the development of opportunistic infections, impairment of the central nervous system, chronic wasting, and often malignancy. Initial symptoms include lymphadenopathy, extreme fatigue, intermittent fever, chills, night sweats, enlarged spleen, anorexia, diarrhea, weight loss, apathy, and depression. As the disease progresses, general malnourishment, decreased energy, and recurrent infections develop. Most people with AIDS are susceptible to malignant neoplasms, especially Kaposi's sarcoma and non-Hodgkin's lymphoma.

Sample Documentation and Diagnoses

FOCUSED HEALTH HISTORY (SUBJECTIVE DATA)

Ms. O, a 25-year-old graduate student, gives a history of headaches for the past 5 months. Headaches have occurred every 2 weeks but are now more frequent. Headaches begin in the late morning to early afternoon. Client describes them as "a tight band around my head with throbbing on the sides" with associated pain and stiffness in the neck and shoulders and slight nausea. Pain is gradual in onset and is typically dull and nagging (5 on a 10-point scale). Occasionally it becomes so severe that she must stop working for 1 to 2 hours. Client denies GI symptoms, photophobia, or changes in vision. Client uses aspirin or acetaminophen q 3 to 4 hours with some relief. Denies allergies to food or drugs, does not smoke, and drinks a glass of wine about twice a month. States she is very concerned about the increasing frequency of the headaches. Is a full-time graduate student and works about 30 hours per week. She is concerned that the headaches are interfering with her ability to study.

FOCUSED PHYSICAL EXAMINATION (OBJECTIVE DATA)

General appearance: Client appears tired and anxious. Neatly groomed.

Physical examination: Scalp is clear of lesions; hair is normally distributed and of medium texture. Temporal artery pulses palpable, nontender.

Eyes: Vision 20/20 in each eye using Snellen; visual fields intact; PERRLA; extraocular movements (EOMs) intact.

Neck: Thyroid not palpable; trapezius muscles stiff and tender to palpation; trapezius and sternocleidomastoid strength good bilaterally. No cervicofacial nodes palpable.

Neurological: Cranial nerves II through XII intact.

DIAGNOSES

HEALTH PROBLEM

Tension headache

NURSING DIAGNOSIS

Pain

Defining Characteristics

- Facial appearance of pain and fatigue
- Verbal report of pain and stiffness at base of head, neck, and shoulders
- Interference with work schedule

Critical Thinking Questions

Review the Sample Documentation and Diagnoses section to answer these questions.

1. What additional history information would be useful to assess thyroid function?
2. What history and physical examination findings would you expect if the problem were a secondary headache caused by sinusitis?
3. Describe the advantages and disadvantages of two methods of thyroid palpation. What are expected findings in the thyroid examination?

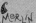 Answers are available on the MERLIN website (www.harcourthealth.com/MERLIN/Barkauskas/). And be sure to check the website regularly for additional learning activities!

Remember to check out the Online Study Guide!
www.harcourthealth.com/MERLIN/Barkauskas/

Eyes

Learning Objectives

On successful study of this chapter and completion of related learning experiences, the learner will be able to:
• Describe the purposes of the eye examination.
• Describe the physiology of vision.

• Identify anatomical structures assessed during the eye examination.
• Demonstrate techniques of examination of the eye.

Outline

Purpose of Examination

Vision is one of our most important mechanisms for experiencing the world. The eyes are complex and delicate structures. They receive visual stimuli and transmit that stimuli to the visual cortex in the brain. The optic nerve (cranial nerve [CN] II) directly connects the eye and the brain. Six of the 12 cranial nerves are involved with the eyes. The eyes are balanced and held in place by six sets of extraocular muscles.

A thorough examination of the eyes can reveal a wealth of information about both local and systemic health, such as neurological status and hepatic function. In conjunction with observation of facial expression and body posture, observation of the eyes frequently provides information about the client's emotional status.

The examination of the eyes includes measurement of visual acuity, evaluation of visual fields, testing of ocular movements, inspection of ocular structures, testing of nerve reflexes, and the ophthalmoscopic examination.

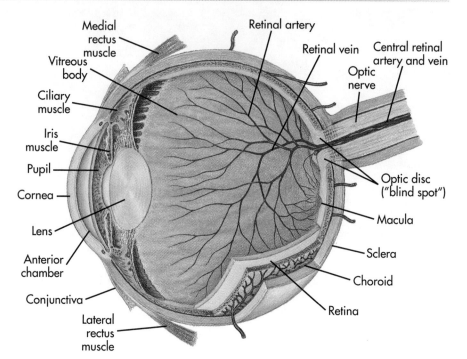

Figure 12-1   Lateral view of structures of the eye. (From Seidel HM et al: *Mosby's guide to physical examination,* ed. 4, St. Louis, 1999, Mosby.)

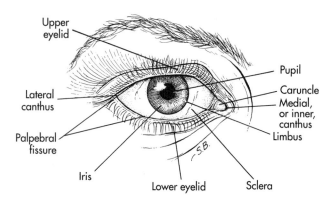

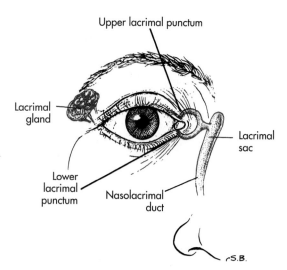

Figure 12-2   Anterior view of the eye and lacrimal system.

ANATOMY AND PHYSIOLOGY

The eyes are located within the bony orbital cavity. The anterior aspect of the eye is exposed, and the remainder is protected within the skull. The structures of the eye described in this chapter include the following:

Eyelids and eyelashes
Conjunctiva
Sclera
Cornea
Anterior chamber
Lacrimal apparatus
Iris
Pupils
Lens
Vitreous body
Retina
Ocular muscles
Optic nerve

Portions of the retina that are described here include the following:

Optic disc
Retinal vessels
Macula
Retinal background

The structures of the eyelid and the globe of the eye are illustrated in Figures 12-1 and 12-2.

Ocular Structures

Eyelids and Eyelashes

The eyelashes are distributed along the margin of each eyelid and curve outward. The eyelids, or **palpebrae,** serve a protective function, covering the anterior aspect of the eye and distributing tears across the surface of the eye to keep it moist and lubricated. The eyelids also limit the amount of light that enters the eyes and protect the eyes from foreign objects. When the eyes are open, the upper eyelid normally covers a small portion of the iris and the cornea overlying it, located about midway between the limbus and the pupil. The margin of the lower eyelid lies at or just below the limbus. The **limbus** is the junction line of the cornea and the sclera. The distance between the upper and the lower eyelid margin is called the **palpebral fissure**. The tarsal plates are thin strips of connective tissue that lie within the eyelid and give it form and consistency.

Conjunctiva

The **conjunctiva** lines the eyelids and covers the anterior portion of the eyeball. This continuous transparent lining is divided into two portions: palpebral and bulbar. The palpebral portion lines the eyelids; it appears shiny pink or red because it overlies the fleshy vascular structures of the lids. The palpebral conjunctiva is continuous with the bulbar conjunctiva, which rests loosely over the sclera to the limbus, where it merges with the corneal epithelium. This portion of the conjunctiva is normally clear; the white color comes from the sclera below. The bulbar portion does, however, contain many small blood vessels. These vessels are normally visible and may become dilated, producing varying degrees of redness. A small fleshy elevation, the **caruncle**, is located in the nasal corner of the conjunctiva (see Figure 12-2). The **meibomian** glands, which secrete an oily lubricating substance, appear as vertical yellow striations on the palpebral conjunctiva.

Sclera

The globe of the eye is surrounded by three coats: sclera, **choroid**, and retina. The **sclera** is the outer fibrous layer. It is visible anteriorly as the white portion of the eye. Several small, distinct conjunctival vessels lie over the sclera, particularly around the periphery. In some dark-skinned persons, small dark-pigmented dots are located on the sclera near the limbus.

Cornea

The **cornea** is a smooth, moist tissue that covers the area over the pupil and the iris. It is continuous with the conjunctiva. Like the bulbar conjunctiva, the cornea is transparent and permits the passage of light inward toward the retina. The cornea merges with the conjunctiva at the limbus. It separates fluid in the anterior chamber from the external environment. The cornea is sensitive to touch. This sensation is transmitted by the ophthalmic branch of the trigeminal nerve (CN V).

Anterior Chamber

The anterior chamber lies posterior to the cornea. It is filled with **aqueous humor**, a fluid that is continuously produced by the ciliary body. The relationship between the rate of production of aqueous humor and the resistance to aqueous outflow at the anterior chamber angle determines the intraocular pressure, which is normally 15 mm Hg ± 3 mm Hg.

Lacrimal Apparatus

The following are the components of the lacrimal apparatus:
Lacrimal gland
Lacrimal puncta
Lacrimal sac
Nasolacrimal duct

The lacrimal gland is located above and slightly lateral to the eye (see Figure 12-2). It produces tears, which moisten and lubricate the conjunctiva and the cornea. The tears wash across the eye and drain through the upper and lower lacrimal **puncta**, which are small openings located at the nasal side of both the upper and lower eyelid margins. The tears then pass into the nasolacrimal sac, which is located medial to the eye. From the nasolacrimal sac, the tears pass into the nasolacrimal duct and the nasal meatus. Tearing is also referred to as **lacrimation**.

Iris

The iris is the circular disc containing pigmented fibrils that give the eye its distinctive color. It is located in front of the lens and behind the anterior chamber. The iris, the ciliary body, and the suspensory ligament form the interior portion of the choroid layer of the eye. Posterior to the layer of fibrils are two groups of muscles, dilator and sphincter muscles. These muscles function in a manner similar to that of the diaphragm of a camera within the image-forming portion of the eye.

Pupil

The **pupil** is the opening in the iris through which light passes. The size of the pupil is determined by the amount of light entering the eye and the closeness of the object being visualized. It is regulated by the constriction and dilation of the muscles of the iris. This muscular activity is controlled by the autonomic nervous system. Stimulation of the parasympathetic fibers leads to constriction of the pupils; stimulation of the sympathetic fibers produces dilation of the pupils. Increasing the amount of light causes pupillary constriction. Diminishing the light causes dilation. These changes represent **adaptation**. The pupils also constrict in response to **accommodation**, which is the change in focus from a distant to a near object.

The constricting response of the pupils to a bright, direct light is a pupillary reflex. This reflex consists of two aspects: the direct reaction and the consensual reaction, or the consensual light reflex. The direct reaction refers to the constriction of the pupil receiving the increased illumination. The constriction of the pupil that is not receiving increased light is the consensual reaction. The optic nerve (CN II) transmits the stimulus from the eye to the brain. The oculomotor nerve (CN III) transmits the reflex from the brain to both eyes. The presence of both direct and consensual responses indicates the functioning of these two cranial nerves.

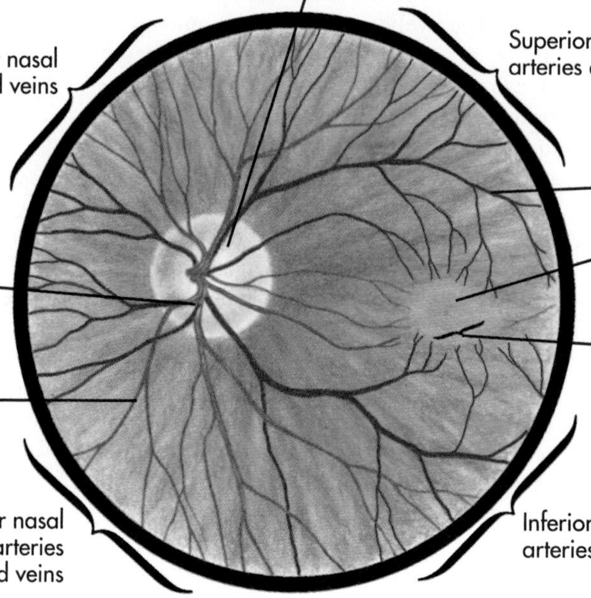

Figure 12-3 Retinal structures of the left eye. (Modified from Seidel HM et al: *Mosby's guide to physical examination,* ed. 4, St. Louis, 1999, Mosby.)

Key: Dark red: veins
Light red: arterioles

Physiologic cup

Superior nasal arteries and veins

Superior temporal arteries and veins

Vein

Fovea centralis

Optic disc

Macula

Arteriole

Inferior nasal arteries and veins

Inferior temporal arteries and veins

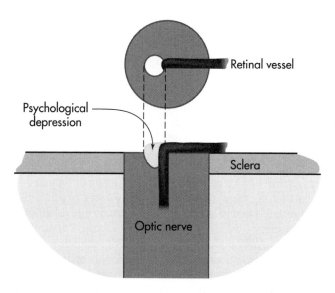

Retinal vessel

Psychological depression

Sclera

Optic nerve

Figure 12-4 The physiologic depression, or physiologic cup, is entirely surrounded by a rim of normal tissue. (From Prior JA, Silberstein JS, Stang JM: *Physical diagnosis: the history and examination of the patient,* ed. 6, St. Louis, 1981, Mosby.)

Lens

The **lens** is located directly behind the iris at the pupillary opening. It is the center of the refracting system of the eye. The lens is composed of epithelial cells within an elastic membrane, the lens capsule. The lens is transparent and has no blood vessels, nerves, or connective tissue. The thickness of the lens is controlled by the muscles of the **ciliary body.** Changes in lens thickness enable the eye to focus on near and distant objects. The coordinated function of the muscles of the iris and the muscles of the ciliary body acting on the lens controls the amount of light permitted to reach the retina and the focusing of objects on the retina.

Vitreous Humor

The **vitreous humor** is a transparent fluid that occupies the area posterior to the lens, which is called the posterior chamber. The vitreous humor is surrounded by the retinal layer of the globe of the eye.

Retina and Retinal Structures

The **retina** is the inner coat of the globe of the eye. It contains the neurosensory elements that transform light impulses into the electrical impulses that are carried to the visual cortex by way of the optic nerve and the optic tract. Several important structures are located on the retina, including (1) the optic disc, which is the head of the optic nerve; (2) four sets of retinal vessels, which emerge from the optic disc and travel medially and laterally around the retina; and (3) the macula, where central vision is concentrated (Figure 12-3).

Optic Disc and Physiologic Cup. The optic disc is located on the nasal half of the retina. This round structure is creamy yellow to pink and is lighter than the surrounding retina. The color of both the disc and the retinal background varies from one individual to another; it is somewhat lighter in fair-complexioned, light-haired people and slightly darker in dark-complexioned, dark-haired people.

The physiologic cup, or physiologic depression, is a small depression within the disc just temporal to the center of the disc. It is yellowish white and slightly lighter in color than the rest of the disc. The physiologic cup does not extend to the disc margins; it occupies one fourth to one third of the area of the disc (Figure 12-4).

Retinal Vessels. Four sets of retinal vessels emerge from the optic disc and extend outward, becoming smaller at the periphery (see Figure 12-3). Each set of vessels, which

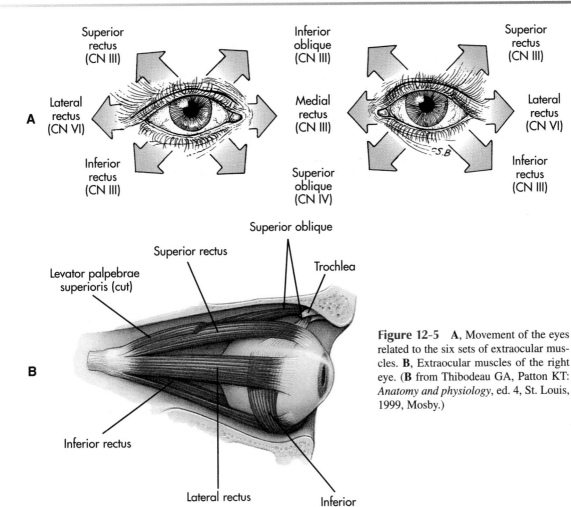

Figure 12-5 A, Movement of the eyes related to the six sets of extraocular muscles. **B**, Extraocular muscles of the right eye. (**B** from Thibodeau GA, Patton KT: *Anatomy and physiology*, ed. 4, St. Louis, 1999, Mosby.)

includes an arteriole and a vein, is named according to the quadrant of the disc in which it is located: superior nasal, inferior nasal, superior temporal, and inferior temporal. The arterioles are brighter red than the veins because they carry oxygenated blood. The veins are darker red because they carry deoxygenated blood. Since the arterioles are approximately 25% smaller than the veins, there is an arteriole/vein ratio (A:V ratio) of about 2:3 or 4:5.

Macula and Retinal Background. The rods and the cones are neurosensory elements located in the retina. The rods mediate black-and-white vision, and the cones mediate color vision. At a point temporal to the optic disc at the posterior pole of the eye, the retina has a slight depression called the **fovea centralis**. The cones are most heavily concentrated in this area, making it the point of central vision and most acute color and daylight vision. The retinal area immediately around the fovea centralis is called the macula. The retinal background is reddish orange.

Extraocular Muscles and Cranial Nerves

Six muscles of each eye, working in a coordinated, or yoked, fashion with those of the other eye, control eye movement. The movements of the two eyes normally occur in conjugate, parallel fashion except during **convergence**. The eyes converge, or come toward each other, when the person focuses on a very close object. The six extraocular muscles are shown in Figure 12-5.

The parallel movement of the eyes makes it possible to have single-image binocular vision. The yoked muscles are the muscles in each eye that work together to move the eyes in parallel motion to any position of gaze (see Figure 12-5, *A*). For example, the left lateral rectus and the right medial rectus are yoked muscles that work concurrently to move the gaze to the left.

The six eye muscles are innervated by three cranial nerves. The oculomotor nerve (CN III) supplies four muscles: the superior, inferior, and medial rectus muscles and the inferior oblique muscle. The trochlear nerve (CN IV) innervates the superior oblique muscle. The abducens nerve (CN VI) supplies the lateral rectus muscle.

■ HELPFUL HINT

A mnemonic device useful for remembering the innervation of the six eye muscles is LR_6SO_4. The lateral rectus is innervated by CN VI, and the superior oblique is innervated by CN IV. The four remaining eye muscles are innervated by CN III.

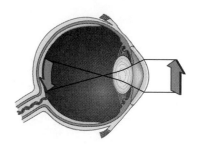

Figure 12-6 Formation of a retinal image. In the normal eye, light rays from an object are refracted by the cornea, aqueous humor, lens, and vitreous humor; those rays converge on the fovea of the retina, where an inverted image is clearly formed. (From Thibodeau GA, Patton KT: *Anatomy and physiology*, ed. 4, St. Louis, 1999, Mosby.)

TABLE 12-1	Relationship of Cranial Nerves to Eye Structures and Functions	
Cranial Nerve	**Function**	
II Optic	Mediates vision	
III Oculomotor	Innervates medial, superior, and inferior rectus muscles; inferior oblique muscle; muscles elevating eyelid (levator palpebrae); and muscles of iris and ciliary body	
IV Trochlear	Innervates superior oblique muscle	
V Trigeminal (ophthalmic division)	Innervates sensory portion of corneal reflex	
VI Abducens	Innervates lateral rectus muscle	
VII Facial	Innervates lacrimal glands and muscles involved in lid closure (orbicularis oculi)	

Six of the 12 cranial nerves and parti of the cerebral hemispheres are involved in the total neurological innervation of the eye and related structures. Table 12-1 summarizes the relationship of the six cranial nerves to the eye structures and their functions (see also Table 19-1).

Physiology of Vision

For someone to perceive a clear visual image, light reflected from an object must pass through several transparent structures: the cornea, anterior chamber, lens, and vitreous fluid. Then the light must focus on the retina, where the neural receptors, the rods and cones, are activated and carry the impulse along the optic nerve and tract to the visual cortex of the brain, which is located in the occipital lobes.

Formation of Retinal Image

The following four processes lead to the formation of a clear image on the retina:
1. Refraction, or light-bending power of a client's eye
2. Accommodation, or change in curvature, of the lens
3. Constriction of the pupil
4. Convergence of the eyes

Refraction is the bending or deflecting of light rays that occurs when the rays pass obliquely from one transparent medium into another of a different density. In the eye these media are the cornea, the aqueous humor, the lens, and the vitreous humor. All of these structures work in conjunction to bring an object into focus on the retina (Figure 12-6).

Accommodation for near vision enables the eye to focus on near objects by increasing the curvature of the lens, constriction of the pupils, and convergence of the eyes. Light rays from close objects are divergent and must be bent to fo-

cus on the retina. The curvature of the lens increases to accomplish this result. Contraction of the ciliary muscle causes the elastic lens to bulge.

The pupils constrict as a result of contraction of the circular fibers of the iris. This constriction prevents divergent light rays from coming into the eye through the peripheral portions of the cornea and the lens. The pupil constricts both for near vision and in the presence of bright light.

Convergence is the movement of the eyes inward to bring together the visual axes on the object being viewed. Single binocular vision requires that light rays from an object fall on corresponding points of the two retinas so that a person sees one object instead of two. The extraocular muscles hold the visual axes of the two eyes parallel.

Visual Pathways and Visual Fields

The relationship of visual pathways and fields of vision is illustrated in Figure 12-7. The field of vision is the area that can be visualized when the eye is not moving. The images formed on the retina are reversed right to left and are upside down. Thus an object in the upper nasal field of vision is formed on the lower temporal quadrant of the retina.

The arrangement of the nerve fibers in the retina is continued in the optic nerve: temporal (lateral) fibers follow the lateral side of the nerve, and nasal (medial) fibers run along the medial portion of the nerve. At the optic chiasm, however, the nasal or medial fibers cross over and join the temporal fibers of the opposite optic tract. Thus the left optic tract contains fibers from only the left half of each retina or only the right half of each field of vision. The right optic tract contains fibers from only the right half of each retina or only the left half of each field of vision. This sequence of pathways and events produces vision.

Visual fields

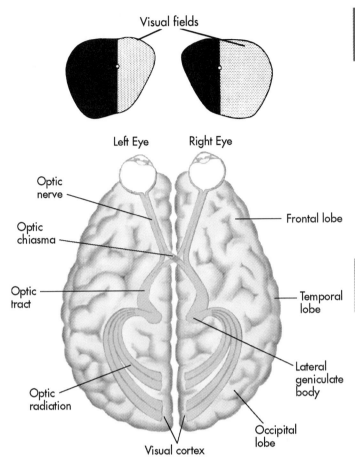

Figure 12-7 The visual pathway. (From Seidel HM et al.: *Mosby's guide to physical examination*, ed. 4, St. Louis, 1999, Mosby.)

EXAMINATION

Focused Health History

Present Health/Illness Status

1. Adequacy of vision in each eye, use of corrective lenses, date of last eye examination, and results of that examination
2. Difficulty with vision
   a. Near or distant
   b. Central, peripheral, or specific area
   c. Constant or intermittent
   d. Day or night
   e. Presence of floaters, halos around lights
   f. Double vision
3. Abnormal eye or lid movements
4. Medications: type and purpose; frequency and duration of use
5. Exposure to irritating chemicals, gases
6. Activities: participation in sports that could endanger the eyes
7. Use of protective devices when participating in activities that could endanger the eyes

Risk Factors
Glaucoma

Glaucoma is the second leading cause of new cases of blindness in the United States. Open-angle glaucoma is the most common form. When symptoms are not present, it may progress until irreversible visual field loss occurs.

Risk factors for glaucoma include diabetes mellitus, myopia, and a family history of glaucoma. African-Americans are at increased risk for glaucoma, which is the leading cause of blindness in this group. Persons older than 75 years are also at increased risk for glaucoma.

Clients who are at risk for glaucoma should be referred to an eye specialist for further assessment.

Cultural Considerations
Eye Distinctions

Persons of Asian heritage have a characteristic shape of upward slanting and narrowed palpebral fissures. In non-Asian individuals this finding may indicate Down syndrome. In a dark-skinned person the sclera, iris, and fundus are typically darker than in a light-skinned person.

8. Presence of other conditions that may affect vision or eye structures (hypertension, diabetes, thyroid disorder, glaucoma, cataract)

Past Health History

1. Trauma to eye(s): efforts to correct damage and degree of success
2. History of eye surgery
3. History of eye infection or red eye

Family Health History

1. Nearsightedness (myopia), farsightedness (hyperopia), strabismus
2. Retinoblastoma (cancer of the retina)
3. Color blindness, cataracts, glaucoma, retinitis pigmentosa, macular degeneration, diabetes, hypertension, thyroid disorder
4. Conditions similar to that of client

Specific Problems/Symptom Analysis

Eye Pain

1. **Onset:** abrupt or gradual
2. **Course since onset:** precipitating events, change in symptoms
3. **Location:** in or around eye, superficial or deep
4. **Quality:** stabbing, dull, ache, tension, pressure
5. **Quantity:** rating of pain severity or intensity
6. **Setting:** relationship to environmental settings such as home, work, leisure activities

7. **Associated phenomena:** itching, burning, photophobia, injection or blood-shot eyes, erythema, other sensations
8. **Alleviating and aggravating factors:** effects of analgesics, application of heat or cold, exposure to light
9. **Underlying concerns:** discomfort, concern about vision

Abnormal Secretions

1. **Onset:** abrupt or gradual
2. **Course since onset:** change in or pattern of symptoms
3. **Location:** bilateral, unilateral
4. **Quality:** color (clear, purulent), consistency (watery, mucoid, grainy)
5. **Quantity:** estimate amount of secretions
6. **Setting:** relationship to time of day, work, home
7. **Associated phenomena:** excessive tearing, pain, upper respiratory infection, allergy exposure, impaired vision
8. **Aggravating and alleviating factors:** effects of medications, heat or cold, reaction to light
9. **Underlying concerns:** eye infection

Trauma or Foreign Body

1. **Onset:** abrupt or gradual, nature of injury (blunt or piercing trauma, thermal burn, chemical exposure)
2. **Course since onset:** change in the timing, duration, or frequency of symptoms, especially pain and vision
3. **Location:** exact location of lesion or object
4. **Quality:** type of injury (trauma, foreign body, abrasion, burn)
5. **Quantity:** extent and severity of injury, especially any change of vision

Preparation for Examination

EQUIPMENT

Item	Purpose

Visual acuity charts
  Snellen or E
    (for distant vision)
  Rosenbaum
    (for near vision)
	To assess visual acuity

Opaque card or eye cover	To assess visual acuity, visual fields, and muscle function
Penlight	To assess pupillary light reflex and external structures of eye
Cotton-tipped applicator	To evert upper eyelid
Ophthalmoscope	To assess transparent ocular media and perform retinal examination

CLIENT AND ENVIRONMENT

The examination room must have lighting that can be controlled and comfortable seating for the client. An area for testing visual acuity is needed that allows the client to be 20 feet from the Snellen chart.

6. **Setting:** environmental exposure
7. **Associated phenomena:** restricted eye movement, tearing, pain, any loss of consciousness or other symptoms related to trauma
8. **Aggravating and alleviating factors:** effects of systemic or topical medications, heat or cold, reaction to light
9. **Underlying concerns:** loss of vision

Preparation for Examination: Client and Environment

The examination should be conducted in a room where the lighting can be controlled. A well-lighted room is needed for the visual acuity tests, and it must be possible to darken the room to assess the pupillary reflexes and to perform the ophthalmoscopic examination. A room or hallway where the client can be 20 feet away from the Snellen chart is required for testing visual acuity.

The eye examination involves multiple components. The order in which the examination is performed should focus on completeness and the comfortable positioning of the client. The client will remain seated during most of the examination. The assessment begins with visual acuity, visual fields, and ocular function. Then the external eye structures are examined. The ophthalmoscopic examination is done last.

Technique for Examination and Expected Findings

In the eye examination the range of normal findings is broad and variations are numerous. Much time, patience, and practice are needed to learn assessment of the many structures and functions of the eyes. Inspection is the main technique used to examine the eye. Palpation should be done only if a symptom or sign requires further investigation, such as palpating the lacrimal sac if blockage or infection is suspected. A description of the procedures that involve palpation is integrated into the discussion of inspection that follows. NOTE: Abbreviations from Latin are used to refer to the right eye and left eye. *Oculus dexter* (OD) refers to the right eye, *oculus sinister* (OS) refers to the left eye, and *oculus uterque* (OU) refers to both eyes.

Inspection

The components of the examination that involve inspection include the following:
Visual acuity
Visual fields
Extraocular muscle function
External ocular structures
Ophthalmoscopic examination

Visual Acuity.   The assessment of visual acuity is a simple test of ocular function. Findings in the normal range of visual acuity give an indication of the clarity of the transparent structures (cornea, anterior body, lens, and vitreous humor), the adequacy of macular (central) vision, and the functioning of the nerve fibers from the macula to the occipital cortex.

The Snellen alphabet chart (Figure 12-8, *A*), which has various sizes of letters, is traditionally used to test visual acuity. For clients who are illiterate or those who are unfamiliar with the English alphabet, the E chart is useful. The letter E is shown in different directions, and the client can state or point to which side is open (Figure 12-8, *B*).

The Snellen chart has standardized numbers at the end of each line of letters. These numbers indicate the degree of visual acuity demonstrated when the client reads the chart from a standard distance of 20 feet. Results are recorded as a fraction with a numerator of 20 and a denominator that refers to the last full line the client can read. If some errors are made on the last line, indicate this by using a minus sign for the number of incorrect letters or figures. For example, in Figure 12-8, *A*, if line number 5 were read with 2 errors,

the results would be recorded as 20/40 −2. The greater the number below the line or to the right, the poorer the visual acuity. For example, 20/20 vision is better than 20/40 vision.

Measurement of 20/20 vision in a client indicates normal visual acuity and a functional optic pathway. Measurement of less than 20/20 vision, such as 20/15, indicates either a refractive error or some other optic disorder.

Be sure that the room is well-lighted for the visual acuity test. Have the client stand or sit 20 feet from the Snellen chart. The chart should be located approximately at eye level. To assess visual acuity, initially test only one eye at a time. Cover the other eye with an opaque card or an eye cover to prevent the client from peeking between his or her fingers. Alternatively, both eyes may be tested together, since binocular vision is the client's functional vision. Test a

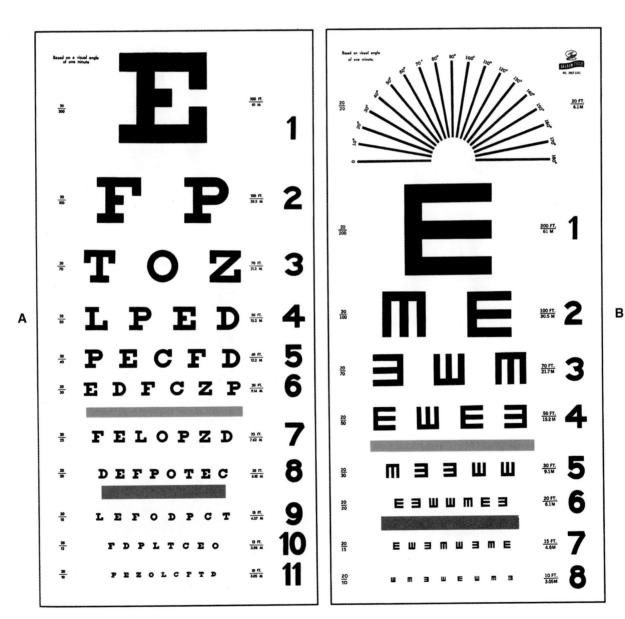

Figure 12-8 **A**, Snellen chart for testing distance vision. **B**, E chart for testing distance vision.
(From Seidel HM et al: *Mosby's guide to physical examination*, ed. 4, St. Louis, 1999, Mosby.)

client who wears corrective lenses both with and without them. This approach allows for an assessment of the adequacy of correction. Since reading glasses blur distant vision, the client should not wear them for this test.

If a client cannot see the largest letter on the chart (20/200), check to see whether he or she can perceive the movement of your hand at about 12 inches from the eyes or can perceive the light of a penlight directed into the eyes.

Perform a gross assessment of near vision for the client who has difficulty reading. Ask the client to read the letters on a Rosenbaum chart (Figure 12-9) or a newspaper with various sizes of print. Have the client hold the reading material at a distance of approximately 12 to 14 inches (Figure 12-10).

Visual Fields Confrontation Test.   The assessment of visual acuity indicates the functioning of the macular area,

the area of central vision. It does not test the sensitivity of the other areas of the retina, which perceive the peripheral stimuli. The visual fields confrontation test (Figure 12-11) provides a gross assessment of peripheral vision. In this test you use your own visual fields to make comparisons with the client's visual fields. For this test to be useful, your own visual fields must be normal.

You and the client sit or stand opposite each other about 30 to 45 cm (12 to 18 inches) apart with your eyes at the same level. The client covers one eye with an opaque card or eye cover, and you cover your own eye that is opposite the client's covered eye. For example, if the client's right eye is covered, then your left eye is covered. This method leaves the same field of vision open for assessment. You and the client stare directly into each other's open eye. Tell the client not to look at the object approaching from the periphery. Hold a small object, such as a penlight or a pen, and gradually move it in from the periphery toward the center from eight directions: right and left, above and below, and at the midpoints between each of these directions. At first, the object should be outside the field of vision. Hold the object equidistant between yourself and the client. Bring it in gradually toward the center. You and the client should be able to see the object enter the field of vision at the same time.

ROSENBAUM POCKET VISION SCREENER

	distance equivalent
95	20/800
874	

			Point	Jaeger	
2 8 4 3			26	16	20/200
6 3 8 E Ш Ɛ X O O			14	10	20/100
8 7 4 5 Ɛ M Ш O X O			10	7	20/70
6 3 9 2 5 M E Ɛ X O X			8	5	20/50
4 2 8 3 6 5 Ш E M o x o			6	3	20/40
3 7 4 2 5 8 Ɛ Ш Ɛ x x o			5	2	20/30
9 3 7 8 2 6 Ш m E x o o			4	1	20/25
4 2 8 7 3 9 E Ш m o o x			3	1+	20/20

Card is held in good light 14 inches from eye. Record vision for each eye separately with and without glasses. Presbyopic patients should read thru bifocal segment. Check myopes with glasses only.

DESIGN COURTESY J. G. ROSENBAUM, M.D.

PUPIL GAUGE (mm.)

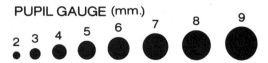

2 3 4 5 6 7 8 9

Figure 12-9   Rosenbaum chart for testing near vision. (From Seidel HM et al.: *Mosby's guide to physical examination*, ed. 4, St. Louis, 1999, Mosby.)

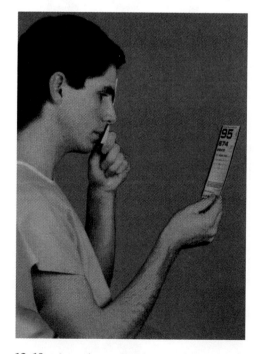

Figure 12-10   Assessing a client's near vision with the Rosenbaum chart.

This test provides only a crude estimate of visual fields. Although it may demonstrate large field defects, it does not usually detect small changes. Therefore clinical use of this test is limited. If you suspect decreased peripheral vision or loss of vision in certain areas, refer the client to an eye specialist for further testing.

Extraocular Muscle Function. The assessment of extraocular muscle function has these three components:
Six cardinal positions of gaze
Corneal light reflex
Cover-uncover test

Basic to each of these components is the observation of the parallelism of the eyes and ocular movements.

Six Cardinal Positions of Gaze. To assess the six cardinal positions of gaze (Figure 12-12, *A*), stand in front of the client and ask him or her to watch your finger or a small object as you move it through the six cardinal positions of gaze. Ask the client to hold the head still and to move only the eyes. Move your finger or the object clockwise to each of the six positions shown in Figure 12-12, *B*. Ask the client to hold the gaze briefly at each position. Observe for parallel movements and for slight oscillating movements of the eyes, called **nystagmus**. A small amount of end-position lateral nystagmus is normal. However, in any other position, nystagmus is abnormal. The eyes should move together in parallel fashion to each position.

After you have examined the extraocular muscles in the six cardinal positions, ask the client to look straight up and then down without moving the head. Observe the relationship of the upper eyelid to the iris as the client's gaze moves. The upper eyelid should overlap the iris slightly throughout this movement. If sclera does show between the iris and the upper eyelid, this is called **lid lag** and may indicate increased intraocular volume or pressure.

Corneal Light Reflex. You can assess the parallelism of the anterior and posterior axes of the two eyes by observing the reflection of light from the cornea. Ask the client to stare straight ahead while you shine a penlight toward the bridge of the nose from a distance of 12 to 15 inches. The bright dot of light reflected from the shiny surface of the corneas should be located symmetrically (e.g., at the 12 o'clock position in both eyes). If the reflected dot of light is not symmetrical, perform the cover-uncover test.

Cover-Uncover Test. Maintenance of parallelism of the eyes is a result of the fusion reflex that makes binocular vision possible. Normally, both eyes are aligned and centrally fixed and there is no movement of the eyes when they are covered or uncovered. If a muscle imbalance is present and the fusion reflex is blocked when one eye is covered, this weakness can be observed.

Ask the client to look at a specific fixed point, such as the corner of a picture or door frame. Then cover one of the client's eyes with an opaque card or eye cover; while doing so, observe the uncovered eye to see whether it moves to fix on the object (Figure 12-13, *A*). Then remove the cover and observe for any movement of the eye that was just uncovered (Figure 12-13, *B*). When an eye is covered, the appearance of an object on that retina is suppressed, and the eye relaxes. If there is a weakness in one of the extraocular muscles, the eye drifts to another resting position. Then, when the eye is uncovered, it pulls back into alignment. Perform this procedure on both eyes.

External Eye Structures

Eyelids and Eyelashes. Inspect the eyelashes to see that they are present and curve outward. The palpebral fissures (distance between the upper and lower lids) should be equal. The margin of the upper eyelid is normally between the upper margin of the pupil and the upper margin of the limbus. Check to see that the client can close the lids completely. Note the position of the globe of the eye: normal, prominent, or sunken. Raised yellow plaques, or xanthelasma, may appear on the lids near the inner canthi. These plaques can be

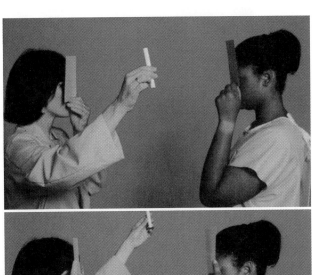
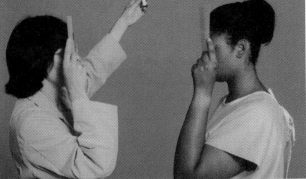
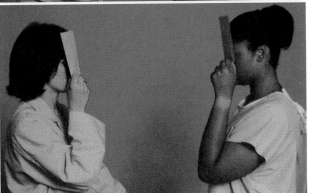

Figure 12-11 Visual fields confrontation test. The examiner assesses the client's right field of vision from the nasal direction (**A**), superior direction (**B**), and inferior direction (**C**). (Also tested but not shown: temporal direction.)

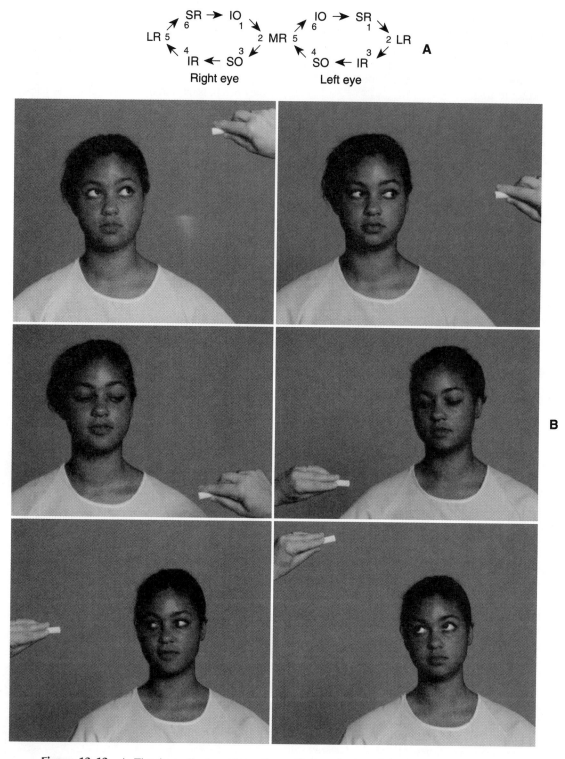

Figure 12-12   **A**, The six cardinal positions of gaze. **B**, Examination of the six cardinal positions of gaze.

normal variations that grow slowly and may disappear spontaneously.

Conjunctiva.   Inspect the bulbar and palpebral portions of the conjunctiva by separating the eyelids widely and having the client look up, down, and to each side. When separating the eyelids, do not exert pressure against the eyeball.

■ HELPFUL HINT

If an eyelid infection is present or suspected, you may gently palpate the eyelid surface. Never exert pressure on the eyeball. Use only the bony orbital rims as points over which to slide the eyelids.

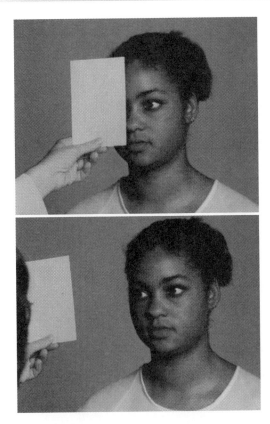

Figure 12-13 Cover-uncover test.

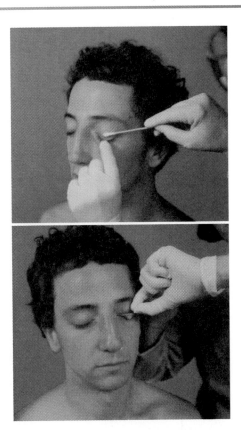

Figure 12-15 Examination of the conjunctiva.

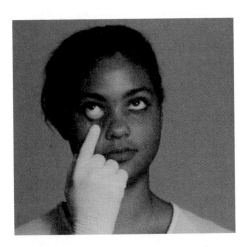

Figure 12-14 Eversion of the eyelid.

Hold the eyelid against the ridge of the bony orbit surrounding the eye (Figure 12-14). Normally, many small blood vessels are visible through the clear conjunctiva. The white sclera is visible through the bulbar conjunctiva.

Although eversion of the upper eyelid is not a necessary part of the physical examination it may be indicated, for example, when you suspect a foreign body in the upper eyelid. Explain the entire procedure to the client before you begin, and provide reassurance as you do it. If you do not show gentleness and care and give reassurance, the client is very likely to become tense when you manipulate the eyelid. When you are everting the eyelid, be aware of those techniques that promote relaxation rather than contraction of the muscles. Perform eversion of the upper eyelid (Figure 12-15) in the following way:

1. Ask the client to look down but keep the eyes slightly open. This maneuver relaxes the levator muscle. Closing the eyes contracts the orbicularis muscle, preventing lid eversion.
2. Gently grasp the upper eyelashes and pull them gently downward. Do not pull the lashes outward or upward, since this action causes muscle contraction.
3. Place a cotton-tipped applicator about 1 cm above the eyelid margin and gently push downward with the applicator while still holding the lashes. This maneuver everts the lid.
4. Hold the lashes of the everted eyelid against the upper ridge of the bony orbit, just beneath the eyebrow. Do not push against the eyeball.
5. Inspect the eyelid for a foreign object, lesion, swelling, or infection.
6. To return the eyelid to its normal position, move the lashes slightly forward and ask the client to look up and then blink. The lid should return easily to a normal position.

Sclera. Inspect the sclera while you are inspecting the bulbar conjunctiva. The sclera is normally white. However, some pigmented deposits are within the ranges of normal findings.

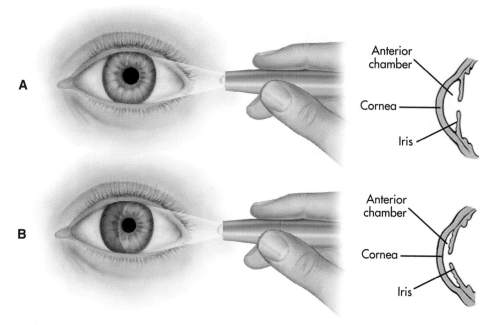

Figure 12-16   Evaluation of the depth of the anterior chambers. **A,** Normal anterior chamber and cross-section. **B,** Shallow anterior chamber and cross-section. (Modified from Seidel HM et al: *Mosby's guide to physical examination*, ed. 4, St. Louis, 1999, Mosby.)

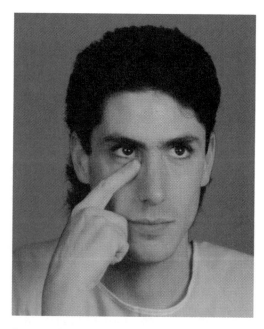

Figure 12-17   Examination of the nasolacrimal sac.

Cornea.   Inspect the cornea by directing the light of a penlight at it obliquely from several positions. The cornea should be transparent, smooth, shiny, and bright. The surface should have no irregularities. The features of the iris should be fully visible through the cornea. In older persons the appearance of arcus senilis may be considered normal.

Anterior Chamber.   Inspect the anterior chamber while you are inspecting the cornea. Use the oblique light from a penlight or the light of the ophthalmoscope. The anterior chamber is a transparent structure. Any visible material is abnormal. Assess the depth of the anterior chamber, which is the distance between the cornea and the iris. Look at the eye from the side, rather than from directly in front, and shine the light across the eye from the opposite side. From a side view, the iris should appear flat and should not be bulging forward (Figure 12-16).

Lacrimal Apparatus.   Of the several components of the lacrimal apparatus (lacrimal gland, puncta, lacrimal sac, and nasolacrimal duct), you can normally inspect only the puncta. These pinpoint openings are located near the inner canthus on the upper and lower eyelid margins. They should be just barely visible, with no swelling or redness noted. Check for blockage of the nasolacrimal duct by pressing against the lacrimal sac with your index finger or with a cotton-tipped applicator. Press in toward the lower inner orbital rim, not against the side of the nose (Figure 12-17). Then pull the lower lid down gently over the lower margin of the orbital rim to check for regurgitant material. Normally, there is no regurgitation of material through the puncta.

Iris.   Inspect the iris for regular round shape. As noted in the discussion of the anterior chamber, the iris should be flat, not bulging into the anterior chamber.

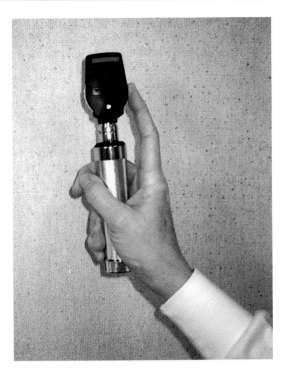

Figure 12-18 Holding the ophthalmoscope.

BOX 12-1

OPHTHALMOSCOPE

The ophthalmoscope (Figures 12-18 and 12-19) is an instrument designed to permit evaluation of certain internal structures of the eye. These structures include the lens, the vitreous humor, and the retinal structures. The ophthalmoscope contains a bright light and lenses of varying magnification that are used to bring the various structures of the eye into focus.

Bring the structures into focus by rotating the lens selector dial until the image becomes clear. You can hold and focus the instrument with one hand (see Figure 12-18). Look through the viewing aperture near the top of the ophthalmoscope to focus on the eye structures. Below the viewing aperture is another aperture that shows the number of the lens. The lens numbers go from 0 to +40 when the lens selection dial is rotated clockwise. (These numbers appear in black.) The numbers go to −25 when the lens selection dial is rotated counterclockwise. (These numbers appear in red.) The plus and minus lenses can compensate for nearsightedness or farsightedness in both the examiner and the client. The lens selection dial is located on the side of the ophthalmoscope head. Of the several different apertures, the large full circle of light is used most frequently because it works best for illuminating most of the structures of the eye. (Other apertures that are used less frequently are described in Table 12-2.)

■ HELPFUL HINT

If you are having difficulty seeing the pupillary response, darken the room for a few moments so that the client's pupils will dilate. Shining the light into the client's eye should then show the pupillary constriction more clearly. A bright, room makes it difficult to see the pupils constrict.

Pupils. Inspection of the pupils includes assessment of the following four components: size, shape, reaction to light, and accommodation. The pupils are normally round and equal in size. Approximately 5% of people have a slight but noticeable difference in the size of their pupils. Inequality in the size of the pupils is called **anisocoria**. Although this condition may be normal, regard the finding with some suspicion until you have completely assessed the health status of the client's eyes. The normal pupil is between 2 and 6 mm in diameter. The size of the pupils varies among individuals exposed to the same amount of light. The pupils tend to be smaller in infancy and older age. Nearsighted persons tend to have larger pupils, whereas farsighted persons tend to have smaller pupils. Pupils of less than 2 mm in diameter are called *miotic*; pupils more than 6 mm in diameter are called *mydriatic*.

To assess the pupillary response to light, bring the beam of a penlight in from the side of the client's head and direct it at one eye at a time. First, observe the pupil toward which you are directing the light. Then glance quickly at the pupil of the other eye. Perform this assessment on each eye. The pupils normally constrict in response to light. The pupil toward which the light is directed should constrict; this reaction is the *direct pupillary response to light*. The other pupil should also constrict; this reaction is the *consensual response to light*. Observe each eye for both direct and consensual response. The rapidity with which the pupils respond varies among individuals.

The accommodation response of the pupils consists of convergence of the eyes and constriction of the pupils as the client shifts the glance from a distant to a near object. Ask the client to stare for several moments at an object across the room or at your finger held several feet away from the client. Visualizing a distant object normally causes the pupils to dilate. Then ask the client to switch the gaze to your finger, which you have placed about 6 inches from the client's nose. The normal response is pupillary constriction and convergence of the eyes. The rapidity of the pupillary response varies; it is slower in older persons.

Ophthalmoscopic Examination. You can inspect the lens, vitreous humor, and retina with the ophthalmoscope (Box 12-1). Darkening the room so that the client's pupils will dilate makes the examination easier to perform. If the client wears corrective lenses, they may be left in place or removed. Try both ways to see which works most effectively for you.

Explain this portion of the examination to the client before you begin. The client's cooperation is essential, since you will be asking him or her to hold the gaze constant and, for part of the examination, to stare into the bright light of the ophthalmoscope.

Ask the client to stare at a fixed point at eye level over your shoulder, such as a light switch or the corner of a picture. Staring at a distant object also helps to dilate the pupils. Tell the client that it is all right to blink, but no more than necessary. If blinking becomes too frequent, you may need to elevate the upper lid and hold it against the upper orbital rim with your free hand. If you elevate the lid, do so for only a few seconds because the cornea can become dry, causing the client discomfort.

Turn on the ophthalmoscope light. Set the lens on 0 diopters. Begin by holding the ophthalmoscope in your right hand with your right index finger on the selector wheel. Hold the aperture of the ophthalmoscope up to your right eye. At a distance of about 12 inches, direct the light toward the client's right eye (Figure 12-20, *A*). When the beam of

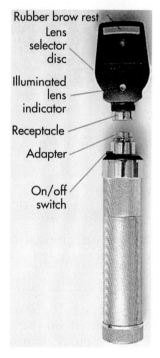

Figure 12-19 Ophthalmoscope. (From Seidel HM et al.: *Mosby's guide to physical examination*, ed. 4, St. Louis, 1999, Mosby.)

TABLE 12-2	**Apertures of the Ophthalmoscope**
Aperture	Description
Full aperture	Used most frequently because it provides a wide field of light for retinal examination
Small aperture	Especially useful for examining retina through a small pupil
Red-free filter	A green beam of light is used to examine optic disc for pallor and retina for small hemorrhages
Grid	Used to estimate size of retinal lesions
Slit	Used to examine anterior portion of eye and to determine elevation of retinal lesions

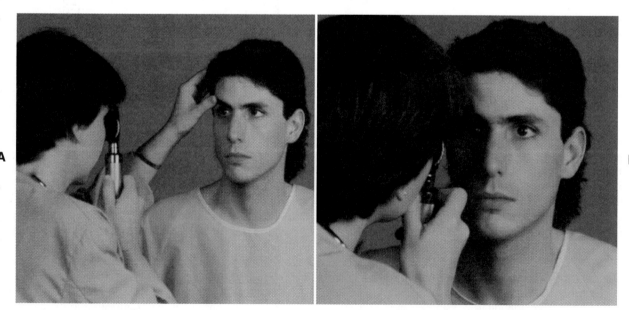

Figure 12-20 **A**, Ophthalmoscopic examination: finding the red reflex. **B**, Examining the retinal structures.

light falls on the client's pupil, you will see a red reflex, which is a reflection of the color of the retina.

> ### ■ HELPFUL HINT
>
> If you lose sight of the red reflex, you are no longer directing the light through the pupil. Instead, you are directing it on the iris or sclera or away from the eye. If this situation occurs, move your head back from the ophthalmoscope, redirect the beam of light to the pupil, and bring your eye back to the aperture.

Gradually move in closer to the client's eye until the ophthalmoscope is just a few inches away from the client's eye (Figure 12-20, *B*). Keep the red reflex in your line of vision while turning the selector wheel clockwise toward the positive numbers. This approach enables you to focus on the more anterior structures—the lens and the vitreous body. Both structures should be clear, with no opacities or clouding. Gradually rotate the selector wheel counterclockwise toward the negative numbers. Look for a structure on the retina, such as the disc or a vessel. When you have found a certain structure, turn the wheel until it is in focus and you can visualize that structure clearly. With a nearsighted person, whose eyeball is more elongated than normal, you will need the more negative lenses to focus farther back. With a farsighted client, rotate the wheel toward 0. Focusing has individual variations and depends on the refractive state of both you and the client. If you locate the optic disc first, begin your inspection there. If you find a vessel first, follow that vessel in toward the optic disc. Examine the retinal structures in this order:

1. Optic disc
2. Retinal vessels
3. Retinal background
4. Macular area

Optic Disc. Examine the optic disc for size, shape, color, distinctness of its margins, and the physiologic cup. The disc is normally approximately 1.5 mm in diameter and round or slightly oval. It ranges in color from creamy yellow to pink and is lighter than the surrounding retina (see Figure 12-3). The color varies somewhat from one individual to another. The margins of the optic disc are usually sharp and clearly demarcated from the surrounding retina. However, several normal variations occur. Dense pigment deposits may be situated around the disc margins, particularly in dark-skinned people. A whitish to grayish crescent of scleral tissue may be located immediately adjacent to the disc, particularly on the temporal side. Note the physiologic cup, or physiologic depression.

> ### ■ HELPFUL HINT
>
> The scleral crescent, a normal finding, is a pale crescent-shaped area around the rim of the disc only. Do not mistake it for disc atrophy.

The optic disc is a standard measurement device for findings on the retina. For example, a finding can be described as being 2 disc diameters (DDs) away from the disc itself. Also, the size of the finding can be described in terms of the disc diameter. For example, an abnormality may measure one half of the disc diameter (Figure 12-21).

Retinal Vessels. Use the light from the ophthalmoscope to follow each of the four sets of vessels out from the optic disc to the periphery. Inspect the retinal vessels for the following four characteristics:

Color
Arteriolar light reflex
Arteriole/vein (A:V) ratio
Arteriovenous crossing changes

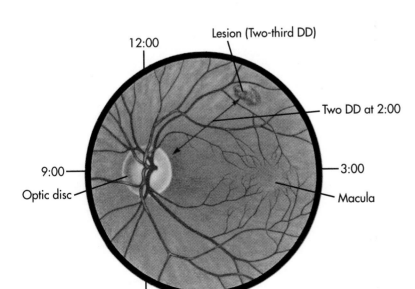

Figure 12-21 Method of describing the position and dimension of a retinal lesion in terms of the disc diameter (DD). (Modified from Seidel HM et al: *Mosby's guide to physical examination,* ed. 4, St. Louis, 1999, Mosby.)

The arterioles are a brighter red and smaller than the veins. Usually, the arterioles will have a narrow light reflex from the center line of the vessel. Veins do not show a light reflex. Normally, both arterioles and veins show a gradually and regularly diminishing diameter as they go from the disc to the periphery. The A:V ratio is between 2:3 to 4:5. Vessels normally cross and intertwine, but where they cross one another, there should be no change in the course or caliber of either vessel. Pulsations are sometimes visible in the veins near the optic disc.

■ HELPFUL HINT

To follow the course of the retinal vessels out to the periphery and to see more of the retinal background, ask the client to shift the gaze upward, downward, and to each side. This maneuver brings more of the retina into view.

Retinal Background.   Inspect the retinal background. It is normally fairly regular in color. Look for any areas that are darker or lighter.

Macular Area.   Inspection of the macular area should be done at the end of the ophthalmoscopic examination. Ask the client to stare directly at the bright light of the ophthalmoscope. You will then be looking at the macular area. The macula may be so similar in color to the rest of the retinal background that it will be difficult to visualize it as a separate structure, or it may be slightly darker. Learn to do this portion of the retinal examination quickly because the client may feel quite uncomfortable as you direct the bright light at the area of most acute color vision.

The macular area, which is approximately 1 DD, is located about 2 DDs temporal to the optic disc. At the center of the macula is the fovea centralis. The macula appears as a regularly colored area. A bright spot of light may be reflected from the fovea centralis. The macular area usually has no visible retinal vessels. It is nourished by choroidal vessels and appears slightly darker than the rest of the retinal background.

The retina appears reddish orange because of its deep vascular supply and deeply pigmented layers. The pigment in the posterior layers of the retina also accounts for its

Examination Step-by-Step

Perform examination of the eyes with the client sitting or standing. Equipment needed includes:
Snellen chart
Rosenbaum chart or newspaper
Opaque card or eye cover
Penlight
Cotton-tipped applicator
Ophthalmoscope
A. Measure visual acuity (CN II).
   1. Distant vision using Snellen chart
   2. Near vision using Rosenbaum chart or newspaper
B. Assess visual fields (CN II) using visual fields confrontation test.
C. Assess extraocular muscle function (CN III, IV, VI).
   1. Six cardinal positions of gaze
   2. Corneal light reflex
   3. Cover-uncover test
D. Inspect external eye structures.
   1. Position of globe—normal, protruding, or sunken
   2. Eyelids and eyelashes
      a. Position of eyelids and eyelashes, palpebral fissures
      b. Ability to close lids
      c. Redness, swelling, lumps
   3. Conjunctiva and sclera
      a. Clarity
      b. Eversion of eyelid, if indicated
      c. Redness, discharge
   4. Cornea
      a. Light reflex
      b. Arcus senilis
   5. Anterior chamber
      a. Clarity
      b. Depth
6. Lacrimal apparatus
   a. Puncta
   b. Swelling or redness
   c. Regurgitation of material from lacrimal sac
7. Iris
   a. Shape
   b. Fluttering movements
8. Pupil
   a. Size
   b. Shape
   c. Response to light and accommodation
9. Ophthalmoscopic examination
   a. Lens clarity
   b. Red reflex
   c. Optic disc
      (1) Size and shape
      (2) Color
      (3) Margins
      (4) Physiologic cup
   d. Retinal vessels
      (1) Color
      (2) Arteriolar light reflex
      (3) Arteriole/vein ratio
      (4) Arteriovenous crossing characteristics
   e. Retinal background
      (1) Regularity
      (2) Color
      (3) Presence of microaneurysms, hemorrhages, exudates
   f. Macula and fovea centralis
      (1) Regularity
      (2) Color

slightly stippled appearance. Normally, the color of the retina is uniform, with no patches of light or dark discoloration present.

Screening Tests and Procedures

The following are United States Preventive Services Task Force (1996) recommendations:

1. Vision screening to detect amblyopia, or double vision, and strabismus, or misalignment of the eyes, once for all children before entering school, preferably between ages 3 and 4. Screening tests include simple inspection, cover test, and visual acuity. The adult Snellen chart can be used on children as young as 6 years. The Snellen E chart can be used if the child cannot read the alphabet.
2. Screening for diminished visual acuity in the elderly with the Snellen visual acuity chart.
3. There is insufficient evidence to recommend routine asymptomatic vision screening for schoolchildren. In many settings, vision screening with the Snellen chart is performed as part of the school physical at required intervals.
4. There is insufficient evidence to recommend routine performance of tonometry by primary care practitioners as an effective screening test for glaucoma. It may be clinically prudent, however, to advise clients at high risk, such as those age 65 or older, to be tested periodically for glaucoma by an eye specialist.

VARIATIONS FROM HEALTH
Variations of Visual Function

Diminished Visual Acuity

An error of refraction is a common variation from normal vision. It is an inability to focus rays of light on the retina.

Common errors of refraction include nearsightedness (myopia), farsightedness (hyperopia), and astigmatism.

Nearsightedness (Myopia).   In **myopia**, the eye focuses the image in front of the retina. This situation can occur when the eyeball is too long or the lens is too thick (Figure 12-22, *A* and *B*). Nearsighted individuals can see objects that are nearby, but not objects that are far away.

Farsightedness (Hyperopia).   In **hyperopia**, the eye focuses the image at a hypothetical distance behind the retina. This situation can occur when the eyeball is too short or the lens is too thin (Figure 12-22, *C* and *D*). Farsighted individuals can see objects that are far away but not those that are nearby. As people age, they typically become farsighted as the lens of the eye becomes more rigid, losing its elasticity. The ciliary muscles also become weaker, and the lens cannot bulge to accommodate for near vision. This condition is known as **presbyopia**.

Astigmatism.   **Astigmatism** occurs with uneven curvature of the cornea. Vision is blurred because the refraction of a ray of light is spread over a diffuse area rather than sharply focused on the retina.

Decreased Vision

Defects in the field of vision may be caused by lesions of the retina, along the optic nerve, at the optic chiasm (where portions of each nerve cross over to the opposite side), along the optic tract, or in the occipital lobes (Figure 12-23). The resulting defect in vision may be central, peripheral, or specific to portions of the visual fields, depending on the nature and location of the lesion. Visual field defects are described according to their location: temporal, nasal, superior, or inferior. The visual field reflects the visual function in the opposite areas of the retina involved. For example, a temporal visual field defect reflects a defect of the nasal retina. A superior field defect reflects an inferior retinal defect. Likewise, an inferior nasal retinal defect would cause a defect in the superior temporal field of vision. The effects of such lesions on the field of vision are illustrated in Figure 12-23.

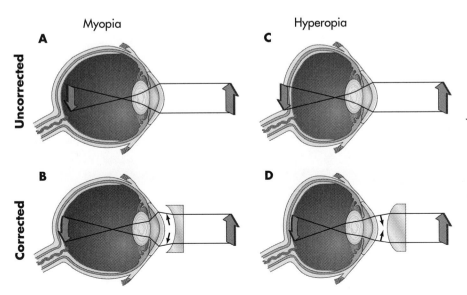

Figure 12-22   Correcting refraction disorders. **A,** In myopia, an elongated eyeball causes the image to focus *in front* of the retina. **B,** An external lens can refocus the image on the retina, correcting the effects of myopia. **C,** In hyperopia, a flattened eyeball causes the image to focus *behind* the retina. **D,** An external lens can refocus the image on the retina. (From Thibodeau GA, Patton KT: *Anatomy and physiology*, ed. 4, St. Louis, 1999, Mosby.)

Monocular Visual Defects.   If the lesion is located in the retina of one eye or along one optic nerve anterior to the optic chiasm, it affects the vision in that eye.

Bitemporal Hemianopsia.   Lesions that are found at the optic chiasm, along the optic tract, or in the occipital lobes affect the visual fields of both eyes. This situation occurs because of the crossing and mixing of fibers from both eyes at the chiasm. A lesion at the optic chiasm may be caused by a pituitary tumor. A tumor would produce a loss of vision from the nasal portion of each retina, resulting in a loss of both temporal fields of vision. This condition is called **bitemporal hemianopsia**.

Homonymous Hemianopsia.   Nerve fibers from both eyes mingle behind the chiasm in the optic tracts and in the brain. Lesions along the optic tract or in the temporal, parietal, or occipital lobes will impair the same half of the field of vision in both eyes. For example, a lesion of the right optic tract or the right side of the brain results in visual field defects in the right nasal field and in the left temporal field.

Called **homonymous hemianopsia**, this condition may be caused by occlusion of the middle cerebral artery.

The location of disease on the retina determines the type of resultant visual field defects. Macular defects lead to a central blind area. Localized damage in other areas of the retina causes a loss of vision corresponding to the involved area. A blind spot is called a **scotoma**. It is an area of blindness surrounded by an area of vision. Advanced diabetic retinopathy may cause macular damage, resulting in a loss of central vision. Increased intraocular pressure, commonly associated with glaucoma, causes decreased peripheral vision. As glaucoma advances, it may also cause a loss of central vision. A retinal detachment causes loss of vision from that portion of the retina where the detachment occurs.

Blindness

A person is considered legally blind when the best visual acuity that can be achieved with corrective lenses in the bet-

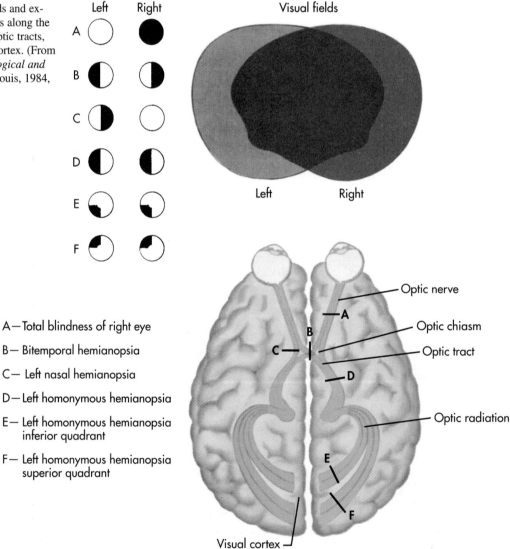

Figure 12-23   Visual fields and examples of visual field defects along the optic nerve, optic chiasm, optic tracts, and optic radiations in the cortex. (From Rudy EB: *Advanced neurological and neurosurgical nursing*, St. Louis, 1984, Mosby.)

Left   Right

A

B

C

D

E

F

Visual fields

Left   Right

A—Total blindness of right eye

B— Bitemporal hemianopsia

C— Left nasal hemianopsia

D—Left homonymous hemianopsia

E— Left homonymous hemianopsia inferior quadrant

F— Left homonymous hemianopsia superior quadrant

Optic nerve

Optic chiasm

Optic tract

Optic radiation

Visual cortex

ter eye is 20/200 or less, or when the peripheral visual field is constricted to within 20 degrees. Major causes of blindness in North America are glaucoma, unoperated cataracts, and retinal disorders (mainly diabetic retinopathy and macular degeneration).

Defects in Color Vision

A variety of conditions may disturb color vision, including diseases of the optic nerve, diseases of the fovea centralis and macular area (where the cones are most concentrated), and nutritional disturbances. In macular degeneration, the decrease in color vision parallels the loss of visual acuity. The person who is deficient in color vision is unable to see the figures on color plates, which are easily recognizable to the person with normal color vision.

Diplopia

Diplopia, or double vision, occurs whenever the visual axes, the parallel lines of vision, are not directed simultaneously at the same object. It is a cardinal sign of weakness of one or more of the extraocular muscles. Diplopia can be a sign of pressure from a brain tumor or of increased intracranial pressure.

Faulty Adaptation to the Dark

Night blindness is caused by pigmentary degeneration of the retina, optic nerve disease, glaucoma, or vitamin A deficiency. Deficiency in vitamin A may occur because of inadequate nutrition or cirrhosis of the liver. A client may experience slow recovery of vision during nighttime driving after the headlights of a passing car shine in the eyes.

Visualization of Objects Within the Eye

Translucent specks of various shapes and sizes that float across the visual field and are visible only when the eye is open are called **floaters**. They are small remnants of the hyaloid vascular system in the vitreous humor. Floaters are visualized as small specks that appear to dart away as the client tries to look at them. Many people experience occasional floaters that have no pathological significance. However, sudden showers of floaters may occur in the periphery of the visual field with vitreous hemorrhage. This occurrence may be the initial symptom of hole formation that precedes retinal separation. The location of the floaters may be helpful in finding the retinal tear. The sudden appearance of a moderately large floater is the main symptom of vitreous detachment. It is important to note that any sudden appearance of floaters is cause for immediate referral to an eye care specialist.

Iridescent Vision

Iridescent vision refers to the halos or rainbows that a client sees surrounding bright lights when he or she has corneal edema. This condition may follow a rapid increase in intraocular pressure with acute glaucoma, after prolonged wearing of hard contact lenses, with corneal abrasion, and with cataracts.

Extraocular Neuromuscular Function Variations

Signs of weakness or paralysis of an extraocular muscle or a defect in the nerve supplying it include the following:
Asymmetrical corneal light reflex
Inability of the eyes to move in a parallel fashion to the six cardinal positions of gaze
Abnormal cover-uncover test
Table 12-3 shows which muscles and cranial nerves are involved when the eye is unable to move to one of the six cardinal positions of gaze.
The following are examples of the effects of nerve lesions:
Oculomotor paralysis (CN III): the eye turns down and out, with drooping of the upper lid
Abducens paralysis (CN VI): the eye turns in toward the nose because of unopposed action of the medial rectus
Asking the client to look out to the endpoint of the six cardinal positions will exaggerate a defect if one is present. (REMEMBER: The rhythmic twitching motion of nystagmus may be normal at the end of the lateral position, but it is abnormal when the eyes are in any other position.)
The following terms are used to describe weakness of the extraocular muscles:
Phoria: mild weakness of the extraocular muscles that appears as a deviation of the axes with the cover-uncover test
Exophoria, exotropia: outward (temporal) deviation of the eye
Esophoria, esotropia: inward (nasal) deviation of the eye
Strabismus (also termed **tropia**): constant disparity of the eye axes; the two eyes do not focus on an object simultaneously

Variations of the Eye and Ocular Structures

Position of the Globe of the Eye

Exophthalmos. **Exophthalmos** is a protrusion of the eyeball anteriorly that may be bilateral or unilateral. Bilateral exophthalmos is most commonly caused by hyperthy-

TABLE 12-3	Muscles and Cranial Nerves Involved When the Eye Is Unable To Move to Cardinal Positions of Gaze	
Position to Which Eye Will Not Turn	**Muscle**	**Cranial Nerve**
Straight nasal	Medial rectus	III
Up and nasal	Interior oblique	III
Down and nasal	Superior oblique	IV
Straight temporal	Lateral rectus	VI
Up and temporal	Superior rectus	III
Down and temporal	Inferior rectus	III

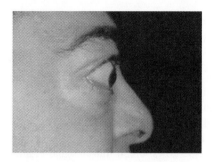

Figure 12-24 Exophthalmos. (From Stein HA, Slatt BJ, Stein RM: *The ophthalmic assistant: a guide for ophthalmic medical personnel*, ed. 6, St. Louis, 1994, Mosby.)

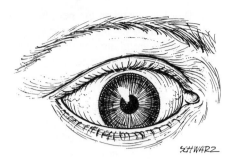

Figure 12-26 Lid lag.

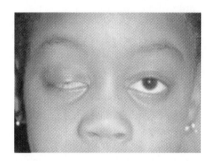

Figure 12-25 Ptosis: drooping upper eyelid. (From Stein HA, Slatt BJ, Stein RM: *The ophthalmic assistant: a guide for ophthalmic medical personnel*, ed. 6, St. Louis, 1994, Mosby.)

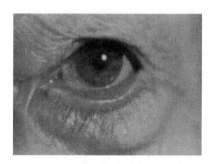

Figure 12-27 Ectropion. (From Stein HA, Slatt BJ, Stein RM: *The ophthalmic assistant: fundamentals and clinical practice*, ed. 5, St. Louis, 1988, Mosby.)

roidism (Figure 12-24). Unilateral exophthalmos may be caused by a tumor located behind the eye. People of Mediterranean or African descent may normally have greater protrusion of the eyes than do Caucasians.

Enophthalmos. **Enophthalmos** is the backward displacement of the eye in the bony socket, which gives the eyes a sunken appearance. This condition is caused by trauma, starvation, or chronic wasting illness.

Eyelids and Eyelashes

Ptosis. With **ptosis**, the eyelid margin is at or below the pupil, and the eyelid appears to be drooping (Figure 12-25). This variation may indicate an oculomotor nerve (CN III) lesion, neuromuscular weakness, or a congenital condition.

Lid Lag. When lid lag is present, the eyelid margin is above the limbus, and some sclera is visible (Figure 12-26). This condition may indicate thyroid disease.

Ectropion. In **ectropion**, the eyelids are loose and roll outward, and the conjunctiva is exposed (Figure 12-27). Tears do not drain through the puncta, and **epiphora** (tearing) results.

Entropion. In entropion, the eyelids roll inward because of spasm or scar tissue. The lashes may produce corneal irritation. The lower eyelid is usually involved.

Periorbital Edema. With **periorbital edema**, tissue within the eyelid is loosely connected and readily collects excess fluid. The eyelids appear swollen and puffy. This condition may be caused by crying, allergies, heart failure, nephrosis, or thyroid deficiency.

Blepharitis. **Blepharitis** is a chronic inflammation of the eyelid margins that may begin in childhood and continue intermittently throughout life. It is caused by staphylococcal infection and seborrheic dermatitis. The blood vessels in the eyelid margins become dilated, and the eyelashes become thin, broken, small, and white. Blepharitis is often associated with sties, chalazia, and conjunctivitis.

Hordeolum (sty). A **hordeolum (sty)** is an infection of the gland of the eyelid. It is located in the hair follicle at the eyelid margin (Figure 12-28). The sty appears painful, red, and swollen.

Chalazion

Chalazion is an infection or retention cyst of the meibomian glands that lies within the posterior portion of the eyelid (Figure 12-29). It is swollen, nontender, firm, and discrete. The skin over the chalazion moves freely.

Xanthelasma. **Xanthelasma** are raised yellow plaques on the eyelids. They may be a normal variation or may be associated with hypercholesterolemia.

Conjunctiva

Conjunctivitis. **Conjunctivitis** is an infection or inflammation of the conjunctiva that typically produces engorgement of the conjunctival vessels and/or a discharge. Clients often experience a foreign body sensation or sensitivity to bright lights. A change in visual acuity is unusual; if present, it is probably due to ocular discharge. Redness of the eye is typically peripheral, not around the limbus. Conjunctivitis

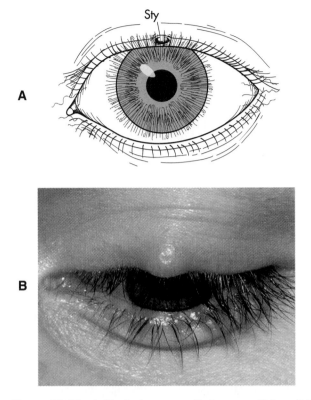

Figure 12-28 **A**, Hordeolum, or sty. **B**, Acute sty. (**B** from Palay DA, Krachmer JH: *Opthalmology for the primary care physician*, St. Louis, 1997, Mosby.)

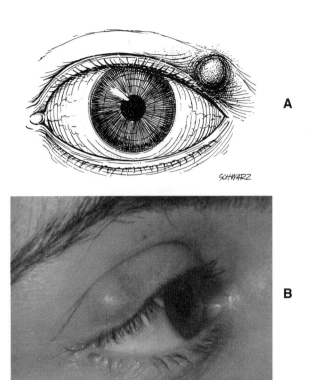

Figure 12-29 **A**, Chalazion. **B**, Chalazion of the right upper eyelid. (**B** from Newell FW: *Ophthalmology: principles and concepts*, ed. 7, St. Louis, 1992, Mosby.)

may be due to bacterial or viral infections or to allergies. Bacterial conjunctivitis produces a thick, purulent discharge. Viral conjunctivitis typically produces a clear, watery discharge; a burning sensation; photophobia; and sometimes swelling of the lids. Allergic conjunctivitis produces a clear or stringy mucoid discharge and swollen eyelids.

Subconjunctival Hemorrhage. This type of hemorrhaging may occur spontaneously or may result from trauma, sneezing, coughing, or lifting. The hemorrhage has sharp borders and appears bright red against the white sclera (Figure 12-30).

Pterygium. **Pterygium** is an abnormal growth of bulbar conjunctival tissue that usually occurs from the nasal side toward the center of the cornea (Figure 12-31). It may interfere with vision if it covers the pupil.

Lacrimal Apparatus

Dacryocystitis. **Dacryocystitis** is an inflammation of the lacrimal sac. Infection and blockage of the lacrimal sac and duct lead to swelling, redness, warmth, and pain below the inner canthus. Pressure on the sac produces purulent discharge through the puncta. To examine for infection in the lacrimal sac, use the examining finger to press against the inner orbital rim, not the nose. Then gently pull the lower eye-

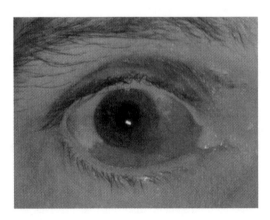

Figure 12-30 Subconjunctival hemorrhage. (From Newell FW: *Ophthalmology: principles and concepts*, ed. 8, St. Louis, 1996, Mosby.)

lid over the lower orbital rim to observe for regurgitation of fluid through the puncta. Dacryocystitis is usually unilateral.

Dacryoadenitis. **Dacryoadenitis** is an inflammation of the lacrimal gland characterized by pain, redness, and swelling developing in the outer third of the upper eyelid. This condition may be associated with mumps, measles, and infectious mononucleosis.

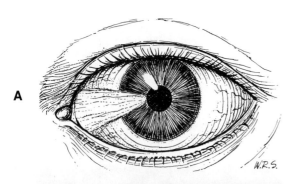

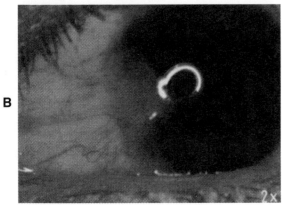

Figure 12-31   **A** and **B,** Pterygium. (**B** from Newell FW: *Ophthalmology: principles and c*oncepts, ed. 8, St. Louis, 1996, Mosby.)

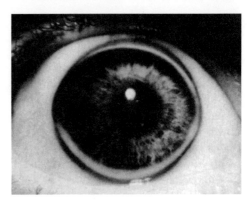

Figure 12-32   Arcus senilis. (From Newell FW: *Ophthalmology: principles and concepts*, ed. 8, St. Louis, 1996, Mosby.)

Epiphora.   **Ectropion**, the outward turning of the eyelid, may cause epiphora, or tearing, because of inadequate drainage. Persistent tearing of an infant's eye suggests a blocked tear duct or congenital glaucoma.

Sclera

Changes in the color of the sclera indicate systemic disease.

Scleral Icterus.   Jaundice manifests its presence in the eyes as a yellow discoloration of the sclera. Excessive bilirubinemia may be evident as scleral icterus before jaundice of the skin becomes apparent.

Bluish Sclera.   This change is associated with osteogenesis imperfecta, a genetic disorder that involves defective development of the connective tissue and is characterized by abnormally brittle and fragile bones.

Cornea

The cornea is an extremely sensitive structure. Pain and photophobia (sensitivity to light) are common manifestations of corneal disease. Any dullness, irregularities, or opacities of the cornea are abnormal.

Corneal Abrasion.   This loss of the outer layer of cells of the cornea usually causes severe pain and photophobia. An abrasion may cause the surface to look irregular, but it is usually invisible. The abrasion results from a scratch to the cornea or from improper (usually prolonged) wearing of contact lenses. Since the cornea is richly supplied with nerve endings, the client with an abrasion feels intense pain and the sensation of a foreign body. Associated signs include lacrimation, redness, and photophobia. If corneal abrasion is suspected, the client should be referred to an eye care specialist.

Arcus Senilis.   This extracellular lipid infiltration occurs at the corneal periphery (Figure 12-32). It appears as a grayish white ring around the edge of the cornea that is separated from the white sclera by a clear interval of 1 mm. Arcus senilis is normal in older people, but in younger clients it may be associated with abnormal lipid metabolism.

Anterior Chamber

Abnormalities of the anterior chamber include a decrease in the depth of the chamber and any foreign material that interrupts the normal transparency of the chamber.

Shallow Anterior Chamber.   This characteristic may be a sign of glaucoma, or it may predispose the eye to glaucoma. As increased intraocular pressure causes the iris to become displaced anteriorly, there is less distance between the cornea and the iris. Because of the anterior displacement, light directed obliquely from the temporal side illuminates only the temporal side, and the nasal side appears darker or shadowed (see Figure 12-16).

Hyphema.   **Hyphema** is an accumulation of blood in the aqueous fluid. It may be caused by trauma or may result from spontaneous hemorrhage. If the hyphema is mild, the red blood cells settle out inferiorly by gravity to a height of a few millimeters. In severe hyphema, the entire anterior chamber may be filled with blood. The blood is bright red.

Hypopyon.   An accumulation of purulent material in the anterior chamber is called **hypopyon**.

Iris

Iritis.   **Iritis** is an inflammation of the iris. Associated findings include circumcorneal injection (a deep pink to red flush around the cornea), a bulging iris, inequality in the size of the pupils, throbbing pain, photophobia, visual blurring, and a constricted or irregularly shaped pupil. The affected client should be referred to an eye care specialist immediately.

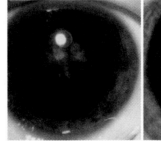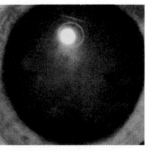

Figure 12-33 Cataract. **A,** Snowflake cataract. **B,** Senile cataract. (**A** from Donaldson DD: *Atlas of diseases of the eye*, vol 5, *The crystalline lens*, St. Louis, 1976, Mosby; **B** from Seidel HM et al.: *Mosby's guide to physical examination*, ed. 4, St. Louis, 1999, Mosby.)

Fluttering Motion of Iris. Removal of the lens takes away the normal support of the iris, leaving it with a tremulous or fluttering motion.

Pupils

Abnormalities of the pupils include alterations in size, shape, and reflexes.

Variations in Size and Shape

Anisocoria. A difference in the size of the pupils is called anisocoria. Approximately 5% of the population has a slight but noticeable difference in pupil size. Although this finding may be normal, until the cause is known, it should be regarded with some suspicion because it can be an indication of central nervous system disease.

Dyscoria. **Dyscoria** is a congenital abnormality affecting the shape of the pupils.

Mydriasis. **Mydriasis** is an enlargement of the pupils that may result from emotional influences, recent or old trauma, acute glaucoma, a systemic reaction to parasympatholytic or sympathomimetic drugs, or the local use of dilating drops. A unilateral fixed and enlarged pupil may be caused by local trauma to the eye or the head. Oculomotor nerve (CN III) damage results in a pupil that is dilated and fixed; the eye deviates downward and laterally, and the eyelid droops. Fixed dilation of both pupils occurs with deep anesthesia, central nervous system injury, and circulatory arrest.

Miosis. **Miosis** is constriction of the pupils that is associated with iritis, the use of narcotics, and the use of pilocarpine drops for the treatment of glaucoma.

Variations in Reflexes

Argyll Robertson Pupil. This condition is a failure of the pupils to react to light with preservation of the accommodation response. It is associated with chronic alcoholism, meningitis, and brain tumor.

Adie's Pupil. With this condition, the pupil is dilated and constricts little to light and accommodation. It is often associated with absent deep tendon reflexes in the extremities. The cause of this condition is unknown.

Horner's Syndrome. This condition involves sympathetic paralysis of the eye, which includes constriction of the pupil, drooping of the eyelid, and lack of tearing. The paralysis is caused by interruption of the cervical sympathetic chain.

Monocular Blindness. In monocular blindness, when light is directed at the blind eye, there is no response to light in either eye. However, when the seeing eye receives illumination, both pupils constrict; this situation occurs because the efferent pupil constriction stimulus via the oculomotor nerve is distributed to both eyes.

Lens

Cataract. A **cataract** is a gray-white opacity within the lens. On ophthalmoscopic examination, the cataract is seen as a dark shadow or black spots within the red reflex or as an absent red reflex because the opacity prevents light from being reflected back to the examiner's eye. Cataracts vary in appearance. They may look like pieces of coral or crystals, or they may have a starlike (stellate) appearance (Figure 12-33, *A*). Cataract formation may accompany aging, or it may be associated with systemic disorders or congenital syndromes.

Senile cataracts occur as a result of various degenerative processes within the lens. These cataracts are the most common type and occur most often after age 50 years (Figure 12-33, *B*). The tendency to develop cataracts is inherited.

In cataracts associated with diabetes mellitus, the metabolic disturbance results in formation of abnormal lens fiber. These cataracts occur more frequently in young people, are bilateral, progress rapidly, and have a classic snowflake appearance.

Congenital cataracts are usually hereditary. However, they may be caused by viral infection during the first trimester of gestation.

Typical symptoms of cataracts include blurred or cloudy vision; sensitivity to bright light; and, later, distorted or double vision. Untreated cataracts lead to loss of vision.

Retinal Structures

Optic Disc

Papilledema. **Papilledema** is a condition characterized by swelling of the optic nerve head that causes the margins of the disc to become blurred and indistinct (Figure 12-34). It is a sign of increased intracranial pressure. This pressure causes decreased venous drainage from the eye and accumulation or leakage of fluid. Papilledema is associated with malignant hypertension, eclampsia of pregnancy, brain tumor, and hematoma.

The nerve head appears to be out of focus with the surrounding retina. The degree of elevation of the optic disc can be assessed by focusing first on the disc and then on the surrounding retina and noting the difference in diopters on the ophthalmoscope.

Cupping of the Optic Disc. The increased intraocular pressure of glaucoma gradually exerts pressure posteriorly against the optic disc. This pressure causes **cupping,** an increased posterior curvature of the disc. It may also produce an increase in the cup/disc ratio. The cup may enlarge to more than one half the disc diameter. The pressure of glaucoma may also cause pallor of the disc, a sign of optic atrophy.

On ophthalmoscopic examination, cupping may be observed by following carefully the course of the vessels as they emerge over the margin of the optic disc. The increased intraocular pressure causes a vessel to seem to disappear from sight at the disc rim and then to reappear at a slightly different site just past the rim (Figure 12-35).

Cupping of the optic disc and optic atrophy are both late findings of glaucoma. If there is any suspicion of the dis-

ease, the client should be referred to an eye care specialist for further testing.

Optic Atrophy.   Death of the optic nerve fibers leads to the disappearance of the tiny disc vessels that give the disc its normal pinkish color. The affected disc is seen as pale and white, either in a portion of or throughout the disc.

Retinal Vessels

Variation in Caliber.   Variation in the caliber of retinal vessels may occur with hypertension. Since caliber changes may not be evenly distributed along the course of the vessel, it is necessary to follow the vessels out from the disc to the periphery. Arterioles are normally about two thirds to three fourths of the diameter of the corresponding veins. With hypertension, the arterioles may decrease in diameter so that they are only about one half the size of the corresponding vein.

Variation in Color.   Normally, the color of the vessel is determined by the color of the blood within it. With hypertension, the arterioles may develop sclerotic or sheathing changes, causing them to become opaque and lighter. With arteriosclerosis, the width of the light reflex from the arteriolar wall also increases to one third or more of the width of the vessel. In advanced stages the vessels may appear as fine, silvery lines.

Vessel Crossing Variations.   Changes at arteriovenous crossings include an apparent narrowing or blocking of the vein, called **nicking**, at the point where an arteriole crosses over it (Figure 12-36). This appearance, which is the result of some degree of concealment of the underlying veins by an abnormally opaque arteriole wall, occurs with longstanding hypertension. It is initially apparent as a narrowing or tapering of the vessel at the crossing. Later it appears as a more complete interruption of the vessel.

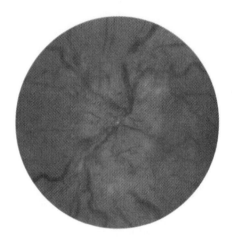

Figure 12-34   Papilledema. (Modified from Newell FW: *Ophthalmology: principles and concepts*, ed. 8, St. Louis, 1996, Mosby.)

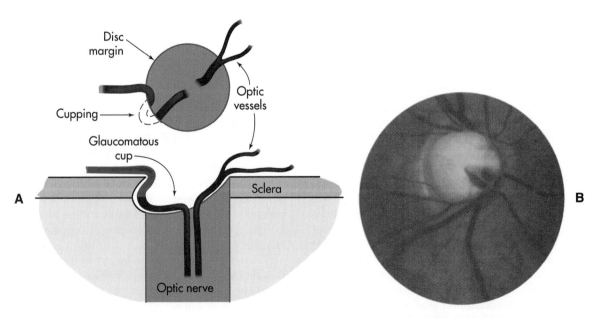

Figure 12-35   **A,** Glaucomatous cupping. **B,** Advanced glaucomatous optic atrophy with cupping of the disc and displacement of the retinal vessels within the optic cup. (**A** from Prior JA, Silberstein JS, Stang JM: *Physical diagnosis: the history and examination of the patient*, ed. 6, St. Louis, 1981, Mosby; **B** from Newell FW: *Ophthalmology: principles and concepts*, ed. 8, St. Louis, 1996, Mosby.)

An embolus in a retinal vessel abruptly impedes the flow of blood and results in the sudden narrowing of an arteriole or dilation of a vein.

RETINAL BACKGROUND VARIATIONS

MICROANEURYSMS. **Microaneurysms** are outpouchings in the walls of the capillaries that appear as tiny bright red dots on the retina (Figure 12-37). They are commonly associated with diabetes mellitus.

RETINAL EXUDATES. Retinal exudates are whitish yellow infiltrates on the retina (see Figure 12-37; Figures 12-38, and 12-39). Both "soft" and "hard" exudates exist. The soft exudates, which look somewhat like a cumulus cloud, are also called "cotton-wool" patches or exudates. Hard exudates have more distinct edges. Retinal exudates are associated with systemic diseases, including diabetes mellitus and hypertension. In addition, they may be associated with inflammatory or degenerative diseases of the retina. Cotton-wool exudates are a common retinal finding in clients with

acquired immunodeficiency syndrome (AIDS). Some exudates are resorbed over time.

HEMORRHAGES OF THE RETINA. Retinal hemorrhages are bright to dark red. They may be small and round, as commonly occur with diabetes, or linear and flame shaped, as noted with hypertension (see Figures 12-37 and 12-38).

PROLIFERATIVE DIABETIC RETINOPATHY. Numerous new vessels (neovascularization) may proliferate on the retina of a diabetic client (Figure 12-40). Bleeding from these vessels can lead to blindness.

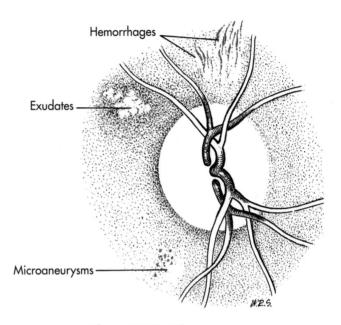

Figure 12-37 Microaneurysms.

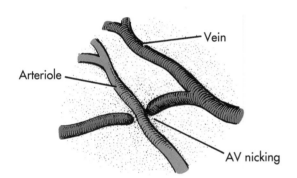

Figure 12-36 Arteriovenous nicking.

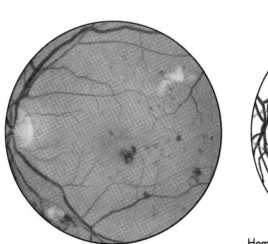

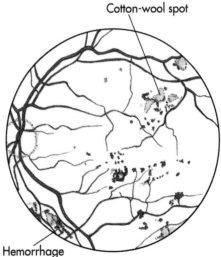

Figure 12-38 Nonproliferative diabetic retinopathy with flame-shaped and dot-blot hemorrhages, cotton-wool spots, and microaneurysms. (From Yannuzzi LA, Guyer DR, Green WR: *The retina atlas*, St. Louis, 1995, Mosby; courtesy Drs. George Blankenship and Everett Ai and the Diabetes 2000 Program.)

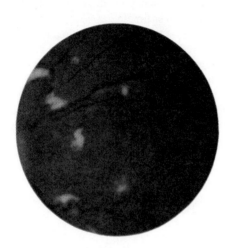

Figure 12-39 Cotton-wool patches, or exudates, and narrowed arterioles in severe vascular hypertension. (Modified from Newell FW: *Ophthalmology: principles and concepts*, ed. 7, St. Louis, 1992, Mosby.)

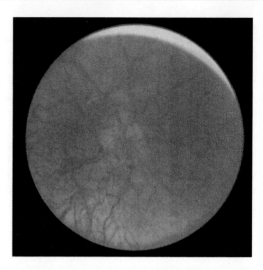

Figure 12-40 Proliferative diabetic retinopathy. (From Seidel HM et al: *Mosby's guide to physical examination*, ed. 4, St. Louis, 1999, Mosby; courtesy John W. Payne, MD, The Wilmer Ophthalmological Institute, The Johns Hopkins University and Hospital, Baltimore, Md.)

Retinal changes may affect any part of the retinal background, including the macular area. Changes in central or peripheral vision depend on the location of the lesion.

Variations in Comfort

Many minor ocular variations are accompanied by itching, burning, or discomfort of the eyes. These symptoms may result from fatigue, allergy, conjunctivitis, or inadequately corrected refractive error.

Superficial eye pain may be caused by any of the following factors:
Dryness of eyes
Lesion in the eyelid
Foreign body on the cornea or conjunctiva
Loss of corneal or conjunctival epithelium

Deep, severe pain within the eye may result from either of these two conditions:
Inflammation of the iris or ciliary body
Rapid increase in intraocular pressure

Findings accompanying deep eye pain include redness and decreased vision. Immediate referral to an ophthalmologist is required.

Variation in Intraocular Pressure: Glaucoma

Acute glaucoma occurs with a sudden increase in intraocular pressure caused by blocked drainage of aqueous fluid from the anterior chamber.

Findings associated with acute glaucoma include the following:
Intense pain
Photophobia
Blurred vision or halos around lights
Unilateral headache
Diffuse conjunctival injection with a limbal flush
Decreased visual acuity
Dilated pupil that is poorly reactive to light
Cloudy cornea
Shallow anterior chamber

The client should be referred to an eye care specialist immediately.

Glaucoma may also be a chronic condition. In this situation symptoms are absent, except for the gradual loss of peripheral vision over a long period of time.

Sample Documentation and Diagnoses

■ FOCUSED HEALTH HISTORY (SUBJECTIVE DATA)

Mrs. S, a 75-year-old retired counselor, states she has noticed that her vision, particularly distant vision, has become increasingly blurred in her right eye over the past 18 to 24 months. Vision in the left eye is unchanged. Reports no pain, itching, inflammation, drainage, or redness in either eye. Wears bifocals—vision is corrected for myopia and presbyopia. Sees an optometrist regularly for eye examinations. Her last eye examination, including a lens prescription, was 2 years ago; new lenses did not correct vision in the right eye as much as previously. Glaucoma testing at that time was normal. Is concerned that her diminished visual acuity is beginning to affect her driving and thus her ability to get together with family and friends and her ability to read and perform other activities she has enjoyed for many years. She lives alone and is able to care for her own home. History of mild hypertension for 15 years, controlled by diet and medication.

■ FOCUSED PHYSICAL EXAMINATION (OBJECTIVE DATA)

Visual acuity: distant vision (with correction)—OD: 20/100 and OS: 20/30; near vision (with correction)—OD: 20/200 at 14 inches on Rosenbaum and OS: 20/25.
Visual fields: intact with confrontation test.
Extraocular muscles: extraocular movements (EOMs) intact; no nystagmus; corneal light reflex—symmetrical; cover-uncover test—eyes aligned; no deviation.
External eye: palpebral fissures equal; lids and lashes asymmetrical.
Conjunctiva: clear, except for several small blood vessels at cornices.
Sclera: white.
Cornea: clear, bright; arcus senilis present bilaterally.
Lacrimal apparatus: no excessive tearing; no tenderness.
Anterior chamber: iris flat.
Pupils: equal; round; react to light and accommodation (PERRLA), though response is somewhat slow.

Ophthalmoscopy
Red reflex: OS—present; OD—not present (obscured by opacity).
Lens: OS—clear; OD—cloudy.
Optic disc: OD—retinal features obscured; OS—optic disc: round, yellowish pink; margins distinct.
Vessels: OS—arterioles: silver wire appearance; slight nicking of superior temporal vessels, 2 DDs from optic disc; A:V ratio, 2:4.
Retinal background: OS—color regular, no hemorrhages or exudates.

■ DIAGNOSES

HEALTH PROBLEM
Decreased visual acuity in right eye, possibly due to cataract

NURSING DIAGNOSIS
Disturbed Sensory Perception (Visual) Related to Cataract
Defining Characteristic
• Presence of uncompensated visual deficits

Related Factors
• Uncompensated visual loss
• Early-stage restricted environment

Critical Thinking Questions

Review the Sample Documentation and Diagnoses box to answer these questions.

1. What retinal findings might be related to Mrs. S's 15-year history of hypertension?
2. What specific history and examination findings might lead the examiner to identify the problem as a cataract?

3. You are counseling a 25-year-old male about health promotion behaviors related to vision. His hobbies are downhill skiing and bicycling. He works as a carpenter apprentice. What guidelines would you discuss?

Answers are available on the MERLIN website (www.harcourthealth.com/MERLIN/Barkauskas/). And be sure to check the website regularly for additional learning activities!

Remember to check out the Online Study Guide!
www.harcourthealth.com/MERLIN/Barkauskas/

Chapter 13

Ears, Nose, Mouth, and Throat

Learning Objectives

On successful study of this chapter and completion of related learning experiences, the learner will be able to:
- Describe the anatomy and physiology of the ears, nose, mouth, and throat.

- Identify relevant history information to assess these regions.
- Explain the rationale for and demonstrate assessment techniques used to examine these structures.
- Recognize variations from expected findings.

Outline

Purpose of Examination

The examination of the ears, nose, mouth, and throat provides the opportunity to inspect, directly or indirectly, most parts of the upper respiratory system and the first division of the digestive system. Examination of these body orifices provides information about the client's general health and the presence of any local disease. This chapter focuses on three areas: the ears, the nose and paranasal sinuses, and the mouth and oropharynx.

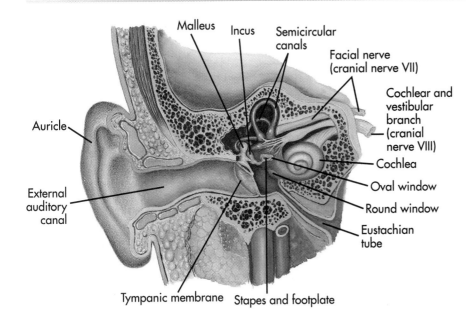

Figure 13-1 External auditory canal, middle ear, and inner ear. (From Seidel HM et al.: *Mosby's guide to physical examination*, ed. 4, St. Louis, 1999, Mosby.)

ANATOMY AND PHYSIOLOGY

Ears

The ear is a sensory organ that functions both in hearing and in equilibrium. It is composed of three parts: the external ear, the middle ear, and the inner ear. Figure 13-1 illustrates the structures of the ear.

External Ear

The external ear has two divisions: the flap called the **auricle**, or **pinna**, and the canal called the external auditory canal, or **meatus**. Stretching across the proximal portion of the canal is the tympanic membrane (eardrum), which separates the external ear from the middle ear. The auricle is composed of cartilage and skin. The main components of the auricle are the **helix**, antihelix, crus of the helix, **lobule**, **tragus**, antitragus, and **concha** (Figure 13-2). The **mastoid process** is not part of the external ear; it is a bony prominence found posterior to the lower part of the auricle (see Figure 11-4).

The external auditory canal, which is approximately 2 cm long, has a skeleton of cartilage in its outer third and a skeleton of bone in its inner two thirds. In adults this skeleton curves slightly with the outer one third of the canal and is directed upward and toward the back of the head; the inner two thirds is directed downward and forward. The skin of the outer portion of the auditory canal is hairy and contains **cerumen** (earwax)-producing glands. Cerumen is produced by the sebaceous and apocrine (sweat) glands in the outer third of the lateral auditory canal. The skin of the inner portion of the canal is very thin and sensitive.

Tympanic Membrane

The **tympanic membrane,** which covers the proximal end of the auditory canal, is made up of layers of skin, fibrous tissue, and mucous membrane (Figure 13-3). The mucous

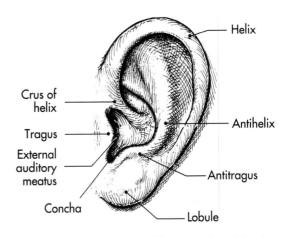

Figure 13-2 Structures of the external ear (pinna).

membrane is shiny, translucent, and pearl gray. The position of the eardrum is oblique with respect to the ear canal. The anteroinferior quadrant is most distant from the examiner. This positioning results in a reflex of light when a light is directed into the ear. This cone of light is located at the 5 o'clock position in the right ear and at the 7 o'clock position in the left ear.

The tympanic membrane, which is slightly concave, is pulled inward at its center by one of the ossicles of the middle ear, called the **malleus**. The short process of the malleus protrudes into the eardrum superiorly, and the handle of the malleus extends downward from the short process to the **umbo**, the point of maximum concavity. Most of the tympanic membrane is taut and is known as the **pars tensa**. A small part located superiorly is less taut and is called the **pars flaccida.** The dense fibrous ring surrounding the tympanic membrane, except for the anterior and posterior malleolar folds superiorly, is the **annulus.**

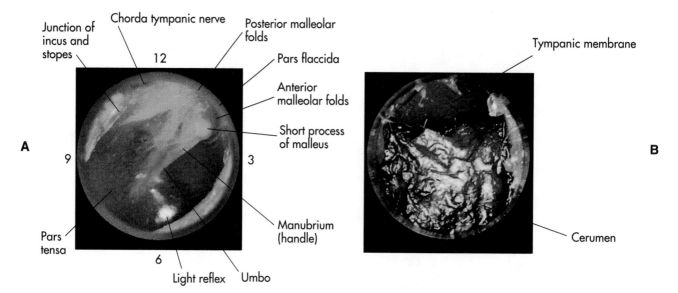

Figure 13-3   **A,** Usual landmarks of the right tympanic membrane with a "clock" superimposed. **B,** External ear canal partially occluded with cerumen. (Courtesy Dr. Richard A. Buckingham, Clinical Professor, Otolaryngology, Abraham Lincoln School of Medicine, University of Illinois, Chicago, Ill.)

Middle Ear

The middle ear is an air-filled cavity located in the temporal bone. It contains three small bones—the malleus, **incus,** and **stapes**—which make up the **auditory ossicles.** The middle ear cavity contains several openings. One, which is from the external auditory meatus, is covered by the tympanic membrane. The two openings into the inner ear are the oval window, into which the stapes fits, and the round window, which is covered by a membrane. Another opening connects the middle ear with the eustachian tube.

The middle ear performs the following three functions:
1. Transmits sound vibrations across the ossicle chain to the inner ear's oval window.
2. Protects the auditory apparatus from intense vibrations.
3. Equalizes the air pressure on both sides of the tympanic membrane to prevent the membrane from being ruptured.

Inner Ear

The two components of the inner ear are the bony **labyrinth** and, inside this structure, a membranous labyrinth. The bony labyrinth consists of three parts: the **vestibule,** semicircular canals, and cochlea. The vestibule and the semicircular canals are the organs of equilibrium. The cochlea is the organ of hearing. The **cochlea** is a coiled structure that contains the organ of Corti and transmits stimuli to the cochlear branch of the auditory nerve (cranial nerve [CN] VIII) (see Figure 13-1).

Pathways of Hearing

Hearing occurs when sound waves enter the external auditory canal and strike the tympanic membrane, causing it to vibrate. The auricle does not direct or amplify sound. Its ma-

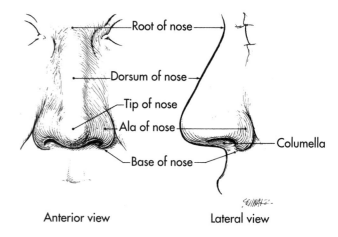

Figure 13-4   External structure of the nose.

jor function is to help perceive the direction of the source of sound (e.g., from behind or ahead). The vibrations are transmitted through the auditory ossicles of the middle ear to the oval window. From the oval window the vibrations travel through the fluid of the cochlea, eventually reaching the round window, where they are dissipated. The vibrations of the membrane cause the delicate hair cells of the organ of Corti to beat against the membrane of Corti, acting as stimuli for impulses carried by the sensory endings of the cochlear branch of the acoustic nerve (CN VIII) to the brain.

Nose and Paranasal Sinuses

The nose is the sensory organ for smell. It also warms, moistens, and filters the inspired air. The **paranasal sinuses** are air-filled cavities that make the skull lighter than it would otherwise be and perform the same functions as the

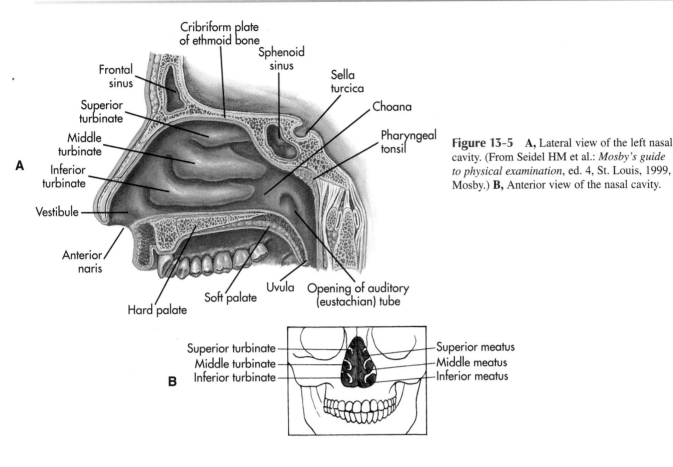

Figure 13-5   A, Lateral view of the left nasal cavity. (From Seidel HM et al.: *Mosby's guide to physical examination*, ed. 4, St. Louis, 1999, Mosby.) **B,** Anterior view of the nasal cavity.

nose—warming, moistening, and filtering air. These sinuses also aid in voice resonance.

The nose is composed of two parts: external and internal (nasal cavity) (Figure 13-4). The upper third of the nose is bone, and the remainder is cartilage. The nasal cavity is divided into two narrow cavities by the septum (Figure 13-5). The cavities have two openings. The anterior opening, which is the vestibule where the naris is located, is thickly lined with small hairs. The posterior opening, or **choana**, leads to the throat. The nasal septum forms the medial walls. The lateral walls are divided into the inferior, middle, and superior turbinate bones, which protrude into the nasal cavity. A highly vascular mucous membrane covers the turbinates. Below each turbinate is a meatus named according to the turbinate above it. The nasolacrimal duct drains into the inferior meatus, and most of the paranasal sinuses drain into the middle meatus. A plexus of blood vessels is located in the mucosa of the anterior nasal septum, which is a common site for **epistaxis** (nose bleeding).

The receptors for smell are located in the olfactory area, which is in the roof of the nasal cavity and the upper third of the septum. The receptor filament cells pass through openings of the cribriform plate, becoming the olfactory nerve (CN I), which transmits neural impulses for smell to the temporal lobe of the brain.

The paranasal sinuses are paired extensions of the nasal cavities within the bones of the skull. They are the frontal, maxillary, ethmoidal, and sphenoidal sinuses (Figure 13-6).

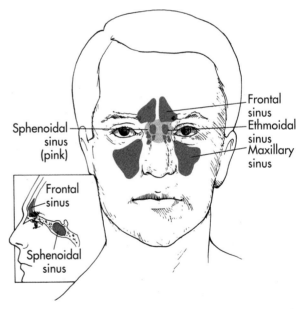

Figure 13-6   Anterior and lateral views of the paranasal sinuses.

Their openings into the nasal cavity are narrow and easily obstructed. The frontal sinuses are located in the anterior part of the frontal bone. The maxillary sinuses, the largest of the paranasal sinuses, are located in the body of the maxilla. The ethmoidal sinuses are small and occupy the ethmoidal

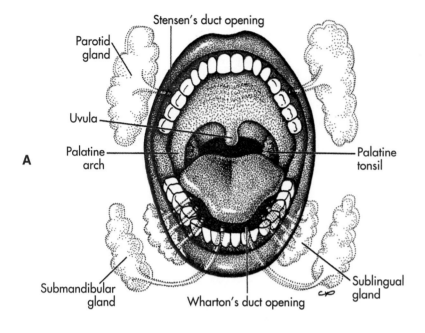

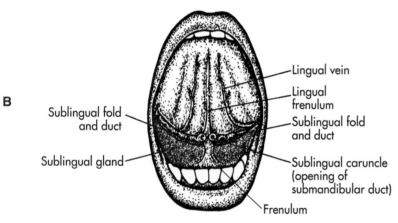

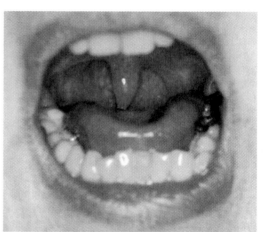

Figure 13-7 **A** and **B**, Structures of the mouth. **C**, The mouth and oropharynx.

labyrinth between the orbit of the eye and the upper part of the nasal cavity. The sphenoidal sinuses are found in the body of the sphenoid.

Mouth and Oropharynx

Mouth

The **oropharynx** conducts air to and from the larynx and food from the mouth to the esophagus. The structures of the mouth and the oropharynx are illustrated in Figure 13-7. The boundaries of the mouth are the lips (anteriorly) and the soft palate and **uvula** (posteriorly). The mandibular bone, which is covered by loose, mobile tissue, forms the floor of the mouth. The hard and soft palates comprise the roof of the oral cavity. The soft palate is pink, and the hard palate is lighter. The uvula is a muscular organ that hangs down from the posterior margin of the soft palate. The muscles of **mastication** (chewing) are innervated by two main nerves: the trigeminal nerve (CN V) and the facial nerve (CN VII). The mouth contains the tongue, gums, teeth, and salivary glands.

Tongue

The tongue is composed of a mass of striated muscles interspersed with fat and many glands. The dorsal surface is rough because of the presence of papillae. The ventral surface toward the floor of the mouth is smooth and shows large veins. The fold of mucous membrane that joins the tongue to the floor of the mouth is called the **frenulum**. The tongue is innervated by the hypoglossal nerve (CN XII). The sensory receptors for taste are the glossopharyngeal nerve (CN IX) for the posterior third of the tongue and the facial nerve (CN VII) for the anterior two thirds of the tongue.

Gums and Teeth

The gums, fibrous tissue covered with a smooth mucous membrane, are attached to the alveolar margins of the jaws and to the necks of the teeth. An adult normally has 32 teeth, 16 in each arch (Figure 13-8; see also Figure 25-46).

Salivary Glands

Three pairs of salivary glands—parotid, submandibular, and sublingual—secrete into the oral cavity. The largest is the

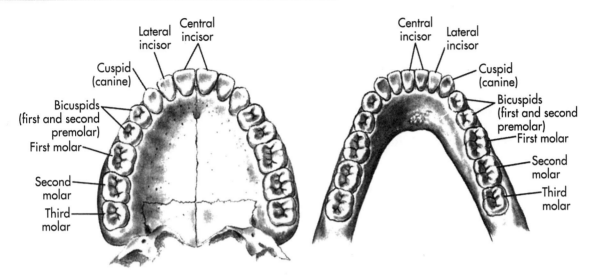

Figure 13-8   Upper and lower permanent teeth. (From Seidel HM et al.: *Mosby's guide to physical examination*, ed. 4, St. Louis, 1999, Mosby.)

parotid gland, which lies in front of and below the external ear. The parotid (Stensen's) duct opens into the buccal membrane opposite the second molar. The submandibular gland lies below and in front of the parotid gland. The submandibular (Wharton's) duct opens at the side of the frenulum on the floor of the mouth. The sublingual gland, the smallest salivary gland, lies in the floor of the mouth and covers its superior surface to form the sublingual fold. The sublingual gland has numerous small openings, which open onto the sublingual fold (see Figure 13-7, *A* and *B*).

Oropharynx

The oropharynx is posterior to the oral cavity and most accessible to examination (see Figure 13-7, *C*). The nasopharynx lies behind the nasal cavities and is superior to the oropharynx. The laryngopharynx is inferior to the oropharynx. Along both lateral walls of the oropharynx are two palatine arches, and between these arches lie the tonsils. The tonsils are usually the same color as the surrounding tissue and do not normally extend beyond the pillars. Tonsillar tissue in children enlarges until puberty, when it shrinks back into the folds of the arches. Consequently, a child's tonsils may normally be larger than an adult's. The posterior pharyngeal wall that is visible during the clinical examination may show many small blood vessels and small areas of pink or red lymphoid tissue.

EXAMINATION

Focused Health History

Present Health/Illness Status

1. Usual state of health
2. Pain or discomfort in ears, nose, mouth, or throat; pain or pressure around eyes, cheeks, or forehead
3. Drainage from ears or nose
4. Seasonal allergies or allergies to medications or food

5. Condition of teeth and gums—presence of dentures or braces, bleeding gums, ability to chew
6. Ability to hear, exposure to loud noise
7. Ability to smell, presence of unusual odors
8. Unusual tastes or reduced ability to taste
9. Difficulty swallowing
10. Dental hygiene practices; frequency of dental checkups
11. Earwax buildup
12. Environmental exposures to fumes, dust, allergens
13. Use of protective gear for work or hobbies—earwear, safety goggles, face mask
14. Smoking status or exposure to second-hand smoke

Past Health History

1. Injury to nose, ears, mouth, or teeth
2. Previous surgery of ears, nose, mouth, or teeth, including tonsillectomy
3. Ringing in ears or dizziness
4. History of frequent nose bleeds
5. History of ear infections, strep throat, upper respiratory infections
6. History of exposure to infection, second-hand smoke

Family Health History

1. Family history of hearing loss or disorders of the ears, nose, mouth, and throat
2. Family history of nose, throat, or sinus cancer

Specific Problems/Symptom Analysis

Earache

1. **Onset:** sudden or gradual
2. **Course since onset:** constant or intermittent symptoms, duration
3. **Location:** bilateral, unilateral, radiating symptoms; deep or superficial

4. **Quality:** sharp, dull, stabbing
5. **Quantity:** rating of pain severity
6. **Setting:** environmental effects such as recent air travel, swimming, exposure to allergens
7. **Associated phenomena:** fever, pain, discharge, injury
8. **Alleviating and aggravating factors:** effects of medications and other efforts to treat, swallowing, movement of earlobe
9. **Underlying concern:** ear infection, discomfort

Sore Throat

1. **Onset:** sudden or gradual; any known exposures
2. **Course since onset:** constant or intermittent, change in symptoms
3. **Location:** exact location of pain or radiation of pain
4. **Quality:** scratchy, raw
5. **Quantity:** rating of pain severity
6. **Setting:** environmental effects of home, work, outdoor settings
7. **Associated phenomena:** fever, earache, runny nose, swollen lymph nodes in the neck, allergies
8. **Alleviating and aggravating factors:** effects of swallowing, eating, hot or cold liquids, topical or oral medications
9. **Underlying concern:** infection, discomfort

Nasal Congestion

1. **Onset:** sudden or gradual; known exposure to allergens
2. **Course since onset:** change in symptoms
3. **Location:** bilateral, unilateral, postnasal drip
4. **Quality:** character of nasal drainage—purulent, clear, thick, watery, bloody
5. **Quantity:** rating of degree of congestion, ability to smell, amount of discharge
6. **Setting:** environmental effects on symptoms
7. **Associated phenomena:** headache, watery eyes, earache, sore throat, sneezing, fever
8. **Alleviating and aggravating factors:** effects of medication or self-care measures (humidity, fluids, positioning) on symptoms
9. **Underlying concern:** viral infection, allergies

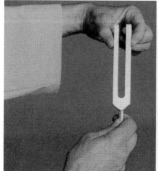
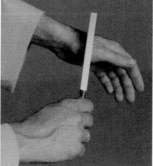

A   **B**

Figure 13-9 Activating the tuning fork. **A,** Stroking the fork. **B,** Tapping the fork on the knuckle.

Preparation for Examination: Client and Environment

The methods of examination for the ears, nose, mouth, and throat are primarily inspection and palpation.

The client should be seated for this examination. The examiner's head should be at approximately the same level as that of the client. A good light source, such as a gooseneck lamp with a 100- to 150-watt bulb, is helpful.

Tuning fork tests are useful in determining whether the client has a conductive or a perceptive (sensorineural) hearing loss. A fork with frequencies of 512 to 1024 hertz (Hz) is used because it provides an estimate of hearing loss in the speech frequencies of roughly 300 to 3000 Hz. The tuning fork should be held by the base without the fingers touching either of the two prongs. The sound vibrations are softened or stopped entirely when the prongs of the fork are touched or held. The fork is activated by stroking it between the thumb and index fingers (Figure 13-9, *A*) or by tapping the tines on the knuckles of the opposite hand (Figure 13-9, *B*). The fork should be made to ring softly.

Technique for Examination and Expected Findings

Ears

External Ear. Begin the examination of the external ear with an inspection of both auricles to determine their horizontal and vertical position, size, and symmetry. The helix should be at or slightly above a line extending from the eye to the occipital area. Next inspect the lateral and medial surfaces of each auricle and the surrounding tissues for skin color and the presence of deformities, lesions, or nodules. Palpate the auricles and mastoid areas for evidence of swelling, tenderness, or nodules.

Preparation for Examination

EQUIPMENT

Item	Purpose
Otoscope with various-size speculums	For inspection of tympanic membrane and external auditory canal
Tongue blade	To help visualize oropharynx
4- × 4-inch gauze sponges	To grasp tongue for inspection
Disposable gloves	For palpation of mouth
Tuning fork (512 cycles/sec [cps])	To assess hearing
Penlight	To visualize mouth, nasal turbinates, and oropharynx

OPTIONAL EQUIPMENT

Item	Purpose
Dental mirror	To visualize teeth and gums
Nasal speculum	To visualize nasal turbinates

CLIENT AND ENVIRONMENT

The client should be seated near a good light source.

Manipulation of the auricle can be helpful in detecting tenderness. If pressure on the tragus or gently pulling on the auricle causes pain, the client may have external otitis. Although fairly simple, this part of the examination is frequently neglected (Figure 13-10, *A*).

External Auditory Canal. Examination of the external auditory canal and tympanic membrane requires an otoscope for additional lighting (Box 13-1). Before inserting the speculum in the client's ear, carefully inspect the meatus and the auditory canal for cerumen, erythema (redness), swelling, narrowing of the canal, a foreign body, or discharge. Describe the appearance and odor of any discharge.

> ### ■ HELPFUL HINT
>
> For the otoscope to be effective, the batteries should be changed or recharged frequently to ensure good light.

Inspect the auditory canal for cerumen, erythema, foreign bodies, or swelling. The appearance of the normal canal varies in diameter, shape, and growth of hairs (Figure 13-10, *B*). A small amount of cerumen will not interfere with the examination. You can look past it and visualize the tympanic membrane. However, if cerumen is excessive, removing it may be necessary.

> ### ■ HELPFUL HINT
>
> Variations in the color of cerumen occur. Dark-skinned clients may have black or brown cerumen. Fresh cerumen is light yellow or even pink in color, as compared with older, drier cerumen, which is dark brown to black.

BOX 13-1

STEPS IN USING AN OTOSCOPE

1. Use the largest speculum that can be inserted in the ear without causing pain.
2. Tip the client's head away from you for easy examination of the canal and the tympanic membrane.
3. In adults, straighten the ear canal by pulling the auricle upward and backward. In young children and infants, straighten the canal by pulling the auricle downward (see Figure 26-41).
4. The inner two thirds of the external meatus is very sensitive to pressure. Insert the speculum gently to minimize discomfort.
5. Vary the angle at which you insert the speculum into the meatus to obtain the best view of the tympanic membrane.

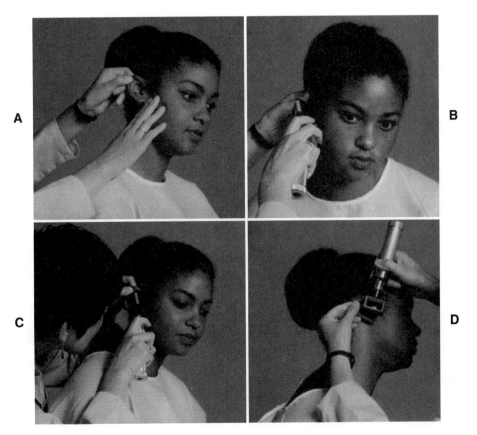

Figure 13-10 Examination of the ear with the otoscope. **A,** Inspection of the meatus. **B,** The client's head is tipped toward the opposite shoulder. **C** and **D,** Two ways of holding the otoscope.

Tympanic Membrane. The examination of the tympanic membrane (see Figure 13-3, *A*) requires a careful assessment of the color of the membrane and the identification of landmarks. The membrane is usually translucent pearl gray, but when disease is present, it may be yellow, white, red, or dull gray. Some membranes have white flecks or dense white plaques, which are the result of healed inflammatory disease.

Identify landmarks, beginning with the light reflex, which is a triangular cone of reflected light seen in the anteroinferior quadrant of the membrane. This landmark is at the 5 o'clock position on the right tympanic membrane and at the 7 o'clock position on the left. At the top point of the light reflex toward the center of the membrane is the umbo, the inferior point of the handle of the malleus. Anterior and superior to the umbo lies the long process of the malleus, which appears as a whitish line extending from the umbo to the malleolar folds, where the short process of the malleus can be seen. The malleolar folds and the pars flaccida, the relaxed portion of the membrane, are superior and lateral to the short process, respectively. Finally, observe the periphery of the pars tensa. Perforations are frequently noted in the areas close to the annulus.

Tympanic membranes vary in size, shape, and color. By examining many healthy membranes, an examiner acquires the ability to recognize the abnormal membrane.

Testing Auditory Function. Testing of auditory function starts early in the physical examination. Because the client's understanding of the spoken word is the principal use of hearing, an impairment of auditory function may become apparent during the interview. Although the precise measurement of hearing requires the use of the audiometer, a good estimate of hearing during the physical examination can be made by using the tests discussed in the following sections.

Auditory Acuity. Simple assessment of auditory acuity requires that only one ear be tested at a time. Therefore it is necessary to mask the hearing in the ear not being tested. Occlude (or have the client occlude) one of the client's ears by gently placing a finger against the opening of the auditory canal.

Voice tests are commonly used to estimate the client's hearing. Begin testing with a very low whisper. Your lips should be 30 to 60 cm (1 or 2 feet) away from the client's unoccluded ear. Softly whisper numbers that the client is to repeat. If necessary, increase the intensity of the whispered voice. To prevent lipreading during the voice tests, stand behind the client. If being in front of the client is more convenient, ask the client to close his or her eyes.

Air conduction is the transmission of sound through the ear canal, tympanic membrane, and ossicles to the cochlea and the auditory nerve. Bone conduction is sound transmitted through the bones of the skull to the cochlea and the auditory nerve. The client with normal auditory function will hear sound twice as long by air conduction, when the tuning fork is held near the external meatus, than by bone conduction, when the base of the tuning fork is placed on the mastoid bone. Explain these tests to the client before the examination so that he or she can fully cooperate.

Tuning Fork Tests. To conduct the **Weber test,** which makes use of bone conduction, place the base of the vibrating tuning fork on the vertex of the skull or on the forehead (Figure 13-11). Ask the client if the sound is clearer in one ear or in the other. In a Weber test, the client reports hearing sound equally in both ears. In lateralization, sound is detected differently in each ear. In conductive deafness, the sound is lateralized (heard louder) to the deafer ear (Table 13-1). This situation occurs because extraneous sounds in the environment will not disturb the cochlea on the weaker side. Sound is not transmitted because of a problem or defect in the ear canal or middle ear. In sensorineural hearing loss, the sound lateralizes to the better ear because the cochlea or auditory nerve is functioning.

The **Rinne test** makes use of air conduction and bone conduction. The tuning fork is used to compare the conduction of sound through the mastoid process (bone conduction) and the auditory meatus (air conduction) (see Table 13-1). The client who has no **conductive hearing loss** will hear the sound twice as long (2:1) by air conduction (AC) as by bone conduction (BC). This normal pattern is called a positive Rinne test, recorded as AC > BC or AC : BC = 2 : 1.

To perform the Rinne test, place the activated tuning fork against the mastoid bone until the client can no longer hear the sound. Then move the fork close to the auditory meatus. The client with no conductive hearing loss will continue to hear the sound by air conduction. A negative Rinne test, a finding in conductive hearing loss, occurs when the client hears sound through bone conduction as long as or longer than air conduction (AC = BC or AC < BC) (Figure 13-12).

Data from both tests need to be considered together to determine conductive or sensorineural loss. Tuning fork test results are difficult to interpret when hearing loss is mixed.

Nose and Paranasal Sinuses

Inspect the external portion of the nose for any deviations in shape, size, or color. Check the nares for flaring or discharge. Palpate the ridge and soft tissues of the nose for displacement of the bone and cartilage and for tenderness or masses (Figure 13-13).

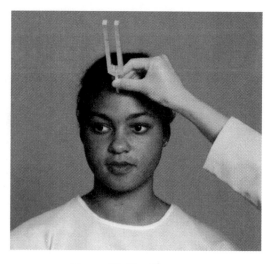

Figure 13-11   Weber test.

TABLE 13-1	**Hearing Tests Using a Tuning Fork**	
Hearing	Weber (Bone Conduction)	Rinne (Air and Bone Conduction)
Normal	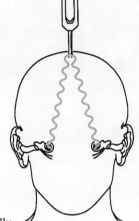 Sound is heard equally well in both ears; no lateralization	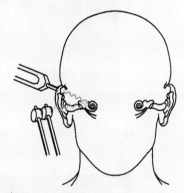 Air conduction (AC) is heard twice as long as bone conduction (BC); AC:BC 2:1
Conduction loss (problem of external or middle ear [e.g., cerumen buildup or otitis media])	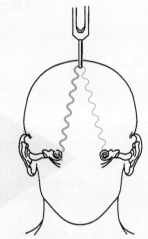 Sound lateralizes to defective ear because it is transmitted through bone rather than air.	Bone conduction is heard longer than air conduction; BC > AC
Sensorineural loss (perceptive problem of inner ear or nerve)	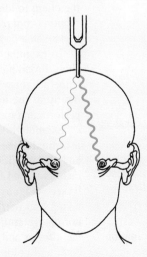 Sound lateralizes to better ear	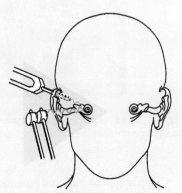 Air conduction is heard longer than bone conduction (AC > BC) but duration is less than 2:1

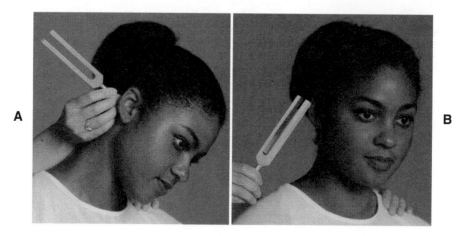

Figure 13-12   Rinne test. **A**, Bone conduction. **B**, Air conduction.

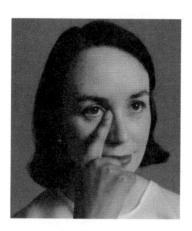

Figure 13-13   Palpation of the external nose.

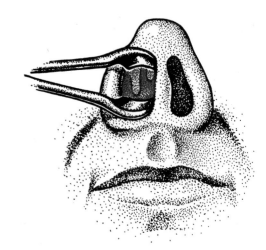

Figure 13-15   Examination of the anterior nasal cavity—view of the inferior and middle turbinates.

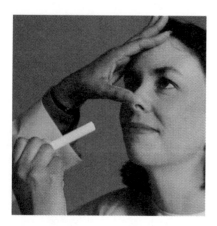

Figure 13-14   Examination of the anterior nasal cavity. Examiner thumb pressure on the tip of the nose enhances visualization.

Examination of the nasal function includes determination of the ability to smell and the patency of the nasal cavities. To determine patency, ask the client to breathe in through the nose while you occlude one naris with a finger. Repeat the procedure to determine the patency of the opposite naris.

To determine the ability to smell, ask the client to close the eyes. Occlude one naris again. Place an aromatic substance, such as coffee or alcohol, close to the client's nose and ask the client to identify the odor. Test each side separately. Olfaction is not routinely tested in a screening examination unless a client describes a change or loss in the ability to smell.

To examine the nasal cavities, use an otoscope with the short, broad nasal speculum. Alternatively, use a penlight to shine a light while using your nondominant thumb to push the tip of the nose upward. The second method is easier to perform and more comfortable for the client (Figure 13-14).

Examination of the nasal cavity through the anterior naris is limited to the vestibule, the anterior portion of the septum, and the inferior and middle turbinates. When the client's head is tipped back, the inferior and middle turbinates can be seen (Figure 13-15). Inspect the septum for deviation, exudate, and perforation. Asymmetry of the nasal septum is normal. Examine the lateral walls of the nasal cavities and the inferior and middle turbinates for polyps, swelling, exudate, and color. The nasal mucosa is normally redder than the oral mucosa. Increased redness indicates infection. Pale turbinates are typical of allergy, whereas redness with edema may indicate localized irritation.

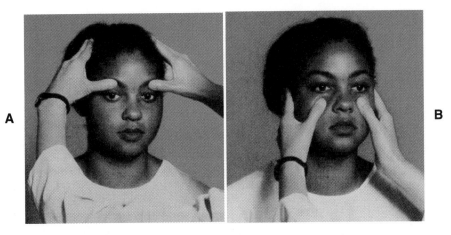

Figure 13-16 Palpation of the frontal (**A**) and maxillary (**B**) sinuses.

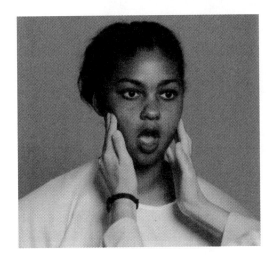

Figure 13-17 Palpation of the temporomandibular joint.

Describe any drainage from the middle meatus, which drains several of the paranasal sinuses. Carefully inspect the floor of the vestibule for evidence of a foreign body. Note the character of nasal secretions. The normal nasal secretion is mucoid. Watery secretions may indicate an acute upper respiratory tract infection or an allergic rhinitis. Purulent, crusty, or bloody secretions are abnormal.

Examination of the paranasal sinuses is performed indirectly. Inspection, percussion, and palpation of the overlying tissues and transillumination are used. Only the frontal and maxillary sinuses are accessible for examination. Palpate or percuss the maxillary sinuses over the maxillary areas of the cheeks to elicit any tenderness. By palpating both cheeks simultaneously, it is possible to determine differences in tenderness. Palpate the frontal sinuses by applying finger pressure below the eyebrows (Figure 13-16). Then percuss both the maxillary and the frontal sinuses for tenderness by lightly tapping the area with the index finger.

Mouth and Oropharynx

Inspect the lips for symmetry, color, edema, or surface abnormalities. Ask the client to open and close the mouth to demonstrate the mobility of the mandible and the occlusion

of the teeth. While the client's mouth is opened wide and then closed, palpate the temporomandibular joint for tenderness, crepitus, or deviation (Figure 13-17). Pressure applied to the joint during closing of the mouth may result in referred pain to the ear, often caused by malocclusion. Palpate the lips for induration.

The oral mucosal surfaces are normally light pink and moistened by saliva. Examine the surfaces systematically to ensure that you inspect all areas (Figure 13-18). Use a tongue depressor or your fingers as retractors. With the client's mouth partially open, inspect the mucosa in the anteroinferior area between the lower lip and gum. With the client's mouth wide open, examine the buccal mucosa and Stensen's duct (the opening to the parotid gland, opposite the upper second molar) of each cheek for patency or inflammation. Next examine the maxillary mucobuccal fold between the upper lip and gum.

■ HELPFUL HINT

A good source of additional light is essential for examination of the mouth and throat. If the client wears dentures, ask him or her to remove them for this part of the examination.

Inspect the tongue for swelling, variation in size or color, coating, or ulceration. To test the function of the hypoglossal nerve (CN XII), ask the client to extend the tongue and observe for deviation, tremor, or limitation of movement. To inspect the posterior and lateral areas of the tongue, hold the extended tongue with a gloved hand (Figure 13-19). A 4- × 4-inch piece of gauze wrapped around the tip of the tongue will make this step easier. Move the tongue to each side to inspect the lateral borders. Release the tongue and ask the client to touch the tip of the tongue to the palate. Observe the ventral surface for swelling or varicosities. Inspect the floor of the mouth for abnormalities or swelling. Identify Wharton's ducts (the openings of the submandibular glands), the frenulum, and the sublingual ridge. Because some abnormalities cause little change in the surface and can be detected only by palpation, use a gloved hand to palpate the entire tongue and floor of the mouth carefully.

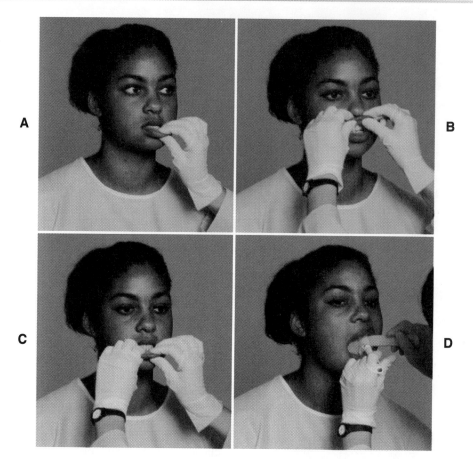

Figure 13-18   Examination of the lips and oral mucosa. **A,** Palpation of the lips. **B** and **C,** Inspection of the mucosa of the upper and lower anterior areas. **D,** Inspection of the mucosa of each cheek with identification of Stensen's duct opening.

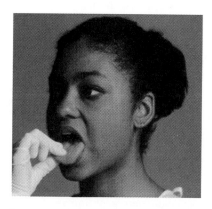

Figure 13-19   Examination of the tongue.

head tipped back, inspect the palate and the uvula. Depressing the base of the tongue with a tongue blade may be necessary to visualize these structures better. Note the difference in color of the hard and the soft palates and any abnormality of architecture. Ask the client to say, "ah," and note the rise of the soft palate and uvula. Any lack of, or asymmetry of, movement indicates impairment of the vagus nerve (CN X) or the glossopharyngeal nerve (CN IX).

These cranial nerves are also tested by touching the posterior wall of the pharynx on each side to elicit a gag reflex. The second method is usually not done in a screening examination.

The examination of the teeth and gums is not a substitute for a dental examination, but inspection should reveal gross problems that need attention. Any soft discolorations on the crown of a tooth should be suspected as carious. Inspect the gums for signs of inflammation and hemorrhage (**gingivitis**). Use a dental mirror to reflect the surfaces of the teeth and gums that are not readily visible such as tooth decay (**caries**), missing teeth, and malocclusions. With the client's

■ **HELPFUL HINT**

When examining the throat, ask the client to open wide and say "ah" with the tongue extended. Most people will be able to lower the tongue and open sufficiently to allow visualization of the pharynx. Use a tongue blade only if necessary because many clients will involuntarily gag when an object is placed in the mouth. Ask a child to take a deep breath with the mouth open to flatten the tongue.

Examination Step-by-Step

EARS

Inspection

1. Observe the position and shape of the auricle.
2. Whisper in each ear separately at a distance of 30 to 60 cm and have the client repeat what you whispered.
3. Apply a vibrating tuning fork to the middle of the forehead, asking the client to identify in which ear the sound or vibration is heard louder (Weber test) or if it is heard equally in both ears.
4. Apply the vibrating tuning fork to the mastoid process and instruct the client to tell you when the sound stops. Then move the tuning fork close to the auditory meatus. Time the duration in seconds or by the ratio of sound perceived by bone and air conduction (Rinne test). For example, if the bone conduction was heard for 30 seconds and air conduction was heard for 60 seconds, record "AC:BC 2:1 or AC > BC."

Palpation

1. Palpate the pinna, tragus, and mastoid processes for tenderness, lesions, or masses.

Otoscopic Examination

1. Observe the condition of the auditory canal.
2. Note the color of the tympanic membrane.
3. Locate landmarks on the tympanic membrane (e.g., cone of light reflex, umbo, long and short processes of malleus, pars tensa, pars flaccida, and annulus).

NOSE AND PARANASAL SINUSES

Inspection

1. Observe the face for symmetry or swelling from a front and profile view.

Percussion

1. Directly percuss over the maxillary areas of both cheeks and over the middle of each eyebrow to assess tenderness.

Palpation

1. Apply pressure over the maxillary areas of both cheeks and below the eyebrows to assess tenderness.

MOUTH AND THROAT

Inspection

1. Using a tongue blade, penlight, and gloves, inspect the lips, gums, teeth, buccal mucosa, sublingual areas, tongue, parotid duct openings, hard palate, pharnyx, and tonsils for color, condition, and presence of lesions.
2. Observe movement of the soft palate and uvula when the client says "ah."

Palpation

1. With gloved hands, palpate with fingers over the lips and sublingual area to assess for tenderness or lumps.

Inspect the oropharynx and anterior and posterior arches for inflammation or swelling. Describe the size of the tonsils, and note any exudate or postnasal discharge. Note the color of the posterior wall of the oropharynx.

Throughout the examination of the mouth and throat, note any mouth odors, which may result from systemic or oral disease.

Special Maneuvers

Cerumen Removal

Irrigation is the preferred method for removing cerumen (earwax) buildup. Curettage is indicated if the cerumen is soft or if the tympanic membrane might be perforated. However, this maneuver should be done only by a skilled clinician using an instrument called a curette or a cerumen spoon. The closeness of blood vessels and nerves to the surface of the auditory canal makes it easy to cause bleeding and pain. The risk also exists of perforating the tympanic membrane if the client moves or if the curette is used too vigorously. Use irrigation when the cerumen is dry and hard, but do not irrigate if the tympanic membrane might be perforated. Use lukewarm water or a 1:1 solution of hydrogen peroxide and water for the irrigation, which is done by injecting the water from a syringe toward the posterosuperior canal wall until cerumen is removed. This procedure may make the client feel dizzy.

Nasal Speculum

To use a nasal speculum for inspection of the nasal mucosa and the turbinates, hold the instrument in the nondominant hand and place the index finger on the side of the client's nose to stabilize the position of the speculum. Use the dominant hand to position the client's head and hold the light. Be careful not to apply pressure on the nasal septum because of its great sensitivity. However, open the blades of the nasal speculum as far as possible (see Figure 13-15). Ask the client to tilt the head back. This change in position increases visualization of the middle turbinate.

Pneumatic Otoscopy

Because the normal eardrum moves to slight pressure changes, the insufflation of air tests the mobility of the tympanic membrane. To perform insufflation, use a large ear speculum to create a seal and introduce a small amount of air into the external ear. The examiner uses a pneumatic bulb and tubing that is attached to an otoscope. A normal tympanic membrane will move slightly. A tympanic membrane that is retracted or bulging due to air or fluid in the middle ear will be immobile (see also Chapter 26).

VARIATIONS FROM HEALTH

External Ear

Otitis externa, or "swimmer's ear," is an inflammation of the external auditory canal. It is most often caused by trauma to the ear canal from cleaning ears with sharp objects or from a moist environment, such as swimming, which favors bacterial or fungal growth. It can occur unilaterally or bilaterally. The meatus of the external ear canal is often swollen shut, and foul-smelling discharge may be present. Manipulation of the pinna of the affected ear causes pain.

Tympanic Membrane

Fluid in the middle ear may sometimes be identified by air bubbles or a fluid level seen through the tympanic membrane (Figure 13-20, *A*).

Bulging of the tympanic membrane may occur when fluid forms in the middle ear. The pressure increases, and the membrane may bulge outward, obliterating some or all of the landmarks. The light reflex may be lost or displaced, and the membrane appears amber or a dull blue-gray (Figure 13-20, *B*).

Increased pressure in the middle ear or trauma can cause a perforation of the membrane (Figure 13-20, *C* and *D*).

Retraction of the tympanic membrane occurs when pressure is reduced from obstruction of the eustachian tube, usually associated with an upper respiratory system infection or allergies. The retraction of the membrane accentuates the landmarks. The light reflex may appear less prominent.

Acute otitis media (AOM) (Figure 13-20, *B*) is the most common cause of ear pain in children younger than 6 years. AOM with effusion refers to inflammation of the tympanic membrane with a collection of fluid in the middle ear that results in a visible fluid line or bulging of the tympanic membrane. AOM often occurs after an upper respiratory tract infection. Symptoms include severe earache of sudden onset. Pain may be suddenly relieved if the pressure creates a rupture of the tympanic membrane with drainage of the fluid from the middle ear (also see Figure 26-46 for other examples of common conditions of the middle ear).

Inner Ear Disorders

Meniere's disease affects the vestibular labyrinth, leading to **sensorineural hearing loss**. Symptoms are episodic and include a sensation of fullness in one ear with some hearing loss, tinnitus, and severe vertigo. Hearing improves after an attack but deteriorates over time.

Labyrinthitis is an inflammation of the labyrinthine canal of the inner ear and occurs as a complication of an upper respiratory tract infection. Symptoms include **vertigo**, a sensation of the body or the room revolving, that is more severe with head movement.

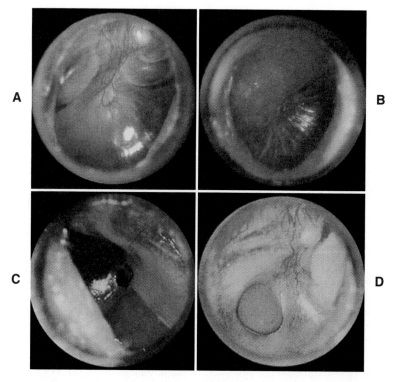

Figure 13-20 **A**, Air fluid levels in the upper middle ear. **B**, Acute otitis media—red, bulging membrane with loss of bony landmarks and light reflex. **C**, Centrally perforated tympanic membrane. **D**, Perforated membrane that has healed. (Courtesy Dr. Richard A. Buckingham, Clinical Professor, Otolaryngology, Abraham Lincoln School of Medicine, University of Illinois, Chicago, Ill.)

Nose

Allergic rhinitis is a recurrent pattern of symptoms of rhinorrhea, sneezing, and **pruritus** caused by exposure to an allergen. Nasal turbinates are pale and swollen (Figure 13-21). Nasal discharge is clear and watery.

Mouth

Pyorrhea is a serious periodontal disease involving the bones and ligaments that anchor the tooth in its socket (Figure 13-22). Note stains, tartar (calculus), or loose teeth as signs of periodontal disease.

Malocclusion is present when two teeth occupy the space for one, teeth overlap, and/or missing teeth create wide spaces. As a result, the lower front teeth are positioned outside the upper front teeth (underbite), or the upper front teeth protrude and hang over the lower front teeth (overbite). Normal occlusion or malocclusion can be demonstrated at oral examination while palpating the temporo-mandibular joint during opening and closing of the mouth (Figure 13-23).

An **exostosis** (torus palatinus) is commonly found in the midline of the posterior two thirds of the hard palate (Figure 13-24). This smooth, symmetrical bony structure results from the down-growth of the palatine processes. This type of growth is benign.

The uvula may be bifid and part of a submucosal cleft palate.

Additional variations from health noted in the mouth are shown in Figures 13-25 through 13-27.

Pharynx

Pharyngitis is an inflammation of the mucous membranes of the pharynx, usually of viral or bacterial origin. The posterior pharynx is erythematous and sometimes has a white coating (exudate) (Figures 13-28 and 13-29), and may have a "cobblestone" appearance secondary to lymphedema

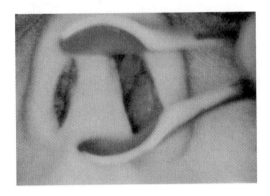

Figure 13-21 Allergic rhinitis.

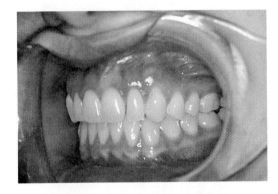

Figure 13-23 Malocclusion. (From Seidel HM et al.: *Mosby's guide to physical examination*, ed. 4, St. Louis, 1999, Mosby; courtesy Drs. Abelson and Cameron, Lutherville, Md.)

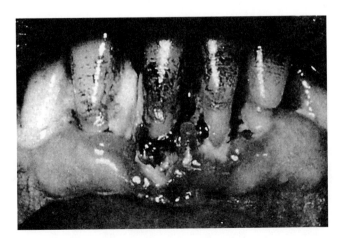

Figure 13-22 Advanced pyorrhea. (From DeWeese DD et al.: *Otolaryngology—head and neck surgery*, ed. 7, St. Louis, 1988, Mosby.)

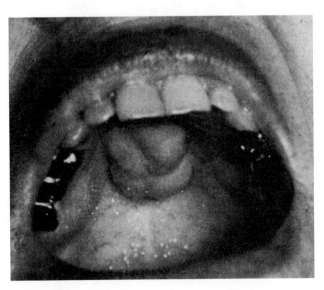

Figure 13-24 Exostosis. (From Prior JA, Silberstein JS, Stang JM: *Physical diagnosis: the history and examination of the patient*, ed. 6, St. Louis, 1981, Mosby.)

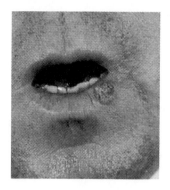

Figure 13-25   Epidermal carcinoma—lip. (Courtesy Dr. Edward L. Applebaum, Head, Department of Otolaryngology, University of Illinois Medical Center, Chicago, Ill.)

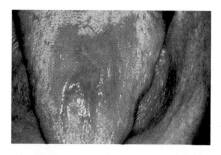

Figure 13-26   Drug reaction—tongue. (Courtesy Dr. Edward L. Applebaum, Head, Department of Otolaryngology, University of Illinois Medical Center, Chicago, Ill.)

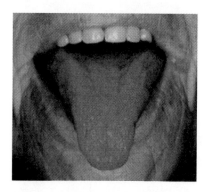

Figure 13-27   Smooth tongue resulting from vitamin deficiency. (From Seidel HM et al.: *Mosby's guide to physical examination*, ed. 4, St. Louis, 1999, Mosby.)

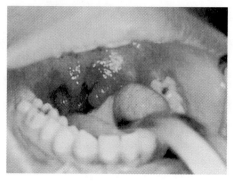

Figure 13-28   Acute viral pharyngitis. (Courtesy Dr. Edward L. Applebaum, Head, Department of Otolaryngology, University of Illinois Medical Center, Chicago, Ill.)

(lymph tissue enlargement). Enlarged tonsils can be graded using a scale from 1⁺ to 4⁺ (Figure 13-30).

Paranasal Sinuses

Sinusitis is an infection or inflammation of one or more of the paranasal sinuses. Examination reveals tenderness to palpation or percussion over one or more of the sinuses. The nasal mucosa is swollen, pale, or dull red.

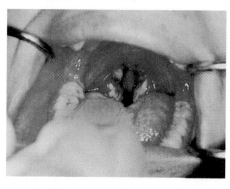

Figure 13-29   Tonsillitis, pharyngitis. (Courtesy Dr. Edward L. Applebaum, Head, Department of Otolaryngology, University of Illinois Medical Center, Chicago, Ill.)

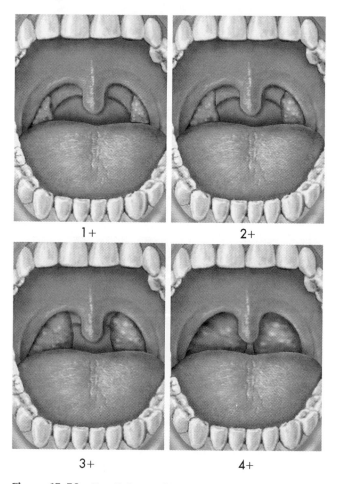

Figure 13-30   Tonsil size grading. Enlarged tonsils are graded to describe their size: 1+, visible; 2+, halfway between tonsillar pillars and uvula; 3+, nearly touching the uvula; 4+, touching the uvula. (From Seidel HM et al.: *Mosby's guide to physical examination*, ed. 4, St. Louis, 1999, Mosby.)

Sample Documentation and Diagnoses

FOCUSED HEALTH HISTORY (SUBJECTIVE DATA)

Mr. B, a 19-year-old African-American male, complains of a sore throat for the past 2 days. The discomfort is described as a dull ache that increases in intensity with swallowing. Client has also noticed clear mucus draining from his nose since yesterday. Has taken acetaminophen 650 mg prn for symptoms but without relief. Discomfort is slightly relieved with throat lozenges. Denies earaches, otorrhea, lethargy, or cough. Reports that his girlfriend has had similar symptoms for the past week.

FOCUSED PHYSICAL EXAMINATION (OBJECTIVE DATA)

Ears: Auricles properly positioned without lesions or tenderness on palpation. Able to hear whispered voice bilaterally at 15 feet. Weber and Rinne tests not done. Otoscopic examination reveals small amount of yellow cerumen in each ear; tympanic membranes pearly gray with slight injection. Cone of light in proper position bilaterally.

Nose: Nasal septum slightly deviated to left. Nostrils patent bilaterally. Mucosa of inferior and middle turbinates pale pink with clear liquid mucus present. Frontal and maxillary sinuses nontender to percussion and palpation.

Mouth and throat: Lips dry and cracked. Gums pink and firm. Teeth are in good repair and alignment. Tongue midline with thin white coating, no lesions. Buccal mucosa is pink without lesions. Parotid and submaxillary gland orifices are without swelling. Tonsils absent. Soft palate rises symmetrically on phonation. Uvula midline. Oropharynx reveals erythematous mucosa with cobblestone lymphedema of posterior pharynx. No exudate is visible.

DIAGNOSES

HEALTH PROBLEM

Pharyngitis

NURSING DIAGNOSES

Impaired Swallowing Related To Irritated Oropharyngeal Cavity

Defining Characteristics

• Observed evidence of difficulty in swallowing
• Complaints of pain when swallowing
• Edema of oropharyngeal cavity

Acute Pain Related To Biological Injuring Agent Of Oropharyngeal Cavity (Pharyngitis)

Defining Characteristic

• Communication of pain when swallowing

Critical Thinking Questions

Review the Sample Documentation and Diagnoses box to answer questions 1 and 2.

1. If Mr. B had a conductive hearing loss on his right side, what would you expect to find when performing the Weber and Rinne tests?
2. How would you proceed during the otoscopic examination if both of Mr. B's ear canals were obstructed with cerumen?

3. A client states that she has symptoms of nasal congestion and fullness in her ears. What history questions and physical examination would you perform to assess the condition of her sinuses?

Answers are available on the MERLIN website (www.harcourthealth.com/MERLIN/Barkauskas/). And be sure to check the website regularly for additional learning activities!

Remember to check out the Online Study Guide!
www.harcourthealth.com/MERLIN/Barkauskas/

Chapter **14**

Breasts and Regional Lymphatics

Learning Objectives

On successful study of this chapter and completion of related learning experiences, the learner will be able to:
- Describe the anatomy and physiology of the breasts throughout the lifespan.
- Outline the history relevant to breast examination.
- Describe the rationale for and purposes of breast examination and regional lymphatics examination.

- Demonstrate physical examination of the breasts and regional lymphatics, using inspection and palpation techniques.
- Recognize abnormalities and common deviations of breasts in women and men.
- Describe procedures used to evaluate breast masses.
- Identify breast cancer risk factors.

Outline

Purpose of Examination

Breast examination is part of the assessment of sexual development and reproductive function. Breast examination and the teaching of breast self-examination are essential components of health assessment for all women after puberty. Breast examination offers an excellent opportunity for breast and reproductive health education and for the identification of minor problems that would be amenable to early intervention, as well as the identification of breast cancer, which can occur in women of all ages.

Because cancer of the breast is a major cause of morbidity and mortality in women and because early detection and treatment of breast cancer improve survival rates, the breast examination is an important component of screening for cancer and an opportunity to teach breast self-examination. Screening for breast cancer is the focus of one of the national health promotion and disease prevention objectives proposed in *Healthy People 2010* (2000).

ANATOMY AND PHYSIOLOGY

Breasts

The breast is a modified sebaceous gland. The breasts are located on the anterior chest wall between the second and third ribs (superiorly), the sixth and seventh costal cartilages (inferiorly), the anterior axillary line (laterally), and the sternal border (medially). The breast is composed of three types of tissue: (1) glandular tissue; (2) fibrous tissue, including suspensory ligaments; and (3) adipose tissue. Subcutaneous and retromammary fat compose much of the bulk of the breast. The breast, which is fairly mobile, is supported by a layer of subcutaneous connective tissue and by Cooper's ligaments (Figure 14-1, *B*). The latter are multiple fibrous bands that begin at the breast's subcutaneous connective tissue layer, run through the breast, and are attached to muscle fascia.

The functional components of the female breast are the **acini** (milk-producing glands), a ductal system, and a nipple (Figure 14-1, *A*). The glandular tissue units, called **lobes**, are situated in a circular, spokelike fashion around the nipple and are embedded in adipose tissue. Each breast has 15 to 25 lobes. A lobe is composed of 20 to 40 lobules, each containing 10 to 100 acini. Lactiferous ducts drain milk or other fluid from the lobes to the surface of the nipples. The nipples, composed of epithelium intertwined with circular and longitudinal smooth muscle fibers, are located centrally on the breasts. These muscle fibers contract in response to tactile, sensory, and autonomical stimuli, producing erection of the nipple and emptying of any material in the lactiferous ducts. The nipples are round, hairless, pigmented, protuberant structures. Their size, color, and shape vary among women and in an individual woman, depending on the state of contraction. Usually nipples are directed, "pointing" slightly upward and laterally. This position of the nipples places them in an ideal angle for breast-feeding an infant.

Inversion of the nipple is an invagination or depression of its central portion. Inversion can occur congenitally or as a response to an invasive process. The **areolae** are pigmented areas surrounding the nipples. Their color varies from pink to brown, and their size differs greatly among individuals. Several to many sebaceous glands, termed **Montgomery's glands** (also called *tubercles* or *follicles*), appearing as small bumps, may be present on the areolar surface.

The largest portion of glandular breast tissue is found in the upper lateral quadrant of each breast. From this quadrant there is a cone-shaped anatomical projection of breast tissue into the axilla. This projection is termed the **axillary tail of Spence** (Figure 14-2). The majority of breast tumors are located in the upper lateral breast quadrant and in the tail of Spence.

On general appearance, the normal breasts are reasonably symmetrical in size and shape, although they are not usually identical. This symmetry remains constant at rest and with movement. The skin of the breast is the same as that of the abdomen or back. In adults a small number of hair follicles may be scattered around the areola. In persons with light complexions, a horizontal or vertical vascular pattern may be observed. This pattern, when normally present, is symmetrical.

During early embryonic development, longitudinal ridges appear, extending from the axilla to the groin. Called "milk lines" (Figure 14-3), these ridges usually atrophy, except at the level of the pectoral muscles, where a breast will eventually develop. In some women, the ridges do not entirely disappear, and portions of the milk lines persist. This occurrence is manifested by the presence of a nipple, a nip-

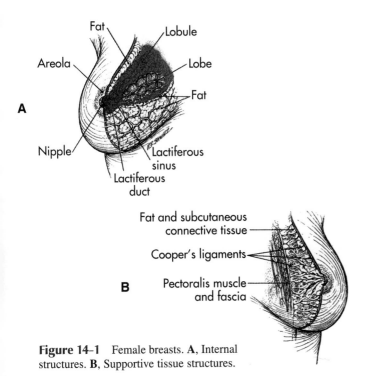

Figure 14-1 Female breasts. **A,** Internal structures. **B,** Supportive tissue structures.

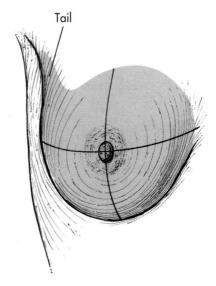

Figure 14-2 Four breast quadrants and the axillary tail of Spence.

ple and a breast, or glandular breast tissue only. This congenital anomaly is called a *supernumerary breast* or *nipple*.

Regional Lymphatics

Knowledge of the lymphatic drainage of the breast is important because of the common metastasis of breast cancer throughout this system. Lymph drainage from the breast is directed toward numerous groups of nodes, with most of the drainage routed to the ipsilateral axillary nodes. However, depending on the site of the lesion, drainage might also be directed into the infraclavicular and supraclavicular nodes, the chest, the abdomen, or the opposite breast.

Two sets of lymph nodes are examined in conjunction with the breast examination: axillary lymph nodes and supraclavicular lymph nodes. Five groups of lymph nodes are located in the axillary fossa (Figure 14-4). All drain upward and medially toward the main lymph-collecting channels. The central axillary nodes are the most frequently palpable. Nomenclature commonly used describes either the area of the axilla in which the nodes are located or their location in relation to one of the adjacent bones or blood vessels.

1. *Anterior axillary (pectoral) nodes* lie in the anterior aspect of the axilla and include a superior group of several nodes found in the region of the third rib and the second and third intercostal spaces, and an inferior group located over the fourth to sixth ribs. The ducts entering these nodes are from the breast and front and side of the costal wall, and from the skin and muscles of the abdominal wall above the umbilicus. They lie along the lateral edge of the pectoralis major muscle, just inside the anterior axillary fold.
2. *Lateral axillary (brachial) nodes* lie along the humerus, inside the upper arm. They receive lymph from the upper extremity; deltoid region; and anterior wall of the chest, including part of the breast.
3. *Posterior axillary (subscapular) nodes* lie in the posterior aspect of the axilla along the lateral edge of the scapula. They drain the posterior wall of the chest and the lower posterior aspect of the neck.
4. *Central axillary (intermediate) nodes* lie high in the middle of the axilla over the ribs. They receive

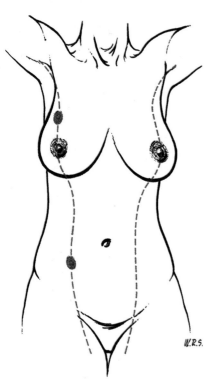

Figure 14-3   Milk lines.

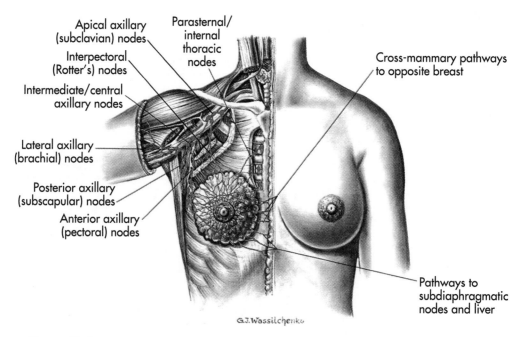

Figure 14-4   Lymphatic drainage of the breast. (From Bobak IM, Jensen MD, Zalar MK: *Maternity and gynecologic care: the nurse and the family*, ed. 4, St. Louis, 1989, Mosby.)

ducts from the anterior axillary (pectoral), lateral axillary (brachial), and posterior (subscapular) lymph nodes draining the chest wall, breast, and arm. Lymph drains from them into the infraclavicular and supraclavicular nodes.

5. *Apical axillary (infraclavicular or subclavian) nodes* lie below the clavicle and receive ducts from the arm, breast, and chest wall.

Drainage flows from the central axillary nodes into the apical axillary (infraclavicular) and supraclavicular nodes. (See also Chapter 11 for additional information about infraclavicular and supraclavicular lymph nodes.) A small amount of lymphatic drainage goes directly to the apical axillary (infraclavicular) nodes, deep into the chest or abdomen, or directly across to the opposite breast. Depending on the location of a lesion in the breast tissue, drainage may go to the axillary nodes, to the infraclavicular nodes, into deep channels in the chest or abdomen, or even to the opposite breast. Some nodes are deep and not accessible to examination. The following are accessible to examination. Note that the first five groups are axillary lymph nodes, and the sixth is in another area.

1. Anterior axillary (pectoral) nodes
2. Lateral axillary (brachial) nodes
3. Posterior axillary (subscapular) nodes
4. Central axillary (intermediate) nodes
5. Apical axillary (infraclavicular) nodes
6. Supraclavicular nodes

Other groups that receive lymphatic drainage (but are not palpable) from the breast include the following:

1. Interpectoral (Rotter's or mammary) nodes, which lie within the pectoral muscle and are diffusely distributed about the breast
2. Parasternal (internal thoracic) nodes, which lie next to the sternum

Breast Development

The gross appearance and size of the normal female breast vary both among individuals and for an individual at various phases of development. The following paragraphs describe breast development throughout a woman's lifespan (Figure 14-5). The presented stages of breast development are referred to *Tanner's stages*. (See also Chapter 26 for additional discussion of sexual development in children and adolescents.)

1. *Appearance before age 10 (approximate age).* Gross appearance of male and female breasts differs little. The nipples are small and slightly elevated. No palpable glandular tissue or areolar pigmentation exists.
2. *Appearance between ages 10 and 14.* The mammary tissues adjacent to and beneath the areola grow, resulting in an increased diameter of the areola and the formation of a "mammary bud." The nipple and breast protrude as a single mound. Breast development may begin bilaterally or may occur unilaterally. Next, the general mammary growth and increases in diameter and pigmentation of the areola continue, resulting in further elevation of the breasts. The nipple begins to separate from the areola. Growth continues in the

mammary tissues. The nipple and areola form a mound that is distinct from the globular shape of the rest of the breast.

3. *Appearance after age 14 (approximate age).* The shape of the adult female breast gradually forms. The areola recedes into the general contour of the breast, and only the nipple protrudes. Heredity, individual sensitivity to hormones, and nutrition influence the ultimate size of the adult female breast.
4. *Appearance during reproductive years.* In response to hormonal changes during the menstrual cycle, a cyclic pattern of breast size change, nodularity, and tenderness occurs. These changes are maximal just before menses. The breast is smallest in days 4 through 7 of the menstrual cycle. Three to 4 days before the onset of menses, many women experience mammary tenseness, fullness, heaviness, tenderness, and pain because of hormonal changes and fluid retention. Total breast volume is significantly increased at this time.
5. *Changes in pregnancy.* Changes in the breast are noted as early as the second month of pregnancy. The breast increases in size, sometimes reaching two to three times the usual size. The areolae and nipples become more prominent and more deeply pigmented. The veins become engorged, Montgomery's glands become more apparent, and **striae** often develop. During palpation the breasts feel more nodular, and

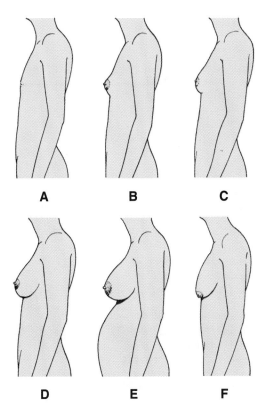

Figure 14-5 Appearance of the female breast in various life periods. **A,** Appearance before age 10. **B** and **C,** Appearance between ages 10 through 14. **D,** Appearance of the nulliparous, adult breast. **E,** Appearance of the breast during pregnancy. **F,** Appearance of the breast after menopause.

after the fourth month, colostrum can be expressed from the nipples.

6. *Menopausal changes.* After menopause the breast's glandular tissue gradually involutes, and fat is deposited in the breasts. The flattening of structures and decreased elasticity make structures more palpable. The lactiferous ducts especially are more distinctly palpable, feeling firm and stringy. The breast formation becomes flabby and flattened.

The male breast contains a small nipple and a relatively well-developed areola. Beneath the nipple is a small amount of breast tissue, which usually cannot be clinically differentiated from the other subcutaneous tissues.

EXAMINATION

Focused Health History

The foci of the health history are identification of problems that require further assessment and to review, teach, and support self-examination practices.

Risk Factors
Breast Cancer in Women

HIGH RISK*

Family history of breast cancer in first-degree relatives (e.g., mother or sister)
Personal history of breast cancer
Atypical hyperplasia in breast biopsy or aspirated sample

MODERATE RISK†

Family history of breast cancer in second-degree relatives (e.g., grandmother or aunt)
Mutations in the BRCA 1 and BRCA 2 genes
Hyperplasia without atypia in breast biopsy or aspirated sample
Older, Caucasian women

LOW RISK‡

Family history of postmenopausal breast cancer in first-degree relative
Previous cancer of the ovary or uterine endometrium
Predominant nodular densities in mammogram
Obesity (in women older than 50)
High-fat diet
High alcohol consumption
High socioeconomic status
Never pregnant (women younger than 40)
Delayed first childbirth
Short duration of breast-feeding
Onset of menstruation before age 12
Onset of menopause after age 49
Prolonged use of oral contraceptives (women younger than 45)
Excess ionizing radiation to chest wall or breasts
Prolonged estrogen replacement therapy

Data from Stoll BA, editor: *Reducing breast cancer risk in women*, Boston, 1995, Kluwer Academic.
* Risk increased more than 4 times.
† Risk increased 2 to 4 times.
‡ Risk increase is up to 2 times or findings inconsistent among studies.

Present Health/Illness Status

1. Breast self-examination
   a. Frequency
   b. Timing with menstrual cycle
2. Changes in breast characteristics and their relationship to menstrual cycle—pain, tenderness, heaviness, swelling, lumps, discharge, and changes in appearance, size, or shape
3. Mammography patterns
   a. Age at first mammography
   b. Date of last mammography and findings
4. Risk factors for breast cancer
5. Menstrual history (relative to breast changes) (refer to Chapter 21 for a complete discussion of menstrual history data collection)
   a. Date of last menstrual period
   b. If menopause—onset, course, associated symptoms
6. Reproductive status
   a. Number of pregnancies
   b. Breast-feeding patterns
7. Medications taken—especially hormones—name, length of use, purpose of therapy

Past Health History

1. Previous diagnoses of breast disease and injuries, age at onset, treatment, and treatment outcomes
2. Previous breast surgeries, biopsies, aspirations, implants, reductions
3. Lactation history: number of children breast-fed, duration of breast-feeding
4. Past use of hormonal medications: name, length of use, purpose of therapy
5. Cancers in other sites
6. Problems in axillary areas

Family Health History

1. Breast cancer in female relative: age at onset, relationship to client, and type of cancer; treatment and treatment outcomes

Personal and Social History

1. Risk factors (see the Risk Factors box on this page)
2. Reproductive and menstrual history
3. Medication history, especially hormones
4. Nutrition history, especially fat and caffeine intake

Symptom Analysis

Breast Discomfort or Pain

1. **Onset:** specific date, sudden or gradual, pattern of discomfort
2. **Course since onset:** lessening or worsening, other changes, relationship to menstrual cycle, pattern of changes
3. **Location:** exact location(s), radiation
4. **Quality:** stinging, burning, pulling, stabbing, aching, throbbing
5. **Quantity:** severity, disability assessment

6. **Setting:** time of day; clothing worn, especially bra
7. **Associated phenomena:** exercise, other health problems or changes
8. **Alleviating and aggravating factors:** use of analgesics or herbal remedies, changes with variations in bras worn
9. **Underlying concern:** discomfort, cancer

Swelling and Lumps

1. **Onset:** exact date of discovery
2. **Course since onset:** always present or does it come and go, change in size, relationship to menstrual cycle
3. **Location:** actual location
4. **Quality:** characteristics, pain with palpation or at rest
5. **Quantity:** size, number of lumps
6. **Associated phenomena:** pain, skin changes, changes in nipple, nipple discharge, tenderness or redness in lump area or lymph node areas, change in skin color
7. **Alleviating and aggravating factors:** recent injury, unusual manipulation of breasts, changes with change in caffeine intake
8. **Underlying concern:** fear of breast cancer

Nipple Discharge

1. **Onset:** date of onset
2. **Course since onset:** pattern of discharge, relationship to menstrual cycle
3. **Location:** exact nipple and nipple area
4. **Quality:** color, consistency, odor, presence of blood, pain
5. **Quantity:** amount
6. **Associated phenomena:** nipple changes; tenderness in lymph node areas; recent breast injury; relationship to activity, especially sexual activity that involves breast stimulation
7. **Alleviating and aggravating factors:** medications, previous breast-feeding
8. **Underlying concern:** pregnancy, fear of cancer

Preparation for Examination: Client and Environment

Some girls and women are embarrassed while undergoing a breast examination. Their reasons for embarrassment may include a sense of modesty or dissatisfaction with their breast development. Take care to ensure privacy during the examination and avoid unnecessary exposure of the breasts. With young adolescents, teaching about the normal sequence of breast development may be reassuring. (See Chapter 26 for additional discussion of assessing young women and advising about sexual development.) Avoid making comments about the client's breast development that could be misinterpreted. Explain the components of the examination to relieve the client's discomfort and provide important health education.

During the health history preceding the physical examination, assess the woman's level of knowledge and practice regarding breast self-examination. The examination provides an excellent opportunity for reviewing the client's technique or for teaching breast self-examination.

Some adolescent or adult male clients may not have had a breast examination previously and may be concerned that the examiner will notice a problem. Explaining to male clients that breast lesions are possible in men and that the breast examination is a routine component of a complete health assessment will help to alleviate any worry and embarrassment. See the Helpful Hints and the Preparation for Examination boxes for performing the male breast examination, a list of equipment needed for the examination, and the recommended approaches for setting up the examination and approaching the client.

■ HELPFUL HINT

Some male clients have perspiration in the axilla and may be embarrassed when an examiner palpates this dampened area; it is helpful to offer the male client a tissue for drying the area before the examination is begun.

Preparation for Examination

EQUIPMENT

Item	Purpose
Small pillow or folded towel	For placement under back of side being examined to spread breast tissue more evenly on chest
Drape	To cover areas not being examined
Centimeter ruler	To measure position and size of any masses located
Glass slides, cytological fixative	To prepare specimen of any nipple drainage for microscopic examination (drainage, which is often thin and acellular, is most effectively collected on a frosted or albumin-coated slide to prevent runoff)
Culture plates and slides	To prepare specimens of nipple drainage when infection is suspected
Teaching aids	For instruction regarding breast self-examination

CLIENT AND ENVIRONMENT

Setting
Well-lit
Private
Warm

Client
Stripped to waist
Seated for first portion of examination; lying down for second portion

Examiner
Standing at front of client for first portion; at right side of client for second portion

Technique for Examination and Expected Findings

Inspection

Inspection and palpation are the techniques used to examine the breast. For initial inspection, the client is seated on the side of the examination table and is uncovered to the waist. If the client reports that she or he has noticed a lump or a change in one of the breasts, ask her or him to point out the area and demonstrate the technique she or he used to feel the lump or change. Take special note of that area during the examination.

Observe the breasts, including the nipples and areolae, for symmetry of shape and size, surface characteristics, and abnormal amount or distribution of hair. As with inspection of all paired organs, use the client as her or his own control and compare both breasts to determine what is "normal" for that individual and to detect any unusual findings for a given individual. Distinct asymmetry always indicates a need for additional assessment.

Cultural Considerations
Biocultural Breast Variations

Breast size, color, and configuration vary widely among women. Women of Asian origin tend to have smaller breasts than other groups. Women of African heritage have a higher prevalence of supernumerary nipples than others. Breast development initiates earlier for African-American girls (average age 8.9 years) than for Caucasian girls (average age 10 years).

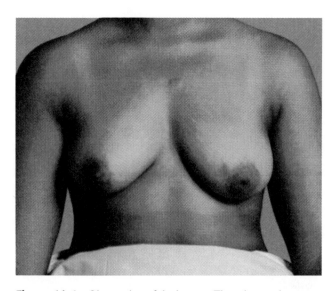

Figure 14-6 Observation of the breasts. These breasts have several characteristics that are deviations within normal limits: (1) the left breast is slightly larger than the right; (2) the nipples are directed in slightly different directions; (3) the left breast has a superficial skin lesion appearing as a dark area medial to the areola; and (4) striae are visible in the upper, inner quadrant of the left breast.

Symmetry of Shape and Size.   Observe the breasts for shape, symmetry, and size. Normal female breasts are bilaterally similar in shape and size and are reasonably symmetrical. However, commonly one breast is somewhat smaller than the other (Figure 14-6). In males, the breasts are normally even with the chest wall, except for obese men, whose breasts assume a bilaterally convex shape similar to that of female breasts.

Surface Characteristics.   Observe the skin and surface characteristics of the anterior thorax and breasts. The surface characteristics of breasts may include hyperpigmentation, moles and nevi, edema, retraction, dimpling, focal vascularity, and lesions. The skin of the breasts should appear smooth, and the surface contour should be even and uninterrupted. Normally, only the areola and the nipple are hyperpigmented. Other portions of the breast are normally a color that is uniform with the individual's skin in other covered parts of the body. Focal hyperpigmentation is an abnormal finding. Moles and nevi are common. The client should be questioned about changes or problems, with any skin lesion noted.

Edema of the breast, usually caused by blocked lymph drainage, produces exaggeration of the skin pores, creating an orange-peel appearance called **peau d'orange** (Figure 14-7, *B*).

Retraction, or dimpling, appears as a depression or pucker on the skin (Figure 14-7, *A*). The fibrotic shortening and immobilization of Cooper's ligament usually cause dimpling or retraction by invasive processes.

Vascular patterns should be diffuse and symmetrical. Hypervascular patterns may be noted in pregnant, obese, and very fair-skinned individuals. Focal or unilateral patterns are abnormal and may be produced by dilated superficial veins from increased blood flow to a malignancy (Figure 14-7, *A*).

The elastic fibers of the dermis may be damaged whenever the skin of the breasts is stretched rapidly, and observable striae, or stretch marks, are produced. Newly created striae are reddish, but they become white with age.

Areolar and Nipple Characteristics.   The areolar area can range from light pink to dark brown, depending on the client's genetic skin color and hormonal influences. In pregnancy, the areolae enlarge and darken. The areolar area is normally round or oval and bilaterally similar. Irregular placement of Montgomery's tubercles is common and normal.

After puberty, women may normally have a scattering of coarse, curly hair on the breasts, mostly near the areola. After puberty, males often have a dense mass of chest hair around the areola. Male hair patterns in female clients are abnormal. The areolar areas should be inspected for size, shape, symmetry, color, surface characteristics, bulging, and lesions. Size, shape, and color can normally vary greatly in symmetrical patterns. Any asymmetry, mass, or lesion should be considered abnormal.

If the breasts are symmetrical, both nipples should be pointing laterally in the same way. The nipples should be inspected for size, shape, ability to become erect, color, discharge, and lesions. The nipples should be round; equal in size; homogeneous in color; and have convoluted surfaces, which produce a wrinkled appearance. They should appear soft and smooth and have no crusting, cracks, or discharge.

Inversion of one or both nipples, if present from puberty, is normal. However, this condition may interfere with breast-feeding. Recent inversion of the nipple is probably retraction (see Figure 14-7, *A*) and should be investigated.

Supernumerary nipples and areolae may appear along the milk lines in about 1% of the population (see Figure 14-3). These lesions can vary in size. They are the color of the individual's actual areolae and are often mistaken for moles. Occasionally, glandular tissue may accompany these lesions.

Paget's disease, a malignant condition requiring prompt therapy, appears as a red glandular erosion of the nipple or as a nipple that is dry, scaly, or friable. The areola may also be affected.

Breast secretions are normal in pregnancy or lactation. Other causes of discharge are mechanical nipple stimulation, drug influence, hypothalamic and pituitary disorders, and malignant and benign breast lesions. The discharge can be milky, watery, purulent, serous, or bloody. The method for determining the origin of discharge production is discussed in the section on palpation.

Sitting Positions for Breast Inspection.   There are four basic sitting positions used for breast inspection. Every adult female client should be examined in each of the following positions:

1. *Client seated with arms at sides* (see Figure 14-6). Observe the breasts at rest and without movement to establish a baseline for comparison. Observe men in this position only, unless they have unusually large breasts, in which case the other inspection positions are also used.
2. *Client seated with arms abducted over head* (Figure 14-8, *A*). This maneuver creates tension on the suspensory ligaments and may accentuate asymmetry, retraction, and fixation.
3. *Client seated and pushing hands into hips* (or pushes palms together) (Figure 14-8, *B* and *C*). This action contracts the pectoral muscles and can reveal dimpling and deviations in symmetry.
4. *Client seated and leaning over* (Figure 14-8, *D*). The examiner assists in supporting and balancing the client during this maneuver. The breasts should hang evenly and symmetrically. This approach is especially useful in examining the movement and contour of large breasts.

While the client is performing these maneuvers, carefully observe the breasts for asymmetry, bulging, retraction, and fixation. An abnormality may not be apparent in the breasts at rest (Figure 14-9, *A*), but a mass may cause a breast, through invasion of suspensory ligaments, to fix, preventing it from upward or forward movements or creating an asymmetrical flattening of one portion of one breast (Figure 14-9, *B*). Tension in the breasts through contraction of the pectoral muscles assists in eliciting dimpling if a mass has infiltrated and shortened suspensory ligaments.

Finally, observe the breasts while the client is lying down, before performing palpation.

Palpation

This portion of the breast examination begins with palpation for axillary, subclavicular, and supraclavicular lymph nodes. This step is most effectively performed with the client in a sitting position.

The underlying tissues in the axilla can be best appreciated if the area muscles are relaxed. Contracted muscles may obscure slightly enlarged nodes. To achieve this relaxation while abducting the arm, support the ipsilateral arm (Figure 14-10). Visualize the axilla as a four-sided pyramid and thoroughly palpate the following areas:

1. *Anterior axillary nodes* (pectoral) lying in the anterior aspect of the axilla and including several nodes found in the region of the third rib and the second and third intercostal spaces and over the fourth and sixth ribs
2. *Lateral axillary nodes* (brachial) along the inside of the humerus (upper arm)
3. *Posterior axillary nodes* (subscapular) lying in the posterior aspect of the axilla along the lateral edge of the scapula

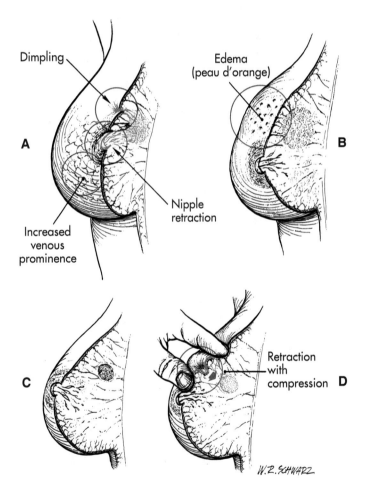

Figure 14-7 Abnormalities of the breast. **A**, Breast with dimpling, nipple retraction, and increased venous prominence. **B**, Breast with edema (peau d'orange or pigskin appearance). **C**, Breast with tumor; no retraction is apparent. **D**, Breast with tumor; retraction is apparent with compression.

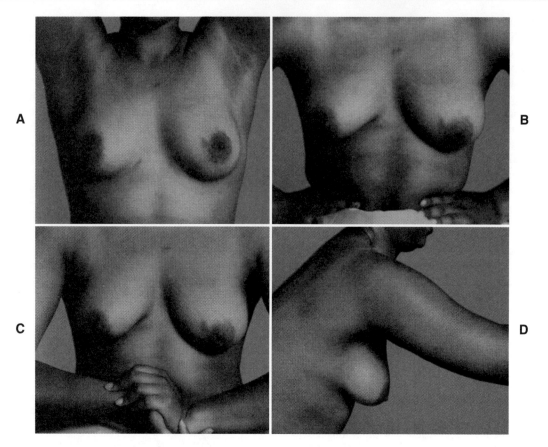

Figure 14-8   Observation of the breasts in several positions. **A,** Observation with the client's arms overhead. **B,** Observation with the client contracting her pectoral muscles by pressing her hands into her waist. **C,** Alternate method of observing the client with pectoral muscle contraction—the client's hands are pressed together in front. **D,** Observation with the client leaning forward.

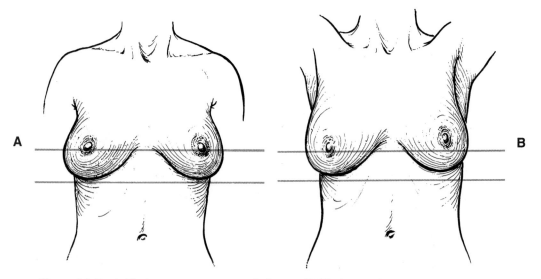

Figure 14-9   **A,** The breasts appear symmetrical at rest. **B,** The breasts do not move symmetrically with arm elevation. The right breast is immobilized.

4. *Central axillary nodes* (intermediate) lying high in the middle of the axilla over the ribs
5. *Apical axillary nodes* (infraclavicular or subclavian) located below the clavicle

Develop a routine system for axillary node examination. Palpate the apical nodes last, since their deep location will require extra pressure in examination. Normally, nodes should not be palpable.

The primary purpose of the palpation of the breasts is to discover masses. If a mass is discovered, assess it according to the characteristics noted in Box 14-1 and shown in Figures 14-11 and 14-12.

The range of normal breast consistency is wide. The normal breast feels somewhat granular and "lumpy." This granularity is generalized and becomes more prominent with age. Breast lumpiness results from the configuration of the breast lobes, the fat and connective tissue between and supporting the lobes and other structures, and the irregular density of lobules. Thus the consistency of breasts is not uniform. However, this variation in consistency should be noted uniformly throughout the breasts of an individual client.

The breasts feel relatively homogeneous in the young adolescent. After menarche the presence of progesterone in pregnancy and premenstrually causes the breasts to feel gen-

BOX 14-1

ASSESSMENT OF BREAST MASSES

1. **Location**: Masses are designated according to the quadrant in which they lie: upper outer, lower outer, upper inner, or lower inner (see Figure 14-11, *A*). To describe the mass in the client's record, it may be helpful to draw the mass within a diagram of the breast (see Figure 14-11, *B*). Another method of describing location is to visualize the breast as the face of a clock with the nipple at the center. For example, in Figure 14-11, *B*, the mass could be described as being 3 cm from the nipple in the 2 o'clock position.
2. **Size**: The size should be approximated in centimeters in all its planes. For example, a mass may be ovoid, 3 cm wide, 2 cm long, and 1 cm thick.
3. **Shape**: The shape may be round, ovoid, irregular, or matted. Matting occurs in the presence of multiple lesions.
4. **Consistency**: The palpable consistency of a breast lesion may be soft, hard, solid, or cystic. One way to evaluate the consistency of a breast lesion is to palpate over the lesion with the pads of the index and middle fingers of the palpating hand (see Figure 14-12, *A*).
5. **Discreteness**: The borders of a mass are assessed to determine whether they are sharp and well defined or irregular. To assess discreteness, an attempt is made to palpate all the borders of the mass with the thumb and index finger of the palpating hand (see Figure 14-12, *B*).
6. **Mobility**: The mobility of the mass within the breast is assessed as freely movable or fixed. To assess mobility, the thumb and index finger of the examining hand are used to "hold" the mass, and then the mass is moved in all directions possible (see Figure 14-12, *C*).
7. **Tenderness**: The client is questioned regarding any discomfort with palpation.
8. **Erythema**: The area of skin overlying the mass is inspected for erythema.
9. **Dimpling over the mass**: The tissue over the mass is compressed to determine whether this maneuver produces dimpling (see Figure 14-7, *D*).
10. **Depth of mass**: The location of the mass is determined in reference to the surface of the breast. Is the mass close to the surface at midlevel or deep against the chest wall?

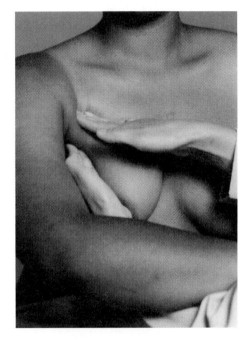

Figure 14-10 Palpation of the axillary lymph nodes. (Note that the client's arm is supported on the examiner's arm.)

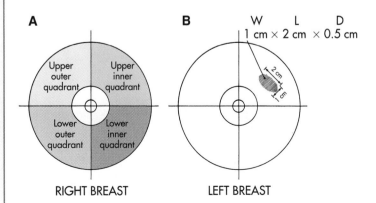

Figure 14-11 **A**, The four quadrants of the breast. **B**, Diagram of a mass within a breast.

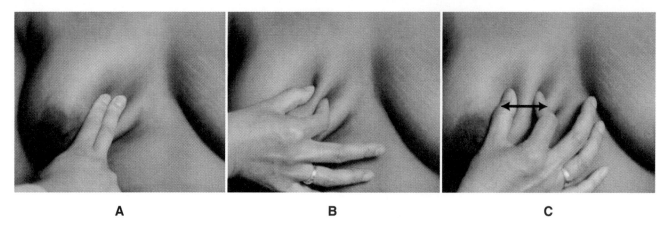

A   **B**   **C**

Figure 14-12 **A**, Palpating for consistency of breast lesion. **B**, Palpating for delineation of borders of breast mass. **C**, Palpating for mobility of breast mass.

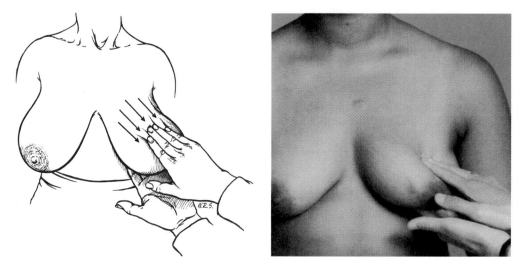

Figure 14-13 Bimanual palpation of the breasts.

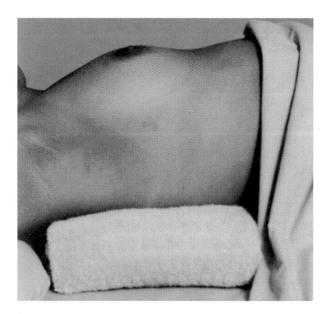

Figure 14-14 Use of a towel to shift breast tissue evenly over the chest for effective palpation.

erally nodular. Hormonally induced nodularity is bilateral and diffuse.

The breasts are palpated most effectively with the client in a supine position. Because of time constraints on most physical examinations, it is not advised that all clients also undergo palpation in a sitting position. However, certain groups of clients should also have breast palpation done in the sitting position: women with present or past complaints of breast masses, women at high risk of breast cancer, and women with large and/or pendulous breasts.

If the breasts are to be examined with the client in a sitting position, small breasts can be examined by using one hand to support the breast and the other hand to palpate the tissue against the chest wall. For palpation of pendulous breasts, use a bimanual technique (Figure 14-13). Support the inferior portion of the breast in one hand while using the other hand to palpate breast tissue against the supporting hand.

With the client lying down, palpate the breasts while they are flattened against the rib cage. If the breasts are large, several methods can be used to enhance flattening. A small pillow or a rolled towel can be placed under the ipsilateral up-

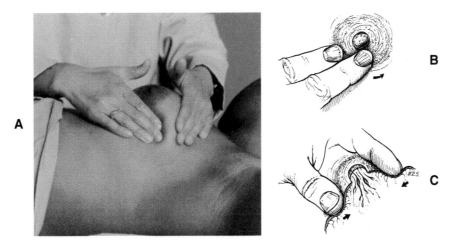

Figure 14-15   Palpation of the breasts. **A**, Glandular areas. **B**, Areolar area. **C**, Compression of the nipple.

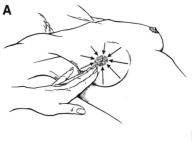

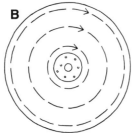

Figure 14-16   Two methods of systematic breast palpation. **A**, Palpation in wedge sections from breast periphery to center. **B**, Palpation along concentric circles from periphery to center.

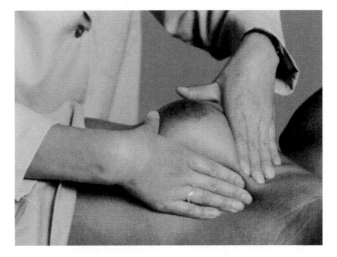

Figure 14-17   Palpation of the axillary tail of Spence.

per back, or the client can abduct the ipsilateral arm and place her hand under her neck (Figure 14-14). Both maneuvers shift the breast medially. For all clients, the humerus should be at least slightly abducted to allow for thorough palpation of the tail of Spence.

Thoroughly palpate the breasts and the tail of Spence areas with the palmar surfaces of the three middle fingers held together (Figure 14-15, *A*). The movements should be smooth and should be done in a back-and-forth or circular motion. Press firmly enough to fully appreciate the underlying tissue, but not so firmly that the tissue is compressed against the rib cage.

Develop a system of breast examination and habitually start and end at a fixed point on the breasts. The important principle is development of a system that ensures a thorough examination of all breast tissues. Several examination patterns have been recommended:

1. The breast is visualized as a round wheel with multiple spokes. Palpation is done along each spoke until the breast has been thoroughly surveyed (Figure 14-16, *A*).

2. The breast is viewed as a group of concentric circles with the nipple as the center. Palpation is performed along the circumferences of the circles, starting at the outermost circle, until the total breast area has been adequately surveyed (Figure 14-16, *B*).

3. Palpation of the breast is done in vertical or horizontal sections, starting immediately below the clavicle at the sternal border and proceeding downward and upward, parallel to the sternal border, or side-to-side until the entire breast has been surveyed.

Whatever system and sequence of examination is used, a thorough examination of all breast tissue and the tail of Spence is critical. Special attention should be focused on the upper outer quadrant area and the tail of Spence because approximately half of all breast cancers develop in those areas (Figure 14-17).

Carefully palpate the areolar areas to determine the presence of underlying masses (see Figure 14-15, *B*). Gently compress each nipple to assess for the presence of masses and discharge (see Figure 14-15, *C*). If discharge is noted, milk the breast along its radii to identify the lobe from which the discharge is originating. Compression of the discharge-producing lobe will cause discharge to exude from the nipple. If the nipple discharge is not associated with expected changes in pregnancy or the postpartum period, collect a specimen of the discharge on a slide according to local health care system protocols. Nipple discharge, which is often thin and cellular, is most effectively collected on a frosted or albumin-coated slide to prevent runoff. When discharge is present on the nipple, bring the slide in contact with the nipple and rub it across the nipple, allowing the discharge to collect across the slide. Immediately apply cytology fixative to the slide. In addition, if infection is suspected, a culture and slide for infective organism identification may be prepared.

If a client reports a breast mass, examine the "normal" breast first so that the baseline consistency of that breast will serve as a control for palpation of the reportedly abnormal one.

Mammary folds, or crescent-shaped ridges of breast tissue found at the inferior portions of very large or pendulous breasts, may be confused with breast masses, but they are nonpathological. They are palpated as somewhat superficial thickened ridges of breast tissue bilaterally along the undersides of the breasts.

The complete sequence of the breast examination is illustrated in Figure 14-18.

Special Breast Examinations

The Male Breast

The routine male breast examination consists of the following steps:
1. Inspection of the breast areas, nipples, and areolae for nodules, swelling, and lesions while the client is in a *sitting position*
2. Palpation of the axillary nodes
3. Palpation of the breast areas, areolae, and nipples while the client is *lying down*

Observe the breast areas with the client sitting with arms at rest for swelling and lesions. The other sitting positions that are used to examine the woman are unnecessary unless the man has large breasts. Perform the axillary examination using the same technique as described for women. Palpate the breasts, nipples, and areolae for nodules while the client is supine, as with the female client.

Male breast cancer, which occurs most commonly in the areolar area, accounts for approximately 1% of all breast cancers. Every male client should be given a thorough breast examination with an adaptation of the technique used for female clients.

Gynecomastia, or enlargement of the male breast, is a commonly occurring, multicausal condition. Causes include pubertal changes, hormonal administration, cirrhosis, leukemia, thyrotoxicosis, and drugs.

Client Who Has Had a Mastectomy

The client who has had a mastectomy has special examination needs. This client may be embarrassed about the condition of the surgical site and apprehensive about the examination of the remaining breast. Perform the inspection and palpation portions of the examination on the unaffected side as described for the routine examination. Inspect the mastectomy scar; surrounding areas; and axilla for swelling, lumps, redness, color changes, and skin lesions. Note the extent of muscle mass and edema and the general appearance and condition of the scar. Palpate the scar with the palmar surface of two fingers of the examining hand with a back-and-forth or circular motion to detect any swelling, lumps, and tenderness. Then systematically and thoroughly palpate the axillary and chest lymph node areas and surrounding tissue. Emphasize the importance of breast self-examination with these clients.

Client Who Has Had Beast Reconstruction, Augmentation, or a Lumpectomy

Examine the breasts in the usual manner, giving special attention to scars. Emphasize the need for breast self-examination with these clients.

Screening Tests and Procedures

Mammography

Mammography is the major method of detecting nonpalpable breast lesions as well as the differential diagnosis of palpable breast lesions. Since nonpalpable cancerous lesions are generally small, and local when found early, survival rates are increased through early detection and intervention. The performance and interpretation of mammograms require specialized skill.

The recommendations for mammography screening tests vary somewhat among health authorities. *Healthy People 2010* (2000) has established the following objective for the year 2010: That 70% of women ages 40 and older will have received a mammogram within the preceding 2 years. The 1998 baseline for this percentage was 68%.

The U.S. Preventive Services Task Force (1996) recommends the following schedule for routine breast cancer screening:

Women ages 40 to 49 or age 70 and older: Insufficient evidence exists to recommend for or against the use of clinical breast examination (CBE) alone or the teaching of breast self-examination. Women with increased risk may require more frequent or additional screening.

Women ages 50 to 69: Routine screening for breast cancer every 1 to 2 years with mammography alone or mammography and annual CBE.

The American Cancer Society recommends yearly mammograms for women starting at age 40. At present, the following screening schedule is recommended in clinical practice:

Mammogram:	From ages 40 to 50, once every 1 to 2 years
	From age 50 on, every year
CBE:	Same schedule as mammogram and performed in conjunction with the mammogram
Self-examination:	Monthly

Since the initiation of mammography screening services, recommended schedules for mammography have changed as research has produced new knowledge related to the risk

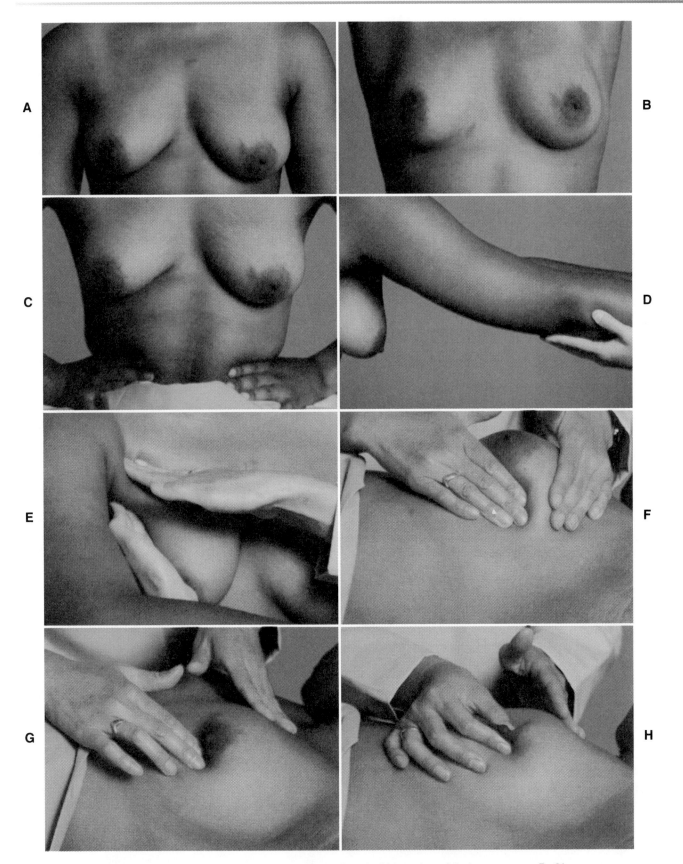

Figure 14-18 Sequence of the breast examination. **A**, Observation of the breasts at rest. **B**, Observation with client's arms overhead. **C**, Observation with client contracting pectoral muscles by pressing hands into waist. **D**, Observation with client leaning forward. **E**, Palpation of axillary nodes. **F**, Palpation of the glandular area. **G**, Palpation of the areolar area. **H**, Palpation of the nipple.

for and detection of breast cancer, as well as the cost-benefit of screening various populations. New knowledge about the development of breast cancer and safe mechanisms for early detection and treatment may affect future guidelines for mammography screening schedules. The practitioner working with adult women clients should be alert to possible changes in screening guidelines.

Genetic Testing

The field of genetic testing for genetic susceptibility to various diseases is a rapidly growing field. The practitioner should keep up with this literature and refer high-risk clients for genetic counseling regarding breast cancer risk.

Examination Step-by-Step

Client: Seated and uncovered to waist
Examiner: Standing in front of client

INSPECTION

1. Skin of anterior thorax—color, vascular patterns, bulging, lesions, and symmetry
2. Breast and areolar size—symmetry, configuration, and surface characteristics
3. Nipple configuration and plane
4. Symmetry of movement when arms are raised over head
5. Retraction of breast tissue through contraction of pectoral muscles
6. Symmetry of movement and retraction when client leans forward
7. Skin of axilla

PALPATION

1. Axillary nodes: Begin along inner aspect of arm and proceed to chest wall, anterior axilla, posterior axilla, and apex of axilla. (Supraclavicular and infraclavicular nodes can be palpated in conjunction with axillary nodes or with the head and neck examination.)
2. Palpate breasts (1) if unusual symptoms or inspection findings are noted, (2) if client is at risk for breast disease, or (3) if breasts are unusually large.

Client: Lying on back
Examiner: To right of client

INSPECTION

1. Skin of thorax
2. Surface characteristics of breasts

PALPATION

1. Palpate breasts to determine consistency of tissue and presence of masses.
2. Palpate areolar areas for masses.
3. Palpate nipples and compress to determine presence of discharge.

TEACHING

1. Review client's technique of breast self-examination or teach breast self-examination.

VARIATIONS FROM HEALTH

The most common variations in breast health are noted in the form of breast lumps. The various causes of breast lumps are listed in Table 14-1, and the most common causes are discussed in this section. See Figure 14-19 for a visual representation of the common characteristic of breast masses. However, be advised that diagnosis is made by mammography and laboratory techniques rather than clinical examination.

Benign Lesions

The most commonly seen benign breast lesions are those associated with fibrocystic disease (also known as benign breast disease) and **fibroadenomas**.

Fibrocystic disease, noted as an exaggeration of the normal changes in the breasts during the menstrual cycle, is eventually characterized by the formation of single or multiple cysts in the breasts. Fibrocystic disease develops in the following three stages:

1. The first stage, called *mazoplasia*, occurs in the late teens and early 20s. It is characterized by painful, tender, premenstrual breast swelling (chiefly in the axillary tails) that subsides after menses.
2. The second stage occurs in the late 20s and early 30s. The breasts exhibit multinodular changes, and sometimes a dominant mass occurs, which is usually described as a thickness rather than a lump.

TABLE 14-1   Common Causes of Breast Lumps

Origin	Lesion Type
Normal structures	Nodularity
	Prominent fat lobule
	Prominent rib
	Edge of biopsy wound
Aberrations of normal development and involution	Fibroadenoma
	Cyclical nodularity
	Cyst
	Sclerosing adenosis
Inflammatory processes	Chronic infected abscess
	Fat necrosis
	Foreign body granuloma
Benign tumors	Duct papilloma
	Giant fibroadenoma
	Lipoma
	Granular cell myoblastoma
Malignant tumors	Carcinoma in situ
	Primary tumor
	Secondary tumor
Lesions of nipple and areola	Squamous papilloma
	Leiomyoma
	Retention cyst
	Papillary adenoma
Skin lesions	Sebaceous cyst
	Benign and malignant skin tumors

Modified from Hughes LE, Mansel RE, Webster DJT: *Benign disorders and diseases of the breast*, London, 1989, Baillière Tindall.

3. The third stage involves the development of cysts. A sudden dull pain, a full feeling, or a burning sensation in the breast often precedes the onset of cyst formation.

The lesions of fibrocystic disease are commonly bilateral, multiple, painful, tender, well delineated, and slightly mobile. The associated tenderness and the size of the lesions increase premenstrually.

Fibroadenomas are benign lesions that contain both fibrous and glandular tissues. They are usually solitary and unilateral. In general, they are palpated as round, mobile, solid, firm, rubbery, regular, well-delineated, nontender, and painless lumps. Fibroadenomas are usually found in women between the ages of 15 and 35 and do not change with the menstrual cycle.

Breast Cancer

Although certain breast lesions have characteristic findings on inspection and palpation, diagnosis is not made by clinical examination but by surgical procedures, laboratory examinations, and mammography. Therefore the practitioner is encouraged to learn the distinguishing characteristics of breast lesions but not to rely on them for diagnosis.

The lesions of breast cancer are often solitary, unilateral, solid, hard, irregular, poorly delineated, nonmobile, painless, nontender, and located in the upper outer quadrants. In advanced stages, breast cancer is accompanied by retraction of breast tissue or nipples on observation or with tissue compression, dimpling, edema, variations of contour, unilateral nipple inversion, and scaly nipple lesions. Breast cancer is a leading cause of death in women in the United States and also a leading cause of cancer morbidity. On average, 1 of every 8 to 10 women will develop breast cancer. Knowledge of the factors indicating that a woman is at a higher-than-usual risk of cancer can assist in decision-making about screening programs and the frequency of general physical examinations.

See the Risk Factors box regarding breast cancer in women on p. 298. For women at increased risk, monthly self-examination should be emphasized. Such women should receive a thorough breast screening examination at least once a year.

TEACHING SELF-ASSESSMENT
Breast Self-Examination and Health Promotion

Despite improved mammography techniques and their availability, a substantial portion of malignant breast lesions are found by women themselves. Women who perform regular breast self-examinations become very familiar with the inspection and palpatory findings within their own breasts and can note any changes immediately. Therefore the health-oriented examiner should assess each client's level of knowledge and practices related to monthly breast self-examination and encourage monthly self-examination. During examination of the breasts, the examiner describes the steps of the examination and the rationale for each step. Use of visual aids, models, pamphlets, and other materials can be valuable additions to demonstrations. A return demonstration by the client on her own breasts reinforces the client's learning and memory of the procedure. See the Teaching Breast Self-Examination box for tips and a procedure for teaching breast self-examination.

In addition to breast self-examination, clients should be advised about the following general activities for breast health promotion:
1. Maintain normal body weight
2. Reduce dietary fat
3. Have an annual breast examination by a health care professional
4. Have mammograms as appropriate for age and risk

Women at high risk should be counseled about chemoprevention and genetic screening.

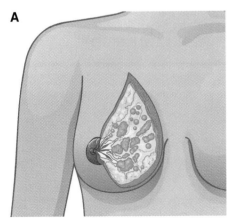
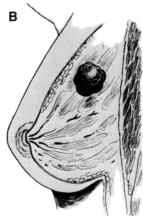

Figure 14-19 Illustration of the common presentation of breast masses. **A,** Benign breast disease (fibrocystic breast disease). **B,** Fibroadenoma. (From Wilson SF, Giddens JF: *Health assessment for nursing practice,* ed. 2, St. Louis, 2001, Mosby.)

Teaching Self-Assessment

BREAST SELF-EXAMINATION

The following points should be emphasized in the teaching of breast self-examination:

1. The majority of breast lumps are not cancerous.
2. The majority of cancerous breast lesions are curable.
3. Breasts should be examined each month between the 4th through the 14th days of the menstrual cycle, when the breasts are least congested. If, for any reason, menses are not present, a specific date of each month should be chosen for the monthly breast examination (e.g., the date of the client's birthday).
4. Visual inspection and palpation should be done.
5. Visual inspection should be done in four arm positions with the woman stripped to the waist and looking at herself in a mirror. The four arm positions are arms at rest; hands on hips and pressed into hips, contracting chest muscles; hands over head; and arms forward with the torso leaning forward.
6. Many women prefer to do palpation in the shower because the soap and water help the hands to glide easily over the skin. However, the examination of large breasts and the axilla are better done in a supine than in a standing position; therefore an examination done in the supine position is recommended in addition to the examination done in the bath or shower.
7. Each entire breast should be palpated in a systematic way.
8. Specific palpation of the nipple (through compression for discharge) and the areola (through palpation) should not be forgotten.
9. Any change should be reported to a health care provider as soon as possible.

Additional Information For Special Situations

Client with a unilateral or bilateral mastectomy: Palpate the area of the scar and the surrounding tissue monthly for any changes.

Client with breast implants: Do the breast examination monthly. Get a sense of the feel of the breasts with implants and report any changes to the primary care provider.

Sample Documentation and Diagnoses

FOCUSED HEALTH HISTORY (SUBJECTIVE DATA)

Mrs. R., a 40-year-old white female, noted a small lump, about the "size of a dime," in the areolar area of the right breast 2 weeks ago in breast self-examination, routinely done on day 7 of the menstrual cycle. No change in the lump since discovery. Denies pain, swelling, change in appearance of the breast, or discharge. No history of breast lesions. No hormonal medications taken. Last clinical breast examination was 9 months ago. Has never had a mammogram. Menses are regular; onset was at age 13. Had two pregnancies, delivered at full term 7 (age 33) and 5 (age 35) years ago, and successfully breast-fed each baby for 6 months. One maternal aunt had breast cancer at age 50 and died within 1 year of diagnosis. Is very concerned about breast cancer.

FOCUSED PHYSICAL EXAMINATION (OBJECTIVE DATA)

Inspection: Right breast slightly larger than left breast. Bilaterally similar in surface characteristics, plane of nipple, and mobility. Skin smooth with no unusual vascular patterns. No lesions, erythema, dimpling, or retraction.

Palpation: Right breast—regular, round, movable mass, approximately 0.25 × 0.25 × 0.5 cm, palpated in left lower quadrant at 5 o'clock position approximately 1 cm from center of nipple. Borders are well defined; mass is soft and cystic. Appears to be very close to skin surface. Not tender on palpation or movement. Left breast—soft, slightly nodular throughout. No masses or tenderness.

Lymph nodes: No axillary, infraclavicular, or supraclavicular nodes palpated. No tenderness in lymph node areas.

DIAGNOSES

HEALTH PROBLEM

Mass in right breast

NURSING DIAGNOSIS

Anxiety Related to Concern About Breast Cancer

Defining Characteristics

- Fear of diagnosis of cancer
- Concern about family history of breast cancer

? Critical Thinking Questions

Review the Sample Documentation and Diagnoses box to answer questions 1 and 2.

1. What is the risk for breast cancer in this client?
2. Given the breast lump characteristics outlined, what is the most likely diagnosis?
3. While examining a male client, he shares that both of his sisters have been recently diagnosed with breast cancer. He asks about his risks for the disease and mechanisms of prevention. What would you tell him?
4. A 14-year-old client has a small nipple, which is flush with the breast. The breast and areolar areas are very slightly developed. She asks whether her development is normal. How would you respond?

MERLIN   Answers are available on the MERLIN website (www.harcourthealth.com/MERLIN/Barkauskas/). And be sure to check the website regularly for additional learning activities!

Remember to check out the Online Study Guide!
www.harcourthealth.com/MERLIN/Barkauskas/

Respiratory System

Learning Objectives

On successful study of this chapter and completion of related learning experiences, the learner will be able to:
- Describe the anatomy and physiology of the respiratory system.
- Outline the history relevant to the respiratory system, including exploration of common complaints.
- Explain the rationale for and perform the assessment of the respiratory system using inspection, palpation, percussion, and auscultation techniques.

- Recognize characteristics associated with normal and abnormal fremitus, percussion tones, and breath sounds.
- Describe the origin and characteristics of adventitious sounds.
- Describe findings frequently associated with common lung conditions.

Outline

Purpose of Examination

The purpose of the respiratory examination is to assess the organs and structures of the respiratory system and the functioning of the system as a whole. Because the respiratory system functions in close relationship with the cardiovascular system, these systems are often examined together. The physical examination is accomplished through inspection, percussion, palpation, and auscultation.

ANATOMY AND PHYSIOLOGY

The major functions of the respiratory system are to supply the body with oxygen and to eliminate carbon dioxide. These tasks are accomplished through the complex cooperation of many body systems that, in wellness, act in harmony. The actual transfer of oxygen and carbon dioxide between environmental gas and body liquid occurs in the alveoli, which are not accessible to clinical examination. However, assessment of respiratory efficiency is accomplished by direct and indirect appraisal of structures that support alveolar function.

Thoracic Cage

The thoracic cage is a bony, semirigid structure consisting of a skeleton of 12 thoracic vertebrae, 12 pairs of ribs, the sternum, the diaphragm, and the intercostal muscles (Figure 15-1). The skeletal components of the thoracic cage are the ribs, the sternum, and the vertebrae. The ribs are paired. Anteriorly, the costal cartilages of the first seven ribs articulate with the body of the sternum. The costal cartilages of the eighth to the tenth ribs are attached to the costal cartilages immediately superior to the ribs. The eleventh and twelfth ribs, the "floating ribs," are unattached anteriorly. The tips of the eleventh ribs are lo-

cated in the lateral thorax; the tips of the twelfth ribs are found in the posterior thorax. Posteriorly, all ribs articulate with the thoracic vertebrae.

In the adult the sternum is approximately 17 cm long and consists of three parts: the manubrium, the body, and the xiphoid process. The manubrium of the sternum articulates with and supports the clavicle. The manubrium and the body of the sternum articulate with the first seven ribs. None of the ribs articulates with the xiphoid. The angle of Louis, an important anatomical landmark, is the junction of the manubrium and the body of the sternum (manubriosternal junction). The second rib attaches to the sternum at the angle of Louis.

The spaces between the ribs are termed **intercostal spaces**. Each space is named according to the rib immediately superior to it; for example, the space between the second and third ribs is designated as the second intercostal space.

Thoracic Cavity and Contents

The thoracic cavity and contents are divided into two distinct (right and left) pleural cavities, which are separated by the **mediastinum**, which contains the heart and the other structures that connect the head with the abdomen. The pleural cavities are lined by serous membranes—the parietal and visceral pleurae. The parietal pleura lines the chest wall and the diaphragm; the visceral pleura covers the outside of the lung. The potential space between the pleurae contains a small amount of lubricating fluid.

The lungs are paired, asymmetrical, conical organs that conform to the shape of the thoracic cavity. The right lung contains three lobes, and the left lung has two lobes.

Air reaches the lungs through a system of flexible tubes. It enters through the mouth or the nose, passes through the respiratory portion of the larynx, and reaches the trachea. The trachea, approximately 10 to 11 cm long in the adult, begins at the lower border of the cricoid cartilage in the neck and divides into a left and right bronchus, usually at the level of T4 or T5 posteriorly and slightly below the manubriosternal junction anteriorly.

The right bronchus is shorter, wider, and more vertical than the left bronchus. The bronchial structures are subdivided into increasingly smaller bronchi and bronchioles. Each bronchiole opens into an alveolar duct from which multiple alveoli radiate (Figure 15-2). In the adult, the lungs contain approximately 300 million alveoli.

The bronchi have both transport and protective purposes. They form the pathway through which air is transported into and out of the lungs. In addition, they protect the respiratory system by filtering the air. The bronchial cavities contain mucus, which entraps foreign particles. This mucus is continuously swept into the throat by ciliary movement and then is eliminated.

Two types of muscles are used in respiration: primary and accessory (Figure 15-3). The diaphragm and the external intercostal muscles are the primary muscles of respiration. The accessory muscles of respiration can be used to fa-

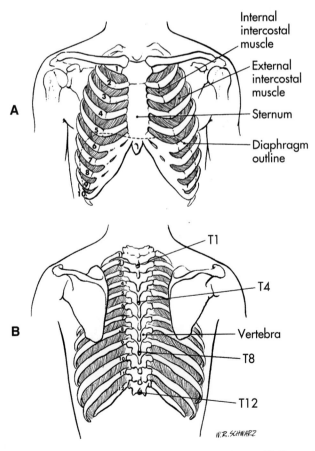

Figure 15-1 Thoracic cage. **A,** Anterior thorax. **B,** Posterior thorax.

cilitate or increase inspiration (i.e., assist in raising the ribs and the sternum) or to force expiration in both health and disease. The accessory muscles of respiration are the scalene muscles and the parasternal intercostal muscles.

The thoracic cage is perpetually moving throughout the inspiratory and expiratory phases of respiration (Figure 15-4).

During inspiration, the diaphragm descends and flattens, and the intercostal muscles contract. Both the diameter and the length of the thorax are increased. These maneuvers produce differences in pressure among the areas of the mouth, the alveoli, and the pleural cavities, and air moves into the lungs. The intrathoracic pressure is decreased, the lungs are ex-

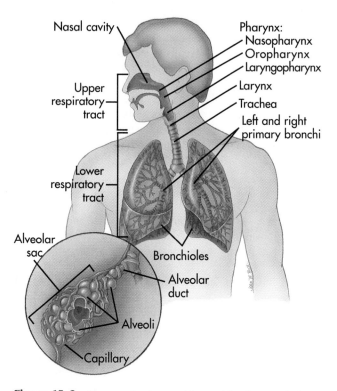

Figure 15-2   Pharynx, trachea, and lungs. Alveolar sacs in *inset*. (From Thibodeau GA, Patton KT: *Anatomy and physiology*, ed. 4, St. Louis, 1999, Mosby.)

BOX 15-1

IMPORTANT LANDMARKS AND LINES

ANTERIOR THORAX

Angle of Louis: junction between the manubrium and the body of the sternum
Midsternal line: vertical, down the midline of the sternum
Midclavicular lines: vertical, parallel to the midsternal line, beginning at the midclavicles
Anterior axillary lines: vertical, parallel to the midsternal line, beginning at the anterior axillary folds
Costal angle: intersection of the costal margins at the sternum, normally < 90 degrees

POSTERIOR THORAX

Vertebra prominens: spinous process of the seventh cervical vertebra
Midspinal line: vertical, down the spinal processes
Scapular lines: vertical, parallel to the midspinal line, through the inferior angle of the scapula when client erect
Posterior axillary lines: vertical, parallel to the midspinal line, beginning at the posterior axillary folds

LATERAL THORAX

Midaxillary lines: vertical, parallel to the anterior and posterior axillary lines, beginning at the midaxilla

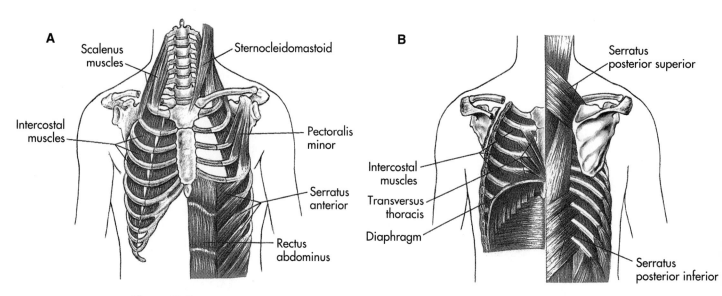

Figure 15-3   Muscles of ventilation. **A**, Anterior view. **B**, Posterior view. (From Seidel HM et al.: *Mosby's guide to physical examination*, ed. 4, St. Louis, 1999, Mosby.)

panded, and the ribs flare, increasing the diameter of the thorax. The second to the sixth ribs move around two axes in a motion commonly termed the "pump handle" movement. The lower ribs move in a "bucket handle" motion. Because of the length and positioning of the lower ribs and because the lower interspaces are wider, the amplitude of movement is greater in the lower thorax.

Expiration is a relatively passive phenomenon. At the completion of inspiration, the diaphragm relaxes and the elastic recoil properties of the lungs expel air and pull the diaphragm to its resting position.

Topographical Anatomy

The topographical, or surface, landmarks of the thorax are helpful in identifying the location of the internal underlying structures and in describing the exact location of physical findings (Figure 15-5; Box 15-1).

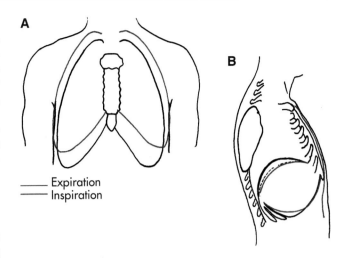

Figure 15-4 Movement of the thorax during respiration. **A,** Anterior thorax. **B,** Lateral thorax.

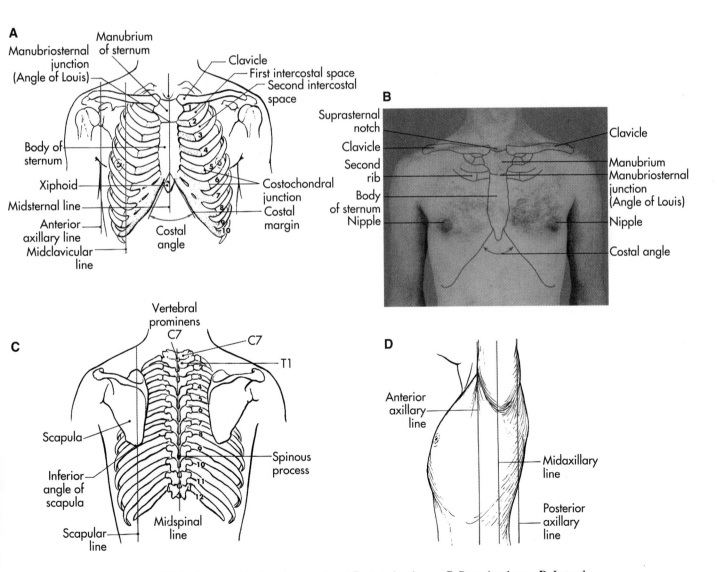

Figure 15-5 Topographical landmarks. **A** and **B,** Anterior thorax. **C,** Posterior thorax. **D,** Lateral thorax.

Manubriosternal Junction (Angle of Louis)

The manubriosternal junction is the articulation between the manubrium and the body of the sternum. Also called the angle of Louis, this junction is a visible and palpable angulation of the sternum. It is an extremely useful aid in the location of underlying structures. Just under the angle of Louis, the trachea bifurcates into the right and left main bronchi.

The superior border of the second rib articulates with the sternum at the manubriosternal junction. Palpation can be started at this junction, with distal ribs and rib interspaces counted from this point. As noted earlier, the number given to an intercostal space corresponds to the number of the rib immediately superior to that space. In palpation done for rib identification, the second intercostal space should first be identified at the sternum. Then palpation should be done along the midclavicular line, rather than at the sternal border, for the remaining ribs and interspaces. The rib cartilages are very close at the sternum and consequently are difficult to differentiate; the cartilages of only the first seven ribs attach directly to the sternum.

Suprasternal Notch

The suprasternal notch is the depression above the manubrium at the top of the sternum.

Costal Angle

The costal angle, which is formed by the intersection of the costal margins, normally measures 90 degrees or less.

Midsternal Line

The midsternal line is an imaginary line drawn through the middle of the sternum.

Midclavicular Lines

The midclavicular lines are left and right imaginary lines drawn through the midpoints of the clavicles and parallel to the midsternal line.

Anterior Axillary Lines

The anterior axillary lines are left and right imaginary lines drawn vertically from the anterior axillary folds, along the anterolateral chest, and parallel to the midsternal line.

Vertebra Prominens (Seventh Cervical Vertebra)

When the client flexes the neck anteriorly and the posterior thorax is noted, a prominent spinous process can be observed and palpated. This structure is the seventh cervical vertebra. If two spinous processes are observed and palpated, the superior one is C7 and the inferior one is T1. The counting of ribs is more difficult on the posterior thorax than on the anterior thorax. The spinous processes of the vertebrae can be counted relatively easily from C7 to T4. From T4 the spinous processes project obliquely, causing the spinous process of the vertebra to lie over the rib below it rather than over its correspondingly numbered rib. For example, the spinous process of T5 lies over the body of T6 and is adjacent to the sixth rib.

Midspinal Line

The midspinal line is an imaginary line that runs vertically along the posterior spinous processes of the vertebrae.

Scapular Lines

The scapular lines are left and right imaginary lines that lie vertically and are parallel to the midspinal line. They pass through the inferior angles of the scapulae when the client stands erect with the arms at the sides.

Posterior Axillary Lines

The posterior axillary lines are imaginary left and right lines drawn vertically from the posterior axillary folds along the posterolateral wall of the thorax when the lateral arm is abducted directly from the lateral chest wall.

Midaxillary Lines

The midaxillary lines are imaginary left and right lines drawn vertically from the apices of the axillae. They lie approximately midway between the anterior and the posterior axillary lines and run parallel to them.

Underlying Thoracic Structures

When examining the respiratory system, it is important to maintain a mental image of the placement of the organs and organ parts of the respiratory system and the other systems located in the thoracic area (Figures 15-6 through 15-9).

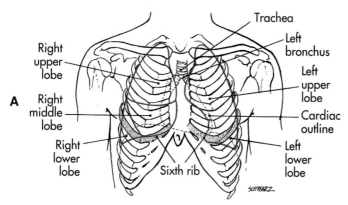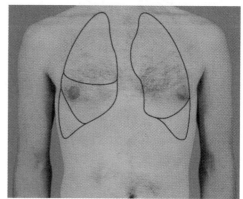

Figure 15-6 Anterior thorax. **A,** Internal organs and structures. **B,** Lung borders.

Lung Borders

In the anterior thorax the apices of the lungs extend approximately 2 to 4 cm above the clavicles. The inferior borders of the lungs cross the sixth rib at the midclavicular line. In the posterior thorax the apices extend to T1. The lower borders vary with respiration and usually extend from the spinous process of T10 on expiration to the spinous process of T12 on deep inspiration. In the lateral thorax the lung extends from the apex of the axilla to the eighth rib of the midaxillary line.

Lung Fissures

The right oblique (diagonal) fissure extends from the area of the spinous process of the third thoracic vertebra laterally and downward until it crosses the fifth rib at the right midaxillary line. It then continues anteriorly and medially to end at the sixth rib at the right midclavicular line. The right horizontal fissure extends from the fifth rib slightly posterior to the right midaxillary line and runs horizontally to the area of the fourth rib at the right sternal border. The left oblique (diagonal) fissure extends from the spinous process of the third thoracic

vertebra laterally and downward to the left midaxillary line at the fifth rib. It continues anteriorly and medially until it terminates at the sixth rib in the left midclavicular line.

Borders of the Diaphragm

Anteriorly, on expiration, the right dome of the diaphragm is located at the level of the fifth rib at the midclavicular line, and the left dome is situated at the level of the sixth rib. Posteriorly, on expiration, the diaphragm is at the level of the spinous process of T10; laterally it is at the eighth rib at the midaxillary line. On nonlabored inspiration, the diaphragm moves approximately 1.5 cm downward, with the right side being slightly higher than the left side because of the placement of the liver. With forced inspiration and expiration, the diaphragmatic excursion can be increased to 3 to 5 cm.

Trachea

The bifurcation of the trachea occurs approximately just below the manubriosternal junction anteriorly and at the spinous process of T4 posteriorly.

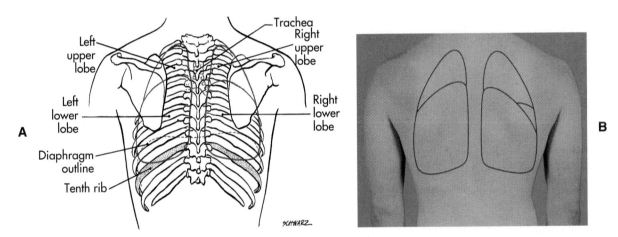

Figure 15-7 Posterior thorax. **A**, Internal organs and structures. **B**, Lung borders.

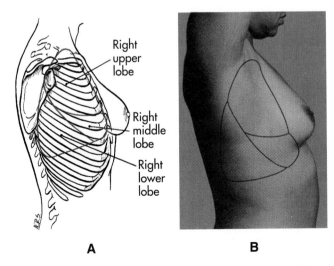

Figure 15-8 Right lateral thorax. **A**, Internal organs and chest structures. (Note the relationship of the breast to chest organs and structures.) **B**, Lung borders.

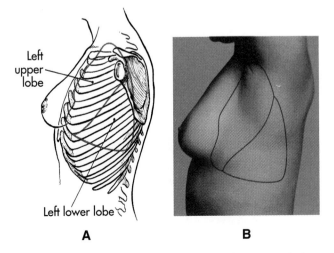

Figure 15-9 Left lateral thorax. **A**, Internal organs and chest structures. **B**, Lung borders.

EXAMINATION

Focused Health History

If a possible respiratory system problem is being investigated, the history of the respiratory system and the cardiovascular system should be taken together because of the symbiotic nature of the two systems, their sharing of the thoracic region of the body, and the potential effect that intervention directed at one system may have on the other system. However, the health history presented here focuses on the respiratory system.

Present Health/Illness Status

1. Allergies, food, plant materials, pets, environmental substances, medications
    a. Specific allergen
    b. Manifestation
    c. Treatment and effect of treatment
2. Tobacco use
    a. Type of tobacco(s) smoked, age at which smoking was started, amount of smoking (packs per day), duration of habit (number of years) (a smoking index can be determined by multiplying the number of years of smoking by the number of packs smoked per day [e.g., 14 yrs x 2 ppd = 28 pack years])
    b. Exposure to smoke of others
    c. History of attempts to quit, and cessation methods tried
3. Medications: types, including prescription and over-the-counter, and patterns of use
4. Recent screening or diagnostic assessments: allergy tests, skin tests, chest x-ray examinations
5. Nutritional data
    a. Sudden weight loss or gain
    b. Adequacy of diet
6. Exercise patterns
7. Use of alcohol and other substances
8. Use of aerosols or inhalants for any purpose
9. Environmental exposures to chemicals or dusts
10. Disabilities
11. Frequent colds or other infections
12. Recent changes in energy

13. Chills, fever, sweats
14. Use of oxygen or any other respiratory assistive devices or medications

Past Health History

1. Respiratory infections and diseases: type, frequency, pattern, and treatment (specific inquiry should include past history of tuberculosis, chronic obstructive pulmonary diseases [e.g., asthma, emphysema, chronic bronchitis])
2. Trauma to respiratory system or area
3. Surgery to respiratory system or area
4. Chronic conditions of other systems: cardiac diseases, malignancies, and renal diseases

Family Health History

1. Tuberculosis
2. Emphysema
3. Lung cancer
4. Allergies, asthma, atopic dermatitis
5. Cystic fibrosis

Personal Health History

1. Place and nature of work; exposure to chemicals, vapors, dust, allergens, animals, and other possible pulmonary irritants; presence of such possible irritants in the home environment (e.g., types of heating, cooling, and ventilation); exposure to viral illnesses (e.g., in a day care center or hospital)
    a. Use of personal protective devices in the case of exposures
    b. Previous work and work environments
2. Hobbies involving dust, chemicals, animals, vapors, or other possible respiratory irritants
3. Leisure time activities and hobbies that might involve exposure to respiratory irritants
4. Stress
5. Current and past residences
6. Travel to places where exposure to uncommon respiratory disease may have occurred
7. Exposure from family members or significant others
8. Any limitation of activities due to respiratory problems

Risk Factors
Respiratory Disease

Smoking: A major risk factor, contributing to a large portion of lung cancer cases
Sedentary lifestyle or recent immobilization
Age: Respiratory problems increase with aging
Sex: Chronic conditions are more common in men
Environmental exposures: Occupational exposure to certain carcinogens
Extreme obesity
Weakened chest muscles for any reason
History of frequent respiratory infections
Family history of respiratory disease
Recent life changes or disruptions
Systemic infections such as human immunodeficiency virus

Symptom Analysis

Cough

A cough is a forceful expiratory maneuver that expels mucus and foreign material from the airways. It occurs when cough receptors in the larynx, trachea, or larger bronchi are stimulated by inflammation, mucus, foreign matter, or other noxious substances.

1. **Onset:** acute or chronic, exact or approximate date
2. **Course since onset:** duration and pattern of symptoms, intermittent or continuous, relationship to activities, time of day, weather, talking, changes by time of year, time of day, eating
3. **Quality:** dry or loose, productive or nonproductive, bubbling, hoarse, hacking, barking, whooping

4. **Quantity:** frequency of coughing, effect on activities of daily living
5. **Setting:** effect of environmental changes or exposures, pattern during sleep, effect of temperature or humidity, exertion, time of day
6. **Associated phenomena:** shortness of breath, chest pain, fever, gagging, choking, changes in respiratory system, sputum production (if sputum is present, fully analyze that symptom as well, see also Sputum Production below), wheezing
7. **Alleviating and aggravating factors:** efforts to treat and patterns of use and effectiveness, home remedies, medications and other interventions, effects of position changes, exercise, exposure to noxious stimuli, humidity, cool air, cool foods
8. **Underlying concerns:** loss of energy, upper respiratory infection

Sputum Production

1. **Onset:** sudden or gradual, exact or approximate date
2. **Course since onset:** pattern of sputum production and changes in pattern
3. **Location:** does the sputum seem to originate from the throat or from deep in the chest after coughing?
4. **Quality:** purulent, color, presence of blood, odor, consistency

> ### ▪ HELPFUL HINT
>
> Mucus from the tracheobronchial tree that has not been mixed with oral secretions is called *phlegm*; mucus that is mixed with oral secretions is called *sputum*.

5. **Quantity:** amount produced daily (normal production is 60 to 90 ml)
6. **Setting:** effects of location on type or amount of production, environmental exposures
7. **Associated phenomena:** shortness of breath, cough, fever, chest pain
8. **Alleviating and aggravating factors:** exposure to cold, smoking, medications, drinking liquids
9. **Underlying concerns:** infection

Shortness Of Breath (Dyspnea) (Box 15-2)

1. **Onset:** sudden or gradual, exact or approximate date
2. **Course since onset:** stable or progressive course, position when condition occurs, most comfortable position, triggers, relationship to exercise and/or other activity, time of day or night, relationship to eating
3. **Location:** differences in symptoms between inhalation and exhalation
4. **Quality:** (1) dyspnea that begins or increases when client lies down (**orthopnea**)—determine number of

---

BOX 15-2

TOOLS FOR ASSESSING DYSPNEA

BORG CATEGORY-RATIO SCALE FOR RATING PERCEIVED BREATHLESSNESS

Score	Code
0	Nothing at all
0.5	Very, very slight
1	Very slight
2	Slight
3	Moderate
4	Somewhat severe
5	Severe
6	
7	Very severe
8	
9	
10	Very, very severe

To use: Enlarge the scale on an 8.5- × 11-inch sheet. Ask the client to identify the number that most closely describes the intensity of dyspnea. This scale may be rated differently by various clients, so it is not useful as a clinical measure across clients. However, the scale may be useful for measuring changes in individual clients as a result of disease or in response to treatment.

ATS-DLD SCALE FOR RATING BREATHLESSNESS
Score

1. Are you troubled by shortness of breath when hurrying on the level or walking up a slight hill?
2. (If yes) Do you have to walk slower than people of your age on the level because of breathlessness?
3. (If yes) Do you ever have to stop for breath after walking at your own pace on the level?
4. (If yes) Do you ever have to stop for breath after walking about 100 yards (or after a few minutes) on the level?
5. (If yes) Are you too breathless to leave the house or breathless on dressing or undressing?

To use: Score by the highest level of breathlessness experienced.

DYSPNEA INDEX DYSPNEA INDEX

Grade	Perceived Breathing Difficulty	Dyspnea with Exertion
0	None	Very little
1	Mild	Slight
2	Moderate	Moderate amount
3	Severe	Pronounced
4	Very severe	Very pronounced

ATS-DLD Scale for Rating Breathlessness: from Hoeman SP: *Rehabilitation nursing: process and application*, ed. 2, St. Louis, 1996, Mosby. Scales modified from Borg G, Holmgren A, Linblad I: Quantitative evaluation of chest pain, *Acta Med Scand* 644:43-45, 1981; and Ferris BG: Recommended respiratory disease questionnaires for use with adults and children, *Am Rev Respir Dis* 118:7-53, 1978. Dyspnea Index: data from Fink JB, Hunt GE: *Clinical practice in respiratory care*, Philadelphia, 1999, Lippincott Williams & Wilkins.

pillows that client uses; (2) sudden onset of dyspnea after a period of lying down that is relieved by sitting upright (**paroxysmal nocturnal dyspnea**); (3) dyspnea that increases when client is upright (Does client feel that he or she can draw in enough air or that he or she cannot breathe fast enough?)

5. **Quantity:** tolerance of activity (e.g., how many flights of stairs can be climbed or blocks walked before dyspnea occurs); effect on ADLs; changes in chest expansion

6. **Setting:** differential effect of setting or particular environmental or interpersonal situations

7. **Associated phenomena:** anxiety, palpitations, leg pain, faintness, cough, wheezing, sweating, pain, discomfort, fever

8. **Alleviating and aggravating factors:** response to any self or professional treatment, use of nebulizers, smoking, exercise, changes in position, changes in air, use of supplemental oxygen, medications, time required for recovery

9. **Underlying concerns:** infection, cardiac disease, asthma

Chest Pain

1. **Onset:** sudden or gradual, comes and goes or present at all times, exact or approximate date of onset

2. **Course since onset:** pattern of chest pain

3. **Location:** exact location of pain, radiation

4. **Quality:** pleuritic (located laterally or posteriorly, worsening when client takes a deep breath and is usually described as sharp or stabbing) or nonpleuritic (usually located in the center of the anterior chest with radiation to the shoulder or back and not affected by breathing), heavy, tight, burning, squeezing, aching, smothering, crushing, deep or superficial

5. **Quantity:** response to pain (e.g., continue activity or need to stop and lie down), rate on a scale of 1 to 10

6. **Setting:** association with exercise, stress, location of onset, temperature of environment, time of day

7. **Associated phenomena:** recent trauma, coughing, infection, fever, anxiety, nausea, vomiting, shortness of breath, weakness, diaphoresis, dizziness, faintness

8. **Alleviating and aggravating factors:** efforts to treat, medications, heat, splinting, rest, position change, food

9. **Underlying concerns:** fear of heart attack

Preparation for Examination: Client and Environment

Adequate respiratory examination requires a warm, well-lighted, quiet room. In addition to adequate room lighting, a mechanism for supplementary lighting is essential to aid in close inspection of specific areas.

Privacy is important because of the need to examine the entire chest area. Female clients may wish to cover their breasts with a gown or towel while the posterior thorax is being examined. Clients with large breasts will be asked to move them to the side so that you will be better able to palpate, percuss, and auscultate the anterior thorax. Male clients can be seated throughout the examination and stripped to the waist.

Preparation for Examination

EQUIPMENT

Item	Purpose
Stethoscope with diaphragm	Auscultation of thorax
Marking pencil	Measurement of diaphragmatic excursion
Metric ruler	Measurement of diaphragmatic excursion

CLIENT AND ENVIRONMENT

Client

Undressed to waist
Gown and sheet covering remainder of body
Covering available for female client to cover chest when anterior thorax is not being examined
Instructed regarding breathing and position for examination of posterior thorax

Setting

Warm
Private
Quiet

Before starting the examination, teach the client how to sit and how to breathe during the auscultation of the posterior thorax. For examination of the posterior thorax, instruct the client to hunch forward slightly and cross the arms over the chest (see Figure 15-16) so that the greatest amount of lung surface is available for examination. Also, instruct the client to breathe deeply and quietly, slowly inhaling and exhaling through the open mouth.

In the event of a respiratory problem, a thorough cardiovascular examination and a general examination, including the examination of nails for clubbing (see Chapter 10), are very important.

The examination of the respiratory system generally is done in the traditional sequence—inspection, palpation, percussion, and auscultation.

Technique for Examination and Expected Findings

Inspection (Box 15-3)

Performed inspection. (1) Measure respirations, (2) assess the pattern of respirations, (3) evaluate the effort required to maintain respiration, (4) assess the skin, and (5) assess the overall configuration, symmetry, and integrity of the thorax.

The approach to the physical examination is regional and integrated. The examination of systems is combined in body regions when appropriate. Because the client is uncovered to the waist during the examination, a large portion of skin and tissue is accessible to inspection. The observation of the skin and underlying tissue provides information about the client's general nutritional state. Common thoracic skin findings are the spider nevi associated with cirrhosis and seborrheic dermatitis (see Chapter 10).

INSPECTION SUMMARY

Skin: color, condition, irregularities, lesions
Thoracic configuration: ribs, interspaces, sternum, spine
Respiratory patterns and effort
Respiratory rate

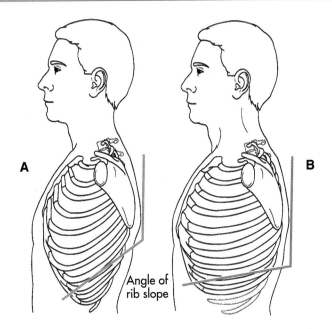

Figure 15-10 **A**, Normal thoracic configuration. **B**, Increased anteroposterior diameter. Note contrast in the angle of the slope of the ribs.

Lips and Nails. Inspection of the respiratory system includes observation of lips and nailbeds for color and observation of the nails for clubbing (see Chapters 10 and 16).

Thoracic Configuration. The first point of observation is the general shape of the thorax and its symmetry. Although no individual is absolutely symmetrical in both body hemispheres, most individuals are reasonably similar from side to side. Using the client as his or her own control whenever paired parts are examined is an excellent habit and often yields important findings. The normal thoracic configuration in adults is oval. The anteroposterior diameter of the thorax in the normal adult is less than the transverse diameter at an approximate ratio of 1:2 to 5:7 (Figure 15-10). In the normal infant, in some adults with pulmonary disease, and in elderly adults, the thorax is essentially round. This condition is called *barrel chest*. The barrel chest is characterized by horizontal ribs, slight kyphosis of the thoracic spine, and a prominent sternal angle. The chest appears as though it is in the continuous inspiratory position.

Other observed abnormalities of thoracic shape include the following (see also Chapter 9):

1. *Retraction of thorax:* The retraction is unilateral, involving only one side.
2. *Pigeon or chicken chest* (**pectus carinatum**): Sternal protrusion anteriorly. The anteroposterior diameter of the chest is increased, and the resultant configuration resembles the thorax of a fowl.
3. *Funnel chest* (**pectus excavatum**): Depression of part or all of the sternum. If the depression is deep, it may interfere with both respiratory and cardiac function.
4. *Spinal deformities (scoliosis, kyphosis, lordosis):* The respiratory examination offers an excellent opportunity to initiate inspection of the spine (see Chapter 18).

Ribs and Interspaces. Retraction of interspaces on inspiration may indicate some obstruction of free air inflow. Bulging of interspaces on expiration occurs when air outflow is obstructed, or it may be a result of tumor, aneurysm, or cardiac enlargement.

Normally the costal angle is less than 90 degrees, and the ribs are inserted into the spine at approximately a 45-degree angle (see Figure 15-1). In clients with obstructive lung disease, these angles are widened.

Pattern of Respiration. Normally, men and children breathe diaphragmatically, and women breathe thoracically or costally. A change in this pattern might be significant.

Respiratory Effort. If the client appears to have labored respiration, it is important to observe for the use of the accessory muscles of respiration in the neck (sternocleidomastoid, scalenus, and trapezius muscles) and for supraclavicular retraction. Impedance to air inflow is often accompanied by retraction of the intercostal spaces during inspiration. An excessively long expiratory phase of respiration is characteristic of outflow impedance and may be accompanied by the use of abdominal muscles to aid in expiration. Clients whose respirations are characteristically labored often sit or stand in a tripod position. In addition to using the accessory muscles of respiration, they support this additional exertion by leaning forward and bracing themselves with their arms or elbows on some stationary object or surface while standing or sitting.

Respiratory Rate. In the normal adult, the resting respiratory rate is 12 to 20 breaths per minute and is regular and unlabored. The ratio of respiratory rate to pulse rate normally is 1:4. **Tachypnea** is an adult resting respiratory rate of more than 20 breaths per minute. **Bradypnea** is an adult respiratory rate of less than 10 breaths per minute. **Dyspnea** is a subjective phenomenon of inadequate or distressful respiration. Many more abnormal patterns of respiration exist. Some of the commonly noted respiratory patterns are listed in Table 15-1.

Palpation (Box 15-4)

Palpation is performed to (1) further assess abnormalities suggested by the health history or by observation, such as tenderness, pulsations, masses, or skin lesions; (2) assess the skin and subcutaneous structures; (3) assess thoracic expansion; (4) assess tactile fremitus; and (5) assess tracheal position.

In examination of the thorax, four parts of the thorax need consideration: the posterior chest, anterior chest, right

TABLE 15-1   Characteristics of Commonly Observed Respiratory Patterns

Type of Respiration	Diagram	Discussion
Normal		12-20 respirations/min in adults; regular in rhythm; ratio of respiratory rate to pulse rate is 1:4
Air trapping		Present in obstructive pulmonary diseases; air is trapped in the lungs; respiratory level rises, and breathing becomes shallow
Biot's breathing (also called ataxic breathing)		Characterized by unpredictable irregularity; respirations may be shallow or deep and interrupted by apnea; seen in some central nervous system disorders
Bradypnea		Slow breathing at a rate of <10 respirations per minute; seen in diabetic coma, drug-induced respiratory depression, and increased intracranial pressure
Hyperventilation or Kussmaul respiration		Increase in both rate and depth; hyperpnea is an increase in depth only; seen in increased exercise, anxiety, and metabolic acidosis; Kussmaul's breathing is hyperventilation due to metabolic acidosis
Periodic respiration		Alternating hyperpnea, shallow respiration, and apnea; sometimes called Cheyne-Stokes respiration; frequently occurs in serious illness, including heart failure, uremia, drug-induced respiratory depression, and brain damage
Sighing respiration		Deep and audible; audible portion sounds like a sigh; seen in hyperventilation syndrome
Tachypnea		Rapid, shallow breathing at a rate of >24 respirations per minute; seen in restrictive lung disease, pleuritic chest pain, and elevated diaphragm

BOX 15-4

PALPATION SUMMARY

General palpation
Assessment of thoracic expansion
Assessment of tactile fremitus
Assessment of tracheal position

and left lateral chest, and apices. During the examination, move from the area of one hemisphere to the corresponding area on the other side (right to left, left to right) until all four major parts have been surveyed. During palpation for assessment of fremitus and all subsequent procedures for examination of the respiratory system, examine all areas meticulously and systematically. It is common for the practitioner to examine the apices, posterior chest, and lateral areas while standing behind the client. However, some examiners prefer to examine apices and lateral chest areas from the front. Either approach is effective. The important point is that no portion of the thorax should be overlooked.

A very helpful landmark for location of points on the thorax, especially the counting of ribs and interspaces, is the angle of Louis—the junction of the manubrium and the body of the sternum. It is also important to remember that the second rib connects with this palpable bony prominence and the second interspace lies immediately below it.

General Palpation.   First, assess the temperature and turgor of the skin. Then palpate the thoracic muscle mass and the thoracic skeleton. If the client has no complaints in relation to the respiratory system, a rapid, general survey of anterior, lateral, and posterior thoracic areas is sufficient. If the client has respiratory complaints, meticulously palpate all chest areas for tenderness, bulges, or abnormal movements. Palpate areas of abnormality or tenderness last so that comparison with apparently normal areas can be made. Clients with complaints of pain or trauma may tend to contract muscles to guard against pain during palpation, making the palpation of the chest very difficult. In these cases, inform the client that you will be palpating painful or injured areas last and will inform the client before palpating sensitive areas to avoid muscle guarding throughout the entire procedure.

Crepitations.   In subcutaneous emphysema, the subcutaneous tissue contains fine beads of air. As this tissue is palpated, audible crackling sounds are heard and popping sensations are noted under the skin. These sounds, elicited by palpation, are termed **crepitations**. Crepitations may be localized or noted diffusely throughout the thorax.

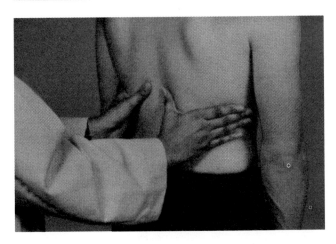

Figure 15-11 Palpation of the thoracic expansion.

Assessment of Thoracic Expansion. The degree of thoracic expansion can be assessed from the anterior or posterior chest (Figure 15-11). Anteriorly, the practitioner places his or her hands over the client's anterolateral chest with the thumbs extended along the costal margin, pointing to the xiphoid process. Posteriorly, the practitioner places the thumbs at the level of the tenth rib and the palms on the posterolateral chest. In either position, the thumbs will be approximately 3 to 5 cm apart before inspiration, depending on the client's size. The amount and symmetry of the thoracic expansion can be felt during quiet and deep respiration. First, feel thoracic expansion during normal, quiet respiration. Next, ask the client to take a deep breath in slowly and then exhale. The symmetry of respiration should be felt between the left and the right hemithoraces as the thumbs are separated an additional 3 to 5 cm during the deep inspiration.

Assessment of Tactile Fremitus. **Fremitus** is vibration that is perceptible on palpation. Tactile (sometimes also called "vocal") fremitus is palpable vibration of the thoracic wall produced by phonation.

Ask the client to repeat "one, two, three" or "ninety-nine" while you systematically palpate the thorax. Use the palmar bases of the fingers, the ulnar aspect of the hand, or the ulnar aspect of the closed fist (Figure 15-12). You can use two hands to assess both sides of the chest simultaneously or one hand moving alternately to compare one side of the chest with the other. See Figure 15-13 for areas of assessment of tactile fremitus. If one hand is used, move it from one side of the chest to the corresponding area on the other side. If two hands are used, place them simultaneously on the corresponding areas of each thoracic side.

Table 15-2 presents information about interpreting tactile fremitus. Fremitus is decreased or absent when the distance between the palpating hand is increased or when there is interference with sound transmission. Distance is increased and sound transmission is decreased in the following conditions: pneumothorax with lung collapse; fluid in the pleural space (pleural effusion); pleural thickening; tumors or masses in the pleural space; emphysema; bronchial obstruction; and a thick, muscular chest wall. Fremitus is increased

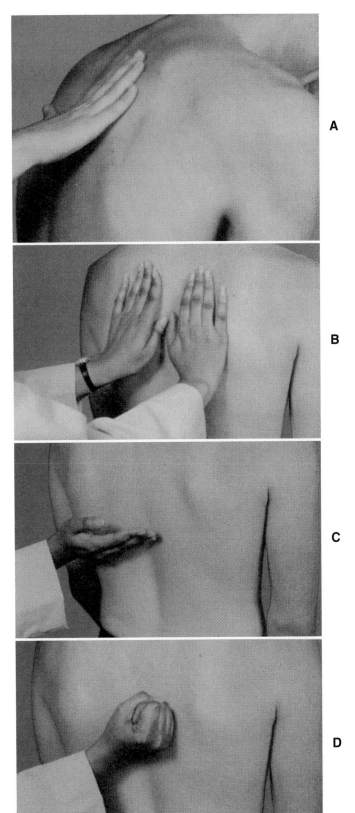

Figure 15-12 Palpation for assessment of tactile fremitus. **A**, Use of the palmar surface of the fingertips. **B**, Simultaneous application of the fingertips of both hands. **C**, Use of the ulnar aspect of the hand. **D**, Use of the ulnar aspect of the closed fist.

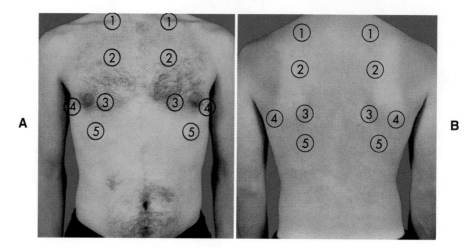

Figure 15-13   Areas of assessment for palpation of tactile fremitus and auscultation of vocal resonance. **A**, Anterior thorax. **B**, Posterior thorax.

in conditions that decrease the distance between the lungs and the palpating fingers and that favor the sound transmission in the chest (e.g., in pneumonia with consolidation, atelectasis [with open bronchus], lung tumors, pulmonary infarction, and pulmonary fibrosis). Before palpating, visually inspect the trachea for a visual shift.

Two other abnormal vibratory changes may be observed during tactile fremitus assessment: pleural friction rub and rhonchal fremitus. Pleural friction rub is produced by inflamed pleural surfaces rubbing together. The sound is produced when inflammation of the pleura results in a decrease in the fluid lubricating the pleural surfaces. On tactic fremitus assessment, pleural friction rub is felt as a grating vibration that is synchronous with respiratory movements, but more prominent on inspiration. Rhonchal fremitus is felt as coarse vibrations produced by the passage of air through exudates in large air passages.

Assessment of Tracheal Deviation.   The trachea is assessed by palpation for lateral deviation. Standing in front of the client, place the index finger of your dominant hand on the trachea in the suprasternal notch, then move the finger laterally left and right in the spaces bordered by the upper edge of the clavicle, the inner aspect of the sternocleidomastoid muscle, and the trachea. These spaces should be equal on both sides. In diseases such as atelectasis and pulmonary fibrosis, the trachea may be deviated toward the abnormal side. The trachea may be deviated toward the normal side in conditions such as neck tumors, thyroid enlargement, enlarged lymph nodes, pleural effusion, unilateral emphysema, and tension pneumothorax.

An alternate method of examining for tracheal deviation is as follows: Stand in front of the seated client, and place both hands around the client's neck with the thumbs in the spaces lateral to the trachea. Normally, both thumbs should palpate the straight borders of the trachea and assess equality of spaces bilaterally.

BOX 15-5

PERCUSSION SUMMARY

General survey
Diaphragmatic excursion

Percussion (Box 15-5)

Percussion is the tapping of an object to set underlying structures in motion and thus produces a sound called a percussion note and a palpable vibration. Percussion penetrates to a depth of approximately 5 to 7 cm into the chest. This technique is used in the thoracic examination to determine the relative amounts of air, liquid, or solid material in the underlying lung and to determine the positions and boundaries of organs. The techniques of percussion, along with other assessment techniques, are discussed thoroughly in Chapter 8.

Mediate (indirect) percussion is used in assessment of the respiratory system. It involves the striking of an object held against the area to be examined. For position in performing mediate percussion on the thorax, see Figure 15-14.

With your forearm and shoulder stationary and all movement done at the wrist, strike the pleximeter sharply with the plexor. Aim the blow at the portion of the pleximeter that is exerting maximum pressure on the thoracic surface, which is usually the base of the terminal phalanx, the distal interphalangeal joint, or the middle phalanx. Execute the blow rapidly, and immediately withdraw the plexor. The plexor strikes with the tip of the finger at right angles to the pleximeter. Strike one or two rapid blows in each area assessed. Avoid bony areas. Use interspaces for percussion. Compare one side of the thorax with the other.

With experience and study, one learns to differentiate among the five percussion tones commonly elicited from the

TABLE 15-2   Characteristics of Normal and Abnormal Tactile Fremitus

Fremitus	Description
Normal (moderate) fremitus	Varies greatly from person to person and depends on intensity and pitch of voice, position and distance of bronchi in relation to chest wall, and thickness of chest wall; is most intense in second intercostal spaces at sternal border near area of bronchial bifurcation
Increased tactile fremitus 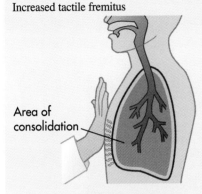 Area of consolidation	Is observed with conditions that increase density of lung tissue; a dense mass (e.g., consolidation of pneumonia) conducts vibrations with greater intensity than a porous medium (e.g., normal lung); for increased fremitus to occur, there must be a patent bronchus, and consolidation must be close to thoracic wall; may be observed in pneumonia, compressed lung, lung tumor, or pulmonary fibrosis
Decreased or absent tactile fremitus 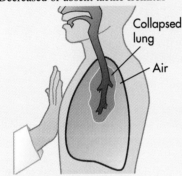 Collapsed lung — Air	Is observed when anything obstructs transmission of vibrations, results in a decreased production of sounds, or creates a barrier between lung and thoracic wall; may be observed in pleural effusion, pleural thickening, pneumothorax, bronchial obstruction, or emphysema
Pleural friction rub 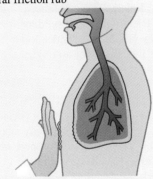	Vibration produced by inflamed pleural surfaces rubbing together; is produced when inflammation of pleura creates a decrease in fluid normally lubricating surfaces; is felt as a grating, is synchronous with respiratory movements, and is more commonly felt on inspiration
Rhonchal fremitus 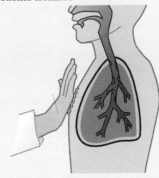	Coarse vibrations produced by passage of air through thick exudates in large air passages; often can be decreased or altered by coughing

TABLE 15-3   Description of Percussion Tones

Tone	Intensity	Pitch	Duration	Quality	Normal Location
Hyperresonance	Very loud	Very low	Long	Booming	Child's lung
Resonance	Loud	Low	Long	Hollow	Peripheral lung
Tympany	Loud	High	Medium	Drumlike	Stomach
Dullness	Medium	High	Medium	Thudlike	Liver
Flatness	Soft	High	Short	Extreme dullness	Muscle

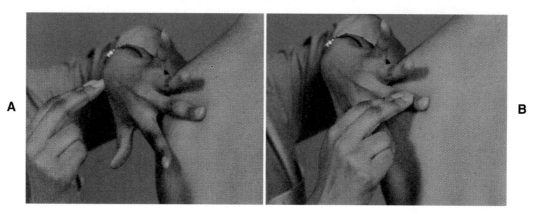

Figure 15-14   Indirect percussion. **A,** Positioning of the hands. **B,** Hand movement.

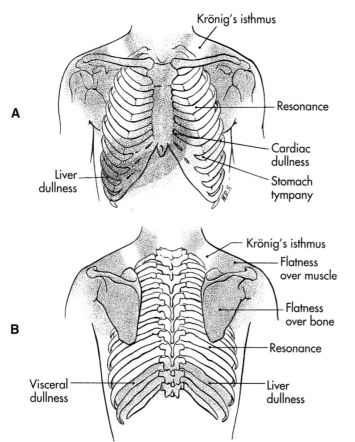

Figure 15-15   Percussion areas. **A,** Normal anterior chest. **B,** Normal posterior chest.

human body. In the study of tones, the determination of the following four characteristics will assist in assessment and labeling:

1. *Intensity (amplitude):* Loudness or softness of the tone.
2. *Pitch (frequency):* Relates to the number of vibrations per second. Rapid vibrations produce high-pitched tones; slow vibrations produce low-pitched tones. The greater the density of an object, the higher the frequency.
3. *Duration:* Amount of time a note is sustained.
4. *Quality:* Subjective phenomena relating to the innate characteristics of the object being percussed.

Table 15-3 lists and explains the commonly used descriptive terms for tones elicited by percussion over the thorax and the normal location of such sounds in the thoracic region. **Hyperresonance** is an abnormal percussion tone in adults. Table 15-6, p. 331, describes clinical assessment findings in several common respiratory system problems and provides examples of abnormal occurrence of the various percussion tones.

General Percussion Survey.   Figure 15-15 is a percussion map for the normal chest. The procedure for thoracic percussion is as follows:

1. Percuss the apices to determine whether the normal area of resonance is present between the neck and the shoulder muscles (see Figure 15-15), an area approximately 3 to 4 cm above the inner third of the clavicles.
2. Position the client with the head bent and the arms folded over the chest (Figure 15-16). With this ma-

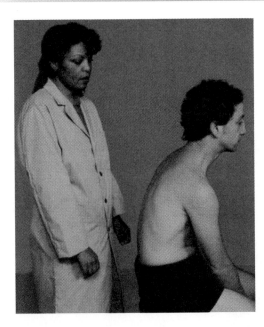

Figure 15-16 Position of the client for examination of the posterior thorax.

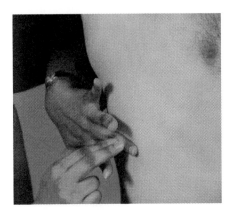

Figure 15-17 Position of the client for percussion of the lateral thorax.

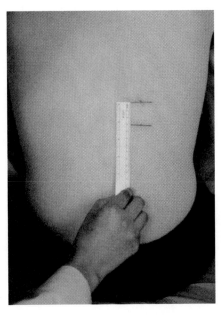

Figure 15-18 Assessment of diaphragmatic excursion.

neuver, the scapulae move laterally and more lung area is accessible to examination. On the posterior chest, percuss systematically at about 5 cm intervals from the upper to lower chest, moving left to right, right to left, and avoiding scapular and other bony areas.

3. Percuss the lateral chest with the client's arm positioned over the head (Figure 15-17).
4. On the anterior chest, percuss systematically, as done for the posterior chest.

Diaphragmatic Excursion. If the client's breathing is shallow or painful, the measurement of diaphragmatic excursion is indicated. Various pulmonary and abdominal lesions, ascites, or trauma may limit the movement of the diaphragm. The following is the procedure for assessing diaphragmatic excursion:

1. Instruct the client to inhale deeply and hold the breath in.
2. Percuss down the scapular line on one side, starting at T7 or at the end of the scapula, until the lower edge of the lung is identified. Sound will change from resonance to dullness.
3. With a skin-marking pencil, mark the point of change at the scapular line. This point is the edge of the diaphragm at full inhalation.
4. Instruct the client to take a few normal breaths.
5. Instruct the client to take a deep breath, exhale completely, and hold the breath at the end of the expiration.
6. Proceed to percuss upward from the previously marked point at the midscapular line. Mark the point where dullness of the diaphragm changes to the resonance of the lung. This point is the level of the diaphragm at full expiration.

7. Repeat the procedure on the opposite side.
8. Measure and record the diaphragmatic excursion— the distance between the upper and lower marks in centimeters for each side of the thorax.

An alternate method of determining the level of the diaphragm at full exhalation is to percuss down along the scapular line and note where the resonance of the lung changes to the dullness of the diaphragm.

The diaphragm is usually slightly higher on the right side because of the location of the liver on that side. Diaphragmatic excursion, which is normally 3 to 5 cm bilaterally, is usually measured only on the posterior chest (Figure 15-18).

In the actual examination, the apices and the posterior and lateral chest would be examined before percussion of the anterior chest is done. A recommended sequence for examination of the posterior, lateral, and anterior thoracic areas is illustrated in Figure 15-19.

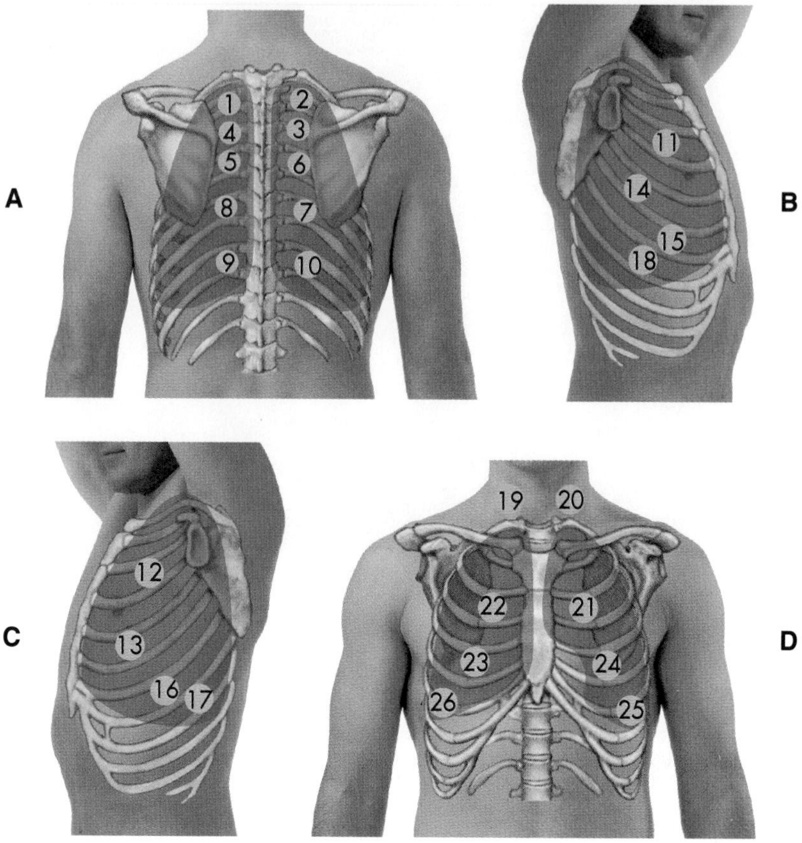

Figure 15-19 Routine for systematic percussion and auscultation of the thorax. Numbers indicate a recommended sequence for percussion and auscultation during a routine screening examination. **A**, Posterior thorax. **B**, Right lateral thorax. **C**, Left lateral thorax. **D**, Anterior thorax. (From Seidel HM et al.: *Mosby's guide to physical examination*, ed. 4, St. Louis, 1999, Mosby.)

BOX 15-6

AUSCULTATION SUMMARY

General survey for breath sounds, adventitious sounds
Assessment of vocal resonance

Auscultation (Box 15-6)

Through auscultation, information can be obtained about the functioning of the respiratory system and about the presence of any obstruction in the passages. For auscultation of the lungs, a stethoscope is used. The diaphragm of the stethoscope is commonly used for the thoracic examination because it covers a larger surface than does the bell. Also, the diaphragm is designed to transmit the usually higher pitch of abnormal breath sounds.

Place the stethoscope firmly, but not tightly, on the skin. Avoid client or stethoscope movement because movements of muscle under the skin or movements of the stethoscope over hair produce confusing extrinsic sounds.

The auscultatory assessment includes (1) analysis of breath sounds, (2) detection of any abnormal sounds, and (3) examination of the sounds produced by the spoken voice, or vocal resonance. As with percussion, use a zigzag approach, comparing the finding at each point with the corresponding point on the opposite hemithorax.

Analysis of Breath Sounds (Box 15-7). Before beginning auscultation, instruct the client to breathe through the mouth and more deeply and more slowly than in usual respiration. Then, systematically auscultate the apices and the posterior, lateral, and anterior chest (see Figure 15-19). At each application of the stethoscope, listen to at least one complete respiration. Observe the client for signs of hyperventilation and alter the procedure if the client becomes light-headed or faint.

Normal Breath Sounds. Breath sounds are produced by the movement of air through the tracheobronchoalveolar system. These sounds are analyzed according to pitch, intensity, quality, and relative duration of inspiratory and expiratory phases. Table 15-4 outlines the types of sounds heard in the thorax.

The sounds heard over normal lung parenchyma are called *vesicular breath sounds.* The inspiratory phase of the vesicular breath sounds is heard better than the expiratory phase and is about 2.5 times longer. These sounds have a low pitch and soft intensity.

Bronchovesicular breath sounds are normally heard in the areas of the major bronchi, especially in the apex of the right lung and at the sternal borders anteriorly and posteriorly between the scapula. Bronchovesicular breath sounds are characterized by inspiratory and expiratory phases of equal duration, moderate pitch, and moderate intensity. When bronchovesicular breath sounds are heard over the peripheral lung of an adult, an underlying pathological condition is likely to be present.

TABLE 15-4   Characteristics of Breath Sounds

Sound	Duration of Inspiration and Expiration	Diagram of Sound	Pitch	Intensity	Normal Location	Abnormal Location
Vesicular	Inspiration > expiration 2.5:1	Rustling quality	Low	Soft	Peripheral lung	Not applicable
Bronchovesicular	Inspiration = expiration 1:1		Medium	Medium	First and second intercostal spaces at sternal border anteriorly; posteriorly at T4 medial to scapulae	Peripheral lung
Bronchial (tracheal)	Inspiration < expiration 1:2	Tubular quality	High	Loud	Over trachea	Lung area

BOX 15-7

CONDITIONS COMMONLY ASSOCIATED WITH BREATH SOUND CHANGES

INCREASED BREATH SOUNDS

Consolidation

Compression

Any condition that increases the density of underlying tissue that increases sound transmission efficiency

DECREASED BREATH SOUNDS

Bronchial tree obstructions

Emphysema (loss of elasticity decreases the force with which air is expired)

Any pathology that obstructs the transmission of sound (e.g., pleurisy or pleural thickening, pnuemothorax, pleural effusion)

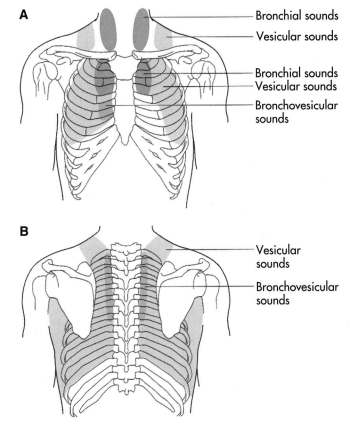

Figure 15-20 Areas for assessing breath sounds of the anterior and posterior thorax. Areas more darkly colored indicate normal point for auscultation of bronchial and bronchovesicular breath sounds.

Bronchial breath sounds are normally heard over the trachea and indicate a pathological condition if heard over lung tissue. They are high-pitched, loud sounds associated with shortened inspiratory and lengthened expiratory phases. A gap of silence audibly separates the inspiratory and expiratory phases.

Figure 15-20 shows the various areas for assessing breath sounds of the anterior and posterior thorax. Absent or decreased breath sounds can occur in (1) any condition that causes the deposition of foreign matter in the pleural space, (2) bronchial obstruction, (3) emphysema, or (4) shallow breathing.

Increased breath sounds, as from vesicular to bronchovesicular or bronchial, can occur in any condition that causes a consolidation of lung tissue.

Adventitious Breath Sounds. Adventitious sounds are not alterations in breath sounds but abnormal sounds superimposed on breath sounds. Classification of these sounds varies among authorities; consequently, the nomenclatures are somewhat inconsistent. The commonly used terms for adventitious sounds are described in Table 15-5.

A **crackle** (or "rale") is a short, discrete, interrupted, crackling or bubbling sound that is most commonly heard

TABLE 15-5   Origin and Characteristics of Adventitious Sounds

Sound	Diagram of Sound		Origin Characteristics
Crackles*—fine to medium		Air passing through moisture in small air passages and alveoli	Discrete, brief, high-pitched, discontinuous; inspiratory; have a dry or wet crackling quality; not cleared by coughing; sound is simulated by rolling a lock of hair near ear
Crackles*— medium to coarse		Air passing through moisture in bronchioles, bronchi, and trachea	Lower in pitch, louder, and more moist and bubbly than fine crackles
Wheezes— sonorous		Air passing through air passages narrowed by secretions, swelling, tumors, and so on	Continuous sounds; originate in large air passages; may be inspiratory and expiratory but usually predominate in expiration; loud, low-pitched, moaning or snoring quality; coughing may alter sounds
Wheezes— sibilant		Same as sonorous wheezes	Continuous sounds; originate in the small air passages; may be inspiratory and expiratory but usually predominate in expiration; high-pitched, wheezing sounds
Friction rubs		Rubbing together of inflamed and roughened pleural surfaces	Creaking or grating quality; superficial sounding; inspiratory and expiratory; heard most often in the lower anterolateral chest (area of greatest thoracic expansion); coughing has no effect

*Previously crackles have been termed rales or crepitations. These terms are still found in older texts.

during inspiration. The sound of crackles is similar to that produced by hairs being rolled between the fingers while close to the ear. The exact mechanism by which crackles are produced is not fully understood. Some crackles are thought to be produced by air passing through moisture in the bronchi, bronchioles, and alveoli or by air rushing through passages and alveoli that were closed during expiration and abruptly opened during inspiration. Other crackles are believed to result from air bubbles flowing through secretions or lightly closed airways during respiration.

The pitch and location in the inspiratory phase of the crackles are thought to indicate their site of production. Low-pitched, coarse crackles occurring early in inspiration are thought to originate in the bronchi, as in bronchitis. Medium-pitched crackles in midinspiration occur in diseases of the small bronchi, as in bronchiectasis. High-pitched, fine crackles are found in diseases affecting the bronchioles and alveoli and occur late in inspiration.

Wheezes (sometimes termed "**rhonchi**") are sounds produced by the movement of air through narrowed passages in the tracheobronchial tree. They predominate in expiration because bronchi are shortened and narrowed during this respiratory phase. However, they can occur in both the inspiratory and the expiratory phases of respiration, suggesting that lumina have been narrowed during both respiratory phases. As with crackles, the pitch and location of wheezes in the expiratory phase are thought to indicate their origins. For example, wheezes heard in early expiration probably originate in the larger bronchi.

A pleural friction rub is a loud, dry, creaking or grating sound indicative of pleural irritation. It is produced by the rubbing together of inflamed and roughened pleural surfaces during respiration (e.g., in pleurisy). Therefore it is heard best during the latter part of inspiration and the beginning of expiration. Because thoracic expansion is greatest in the lower anterolateral thorax, pleural friction rubs are most often heard there.

If the client has crackles, listen for several respirations in the areas in which the crackles are heard to determine the effects of deep breathing. Also, ask the client to cough and note the changes in adventitious sounds after coughing. Crackles and wheezes sometimes clear with coughing, but pleural friction rubs do not. If the client has complained of respiratory difficulty and no adventitious sounds are heard, ask him or her to cough; often, adventitious sounds are noted after coughing.

Vocal Resonance. The same mechanism that produces tactile fremitus produces vocal resonance. Resonance is the transmission of voice sounds as heard through the stethoscope placed on the chest wall. Normal vocal resonance is heard as muffled, nondistinct sounds. It is loudest medially and is less intense at the periphery of the lung.

Vocal resonance should be assessed if any respiratory system abnormality has been detected on observation, palpation, percussion, or auscultation (Table 15-6). The routine is the same systematic one previously used in assessing tactile fremitus (see Figure 15-13). The client says "one, two, three" or "ninety-nine" while the examiner does an auscultatory survey of the thorax.

TABLE 15-6	Voice Sound Assessment Techniques	
Client Vocalization	**Normal Auscultatory Finding**	**Abnormal Auscultatory Finding**
"Ninety-nine" spoken	Muffled, nondistinct sound	"Ninety-nine": bronchophony
"Ninety-nine" whispered	Barely audible, nondistinct sound	"Ninety-nine": whispered pectoriloquy
"e- e- e" spoken	Muffled, nondistinct sound	"a- a- a": egophony

BOX 15-8

GENERAL SCREENING TESTS

SCREENING FOR LUNG CANCER

Routine screening for lung cancer with chest x-ray study or sputum cytology in asymptomatic persons is not recommended. All patients should be counseled against tobacco use.

SCREENING FOR TUBERCULOSIS

Persons at high risk for tuberculosis should be screened for exposure to tuberculosis using the purified protein derivative (PPD). Those at high risk include HIV-positive persons; close contacts of persons with known or suspected tuberculosis; health care workers; persons with medical risk factors associated with tuberculosis; immigrants from countries with high tuberculosis prevalence; medically underserved, low-income populations; alcoholics; injection drug users; and residents of long-term care facilities.

Data from US Preventive Services Task Force: *Guide to clinical preventive services*, ed. 2, Alexandria, Va, 1996, International Medical Publishing.

Cultural Considerations
Chest Volume

Caucasian Americans have a larger chest volume and therefore greater vital capacity and forced expiratory volume than African-Americans and Asian-Americans. The average forced expiratory volume for Caucasian Americans is 3.22 liters compared with 2.53 liters for Asian-Americans, and the forced vital capacity is 4.30 liters for Caucasian Americans but only 3.27 liters for Asian-Americans.

Bronchophony is an increase in loudness and clarity of vocal resonance. Special vocal resonance techniques are used when resonance is increased. These include tests for whispered pectoriloquy and egophony.

Whispered pectoriloquy is exaggerated bronchophony. The client is instructed to whisper a series of words. The words as heard through the stethoscope on the chest wall are distinct and understandable.

In **egophony**, the intensity of the spoken voice, as heard through the stethoscope applied to the chest wall, is increased and the voice has a nasal or bleating quality. If the client says "e- e- e," the transmitted sound will be "a- a- a."

Decreased vocal resonance occurs in the same clinical situations in which tactile fremitus is decreased and breath sounds are absent. Vocal resonance is increased and whispered pectoriloquy and egophony may be present in any condition that causes a consolidation of lung tissue.

Screening Tests and Procedures

A variety of radiological, functional, and chemical diagnostic tests are used in assessing respiratory health (Box 15-8). It is beyond the capabilities of this text to describe these various tests fully. However, some of the major ones are mentioned here.

Chest X-Ray Examination

The chest x-ray examination is a common means of determining the health of lung parenchyma. A chest x-ray also provides information about heart size as well as the condition of the lungs.

Pulmonary Function Tests

Common indications for pulmonary function testing include diagnosing disease, determining the course of a disease, determining the effects of treatment, monitoring pulmonary side-effects of medications, determining preoperative risk, evaluating disability, and providing disease prognosis.

Spirometry

Spirometry requires some respiratory effort by the client. The effort includes blowing air into a spirometer designed to measure lung volumes and flow rates. Specialized technicians in a designated laboratory generally do this assessment. Spirometry readings are commonly expressed in volumes and capacities. Volumes are single compartments in the lung. The addition of two or more volumes together results in a capacity. Volumes and capacities are expressed as a percentage of normal. Generally, the normal range is plus or minus 20% of the predicted value of all volumes and capacities (Figure 15-21).

The following are common spirometric assessments:

Tidal volume (TV): Volume of air exhaled or inhaled during quiet breathing (typically 500 ml).

Inspiratory reserve volume (IRV): The maximum amount of air that can be inspired after normal inspiration (typically 3000 to 3300 ml).

Expiratory reserve volume (ERV): Volume that can be maximally exhaled after a passive exhalation (typically 1000 to 1200 ml).

Residual volume (RV): Amount of gas left in the lung after exhaling all that is physically possible. This

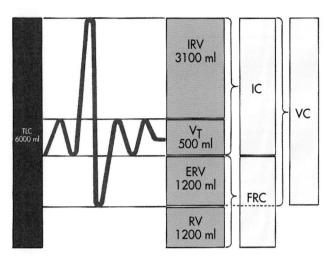

Figure 15-21 Components of lung capacity. *ERV,* Expiratory reserve volume; *IC,* inspiratory capacity; *IRV,* inspiratory reserve volume; *FRC,* functional residual capacity; *RV,* residual volume; *TLC,* total lung capacity; *VC,* vital capacity; *V$_T$, tidal volume.* (From Wilson SF, Thompson JM: *Respiratory disorders,* St. Louis, 1990, Mosby.)

■ **HELPFUL HINT**

FINDING	POSSIBLE EXPLANATION
Increased respiratory rate	Problems that cause loss of lung volume (e.g., pulmonary fibrosis) The increase in rate is proportional to the degree of lung volume reduction
Prolonged expiratory phase	Problems that cause airways to narrow (e.g., asthma)
Prolonged inspiratory phase	Problems that cause the upper airway to narrow (e.g., croup)
Expiratory wheezes and rhonchi	Problems that indicate obstruction of intrathoracic airways (e.g., asthma)
Fine, late inspiratory crackles	Restrictive lung diseases, such as pulmonary fibrosis
Dyspnea	Occurs when the work of breathing is excessive for the level of exertion The work of breathing increases with reduced lung compliance and narrowed airways

measurement is expressed as a ratio of total lung capacity to vital capacity (typically 1200 ml).

Vital capacity (VC): Maximum amount of air a person can exhale (the sum of TV + IRV + ERV, typically 4500 to 5000 ml). It is usually measured after forceful exhalation and termed forced vital capacity.

Inspiratory capacity (IC): Maximum amount of air inspired with one breath (the sum of TV + IRV, typically 3500 to 3800 ml).

Functional residual capacity (FRC): Sum of the residual volume and the expiratory reserve volume (typically 2200 to 2400 ml).

Total lung capacity (TLC): Sum of the vital capacity and the residual volume (typically 5700 to 6200).

Minute volume: Volume of gas expired over 1 minute.

Forced expiratory volume in 1 second (FEV$_1$): Measurement of the maximum volume of air exhaled during the first second of expiration.

FEV$_1$/FVC: Ratio of forced expiratory volume in 1 second to forced vital capacity.

Peak flow: Measurement of the maximum flow rate achieved during the forced vital capacity maneuver.

Diffusing capacity: Ability of gas to diffuse across the alveolar-capillary membrane.

Arterial Blood Gases

The measurement of arterial blood gases provides valuable information about the physiological functioning of the respiratory system. Some of the commonly used tests are listed here.

Oxygenation status is measured by the following values:

Pao$_2$: Partial pressure of oxygen in arterial blood. The normal range at sea level is 80 to 100 mm Hg. Decreased levels may indicate hypoxemia or insufficient oxygenation of the blood.

Sao$_2$: Percent of saturation of oxygen on hemoglobin in arterial blood. The normal level at sea level is greater than 96%.

Cao$_2$: Content of oxygen in arterial blood expressed in ml/100 ml of blood. The normal value is 18 to 20 ml/100 ml of blood (18% to 20%).

Pvo$_2$: Partial pressure of oxygen in mixed venous blood.

Acid-base balance is measured by the following values:

pH: Hydrogen ion concentration in the blood. The normal range is 7.35 to 7.45.

Examination Step-by-Step

The examination described here is for a client who is able to sit during the procedure. The approach would need to be adapted for a client who was unable to sit during the examination. In general, the examiner moves around the client, completing one aspect of assessment before initiating the next. Traditional organization of inspection, palpation, percussion, and auscultation is followed.

The client is stripped to the waist and seated so that all areas of the thorax are visible.

A. Inspect all areas of the thorax, noting especially:
1. Breathing rate, pattern, inspiratory-expiratory ratio, thoracic movement, audible adventitious sounds
2. Use of accessory muscles of respiration
3. Condition of skin and underlying structures
4. Presence of bulging
5. Skin color and superficial venous patterns
6. Size, shape, and symmetry of thorax

B. Examine the posterior, lateral, and apical thorax:
1. Palpate the thorax
   a. General assessment of skin tone, temperature, tenderness, unusual sensations
   b. Thoracic expansion
   c. Tactile fremitus
2. Percuss the thorax
   a. Percussion survey of thorax, including assessment of appropriateness of various tones for their location
   b. Diaphragmatic excursion
3. Auscultate with the diaphragm of the stethoscope from apex to base, from side to side
   a. Appropriateness of type of breath sound for location
   b. Adventitious sounds
   c. Vocal resonance

C. Examine the anterior thorax:
1. Palpate the thorax
   a. General assessment of skin tone, temperature, tenderness, unusual sensations
   b. Position of trachea
   c. Thoracic expansion
   d. Tactile fremitus
2. Percuss the thorax
   a. Percussion survey of thorax, including assessment of appropriateness of various tones for their location
3. Auscultate with the diaphragm of the stethoscope from apex to base, from side to side
   a. Appropriateness of type of breath sound for location
   b. Adventitious sounds
   c. Vocal resonance

EXPECTED FINDINGS

Inspection: no skin or surface abnormalities, symmetry of movement and expansion, absence of retractions
Palpation: trachea midline, symmetrical unaccentuated tactile fremitus, symmetrical thoracic expansion, no masses or tenderness
Percussion: diaphragmatic expansion of 3-5 cm, resonant and symmetrical percussion notes
Auscultation: no adventitious sounds, vesicular breath sounds over lung fields

Paco₂: Partial pressure of carbon dioxide in arterial blood. The normal range at sea level is 35 to 45 mm Hg. Increased levels indicate hypercapnia and respiratory acidosis. Decreased levels indicate respiratory alkalosis.

HCO₃: Plasma bicarbonate concentration. The normal range at sea level is 22 to 26 mEq/L.

Sputum Examination

Sputum contains exfoliated cells and organisms that are being expelled from the lungs. Therefore examination of sputum can be a valuable component of the respiratory assessment. Sputum specimens can be examined with Gram stain, cultures, and culture sensitivity tests for the presence of various organisms and by cytological examination for the presence of malignancies. Sputum specimens should always be collected in a sterile container to avoid contamination.

VARIATIONS FROM HEALTH

Despite the heavy reliance on laboratory and x-ray findings in the diagnosis of respiratory problems, reasonably compiling and analyzing the physical assessment data can derive sound diagnostic probabilities. Table 15-7 outlines the usual assessment findings in a variety of common lung conditions.

TABLE 15-7   Assessment Findings Frequently Associated With Common Lung Conditions

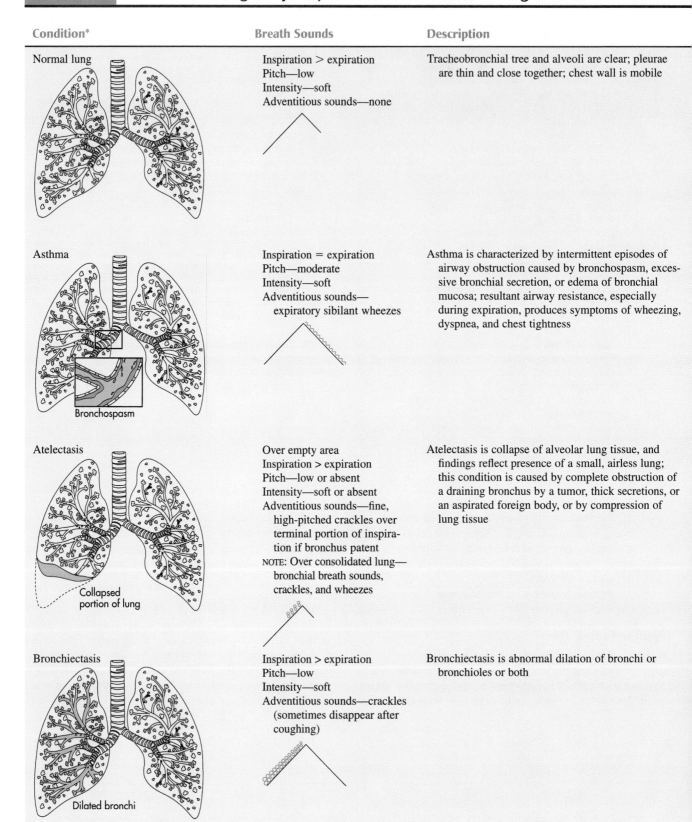

Condition*	Breath Sounds	Description
Normal lung	Inspiration > expiration Pitch—low Intensity—soft Adventitious sounds—none	Tracheobronchial tree and alveoli are clear; pleurae are thin and close together; chest wall is mobile
Asthma Bronchospasm	Inspiration = expiration Pitch—moderate Intensity—soft Adventitious sounds— expiratory sibilant wheezes	Asthma is characterized by intermittent episodes of airway obstruction caused by bronchospasm, excessive bronchial secretion, or edema of bronchial mucosa; resultant airway resistance, especially during expiration, produces symptoms of wheezing, dyspnea, and chest tightness
Atelectasis Collapsed portion of lung	Over empty area Inspiration > expiration Pitch—low or absent Intensity—soft or absent Adventitious sounds—fine, high-pitched crackles over terminal portion of inspiration if bronchus patent NOTE: Over consolidated lung—bronchial breath sounds, crackles, and wheezes	Atelectasis is collapse of alveolar lung tissue, and findings reflect presence of a small, airless lung; this condition is caused by complete obstruction of a draining bronchus by a tumor, thick secretions, or an aspirated foreign body, or by compression of lung tissue
Bronchiectasis Dilated bronchi	Inspiration > expiration Pitch—low Intensity—soft Adventitious sounds—crackles (sometimes disappear after coughing)	Bronchiectasis is abnormal dilation of bronchi or bronchioles or both

*Although some disease conditions are bilateral, one diseased lung and one normal lung are illustrated for each condition to provide contrast. When an abnormality is illustrated, the pathological condition is illustrated on the left side and the normal lung is on the right side of the illustration.

Inspection	Palpation	Percussion	Auscultation	Other Clinical Signs and Symptoms
Good, symmetrical rib and diaphragmatic movement Anteroposterior diameter < transverse diameter Respirations 12-20/min and regular	Trachea—midline Expansion—adequate, symmetrical Tactile fremitus—moderate and symmetrical No lesions or tenderness	Resonant Diaphragmatic excursion—3 to 5 cm	Breath sounds—vesicular Vocal resonance—muffled Adventitious sounds—none, except for a few occasional transient crackles at bases	Not applicable
Cyanosis Air trapping with audible wheezing Use of accessory muscles of respiration Increased respiratory rate Shortness of breath Expiration labored	Tactile fremitus—decreased	Hyperresonant	Breath sounds—distant Vocal resonance—decreased Bilateral adventitious sounds—wheezes	During attacks: Cyanosis Prolonged attacks of dyspnea Difficulty in expiration Profuse diaphoresis
Less chest motion on affected side Affected side retracted, with ribs appearing close together Cough Rapid, shallow breathing	Trachea—shifted to affected side Expansion—decreased on affected side Tactile fremitus—decreased or absent Trachea—midline or deviated toward affected side Expansion—decreased on affected side Tactile fremitus—decreased or absent Expansion—limited	Dull to flat over collapsed lung Hyperresonant over remainder of affected hemithorax	Breath sounds—decreased or absent Vocal resonance—varies in intensity, usually reduced or absent in affected area Adventitious sounds—fine, high-pitched crackles may be heard over terminal portion of inspiration	Cough Cyanosis
If mild, respirations are normal If severe, tachypnea Less expansion of affected side Cough with purulent sputum	Tactile fremitus—increased	Resonant or dull	Breath sounds—usually vesicular Vocal resonance—usually muffled Adventitious sounds—crackles	Chronic productive cough Dyspnea Fever Weight loss Digital clubbing

Continued

| TABLE 15-7 | **Assessment Findings Frequently Associated With Common Lung Conditions—cont'd** |

Condition*	Breath Sounds	Description

Bronchitis – acute 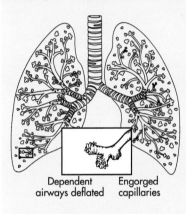 Bronchial inflammation and constriction	Inspiration > or = expiration
	Pitch—low
	Intensity—soft
	Adventitious sounds—
	   localized crackles,
	   expiratory sibilant wheezes
	
		Acute bronchitis is inflammation of bronchial tree characterized by partial bronchial obstruction and secretions or constrictions; it results in abnormally deflated portions of lung

Congestive heart failure (left-sided) with pulmonary edema 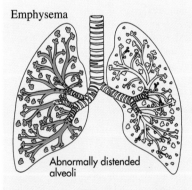 Dependent Engorged airways deflated capillaries	Inspiration > expiration Pitch—low intensity—soft Adventitious sounds—crackles 	Congestive heart failure is primarily a cardiac condition in which the heart is unable to maintain output sufficient to meet the metabolic needs of the body This situation may result in increased pressure in the pulmonary veins, which causes congestion and interstitial edema The bronchial mucosa may also become edematous

Emphysema
 	
Abnormally distended alveoli
	Inspiration = expiration
	Pitch—low to very low
	Intensity—soft to very soft
	Adventitious sounds—
	   occasional sonorous and/or
	   sibilant wheezes; fine
	   inspiratory crackles
	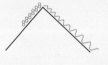
		Emphysema is a permanent hyperinflation of lung beyond terminal bronchioles, with destruction of alveolar walls; airway resistance is increased, especially on expiration

Pleural effusion and thickening   Normal
 	
Fluid in the pleural space
	Inspiration > expiration
	Pitch—low to absent
	Intensity—soft to absent
	Adventitious sounds—
	   occasional pleural
	   friction rub
	
		Pleural effusion is a collection of fluid in pleural space; if pleural effusion is prolonged, fibrous tissue may also accumulate in pleural space; clinical picture depends on amount of fluid or fibrosis present and rapidity of development; fluid tends to gravitate to most dependent areas of thorax, and adjacent lung is compressed

Inspection	Palpation	Percussion	Auscultation	Other Clinical Signs and Symptoms
If severe, tachypnea and cyanosis Rasping cough with mucoid sputum	Tactile fremitus—normal to increased	Resonant	Breath sounds—vesicular Vocal resonance—moderate Adventitious sounds—localized crackles, sibilant wheezes	Hacking, rasping cough Thick mucoid sputum production
Pale or cyanotic Retractions may be present Tachypnea Orthopnea	Tactile fremitus— normal Expansion— may be decreased	Resonant Diaphragmatic excursion— may be decreased	Breath sounds—vesicular Vocal resonance— moderate Adventitious sounds—late inspiratory crackles; may disappear with continued exaggerated respiration	Dyspnea Orthopnea Productive cough Diaphoresis
Dyspnea with exertion Barrel chest (increased anterior-posterior diameter) Tachypnea Use of accessory muscles of respiration Shortness of breath Use of "tripod" posture	Expansion— limited Tactile fremitus— decreased	Resonant to hyper-resonant Diaphragmatic excursion— decreased	Breath sounds—decreased intensity; often prolonged expiration Vocal resonance—muffled or decreased Adventitious sounds—occasional wheezes; often fine crackles in late inspiration	History of heavy smoking Intolerance of normal levels of activity
Tachypnea Decrease in definition of intercostal spaces on affected side Dyspnea	Trachea—deviation toward normal side Expansion— decreased on affected side Tactile fremitus— decreased or absent	Dull to flat No diaphragmatic excursion on affected side	Breath sounds—decreased or absent Vocal resonance—muffled or absent; if fluid compresses lung, sounds may be bronchial over compression, and bronchophony, egophony, and whisper pectoriloquy may be present Adventitious sounds—pleural friction rub sometimes present	Chest pain Dry cough Cyanosis

Continued

TABLE 15-7   Assessment Findings Frequently Associated With Common Lung Conditions

Condition*	Breath Sounds	Description
Pneumonia with consolidation 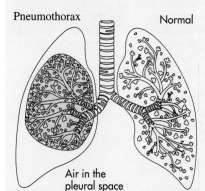 Normal Consolidation	Inspiration = expiration Pitch—high Intensity—loud Adventitious sounds—inspiratory crackles in terminal third of inspiration	Pneumonia with consolidation occurs when alveolar air is replaced by fluid or tissue; physical findings depend on amount of parenchymal tissue involved
Pneumothorax 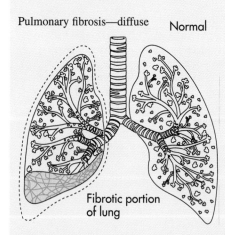 Normal Air in the pleural space	Inspiration > expiration Pitch—low to absent Intensity—soft to absent Adventitious sounds—none	Pneumothorax implies air in pleural space There are three types of pneumothorax: (1) closed—air in pleural space does not communicate with air in lung; (2) open—air in pleural space freely communicates with air in lung; air in pleural space is atmospheric; and (3) tension—air in pleural space communicates with air in lungs only on inspiration; air pressure in pleural space is greater than atmospheric pressure Physical signs depend on degree of lung collapse and presence or absence of pleural effusion
Pulmonary fibrosis—diffuse Normal Fibrotic portion of lung	Inspiration = expiration Pitch—low to absent Intensity—soft to absent Adventitious sounds—crackles	Pulmonary fibrosis is presence of excessive amount of connective tissue in lungs; consequently, lungs are smaller than normal and less compliant; lower lobes are usually affected most

Inspection	Palpation	Percussion	Auscultation	Other Clinical Signs and Symptoms
Tachypnea Guarding and less motion on affected side	Expansion—limited on affected side Tactile fremitus—usually increased, but may be weak if a bronchus leading to the affected area is plugged	Dull to flat over affected area	Breath sounds—increased in intensity; bronchovesicular or bronchial breath sounds over affected area Vocal resonance—increased bronchophony, egophony, whisper pectoriloquy present Adventitious sounds—inspiratory crackles in terminal third of inspiration	Fever Chukks Sputum production Dyspnea
Restricted lung expansion on affected side If large, tachypnea Bulging in intercostal spaces on affected side Cyanosis	Trachea—deviated toward normal side Expansion—decreased on affected side Tactile fremitus—absent	Hyperresonant Decreased diaphragmatic excursion	Breath sounds—usually decreased or absent; if open pneumothorax, have an amorphous quality Vocal resonance—decreased or absent Adventitious sounds—none	Chest pain History of trauma to chest Agitation
Dyspnea on exertion Tachypnea Thoracic expansion diminished Cyanosis	Trachea—deviated to most affected side		Breath sounds—reduced or absent, bronchovesicular or bronchial Vocal resonance—increased, whisper pectoriloquy may be present Adventitious sounds—crackles on inspiration	Nonproductive cough Exposure to environmental contaminants Decreased tolerance to normal activity Digital clubbing Fever

Sample Documentation and Diagnoses

FOCUSED HEALTH HISTORY (SUBJECTIVE DATA)

This is a regular, health maintenance clinic visit for Mr. T, a 65-year-old African-American male with the chief complaint of "low energy." Was diagnosed with emphysema 3 years ago. Is always short of breath, but has been worse for the past 2 days during hot, humid weather. Stays at home with fans, but home is not air-conditioned. Denies chest pain, fever, or change in sputum production. Is unable to climb more than one flight of stairs without resting for 2 to 3 minutes. Has difficulty walking on flat ground for more than two blocks. Uses oxygen at home at 2 L/min after meals, at night, and during physical exertion. Complains of insomnia and restlessness at night—sleeps with three pillows. Has moist cough several times daily that produces about 1 to 2 tablespoons of white or yellow sputum. When sputum is yellow, takes ampicillin as directed. Color of sputum has always cleared after medication. Sputum has been white for the past several months. Smoked two to three packs of cigarettes a day for 50 years, but stopped 3 years ago when emphysema was diagnosed. Diagnosis verified per clinic record. Denies allergies and exposure to lung irritants. Denies TB, cancer, familial lung disease, allergies, heart disease, and renal disease.

FOCUSED PHYSICAL EXAMINATION (OBJECTIVE DATA)

Inspection: Respirations regular at 22/min. After minimal exercise (walking around examination room ×2) 30/min. Respirations deep—uses accessory muscles of respiration. Chest is barrel shaped. Thorax moves symmetrically; no bulges or retractions.

Palpation: Trachea in midline. Thoracic expansion symmetrical at 3 cm. No areas of bulging or tenderness. Percussion tones resonant and symmetrical. Tactile fremitus decreased throughout lung fields.

Percussion: Diaphragmatic excursion 2 cm bilaterally. Percussion sounds hyperresonant throughout thorax.

Auscultation: Diminished vesicular breath sounds throughout throat. Expiration sometimes prolonged. Fine crackles and occasional wheezes noted throughout respiratory cycle in bases of right and left lungs. Expiration > inspiration.

DIAGNOSES

HEALTH PROBLEM

Chronic Emphysema

NURSING DIAGNOSES

Activity Intolerance Related to Imbalances between Oxygen Supply and Demand

Defining Characteristics

• Complains of shortness of breath when walking > 2 blocks or climbing one flight of stairs
• Sleep orthopnea

Ineffective Breathing Pattern Related to Decreased Lung Expansion

Defining Characteristics

• Dyspnea on exertion
• Tachypnea with activity
• Tactile fremitus decreased
• Prolonged expiratory phase
• Increased anteroposterior diameter
• Use of accessory muscles

Ineffective Airway Clearance Related to Tracheobronchial Restriction

Defining Characteristics

• Abnormal breath sounds—crackles throughout all lung fields
• Tachypnea with exercise
• Dyspnea

Anxiety Related to Change in Health Status

Defining Characteristics

• Restlessness
• Insomnia
• Expressed concern regarding changes in life events

Critical Thinking Questions

Review the Sample Documentation and Diagnoses box to answer these questions.

1. If the client complained of fever and dyspnea and if an area of the lung demonstrated increased tactile fremitus and breath sounds and dull percussion sounds, what additional problem would you suspect?
2. What mechanisms might cause the following combination of symptoms:

Trachea shifted toward the side of the thorax without additional symptoms and dull to flat percussion findings?
Trachea shifted toward the side of the thorax with additional symptoms with dull percussion findings?
Trachea shifted toward the unaffected side with hyper-resonant percussion findings?

3. Under what conditions should tactile fremitus be assessed? Under what conditions should vocal resonance be assessed?

Answers are available on the MERLIN website (www.harcourthealth.com/MERLIN/Barkauskas/). And be sure to check the website regularly for additional learning activities!

Remember to check out the Online Study Guide!
www.harcourthealth.com/MERLIN/Barkauskas/

Cardiovascular System

Learning Objectives

On successful study of this chapter and completion of related learning experiences, the learner will be able to:
- Describe the anatomy, physiology, and anatomical landmarks of the cardiovascular system: the heart and great vessels, the neck vessels, and the peripheral vessels.
- Outline the history pertinent to the assessment of the cardiovascular system, including exploration of common complaints.
- Explain the rationale for and demonstrate assessment of cardiovascular structures (the heart and great vessels, the neck vessels, and the peripheral vessels), including use of inspection, auscultation, percussion, and palpation.
- Explain the rationale for and demonstrate special maneuvers used to assess cardiovascular problems.

Outline

Purpose of Examination

The cardiovascular system is composed of the heart and an extensive system of blood vessels. The purpose of examination of this system is to assess the function of the heart as a pump and the function of the arteries and veins throughout the body in their role in transporting oxygen and nutrients to the tissues of the body and in transporting waste products and carbon dioxide from those body tissues.

Assessment of the heart, the vessels of the neck, and some aspects of the peripheral vessels is discussed in this chapter. For assessment of the blood pressure and pulse and their variations from health, see Chapter 9. Assessment of the cardiovascular system is closely related to assessment of the respiratory system, which is discussed in Chapter 15.

ANATOMY AND PHYSIOLOGY

Several chest wall landmarks and lines are used to describe the anatomical position of the heart, its movements, and the sounds produced (Figure 16-1). The area of the chest that overlies the heart and the great vessels is called the **precordium**. The suprasternal notch lies at the top of the sternum. The angle of Louis is the area where the manubrium of the sternum meets the body of the sternum. The ribs and intercostal (between-the-ribs) spaces are numbered from the first rib, with each space taking its number from the rib directly above it.

The imaginary lines used for description (and their abbreviations) include:
- The midsternal line (MSL) down the center of the sternum
- The midclavicular line (MCL) down from the center of the clavicle
- The anterior, middle, and posterior axillary lines (AAL, MAL, PAL) down from the axilla

Other abbreviations commonly used include:
- 2 LICS—second left intercostal space
- 2 RICS—second right intercostal space
- 5 LICS—fifth left intercostal space
- LSB—left sternal border

For a more thorough discussion of thoracic landmarks, see Chapter 15.

Heart and Great Vessels

Location and Position of the Heart

The heart is located behind the sternum and between the lungs in the mediastinum. It lies mostly to the left of the midsternal line, above the diaphragm. It occupies the space from the second to the fifth intercostal spaces and from the right side of the sternum to the left midclavicular line (Figure 16-2).

The position of the heart can vary somewhat according to the body build, chest configuration, and level of the diaphragm. In persons of average build, the heart lies obliquely: one third of it lies to the right of the midsternal line, and two thirds lies to the left of this line. In short, stocky persons, the heart is usually positioned more horizontally. If the diaphragm is positioned higher, as occurs with pregnancy, the heart also lies more horizontally. In tall, slender individuals, the heart hangs more vertically. With the rare condition of **dextrocardia**, the position of the heart is reversed, and the heart lies on the right side of the chest.

The heart is shaped like an inverted cone. The upper portion is broader and is called the base of the heart. The lower portion is narrower and is called the apex.

Structure of the Heart

Pericardium.   The heart is encased in and protected by the **pericardium**, a double-walled fibrous sac of elastic connective tissue. The pericardium contains several cubic centimeters of fluid that permit the smooth, low-friction movement of the heart.

Heart Wall.   The heart wall has three main layers: the epicardium, myocardium, and endocardium (Figure 16-3). The **epicardium** is the thin, outermost serous membrane layer. It covers the surface of the heart and the great vessels. The **myocardium** is the thick, muscular middle layer that forms the bulk of the heart. This layer is the contractile tissue that pumps the blood. The **endocardium** is the thin inner layer of epithelial tissue that lines the inner surface of the heart and heart valves.

Heart Chambers.   The heart is composed of four chambers: the right and left **atria** and the right and left **ventricles** (Figure 16-4). The two atria lie at the top, or base, of the heart. The two ventricles form the lower portion of the heart.

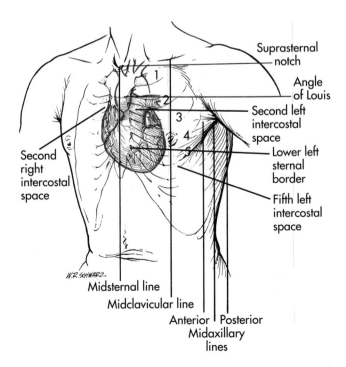

Figure 16-1   Location of the heart and chest wall landmarks of the precordium.

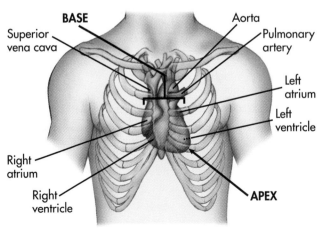

Figure 16-2   Position of the heart and great vessels.

The right atrium and ventricle form the right side of the heart, and the left atrium and ventricle form the left side of the heart. The right and left sides of the heart are separated by a septum; the interatrial septum separates the two atria, and the interventricular septum divides the ventricles. The two atria are thin-walled chambers that receive blood from the body and lungs by way of the major veins. The two ventricles are thick-walled chambers that pump blood out to the body and lungs by way of the major arteries.

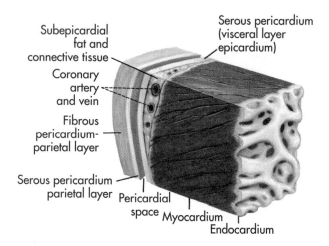

Figure 16-3   Cross section of cardiac muscle. (From Canobbio MM: *Cardiovascular disorders*, St. Louis, 1990, Mosby.)

Within the mediastinum, the heart is rotated so that the right ventricle composes most of the anterior surface of the heart and the left ventricle forms most of the posterior surface. The right ventricle lies behind the sternum and extends to the left of it. The left ventricle is located posterior to the right ventricle and extends farther to the left, forming the left anterior border of the heart. The right atrium lies slightly above and to the right of the right ventricle, and the left atrium occupies a posterior position on the heart (Figure 16-5).

Abbreviations commonly used for the heart chambers are:
- RA—right atrium
- RV—right ventricle
- LA—left atrium
- LV—left ventricle

Heart Valves.   The heart valves are structures through which blood flows either from the atria to the ventricles or from the ventricles to the great vessels. These valves function to permit the forward flow of blood and to prevent the backward flow of blood during the cardiac cycle. Their closure produces the normal heart sounds. The opening of heart valves is normally silent. The heart chambers and great vessels are separated by two sets of valves: **the atrioventricular (AV) valves** and the **semilunar (SL) valves.** The AV valves separate the atria and ventricles; the SL valves separate the ventricles and great vessels (Figure 16-6). The term competent is used to describe a properly functioning valve.

Atrioventricular Valves.   The AV valve on the right side of the heart between the right atrium and right ventricle is

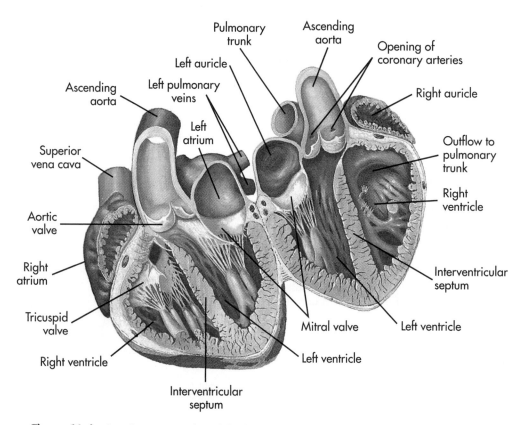

Figure 16-4   Anterior cross section of the heart showing the valves and chambers of the heart. (From Seidel HM et al.: *Mosby's guide to physical examination*, ed. 4, St. Louis, 1999, Mosby.)

called the **tricuspid valve**. It has three cusps, or leaflets. The AV valve on the left side of the heart between the left atrium and left ventricle is called the **mitral valve**. It is a bicuspid valve with two cusps. The AV valves open as a result of lower ventricular pressure during ventricular diastole. During ventricular systole, the pressure in the ventricle builds, and the cusps on each of these valves meet and close to form a seal so that no blood flows back into the atria. The valve cusps are anchored by strong, fibrous strands, the **chordae tendineae**, to the papillary muscles, which are attached to the ventricles. The chordae tendineae prevent prolapse of the AV valves into the atria during ventricular contraction (see Figure 16-4).

Semilunar Valves. The SL valves are located between the ventricles and the great arteries. Each has three cusps. On the right, the **pulmonic valve** separates the right ventricle from the pulmonary artery. On the left, the **aortic valve** separates the left ventricle from the aorta. When the ventricles contract during ventricular systole, these valves open to permit the flow of blood out from the heart into the pulmonary artery and the aorta. During ventricular diastole, when the ventricles are filling with blood, these valves are closed, preventing the backward flow of blood from the pulmonary artery and the aorta into the ventricles.

There are no valves between the venae cavae and the right atrium or between the pulmonary veins and the left atrium. Therefore, abnormally elevated pressure on the right side of the heart leads to congestion in the neck veins and abdomen, and abnormally elevated pressure on the left side of the heart leads to pulmonary congestion.

Great Vessels

The large arteries and veins that lie in a cluster at the base of the heart are called the great vessels. The arteries include the

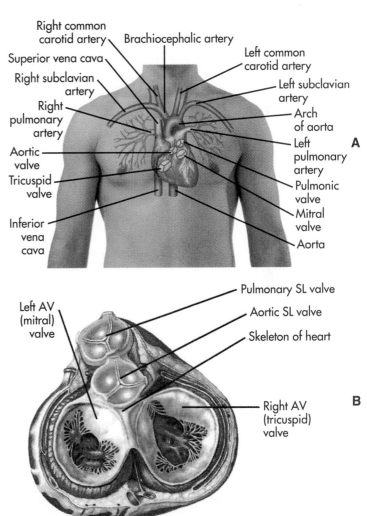

Figure 16-5 **A**, Location of the great vessels. **B**, Heart and great vessels. (**B** from Canobbio MM: *Cardiovascular disorders,* St. Louis, 1990, Mosby.)

Figure 16-6 **A**, Anatomical location of the heart valves and their relationship to the great vessels. **B**, Valves of the heart viewed from above. The atria are removed to show the mitral and tricuspid valves. (**A** from Seidel HM et al.: *Mosby's guide to physical examination,* ed. 4, St. Louis, 1999, Mosby; **B** from Thibodeau GA, Patton KT: *Anatomy and physiology,* ed. 4, St. Louis, 1999, Mosby.)

pulmonary artery and the aorta, and the veins include the superior and inferior venae cavae and the pulmonary veins (see Figure 16-5). These vessels circulate blood to and from the body and lungs. The superior and inferior venae cavae return unoxygenated blood from the upper and lower body to the right atrium. The pulmonary artery leaves the right ventricle, bifurcates almost immediately, and carries the unoxygenated blood from the right ventricle to both lungs. The pulmonary veins return the oxygenated blood from the lungs to the left atrium. The aorta receives the blood from the left ventricle and carries it to the body. The aorta ascends from the left ventricle, arches back at the level of the sternal angle, and descends behind the heart. Several major arteries branch off along the aortic arch. (Blood is supplied to the myocardium by the coronary arteries, which are the first arteries to branch off the aorta.)

Blood Circulation

When blood is ejected from the ventricle, it flows through two circulatory systems—the pulmonary and the systemic—simultaneously (Figure 16-7). Unoxygenated blood returning from circulation throughout the body—the systemic circulation—passes through the superior and inferior vena cavae and enters the heart at the right atrium. From there, it crosses the tricuspid valve and enters the right ventricle. When the ventricles contract, the blood flows from the right ventricle over the pulmonic valve and enters the pulmonary artery. The pulmonary circulation carries blood to the lungs, where it releases carbon dioxide and is reoxygenated. The blood returns to the heart through the pulmonary veins and enters the left atrium. From there, it flows across the mitral valve and into the left ventricle. When the ventricles contract, the blood flows from the left ventricle across the aor-

BOX 16-1

CHEST PAIN

The presence of chest pain suggests heart disease in the minds of both the professional health care worker and the layperson. The variety of causes of chest pain, however, is great. *Angina pectoris* is traditionally described as a pressure or choking sensation substernally, or up into the neck. The discomfort, which can be intense, may radiate as high as the jaw and down the left (and sometimes the right) arm. It often begins during strenuous physical activity or eating and frequently during exposure to intense cold, windy weather. Relief may occur in minutes if the activity can be stopped.

There are, however, myriad variations on this theme, sometimes quite similar, sometimes varying in location, intensity, and radiation—and often arising from sources other than the heart. "The precordial catch," for example, is a sudden, sharp, relatively brief pain that does not radiate, occurs most often at rest, and is unrelated to exertion and may not have a discoverable cause. It will, however, cause concern.

SOME POSSIBLE CAUSES OF CHEST PAIN
Cardiac

Typical angina pectoris
Atypical angina pectoris, angina equivalent
Prinzmetal variant angina
Unstable angina
Coronary insufficiency
Myocardial infarction
Nonobstructive, nonspastic angina
Mitral valve prolapse

Aortic

Dissection of the aorta

Musculoskeletal

Cervical radiculopathy
Shoulder disorder or dysfunction (arthritis, bursitis, rotator cuff injury, biceps tendinitis)
Costochondral disorder
Xiphodynia

Pleuropericardial pain

Pericarditis
Pleurisy
Pneumothorax
Mediastinal emphysema

Gastrointestinal disease

Hiatus hernia
Reflux esophagitis
Esophageal spasm
Cholecystitis with or without gallstones
Peptic ulcer disease
Pancreatitis

Pulmonary disease

Pulmonary hypertension
Pneumonia
Pulmonary embolus
Bronchial hyperreactivity

Psychoneurotic

Illicit drug use (e.g., cocaine)

Unlike in adults, chest pain in children and adolescents is seldom due to a cardiac problem. It is very often difficult to find a cause, but trauma and exercise-induced asthma and, even in a somewhat younger child as in the adolescent and adult, the use of cocaine should be among the considerations.

Data from Samiy, Douglas, Barondess, 1987; Harvey, 1988. From Seidel HM et al.: *Mosby's guide to physical examination,* ed. 4, St. Louis, 1999, Mosby.

tic valve and enters the aorta. The arterial system carries the blood throughout the body. The blood then returns through the venous vasculature to the superior and inferior venae cavae and into the right atrium. To summarize, a single red blood cell that started its route at the right atrium would follow this pathway: right atrium → tricuspid valve → right ventricle → pulmonary valve → pulmonary artery → lung → pulmonary vein → left atrium → mitral valve → left ventricle → aortic valve → aorta → systemic circulation → vena cava → right atrium (Box 16-1).

Cardiac Cycle

The heart contracts and relaxes rhythmically, permitting it to fill and then to eject blood, which circulates throughout the body. This occurs at the rate of about 60 to 100 times per minute. The average time for each cardiac cycle is about 0.8 second. The cardiac cycle describes the events of one complete cycle of the contraction and relaxation of the atria and ventricles. Pressure gradients within the heart and great vessels change with the rhythmic pumping of the heart. Blood flows from areas of higher pressure to areas of lower pressure. There are two phases to the cardiac cycle: **diastole**, or relaxation, and **systole**, or contraction. In general, the terms

diastole and systole refer to the actions of the ventricles, although the atria also have their own phases of relaxation and contraction.

The mechanical events described in this section must be in synchrony with the electrical stimulation of the heart, described in the next section.

Ventricular Diastole (Figure 16-8).   During ventricular diastole the ventricles relax, and the AV valves open. Pressure in the atria is higher than in the ventricles, so blood flows rapidly across the AV valves into the ventricles. This first, passive filling phase is called early or protodiastolic filling. About 70% of the blood in the atria enters the ventricles during this time. Toward the end of this phase, the atria contract (atrial kick) and eject the remaining 30% of the blood out of the atria and into the ventricles. This is called atrial systole.

Ventricular Systole (Figure 16-9).   During systole the ventricles contract, ejecting blood from the right ventricle into the pulmonary artery and from the left ventricle into

---

■ HELPFUL HINT

Note that atrial systole occurs at the same time as ventricular diastole. This may be confusing initially, but it is helpful to remember that the upper chambers—the atria—contract while the lower chambers—the ventricles—relax to receive the blood. Similarly, ventricular contraction occurs at the same time as atrial relaxation and filling.

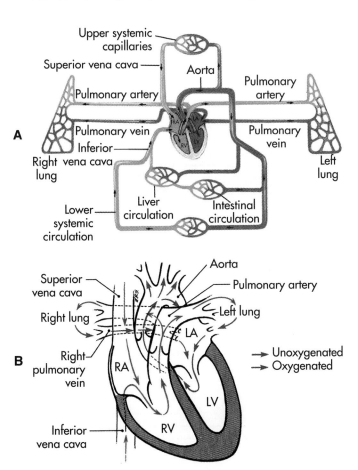

Figure 16-7 **A,** Circulatory system. **B,** Route of blood flow through the chambers of the heart and great vessels (**A** from Canobbio MM: *Cardiovascular disorders*, St. Louis, 1990, Mosby.)

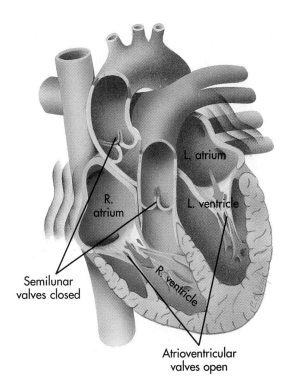

Figure 16-8 Ventricular diastole. The ventricles relax, and the mitral and tricuspid valves open, allowing blood to flow from the atria to the ventricles. (From Thibodeau GA, Patton KT: *Anatomy and physiology*, ed. 4, St. Louis, 1999, Mosby.)

the aorta. When the ventricles have filled with blood, ventricular pressure is higher than atrial pressure. The mitral and tricuspid valves snap shut, preventing any backflow of blood into the atria. Briefly, all four heart valves are closed. The ventricle walls then begin to contract, building pressure inside the ventricles. This is the period of isovolumic (same-volume) contraction: the volume of blood within the ventricles does not change. When the pressure in the ventricles exceeds the pressure in the pulmonary artery and the aorta, the pulmonic and aortic valves open and blood is rapidly ejected into the pulmonary artery and the aorta. After the blood is fully ejected from the ventricles, pressure within the ventricles is less than the pressure in the pulmonary artery and the aorta. The pulmonic and aortic valves close. While the ventricles have been contracting, the atria have been filling again with blood from the lungs and the body. Atrial pressure is again higher than ventricular pressure, the AV valves open, and the cycle begins again.

When the ventricles fill during diastole, they must respond to the force under which filling occurs; this force is called preload. During systole the ventricles eject the blood through the pulmonic and aortic valves against the force in the pulmonary artery and aorta; this force is called afterload.

The relationships of the left ventricular pressure curve, the heart sounds, and the electrocardiogram (ECG) are illustrated in Figure 16-10.

Differences Between Events on the Right and Left Sides of the Heart. Although the same events are occurring simultaneously on both sides of the heart, the pressure relationships are different on each side of the heart. Pressures on the right side are lower than those on the left side. The right side is pumping blood to the lungs while the left side is pumping blood to the rest of the body. As a result, there are two distinct components to each of the heart sounds. The difference is more distinct with the second heart sound (S_2). During the first heart sound (S_1), the mitral valve (M_1) closes just before the tricuspid valve (T_1). With the second heart sound (S_2), the aortic valve closure (A_2) occurs slightly before the pulmonic valve closure (P_2).

The four heart valves produce the normal heart sounds of S_1 and S_2. They are located close to each other anatomically. However, the sound produced by each valve is best heard at various areas of transmission across the precordium. These auscultation sites are described in this chapter under Technique for Examination and Expected Findings.

Electrical Stimulation and Conduction in the Heart

The heart is distinguished by the feature of automaticity, that is, it is stimulated and contracts by itself. The heart contracts in response to an electrical impulse that spreads through the

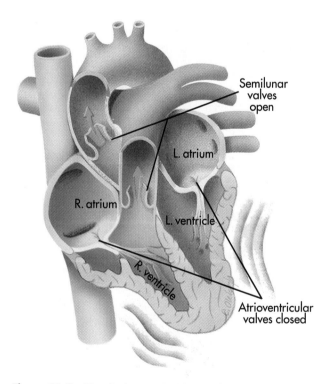

Figure 16-9 Ventricular systole. The ventricles contract, forcing the aortic and pulmonic valves to open; blood flows into the aorta and the pulmonary artery. (From Thibodeau GA, Patton KT: *Anatomy and physiology*, ed. 4, St. Louis, 1999, Mosby.)

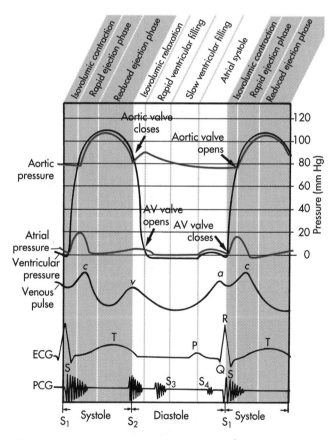

Figure 16-10 Events of the cardiac cycle, showing aortic, atrial, and ventricular pressure curves; the venous pulse wave; and the ECG and phonocardiogram tracings during systole and diastole. (From Seidel HM et al.: *Mosby's guide to physical examination*, ed. 4, St. Louis, 1999, Mosby.)

heart, activating and coordinating the mechanical pumping events of each cardiac cycle. The electrical current depolarizes as it is conveyed along the conduction system. In other words, when in the resting state, the cardiac cell is more positively charged on the outside of the cell and more negatively charged on the inside of the cell. When the electrical current, which is normally initiated in the sinoatrial node, flows across the atria and ventricles, depolarization occurs. As a result, the inside of the cardiac cell becomes more positively charged. Contraction of the atria and then the ventricles follows the electrical stimulation. After contraction, the cardiac cells repolarize, that is, the inside of the cells returns to a more negatively charged state.

The electrical discharge originates at specialized cells in the sinoatrial (SA) node, located near the vena cava in the right atrium (Figure 16-11). This node is also called the pacemaker. The electrical stimulus flows through the heart in an orderly sequence: from the sinoatrial node through the atria to the AV node, located low in the atrial septum. The impulse is briefly delayed at the AV node and then proceeds through the bundle of His and its branches, reaching the Purkinje fibers in the ventricular myocardium, where it stimulates myocardial contraction. The SA node discharges between 60 and 100 electrical impulses per minute.

A small portion of this electrical activity spreads to the skin, where it can be recorded as an ECG (Figure 16-12). The letters *PQRST* stand for the components of the electri-

cal impulse as it spreads through the heart. The relationship of these letters of the ECG to the phases of the cardiac cycle is shown in Table 16-1.

The passage of the electrical impulse as traced by the ECG and its relationship to the pressure curves and heart sounds are illustrated in Figure 16-10.

The electrical stimulation briefly precedes the mechanical response of the myocardium. Because of the pattern in which cardiac depolarization occurs, events on the left side of the heart normally take place slightly before those on the right side of the heart.

Heart Sounds

Events in the cardiac cycle produce sounds that can be heard over the chest wall through a stethoscope. The heart sounds include the S_1 and S_2, extra sounds, and murmurs. In some persons a third or fourth heart sound, S_3 or S_4, is a normal finding, as are certain kinds of murmurs.

Characteristics. All cardiovascular sounds have the following characteristics:

Frequency: The pitch or tone at which a sound is heard. Frequency is a measure of the number of vibrations in cycles per second (cps). Heart sounds are described as high or low pitched. Since all cardiovascular sounds are actually low pitched, these terms are relative.

Intensity: The loudness of the sound, determined by the amplitude of the vibrations, the source generating the

ECG Segment	Correlating Component of the Cardiac Cycle
P wave	Spread of impulse through atria—atrial systole (atrial depolarization)
PR interval	From beginning of P wave to beginning of QRS complex; passage of impulse from SA node through atria to AV node; time from initial stimulation of atria to initial stimulation of ventricles
QRS complex	Spread of impulse through ventricles—ventricular systole (ventricular depolarization)
ST segment and T wave	Ventricular muscle returns to resting state (ventricular repolarization)
QT interval	Period from beginning of ventricular depolarization to moment of repolarization: ventricular contraction

TABLE 16-1 **PQRST Relationship to ECG Phases**

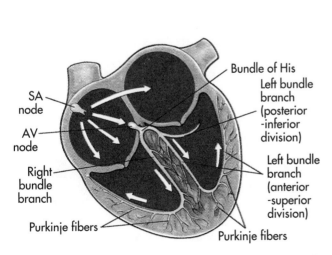

Figure 16-11 Cardiac electrical conduction. (From Canobbio MM: *Cardiovascular disorders*, St. Louis, 1990, Mosby.)

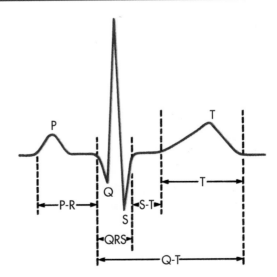

Figure 16-12 Normal ECG waveform. (From Berne RM, Levy MN: *Physiology*, ed. 3, St. Louis, 1993, Mosby.)

sound, the distance the vibrations must travel, and the medium through which they travel. Some cardiovascular sounds can be heard with the stethoscope barely touching the chest wall; others can be heard only with great concentration. The loudness of the sound is modified by the amount of tissue or space that lies between the sound at its origin and the outer chest wall. The heart sounds are typically very clear in a thin-chested individual but seem diminished or distant in the client who is very muscular or overweight or who has emphysema.

Quality: The overtones of a sound determine its quality, such as whether it is musical, blowing, or harsh.

Duration: Normal cardiovascular sounds are of short duration; the silent phases are longer. Abnormal sounds may be of short duration; such as clicks or snaps, or of longer duration, such as some murmurs.

Timing in the cardiac cycle: Sounds are heard either during systole (between S_1 and S_2) or during diastole (between S_2 and S_1).

First Heart Sound: S_1 (Figure 16-13).   The first heart sound results from closure of the AV valves. **S_1** signals the beginning of ventricular systole. S_1 can be heard over the entire precordium, but it is best heard at the apex, where it is usually louder than the second heart sound. Because pressure is higher and depolarization occurs slightly earlier on the left side of the heart, mitral valve closure occurs slightly before tricuspid valve closure. However, both components of S_1 are usually heard as one sound. Occasionally, both components of S_1 will be audible. This is known as a split first sound.

Second Heart Sound: S_2 (Figure 16-13).   The second heart sound results from the closure of the two semilunar valves: the pulmonic and the aortic. When ventricular systole is completed, pressure in the aorta and pulmonary artery exceeds ventricular pressure, and the semilunar valves are forced closed. S_2 signals the end of ventricular systole and the beginning of ventricular diastole. Diastole is normally the longer interval between the heart sounds. S_2 is audible over the entire precordium, but it is best heard at the base of the heart, where it is louder than S_1. S_2 is slightly higher in pitch and longer in duration than S_1. The two components of S_2 are A_2 (aortic valve closure) and P_2 (pulmonic valve closure). Pressure on the left side of the heart is higher than on the right, making aortic valve closure louder than pulmonic valve closure. Closure of the aortic valve is the loudest component of S_2 across the base of the heart, at both the left and right second intercostal spaces. Normally, the sound produced by the pulmonic valve can be heard only in a small area centering around the second left intercostal space. P_2 can be heard separately from A_2 when splitting of the second heart sound occurs. Remember, in the production of S_1, mitral valve closure (M_1) briefly precedes tricuspid valve closure (T_1). Similarly, in the production of S_2, aortic valve closure (A_2) briefly precedes pulmonic valve closure (P_2).

Effect of Respiration on the Second Heart Sound: Splitting of S_2 (Figure 16-14).   Although the volume of the right and left ventricles is about equal, respiration does affect the volume of blood returned to the right atrium from the vena cava. This increases the stroke volume of the right ventricle and delays the P_2 component of S_2. Also during inspiration, a slightly greater amount of blood remains in the lungs, which decreases the amount of blood returned to the left side of the heart from the pulmonary veins. This permits the aortic valve to close a bit sooner. With the aortic valve closing a bit earlier and the pulmonic valve closing a bit later, the two distinct components of the second heart sound—a split S_2—can be heard. This is known as physiological splitting. A split S_2 is most marked at the peak of the inspiratory phase of respiration. In healthy adult clients, A_2 and P_2 are separated by 0.04 to 0.05 of a second during inspiration. During expiration the disparity between the blood return to the two ventricles is equalized, and the semilunar valves close nearly synchronously, producing a single S_2. If the client holds his or her breath during inspiration, the ejection times of both ventricles become nearly equal again and the split sound becomes single. If a split S_2 is audible, it may be so in either the supine or sitting position.

Extra Heart Sounds

Third Heart Sound: S_3 (Figure 16-15).   Diastole is usually a silent phase of the cardiac cycle. Two phases of rapid

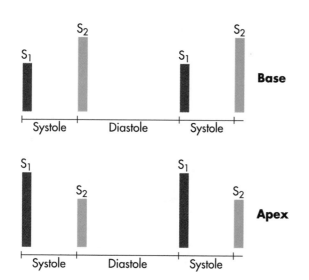

Figure 16-13   Relative loudness of S_1 and S_2 as heard over the base and the apex of the heart.

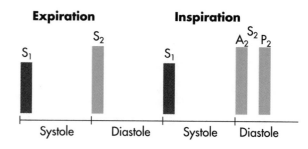

Figure 16-14   Normal splitting of S_2 (heard best at the second left intercostal space).

ventricular filling occur during diastole. The first, which takes place early in diastole, is a passive rapid filling phase. This occurs when the AV valves open after the second heart sound. The blood stored in the atria flows rapidly into the ventricles. This rapid distention of the ventricles causes vibrations of the ventricular walls. These vibrations may produce a third heart sound (S_3). S_3 is low in pitch and loudness and is best heard at the apex of the heart. This sound is common in children and young adults and in such instances is known as a physiological S_3. It is often heard in hyperkinetic states producing increased cardiac output, such as hyperthyroidism, exercise, pregnancy, and anxiety-related tachycardia. When it is heard in middle-aged adults, it is usually abnormal. When the third heart sound originates from the right ventricle, it is diminished during expiration and augmented during inspiration. When it originates from the left ventricle, it is augmented during expiration and diminished during inspiration.

Fourth Heart Sound: S_4 (Figure 16-16). The second phase of rapid ventricular filling that occurs during ventricular diastole results from the contraction of the atria and is the active rapid filling phase. The atrial contraction, or atrial kick, causes the blood remaining in the atria to rapidly enter the ventricles. This can create vibrations that produce a fourth heart sound (S_4). S_4 occurs just before S_1. Like S_3, it is a soft, low-pitched sound. When the fourth heart sound originates from the right ventricle, it is diminished during expiration and augmented during inspiration. When it originates from the left ventricle, it is augmented during expiration and diminished during inspiration. A physiological S_4 may be heard in middle-aged adults with thin-walled chests, especially after exercise, but it is less likely to be found in a well client than is a physiological S_3.

Neck Vessels

Carotid Arteries

The carotid arteries lie in the neck in the groove between the trachea and the sternocleidomastoid muscles. They are lateral to the trachea and medial to and alongside the sternocleidomastoid muscles (Figure 16-17). The pulse wave in the carotid arteries results from ventricular systole. Because of their proximity to the heart, the carotid arteries are easy to palpate, and the pulse wave is commonly visible.

The normal carotid pulse wave consists of a single positive wave followed by a dicrotic notch (Figure 16-18). The curve of the wave is a reflection of left ventricular activity. The upstroke is smooth and rapid, the summit is dome shaped, and the downstroke is less steep than the upstroke. The peak occurs just after the first heart sound. Figure 16-18 illustrates the relationship of the carotid pulse to S_1, S_2, and

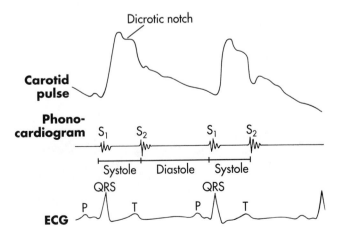

Figure 16-17 Neck vessels.

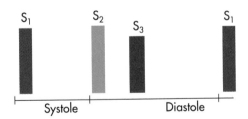

Figure 16-15 S_3, an early diastolic sound.

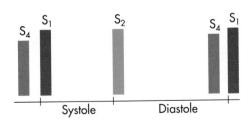

Figure 16-16 S_4, a late diastolic sound.

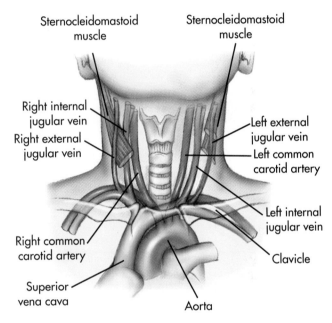

Figure 16-18 Carotid pulse wave in relation to S_1, S_2, and the ECG.

the ECG. The size and amplitude of the carotid pulse are determined by several factors, including the left ventricular stroke volume, ejection rate, peripheral vascular resistance, vessel distensibility, and pulse pressure.

Jugular Veins

The jugular veins empty blood directly into the vena cava. No valves separate the jugular veins from the vena cava or the vena cava from the right atrium. Therefore the jugular veins reflect the activity on the right side of the heart, providing an indication of the competency of right-sided heart function. They reflect changes in right atrial volume and filling pressure.

There are two sets of jugular veins: the external jugular veins and the internal jugular veins (see Figure 16-17). The external jugular veins are smaller; more superficial and discrete; and visible bilaterally above the clavicles, lateral to the insertion of the sternocleidomastoid muscles. The internal jugular veins are larger and lie beneath and medial to the sternocleidomastoid muscles and lateral to the carotid arteries. Because of their superficial location, the external jugular veins are often easier to see and may be particularly prominent in individuals who have chronic elevation of venous pressure (Figure 16-19). The internal jugular veins are less accessible to inspection, but reflection of their activity may be visible as diffuse pulsations on the skin overlying the lower part of the neck.

Jugular Venous Pulse.   Normal **jugular venous pulsations** are low-pressure impulses or waves that resemble the pressure changes in the right atrium. The pulsations are waveforms moving back from the right side of the heart. They indicate the pressure and volume changes as the blood returns to the right atrium and the heart contracts and relaxes. The jugular venous pulse wave has five major components: three upward waves and two descent slopes. These wave components are illustrated in Figure 16-20 and described in Table 16-2.

Jugular Venous Pressure.   Jugular venous pressure is the level at which the jugular veins appear full. In a client with normal right-sided heart function, any filling of the jugular veins is not evident until the person is nearly in a supine position. If the jugular veins appear full when the client's head is elevated to a higher position, this indicates less competent function on the right side of the heart.

TABLE 16-2	Jugular Venous Pulse Wave Components		
Jugular Pulse Component	**Reflects**	**Produced by**	**Timing**
a wave	Atrial contraction	Brief backflow of blood to vena cava during right atrial contraction—normally highest wave in cycle	Peaks just before S_1
c wave	Ventricular contraction	Upward bulging of tricuspid valve early in ventricular systole	Occurs at end of S_1
x descent	Atrial relaxation	Downward pull on right atrium when ventricles contract during systole	Occurs just before S_2
v wave	Atrial filling before tricuspid valve opens	Continuous filling and increased pressure in right atrium	Peaks after S_2
y descent	Passive ventricular filling	Fall in right atrial pressure after tricuspid valve opens; blood flows from right atrium to right ventricle	Follows v wave after S_2

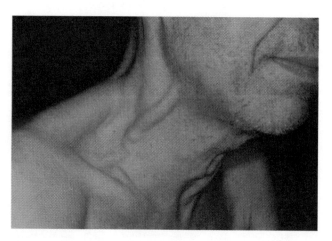

Figure 16-19   Neck vein distention. (From Swartz MH: *Textbook of physical diagnosis: history and examination*, ed. 3, Philadelphia, 1998, WB Saunders.)

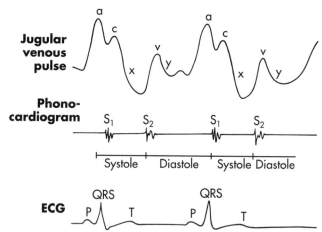

Figure 16-20   Jugular venous pulse waves in relation to S_1 and S_2, and the ECG.

Venous hum. The venous hum is a continuous, low-pitched humming sound heard over the major veins at the base of the neck in many children and in some adults. It usually has no pathological significance. It is produced by turbulent blood flow in the internal jugular veins. The venous hum is most audible over the supraclavicular spaces, more commonly on the right.

Peripheral Vessels

The arteries and veins of the peripheral vascular system are illustrated in Figure 16-21.

Arteries and veins differ somewhat in their structure, which reflects their functions. Arteries are subject to higher pressures; their walls are tougher and less distensible. The venous system involves lower pressures; the vein walls are less tough and more distensible. Lower extremity veins contain valves to prevent the backflow of blood. If blood volume increases, the veins can become distended to hold some of the excess blood; this decreases the workload of the heart. Because of their ability to stretch and accommodate the majority of the total blood volume, veins are also known as capacitance vessels. Veins lie closer to the surface of the skin than do arteries. The variation in structure between veins and arteries is illustrated in Figure 16-22.

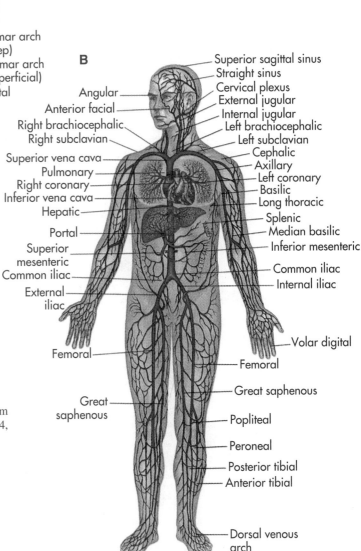

Figure 16-21 Systemic circulation. **A**, Arteries. **B**, Veins. (From Seidel HM et al: *Mosby's guide to physical examination*, ed. 4, St. Louis, 1999, Mosby.)

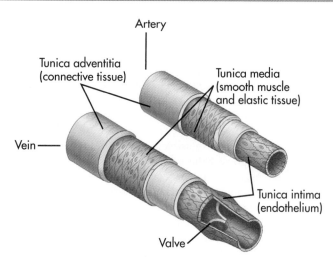

Figure 16-22 Drawings of sectioned artery and vein (note valve in vein). (From Thibodeau GA, Patton KT: *Anatomy and physiology*, ed. 4, St. Louis, 1999, Mosby).

EXAMINATION

Focused Health History

For each symptom, describe the following characteristics in the health history: onset, course since onset, location, quality, quantity, setting in which the symptoms occur, associated phenomena, alleviating and aggravating factors and efforts to treat, and underlying concern or meaning.

Special areas to assess for risk for and existing problems of the cardiovascular system are included in the history outline that follows. Always try to have the client explain or describe the situation in his or her own words before suggesting descriptive terms of your own. Information from family members and/or friends may also be useful in understanding the client's level of health or disability and can provide a broader perspective on the impact of a cardiovascular problem on both the client and the family.

Present Health/Illness Status

1. Activity pattern: normal level of activity, type, pattern, frequency, duration, intensity, regularity, any recent changes
2. Nutritional status
   a. Usual diet: proportion of fat, use of salt, intake of caffeine products, food preferences (a dietary log may be useful in gathering this information over time or 24-hour recall), cultural influences on eating (foods commonly served or forbidden), lifestyle influences on intake
   b. Weight: loss or gain, history of dieting (type, effectiveness)
3. Tobacco use
   a. Type (cigarettes, cigars, pipe, chewing tobacco, snuff), duration, amount, age started, efforts to quit (NOTE: pack-years of smoking are calculated by

Risk Factors
Cardiovascular Disease

CORONARY ARTERY DISEASE
Principal modifiable risk factors

Elevated serum cholesterol level (greater than 200 mg/dl) and lowered high-density lipo-protein level (less than 35 mg/dl)
Smoking
Hypertension
Obesity
Excessive dietary intake of calories and fat, especially saturated fat
Diabetes mellitus
Sedentary lifestyle
Long-term use of oral contraceptives
Personality characteristics such as intensity, compulsivity, hostility

Principal nonmodifiable risk factors

Increasing age
Gender: Men at greater risk; postmenopausal women at greater risk because of loss of protective effect of estrogen
Family history of cardiovascular disease, diabetes, hyperlipidemia, hypertension, or sudden death in young adults.

CEREBROVASCULAR DISEASE

Hypertension
Obesity
Smoking
Coronary artery disease
Atrial fibrillation
Diabetes mellitus
Increased age

PERIPHERAL ARTERY DISEASE

Smoking
Diabetes mellitus
Age older than 50
Hypercholesterolemia
Obesity
Excessive dietary intake of fat, especially saturated fat
Menopause
Varicose veins
Prolonged standing or sitting
Obesity
Sedentary lifestyle
Gender: Women at greater risk than men, particularly during pregnancy
Increasing age
Race: Caucasians at greater risk than African-Americans

multiplying the number of years of smoking by the number of packs smoked each day)
   b. Exposure to passive smoke (e.g., at home, work)
4. Alcohol consumption: amount per day or week, frequency, duration of current consumption
5. Medications: antihypertensives, beta-blockers, calcium channel blockers, digoxin, diuretics, oral contraceptives, aspirin, anticoagulants, over-the-counter drugs

(OTCs), mood altering drugs, herbal preparations, vitamins, weight loss medications (ask about dosage, frequency, when began and why, side effects, compliance)

Personal and Social History

1. Personality assessment
   a. Perceived level of stress in life
   b. Type and intensity of work (e.g., physical demands, exposure to heat, chemicals, dust)
   c. Compulsive behaviors
   d. Self-description of mood (frequently angry, impatient, frustrated, intense, anxious, easygoing, ability to relax)
2. Relaxation habits
   a. Routine activities
   b. Hobbies
   c. Exercise: type, amount, frequency, intensity
   d. Stress reduction practices
   e. Use of alcohol, illegal drugs (amyl nitrate "poppers," cocaine)
   f. Sexual activity (frequency, number of partners, sexual practices)
   g. Alternative health practices (yoga, Tai Chi, meditation, etc.)
3. Significant others: who is in the home; current support system
4. Recent stressful life events or major life changes (e.g., changes in employment, family events, losses)

Past Health History

1. Hypertension
2. Coronary artery disease (transient ischemic attacks, stroke, etc.)
3. Elevated lipids (cholesterol, triglycerides)
4. Dysrhythmias
5. Previous myocardial infarctions
6. Congenital heart defect or disease
7. Murmurs
8. Cardiac disease
9. Cardiac surgery or hospitalization for cardiac disorder
10. Palpitations
11. Dizziness
12. Dependent leg edema
13. Rheumatic fever, unexplained fever, swollen joints
14. Diabetes mellitus
15. Anemia
16. Most recent ECG, stress ECG, or other heart test

Family History

1. Angina
2. Heart disease (heart failure, valvular disease)
3. Myocardial infarction
4. Stroke
5. Diabetes mellitus
6. Hyperlipidemia
7. Hypertension
8. Obesity

9. Sudden death, particularly of young and middle-aged relatives
10. Congenital heart defects
11. Peripheral vascular disease
12. Symptoms such as dyspnea, fatigue, leg pains after exertion, palpitations, syncope

Symptom Analysis

Dyspnea

Dyspnea, an abnormally uncomfortable awareness of breathing and shortness of breath, is one of the principal symptoms of cardiac disease. Dyspnea is normal in healthy persons when it is caused by moderate to strenuous exertion. It is considered abnormal when it occurs at rest or at a level of physical exertion not expected to cause distress. It is associated with a variety of diseases of the heart, lungs, chest wall, and respiratory muscles, and with anxiety. Therefore it is important to gather a careful and precise history on this symptom.

Dyspnea on exertion (DOE) is usually due to chronic congestive heart failure or severe pulmonary disease. It can be quantified by determining the number of level blocks the client can climb currently and 6 months ago or the number of flights of stairs the client can climb.

Orthopnea is shortness of breath that occurs when a person is lying flat and that is relieved by sitting or standing. **Paroxysmal nocturnal dyspnea** (PND) is shortness of breath that begins several hours after the onset of sleep (due to the inability of a weakened heart to handle the increased vascular load caused by prolonged periods in the supine position) and that is relieved by sitting or rising. The symptom of PND often associated with orthopnea is the need to use more pillows to sleep. Determining the number of pillows the client uses to sleep will help quantify the degree of orthopnea (e.g., four-pillow orthopnea). In particular, comparing the change over a consistent time period, such as 6 months, will help in the assessment of the course of the problem (see also Chapter 15).

When assessing dyspnea, inquire about the following:
1. **Onset:** sudden or gradual
2. **Course since onset:** duration, constant or intermittent; frequency of episodes; pattern of awakening from sleep; interference with activities of daily living or with sleep
3. **Location:** generalized versus localized
4. **Quality:** "strangling" sensation
5. **Quantity:** amount of activity or exertion required to cause shortness of breath (number of blocks walked, number of stairs climbed); compare with 3 and 6 months ago; number of pillows needed to sleep
6. **Setting:** home, work, recreation, other situations where symptom occurs
7. **Associated phenomena:** anxiety, confusion, lightheadedness, cough, fever, wheezing, edema, weight change, sputum (frothy, purulent, bloody), palpitations
8. **Alleviating and aggravating factors:** effect of position, activity, rest, environmental change, medication, smoking, occupational exposures

9. **Underlying concern or meaning:** concerns about cardiac condition, changing life patterns, decreased energy

Chest Pain, Tightness, or Discomfort

Chest pain can be due to problems with noncardiac structures (e.g., thoracic structures, tissues of the neck and thoracic wall, and some abdominal organs) as well as to cardiac problems (see Box 16-1; Box 16-2). The history will be important to make this differentiation.

1. **Onset:** sudden or gradual; triggering factors—eating, physical exertion, rest, stressful situation, emotional experience, coughing, cold temperature, sexual intercourse
2. **Course since onset:** duration (time episode[s] lasted, intervals between episodes), frequency of episodes
3. **Location:** area of chest wall (may occur on both sides of the chest wall and substernally), radiation (note whether pain moves to arms, shoulders, neck, scapula, jaw, teeth, upper abdomen)
4. **Quality:** aching, sharp, dull, tingling, burning, stabbing, cramping, crushing, viselike, pressing, squeezing, strangling, constricting, bursting (note the client's use of the clenched fist over the sternum to describe the character and location of the pain; this is a characteristic sign of angina commonly referred to as Levine's sign)
5. **Quantity:** degree of interference with activity, sleep disruption
6. **Setting:** home, work, during interactions with specific individuals or during stressful situations
7. **Associated phenomena:** diaphoresis; nausea/vomiting; dyspnea; palpitations; dizziness; faintness; fatigue; cold, clammy skin; cyanosis of lips, ears, nailbeds; pallor; anxiety
8. **Alleviating and aggravating factors:** rest; position change; activities that make the pain worse (moving the arms or neck, breathing, lying flat); medications, including nitroglycerin (number of tablets); other cardiac medications, and analgesics
9. **Underlying concern:** fear of heart attack

Palpitations

Described as an unpleasant awareness of the forceful or rapid beating of the heart, palpitations may be caused by changes in cardiac rhythm or rate. Episodes may be described as "skipped beats" or a "flopping sensation" (most commonly due to extrasystoles), or the client may say that the heart has "stopped beating" (often a result of the compensatory pause after a premature contraction).

1. **Onset:** sudden or gradual
2. **Course since onset:** duration (length of episodes, abrupt cessation), frequency of episodes, pattern of episodes
3. **Location:** area of chest felt
4. **Quality:** fluttering, pounding, jumping, stopping
5. **Quantity:** degree of interference with activity; need to stop all activity
6. **Setting:** after strenuous exercise, after a meal
7. **Associated phenomena:** throbbing of the neck, syncope, dizziness, tingling in the hands, flush, sweating, headache, angina, intolerance to heat or cold, relation to exercise
8. **Alleviating and aggravating factors:** rest, position change, vomiting; exertion, excitement, stress, medications, caffeine, smoking, alcohol
9. **Underlying concern:** cardiac condition

BOX 16-2

COMPARISON OF SOME TYPES OF CHEST PAIN

ANGINA PECTORIS	MUSCULOSKELETAL	GASTROINTESTINAL
Presence of cardiac risk factors	History of trauma	History of indigestion
Specifically noted time of onset	Vague onset	Vague onset
Related to physical, emotional, or psychosocial effort	Related to physical effort	Related to food consumption
Disappears if stimulating effort can be terminated	Continues after cessation of effort	May go on for several hours; unrelated to effort
Frequently forces clients to stop effort	Clients can very often continue activity	Clients can very often continue activity
Client may awaken from sleep	Delays falling asleep	Client may awaken from sleep, particularly during early morning
Relief at times with nitroglycerin	Relief at times with heat, aspirin, or rest	Relief at times with antacids
Pain frequently in early morning or after washing and eating	Worse in evening after a day of physical effort	No particular relationship to time of day; related to food, tension
Greater likelihood in cold weather	Greater likelihood in cold, damp weather	Anytime

Data from Samiy, 1987; Harvey, 1988. From Seidel HM et al.: *Mosby's guide to physical examination*, ed. 4, St. Louis, 1999, Mosby.

Fatigue

1. **Onset:** sudden or gradual
2. **Course since onset:** duration (unusual or typical, recent change), pattern (time of day— morning, evening, all day), bedtime earlier than usual, naps
3. **Location:** specific area (arms/legs feel heavy) versus generalized
4. **Quality:** inability to keep up with family, co-workers; limitation of usual activities
5. **Quantity:** degree of interference with activity
6. **Setting:** worse at home, work, or other area
7. **Associated phenomena:** dyspnea, orthopnea, chest pain, palpitations, anorexia, nausea, vomiting, weakness, weight loss, nocturia, visual changes, heavy menstrual flow, anemia, sleep problems, depression
8. **Alleviating and aggravating factors:** medications (prescription and nonprescription), home remedies, exercise, rest, stress
9. **Underlying concern:** systemic illness, leukemia

Dependent Edema

1. **Onset:** sudden or gradual
2. **Course since onset:** duration (changes over 24-hour period—better after a night of sleep), pattern (time of day—morning, end of the day), progressive changes
3. **Location:** one or both legs, abdomen, face, neck, upper arms, generalized
4. **Quality:** pain associated with the swelling, equal amount in both limbs
5. **Quantity:** amount of swelling, tightness of shoes or rings
6. **Setting:** at work, home (situations that require a lot of standing)
7. **Alleviating and aggravating factors:** effects of standing, leg elevation, rest; support hose; weight gain or loss
8. **Associated phenomena:** dyspnea, jaundice, ulceration and pigmentation changes of the skin of the legs
9. **Underlying concern:** cardiac condition

Leg Pain or Cramps

1. **Onset:** gradual or sudden, with activity or rest, effect of leg elevation
2. **Course since onset:** duration (changes over 24-hour period and longer time period) frequency of occurrence (effect of activity), pattern (time of day—morning, end of the day), waking with pain or cramp (wakes at night)
3. **Location:** one or both legs
4. **Quality:** burning in toes; pain when pointing toes; pain in thighs or buttocks; "charley horses"; aching, pain over specific location; character of pain; radiation
5. **Quantity**: amount of pain
6. **Setting:** at work, home, in situations that require a lot of walking
7. **Associated phenomena:** skin changes in extremities (coldness, pallor, hair loss, sores, redness or warmth over vein, visible veins), fatigue or limping (effect of walking)
8. **Alleviating and aggravating factors:** improved or worsened by walking; effect of rest, elevation, medication, home remedies

9. **Underlying concern:** cardiac condition, decreased ability to move freely

Nocturia

1. **Onset:** suddenly awakened at night with an urgent need to urinate
2. **Course since onset:** duration (recent change), frequency of occurrence (every night versus occasionally, number of times during the night), pattern (time of night, relationship to fluid intake or medications)
3. **Quality:** burning or pain, urgency, hesitancy, straining, change in stream
4. **Quantity:** amount of urine each episode
5. **Setting:** home, traveling
6. **Associated phenomena:** fever, pain, dyspnea, orthopnea
7. **Alleviating and aggravating factors:** fluid intake, medication (especially diuretics), home remedies
8. **Underlying concern:** bladder infection, diabetes, interrupted sleep

Syncope

Syncope (loss of consciousness) results most commonly from reduced perfusion of the brain. It may be due to ventricular fibrillation with AV block, other cardiac dysrhythmias, valvular disease, orthostatic hypotension, stroke, vasovagal response, or seizure disorders.

1. **Onset:** sudden or gradual; precipitating factors (exertion, position change, bleeding)
2. **Course since onset:** duration (length of episodes, time taken to regain consciousness), frequency (recurrent)
3. **Quality:** preceding sensations (light-headedness, vertigo, weakness, aphasia, confusion, sudden movements, visual changes, emotional disturbance); loss of consciousness
4. **Quantity:** number and length of episodes
5. **Setting:** hot shower or enclosed room; in a stressful situation, as when giving blood or hearing bad news
6. **Associated phenomena:** nausea, chest pain, diaphoresis, palpitation, confusion, numbness, hunger, extra or unusual exertion, sudden turning of neck (carotid sinus effect), change in posture
7. **Alleviating and aggravating factors:** change in position, temperature, medication
8. **Underlying concern:** seizures, stroke

Preparation for Examination: Client and Environment

A quiet environment is essential for a thorough examination of the cardiovascular system. All heart sounds are quiet and of relatively low pitch. They are very difficult to hear when any extraneous noises are present. A room temperature that is comfortable for the client is also important to prevent chilling and subsequent interference with hearing the heart sounds. For inspection of the subtle motions of the precordium and the neck vessels, good lighting in the room is required, including both standard examination room lighting and a movable light that can be directed at an angle across

Preparation for Examination

EQUIPMENT

Item	Purpose
Examination table large enough for client to change position easily	Client needs to be able to move to left lateral recumbent position for auscultation of the heart
Penlight or lamp with movable arm	Tangential lighting for inspection of precordium and jugular venous pulsations
Sphygmomanometer with appropriate-size cuff	Measurement of blood pressure
Stethoscope with diaphragm and bell	Auscultation of heart and large arteries
Metric ruler	Measurement of jugular venous pressure
Tape measure	Measurement of edematous extremities

CLIENT AND ENVIRONMENT

1. Ensure privacy for the client (provide a drape).
2. Make sure the room, your hands, and the stethoscope are warm during the examination.
3. Ensure a quiet room.
4. Ensure good lighting.

the precordium and neck vessels. Respect the client's need for privacy. Provide a drape, and uncover only those portions of the body being examined as you proceed.

Other Considerations: Components, Sequence, and Integration With Other Systems

The examination of the cardiovascular system includes the following: (1) inspection and palpation of the peripheral pulses; (2) blood pressure measurement (see Chapter 9); (3) inspection and auscultation of the neck vessels—the jugular veins and carotid arteries; (4) inspection, palpation, and auscultation of the heart; and (5) inspection of the peripheral veins.

Several changes of position are required of the client during the cardiovascular examination, so it is very important to organize the various parts of the physical examination in a sequence that is comfortable for the client and that does not involve unnecessary movement. Remember that the judgments about functioning of the cardiovascular system also depend on findings in other body systems, such as crackles in the lungs, engorgement of the liver, hypertensive changes in the vessels of the retina, a barrel chest, or the bruit of an abdominal aortic aneurysm. Consequently, the cardiovascular assessment, in actual practice, may require integration of findings from several systems.

Discussion of the cardiovascular examination in this chapter is divided into three parts: the heart, the neck vessels, and the peripheral vessels.

Technique for Examination and Expected Findings

Begin the cardiovascular examination by assessing the client's general appearance—something which you will have begun to assess while taking the history. Note the client's general build, skin color, respiration pattern, position, and movements.

Examination of the Heart

For a thorough examination of the heart, you must examine the client in the sitting, supine, and left lateral recumbent positions. Inspection and palpation are performed with the client primarily in the sitting and supine positions; auscultation must be performed with the client in the sitting, forward-leaning, supine, and left lateral recumbent (also called left lateral decubitus) positions. Examination of the heart in these various positions improves audibility of heart sounds by bringing the heart closer to the chest wall. Always be aware of the client's ability to move and of his or her comfort in the various positions, particularly when examining the client in the supine and left lateral recumbent positions. Clients with a compromised respiratory or cardiovascular system may not be able to tolerate all positions. Also note the client's posture, breathing patterns, and energy level, which will provide clues to the client's status.

The techniques of inspection, palpation, and auscultation are used to examine the heart. Percussion is not a standard part of the cardiac examination; however, percussion of the heart may be useful to estimate cardiac size and will be addressed briefly.

Although it is tempting to auscultate the heart first, be sure to inspect and palpate the precordium before placing the stethoscope on the chest wall. You will gain much information that will enhance your auscultatory assessment.

All the techniques used for examining the heart are affected by the amount and type of tissue lying between the heart and the chest wall. In clients with more developed musculature, more adipose tissue, or a barrel chest, precordial findings may not be visible or palpable, and the sounds will seem more distant.

Inspection.   With the client in the supine or sitting position, inspect the chest wall. You will need a tangential light to observe the subtle movements of the chest. Observe the chest first for size and symmetry and for any deformities of the thoracic cage. Note the frequency, depth, and regularity of respirations. Then look for any visible pulsations, retractions, heaves, or lifts.

Apical Impulse.   The thrust of the contracting left ventricle may produce a visible pulsation in the area of the left midclavicular line at the fifth intercostal space. This is the **apical impulse**. It occurs nearly synchronously with the carotid pulse and the first heart sound; simultaneous palpation of a carotid artery is helpful in identifying it. When it is visible, the apical impulse helps to identify an area very near the cardiac apex, thus giving some indication of cardiac size. (The apical beat was previously called the point of maximal impulse [PMI]; since other pulsations may be more prominent than the apical beat, this term is no longer used.)

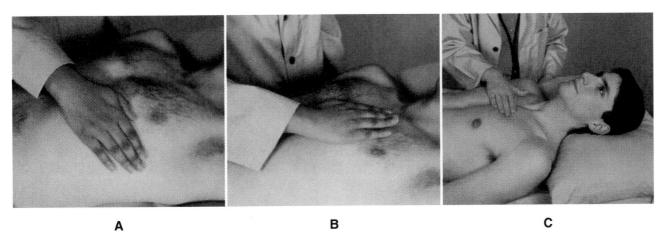

Figure 16-23 Palpation of the precordium. **A**, Apex. **B**, Left sternal border. **C**, Base.

> ■ **HELPFUL HINT**
>
> The apical impulse is visible in only about half of the adult population.

Retraction. A **retraction** is a pulling in of some of the tissues on the precordium related to the position and activity of the heart. A slight retraction of the chest wall just medial to the midclavicular line in the fifth intercostal space is a normal finding. It is more evident when the chest wall is thin.

Lifts and Heaves. A lift is a sustained thrust of the ventricle during systole. A heave is an excessive thrust of the heart against the chest wall. A lift or heave may be present with ventricular hypertrophy as a result of an increased workload. A left ventricular lift or heave is seen or palpated in the apical area; a right ventricular lift or heave is seen or palpated at the left sternal border.

Palpation. Use the technique of palpation to build on and expand the findings obtained during inspection. Take time to "tune in" to the movement over the precordium. Most of these movements are subtle and are better perceived after careful inspection. Varying the hand pressure you apply only slightly, use a light and gentle touch, allowing any movements of the chest to come toward your hand. The sensitivity of your hand decreases as the pressure you use increases. Palpate the precordium while the client is sitting, while the client is lying in the lowest position that he or she is able to tolerate, and while the client is in the left lateral decubitus position.

Stand on the right side of the client. Palpate the precordium in three areas, moving either from the apex to the base or from the base to the apex; develop a methodical system. (In this text the apex-to-base approach is used.) Either way, you will palpate the apical area, along the left sternal border, and at both the left and right second intercostal spaces.

Using the palmar surface of your right hand and fingers, begin at the fifth left intercostal space in the midclavicular line, where the apical impulse is normally located (Figure 16-23, *A*). You will feel this as a slight tap of short duration against your fingers. This pulsation is approximately 1 cm in diameter. On occasion, the apical impulse is located lateral to the midclavicular line (e.g., in association with a high diaphragm, such as occurs with pregnancy). The outward tap of the normal apical impulse is felt only during early systole. Next, place your hand along the left sternal border (Figure 16-23, *B*), move to the base of the heart at the right and then the left sternal borders in the second intercostal space (Figure 16-23, *C*). Palpate in these locations for any pulsations, vibrations, heaves, or thrills. None should be palpable against the palm of your hand.

> ■ **HELPFUL HINT**
>
> A thrill is the rushing sensation of blood moving through the heart or a major artery. It is like the sensation transmitted to your fingers when they are placed over the neck of a purring cat. A thrill may be felt over a large murmur.

The amplitude of the apical impulse may seem to be increased in normal individuals with thin chest walls. In clients with high cardiac output states, such as anemia, anxiety, fever, or hyperthyroidism, the apical impulse often increases in amplitude and duration. In persons who are obese, have thick chest walls, or have emphysema, you are unlikely to be able to palpate the apical impulse. Left ventricular hypertrophy and/or dilation displaces the apical impulse downward and to the left, and may also increase the size of the impulse.

If significant movements are palpable over the precordium, extend palpation beyond the standard areas. Include the left anterior axillary area, the epigastrium, the right sternal border and any area where you note abnormalities. Note the timing of any abnormal palpable movements, using the carotid artery pulsation as a guide.

Percussion. Percussion of the heart is not commonly done since chest x-ray study is a more accurate measure of heart enlargement. However, percussion of the cardiac bor-

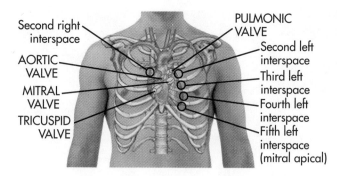

Figure 16-24 Anatomical location of the heart valves and transmission of closure sounds from the heart valves. (From Seidel HM et al.: *Mosby's guide to physical examination*, ed. 4, St. Louis, 1999, Mosby.)

ders may be useful as an estimate of cardiac enlargement in instances where x-ray studies are unavailable or inaccessible (e.g., in an outpatient clinic, in the patient's home).

Standing on the client's right, place your stationary (pleximeter) finger at the fifth intercostal space on the left side of the chest near the anterior axillary line. Slide your stationary hand toward yourself, while continuing to percuss. The sound will change from resonance (over the lung) to dullness (over the heart). Normally, the left border of cardiac dullness (LBCD) is percussed in the fifth interspace at the midclavicular line (approximately 6 cm lateral to the left of the sternum). As you continue percussion, the dullness will slope toward the sternum as you progress upward so that the right border of dullness coincides with the left sternal border at the second interspace. Cardiac enlargement may be due to increased ventricular volume, wall thickness, or a left ventricular mass.

Auscultation. Although heart sounds are described as being "high pitched" or "low pitched," these terms are relative. All heart sounds are of low frequency and in a range that is difficult for the human ear to hear. A quiet room and careful use of the stethoscope make it possible to hear the sounds of the heart.

Stethoscope. Review the material on the use of the stethoscope in Chapter 8. Use both the diaphragm and the bell of the stethoscope to auscultate heart sounds. Use the diaphragm to listen to the high-pitched sounds, such as S_1 and S_2. Use the bell to listen to the low-pitched sounds, such as S_3 and S_4. (See Table 16-3 to learn which sounds are best heard with the diaphragm and which ones are best heard with the bell.)

■ HELPFUL HINT

If you apply too much pressure to the bell of the stethoscope, the underlying skin becomes tight and the skin itself then acts as a diaphragm. Place the bell very lightly on the chest wall, with just enough pressure applied to seal the edge.

Auscultatory Areas. Although the four heart valves are located close to one another in a small area behind the ster-

TABLE 16-3 Use of the Bell and Diaphragm of the Stethoscope for Cardiac Auscultation

Sounds Best Heard with the Diaphragm	Sounds Best Heard with the Bell
High-frequency sounds 　First heart sound 　Second heart sound 　Systolic clicks 　High-pitched murmurs of 　　valvular regurgitation 　Ejection clicks 　Opening snap of mitral valve 　Pericardial friction rub	Low-frequency sounds 　Third heart sound 　Fourth heart sound 　Diastolic murmurs originating from mitral and 　　tricuspid valves

TABLE 16-4 Areas Where Valve Closures Are Best Heard

Valve	Area
Mitral	Fifth left intercostal space at the midclavicular line
Tricuspid	Left sternal border, fourth left intercostal space
Pulmonic	Left sternal border, second left intercostal space
Aortic	Right sternal border, second right intercostal space

num, the areas on the chest wall where their closure sounds are most audible are not located directly over the valves, but rather in the direction of the flow of blood. The area where the closure of each valve can normally be heard best is summarized in Table 16-4 and illustrated in Figure 16-24.

While these are the main areas for auscultation, do not limit auscultation to these areas only. Listen in an area around each of the areas just described. Important findings are sometimes present in other locations, such as the right parasternal region, axilla, neck, and epigastrium.

Complete auscultation includes listening with the client in the sitting, leaning-forward, supine, and left lateral decubitus positions. Begin auscultation by standing on the right side of the client. The client may be in the sitting or supine position as you begin. A systematic method of auscultation is essential, as with palpation. Begin either at the apex or at the base of the heart. (We will begin at the apex in this description.) Start at the fifth left intercostal space in the midclavicular line (Figure 16-25, *A*). Inch your stethoscope toward the lower left sternal border (Figure 16-25, *B*). Inching from area to area allows a full hearing of the sounds. Move upward along the left sternal border to the base of the heart. Listen at the base of both the second left intercostal space at the sternal border (Figure 16-25, *C*) and the second right intercostal space at the sternal border (Figure 16-25, *D*).

Repeat this pattern using first the diaphragm and then the bell of the stethoscope. If any sounds radiate beyond the standard area of auscultation, follow them with the stethoscope by inching the stethoscope along in the direction of

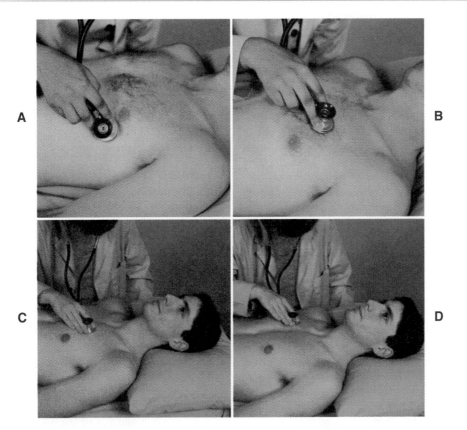

Figure 16-25 Auscultation of the precordium. **A**, Apex. **B**, Left sternal border. **C**, Second left intercostal space. **D**, Second right intercostal space.

the sound. For example, sounds may radiate to the area of the anterior axillary line or up to the carotid arteries.

Listen selectively to one sound at a time. As with palpation, the process of auscultation requires a period of "tuning in." Use the following sequence for listening:

1. Note the rate and rhythm of the heartbeat.
2. Identify S_1 and S_2.
3. Focus on S_1; note the intensity, the effect of respiration, and any variations.
4. Focus on S_2; note the intensity, splitting with respiration, and any variations.
5. Focus on systole, then on diastole, noting any extra sounds or murmurs.

■ HELPFUL HINT

Listen selectively to each sound and phase of the cardiac cycle—both the sounds and the silences. It is impossible to listen for everything at once.

Any variations mentioned in this section are more fully described later in this chapter under Variations from Health. They are mentioned here to give you some idea of what types of sounds you might anticipate hearing.

As you complete auscultation with the client supine, ask him or her to roll to the left side (Figure 16-26). Apply the

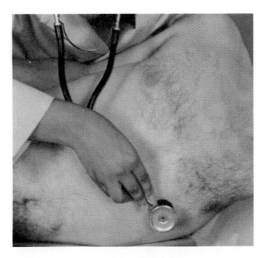

Figure 16-26 Auscultation at the apex of the heart with the client in the left lateral recumbent position.

bell of the stethoscope lightly at the apex and listen for any low-frequency diastolic sounds, such as the following:

• S_3, an early diastolic ventricular filling sound
• S_4, a late diastolic ventricular filling sound
• Mitral valve murmur

As you complete auscultation with the client in the sitting position, ask him or her to lean slightly forward. Press the diaphragm of the stethoscope firmly against the client's chest and listen at both the second left and right intercostal spaces near the sternal border to detect any high-pitched diastolic murmurs of aortic or pulmonic valve insufficiency (Figure 16-27). Listen during normal respiration and then ask the client to hold his or her breath in deep expiration.

Rate and Rhythm. The normal heart rate ranges from 60 to 100 beats per minute. (Review assessment of the pulse in Chapter 9.) The rhythm is normally regular; however, sinus arrhythmia occurs normally in some children and young adults. With sinus arrhythmia, the rhythm varies with breathing, increasing at the peak of inspiration and slowing with expiration. Note any pattern to the irregularity or whether it is totally irregular. If you notice any irregularity, check for a **pulse deficit** by auscultating the apical beat while simultaneously palpating the radial pulse. Each apical beat should be followed by a radial beat. If there are fewer radial pulse beats, count each for 1 minute and subtract the radial rate from the apical rate. The remainder is the pulse deficit.

S_1 and S_2. Distinguish the first and second heart sounds. At heart rates less than 100, S_1 is clearly the first of the pair of sounds making up the "lub-dub" of each heartbeat. S_1 is louder at the apex than S_2; S_2 is louder at the base than S_1 (see Figure 16-13). S_1 is very nearly synchronous with the carotid pulse (see Figure 16-18). Note whether each heart sound is normal, accentuated, diminished, or split.

CHARACTERISTICS OF S_1
• Caused by closure of the AV valves (mitral and tricuspid)
• Beginning of ventricular systole

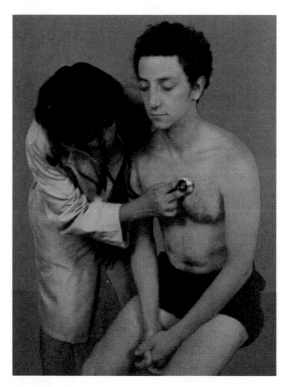

Figure 16-27 Auscultation at the base of the heart with the client leaning forward.

• Can be heard over the entire precordium but is loudest at the apex
• Best heard with the diaphragm of the stethoscope
• Split S_1 (mitral and tricuspid components heard separately) may be normal, but that is rare; split S_1 is best heard along the lower left sternal border—the tricuspid area

CHARACTERISTICS OF S_2
• Caused by closure of the semilunar valves (pulmonic and aortic)
• Beginning of ventricular diastole
• Can be heard over the entire precordium but is loudest at the base
• Best heard with the diaphragm of the stethoscope
• Split S_2 toward the end of inspiration is normal

The split-second sound (split S_2) is heard only in the area where pulmonic valve closure is loudest (i.e., in the second left intercostal space). Inspiration affects the return of blood to the heart, causing the closure of the pulmonic valve (P_2) to be slightly delayed; thus A_2 occurs slightly before P_2. If the S_2 is split, you will hear a brief double sound near the end of inspiration. During expiration, blood return to the heart equalizes, and the two sounds are heard as one. Asking the client to hold his or her breath during inspiration will equalize the blood return and ejection times, and inspiratory splitting will disappear. To help with your timing, focus on the rise and fall of the client's chest during normal respiration.

Note whether S_1 and S_2 are normal, including the normal splitting of S_2. Note whether fixed splitting of S_2 (split remains and is not affected by respiration) or paradoxical splitting (the reverse—S_2 splits on expiration and comes together on inspiration) occurs.

Extra Heart Sounds During Systole and Diastole. Systole is normally silent. The midsystolic ejection click of mitral valve prolapse is the most common extra sound heard during systole. The third and fourth heart sounds, which occur during diastole, may be normal or abnormal.

Venous Hum. A venous hum, caused by turbulent blood flow in the jugular veins, is common in healthy children and is not pathologically significant. Use the bell of the stethoscope to auscultate over the supraclavicular area on the right side. Auscultation can be improved by turning the client's head away and slightly upward from the side being auscultated. The hum is loudest during diastole. Because it is produced by blood flow in the jugular veins, the hum can be stopped by applying gentle pressure over the internal jugular vein in the neck between the trachea and the sternocleidomastoid muscle at approximately the level of the thyroid cartilage (Figure 16-28).

Murmurs. A **murmur** is a blowing, swooshing sound that occurs with turbulent blood flow in the heart or great vessels. Murmurs can be categorized in the following ways:

1. Innocent murmurs, which are always systolic and occur without evidence of physiological or structural abnormalities
2. Functional murmurs, which are associated with physiological alterations such as high cardiac output states (e.g., exercise, anemia, hyperthy-

roidism, or increased blood volume associated with pregnancy)

3. Pathological murmurs, which are always caused by structural abnormalities

Because some murmurs are within the range of normal findings, some basic information on murmurs is presented in this section. Certain murmurs are common in healthy children or adolescents and are termed innocent or functional. The contractile force of the heart is greater in children; this increases blood flow velocity. The increased velocity plus a smaller chest measurement makes a murmur audible. An innocent murmur is generally soft (grade I to II), midsystolic, short, and crescendo-decrescendo, with a vibratory or musical quality. Also, the innocent murmur is heard at the second or third left intercostal space and disappears with sitting. The young person with an innocent murmur has no associated signs of cardiac dysfunction.

Although it is important to distinguish innocent murmurs from pathological ones, it is best to suspect all murmurs as pathological until they are proved otherwise. Diagnostic tests such as the ECG, phonocardiogram, and echocardiogram are needed to establish an accurate diagnosis.

If you hear a murmur, describe it according to the following characteristics:

TIMING IN THE CARDIAC CYCLE.   The timing of a murmur within systole or diastole is the basis for its classification. First, note whether the murmur occurs during systole or diastole, or both. There are three basic categories of murmurs: systolic, diastolic, and continuous. A continuous murmur begins in systole and continues into all or part of diastole.

Note during which portion of systole or diastole the murmur occurs: early, mid-, or late systole or diastole. Early diastolic murmurs are referred to as protodiastolic, and late diastolic murmurs are called presystolic.

DURATION.   The duration of different murmurs varies from short to long, with gradations in between. Does the murmur end before, with, or after S_1 or S_2. Does the murmur occur only in early, mid-, or late systole or diastole? Murmurs occurring throughout systole are called pansystolic or holosystolic. Those that occur throughout diastole are called pandiastolic or holodiastolic.

PITCH (FREQUENCY).   Describe the pitch as high, medium, or low. The pitch depends on the pressure and the velocity of blood flow producing the murmur. Generally, when the rate of flow is rapid, a high pitch results; when the velocity is slower, the pitch is low.

LOUDNESS (INTENSITY).   Describe the intensity in terms of six grades:

Grade I Faintest that can be detected; audible only in a quiet room and then with special effort
Grade II Faint but clearly audible
Grade III Moderately loud; easy to hear (without a thrill)
Grade IV Loud; may be associated with a thrill palpable on the chest wall
Grade V Very loud; heard with one edge of the stethoscope lifted off the chest wall; thrill may be palpable
Grade VI Loudest possible; still audible with the entire stethoscope lifted just enough to remove it from contact with the chest wall; thrill may be palpable

Murmurs are usually described as "grade II/VI" to make it clear what scale is being used. When considering the loudness of the murmur, also note whether it muffles or obscures the heart sounds.

PATTERN (SHAPE, CONFIGURATION).   The terms crescendo and decrescendo describe the pattern of loudness, reflecting changes in the rate of blood flow. The intensity follows a pattern: growing louder (crescendo), tapering off (decrescendo), or increasing to a peak and then decreasing (crescendo-decrescendo). Some murmurs have a flat or nearly flat configuration (see Figure 16-42 on p. 373).

QUALITY.   Several descriptive terms are used to describe the quality, including: "musical," "blowing," "harsh," or "rumbling."

LOCATION.   Describe the area of maximum intensity of the murmur by using the anatomical landmarks of the area where you hear it best. Some murmurs are localized to small areas; others are heard over large portions of the chest wall.

RADIATION.   The murmur may be transmitted downstream in the direction of blood flow and may be heard in another place on the precordium, the neck, the back, or the axilla. Factors affecting radiation include the direction and velocity of the blood flow and the sound transmission through various tissues.

POSITION.   Some murmurs disappear or are enhanced by a change in position, such as standing, leaning forward, or lying supine.

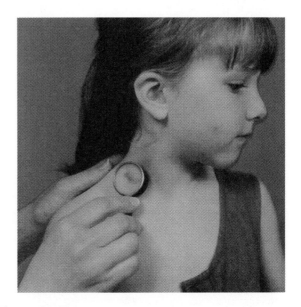

Figure 16-28 Venous hum. A continuous, low-pitched hum noted over the neck in many children; it is often best heard over the right supraclavicular space.

EFFECT OF RESPIRATION. Respiration, with its intrathoracic pressure changes, affects filling on the right side of the heart. Venous return to the right side increases with inspiration and decreases with expiration. Murmurs originating in the right side of the heart may be influenced by these factors.

POSITION CHANGE TO HEAR EXTRA HEART SOUNDS/MURMURS. After auscultating in the supine position, have the client roll on the left side. Listen with the bell at the apex for the presence of any diastolic filling sounds of S_3 or S_4. After auscultating in the sitting position, have the client lean forward slightly and exhale. Listen with the diaphragm firmly pressed at the second right and then left intercostal spaces. Listen for the soft, high-pitched murmurs of aortic or pulmonic regurgitation. S_3, S_4, and the semilunar valve regurgitant murmurs may be heard only with these changes in position.

Examination of the Neck Vessels

The techniques of inspection, palpation, and auscultation are used to examine the carotid arteries. The technique of inspection is used to examine the jugular veins.

Carotid Arteries

Inspection. Inspect the neck for the amplitude of the carotid pulsation. Note unusually large, bounding pulsations.

Palpation (Figure 16-29). Palpate along the medial edge of the sternocleidomastoid muscle for the carotid pulse. Palpate one carotid pulse at a time to avoid reducing blood flow to the brain. Palpate gently, since excessive vagus stimulation can slow down the heart rate and reduce blood pressure. This is particularly important in older adults who may already have compromised cardiovascular function. (Chapter 9 gives a more detailed description of general pulse assessment, including a description of abnormalities found in arterial pulse assessment in Table 9-3.)

Auscultation. A **bruit** is a blowing sound heard over an artery. It indicates increased flow through the artery or stenosis of the artery. Use the bell of the stethoscope to lis-

ten for bruits over the carotid arteries (Figure 16-30). Normally no sound is present. For middle-aged or older individuals or those with signs or symptoms of cardiovascular problems, it important to assess for the presence of a bruit.

Jugular Veins

Jugular Venous Pulse. Position the supine client's head and thorax at about a 30- to 45-degree angle or at the level where venous pulsations are best visible. Have the client turn the head slightly away from the side to be examined. Direct tangential lighting across the neck where the jugular veins are located (Figure 16-31). The jugular venous pulse (JVP) can be recognized by its location in the neck and by its characteristic pulsation. However, the distinct a, c, and v waves are not always clearly visible.

The jugular venous pulse may appear as a gentle, undulant wave. In the client with a healthy cardiovascular system, the venous pulse will not be visible until the client is in, or nearly in, the supine position. To evaluate the JVP, lower the client's head and thorax until the venous pulsations are visible.

The jugular veins lie close to the carotid arteries, and their pulsations need to be distinguished from each other. There are five ways to distinguish venous from arterial pulsations:

1. *Character of the pulse.* The venous pulse is more undulating than the brisk arterial pulse. The carotid pulse has one upstroke, whereas the venous pulse has three. Palpate the carotid pulse on one side of the neck while observing the jugular pulse on the other side.

2. *Effect of position.* Arterial pulsations do not change when the client's position changes. In the healthy individual, the venous pulsations are normally visible only in the supine position.

3. *Effect of respiration.* Venous pulsations change with respiration; arterial pulsations do not. With inspira-

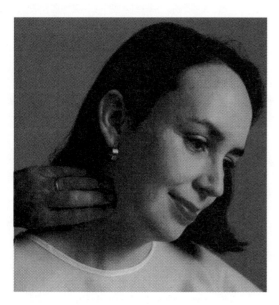

Figure 16-29 Palpation of the carotid artery pulse.

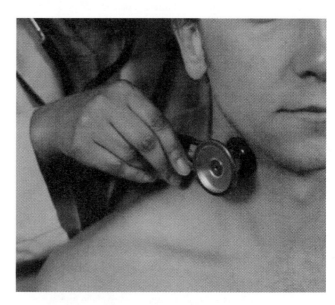

Figure 16-30 Auscultation of the carotid artery.

tion, intrathoracic pressure decreases, blood flow into the right atrium increases, and the level of the pulsation in the neck veins descends. During expiration, it rises.

4. *Effect of venous compression.* You can easily eliminate the pulsation of the jugular veins by applying gentle pressure over the external jugular vein at the base of the neck above the clavicle. This maneuver blocks the transmission of the venous pulse wave, leaving only the arterial pulsation.

5. *Effect of abdominal pressure (hepatojugular reflux).* The hepatojugular reflux technique may reveal some degree of heart failure when the jugular veins are not obviously distended. With the client in the supine or low Fowler's position with the mouth open (to prevent a Valsalva maneuver) but otherwise breathing normally, apply moderate pressure over the upper right quadrant of the abdomen for about 30 seconds. In the client with normal heart function, a slight rise in the venous pulsation may occur but diminishes quickly. In an individual with right-sided heart failure, the jugular venous pressure increases as venous return to the heart increases. Sustained distention suggests right-sided heart failure or chronic lung disease. If performed incorrectly with the client's mouth closed, a Valsalva maneuver will result, giving false-positive results. (The hepatojugular reflux is further described under Variations from Health.)

Jugular Venous Pressure

INSPECTION. Inspecting the jugular veins for the height of the column of blood provides a gross estimate of right-sided heart pressure. When a healthy client is in the sitting position, no neck veins are visible. They become visible only when the client is in the supine position. When the venous pressure is greatly elevated, the jugular veins become evident when the client is sitting (see Figure 16-19).

ESTIMATION OF JUGULAR VENOUS PRESSURE. One method of measuring the height of the venous column is illustrated in Figure 16-32. Before attempting to do this assessment, determine the client's comfort level and ability to have his or her head and chest lowered while in a supine position.

Position the client's head and thorax at the level needed to see the upper level of venous pulsations. Use the sternal angle (angle of Louis), the juncture of the manubrium, and the body of the sternum as a reference point. Place a centimeter ruler at the sternal angle and place another ruler perpendicular to the first at the top of the level of jugular venous distention. Note the angle of the client's head and thorax and the level in centimeters of the pulsation. The lower you place the client's head before the pulsations are visible, the lower the pressure; the higher the client's head when you can identify the upper level of pulsation, the higher the pressure.

Examination of the Peripheral Vascular System

The techniques of inspection, palpation, and auscultation are used to examine the peripheral vascular system. The peripheral vasculature is examined over the entire body during the course of the complete physical examination; develop a systematic way of integrating this assessment into the complete examination.

Inspection. There are some general considerations when inspecting the peripheral vasculature of the body. These are also discussed in chapters related to the specific regional examinations but will be summarized here. Inspection of peripheral vasculature should include the following:

1. *Skin color changes:* Pallor, cyanosis, rubor (redness).

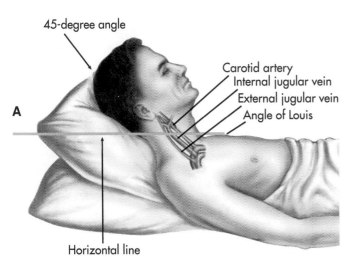

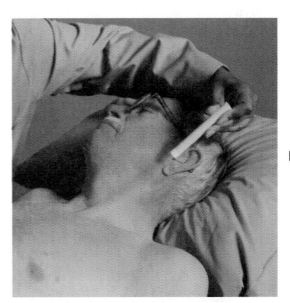

45-degree angle

A

Carotid artery
Internal jugular vein
External jugular vein
Angle of Louis

Horizontal line

B

Figure 16-31 Inspection of the external jugular vein, directing the light across the neck to see the venous pulse wave. (**A** from Thompson JM at al.: *Mosby's clinical nursing*, ed. 4, St. Louis, 1997, Mosby.)

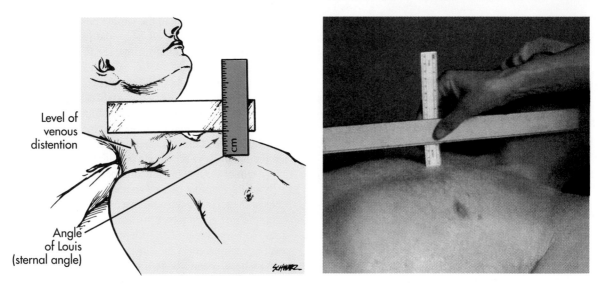

Figure 16-32   Measurement of jugular venous pressure. *Arrows* indicate the height of the jugular venous pressure in centimeters.

2. *Hair distribution*: Lack of hair growth may indicate inadequate circulation.
3. *Size and symmetry of extremities:* Atrophy, swelling, edema. If swelling or edema is present, measure both legs (or arms) at the widest part with a tape measure, noting differences in size and at precisely what distance from a bony landmark (such as the patella or medial malleolus) the measurement is taken. Inspect for pretibial edema. Normally, none is present, although mild edema may be noted in a healthy client who is pregnant or who has been standing all day.
4. *Venous patterns:* The venous pattern is normally flat and only slightly visible; look for varicosities.
5. *Lesions, ulcerations:* None are present on healthy skin; if present, they may be due to an inadequate blood supply.
6. *Nails:* Color, clubbing.
   a. Nail color should be pink. Pale or bluish color may indicate decreased circulation due to cold temperature or circulatory problems.
   b. Check for clubbing of the fingernails by inspecting the fingers from the side. The normal nailbed angle is 160 degrees. With clubbing, the nail becomes thickened, hard, shiny, and curved at the free end (see Figure 10-9). In advanced cases the entire nail is pushed away from the base at an angle greater than 180 degrees and feels "spongy."

Palpation.   Palpation of the peripheral pulses of the upper and lower extremities is described in Chapter 9. Palpation of the aorta is described in Chapter 17. After palpating the pulses, palpate the extremities for skin temperature and turgor (see Chapter 10). Other indicators of function of the peripheral vascular system that require palpation include assessment of edema in the lower extremities and assessment of capillary refill in the nails, as described in the following.

1. *Edema.* Edema or a buildup of fluid in the interstitial tissues is commonly caused by systemic cardiovascular problems such as congestive heart failure or by local vascular problems such as venous stasis or prolonged dependency. Other causes of edema may be systemic causes such as hypoalbuminemia or excessive renal retention of salt and water or local as with lymphatic stasis. When palpating the lower extremities always check for edema. Compare one foot and leg with the other. Firmly depress the skin over the dorsum of each foot, behind the medial malleolus and on the shins for at least 5 seconds. Look for "pitting" or a depression caused by the pressure of your fingertips (Figure 16-33). The degree of edema can be graded on a scale of 1 to 4+ as follows (Figure 16-34):

   1+   Slight pitting; no visible change in the shape of the extremity; disappears rapidly
   2+   Somewhat deeper pitting; no marked change in the shape of the extremity; disappears in 10 to 15 seconds
   3+   Noticeably deep pitting; full and swollen extremity; may last for more than 1 minute
   4   Very deep pitting; very swollen and distorted extremity; lasts as long as 2 to 5 minutes

---

■ **HELPFUL HINT**

If there is edema without pitting, the cause may be arterial disease and arterial occlusion. Unilateral edema is likely due to occlusion of a major vein.

---

2. *Nails: capillary refill time.* Assess capillary refill time by placing the client's hands near the level of the heart; depress and blanch the nailbeds, then release and note the time it takes for normal color

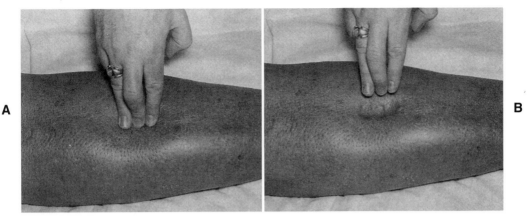

Figure 16-33 Technique for testing for pitting edema. **A**, Press fingertips into the shin area. **B**, Note the indentation that occurs after fingers are lifted with pitting edema. (From Swartz MH: *Textbook of physical diagnosis: history and examination*, ed. 3, Philadelphia, 1998, WB Saunders.)

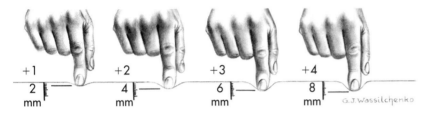

Figure 16-34 Assessing degree of pitting edema. (From Canobbio MM: *Cardiovascular disorders*, St. Louis, 1990, Mosby.)

to return. This should occur in less than 1 to 2 seconds. Remember that a cool room can increase refill time.

Auscultation. Auscultate the blood pressure. Assessment of the blood pressure that involves auscultation is discussed in detail in Chapter 9 (for adults) and in Chapter 26 (for children).

Screening Tests and Procedures

Screening for Asymptomatic Coronary Artery Disease

1. Measure blood pressure.
2. Assess modifiable cardiac risk factors, such as cigarette smoking, physical inactivity, and excessive dietary intake of fat and cholesterol (see also Risk Factors box on p. 354).

Screening for High Blood Cholesterol

The National Cholesterol Education Program guidelines (NCEP) recommend measuring a random total and high-density lipoprotein (HDL) cholesterol in all adults (ages 20 and older) every 5 years with additional testing determined as a result of those findings. Nonlipid coronary heart disease (CHD) risk factors should also be assessede. CHD risk factors include age ≥45 years in men and ≥55 years in women (or premature menopause without estrogen replacement therapy), family history of very high cholesterol

---

Cultural Considerations
Cardiovascular Disease

Heart disease and stroke are two of the major causes of death among people from various cultural backgrounds, accounting for about 30% of mortality.

HEART DISEASE

Among African-Americans and Native Americans, the incidence of death from heart disease is approximately twice as high as that for all other Americans.

STROKE

African-American males are twice as likely to die of a stroke as are Caucasian males, and among all African-American adults, death from coronary artery disease is higher than among other Americans.

DIABETES MELLITUS

Diabetes mellitus is ranked as the seventh leading cause of death in the United States. It is a major factor in heart disease. The incidence of diabetes mellitus varies greatly among various cultural groups. It is high among some Native American groups, African-Americans, Hispanics, and Chinese-Americans, Japanese-Americans, and Filipino-Americans.

VARICOSE VEINS

Caucasians are at greater risk for varicose veins than African-Americans because African-Americans have more venous valves in the lower legs than do Caucasians.

Data from U.S. Preventive Services Task Force: *Guide to clinical preventive services: an assessment of the effectiveness of 169 interventions*, ed. 2, Baltimore, 1996, Williams & Wilkins.

Examination Step-by-Step

1. Before beginning the examination, be sure that the room is quiet and the temperature is comfortable for the client.
2. Have equipment ready: stethoscope, penlight or flashlight for tangential lighting; metric ruler; tape measure; sphygmomanometer.
3. Explain the examination to the client.
4. If possible, position the client in the sitting position to begin the examination. Be sure to examine the client in the sitting, leaning-forward, supine, and left lateral recumbent positions. Proceed from neck to precordium to peripheral vasculature. (The sequence may vary but must include all components.)

NECK VESSELS

1. Carotid arteries
   a. Inspection: Amplitude of pulsations
   b. Palpation: Check pulse in each carotid artery separately
   c. Auscultation: Bruits
2. Jugular veins
   a. Inspection: Pulsations and pressure level

PRECORDIUM-HEART

1. Inspection: Pulsations, heaves, retractions
2. Palpation: Fifth left intercostal space, left sternal border, and second left and right intercostal spaces; for apical impulse, lifts, heaves, thrills
3. Auscultation: Fifth left intercostal space, left sternal border, second left and right intercostal spaces, and other areas of the precordium as indicated by the history or findings; for normal heart sounds, extra heart sounds, and murmurs (Use both the diaphragm and the bell to auscultate all areas.)

PERIPHERAL VASCULAR SYSTEM

1. Inspection: Venous vasculature, varicose veins, skin, and peripheral tissues for adequacy of vascular delivery of nutrients and clearance of metabolic by-products and fluids
2. Palpation: Peripheral pulses

levels, family history of premature CHD in a first-degree relative (before age 50 in men or age 60 in women), HDL cholesterol <35 mg/dl, cigarette smoking, hypertension, diabetes.

Periodic screening is most important when cholesterol levels are increasing (e.g., in middle-aged men, perimenopausal women, and persons who have gained weight). All clients should receive periodic assessment regarding dietary intake of fat, especially saturated fat, weight control, and exercise.

Serum cholesterol levels normally undergo substantial physiological fluctuations; therefore a single blood test may not be representative. Levels of serum cholesterol are described as:

- *High:* 240 mg/dl and above
- *Borderline:* 200 to 239 mg/dl
- *Normal:* <200 mg/dl

Screening for Hypertension

Screening for hypertension is discussed in detail in Chapter 9.

VARIATIONS FROM HEALTH

Heart

Variations With Inspection

Finding	Possible Cause(s)
1. Prominent pulsations in:	Enlargement of:
Apex	Left ventricle
Left parasternal region	Right ventricle
Second left intercostal space	Pulmonary artery
Second right intercostal space	Aorta
2. Thrusting apex exceeding 2 cm in diameter	Left ventricular enlargement
3. Retraction of tissues around apex	Constrictive pericarditis
4. Pulsations visible lateral to and/or inferior to midclavicular line	Cardiac enlargement
5. Shaking of entire precordium with each heartbeat	Severe valvular regurgitation, large left-to-right shunts, complete AV block, hypertrophic obstructive cardiomyopathy, various hyperkinetic states

Variations With Palpation

REMINDER: Palpate with the client in both the supine and left lateral decubitus positions.

Finding	Possible Cause(s)
1. Prolonged apical thrust during systole; may be accompanied by retraction in left parasternal area	Moderate-to-severe left ventricular hypertrophy Aortic regurgitation
2. Systolic impulse displaced laterally and downward into the sixth or seventh intercostal space	Left ventricular enlargement
3. Apical impulse not palpable	Hypovolemia, pericardial effusion, acute myocardial infarction
4. Systolic movement along left sternal border	Right ventricular enlargement, pulmonary hypertension, pulmonic stenosis
5. Exaggerated motion of entire parasternal area	Atrial septal defect, tricuspid regurgitation
6. Prominent systolic impulse in second left intercostal space	Pulmonary hypertension, increased pulmonary blood flow
7. Left parasternal movement	Enlarged left atrium, large posterior left ventricular aneurysm, severe mitral regurgitation with expanding left atrium
8. Right parasternal movement	Aneurysm of aorta, marked enlargement of right atrium
9. Thrill	Loud, harsh heart murmur of grade IV or greater

The degree of displacement of the apical impulse generally correlates with the extent of cardiac enlargement. Displacement tends to be maximal when both hypertrophy and dilation of the ventricle are present. Conditions associated with volume overload, such as mitral and aortic regurgitation and left-to-right shunts, tend to produce hypertrophy and dilation.

Variations With Auscultation

Variations that are audible with auscultation include changes in heart sounds (S_1 and S_2), extra heart sounds, and murmurs.

Normal first and second heart sounds are largely the result of competent heart valves. Valves that fail to prevent the backflow of blood are described as incompetent, insufficient, or regurgitant. Valves that restrict the forward flow of blood are described as stenosed.

The position of the client has an effect on which abnormal sounds can be heard. Most murmurs and gallop rhythms are louder in the recumbent position because of increased venous return to the heart. They can be further increased by raising the client's legs. Mitral murmurs and early and late diastolic gallop rhythms become more audible when the client is in the left lateral recumbent position because this brings the apex closer to the chest wall.

Variations in the carotid artery pulse are discussed in Chapter 9.

Variations in the Heart Sounds: S_1 and S_2

Variations in S_1. Variations in the first heart sound include splitting (discussed earlier in this chapter under Anatomy and Physiology) and changes in loudness. Changes in S_1 depend on the following:

1. The status of the pulmonary and systemic circulation
2. Structure of the heart valves
3. Valve leaflet position when ventricular contraction begins
4. The force of the contraction

INCREASED S_1. If systole begins with the mitral valve completely open, the valve closes shut more vigorously, producing a louder S_1. This occurs with the following:

- Increased blood velocity found with hyperkinetic states, such as anemia, anxiety, fever, hyperthyroidism, and exercise
- Stenosis of the mitral valve where greater ventricular pressure is needed to overcome the increase in atrial pressure (increased closing pressure and more abrupt closure result)

DIMINISHED S_1. Causes include the following:

- A mitral or tricuspid valve that is so fibrosed or calcified that only limited motion is possible, producing closure with less force; this may result from rheumatic fever
- Systemic or pulmonary hypertension leads to more forceful atrial contraction. If the ventricle is noncompliant, the contraction may be delayed or diminished
- An increase in the overlying substance—including fat, fluid, or air, such as occurs with obesity, pericardial fluid, and emphysema—obscures S_1

VARYING S_1. The loudness of S_1 varies when the valves are in varying positions at the beginning of each beat. Changes in the loudness of S_1 are produced by the following:

- Incomplete heart block in which the PR interval is changing, the atria and ventricles beat independently, and the position of valves changes from beat to beat
- Gross disruption of rhythm, such as occurs during fibrillation

Variations in S_2. Variations in S_2 include changes in loudness and splitting that is not normal physiological splitting.

INCREASED S_2. Louder closure sounds result from the following:

- Higher closing pressure due to systemic hypertension—may result in S_2 having a ringing sound.
- Exercise and excitement—increased pressure in the aorta, producing an increase in the A_2 component of S_2.
- Conditions associated with pulmonary hypertension, such as mitral valve stenosis and congestive heart failure—may produce an increase in the P_2 component of S_2.
- Semilunar valves that are injured but still flexible; the component of S_2 affected depends on which valve is injured.

DIMINISHED S_2. Quieter closure results from the following:

- A decrease in systemic blood pressure, such as occurs with shock; A_2 is diminished.
- Injured valves that are thickened, calcified, and less mobile; the component of S_2 affected depends on which valve is compromised—aortic stenosis affects A_2; pulmonic stenosis affects P_2.
- Overlying fat, fluid, or air mutes S_2.

VARIATIONS IN THE SPLITTING OF S_2. Variations in the splitting of S_2 include wide splitting, fixed splitting, and paradoxical splitting (Figure 16-35).

WIDE SPLITTING. With wide splitting of S_2, splitting is present with expiration and is even wider with inspiration. Conditions causing delayed electrical stimulation of right ventricular contraction or delayed emptying of the right ventricle result in delayed closure of the pulmonic valve. This occurs with right bundle-branch block, which splits both S_1 and S_2, causing a delay in pulmonic valve closure. Wider splitting also exists with pulmonary hypertension, which delays ventricular emptying.

FIXED SPLITTING. Splitting of S_2 is described as fixed when it is unaffected by respiration. It is associated with atrial septal defect and right ventricular failure. Pulmonic closure is delayed because with each beat the right ventricle is ejecting a larger volume than is the left ventricle. Right-sided filling cannot be further increased by inspiration, so the split sound remains fixed.

PARADOXICAL SPLITTING. Delayed closure of the aortic valve in left bundle-branch block results in narrowed splitting, or splitting where the normal sequence of sounds is reversed: pulmonic closure precedes aortic valve closure. Paradoxically, inspiration results in the two sounds coming closer together and even fusing into a single sound, and expiration results in more widely separated sounds.

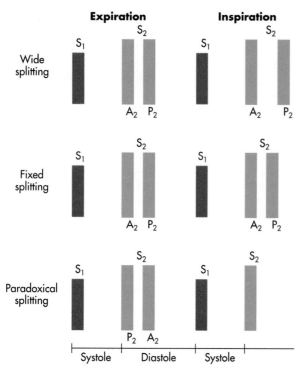

Figure 16-35 Variations in splitting of S₂.

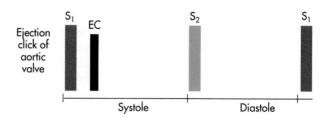

Figure 16-36 Ejection click of the aortic valve following S_1.

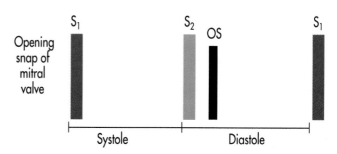

Figure 16-37 Opening snap of the mitral valve following S_2.

Extra Heart Sounds

Extra Heart Sounds During Systole	Extra Heart Sounds During Diastole
Ejection click of aortic and pulmonic valve	Opening snap of mitral or tricuspid valve S₃ S₄

Extra Sounds in Systole. Extra sounds are not normally present during systole. Therefore hearing any sound after the first heart sound should cause you to consider whether a client has heart disease.

AORTIC OR PULMONIC EJECTION SOUNDS. (Figure 16-36). Semilunar valve ejection sounds are sharp, high-pitched, and clicking; they are best heard with the diaphragm of the stethoscope. They occur just after the first heart sound, early in systole at the end of isovolumic contraction when the semilunar valves open. Ejection clicks are caused by opening of the stenotic semilunar valves or from the ejection of blood into a dilated aorta or pulmonary artery. They may also be due to systemic or pulmonary hypertension.

Aortic valve ejection clicks are more common than pulmonic valve ejection clicks. The aortic ejection sound is often well heard at the cardiac apex and second right intercostal space. Its intensity does not significantly change with respiration.

The pulmonic ejection sound also is a sharp sound following the first heart sound and is often best heard at the second and third left intercostal spaces along the sternal border. It may decrease in intensity during inspiration and increase during expiration.

Extra Sounds in Diastole

OPENING SNAPS (Figure 16-37). A mitral or tricuspid valve that is stenotic but mobile produces an opening snap as the valve opens at the beginning of diastole. It may be heard at the apex and second right intercostal space. Opening snaps are high pitched and best heard through the diaphragm. Opening snaps precede third heart sounds and are higher pitched. Their earlier timing and higher frequency can prevent their being misinterpreted as a physiological third heart sound.

THIRD AND FOURTH HEART SOUNDS. Although they may be normal heart sounds, when S₃ and S₄ are abnormal, they produce a gallop **rhythm**. Third and fourth heart sounds are low-pitched sounds best heard with the bell of the stethoscope. They are intensified by the recumbent position and by exercise. At heart rates greater than 100 beats/min, when both S₃ and S₄ sounds are present, they may fuse, producing a loud sound called a summation gallop.

S₃ (see Figure 16-15) occurs as passive ventricular filling begins. It is best heard with the client in the left lateral recumbent position and during expiration. Left-sided S₃ sounds are best heard at the apex; those originating from the right ventricle are best heard at the left sternal border and are accentuated with inspiration.

Auscultate at the apex, placing the bell of the stethoscope lightly against the skin, with just enough pressure to form a seal. Then move to the left sternal border. The pathological S₃ indicates decreased compliance of the ventricles, such as with congestive heart failure, and may also occur with conditions of volume overload, such as with mitral, tricuspid, or aortic regurgitation.

TABLE 16-5	Characteristics of Extra Heart Sounds			
Sound	Timing in Cardiac Cycle	Location—Bell/ Diaphragm	Qualities	Causative Factors
Ejection click of aortic or pulmonic valve	Early systole, after S_1	Apex and second right intercostal space Diaphragm	Sharp, high pitched, clicking	Stenotic aortic or pulmonic valve; or ejection of blood into dilated aorta or pulmonary artery
Opening snap of mitral valve	Early diastole, after S_2, before S_3	Medial to apex and second right intercostal space Diaphragm	High pitched	Stenotic but still mobile mitral valve
S_3	Early to mid-diastole	Apex, left lateral position, during expiration Bell	Low pitched	Heart failure, volume overload, pulmonary or systemic hypertension; also heard in hyperkinetic states
S_4	Late diastole/presystole	Apex, supine or left lateral position Bell	Low pitched	Increased resistance to ventricular filling due to decreased compliance of ventricle or obstruction to outflow due to valve stenosis, systemic or pulmonary hypertension
Summation gallop	Mid-diastolic	Apex, supine or left lateral recumbent Bell	Intense	S_3 and S_4 with tachycardia
Pericardial friction rub	May occupy all of systole and diastole	Apex to left sternal border Diaphragm	Intense, grating, grating, to-and-fro scratching like shoe leather; may obliterate heart sounds	Inflammation of pericardium

S_4 (see Figure 16-16) occurs late in diastole when the atria contract—the rapid ventricular filling phase. Vigorous atrial contraction is necessary to produce an audible S_4. It is best heard with the client in the left lateral recumbent position and with the bell of the stethoscope gently applied to the chest wall. An S_4 originating from the right ventricle as a result of tricuspid regurgitation or right ventricular failure is heard best along the lower left sternal border. An abnormal S_4 results from an increased resistance to filling secondary to decreased compliance of the ventricle, such as follows a myocardial infarction, or from systolic overload, including obstruction to outflow from the ventricle, such as occurs with aortic stenosis and systemic hypertension.

When both phases of rapid ventricular filling become audible events as S_3 and S_4, a quadruple rhythm with four audible components results. If the heart rate increases and diastole is shortened, S_3 and S_4 come closer together and may be heard as one sound during diastole—the summation gallop. It may be louder than S_1 and S_2.

Sounds That May Occur During Both Systole and Diastole
PERICARDIAL FRICTION RUB. Inflammation of the pericardial sac causes the parietal and visceral surfaces of the roughened pericardium to rub against each other. This action produces an extra cardiac sound having a to-and-fro character and both systolic and diastolic components. This sound is high pitched and can be best heard with the diaphragm. It resembles the sound of squeaky leather and is often described as grating, scratching, or rasping. The sound seems very close to the ear and may seem louder than, or even

TABLE 16-6	Differentiating a Split S_2 from S_3	
Split S_2		S_3
Heard best at base		Heard best at apex or lower left sternal border
High pitched; heard best with diaphragm		Low pitched; heard best with bell
Varies with respiration		Not affected by respiration

mask, the other heart sounds. Pericardial friction rubs can usually be heard best between the apex and the sternum, where the pericardium comes in close contact with the chest wall. A pericardial friction rub is common after a myocardial infarction.

Differentiating heart sounds is difficult and challenging. Tables 16-5 through 16-8 present some of the differentiating characteristics of the extra heart sounds, some of which are very close to each other in the cardiac cycle. Table 16-5 summarizes the characteristics of the extra heart sounds. Tables 16-6 through 16-8 highlight the auscultatory differences between a split S_2, S_3, and the opening snap of mitral stenosis.

Murmurs. Heart murmurs are relatively prolonged sounds that occur during systole or diastole. Some murmurs occur in the presence of normal structures when blood flow is increased because of a hyperkinetic condition. Others are caused by defects in the heart valves, major vessels, or blood flow through an abnormal opening. The abnormal sounds are produced by some turbulence of the blood flow as it enters, passes through, or leaves the heart. The sounds heard on auscultation of a murmur depend on numerous cardiovascular components, including the adequacy of valve function, the size of openings between structures, the rate of blood flow, and the health of the myocardium, and on extracardiac factors, such as the thickness and consistency of the overlying tissues through which the sound of the murmur travels. Four mechanisms of murmur production are illustrated in Figure 16-38.

Diseased valves that either do not open or do not close well are a common cause of murmurs. Stenosis is the condi-

tion in which the leaflets are thickened and the passage is narrowed, thus restricting the forward flow of blood. **Regurgitation** is the condition in which the valve leaflets, which are intended to fit together snugly, no longer do so and the incompetent (or insufficient) opening allows the backward flow of blood.

In general, systolic murmurs caused by valvular disease are due to stenotic aortic or pulmonic valves (Figure 16-39) or incompetent mitral or tricuspid valves (Figure 16-40), and in general, diastolic murmurs caused by valvular disease are due to incompetent aortic or pulmonic valves (Figure 16-41) or

TABLE 16-7	Differentiating S₂ From an Opening Snap of the Mitral Valve

S_2	Opening Snap
Occurs before opening snap	Occurs after S_2, during diastole
Heard best at base	Heard best at apex to lower left sternal border; may radiate toward base
Lower pitch than opening snap	Higher pitch than S_2
Varies with respiration	Does not vary with respiration

TABLE 16-8	Differentiating S₃ From an Opening Snap of the Mitral Valve

S_3	Opening Snap
Occurs after opening snap	Occurs earlier than S_3
Heard best with bell	Heard best with diaphragm

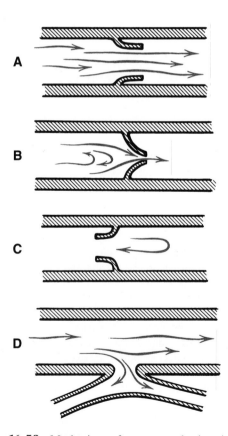

Figure 16-38   Mechanisms of murmur production. **A,** Increased flow across a normal valve. **B,** Forward flow through a stenotic valve. **C,** Backflow (regurgitation) through an incompetent valve. **D,** Flow through an abnormal opening, such as a septal defect or an arteriovenous fistula (patent ductus arteriosus).

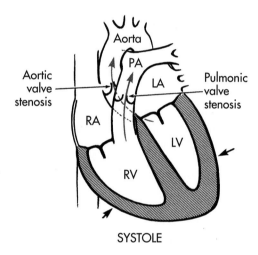

Figure 16-39   Aortic or pulmonic valve stenosis.

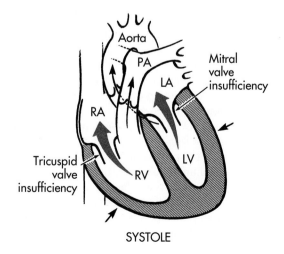

Figure 16-40   Mitral or tricuspid valve insufficiency.

stenotic mitral or tricuspid valves (Figure 16-42). Stenosis or incompetence can affect any of the four heart valves, but problems with the aortic and mitral valves are the most common.

The blood flow patterns of the various murmurs produce murmurs of the following three basic shapes (Figure 16-43):

1. The crescendo-decrescendo, or diamond-shaped, pattern of systolic functional murmurs and murmurs of aortic or pulmonic stenosis
2. The decrescendo pattern of the diastolic murmurs of aortic or pulmonic regurgitation

3. The flat pattern of the pansystolic (holosystolic) murmurs of mitral and tricuspid regurgitation

The greater the blood flow, the greater the intensity of the murmur.

Table 16-9 summarizes the characteristics of six systolic murmurs. Table 16-10 summarizes the characteristics of four diastolic murmurs. Table 16-11 reviews the extra heart sounds and murmurs heard during systole and diastole, and the Box 16-3 reviews the sounds to listen for over each area of the precordium. *Text continued on p. 378*

BOX 16-3

SOUNDS TO LISTEN FOR OVER EACH AREA OF THE PRECORDIUM

APEX

First and second heart sounds
Aortic ejection click
Opening snap of mitral stenosis
Systolic murmur of mitral regurgitation
High-pitched murmur of aortic regurgitation
Diastolic murmur of mitral stenosis (left lateral recumbent position)

LOWER LEFT STERNAL BORDER—FOURTH AND FIFTH INTERCOSTAL SPACES

First and second heart sounds
Aortic ejection click
Opening snap of mitral or tricuspid stenosis
Diastolic murmur of tricuspid stenosis (left lateral recumbent position)

Systolic murmurs of aortic stenosis, tricuspid regurgitation, and ventricular septal defect

LEFT STERNAL BORDER—SECOND AND THIRD INTERCOSTAL SPACES

Both components of second heart sound
Pulmonary ejection click
Systolic murmur of pulmonic stenosis
Diastolic murmurs of aortic and pulmonic valve regurgitation
Systolic murmur of atrial septal defect

RIGHT STERNAL BORDER—SECOND INTERSPACE

First and second heart sounds
Systolic murmur of aortic stenosis

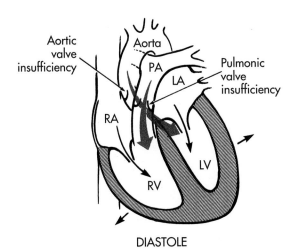

DIASTOLE

Figure 16-41 Aortic or pulmonic valve insufficiency.

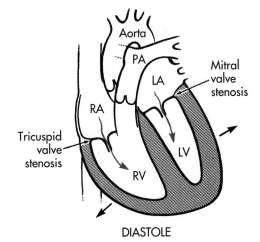

DIASTOLE

Figure 16-42 Mitral or tricuspid valve stenosis produces a diastolic murmur.

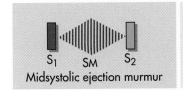
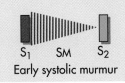
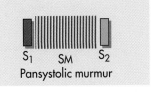

Figure 16-43 Shapes of murmurs.

TABLE 16-9 Systolic Murmurs

Type	Description of Murmur	Other Examination Findings	Mechanism of Production

Midsystolic Murmurs*

Systole Diastole

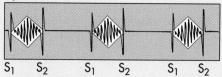

S₁ S₂ S₁ S₂ S₁ S₂

Aortic stenosis 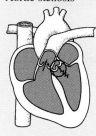	Heard best with diaphragm at second right intercostal space or at third left intercostal space with client sitting up and leaning forward, breath held in expiration; may radiate to carotids or left sternal border; loudness varies; medium pitch; harsh; midsystolic; crescendo-decrescendo; intensifies when client lies flat; if murmur is loud, may be heard over entire thorax; the more severe the stenosis, the later the crescendo of the murmur during systole	May be accompanied by a thrill; S₁ may disappear if stenosis is severe; S₂ diminished; S₄ may be present; early ejection sound at second right intercostal space; slowly rising carotid pulse wave; narrow pulse pressure; with left ventricular hypertrophy, apical impulse is prolonged and shifts downward and to left	Fibrosed or calcified aortic valve cusps make it difficult for blood to flow from left ventricle to aorta; caused by congenitally defective valves, rheumatic heart disease, atherosclerosis
Pulmonic stenosis 	Heard best at second or third left intercostal space; may radiate to left side of neck; louder on inspiration; systolic; medium pitch; coarse; crescendo-decrescendo	Thrill may be present; S₁ often followed by ejection click; S₂ widely split and often diminished; P₂ soft or absent; S₄ common in right ventricular hypertrophy	Calcification of pulmonic valve restricts forward flow of blood; usually congenital
Atrial septal defect 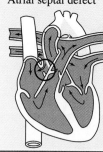	Heard best at base, second left intercostal space; systolic; medium pitch (this murmur is not caused by the shunt, but by the increased blood flow through the pulmonic valve)	Sternal lift; S₂ has fixed split; P₂ often louder than A₂	Abnormal opening in atrial septum resulting in left-to-right shunt, causing large increase in pulmonary blood flow

Illustrations for atrial septal defect and ventricular septal defect are from Wong DL et al.: *Whaley and Wong's nursing care of infants and children,* ed. 6, St. Louis, 1999, Mosby; all other illustrations are from Wilson SF, Giddens JF: *Health assessment for nursing practice,* ed. 2, St. Louis, 2001, Mosby.
*Caused by the forward flow of blood through the semilunar valves.

TABLE 16-9 Systolic Murmurs—cont'd

Type	Description of Murmur	Other Examination Findings	Mechanism of Production
Pansystolic Murmurs*			

Systole Diastole

S₁ S₂   S₁ S₂   S₁ S₂

Type	Description of Murmur	Other Examination Findings	Mechanism of Production
Mitral regurgitation	Heard best around apical area with diaphragm; high pitched; harsh or blowing quality; often loud; radiates from apex to base or to left axilla; does not vary with respiration	Apical impulse displaced down and to left; apical lift; thrill may be palpable at apex; S_1 diminished; S_2 more intense, with P_2 often accentuated; S_3 at apex often present; S_3-S_4 gallop common in late disease	Mitral valve incompetence permits backflow of blood from left ventricle to left atrium; results from rheumatic fever, myocardial infarction, rupture of chordae tendineae, or papillary muscle
Tricuspid regurgitation	Heard best at lower right and left sternal borders; increases with inspiration; pansystolic; soft, blowing	Enlarged jugular veins with large wave, enlarged liver; lift at sternum if right ventricular hypertrophy present; may be thrill at left lower sternal border; S_3 may be present	Incompetent tricuspid valve permits backflow of blood from right ventricle to right atrium; caused by pulmonary hypertension, cardiac trauma, congenital defects, or bacterial endocarditis
Ventricular septal defect	Heard best at lower left sternal border; loud; harsh; pansystolic; large defects also have soft diastolic murmur at apex because of increased blood flow through mitral valve	May be accompanied by a thrill	Abnormal opening in septum between ventricles; size and location vary

*Caused by backward flow of blood from area of higher pressure to one of lower pressure across incompetent AV valves.

TABLE 16-10   **Diastolic Murmurs**

Type	Description of Murmur	Other Examination Findings	Mechanism of Production

Early Diastolic Murmurs

Systole Diastole

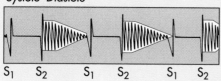

S₁   S₂   S₁   S₂   S₁   S₂

Type	Description of Murmur	Other Examination Findings	Mechanism of Production
Aortic regurgitation 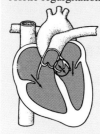	Heard best with diaphragm at second or third left intercostal space at base, with client sitting up and leaning forward; ask client to hold breath at end of expiration; early diastolic (starts almost simultaneously with S₂); decrescendo; high pitched; soft; blowing; radiates down; duration varies; low-pitched, rumbling murmur at apex is common (Austin-Flint murmur)	Early ejection click sometimes present; S₁ soft; S₂ may have tambourlike quality; S₃-S₄ gallop common; with left ventricular hypertrophy, prominent prolonged apical impulse displaced down and to left; bounding water-hammer pulse in carotid, brachial, and femoral arteries; pulse pressure wide; pulsations in cervical and suprasternal area; aortic stenosis often a concurrent problem	Incompetent aortic valve permits blood to flow back from aorta to left ventricle during diastole; decrescendo pattern of murmur reflects progressive decline in volume and rate of backflow during course of diastole; left ventricle dilates and hypertrophies as a result of increased stroke volume; caused by rheumatic heart disease, hypertension, endocarditis, congenital heart disease, syphilis, or cardiac trauma
Pulmonic regurgitation	Murmur has similar timing and characteristics as that of aortic regurgitation: high pitched, blowing, and decrescendo; heard best at second left intercostal space; may radiate to left lower sternal border, increases with inspiration		Incompetent pulmonic valve permits backflow of blood from pulmonary artery to right ventricle; caused by pulmonary hypertension or bacterial endocarditis

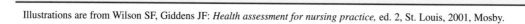

Illustrations are from Wilson SF, Giddens JF: *Health assessment for nursing practice,* ed. 2, St. Louis, 2001, Mosby.

TABLE 16-10	**Diastolic Murmurs—cont'd**		
Type	Description of Murmur	Other Examination Findings	Mechanism of Production

Mild- to Late Diastolic Murmurs

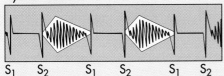

Systole Diastole

S_1 S_2 S_1 S_2 S_1 S_2

Mitral stenosis 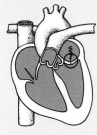	Heard best with bell held lightly at apex, with client in left lateral position; low-pitched diastolic rumble, more intense in early and late diastole; does not radiate; with increased stenosis, atrial contraction may force more blood across valve at end of ventricular diastole, giving murmur a late diastolic (presystolic) pattern	Systole usually quiet; diastolic thrill commonly palpable at apex in late diastole; apical lift; S_1 increased; S_2 split often with accentuated P_2, heard over wide area of precordium; opening snap follows P_2 closely, followed by murmur arterial pulse amplitude decreased; pulse often irregular; often occurs with systolic murmur of mitral regurgitation	Calcified mitral valve does not open adequately, thus restricting forward flow of blood from left atrium to left ventricle during diastole; left atrium becomes enlarged; caused by rheumatic fever or calcification
Tricuspid stenosis 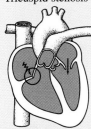	Heard best with bell at lower left sternal border with client in left lateral position; low-pitched diastolic rumble; louder with inspiration; does not radiate; similar to murmur of mitral stenosis; may be hard to differentiate	Diminished arterial pulse, prominent jugular venous pulse	Calcified tricuspid valve restricts forward flow of blood from right atrium to right ventricle during diastole; caused by rheumatic heart disease

Continuous Murmurs

Result of abnormal link between two parts of circulatory system, such as patent ductus arteriosus; with exception of normal venous hum, continuous murmurs are always pathological; typical continuous murmur begins in systole and spills over into diastole, thus sounding like a single murmur; best heard in second left intercostal space lateral to pulmonary area and may radiate down sternal border

TABLE 16-11	**Timing of Cardiac Sounds: Sounds Heard During Systole, Diastole, or Both**	
Systolic Sounds	Diastolic Sounds	Both
Aortic and pulmonic ejection clicks	Third heart sound	Pericardial friction rub
Click of mitral valve prolapse	Fourth heart sound	
Functional murmur	Mitral stenosis murmur	
Aortic stenosis murmur	Tricuspid stenosis murmur	
Pulmonic stenosis murmur	Aortic regurgitation murmur	
Mitral regurgitation murmur	Pulmonic regurgitation murmur	
Tricuspid regurgitation murmur	Summation gallop	

Other Cardiac Disorders

Left Ventricular Hypertrophy. Increased resistance to the emptying of blood from the left ventricle into the aorta occurs with systemic hypertension, aortic stenosis, and volume overload. The left ventricle hypertrophies as a result of the extra workload. It is sometimes displaced laterally and downward, and the apical impulse may be palpable over a larger area than usual.

Myocardial Infarction. Ischemia and necrosis of the myocardium are caused by an abrupt obstruction of circulation to some portion of the heart. The left ventricle is most frequently affected, but damage may extend to either the right ventricle or either atrium. Infarction is characterized by severe pain involving the central area of the chest, commonly with radiation to the left arm, jaw, neck, back, or abdomen. Associated symptoms may include sweating, weakness, nausea, vomiting, dyspnea, lightheadedness, restlessness, coolness of the extremities, and anxiety. Underlying causes include atherosclerotic coronary disease and embolus to the coronary arteries.

Physical examination findings vary but may include the following:
- Pulse: Thready
- Blood pressure: Variable
- Heart: Dysrhythmias; normal or diminished heart sounds; S_4, sometimes an S_3; soft, systolic, apical murmur of mitral regurgitation; pericardial friction rub

Congestive Heart Failure. Congestive heart failure (CHF) is a condition in which the heart cannot pump blood forward in the normal pattern, resulting in congestion of the pulmonary or systemic circulation. It may result from some defect in the heart or in the rhythmicity pattern. Heart failure may be predominantly right sided or left sided. Right-sided failure leads to peripheral edema, liver congestion, and jugular venous distention. Left-sided failure leads to pulmonary congestion and dyspnea. Pulmonary hypertension can lead to right-sided hypertrophy and right ventricular failure. This condition is known as **cor pulmonale**. Heart dysfunction produces changes in other organs, including the lungs, kidneys, and liver. It may develop gradually, such as with hypertension, or suddenly as a result of myocardial infarction.

Symptoms may include dyspnea, orthopnea, paroxysmal nocturnal dyspnea, edema, cough, fatigue at rest, and frequent nocturnal urination.

Physical examination findings may include the following:
- *Pulse:* Weak, rapid
- *Blood pressure:* Varies
- *Skin:* Cool, moist, pale, or cyanotic
- *Neck:* Jugular venous distention
- *Heart:* Tachycardia, lifts, heaves, displacement of the apical impulse downward and to the left; S_3, S_4
- *Lungs:* Moist rales, crackles, bronchial wheezing
- *Abdomen:* Ascites, liver enlargement
- *Extremities:* Dependent, pitting edema in the legs and sacral area

Jugular Venous Pulse

Variations in the Jugular Venous Pulse Waves

Variations in the a Wave. The *a* wave is the highest of the venous waves. It is increased when it is more difficult for the contracting right atrium to empty into the right ventricle. This occurs with tricuspid valve stenosis or decreased compliance of the right ventricle due to right ventricular hypertrophy, pulmonary hypertension, or pulmonic stenosis. Intermittently enlarged *a* waves, called cannon *a* waves, result when the atrium contracts against a closed tricuspid valve. This can occur during a premature ventricular beat or during complete AV block.

Variations in the x Descent and in the c and v Waves. An incompetent tricuspid valve permits backflow of blood from the right ventricle to the right atrium during atrial filling and ventricular systole. This increased backflow obliterates the x slope, which is replaced by an enlarged combined *c-v* wave. With severe disease, the wave may become as large as a bounding carotid pulsation.

Variations of the y Descent. The tricuspid valve opens shortly after S_2, and the rapid filling phase of ventricular diastole begins. The characteristics of the y descent depend on right-sided pressure and volume and on resistance to flow across the tricuspid valve. Tricuspid stenosis produces a slow y descent because it obstructs right atrial emptying. In clients with severe heart failure in whom the right atrial pressure is extremely high, an exaggerated y wave is produced.

Peripheral Vasculature

Arterial Occlusion and Insufficiency

Arteries in any location can become occluded or traumatized, making them unable to perform their task of deliver-

BOX 16-4

COMPARISON OF PAIN FROM VASCULAR INSUFFICIENCIES AND MUSCULOSKELETAL DISORDERS

ARTERIAL	VENOUS AND MUSCULOSKELETAL
Comes on during exercise	Comes on during or often several hours after exercise
Quickly relieved by rest	Relieved by rest but sometimes only after several hours or even days; pain tends to be constant.
Intensity increases with the intensity and duration of exercise	Greater variability than arterial pain in response to intensity and duration of exercise.

From Seidel HM et al.: *Mosby's guide to physical examination,* ed. 4, St. Louis, 1999, Mosby.

ing blood and other nutrients to the tissues. Arterial occlusive disease can be an acute condition in which a thrombus or an embolus suddenly occludes an artery, or a chronic condition caused by the buildup of atherosclerotic plaque and resulting in arterial wall thickening, hardening, and loss of elasticity; it can lead to arterial obstruction.

> ### ■ HELPFUL HINT
>
> The signs of an acute arterial occlusion can be remembered as the five *P*s. They are: *P*ain, *P*allor, *P*aresthesia, *P*aralysis, and *P*ulselessness.

A decrease in arterial circulation results in findings related to the following:
1. Site of the problem
2. Degree of occlusion or trauma
3. Ability of collateral channels to compensate
4. Rapidity with which the problem develops

Arterial disease pain can be acute or chronic.

Arterial Insufficiency

Pain or a sharp, cramplike sensation distal to the affected artery is the first symptom that results from inadequate blood supply to the muscle. With chronic insufficiency, intermittent claudication is experienced as a dull ache with muscle fatigue and cramping. It typically appears during sustained exercise, such as walking or climbing stairs. A brief rest usually relieves it. Box 16-4 presents a comparison of the pain caused by arterial insufficiency and that caused by venous insufficiency

Other characteristics of chronic arterial insufficiency may include localized pallor and cyanosis; weak, thready, or absent pulses; ulceration; hair loss; trophic changes of the toenails; diminished sensation; and some degree of atrophy. With more severe insufficiency, pain may occur when the person is supine and may be relieved by lowering the feet, which improves the perfusion pressure and oxygen supply to the distal tissues.

Arterial Occlusion. Arterial occlusion is due to either a thrombus or an embolus. The development of a thrombus can follow chronic insufficiency in the area as a result of the atherosclerotic process. An arterial embolism can be due to stagnant blood flow within the heart, such as occurs with a diseased mitral valve, from bacterial endocarditis, or with atrial fibrillation. An acute obstruction results in excruciating pain that is more severe distally and is followed after several hours by numbness and cold. Distal pallor and cyanosis are present when the extremity is raised above the level of the heart, and pulses are weak or absent distal to the occlusion.

Increased Capillary Refill Time. Capillary refill time lasting more than 2 seconds can be due to anemia, peripheral edema, or vasoconstriction or decreased cardiac output due to hypovolemia, shock, or CHF.

Arterial Aneurysm. An **aneurysm** is a localized dilation of an artery resulting from weakness of the arterial wall. The aorta is the most common site for an aneurysm, but an aneurysm may also occur in other peripheral vessels. A bruit, thrill, or visible pulsation may be present over the site of the aneurysm, or it may be palpated as a pulsating mass. Atherosclerosis, which weakens the middle layer of the arterial wall, is a common cause of an aneurysm.

Coarctation of the Aorta. Coarctation is a localized narrowing of the aorta. It results in increased pressure proximal to the narrowing and decreased pressure distal to the narrowing. Other symptoms and signs include dizziness, headaches, fainting, epistaxis, reduced or absent femoral pulses, and muscle cramps in the legs. Blood pressure in the arms is higher than in the legs.

Raynaud's Syndrome. In **Raynaud's phenomenon,** intermittent spasm of the arterioles causes ischemia of the extremities, especially the fingers, toes, ears, and nose (Figure 16-44). There is a classic tri-colored sequence of events in Raynaud's attack. Exposure to cold, vibrating tools, certain repetitive motions, smoking, or emotional stress causes spasm of the local arteries and arterioles, resulting in severe pallor due to decreased capillary perfusion. The pallor is followed by cyanosis as the small vessels dilate somewhat, allowing a small amount of blood into the capillary bed. Redness follows as an increasing amount of blood enters the area, and the attack terminates with the relaxation of arterial spasm and the return of normal blood flow and perfusion.

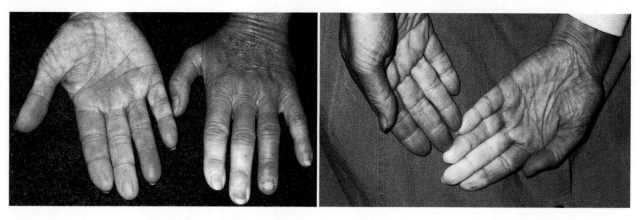

Figure 16-44 Raynaud's phenomenon.

TABLE 16-12	**Signs of Venous and Arterial Insufficiency**	
Assessment Criterion	Venous	Arterial
Color	Normal or cyanotic	Pale; worsened by elevation of extremity; dusky red when extremity lowered
Temperature	Normal	Cool (blood flow blocked to extremity)
Pulse	Normal	Decreased or absent
Edema	Often marked	Absent or mild
Skin changes	Brown pigmentation around ankles	Thin, shiny skin; decreased hair growth; thickened nails

From Potter PA, Perry AG: *Fundamentals of nursing*, ed. 5, St. Louis, 2001, Mosby.

This condition may be accompanied by numbness, tingling, burning, and pain. The attack may last from minutes to hours. The skin may eventually become smooth, shiny, and tight, and ulcers may appear on the fingertips. When the condition is a benign primary disease, it is called Raynaud's disease; when it is secondary to another disease, such as lupus or scleroderma, it is called Raynaud's phenomenon.

Venous Insufficiency and Obstruction

Venous disease results from incompetence of the venous valves or from obstruction. Table 16-12 compares the signs of venous and arterial insufficiency.

Venous Insufficiency. Incompetent valves lead to overstretched veins and increased venous pressure and stasis. Clients with this condition experience aching, throbbing discomfort during the day, particularly when the legs are in a dependent position. Accumulation of metabolic wastes in the tissues can lead to aching or cramping pain at night. Pain is a frequent symptom and is typically described as diffuse, dull, and aching; it increases as the day progresses. Long periods of standing exacerbate it, whereas leg elevation and the use of support hose may relieve it (see Box 16-2). Swelling may develop toward the end of the day and be resolved by elevating the legs.

Physical examination findings typically include edema, cyanosis of the affected leg, brown discoloration, and varicosities of the greater and lesser saphenous veins. Pulses are

usually normal, although they may be difficult to palpate if edema is present.

Thrombophlebitis. **Thrombophlebitis** is inflammation of a superficial vein. It is characterized by redness, thickening, and tenderness along the vein. It occurs most commonly as a result of trauma to the vessel wall; hypercoagulability of the blood; infection; chemical irritation; postoperative venous stasis; prolonged sitting, standing, or immobilization; or a long period of intravenous catheterization.

Deep Vein Thrombosis. Thrombus formation is the main cause of obstructed venous flow. The following are three causative factors of deep vein thrombosis (DVT):

1. Changes in the lining of the vessel
2. Changes in blood flow (stasis)
3. Changes in blood constituents (hypercoagulability)

Signs and symptoms include local tenderness, pain, increased tissue turgor, swelling, and increased skin temperature. Swelling of the legs, or ankle edema, may also be noted (Figure 16-45). Test for a positive Homan's sign by flexing the client's knee slightly with one hand while dorsiflexing the foot with the other hand. Calf pain is a positive Homan's sign indicating thrombosis. However, this calf pain can be confused with Achilles tendon pain.

Edema. **Edema** is an accumulation of fluid in the tissues that changes the shape of the area affected. Right-sided heart failure leads to increased fluid volume, which in turn leads to edema in dependent parts of the body. Edema caused by CHF

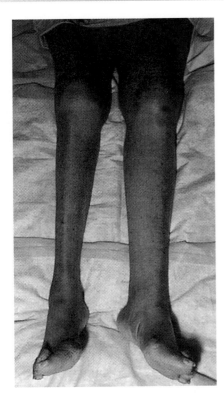

Figure 16-45 Deep vein thrombosis. (From Swartz MH: *Textbook of physical diagnosis: history and examination*, ed. 3, Philadelphia, 1998, WB Saunders.)

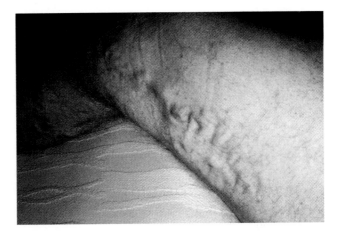

Figure 16-46 Varicose veins.

is bilateral. Pitting edema is not usually accompanied by thickening or pigmentation of the overlying skin. Edema accompanied by some thickening and ulcerations of the skin is associated with deep venous obstruction or valvular incompetence.

Varicose Veins. **Varicose** veins result from incompetent venous valves, weakened vessel walls, or obstruction in a proximal vein (Figure 16-46). Inside the veins there is a decreased flow rate and an increased intravenous pressure. Superficial varicosities are readily visible on inspection, especially when the client is standing. The veins look dilated, swollen, and tortuous.

The Trendelenburg test is used to evaluate venous incompetence when varicose veins are present. Start with the client in the supine position. Lift the affected leg above the level of the heart until the veins empty, then tie a tourniquet around the upper thigh. Ask the client to stand, and observe the venous filling pattern. Normally, the superficial veins should fill from below, taking about 35 seconds for the blood to flow through the capillary bed to the venous system. With incompetent valves, the veins will fill rapidly from above. Remove the tourniquet and check to see whether the veins fill rapidly from above. Normally, they do not—sudden filling indicates incompetent valves.

Clubbing. Clubbing of the distal portions of the fingers is characterized by a flattening of the normal nailbed angle from a 160-degree angle to a 180-degree angle. It occurs in subacute bacterial endocarditis, cor pulmonale, and cyanotic congenital heart disease (see also Figure 10-9).

Sample Documentation and Diagnoses

FOCUSED HEALTH HISTORY (SUBJECTIVE DATA)

Mr. Y, a 58-year-old Native American male, complains of shortness of breath with exertion after walking two to three blocks or up two flights of stairs; also has swollen ankles. Symptoms have been increasing gradually over the past 2 months. This is a significant change for him, since he is a carpenter accustomed to heavy work, and until several months ago, jogged during his leisure time. Dyspnea is relieved after about 10 minutes of rest; swelling is relieved by elevating his feet overnight. Gets up two or three times during the night to urinate. Sleeps well using one pillow. States that he is very concerned about these symptoms and about feeling more fatigued than usual. No chest pain or discomfort, palpitations, cough, leg cramps, or cyanosis. Usual weight about 175 lb.

History of: Diabetes—onset at age 49, controlled with daily insulin injection and diet. Cholesterol—250 3 years ago, 210 1 year ago, monitors his saturated fat consumption carefully. Hypertension—takes beta-blocker bid. No myocardial infarctions (MIs), murmurs, other cardiac diseases, or surgery. Family history of heart disease and diabetes mellitus. Father died of MI at age 59; paternal uncle died of MI at age 64.

FOCUSED PHYSICAL EXAMINATION (OBJECTIVE DATA)

Vital signs: BP 150/96; pulses—radial: 80, strong, rhythm regular; brachial, ulnar, and femoral: strong; posterior tibial and pedal: slightly diminished.

Weight: 180 lb., height 5 ft, 11 in.

Skin: Good turgor, no cyanosis, no lesions of lower extremities.

Heart: Left ventricular heave palpable—apical area. Apical impulse 2 cm left of MCL, 5 LICS. S_1 loudest at apex; S_2 loudest at base, split at 2 LICS. No S_3 or S_4. No extra sounds or murmurs.

Lungs: Clear to percussion and auscultation.

Neck vessels: Carotid pulsations visible, no bruits. Jugular pulse wave visible when client supine; pattern normal; disappears when sitting.

Hepatojugular reflux: No jugular venous distention on compression of liver.

Extremities: 1+ edema bilaterally over medial malleoli.

DIAGNOSES

HEALTH PROBLEM

Shortness of breath on exertion and peripheral edema, probably caused by congestive heart failure

NURSING DIAGNOSES

Fluid Volume Excess Related to Increased Preload, Decreased Contractility, and Decreased Cardiac Output Secondary to Congestive Heart Failure

Defining Characteristics

• Edema
• Shortness of breath

Activity Intolerance Secondary to Congestive Heart Failure

Defining Characteristic

• Verbal report of dyspnea on exertion and fatigue

Health-Seeking Behaviors

Defining Characteristics

• Verbal report of attempts to modify diet
• Verbal report of concern about health situation and desire to improve it

Critical Thinking Questions

Review the Sample Documentation and Diagnoses box to answer these questions.

1. What specific components of Mr. Y's history demonstrate risk factors for cardiovascular disease?
2. What additional history information would be helpful in helping him address his cardiovascular problem?
3. How would his risk change if he were of a different race? Would age or gender make a difference? If so, in what way?
4. What other specific physical examination techniques and/or tests could have been done to more thoroughly assess his condition, and why would you want to do them?

Answers are available on the MERLIN website (www.harcourthealth.com/MERLIN/Barkauskas/). And be sure to check the website regularly for additional learning activities!

Remember to check out the Online Study Guide!
www.harcourthealth.com/MERLIN/Barkauskas/

Abdomen

Learning Objectives

On successful study of this chapter and completion of related learning experiences, the learner will be able to:
- Describe the anatomy and physiology of and anatomical landmarks related to the vital organs contained in the abdomen.
- Outline the history pertinent to the assessment of the abdominal region, including exploration of common complaints.
- Explain the rationale for and demonstrate assessment of abdominal structures, including use of inspection, auscultation, percussion, and palpation.
- Explain the rationale for and demonstrate special maneuvers used to assess for problems in specific abdominal structures.

Outline

Purpose of Examination

Because the abdominal cavity contains many of the body's vital organs, the abdominal examination provides information about a variety of systems. It yields direct and indirect information about the functioning of the gastrointestinal and the genitourinary systems. The examination may also reveal specific vascular anomalies, such as an aortic aneurysm, and inflammatory processes affecting various organs.

The screening examination includes a general survey of the organs for signs of tenderness, enlargement, masses, and other indications of dysfunction. Specific maneuvers allow the examiner to determine the source of symptoms, such as abdominal pain, and to delineate more clearly the characteristics of masses and other abnormal findings. Although it is difficult to directly examine many of the abdominal organs, some of the examination techniques provide indirect information about organ function. When abnormal findings are present, further diagnostic studies and laboratory tests need to be conducted.

This chapter focuses on the abdominal portion of the gastrointestinal system. Chapter 6 describes nutritional assessment, Chapter 13 addresses the mouth and throat examination, and Chapter 22 describes assessment of the anus and rectum.

ANATOMY AND PHYSIOLOGY

The abdomen, the largest body cavity, extends from the diaphragm to the lesser pelvis. It is bounded anteriorly by the abdominal muscles, the costal border, and the superior border of the pelvis and posteriorly by the vertebral column and the lumbar muscles. The abdomen contains many of the body's vital organs—the stomach, small and large intestines, liver, gallbladder, pancreas, spleen, kidneys, bladder, adrenal glands, uterus, fallopian tubes and ovaries (in women), and major blood vessels (Figure 17-1). Because many major body organs are contained in this single cavity, susceptibility to organ dysfunction is increased. Methodical and systematic evaluation is vital to distinguish variations from the norm.

Stomach

The stomach is located in the left upper quadrant of the abdomen, directly below the diaphragm. It is separated into three areas: (1) the fundus, located above and to the left of the cardiac sphincter; (2) the body, found directly below the fundus; and (3) the pyloric antrum, positioned proximal to the pyloric sphincter.

Two sphincters regulate the flow of substances into and out of the stomach. The cardiac sphincter controls the inflow of food from the esophagus into the stomach. The pyloric sphincter regulates the outflow of chyme to the duodenum.

The primary functions of the stomach are to store food, to mix digestive enzymes and hydrochloric acid, and to liquefy food into chyme. Protein breakdown is initiated with the conversion of protein to peptones.

Intestines

The small intestine fills a major section of the abdominal cavity and extends from the pyloric sphincter to the ileocecal valve. It consists of three segments: the duodenum, the top portion; the jejunum, the middle portion; and the ileum, the lower portion. At the duodenum, bile and pancreatic secretions are received from the common bile duct for digestion. Absorption then takes place through the walls of the small intestine.

The large intestine extends from the ileocecal valve to the anus. It is composed of three segments: the cecum (with the vermiform appendix), the colon, and the rectum.

The cecum is located in the lower right quadrant of the abdomen. The vermiform appendix is a process extending from the lower part of the cecum. It is subject to infection and inflammation that can cause a rupture, expelling bacteria-laden substances into the abdominal cavity.

The colon frames the abdominal cavity. The ascending colon advances upward on the right side to the hepatic flexure. The transverse colon passes along the top of the abdominal cavity anterior to the liver and the stomach. The colon curves downward at the splenic flexure. The descending colon progresses to the brim of the pelvis, where it unites with the sigmoid colon and proceeds to the rectum and anus.

Liver

The liver lies primarily within the right hypochondrium and epigastrium, with a small portion situated in the left hypochondriac region. It is situated beneath the diaphragm. The rib cage covers a substantial part of the liver, with only the lower margin exposed. The liver spans the upper quadrant of the abdomen from the fifth intercostal space to slightly below the costal margin.

The liver performs the following functions:
1. Produces and secretes bile
2. Plays a major role in regulating blood glucose levels
3. Maintains protein, carbohydrate, and lipid metabolism
4. Stores vitamins—A, B_{12}, other B-complex vitamins, and D—and various minerals such as iron and copper
5. Synthesizes most plasma proteins, such as serum albumin, serum globulin, fibrinogen, and blood-clotting factors
6. Detoxifies many substances, including drugs

Gallbladder

The gallbladder is located on the inferior surface of the liver. A pear-shaped sac, it acts as a reservoir for bile secreted from the liver. The gallbladder concentrates the bile by absorbing excess water through its walls. The gallbladder is drained by the cystic duct. The cystic duct unites with the hepatic duct to form the common bile duct, which passes downward into the duodenum.

Pancreas

Immediately below the liver lies the pancreas. The pancreas is situated posterior to the greater curvature of the stomach in front of the first and second lumbar vertebrae.

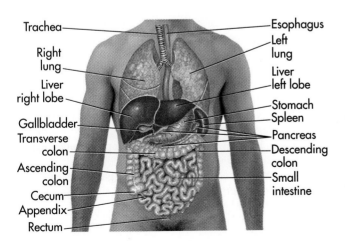

Figure 17-1 Anatomy of the gastrointestinal system. (From Wilson SF, Giddens JF: *Health assessment for nursing practice,* ed. 2, St. Louis, 2001, Mosby.)

The pancreas has both an exocrine and an endocrine function. The endocrine secretions from the islets of Langerhans produce insulin, glucagon, and gastrin, which are used in carbohydrate metabolism. The exocrine secretions from the acinar cells produce bicarbonate and pancreatic enzymes necessary for digestion and absorption in the small intestine.

Spleen

The spleen is located in the left upper abdominal quadrant. It lies to the left of the stomach directly above the kidney. The spleen has numerous functions, but its four primary ones are as follows:

1. Acts as a blood reservoir for 1% to 2% of the red blood cell mass
2. Removes old or agglutinated red blood cells and platelets
3. Is partially responsible for iron metabolism
4. Helps produce erythrocytes outside the bone marrow in the fetus and during bone marrow depression

Kidneys, Ureters, and Bladder

Covered by peritoneum and embedded in fat, the kidneys are located in the dorsal part of the abdomen between the twelfth thoracic and third lumbar vertebrae. The right kidney is slightly lower than the left one. The kidneys measure approximately 11 cm long, 5 to 7.5 cm wide, and 2.5 cm thick.

The nephron is the working unit of the kidney. Its structure consists of the glomerulus and the tubular system. Filtration occurs at the glomerular membrane, whereas reabsorption and secretion of essential materials take place in the tubular system.

The kidneys are drained by the ureters and empty into the bladder. The ureters pass anteriorly along the psoas major muscles toward the pelvis. These tubes enter the bladder at the posterolateral aspect. Peristaltic action propels the urine downward to the bladder.

The urinary bladder is located behind the symphysis pubis in the anterior half of the pelvis. The bladder has a maximum storage capacity of 1000 to 1800 ml. Moderate distention is felt when the bladder contains approximately 250 ml of urine, and discomfort is experienced with 400 ml. When distended, the bladder will rise above the level of the pubic bone.

Peritoneum

The peritoneum is a serous membrane that covers and protects the abdominal cavity. It is divided into two layers: the parietal and the visceral peritoneum. The parietal peritoneum lines the abdominal wall, and the visceral peritoneum covers the organs in the abdomen. The mesentery and the omentum are two folds of the peritoneum. The mesentery encircles the jejunum and the ileum and attaches them to the posterior abdominal wall. In addition, it supports blood vessels, lymphatic vessels, lymph nodes, and nerves. The greater omentum is connected to the upper border of the duodenum, to the lower edge of the stomach, and to the transverse colon. Its function is to protect and insulate. The lesser omentum is attached between the liver and the stomach. **Peritonitis** is an inflammation of the peritoneum, often associated with rupture of an intra-abdominal viscus such as the appendix.

EXAMINATION
Focused Health History

The health history related to the abdominal examination focuses on concerns related to the digestive system. The interviewer needs to ask both general questions about the client's health and specific questions that will vary according to the client's symptoms and the organs affected. Determining the client's primary concern is important because it guides the interview and will also influence the client's receptiveness to care. Because a client's nutritional practices, habits, and level of stress influence many gastrointestinal complaints, eliciting information about the client's lifestyle, perceived level of stress, and means of coping with stress is also important.

Present Health/Illness Status

1. Nutrition: appetite, recent change in eating pattern or foods, recent (intentional or unintentional) weight loss or gain, food preferences, food intolerances, cultural influences on eating (foods commonly served or forbidden), lifestyle influences on intake, special diets, 24-hour dietary recall (see Chapter 6 for a more detailed discussion)
2. Allergies: food, medications
3. Medications: prescription and over-the-counter drugs— laxatives, antiemetics, stool softeners, antidiarrheal agents, antacids, histamine$_2$- antagonists, lactulose, antiflatulents, antiparasitics; high doses of aspirin, acetaminophen, or nonsteroidal anti-inflammatory agents; antibiotics, corticosteroids, diuretics, antihypertensives, insulin
4. Cigarette smoking status: number of packs/day and number of years of habit
5. Alcohol intake: usual amounts, frequency
6. Use of recreational drugs: type, needle exposure
7. Stool characteristics: frequency, consistency, color, odor
8. Urinary characteristics: frequency, urgency, color, odor, pain (dysuria, suprapubic, flank), ease of starting stream, force of stream, ability to empty bladder, dribbling, episodes of incontinence
9. Exposure to infectious diseases: flu, gastroenteritis, family members or companions with similar symptoms, travel history, hepatitis
10. Recent stressful life events: social, psychological, and physical changes
11. Possibility of pregnancy: first day of last menstrual period, use of contraceptives, unprotected intercourse

Past Health History

1. Previous gastrointestinal problems, such as peptic ulcer, ulcerative colitis, polyps, intestinal obstruction, pancreatitis, gallbladder disease, hepatitis, cirrhosis of the liver, parasitic infections, diverticulosis
2. Abdominal or urinary tract surgery or injury
3. Past history of urinary tract infections (number, how many in the past year, treatment) or renal calculi (number, treatment)
4. History of major illnesses, such as cancer (type), arthritis (specify steroid or aspirin use), kidney disease, cardiac disease, respiratory disease (steroid use), reproductive system problems
5. Any blood transfusions, needle exposure
6. Hepatitis vaccination status (see Risk Factors box on hepatitis)

Family Health History

1. Kidney problems (renal stones, polycystic disease, renal tubular acidosis, renal or bladder cancer)
2. Colon cancer (see Risk Factors box on colon cancer)
3. Malabsorption syndromes (cystic fibrosis, celiac disease)
4. Gallbladder disease
5. Colitis
6. Familial polyposis

Personal and Social History

1. Significant others: who is in the home, current support system
2. Usual activities: work, school, day care; hobbies

Risk Factors
Hepatitis B

The following individuals are at risk for infection and should consider vaccination against hepatitis B virus (HBV):

Persons with occupational risk, such as health care workers and public safety workers who may be exposed to blood or other body fluids

Clients and staff in institutions for the developmentally disabled

Hemodialysis clients

Recipients of blood or blood products

Household contacts and sexual partners of persons with an active or ongoing case of HBV or HBV carriers

Adoptees from countries where HBV is endemic (e.g., China, Southeast Asia)

International travelers, particularly those visiting regions where HBV is endemic

Injecting drug users

Sexually active homosexual and bisexual men

Sexually active heterosexual men and women with a history of (1) more than one partner in 6 months, (2) sexually transmitted diseases, or (3) prostitution

Inmates of long-term correctional facilities

Children and household contacts or populations of high HBV endemicity

3. Recent life changes: (positive and negative), stresses, losses, anniversaries of losses
4. Cultural practices: folk remedies

Symptom Analysis

Abdominal Pain

1. **Onset:** specific date, sudden or gradual
2. **Course since onset:**
   Frequency: previous occurrence or progressive problem; give specific time interval
   Timing: relationship of symptoms to specific events or other symptoms, specific time of day; preprandial or postprandial; night time, seasonal, stressful situations, relation to menstrual cycle, urination, defecation, trauma
   Duration: how long has client experienced problem, recurrent or persistent
3. **Location:** at onset, radiation to another area, change in location over time, superficial or deep
4. **Quality:** burning, knifelike, cramping (severe cramping is called colic pain), aching, dull, gnawing, sharp
5. **Quantity:** how bad is pain on a scale of 1 to 10 (with 10 being the worst pain); does it interfere with daily activities
6. **Setting:** home, school, work; during mealtimes, social or recreational activity
7. **Associated phenomena:** vomiting, diarrhea, bleeding, constipation, flatulence, belching, jaundice, fever, weight loss, change in abdominal girth, vaginal discharge
8. **Alleviating and aggravating factors:** change in body position, passage of flatus or stool, belching, food or alcohol intake
9. **Underlying concern:** new symptom, sexually transmitted infection (STI), cancer, ulcer, appendicitis, pregnancy

Nausea

1. **Onset:** date of onset; sudden or gradual
2. **Course since onset:**
   Frequency: how often it occurs
   Timing: relationship to particular stimuli (odors, time of day); relationship to food intake; menstrual cycle, date of last menstrual period

Risk Factors
Colon Cancer

Age older than 50 (risk increases markedly after age 40, but 90% of cancers occur after age 50)

First-degree family member (parent or sibling) with colorectal cancer

Personal history of endometrial, breast, or ovarian cancer

Previous diagnosis of inflammatory bowel disease, adenomatous polyps, or colorectal cancer

Family history of hereditary polyposis or hereditary nonpolyposis colorectal cancer

Duration: how long has client experienced problem, recurrent or persistent

3. **Quality:** waves of nausea versus queasiness
4. **Quantity:** slight perception versus severe
5. **Setting:** emotional state; specific location such as home, school, work; mealtime; social or recreational activity
6. **Associated phenomena:** vomiting, dizziness, headache, pregnancy
7. **Alleviating and aggravating factors:** change in body position, ingestion of specific foods or alcohol, response to odors
8. **Underlying concern:** pregnancy, infectious disease

Vomiting

1. **Onset:** sudden or preceded by nausea; time elapsed since last meal
2. **Course since onset:**
   Frequency: number of occurrences; specific time intervals
   Timing: relationship to specific event or time of day, medication, diarrhea, constipation, fever, abdominal pain, missed period, number of hours after a meal
   Duration: how long has problem persisted, recurrent or persistent
3. **Quality:** nature of emesis (coffee grounds or fresh blood, color, undigested food), ability to keep fluids or solids in stomach, force (projectile)
4. **Quantity:** amount of emesis per episode
5. **Setting:** emotional state; specific location such as home, school, work; mealtime; social or recreational activity
6. **Associated phenomena:** nausea, fever, headache, previous meal, weight loss, abdominal pain, family members or companions experiencing similar symptoms, medication, pregnancy
7. **Alleviating and aggravating factors:** change in body position, ingestion of specific foods or alcohol, passage of flatus, belching
8. **Underlying concern:** food poisoning, appendicitis

Indigestion

1. **Onset:** sudden or gradual
2. **Course since onset:**
   Frequency: previous occurrence or progressive problem; give specific time interval
   Timing: relationship of symptoms to specific events, specific time of day; meals, night time, stressful situations, menstrual cycle
   Duration: how long has problem persisted, recurrent or persistent
3. **Location:** specific region (e.g., substernal, right upper quadrant, epigastrium), radiation to another area
4. **Quality:** bloated feeling after eating, excessive belching or flatulence, heartburn, loss of appetite, severe pain
5. **Quantity:** How bad is pain, gradual increase or steady; does it interfere with daily activities
6. **Setting:** emotional state; specific location such as home, school, work; mealtime; social or recreational activity
7. **Associated phenomena:** vomiting, headache, diarrhea, nausea associated with vomiting, date of last menstrual period

8. **Alleviating and aggravating factors:** association with type or quantity of food, smoking; response to antacids, histamine$_2$- antagonists, other prescription or nonprescription medications; rest, activity, self-care measures
9. **Underlying concern:** ulcer, heart attack

Diarrhea

1. **Onset:** gradual or sudden
2. **Course since onset:**
   Frequency: stool frequency, number/day, change in usual pattern of bowel movements, alternation with constipation, previous occurrence or progressive problem
   Timing: relationship to timing and nature of food intake, stressful situations, menstrual cycle
   Duration: how long has problem persisted, recurrent or persistent
   Course: improving or getting worse
3. **Quality:** watery; explosive; color; presence of mucus, blood, undigested food, or fat; odor
4. **Quantity:** copious, scant
5. **Setting:** home, school, work, during mealtimes, social or recreational activity
6. **Associated phenomena:** fever, chills, weight loss, abdominal pain, thirst, recent course of antibiotics
7. **Alleviating and aggravating factors:** food intake, stressful encounters, medications, self-care measures
8. **Underlying concern:** food poisoning, gastroenteritis

Constipation

1. **Onset:** recent occurrence or long-standing problem, sudden or gradual, last bowel movement
2. **Course since onset:**
   Frequency: number of bowel movements per week, any change in usual pattern of bowel movements
   Timing: relation to nature of food, alternates with diarrhea
   Duration: how long has problem persisted, continuous or intermittent problem
   Course: improving or getting worse
3. **Location:** abdominal discomfort, rectal pressure or pain
4. **Quality:** stool consistency (dry, hard); change in size or pattern of stools; black or tarry or associated with bright blood; accompanied by abdominal or rectal pain
5. **Quantity:** copious, scant
6. **Setting:** home school, work, during mealtimes, social or recreational activity
7. **Associated phenomena:** abdominal pain, depression
8. **Alleviating and aggravating factors:** diet—recent change in intake, increase or decrease in fiber, fluid intake; use of enemas, laxatives, stool softeners; prescription or nonprescription medications
9. **Underlying concern:** impaction, cancer

Preparation for Examination: Client and Environment

Helping the client to relax is an important prerequisite to performing a thorough examination of the abdomen. The client should have an empty bladder before the examination begins. He or she needs to be in a comfortable supine position with arms at the sides. To help the client to relax the stomach muscles, place a small pillow under the head and ask the client to flex the knees slightly. A pillow can also be placed behind the knees to support them in a slightly flexed position. The examination room should be warm enough so that the client will not shiver (thereby tensing the abdomen). The abdomen must be fully exposed. For both warmth and modesty, drape the client's chest and groin area.

Have the client breathe quietly and slowly through the mouth. Your hands and the diaphragm of the stethoscope should be warm, and your fingernails should be short. Talk to the client slowly and gently. Avoid sudden movements. Explain what you will be doing during the examination. Have the client point to tender areas, and tell the client that you will examine those areas last. Observe the client's facial expression as you conduct the examination. The stoic client may not admit to discomfort, but the facial expression may show when that person feels tenderness. You can then confirm this observation with the client and modify the examination accordingly.

Technique for Examination and Expected Findings

Physical assessment of the abdomen includes all four methods of examination (inspection, auscultation, percussion, and palpation). In the abdominal examination, auscultation is done before percussion and palpation because stimulation by pressure on the bowel can alter bowel motility and heighten bowel sounds. Palpation is the technique most useful in detecting pathological conditions of the abdomen.

Preparation for Examination

EQUIPMENT

Item	Purpose
Stethoscope (with bell and diaphragm)	To listen to bowel and vascular sounds
Metric ruler	To measure liver span
Marking pen	To mark borders of organs
Small pillows	To position client

CLIENT AND ENVIRONMENT

1. Assemble needed equipment (stethoscope, ruler, marking pen, pillows).
2. Make sure that the room is comfortably warm.
3. Explain the steps of the examination to the client.
4. Position the client in a comfortable supine position with arms at the sides, head supported by a pillow, and knees slightly flexed.
5. Completely expose the abdomen from the costal border to the symphysis pubis, draping the client's chest and pubic area for modesty and warmth.
6. Ask the client to point to any tender areas and reassure him or her that you will examine those areas last.
7. Watch the client's facial expressions for signs of discomfort during the examination.

Anatomical Mapping

To describe clearly the location of organs and the areas of pain or tenderness, the abdomen can be divided into either four quadrants or nine regions. The most frequently used method is division into four quadrants (Figure 17-2). An imaginary vertical line is drawn from the sternum down to the pubic bone through the umbilicus, and a second line is drawn perpendicular to the first line through the umbilicus. In general, abdominal structures will be located in one of these quadrants (Box 17-1). Loops of the small bowel are

BOX 17-1

ANATOMICAL CORRELATES OF THE FOUR QUADRANTS OF THE ABDOMEN

RIGHT UPPER QUADRANT

Liver and gallbladder
Pylorus
Duodenum
Head of pancreas
Right adrenal gland
Portion of right kidney
Hepatic flexure of colon
Portions of ascending and transverse colon

LEFT UPPER QUADRANT

Left lobe of liver
Spleen
Stomach
Body of pancreas
Left adrenal gland
Portion of left kidney
Splenic flexure of colon
Portions of transverse and descending colon

RIGHT LOWER QUADRANT

Lower pole of right kidney
Cecum and appendix
Portion of ascending colon
Bladder (if distended)
Ovary and salpinx
Uterus (if enlarged)
Right spermatic cord
Right ureter

LEFT LOWER QUADRANT

Lower pole of left kidney
Sigmoid colon
Portion of descending colon
Bladder (if distended)
Ovary and salpinx
Uterus (if distended)
Left spermatic cord
Left ureter

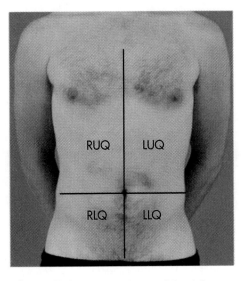

Figure 17-2   Four quadrants of the abdomen.

found in all four quadrants. The bladder and the uterus are located at the lower midline.

The second, less frequently used method divides the abdomen into nine zones (Figure 17-3). This is accomplished by drawing two imaginary vertical lines from the midclavicle to the middle of Poupart's (inguinal) ligament, approximating the lateral borders of the rectus abdominis muscles. At right angles to these lines, two imaginary parallel lines cross the border of the costal margin and the anterosuperior spine of the iliac bones. The abdominal structures correlated with the zones are shown in Figure 17-3 and described in Box 17-2. Mentally visualize the underlying structures and organs in each zone as you conduct the examination.

Certain anatomical structures are used as landmarks to facilitate the description of abdominal signs and symptoms (Figure 17-4). The following landmarks are useful for this

BOX 17-2

ANATOMICAL CORRELATES OF THE NINE REGIONS OF THE ABDOMEN

RIGHT HYPOCHONDRIAC

Right lobe of liver
Gallbladder
Portion of duodenum
Hepatic flexure of colon
Portion of right kidney
Suprarenal gland

EPIGASTRIC

Pyloric end of stomach
Duodenum
Pancreas
Portion of liver

LEFT HYPOCHONDRIAC

Stomach
Spleen
Tail of pancreas
Splenic flexure of colon
Upper pole of left kidney
Suprarenal gland

RIGHT LUMBAR

Ascending colon
Lower half of right kidney
Portion of duodenum and jejunum

UMBILICAL

Omentum
Mesentery
Lower duodenum
Jejunum and ileum

LEFT LUMBAR

Descending colon
Lower half of right kidney
Portions of jejunum and ileum

RIGHT INGUINAL

Cecum
Appendix
Ileum (lower end)
Right ureter
Right spermatic cord
Right ovary

HYPOGASTRIC

Ileum
Bladder
Uterus (in pregnancy)

LEFT INGUINAL

Sigmoid colon
Left ureter
Left spermatic cord
Left ovary

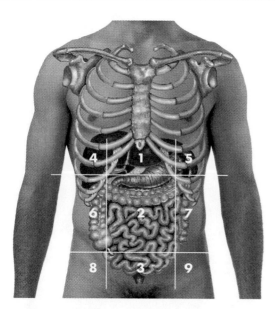

Figure 17-3 Nine regions of the abdomen. 1, Epigastric; 2, umbilical; 3, hypogastric (pubic); 4 and 5, right and left hypochondriac; 6 and 7, right and left lumbar; 8 and 9, right and left inguinal. (From Wilson SF, Giddens JF: *Health assessment for nursing practice,* ed. 2, St. Louis, 2001, Mosby.)

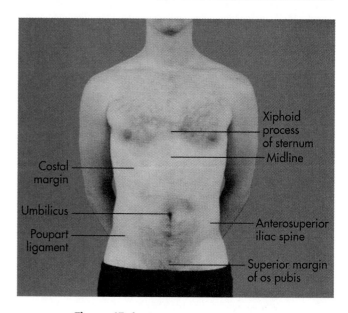

Figure 17-4 Landmarks of the abdomen.

purpose: the ensiform (xiphoid) process of the sternum, the costal margin, the midline (drawn from the tip of the sternum through the umbilicus to the pubic bone), the umbilicus, the anterosuperior iliac spine, Poupart's (inguinal) ligament, and the superior margin of the pubic bone.

Abdominal structures protected by the rib cage that are examined in health assessment are the liver, stomach, and spleen (Figure 17-5). These structures are evaluated by palpation and percussion.

Inspection

A good source of light is necessary for inspection of the abdomen. Direct the light at a right angle to the long axis of the client, or focus the light lengthwise over the client, shining it from the foot to the head. Ideally, you should sit at the right side of the client with your head only slightly higher than the client's abdomen. This will enhance shadows. Shadows highlight small changes in contour, thus increasing the likelihood of detecting a pathological condition.

When the client is on the examining table, note the position that he or she assumes voluntarily. The individual with abdominal pain commonly draws up the knees to reduce tension on the abdominal muscles and to alleviate intraabdominal pressure. The client with generalized peritonitis lies almost motionless with the knees flexed. Marked restlessness has been associated with biliary and intestinal colic, renal colic, and intraperitoneal hemorrhage.

Become familiar with the normal topography of the abdomen to avoid identifying normal contours as masses (Figure 17-6). Describe the presence or absence of symmetry, distention, masses, visible peristaltic waves, and respiratory movements. If the presence of peristalsis is in question, carefully study the abdomen for several minutes.

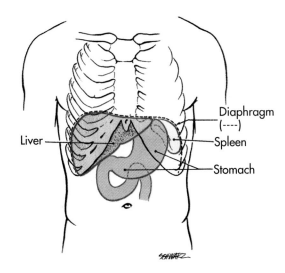

Figure 17-5 Abdominal structures protected by the rib cage. Palpation and percussion are used for examination of the liver, stomach, and spleen.

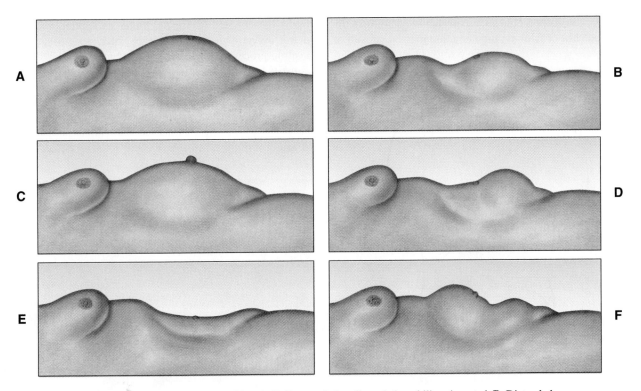

Figure 17-6 Abdominal profiles. **A,** Fully rounded or distended, umbilicus inverted. **B,** Distended lower half. **C,** Fully rounded or distended, umbilicus everted. **D,** Distended lower third. **E,** Scaphoid. **F,** Distended upper half. (From Seidel HM et al.: *Mosby's guide to physical examination,* ed. 4, St. Louis, 1999, Mosby.)

To detect masses, such as an enlarged liver or spleen, ask the client to take a deep breath. This action forces the diaphragm downward and decreases the size of the abdominal cavity, which makes masses become more obvious.

The rectus muscles are prominent landmarks of the abdominal wall (Figure 17-7). **Diastasis recti abdominis** is a separation of the rectus abdominis muscles. The separation may be palpated and observed as a ridge between the muscles by having the client raise the head and shoulders, which increases the intra-abdominal pressure. This defect does not pose a threat to the functions of the abdominal structures. Diastasis recti abdominis generally occurs as a result of pregnancy or marked obesity.

Next, inspect the abdomen from a standing position at the foot of the bed or examining table. Asymmetry of the abdominal contour may be more readily detected from this position.

Skin. The abdomen is an especially valuable area for dermatological observation because it encompasses a relatively large expanse of skin. Inspect the abdominal skin for pigmentation (particularly jaundice), lesions, striae, scars, dehydration, general nutritional status, venous patterns, and the condition of the umbilicus. This can yield valuable information about the client's general state of health.

Pigmentation. Because the skin of the abdomen is frequently protected from the sun by clothing, abdominal skin may serve as a baseline for comparison with more tanned areas. Jaundice is more readily observed in this less exposed skin. When assessing for jaundice it is important to use natural light, since incandescent light may mask the presence of jaundice. Skin color on the abdomen should be uniform. Irregular patches of faint tan pigmentation may be a result of

von Recklinghausen's disease. A bluish tint at the umbilicus (Cullen's sign) suggests periumbilical bleeding.

Lesions. The observation of skin lesions or nodules is of particular significance because gastrointestinal alterations are frequently associated with skin changes. A pearl-like enlarged umbilical node may be related to intra-abdominal lymphoma. Tense and glistening skin is often correlated with ascites or edema of the abdominal wall. Spider angiomas may be related to alcoholic cirrhosis; however, they also occur in pregnancy and collagen vascular disorders.

Striae. **Lineae albicantes (striae)** are atrophic lines or streaks that may be seen in the skin of the abdomen after rapid or prolonged stretching (Figure 17-8). This disrupts the elastic fibers of the reticular layer of the cutis. Striae of recent origin are pink or blue but progress to silvery white. Striae occurring as a result of Cushing's disease, however, remain pink-purple. The stretching of abdominal skin may occur as a result of pregnancy **(striae gravidarum)**, an abdominal tumor, ascites, or obesity.

Scars. Inspection of the abdomen for scars may yield valuable data concerning previous surgery or trauma. The size and shape of scars are best described through the use of a drawing of the abdomen on which the landmarks or quadrants are shown and the dimensions are noted in centimeters. If the cause of the scar is not elicited through the history, this information should be sought through inspection. Figure 17-9 shows the locations of common surgical scars.

The fact that the client has experienced a previous surgery should alert the examiner to the possibility that adhesions may be present. Deep, irregular scars may indicate burns (see Figure 10-36, *B*). Some individuals produce a dense overgrowth, or hypertrophy, of fibrous tissue in the healing process. This overgrowth, which is called a **keloid**, consists of large, essentially parallel bands of dense collagenous material separated by bands of cellular fibrous tissue. Keloid formation most commonly occurs after a traumatic injury or burn. Increased prevalence of keloid formation has been noted in African-American individuals and those of Asian origin.

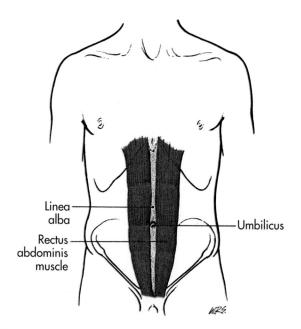

Figure 17-7 Rectus abdominis muscles. Separation of these muscles is called diastasis recti and may be detected by observation or palpation.

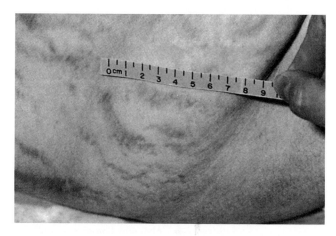

Figure 17-8 Striae. (From Swartz MH: *Textbook of physical diagnosis,* ed. 3, Philadelphia, 1998, WB Saunders.)

Veins. A fine venous network is often seen in the abdominal wall. Dilated veins are observed in vena cava obstruction that is usually related to congested portal circulation.

Umbilicus. The umbilicus should be observed for signs of vena cava obstruction (dilated veins), umbilical hernia, metastatic carcinoma, and dampness or the smell of urine (patent urachus).

Contour. Contralateral areas of the normal abdomen are symmetrical in contour and appearance. The contour is determined by the abdominal profile from the rib margin to the pubic bone as viewed from a right angle to the umbilicus with the client in a recumbent position (see Figure 17-6). The contour of the normal abdomen is described as flat, rounded, or scaphoid.

A flat contour is seen in the muscularly competent and well-nourished individual. A rounded or convex contour is normal in the infant or toddler, but in the adult it is generally caused by poor muscle tone, excessive subcutaneous fat deposits, or both. The rounded abdomen is often called the "spare tire" or "bay window" of middle age (see Figure 17-6, *A*). A scaphoid, or concave, contour may be seen in thin clients of all ages. This type of contour reflects a decrease in fat deposits in the abdominal wall and relaxed or flaccid abdominal musculature (see Figure 17-6, *E*).

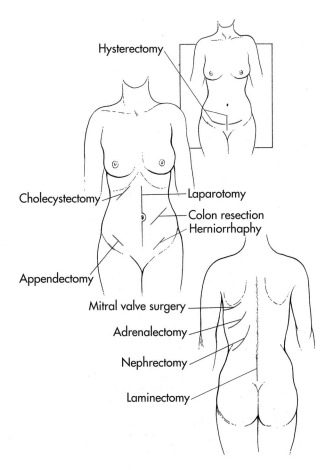

Figure 17-9 Location of common surgical scars. (From Swartz MH: *Textbook of physical diagnosis*, ed. 3, Philadelphia, 1998, WB Saunders.)

Unusual stretching of the abdominal wall is referred to as distention. Abdominal distention may result from fat (obesity), feces or flatus (constipation or intestinal obstruction), a fetus (pregnancy), fluid **(ascites),** a fibroid tumor, or a fatal tumor. The presence of distention generally implies disease and therefore warrants further investigation. Asymmetrical distention of the abdominal wall may be caused by a hernia, tumor, cysts, or bowel obstruction. A mnemonic device for classifying the six most common causes of distention are *f*luid, *f*latulence, *f*at, *f*eces, *f*ibroid tumor, and *f*etus—the six *F*s.

Generalized, or symmetrical, distention of the abdomen with the umbilicus in its normal inverted position is generally a result of obesity or recent pressure of fluid or gas within the hollow viscera. If the umbilicus is in an everted position (umbilical hernia), ascites or an underlying tumor may be the cause (see Figure 17-6, *C*). An ovarian tumor, distended bladder, or pregnancy may be suspected if the distention is confined to the area between the umbilicus and the symphysis pubis (see Figure 17-6, *B*). Distention of the lower third of the abdomen suggests an ovarian tumor, uterine fibroid tumor, pregnancy, or bladder enlargement (see Figure 17-6, *D*). Possible causes of distention of the upper half of the abdominal wall include a pancreatic cyst or tumor and gastric dilation (see Figure 17-6, *F*).

Movement

Respiratory Movement. Observation of respiratory movement has more significance in the male client because men exhibit predominantly abdominal movement with respiration. Women exhibit mainly costal movement. Therefore, limited abdominal respiratory action in the male client may be indicative of peritonitis or other abdominal infection or disease. Abdominal breathing is also common in a child younger than 6 or 7 years old. The presence of abdominal respiratory movements in an older child may indicate respiratory problems. The absence of abdominal respiratory movements in the child who is younger than 6 years suggests peritoneal irritation. Retraction of the abdominal wall on inspiration, called Czerny's sign, is associated with certain central nervous system diseases, such as chorea.

Visible Peristalsis. In lean individuals, motility of the stomach and intestines may be seen as movement of the abdominal wall even in the absence of disease. However, when strong contractions are visible through an abdominal wall of average thickness, investigate the possibility of bowel obstruction. Sit at the client's side and gaze across the abdomen for several minutes. Percussing the abdomen may augment weak peristalsis. Peristaltic waves of the stomach and small intestine may be seen as elevated oblique bands in the upper left quadrant that move downward to the right. Several of these peristaltic waves occurring in rapid succession may produce a series of parallel bands, or a "ladder effect."

Reverse peristalsis, observed in the upper abdomen in an infant, is seen as an undulation moving from left to right. This observation indicates the presence of pyloric stenosis or, less commonly, duodenal stenosis or malrotation of the bowel.

Pulsation. In thin persons, pulsation of the abdominal aorta is visible throughout most of its length. However, in most persons the pulsation is visible only in the epigastrium.

Auscultation

Auscultation of the abdomen precedes percussion because bowel motility, and thus bowel sounds, may be increased by palpation and percussion. Both the stethoscope and the examiner's hands should be warm. If they are cold, they may initiate a contraction of the abdominal muscles.

Auscultatory findings of diagnostic significance are those sounds originating from the viscera, the arterial system, the venous system, muscular activity, or parietal friction rubs. Gently place the stethoscope on the abdomen to auscultate (Figure 17-10). Light pressure on the stethoscope is sufficient to detect bowel sounds and bruits. To listen to the relatively high-pitched abdominal intestinal sounds, use the diaphragm of the stethoscope, which accentuates the higher-pitched sounds. Use the bell of the stethoscope to listen for low-pitched arterial bruits and venous hums.

Peristaltic Sounds. Normal bowel sounds are high-pitched, gurgling noises that occur approximately every 5 to 15 to 20 seconds or roughly one bowel sound for each breath sound. The duration of a single sound may be less than 1 second or may extend over several seconds. The frequency of sounds is related to the presence of food in the gastrointestinal tract or to the state of digestion. Since the passage of fluids and gases through the intestine causes bowel sounds, uninterrupted bowel sounds may be heard over the ileocecal valve 4 to 7 hours after a meal. A silent abdomen (i.e., the absence of bowel sounds) indicates the arrest of intestinal motility. Flick the abdominal wall with a finger (direct percussion) to stimulate peristalsis. Peristaltic sounds may be quite irregular, so it is essential to listen for at least 5 minutes before concluding the absence of bowel sounds. Auscultate each of the four quadrants for at least 1 minute to avoid missing any sounds and to localize specific sounds.

The two significant alterations in bowel sounds are (1) the absence of any sound or extremely soft and widely separated sounds and (2) increased sounds with a characteristically high-pitched, loud, rushing sound (**borborygmi).**

Decreased Bowel Sounds. Diminished or absent bowel sounds accompany inhibition of bowel motility. Decreased motility occurs with inflammation, gangrene, or paralytic ileus. Decreased peristalsis commonly accompanies peritonitis, electrolyte disturbances, the aftermath of surgical manipulation of the bowel, and late bowel obstruction. In addition, diminished bowel sounds are often correlated with lower lobe pneumonia.

Increased Bowel Sounds. Loud, gurgling borborygmi accompany increased motility of the bowel, such as with diarrhea. Sounds of loud volume also are heard over areas of a stenotic bowel. Sounds from an early bowel obstruction are high pitched. These may be splashing sounds, similar to the emptying of a bottle into a hollow vessel. Fine, metallic, tinkling sounds are emitted as tiny gas bubbles break through the surface of intestinal juices. Increased motility may be caused by the use of a laxative or by gastroenteritis. Common pathological conditions associated with increased bowel sounds are gastroenteritis and subsiding ileus.

Vascular Sounds

Arterial Sounds. Bruits are heard when an artery is partially obstructed, causing turbulent flow. A bruit that is heard with the bell of the stethoscope held lightly against the abdomen while the client is in a variety of positions may indicate a dilated, tortuous, or constricted vessel (Figure 17-11). Loud bruits detected over the aorta suggest the presence of an aneurysm. Auscultation of the aorta should be done superior to the umbilicus. The locations of the aorta, renal arteries, and iliac arteries are illustrated in Figure 17-12. Soft, medium- to low-pitched murmurs resulting from renal arterial stenosis may be heard over the upper midline or toward the flank. For the hypertensive client, listen carefully over the center epigastrium and posterior flank for a bruit in the

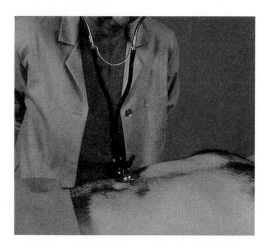

Figure 17-10 Auscultation for bowel sounds. The diaphragm of the stethoscope is used to listen to the relatively high-pitched intestinal sounds.

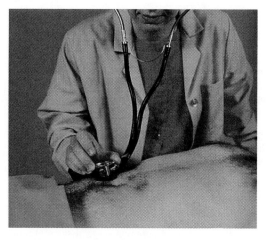

Figure 17-11 Auscultation for bruits is performed with the bell of the stethoscope held lightly against the abdomen.

arterial tree. An epigastric bruit radiating laterally suggests renal artery stenosis.

Venous Hums. A normal hum originating from the inferior vena cava and its large tributaries is continuously audible with a stethoscope. Its tone is medium pitched and is similar to a muscular fibrillary hum. In the presence of obstructed portal circulation, as from a cirrhotic liver, an abnormal venous hum may be detected in the periumbilical region. Pressure on the bell may obscure the hum. A palpable thrill may accompany the hum. Angiomas may produce hums that can be auscultated over the liver.

Peritoneal Friction Rub. Peritoneal friction rub creates a rough, grating sound that resembles two pieces of leather being rubbed together. Because the liver and the spleen have large surface areas that are in contact with the peritoneum, these two structures are most often the originating sites of peritoneal friction rubs.

Common causes of friction rubs include splenic infection, abscess, and tumor. These sounds are heard best over the lower rib cage in the anterior axillary line. Deep respiration may emphasize the sound. Metastatic disease of the liver and abscess are the usual causes of peritoneal friction rubs located over the lower right rib cage.

Muscular Activity Sounds. A fibrillating muscle produces a hum that can be heard with a stethoscope. Both voluntary and involuntary contractions (e.g., muscle guarding of a painful area) produce this sound. Palpation of the tender area often accentuates the hum.

Percussion

Percussion of the abdomen is done to detect fluid, gaseous distention, and masses and to assess the position and size of solid structures within the abdomen. Percussion can be done independently or in conjunction with palpation. For example, in a client with a tumor, percussion should be done before deep palpation to establish a sense of the size and location of the enlarged organ.

Lightly percuss the entire abdomen for a general picture of the areas of tympany and dullness. Tympany predominates because of the presence of gas in the large and small bowels. Solid masses will percuss as dull, as will organs such as a distended bladder.

Establish a systematic pattern or route to use each time you percuss abdominal structures (Figure 17-13). This will lessen the chance of omitting any portion of the examination.

Assessment of the Liver Span. To determine the size of the liver, begin percussion in the right midclavicular line at a level below the umbilicus (Figure 17-14, *A*). Start percussion over a region of gas-filled bowel (tympany) and progress upward toward the liver. The first dull percussion note indicates the lower border of the liver. (Be careful not to confuse the costal border with the liver border. Both are dull, but the costal border is easily palpable.) Mark the lower border on the abdomen. To determine the upper border of liver dullness, start percussion in the midclavicular line and examine from an area of lung resonance down to the first dull percussion note (generally the fifth to seventh interspace [Figure 17-14, *B*]). Mark this spot, and measure the distance between the two marks in centimeters (Figure 17-14, *C*). When the liver appears enlarged, percuss and measure the liver at the anterior axillary line and the midsternal line.

The usual liver span is 6 to 12 cm in the midclavicular line and 4 to 8 cm in the midsternal line (Figure 17-15). A direct correlation exists between body size (lean body mass) and liver span. It is important to remember that men have larger livers than women. The mean midclavicular liver span in men is 10.5 cm, whereas it is 7 cm in women. A midclavicular liver span of 11 cm may indicate hepatomegaly in a 5-foot, 100-pound woman, but it may be within normal limits for a man.

The descent of the liver can also be assessed. Ask the client to take a deep breath and hold it while you percuss upward from the abdomen to detect the lower liver border. The liver normally descends 2 to 3 cm with inspiration. This ma-

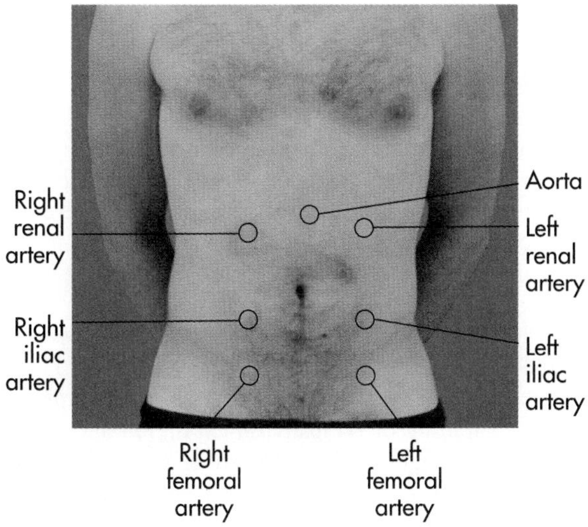

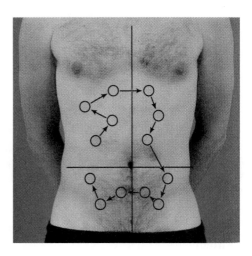

Figure 17-12 Sites to auscultate for bruits: renal arteries, iliac arteries, aorta, and femoral arteries.

Figure 17-13 Systematic route for abdominal percussion.

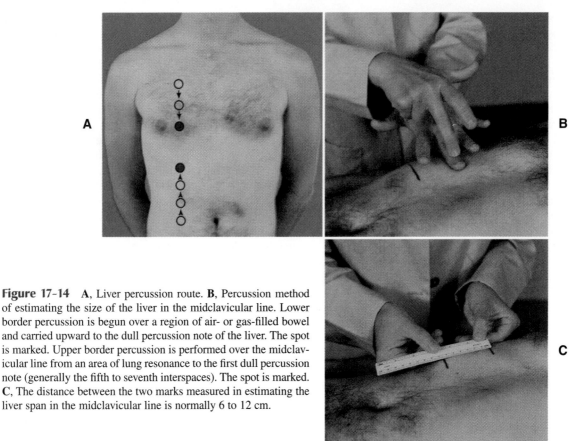

Figure 17-14 **A**, Liver percussion route. **B**, Percussion method of estimating the size of the liver in the midclavicular line. Lower border percussion is begun over a region of air- or gas-filled bowel and carried upward to the dull percussion note of the liver. The spot is marked. Upper border percussion is performed over the midclavicular line from an area of lung resonance to the first dull percussion note (generally the fifth to seventh interspaces). The spot is marked. **C**, The distance between the two marks measured in estimating the liver span in the midclavicular line is normally 6 to 12 cm.

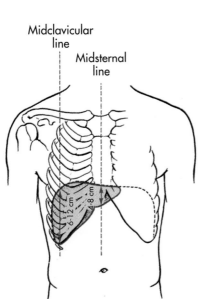

Figure 17-15 The range of liver span in the midclavicular and midsternal lines. The size of the liver shows a direct correlation to lean body mass. Thus the mean clavicular liver span is 10.5 cm in men and 7 cm in women.

neuver can help to guide placement of your hands for palpating the liver border.

Error in estimating the liver span can occur when pleural effusion or lung consolidation obscures the upper liver border or when gas in the colon obscures the lower border. On inspiration, the diaphragm moves downward. This movement shifts the normal span of liver dullness inferiorly 2 to 3 cm. Pulmonary edema may also displace the liver downward. Ascites, massive tumors, or pregnancy may push the liver upward. The liver assumes a more square configuration in cirrhosis of the liver, and the midclavicular and midsternal measurements may approach equality. Liver dullness is decreased when the liver is small. This may indicate atrophy of the liver, such as might occur in acute fulminating hepatitis.

Percussion for Tympany and Dullness

Spleen. Splenic dullness can be percussed from the level of the seventh to the eleventh rib just posterior to or at the midaxillary line on the left side. Begin percussion at the tenth rib just posterior to the midaxillary line. Percuss in several directions from dullness to resonance or tympany to outline the edges of the spleen (Figure 17-16). The span of normal splenic dullness does not exceed 7 cm. When the spleen has normal dimensions, tympany may be percussed over the lowest left intercostal space between the anterior and midaxillary lines during both inspiration and expiration. However, a finding of tympany on expiration and dullness on inspiration suggests splenic hypertrophy. A full stomach, an enlarged kidney, or a colon packed with feces may elicit dullness and therefore can mimic splenic enlargement. Gastric or colonic air may also obscure normal splenic dullness.

Stomach. The percussion note of the gastric air bubble is lower-pitched tympany than that of the intestine. Percuss

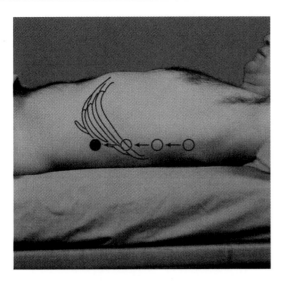

Figure 17-16   Spleen percussion route.

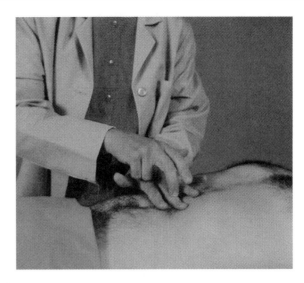

Figure 17-17   Percussion of the abdomen for evaluation of fluid, gaseous distention, and masses within the abdominal cavity.

in the area of the left lower anterior rib cage and in the left epigastric region to define the area occupied by the bubble (Figure 17-17). The percussion sounds of the stomach vary with the time the last meal was eaten.

Fist Percussion.   Another percussion method used in the abdominal examination is fist percussion, which causes the tissue to vibrate rather than produce sound (Figure 17-18). Place the palm of the left hand over the region of liver dullness and strike a light blow to the left hand with the fisted right hand. Tenderness elicited by this method is usually associated with hepatitis or cholecystitis. Fist percussion done at the costovertebral angle (CVA) is also used to assess renal tenderness. Common causes of tenderness are pyelonephritis and renal calculi.

Palpation

Palpation is the most important part of the abdominal examination. It is used to substantiate findings noted from careful inspection, auscultation, and percussion and to further explore the abdomen. Palpation is used to assess the major abdominal organs for shape, position, mobility, size, consistency, tenderness, and tension. Thorough and systematic screening is performed to detect areas of tenderness, muscular spasm, masses, or fluid.

Make sure that the client is comfortable and that your hands are warm. The client's abdominal muscles should be relaxed. You may need to use relaxation techniques to help the client achieve the appropriate level of relaxation. If the client is unable to relax the abdominal muscles despite these maneuvers, try exerting downward pressure on the lower sternum with the left hand while palpating with the other hand. The deeper inspiration that results inhibits abdominal muscle contraction. You can also ask the client to put his or her hand on the abdomen so that you can palpate on top of the client's hand.

Light Palpation.   Light palpation is gentle exploration performed while the client is in the supine position. It helps identify regions of tenderness, large or superficial masses,

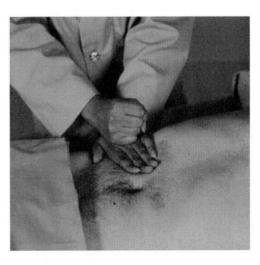

Figure 17-18   Fist percussion of the liver. The palm of the hand is placed over the region of liver dullness, and a light blow is struck with the fisted right hand. Tenderness elicited by this method is usually a result of hepatitis or cholecystitis.

and muscle guarding. Frequently, an enlarged or distended structure may be noted as a sense of resistance. Areas of tenderness or guarding, or both, should alert you to proceed with caution in more vigorous manipulation of these structures during deep palpation.

Begin palpation at a site distant from painful areas or areas expected to be tender. Elicitation of pain may result in the client's refusing further examination. Stand at the client's right side. Place the palm of your hand lightly on the client's abdomen with your fingers extended and approximated (Figure 17-19). Press the fingertips gently into the abdominal wall approximately 1 cm. Use a light dipping motion (avoid a digging action). Move systematically from one quadrant to another. The abdomen should feel smooth and soft. Watch the client's face for signs of pain elicited by palpation and confirm this verbally with the client.

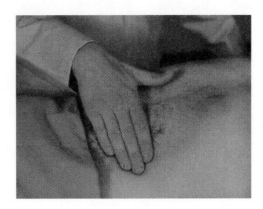

Figure 17-19 Light palpation is performed with the hand parallel to the floor and the fingers approximated. The fingers depress the abdominal wall about 1 cm. This method of palpation is recommended for eliciting slight tenderness, large masses, and muscle guarding.

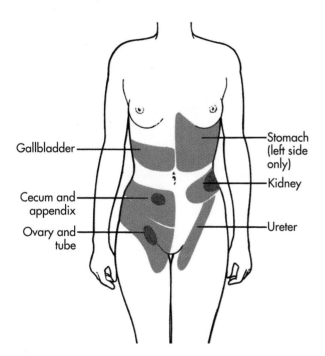

Figure 17-20 Head's zones of cutaneous hypersensitivity. (From Seidel HM et al.: *Mosby's guide to physical examination*, ed. 4, St. Louis, 1999, Mosby.)

Gallbladder

Cecum and appendix

Ovary and tube

Stomach (left side only)

Kidney

Ureter

Tensing of the abdominal musculature may occur because (1) the examiner's hands are too cold or are pressed too vigorously or deeply into the abdomen; (2) the client is ticklish or guards involuntarily; or (3) a subjacent, generally inflammatory, pathological condition exists. If resistance occurs, try to determine whether it is an involuntary spasm or voluntary tensing by feeling for the rectus muscle. The rectus muscle should normally relax as the client exhales. If the

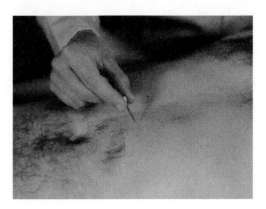

Figure 17-21 Assessment of superficial pain sensation of the abdomen.

rigidity remains unaltered, it is probably an involuntary response to localized or generalized rigidity. Rigidity is a boardlike hardness of the abdominal wall overlying peritoneal irritation. In generalized peritonitis, rigidity may be constant and hard.

> ■ **HELPFUL HINT**
>
> To examine the ticklish client:
> - Ask the client to rest his or her hand on the back of your examining hand and follow it around the abdomen. This method works because tickling yourself is difficult.
> - Exert downward pressure on the lower sternum with the left hand while palpating with the right hand. This distraction may decrease the ticklish response.

Assessment of Cutaneous Hypersensitivity. When tenderness is noted, testing for cutaneous hypersensitivity can help to delineate the areas of peritoneal irritation. Zones of hypersensitivity of sensory nerve fibers of the skin are thought to reflect specific areas of peritoneal irritation (Figure 17-20). Although research has not provided proof for all the zones, the clinical consensus is that hypersensitivity in the area of the appendix is associated with appendicitis and hypersensitivity in the middle epigastrium is associated with an active peptic ulcer.

Hypersensitivity can be evaluated in two ways. One method is to stimulate the skin gently with the sharp end of an open safety pin, a wisp of cotton, or the fingernail (Figure 17-21). The second method is to gently lift a fold of skin away from the underlying musculature (Figure 17-22). The alert client will perceive pain or an exaggerated sensation in response to this stimulation. Look for changes in facial expression (grimacing), which may also indicate the increased sensation that the individual is experiencing.

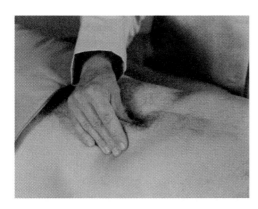

Figure 17-22 Assessment of hypersensitivity by lifting a fold of skin away from the underlying musculature.

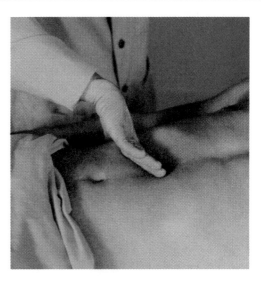

Figure 17-24 Moderate palpation performed with the side of the hand. This method of palpation is particularly useful in assessing organs that move with respiration, such as the liver and spleen.

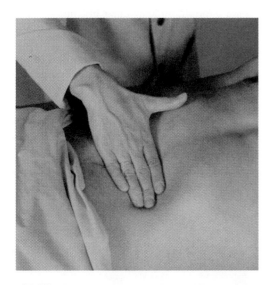

Figure 17-23 Moderate palpation. Use moderate pressure with the palm of the hand to continue to survey the four quadrants.

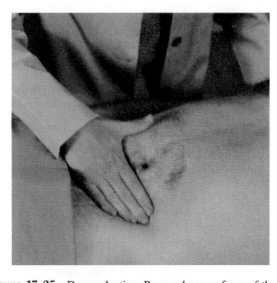

Figure 17-25 Deep palpation. Press palmar surfaces of the extended fingers deeply and evenly into the abdominal wall.

Moderate Palpation. Moderate palpation is an intermediate step for gradually approaching deep palpation. After light palpation, apply moderate pressure with the palm of the hand to continue to survey the four quadrants (Figure 17-23). Alternatively, use the side of the hand rather than the fingertips for moderate palpation (Figure 17-24). This technique avoids the tendency to dig into the abdomen with the fingertips. The sensation produced by palpating with the side of the hand is particularly useful in assessing organs that move with respiration, such as the liver and the spleen. Feel the organ during normal breathing and then as the client takes a deep breath. On inspiration, the organ will be pushed downward against your hand. Tenderness not elicited by gentle palpation may be perceived by the client when moderate pressure

is applied. This stage allows you to gradually prepare the client for deep palpation.

Deep Palpation. To assess abdominal organs thoroughly and to detect masses, use deep palpation. Deeply press the palmar surfaces of the fingers into the abdominal wall (Figure 17-25). Systematically palpate all four quadrants. The abdominal wall may slide back and forth while the fingers are moving back and forth over the organ being examined. Deeper structures, such as retroperitoneal organs (the kidneys), or masses may be felt with this type of palpation. This method may uncover tenderness of organs that cannot be elicited by light or moderate palpation. In the absence of disease, the pressure produced by deep palpation may produce tenderness over the cecum, the sigmoid colon, and the aorta.

Bimanual Palpation

Superimposition of One Hand. Use bimanual palpation when additional pressure is necessary to overcome resistance or to examine a deep abdominal structure. In this method one hand is superimposed on the other so that pressure is exerted by the upper hand while the lower hand remains relaxed and sensitive to the tactile sensation produced by the structure being examined. If you are right-handed, apply pressure with your right (top) hand while concentrating on feeling with your left (bottom) hand (Figure 17-26).

Trapping Technique. Use both hands to determine the size of a mass. Trap the mass between your hands for measurement. Clearly describe a mass in terms of location, size, shape, consistency, tenderness, mobility, pulsation, and movement with respiration.

Detection of a Pulsatile Mass. Place the fingertips of both hands on either side of the mass. Pulsation may be

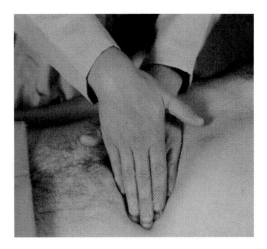

Figure 17-26 Deep bimanual palpation. Apply pressure with the upper hand while concentrating on feeling structures with the lower hand.

sensed in the fingertips as they feel the motion of a pulsatile flow expanding a structure, such as the aorta. This palpatory finding indicates that the structure being felt is pulsating rather than transmitting pulsation.

Examination of Specific Abdominal Structures

Palpation is a useful technique for identification and assessment of the specific abdominal structures. Use a systematic approach, always beginning at the same area, so that you do not skip any part of the abdomen. Because you are approaching the client from the right, the liver may be the most convenient structure to palpate first.

Liver. Two types of bimanual palpation are recommended for examination of the liver. In the first method, place your left hand beneath the client at the level of the eleventh and twelfth ribs. Apply upward pressure with your left hand to throw the liver forward, toward your right hand. Place the examining hand below the costal margin and palpate for the liver border with deep inspiration. There are two methods of positioning your right hand. Either place the palmar surface of your right hand parallel to the right costal margin (Figure 17-27, *A*) or place your right hand on the abdomen, with the fingers pointing toward the head and extended along the right midclavicular line below the level of liver dullness (Figure 17-27, *B*). Ask the client to breathe normally for two or three breaths and then to breathe deeply. The diaphragm is exerted downward on inspiration and will push the liver toward the examining hand (Figure 17-27, *A*).

The liver usually cannot be palpated in the normal adult. However, in extremely thin but otherwise well individuals, it may be felt at the costal margin on inspiration. When the normal liver margin is palpated, it feels smooth, regular in contour, and somewhat sharp. Descriptions of the abnormal liver are provided in Table 17-1.

In the second technique, commonly referred to as the "hooking technique" or "Middleton's technique," place your hands side by side on the client's right costal margin below

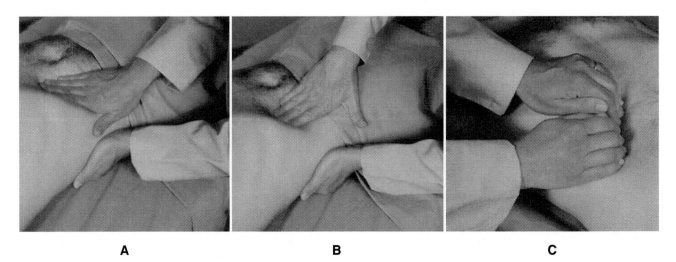

A   **B**   **C**

Figure 17-27 **A,** Palpating the liver with the fingers parallel to the costal margin. **B,** Palpating the liver with the fingers extended along the right midclavicular line. **C,** Palpating the liver with the fingers "hooked" over the costal margin.

the border of liver dullness. Stand on the right side facing the client's feet. Press in with your fingers and up toward the costal margin. Ask the client to take a deep breath. As the client inspires, the liver may be felt to descend toward your fingers (Figure 17-27, *C*). Regardless of the technique that is chosen, palpation of the liver should be done slowly, carefully, and gently so that the liver margin is not missed.

To demonstrate tenderness over the liver, place the palm of one hand over the lateral costal margin and deliver a blow to that hand with the ulnar surface of the other hand, which has been curled into a fist (fist percussion) (see Figure 17-18).

Scratch Test. The scratch test is useful when the usual techniques for determining the lower liver border have been unsuccessful. This test makes use of the difference in sound heard over solid versus hollow organs. Actually a percussion technique, the scratch test can be used to assess the size of the liver. Place the diaphragm of the stethoscope over the liver while using the opposite hand to scratch lightly over the abdominal surface. Use short, transverse strokes moving toward the liver border (Figure 17-28). When the scratch is done over the liver, the sound is magnified. Although this test is of questionable accuracy, it may be of some value in assessing the individual with abdominal distention or spastic abdominal muscles.

Spleen. The spleen is not usually palpable in the normal adult because it is normally soft and is located in the retroperitoneal area. If the spleen is palpable, it is probably enlarged.

To palpate the spleen, stand at the supine client's right side. Extend your left hand and place it beneath the client's left costovertebral angle. Exert an upward pressure with your left hand to displace the spleen anteriorly. Feel for the spleen by pressing your right hand gently under the left anterior costal margin (Figure 17-29). Have the client take a deep breath, and palpate as the client exhales. Repeat the examination with the client lying on the right side with the hips and knees slightly flexed. Turning the client on the right side

uses gravity to bring the spleen downward and forward and thus closer to the abdominal wall.

Remember that the enlarged spleen can rupture with vigorous palpation. If splenic enlargement is suspected, first percuss the splenic area and then palpate very gently and carefully. Splenic enlargement is described by the number of centimeters that the spleen extends below the costal margin:

1. *Slight:* 1 to 4 cm below the costal margin
2. *Moderate:* 4 to 8 cm below the costal margin
3. *Great:* more than 8 cm below the costal margin

As previously mentioned, the spleen may be percussed to assess enlargement. Normally, splenic dullness may be percussed from the seventh to the eleventh ribs in the midaxil-

TABLE 17-1	**Characteristics of Hepatomegaly Related to Common Pathological Conditions**
Description of Liver	**Possible Pathological Condition**
Smooth, nontender	Portal cirrhosis
	Lymphoma
	Passive congestion of liver
	Portal obstruction
	Obstruction of vena cava
	Lymphocytic leukemia
	Rickets
	Amyloidosis
	Schistosomiasis
Smooth, tender	Acute hepatitis
	Amebic hepatitis or abscess
	Early congestive cardiac failure
Nodular	Late portal cirrhosis
	Tertiary syphilis
	Metastatic carcinoma
Hard	Carcinomatosis

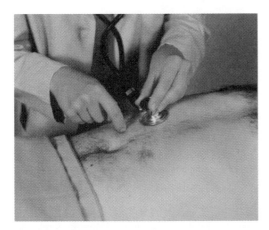

Figure 17-28 Scratch test in assessment of liver size. Place the stethoscope over the liver while the other hand scratches lightly over the abdominal surface with short, transverse strokes; when the scratch is done over the liver, the sound is magnified.

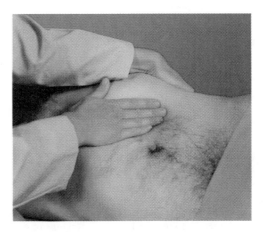

Figure 17-29 Palpation of the spleen

lary line or posterior to the line. To best describe splenic enlargement, draw the anterior abdomen, indicating the relative size and shape of the spleen in relation to the costal border and the umbilicus (Figure 17-30).

Gallbladder. The normal gallbladder cannot be felt. A distended gallbladder can be palpated below the liver margin at the lateral border of the rectus muscle. The cystic nature of the mass helps to identify the gallbladder. However, the location of the left border varies greatly. It may be found either more medially or more laterally.

An enlarged, tender gallbladder indicates cholecystitis, whereas a large but nontender gallbladder suggests obstruction of the common bile duct. Murphy's sign is helpful in determining the presence of cholecystitis. While performing deep palpation, ask the client to take a deep breath. As the descending liver brings the gallbladder in contact with the examining hand, the client with cholecystitis will experience pain and will stop the inspiratory movement (a positive Murphy's sign). Pain may also occur in the client with hepatitis.

Pancreas. The pancreas cannot be palpated in the normal client because of its small size and retroperitoneal position. However, a pancreatic mass may occasionally be felt as a vague sensation of fullness in the epigastrium.

Urinary Bladder. The urinary bladder is not palpable in the normal client unless it is distended with urine. A distended bladder is felt as a smooth, round, and rather tense mass. Percussion can be used to define the outline of the distended bladder, which may extend upward as far as the um-

bilicus. Note that in pregnancy an enlarged uterus may be confused with a distended bladder (see Chapter 25).

Umbilicus. Observe the umbilicus for its relationship to the skin surface, hernia, inflammation, or signs of bleeding. The normal umbilicus is recessed below the skin surface. The umbilical ring should be round and regular. There should not be bulges, granulation, or nodules in the area.

Umbilical Hernia. The umbilical hernia noted in children is seen directly at the umbilical opening, which is centrally located in the linea alba. In the adult, this defect is often apparent above an incomplete umbilical ring and is referred to as paraumbilical. Examine for an umbilical hernia by pressing your index finger into the navel. The fascial opening may feel like a sharp ring with a soft center. The umbilicus may be everted by marked intra-abdominal pressure from masses, pregnancy, or large amounts of ascitic fluid.

Abdominal Reflexes. To elicit the abdominal reflex, use a key, the base end of an applicator, or your fingernail to stroke the abdominal skin gently over the lateral borders of the rectus abdominis muscles toward the midline (Figure 17-31). Repeat this maneuver in each quadrant. With each stroke, observe contraction of the rectus abdominis muscles, coupled with pulling of the umbilicus to the stimulated side. The abdominal reflex may be weak or absent in the individual who has sustained a good deal of stretching of the abdominal musculature. Thus you may be unable to obtain the abdominal reflex in the multiparous or obese client. In addition, the reflex may be absent in the normal aging client. Its absence may also indicate a pyramidal tract lesion. Absence of the upper abdominal reflex suggests problems at the spinal levels of T7, T8, and T9. Absence of lower abdominal reflexes indicates problems at the spinal levels of T10 and T11.

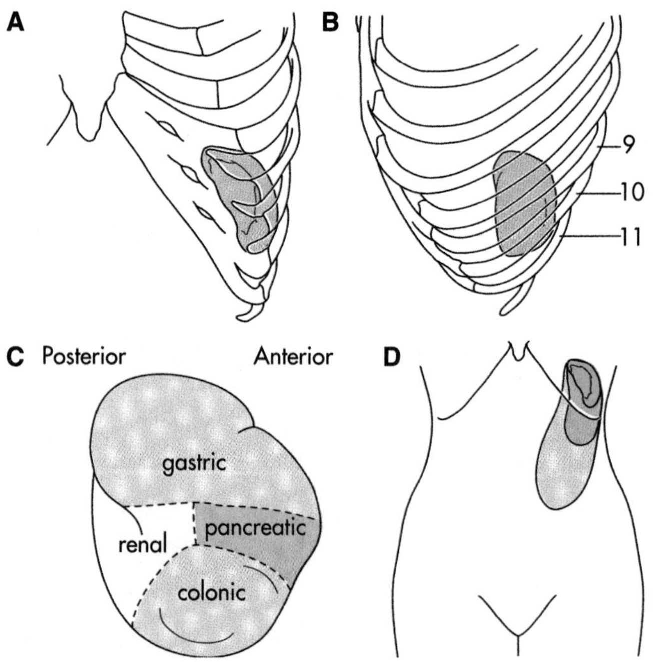

Figure 17-30 Normal (**A, B, C**) and enlarged (**D**) spleen. **A,** Anterior view. **B,** Left lateral view. **C,** Regions of the spleen (anterior view) that touch other viscera. **D,** Directions of splenic enlargement.

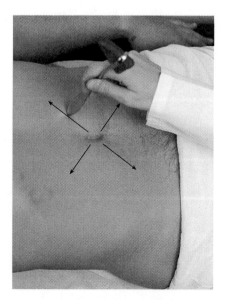

Figure 17-31 Examination of the superficial abdominal reflexes. One of several approaches is illustrated. Stroke the upper abdominal area upward, away from the umbilicus, and the lower abdominal area downward, away from the umbilicus. (From Seidel HM et al.: *Mosby's guide to physical examination,* ed. 4, St. Louis, 1999, Mosby.)

Aorta. With the client in a supine position, press firmly and deeply in the upper abdomen slightly to the left of midline and palpate for aortic pulsations. In an older individual (older than 50 years), try to assess the width of the aorta to screen for an aneurysm. Press deeply in the upper abdomen with one hand on either side of the aorta (Figure 17-32). The normal aorta is approximately 1.3 to 3 cm wide, whereas an aneurysm is much broader (more than 4 to 5 cm). A bruit is generally heard over an aneurysm. The most common physical finding in clients with an abdominal aneurysm is the presence of an expanding, pulsating mass. More than 95% of such masses are located below the renal arteries but generally at or above the umbilicus. Femoral pulses are usually present but are markedly damped in amplitude.

More than half of clients with abdominal aneurysms are asymptomatic; therefore the mass may be discovered during a screening physical examination. Although more than 80% of abdominal aneurysms can be palpated, small aneurysms in the markedly obese client may not be felt. If you observe a pulsating abdominal aortic mass and auscultate a bruit, refrain from palpation.

Changes in Vascular Patterns: Venous Engorgement.
In a healthy person, the veins of the abdominal wall are not prominent. However, in the malnourished individual, the veins are more easily visible because of decreased adipose tissue. The venous return to the heart is cephalad (toward the head) in the veins above the umbilicus and caudal below the navel. The visibility of veins is not useful. However, the direction of flow in visible veins can be helpful to assess obstruction of the vena cava (Figure 17-33).

To demonstrate the direction of flow, place the tips of the index fingers side by side over a vein, pressing laterally and separating the fingers. "Milk" the blood from a section of the vein. Remove one finger and measure the time for filling. Remove the other index finger, and measure the time for filling from this side. The flow of venous blood is in the direction of the faster-filling side. Reversal of flow or an upward venous flow in the veins below the umbilicus accompanies obstruction of the inferior vena cava. Superior vena cava obstruction promotes downward flow in the veins above the navel. A pattern of engorged veins around the umbilicus, called caput medusae, is occasionally seen as an accompa-

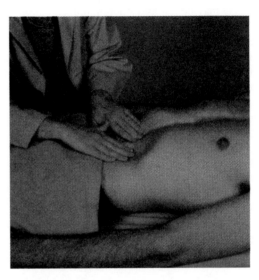

Figure 17-32 Palpation of the aorta. Press fingers deeply with one hand on either side of the aorta and feel for pulsation.

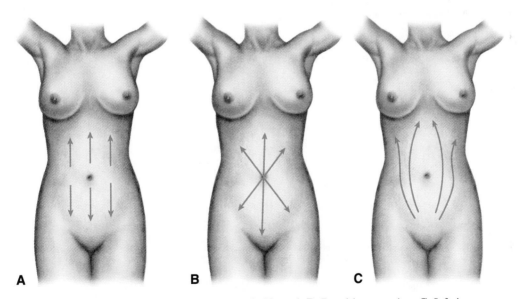

A **B** **C**

Figure 17-33 Abdominal venous patterns. **A,** Normal. **B,** Portal hypertension. **C,** Inferior vena cava obstruction. (From Seidel HM et al.: *Mosby's guide to physical examination*, ed. 4, St. Louis, 1999, Mosby.)

niment to emaciation or to obstruction of the superior or inferior vena cava, the superficial vein, or the portal vein.

Kidney. When palpating the kidneys, stand at the client's right side with the client in a supine position. To examine the left kidney, reach across the client with your left arm and place your hand behind the client's left flank (Figure 17-34). Elevate the left flank with your fingers, displacing the kidney anteriorly. Then use the palmar surface of your right hand to deeply palpate the kidney.

To examine the right kidney, remain on the client's right side. Elevate the right flank with the left hand. Use the right hand to deeply palpate the right kidney. The lower pole of the right kidney may be felt as a smooth, rounded mass that descends on inspiration. The kidneys are usually not palpable in the normal adult. In very thin persons, only the lower pole of the right kidney can be felt. In the elderly, as muscle tone decreases and elastic fibers are lost, the kidneys may be more readily palpated. The left kidney is generally not palpable.

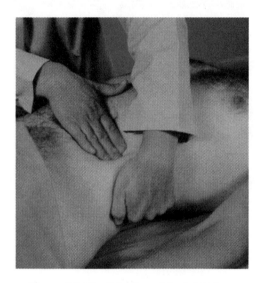

Figure 17-34 Palpation of the left kidney.

Percussion may be used to differentiate between splenic and left kidney enlargement. The percussion note over the spleen is dull because the bowel is displaced downward. Resonance is heard over the kidney because it is located behind the bowel (Figure 17-35). In addition, the free edge of the spleen is sharp in contour and tends to enlarge caudally and to the right.

Back. The final step in the abdominal examination includes inspection and fist percussion of the back for renal problems. The client should be in the sitting position for this portion of the examination. In the normal individual, the flanks are symmetrical. Fullness or asymmetry may be a result of renal disorders. Ecchymoses of the flanks (Grey Turner's sign) are associated with retroperitoneal bleeding and may indicate hemorrhagic pancreatitis. Unilateral flank pain or tenderness suggests renal or ureteral disease, such as a stone, tumor, infection, or infarct.

Fist percussion in each costovertebral angle is done to evaluate kidney tenderness. Figure 17-36 demonstrates the relationship of the kidney to the costovertebral junction. For indirect percussion, place the palm of one hand in the costovertebral angle and strike it with the ulnar surface of the fist of your other hand (Figure 17-37, *A*). Direct percussion is demonstrated in Figure 17-37, *B*. In either type of percussion, use enough force for the client to perceive a painless jarring or a thud. Fist percussion should not cause pain in the normal person. Pressure from your fingertips in the costovertebral angle may be enough to reveal tenderness in the client with a kidney infection. Frequently, this maneuver is integrated into the back examination, or it is done at the end of the posterior lung examination for increased efficiency and client comfort.

Special Maneuvers

Evaluation of Ascites (Free Fluid). Ascites should be considered in the client with a protuberant abdomen and bulging flanks. This condition is caused by (1) diseases of the liver, such as cirrhosis and hepatitis; (2) diseases of the heart, such as congestive failure and constrictive pericardi-

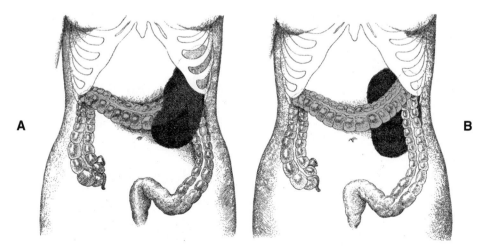

Figure 17-35 Differentiation of enlarged spleen (**A**) from enlarged left kidney (**B**). (From *GI series: physical examination of the abdomen*, Richmond, Va, 1981, Whitehall-Robins Healthcare.)

tis; (3) pancreatitis; (4) cancer, such as peritoneal metastases and ovarian tumors; (5) tuberculous peritonitis; and (6) hypoalbuminemia. A technique for differentiating ascites from cysts or edema fluid in the abdominal wall is the percussion test for shifting dullness. Palpation of a fluid wave is another method to assess for ascites.

Shifting Dullness. Place the client in the supine position. Percuss for areas of dullness and resonance. Ascites will sink with gravity and will produce a dull percussion note in dependent areas (Figure 17-38, *A*). Gas-filled loops of bowel will rise to the upper areas and have a resonant note. Mark the borders between tympany and dullness. Next, test for shifting dullness (Figure 17-38, *B*). After marking the borders, ask the client to turn on one side. The ascites will flow with gravity to shift the line of dullness closer to the umbilicus on the client's dependent side. Percuss and mark a new line, and measure the change in centimeters. In a person without ascites, the borders will remain

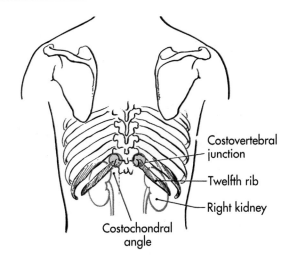

Figure 17-36 Relationship of the kidney to the twelfth rib. Note the costovertebral junction.

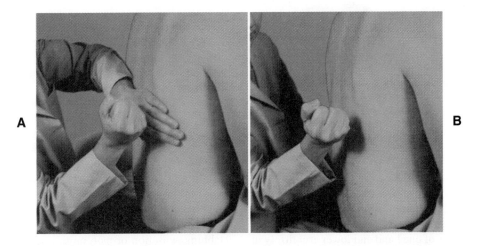

Figure 17-37 **A,** Indirect percussion of the costovertebral angle to elicit tenderness related to the kidney. **B,** Direct percussion of the costovertebral angle to elicit tenderness related to the kidney.

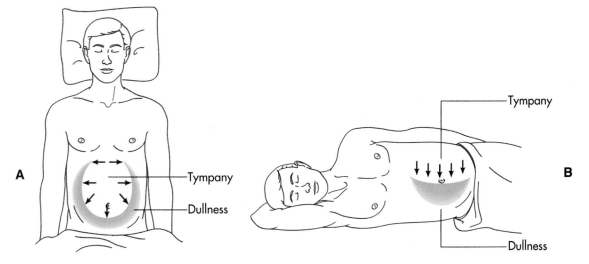

Figure 17-38 Assessment of ascites. **A,** In the supine client, ascites fluid will sink with gravity and give a dull percussion note. Mark borders between tympany and dullness. **B,** To test for shifting dullness, ask the client to turn on one side. Ascites fluid will flow with gravity. Dullness shifts to the dependent side while tympany shifts to the top. Percuss and mark the new line and measure the change.

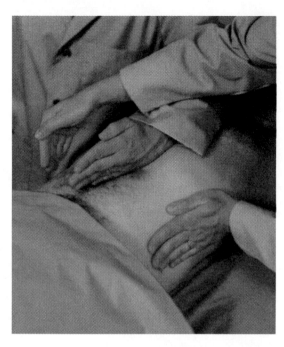

Figure 17-39   Testing for a fluid wave. Place the palmar surface of one hand against the abdominal wall and tap the other side with the other hand. An easily felt fluid wave suggests ascites.

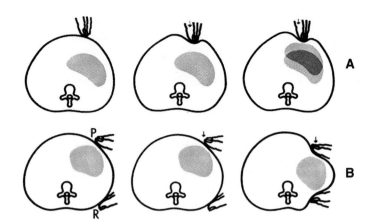

Figure 17-40   Ballottement. **A,** Single-handed ballottement. **B,** Bimanual ballottement. *P,* Pushing hand. *R,* Receiving hand. (From *GI series: physical examination of the abdomen,* Richmond, Va, 1981, Whitehall-Robins Healthcare.)

relatively constant. A volume of free fluid in the peritoneal cavity greater than 2 L can be detected by methods of shifting dullness.

Fluid Wave.   The presence of large amounts of fluid within the peritoneal cavity allows the elicitation of a fluid wave (Figure 17-39). To test for the presence of a fluid wave, place the client in a supine position. Ask the client or an assistant to place the edge of one hand and lower arm firmly in the vertical midline of the client's abdomen. This maneuver will help to stop vibrations that might otherwise be transmitted through fat. Place the palmar surface of one of your hands firmly against the lateral abdominal wall and tap the other side with your other hand. An easily felt fluid wave suggests ascites. However, this sign is often negative until ascites becomes obvious. The fluid wave may sometimes be felt in individuals without ascites.

Ballottement.   Ballottement (Figure 17-40) is an advanced palpation technique used to assess a floating object. Fluid-filled tissue is pushed toward the examining hand so that the object will float against the examining fingers. This abdominal palpation technique is used to determine whether the head or the breech of the fetus is in the fundus of the uterus (Leopold's maneuver).

Single-Handed Ballottement.   Single-handed ballottement is performed with the fingers extended in a straight line with the forearm and positioned at a right angle to the abdomen. Move the fingers quickly toward the mass or organ to be examined and hold them there. As fluid or other structures are displaced, the mass will move upward and be felt at the fingertips. Some examiners prefer this technique for examination of the spleen.

Bimanual Ballottement.   To perform bimanual ballottement, with one hand push on the anterior abdominal wall to displace the contents to the flank while the other hand feels the mass or structure pushed against it and assesses its dimensions.

Palpation to Elicit Rebound Tenderness.   Rebound tenderness is a symptom of peritoneal irritation. To provoke rebound tenderness, hold your hand with the fingers extended at a 90-degree angle. Push your fingers gently but deeply in a region remote from the area of suspected tenderness and then rapidly remove them. The maneuver, when performed over McBurney's point (as illustrated in Figure 17-41), may elicit rebound tenderness related to appendicitis. The rebound of the structures indented by palpation causes a sharp, stabbing sensation of pain on the side of the inflammation. This sensation following the withdrawal of pressure is a sign of peritoneal irritation. The test may be repeated on the side of the suspected disease. It is best performed near the conclusion of the examination because the production of severe pain or muscle spasm may interfere with subsequent examination. Voluntary coughing by the client may produce the same results.

Many examiners consider the elicitation of rebound tenderness by palpation to be a crude and painful technique. The resultant severe pain and muscle spasm not only interfere with subsequent examination but also may adversely affect the element of trust in the client-physician relationship. Light percussion can be used to produce vibration, which causes a mildly uncomfortable response in the presence of peritoneal inflammation. This technique is reputed to be able to localize very small areas of peritoneal inflammation, in some instances an area as small as a quarter.

Palpation for Abdominal Masses.   One of the goals of abdominal palpation is to determine the presence of abdominal masses. (Palpation techniques were described in detail in the preceding sections.) Once a mass is found, carefully describe its characteristics. Of particular importance are consistency, regularity of contour movement with respira-

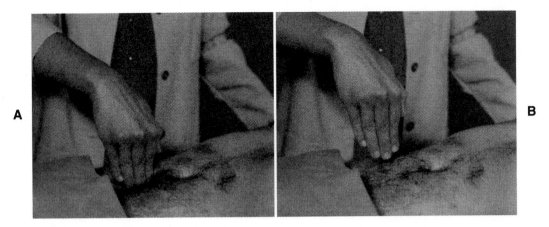

Figure 17-41 Palpation to elicit rebound tenderness. **A**, Deep pressure is applied to the abdominal wall. **B**, On release of pressure, a sensation of pain would indicate peritoneal irritation. This is a test for appendicitis.

TABLE 17-2	**Characteristics of Abdominal Masses Related to Common Pathological Conditions**
Description of Mass	**Possible Pathological Condition**
Descends on inspiration	Liver, spleen, or kidney mass
Pulsatile mass	Abdominal aneurysm, tortuous aorta
Movable from side to side, not head to foot	Mesenteric or small bowel mass
Complete fixation	Tumor of pancreatic or retroperitoneal origin

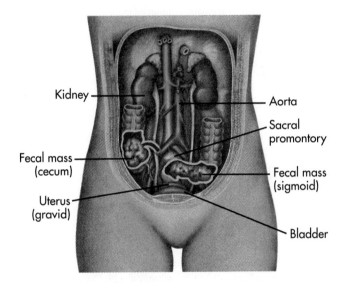

Figure 17-42 Abdominal structures commonly mistaken for masses. (From Seidel HM et al.: *Mosby's guide to physical examination*, ed. 4, St. Louis, 1999, Mosby.)

tion, tenderness, and mobility (Table 17-2). A sketch of the anterior abdominal wall with all its bony landmarks and the umbilicus may be the most efficient way to convey location, shape, and size.

To determine whether a palpable mass is located in the anterior abdominal wall or is situated in an intraabdominal position, ask the client to raise the head and shoulders from a supine position or to flex the abdominal muscles. Masses in the subcutaneous tissue will continue to be palpable, whereas those in the peritoneal cavity will be more difficult to feel or will be pushed out of reach altogether.

Normal abdominal structures that are occasionally mistaken for masses are the following (Figure 17-42):

1. Lateral borders of rectus abdominis muscles
2. Uterus
3. Feces-filled ascending colon
4. Feces-filled descending colon and sigmoid colon
5. Aorta
6. Common iliac artery
7. Sacral promontory

Palpable Bowel Segments. The presence of feces within the bowel frequently contributes to the examiner's ability to palpate the cecum, ascending colon, descending colon, and sigmoid colon. The feces-filled cecum and ascending colon produce a sensation suggestive of a soft, boggy, rounded mass. The client may complain of cramps resulting from stimulation of the bowel by the movements of palpation.

Tests for Peritoneal Irritation—(Commonly Used to Assess for Appendicitis)

Iliopsoas Muscle Test. An inflamed or perforated extrapelvic appendix may cause contact irritation of the lateral iliopsoas muscle. To elicit an indication of involvement, place the client in a supine position. Ask the client to flex the leg at the hip. As the client is flexing, simultaneously exert a moderate downward pressure over the lower thigh (Figure 17-43). With psoas muscle inflammation, the client will describe pain in the lower quadrant. A more sensitive test of psoas muscle irritation is performed with the client lying on the left side.

With inflammation, pain will be elicited through all positions of full extension of the right lower limb at the hip.

Obturator Muscle Test. A perforated intrapelvic appendix or a pelvic abscess adjacent to it can cause irritation of the internal obturator muscle. This pain is demonstrated with the client in the supine position. Ask the client to flex the right extremity at the hip and at the knee to 90 degrees. Grasp the ankle and rotate it internally and externally (Figure 17-44). A complaint of hypogastric pain indicates obturator muscle involvement.

Assessment of Muscle Spasticity. Involuntary muscle contraction or spasticity may indicate peritoneal irritation. Further palpation is done to determine whether the spasticity is unilateral or present on both sides of the abdomen. Generalized and boardlike contraction is thought to be typical of peritonitis. Ask the client to raise the trunk from a hor-

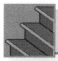

Examination Step-by-Step

INSPECTION

1. Observe the surface of the abdomen for the following factors:
   a. Skin color
   b. Scars
   c. Venous network
   d. Umbilicus—placement, contour, surface characteristics
   e. Symmetry (view from the right side at eye level and from behind the client's head)
   f. Contour
   g. Surface characteristics
   h. Surface motility, peristalsis, pulsations

AUSCULTATION

1. Listen to all four quadrants and the epigastrium using the diaphragm of the stethoscope; note the timing and quality of sounds.
2. Listen for arterial vascular sounds (abdominal aorta, renal and femoral arteries). Use the bell of the stethoscope to pick up low-pitched sounds such as a venous hum.
3. Listen for a friction rub, most commonly heard over the liver or the spleen.

PERCUSSION

1. Lightly percuss all four quadrants.
2. Percuss the liver borders at the midclavicular and midsternal lines. Mark the upper and lower borders with a pen, and measure the liver span.
3. Percuss the spleen at the left midaxillary line.
4. Percuss the "gastric bubble" at the left lower rib cage.

PALPATION

1. Use light palpation with the pads of the fingertips to survey all four quadrants for tenderness, muscle tone, and masses.
2. Use moderate palpation with the palm and the sides of the hands to continue to assess all four quadrants for tenderness, muscle tone, masses, and the general location of major structures.
3. Use deep palpation to survey all four quadrants for tenderness, masses, and the location of deeper structures.
4. Palpate specific organs:
   a. Liver: Deeply palpate by placing the left hand under the eleventh and twelfth ribs and the right hand parallel to the right costal margin. Have the client breathe normally and then take a deep breath. Palpate on inspiration.
   b. Spleen: While standing on the client's right side, extend your left hand and place it beneath the client's left costovertebral angle. Feel for the spleen by pressing your right hand gently under the left anterior costal margin.
   c. Aorta: With the client in the supine position, deeply palpate slightly to the left of midline to feel for the aortic pulsation.
   d. Palpate the umbilicus with the fingertips for bulges, nodules, and the umbilical ring.
   e. Kidneys: With the client supine, palpate each kidney. Left kidney: Extend the left hand across the client to elevate the left flank, then deeply palpate the kidney with the right hand (the left kidney is usually not palpable). Right kidney: Place the left hand under the right flank and palpate deeply with the right hand. To assess kidney tenderness, have the client sit up and use fist percussion at the right and left costovertebral angles.

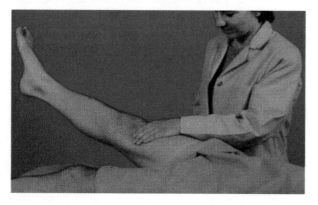

Figure 17-43 Iliopsoas muscle test.

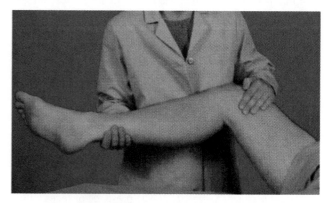

Figure 17-44 Obturator muscle test.

izontal position without arm support. The experience of unilateral pain in response to this maneuver may further pinpoint the areas of spasticity. This mechanism may also help to differentiate muscle contraction from abdominal mass. As the head is raised, the examining hand would be moved away from an abdominal mass. Rigidity and tenderness over McBurney's point, and in some cases over the entire right side, strongly suggest appendicitis. Acute cholecystitis is commonly accompanied by rigidity of the right hypochondrium.

Test for Diastasis Recti or Abdominal Hernia. If an umbilical or incisional hernia or diastasis recti abdominis is suspected, instruct the client to raise the head from the pillow, increasing the intra-abdominal pressure, which may cause the hernia to protrude. Asking the client to cough will also cause a hernia to bulge outward. When the client raises the head from the pillow, the rectus muscles contract and will reveal a separation of the muscles. Diastasis recti may be congenital or may be acquired as a result of weakening of the muscles by conditions such as pregnancy and obesity.

VARIATIONS FROM HEALTH

Tables 17-3 through 17-6 list the history, signs, and symptoms of various conditions associated with the abdomen. The signs and symptoms of intestinal obstruction and of peritoneal irritation are shown in Boxes 17-3 and 17-4.

TABLE 17-3	**Conditions Associated With the Right Lower Quadrant of the Abdomen**		
Condition	**History**	**Symptoms**	**Signs**
Appendicitis	Children (except infants) and young adults	Anorexia Nausea Pain—early, vague epigastric, periumbilical, or generalized pain after 12-24 hours; RLQ at McBurney's point	Signs may be absent early Vomiting Localized RLQ guarding and tenderness after 12-24 hours Rovsing's sign—pain with pressure in RLQ, iliopsoas sign Obturator sign White blood cell count 10,000 mm³ or shift to left Low-grade fever Cutaneous hyperesthesia in RLQ Signs are highly variable
Mesenteric adenitis	Young person with history of respiratory infection	Lower abdominal pain May have normal appetite	Tenderness in RLQ Peritoneal irritation signs rare
Perforated duodenal ulcer	Prior history	Abrupt onset of pain in epigastric area or RLQ	Tenderness in epigastric area or RLQ Signs of peritoneal irritation Heme-positive stool Increased white blood cell count
Cecal volvulus	Seen most commonly in the elderly	Abrupt severe abdominal pain	Distention Localized tenderness Tympany
Strangulated hernia	Any age Women—femoral Men—inguinal	Severe localized pain If bowel obstructed, generalized pain	If bowel obstructed, distention

Ectopic pregnancy (1% of all pregnancies)	Woman of childbearing age
	Previous tubal pregnancy or pelvic inflammatory disease
	Missed menstrual period
	Spotting
		Symptoms of pregnancy (e.g., breast changes)
		Lower abdominal pain
		Referred pain to shoulder
		Nausea
			Unruptured:
			   Tenderness—cervical
			   Mass—adnexal or cul-de-sac
			Ruptured:
			   Shock
			   Distention
			   Rigidity
			Mass—cul-de-sac
			Fever

Pelvic inflammatory disease	Women
	Exposure to infection
		Lower abdominal pain
		Dyspareunia
			Tenderness—adnexal and cervical (chandelier sign)
			Cervical discharge
			Endocervical smear
			   Gonococcus in one third to one half of cases
			   Chlamydial and anaerobic bacteria cause remainder

Tubal abscess	Woman Exposure to infection	Lower abdominal pain Dyspareunia	Fever Mass—adnexal

RLQ, Right lower quadrant.

| TABLE 17-4 | **Conditions Associated With the Right Upper Quadrant of the Abdomen** | | |

Condition	History	Symptoms	Signs
Hepatitis	Any age, often young blood product user	Fatigue Malaise Anorexia	Hepatic tenderness Hepatomegaly Bilirubin elevated Jaundice
	Drug addict	Pain in RUQ Low-grade fever May have severe fulminating disease with liver failure	Lymphocytosis in one third of cases Liver enzymes elevated Hepatitis B or D or antibodies to these viruses may be found
Acute hepatic congestion	Usually elderly with congestive heart failure Pericardial disease Pulmonary embolism	Symptoms of congestive heart failure	Hepatomegaly Congestive heart failure
Biliary stones, colic	"Fair, fat, forty" (90%) but can be 30 to 80 years of age	Anorexia Nausea Pain severe in RUQ or epigastric area Episodes last 15 minutes to hours	Tenderness in RUQ Jaundice
Acute cholecystitis	"Fair, fat, forty" (90%) but may be 30 to 80 years of age	Severe RUQ or epigastric pain Episodes prolonged up to 6 hours	Vomiting Tenderness in RUQ Peritoneal irritation signs Increased white blood cell count
Perforated peptic ulcer	Any age	Abrupt RUQ pain	Tenderness in epigastrium and/or right quadrant Peritoneal irritation signs Free air in abdomen

RUQ, Right upper quadrant.

| TABLE 17-5 | **Conditions Associated With the Left Lower Quadrant of the Abdomen** | | |

Condition	History	Symptoms	Signs
Ulcerative colitis	Family history Jewish ancestry	Chronic, watery diarrhea with blood, mucus Anorexia Weight loss Fatigue	Fever Cachexia Anemia Leukocytosis
Colonic diverticulitis	Older than 39 Low-residue diet	Pain that recurs in LLQ	Fever Vomiting Chills Diarrhea Tenderness over descending colon

LLQ, Left lower quadrant.

TABLE 17-6	Conditions Associated With the Left Upper Quadrant of the Abdomen		
Condition	**History**	**Symptoms**	**Signs**
Splenic trauma	Blunt trauma to LUQ of abdomen	Pain—LUQ pain of abdomen often referred to left shoulder (Kehr's sign)	Hypotension Syncope Increased dyspnea X-ray studies show enlarged spleen
Pancreatitis	Alcohol abuse Pancreatic duct obstruction Infection Cholecystitis	Pain in LUQ or epigastric region radiating to back or chest	Fever Rigidity Rebound tenderness Nausea Vomiting Jaundice Cullens' sign Turner's sign Abdominal distention Diminished bowel sounds
Pyloric obstruction	Duodenal ulcer	Weight loss Gastric upset Vomiting	Increasing dullness in LUQ Visible peristaltic waves in epigastric region

LUQ, Left upper quadrant.

BOX 17-3

SIGNS AND SYMPTOMS OF INTESTINAL OBSTRUCTION

GENERAL SIGNS

Distention
Hyperactive bowel sounds of high-pitched, tinkling character
Minimum rebound tenderness
Pain

SIGNS OF PROXIMAL OBSTRUCTION

Acute onset
Vomiting (marked)
Frequent bouts of pain
Distention (minimal)

SIGNS OF DISTAL OBSTRUCTION

Onset may be more gradual
Less marked vomiting
Less frequent bouts of pain
Distention (marked)

BOX 17-4

SIGNS AND SYMPTOMS OF PERITONEAL IRRITATION

Boardlike, increased rigidity of abdominal wall
Silent bowel sounds
Tenderness and guarding
Severe focal pain
Palpable abdominal rigidity
Positive obturator test
Positive iliopsoas test
Nausea, vomiting
Shock-diaphoresis (requires emergency attention)
Hypotension

Abdominal Pain

Tables 17-7 and 17-8 list possible pathological conditions based on descriptions of abdominal pain and its onset.

Referred Pain or Somatic Pain from Intra-abdominal Structures

Pain related to abdominal structures may be sensed in remote body surface regions (Table 17-9). The explanation for this phenomenon is that as pain is intensified, increased afferent impulses lower the client's pain threshold and excite secondary sensory neurons in the spinal cord. Thus contact may be established between afferent visceral fibers and so-

matic nerves of the same embryological dermatome. An example of this phenomenon is pain sensed in the top of the shoulder that is caused by abdominal lesions or peritonitis. The diaphragm, which is irritated in this situation, originates in the region of the fourth cervical nerve and derives its nerve supply from the third, fourth, and fifth cervical nerves. The shoulder is innervated by the fourth cervical nerve. Thus shoulder pain may be a valuable clue in diagnosing a perforated ulcer, hepatic abscess, pancreatitis, cholecystitis, a ruptured spleen, pelvic inflammation, or hemorrhage into the peritoneum. Other examples of referred pain are noted in Figure 17-45.

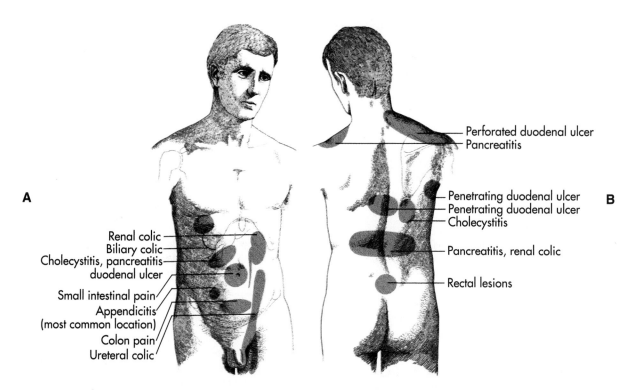

Figure 17-45   **A,** Common areas where abdominal pain is referred or perceived—anterior view. **B,** Common areas where abdominal pain is referred or perceived—posterior view. (From *GI series: physical examination of the abdomen*, Richmond, Va, 1981, Whitehall-Robins Healthcare.)

TABLE 17-7	Nature of Abdominal Pain
Description of Pain	**Possible Pathological Condition**
Burning	Ulceration (peptic)
Cramping	Biliary colic
Severe cramping (colic)	Appendicitis with fecalith
Aching	Appendiceal inflammation
Knifelike	Pancreatitis
Radiation of pain	See Figure 17-45

TABLE 17-8	Onset of Abdominal Pain
Description of Pain	**Possible Pathological Condition**
Gradual onset	Infection
Acute onset—awakening client from sleep	Duodenal ulcer
Loss of consciousness	Acute pancreatitis
	Perforated ulcer
	Ruptured ectopic pregnancy
	Intestinal obstruction (strangulated)

TABLE 17-9	Symptoms or Signs Elicited in Other Systems That May Focus the Abdominal Examination

Symptom or Sign	Possible Pathological Condition	Symptom or Sign	Possible Pathological Condition
Shock	Acute pancreatitis, ruptured tubal pregnancy	Flank tenderness	Renal inflammation, pyelonephritis
			Renal stone
Mental status deficit	Hemorrhage—duodenal ulcer		Renal infarct
	Abdominal epilepsy		Renal vein thrombosis
Hypertension	Aortic dissection	Leg edema	Iliac obstruction, pelvic mass
	Abdominal aortic aneurysm		Renal disease
	Renal infarction		Renal vein thrombosis
	Glomerulonephritis	Lymphadenopathy	Hepatitis
	Vasculitis		Lymphoma
Orthostatic hypotension	Hypovolemia—blood loss, fluid loss		Mononucleosis
		Jaundice	Liver-biliary disease
Pulse deficit	Aortic dissection		Excessive hemolysis
	Aortic aneurysm or thrombosis	Dark yellow to brown urine	Liver-biliary disease
Bruits	Aortic dissection		Blood resulting from kidney stone, infarct, glomerulonephritis, or pyelonephritis
	Aortic aneurysm		
	Dissection or aneurysm of arteries—splenic, renal, or iliac	Fever (39.4° C [103° F]) and chills	Peritonitis
Low-output cardiac symptoms—atrial fibrillation	Ischemia of mesentery		Pelvic infection
			Cholangitis
			Pyelonephritis
Valvular disease, congestive heart failure	Embolus	White blood cell count >10,000 mm³ or shift to left (more than 80% polymorphonuclear cells) >20,000 mm³	Appendicitis (95%)
			Acute cholecystitis (90%)
			Localized peritonitis
Pleural effusion	Esophageal rupture		Bowel strangulation
	Pancreatitis		Bowel infarction
	Ovarian tumor		

Sample Documentation and Diagnoses

FOCUSED HEALTH HISTORY (SUBJECTIVE DATA)

Mr. M, a 45-year-old white male, complains of severe abdominal cramping, nausea, vomiting, and diarrhea since yesterday. States he ate lunch out yesterday at a local restaurant ("some type of pasta salad and fish dish") and 4 to 5 hours later noted cramping, diarrhea, and vomiting. Has had watery, brownish stools about every hour since yesterday. No longer vomiting or crampy. Tried eating bland foods (tea and crackers) without improvement. Denies blood, pus, or mucus in stools. States is usually healthy. No chronic illnesses. Denies history of constipation, indigestion, weight changes, or change in appetite. Has not taken any medications (prescription or over-the-counter) before or after episode. No family history of liver, peptic ulcer, or kidney disease. Smokes 1½ packs/day x 15 years; drinks two to three alcoholic beverages weekly in social setting. Denies increased stress or major life changes; states family situation is good; lives with wife and two children, ages 6 and 10.

FOCUSED PHYSICAL EXAMINATION (OBJECTIVE DATA)

Vital signs: BP 122/80, pulse 88, respirations 18, temperature 37.7° C (99.9° F).
Skin: Turgor somewhat diminished.
Abdomen:
  Inspection: Flat no visible masses, pulsations, or peristalsis.
  Auscultation: Hyperactive bowel sounds in all four quadrants.
  Percussion: Tympany in all four quadrants.
  Palpation: Tenderness over epigastric area; slight tenderness in all four quadrants; no masses or organomegaly; no costovertebral angle tenderness; negative Murphy's sign, negative McBurney's sign.
  Rectal examination: Stool negative for occult blood.

DIAGNOSES

HEALTH PROBLEM

Acute gastroenteritis; rule out food poisoning

NURSING DIAGNOSES

Pain Related to Irritation of Gastric Mucosa

Defining Characteristics

- Subjective communication of pain
- Grimacing of face when abdomen palpated
- Guarding behavior of upper abdomen

Altered Nutrition: Less Than Body Requirement Related to Nausea, Vomiting, and Pain

Defining Characteristics

- Abdominal pain
- Aversion to eating at present time
- Lack of interest in food at present time
- Decreased skin turgor

Diarrhea Related to Irritation of Gastric Mucosa

Defining Characteristics

- Abdominal pain
- Cramping
- Increased frequency of bowel movements
- Increased frequency of bowel sounds

Critical Thinking Questions

Review the Sample Documentation and Diagnoses box to answer question 1.

1. What other history information would be helpful in determining the cause of the client's symptoms?
2. What signs, symptoms, and physical findings would you expect to see if this client had an appendicitis?
3. What signs, symptoms, and physical findings would you expect to see if this client had a cholecystitis?
4. How does your palpation technique differ in the client's situation from a routine abdominal examination?
5. What assessment techniques would you use in the examination of a client with suspected abdominal fluid?

Answers are available on the MERLIN website (www.harcourthealth.com/MERLIN/Barkauskas/). And be sure to check the website regularly for additional learning activities!

Remember to check out the Online Study Guide!
www.harcourthealth.com/MERLIN/Barkauskas/

Chapter 18

Musculoskeletal System

Learning Objectives

On successful study of this chapter and completion of related learning experiences, the learner will be able to:

- Describe the components of the musculoskeletal system.
- Distinguish the seven types of joint motion (flexion, extension, abduction, adduction, internal rotation, external rotation, and circumduction).
- Outline the history pertinent to the assessment of the musculoskeletal system, including exploration of common complaints.
- Explain the rationale for and demonstrate assessment of musculoskeletal structures, including use of inspection and palpation.
- Explain the rationale for and demonstrate special maneuvers used to assess for problems in specific musculoskeletal structures.

Outline

Purpose of Examination

The purpose of the musculoskeletal examination is to perform a systematic functional assessment of the musculoskeletal system as it relates to activities of daily living and detection of common dysfunctions.

The musculoskeletal system provides support for the body, protection for the internal organs, mobility to engage in physical activities, production of red blood cells, and storage of minerals. It includes bones, muscles, ligaments, tendons, cartilage, and joints. Because the central nervous system coordinates muscle and bone function, understanding how these two systems interrelate is important. The neurological examination is detailed in Chapter 19.

Musculoskeletal concerns vary at different ages. Injuries, however, are the most common musculoskeletal disorders seen in clinical practice, particularly in children and young adults. Middle-aged and older adults (and, to a lesser degree, children) are also affected by inflammatory, degenerative, and rheumatic conditions. In addition, neurological problems may also affect the musculoskeletal system. A particular symptom, such as difficulty walking, may be caused by a musculoskeletal injury or a cerebellar defect.

ANATOMY AND PHYSIOLOGY

Skeleton

The skeleton is made up of 206 bones that are shaped according to their function. Bones provide support, allowing the individual to stand erect. They protect the tissues and the internal organs (e.g., skull, rib cage, and pelvis). They assist movement in coordination with muscles and joints. Bones provide storage areas for minerals and serve as sites for the formation of red blood cells **(hematopoiesis).**

The appendicular skeleton consists of the bones of the shoulders, arms, legs, and pelvis. The axial skeleton is composed of the bones of the face, skull, auditory ossicles, hyoid bone, vertebrae, ribs, and sternum (Figures 18-1 and 18-2).

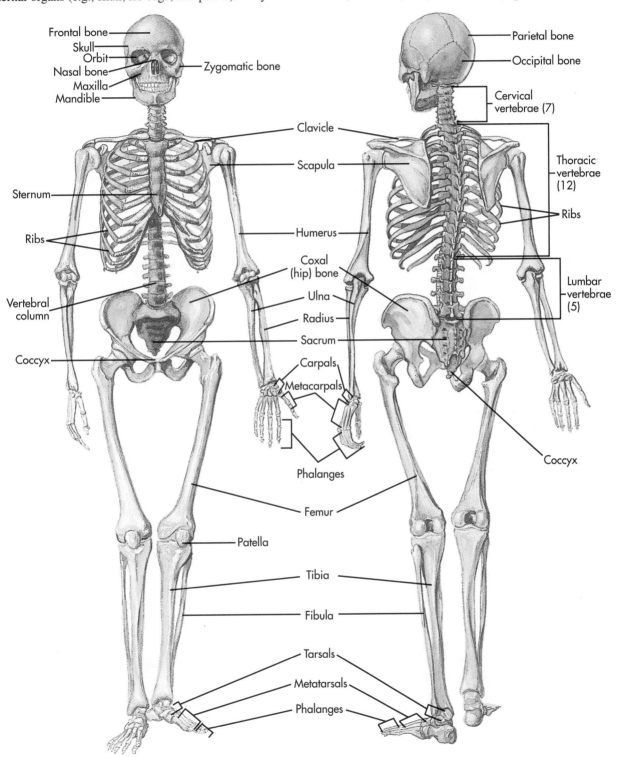

Figure 18-1   Bones that compose the skeleton. (From Thibodeau GA, Patton KT: *Anatomy and physiology,* ed. 4, St. Louis, 1999, Mosby.)

Muscles

The musculoskeletal system is composed of more than 600 voluntary, or striated, muscles (Figures 18-3 and 18-4). It constitutes the principal organ of movement and is a repository for metabolites. There are three types of muscles: visceral (smooth, involuntary); cardiac; and skeletal (striated, voluntary). This discussion concerns only skeletal muscle. Skeletal muscle mass accounts for 40% to 45% of body weight. The partial contracture of skeletal muscle makes possible all the characteristic postures of human beings, including our upright position. Muscles are attached at each end to a bone, tendon, ligament, or fascia. The fixed end of the muscle is called the origin. The more movable end is known as the muscle insertion (Figure 18-5). Muscles are normally full and supple. Aging may bring a loss of muscle fiber and an increase in connective tissue that causes loss of muscle strength. Nutrition, exercise, gender, and genetic constitution account for variations in muscle strength among individuals.

Ligaments

Ligaments are strong, dense, flexible bands of connective tissue that join bone to bone. They may add strength and stability to a joint by encircling it, as with the hip joint, or they may hold on to the joint obliquely or lie parallel to the ends of bones across the joint, as with the knee joint (Figure 18-6, *A* and *B*). Ligaments allow movement in some directions and restrict movement in other directions. They may be injured by partial tears (sprains) or they may become detached from the bones (avulsion).

Tendons

Tendons are strong, dense bands of connective tissue at the end of muscles. They attach muscles to the periosteum, the fibrous membrane that covers the bone (see Figures 18-5 and 18-6). Tendons enable bones to move when skeletal muscles contract. They are capable of transmitting great force from the contractile muscles to the bone or cartilage

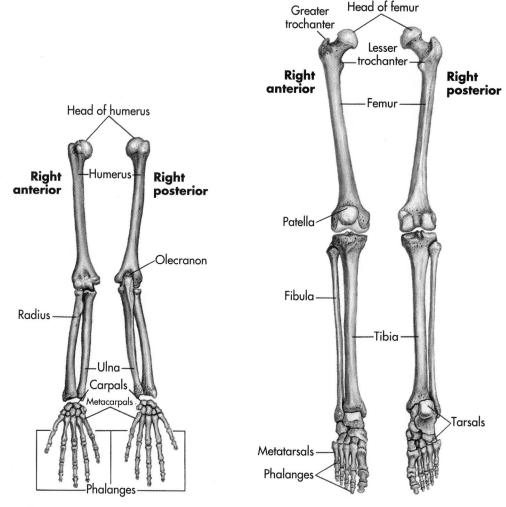

Figure 18-2   Bones of the trunk and pelvis. (From Mourad LA: *Orthopedic disorders,* St. Louis, 1991, Mosby.)

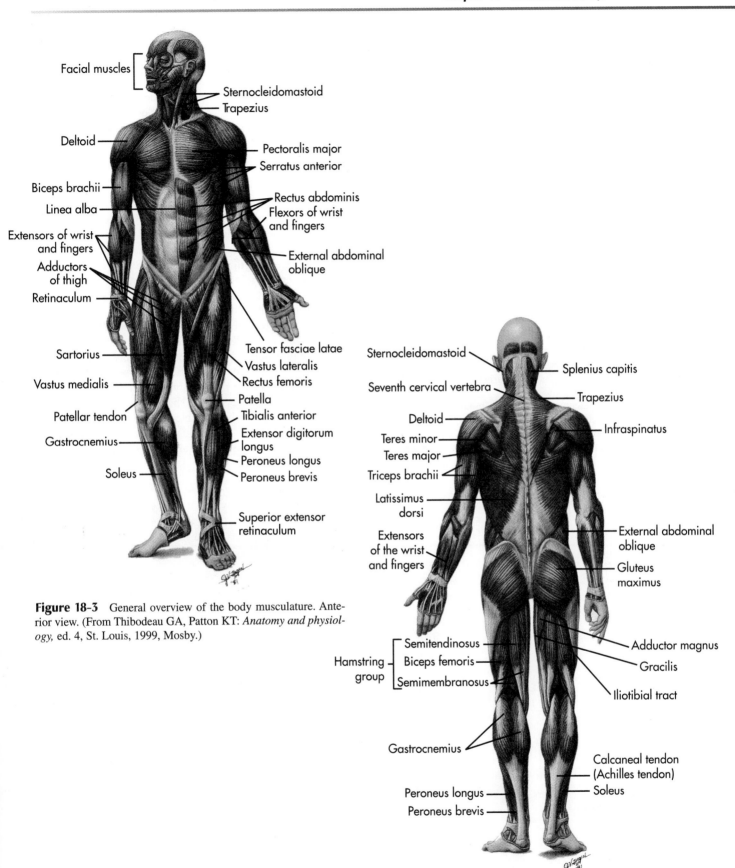

Figure 18-3 General overview of the body musculature. Anterior view. (From Thibodeau GA, Patton KT: *Anatomy and physiology,* ed. 4, St. Louis, 1999, Mosby.)

Figure 18-4 General overview of the body musculature. Posterior view. (From Thibodeau GA, Patton KT: *Anatomy and physiology,* ed. 4, St. Louis, 1999, Mosby.)

without being injured themselves. Most tendons are small (2 to 3 cm in length). The Achilles tendon is the longest and largest in the body (10 to 14 cm long).

Cartilage

Cartilage is a semismooth layer of elastic, gel-like supporting tissue found at the ends of bones. It forms a cap over the

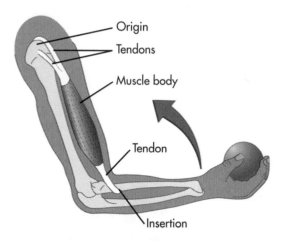

Figure 18-5 Attachments of a skeletal muscle. A muscle originates at a relatively stable part of the skeleton (origin) and inserts at the skeletal part that is moved when the muscle contracts (insertion). (From Thibodeau GA, Patton KT: *Anatomy and physiology,* ed. 4, St. Louis, 1999, Mosby.)

ends of bones to protect and support the bone during weight-bearing activities. The outer layer of cartilage is avascular and receives its nourishment from synovial fluids forced into it during movement and weight-bearing activity. Cartilage must have weight-bearing activity and joint movement to remain healthy. It may fray or wear unevenly if joints are abnormally shaped or unstable.

Joints

Joints are locations where two surfaces of bone come together or where two bones are joined to each other. There are three types of joints, classified by their degree of movement and the material that separates them. Synarthrotic joints are immovable. This type of joint separates bones with a thin layer of cartilage. An example is the cranial suture. Amphiarthrotic joints are slightly movable and separate bones with cartilage, such as the symphysis pubis or the manubriosternal joint, or with a fibrocartilaginous disk, such as the joints between the vertebral bodies (Figure 18-7). These are "gliding" joints. Diarthrotic joints, which are commonly called synovial joints, are freely movable. They are lined with a synovial membrane that secretes a lubricating synovial fluid. Synovial (or diarthrotic) joints include the ankle, wrist, knee, hip, or shoulder joints (Figure 18-8). Most joints are freely movable, or synovial, joints. These joints are supported by a casing that surrounds them, called the joint capsule. Ligaments also add strength by encasing the capsule.

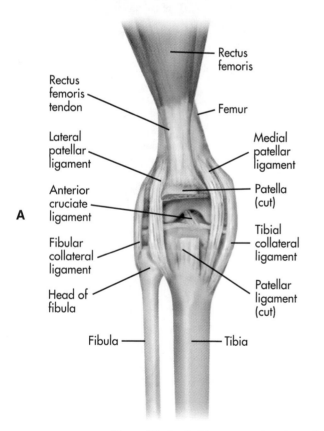

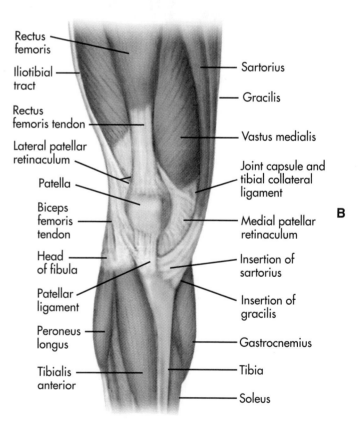

Figure 18-6 **A,** Ligaments and tendons of the knee joint. **B,** Muscles attaching at the knee. (From Seidel HM et al.: *Mosby's guide to physical examination,* ed. 4, St. Louis, 1999, Mosby.)

Range of Motion

The degree of movement of a joint is called its range of motion. Diarthrotic, or freely movable, joints are the only joints that have one or more ranges of motion (Figure 18-9). Seven types of joint motion have been defined as follows:

Flexion—The bending forward of the joint to decrease the angle between the bones that it connects.

Extension—The straightening of a limb to increase the joint angle.

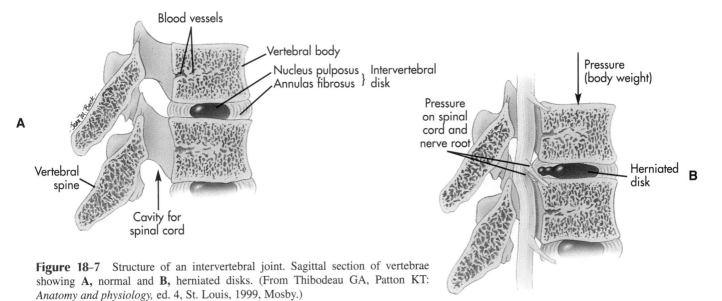

Figure 18-7 Structure of an intervertebral joint. Sagittal section of vertebrae showing **A,** normal and **B,** herniated disks. (From Thibodeau GA, Patton KT: *Anatomy and physiology,* ed. 4, St. Louis, 1999, Mosby.)

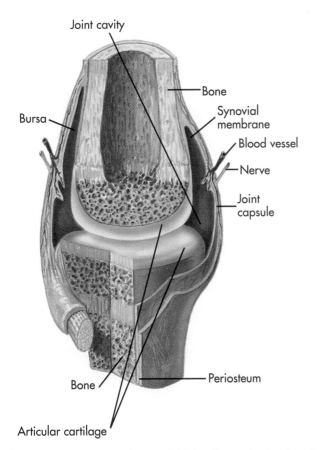

Figure 18-8 Structure of a synovial joint. Composite drawing of a typical synovial joint. (From Thibodeau GA, Patton KT: *Anatomy and physiology,* ed. 4, St. Louis, 1999, Mosby.)

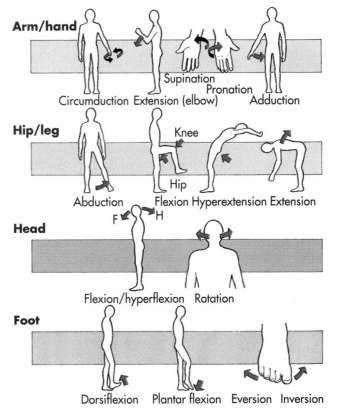

Figure 18-9 Body movements provided by synovial (diarthrotic) joints. (From Mourad LA: *Orthopedic disorders,* St. Louis, 1991, Mosby.)

Abduction—The movement of a limb away from the midline of the body.

Adduction—The movement of a limb toward the central axis of the body or beyond it.

Internal rotation—The turning of the body part inward toward the central axis of the body.

External rotation—The turning of the body part away from the midline.

Circumduction—The movement of a body part in a circular pattern. It is not a singular motion but a combination of motions.

Muscles are categorized according to the type of joint movement produced by their contraction. Therefore, they are called flexors, extensors, adductors, abductors, internal rotators, external rotators, or circumflexors (the example shown in Figure 18-5 is a flexor muscle). Muscles shorten on contraction and in so doing exert pull on the bones to which they are attached. This action moves bones closer together. Most muscles attach to two bones that articulate at an intervening joint. Generally, one bone moves while the other is held stable. This effect is caused by simultaneous shortening of other muscles. The body of the muscle that produces movement of an extremity generally lies proximal to the bone that is moved.

EXAMINATION

Focused Health History

The health history for the musculoskeletal system includes information about the client's current concerns, general health, and specific lifestyle factors that may affect his or her physical condition. Lifestyle factors include information about employment, activity level, and any recent or past injuries. Common complaints include pain, loss of mobility, deformity, swelling, inflammation, and weakness. The client's chief complaint may indicate the direction for emphasis in the physical assessment. The individual with a chief complaint of body deformity, paralysis, weakness, or pain associated with movement prompts the examiner to focus attention on the bones, joints, and muscles as the possible sites of disorder. The client's age is also important to note since many conditions occur within specific age ranges. For example, osteoporosis and osteoarthritis are more likely seen in older individuals, whereas Osgood-Schlatter disease occurs in children and adolescents.

Present Health/Illness Status

1. Usual condition of musculoskeletal system
2. Current and previous employment: risk of accidental injury, lifting, repetitive motion activities, safety precautions
3. Activities of daily living: ability to perform personal care (bathing, dressing, grooming, eating, elimination), household tasks, walking, shopping, communication
4. Exercise: walking, specific regimen of exercise or sports activity (type, frequency, duration, special equipment, safety measures), overall conditioning

5. Weight: recent changes, overweight or underweight
6. Height: maximum height attained, any changes
7. Nutrition: intake of calcium and vitamin D, calories, and protein
8. Cigarette smoking (number of packs/day for number of years)
9. Alcohol intake
10. Medications: calcium supplements, nonsteroidal anti-inflammatory agents, muscle relaxants, hormone replacement therapy, steroids

Past Health History

1. Previous occurrences of the problem(s), their duration and resolution
2. Past history of trauma to bones, joints, nerves, or soft tissue; residual problems; infections
3. Orthopedic surgery
4. Congenital deformities
5. Chronic illnesses: arthritis, osteoporosis, cancer, renal or neurological problems

Family History

1. Arthritis: osteoarthritis, rheumatoid arthritis, gout, ankylosing spondylitis
2. Congenital hip or foot disorders
3. Scoliosis or back problems
4. Osteoporosis

Risk Factors
Osteoarthritis

Age over 50
Family history of osteoarthritis
Obesity
Joint abnormality
History of trauma, rheumatoid arthritis, or other degenerative
   process

Risk Factors
Osteoporosis

Advanced age
Gender (female)
Family history of osteoporosis
Estrogen deficiency caused by menopause, surgical removal of
   the ovaries, or anorexia accompanied by amenorrhea
Small stature
Race (white)
Northern European descent
Heavy cigarette and/or alcohol use
Poor diet with low calcium intake
Periods of immobilization
Use of steroids
Sedentary lifestyle

Cultural Considerations
Differences in Musculoskeletal Characteristics

Differences in musculoskeletal characteristics have been noted between different races, between genders, and even in specific ethnic groups. Awareness of such differences may help the provider identify individuals who are at greater risk for specific health concerns. Following is a compilation of findings related to biocultural variations in the musculoskeletal system and their clinical significance.

COMPONENT	REMARKS
Bone	
Frontal	Thicker in African-American than in white males
Parietal occiput	Thicker in Caucasian than in African-American males
Palate	Tori (protuberances) along the suture line of the hard palate
	Problematic for denture wearers
	Incidence:
	African-Americans — 20%
	Caucasians — 24%
	Asians — Up to 50%
	Native-Americans — Up to 50%
Mandible	Tori (protuberances) on the lingual surface of the mandible near the canine and premolar teeth
	Problematic for denture wearers
	Most common in Asians and Native Americans; exceeds 50% in some Eskimo groups
Humerus	Torsion or rotation of proximal end with muscle pull
	Caucasians > African Americans
	Torsion in African-Americans is symmetrical torsion in Caucasians tends to be greater on right than left side
Radius	Length at the wrist variable
Ulna	Ulna or radius may be longer
	Equal length
	Swedes — 61%
	Chinese — 16%
	Ulna longer than radius
	Swedes — 16%
	Chinese — 48%
	Radius longer than ulna
	Swedes — 23%
	Chinese — 10%
Vertebrae	Twenty-four vertebrae are found in 85% to 93% of all people; racial and sex differences reveal 23 or 25 vertebrae in select groups
	Vertebrae — Population
	23 — 11% of African-American females
	25 — 12% of Eskimo and Native American males
	Related to lower back pain and lordosis

COMPONENT	REMARKS
Pelvis	Hip width is 1.6 cm (0.6 in) smaller in African-American than in Caucasian women; Asian women have significantly smaller pelvises
Femur	Convex anterior — Native American
	Straight — African-American
	Intermediate — Caucasian
Second tarsal	Second toe longer than the great toe
	Incidence:
	Caucasians — 8%–34%
	African Americans — 8%–12%
	Vietnamese — 31%
	Melanesians — 21%–57%
	Clinical significance for joggers and athletes
Height	Caucasian males are 1.27 cm (0.5 in) taller than African-American males and 7.6 cm (2.9 in) taller than Asian males
	Caucasian females = African-American females
	Asian females are 4.14 cm (1.6 in) shorter than Caucasian or African-American females
Composition of long bones	Longer, narrower, and denser in African-Americans than in Caucasians; bone density in whites > Chinese, Japanese, and Eskimos
	Osteoporosis lowest in African-American males; highest in Caucasian females
Muscle	
Peroneus tertius	Responsible for dorsiflexion of foot
	Muscle absent:
	Asians, Native Americans, and Caucasians — 3%–10%
	African-Americans — 10%–15%
	Berbers (Sahara desert) — 24%
	No clinical significance because the tibialis anterior also dorsiflexes the foot
Palmaris longus	Responsible for wrist flexion
	Muscle absent:
	Caucasians — 12%–20%
	Native Americans — 2%–12%
	African-Americans — 5%
	Asians — 3%
	No clinical significance because three other muscles are also responsible for flexion

Based on data reported by Overfield T: *Biologic variation in health and illness: race, age, and sex differences,* New York, 1995, CRC Press. From Andrews MM, Boyle JS: *Transcultural concepts in nursing care,* ed. 3, Philadelphia, 2000, JB Lippincott.

Personal and Social History

1. Significant others: who is in the home, current support system, who can assist if needed
2. Usual activities: work, school, day care; hobbies
3. Recent life changes (positive and negative): stresses, losses, anniversaries of losses, financial difficulties
4. Cultural practices, folk remedies (e.g., ointments, liniments)

Pain Assessment

Pain is the symptom that most commonly causes the client to seek help for musculoskeletal problems. In the assessment of musculoskeletal pain, gathering particular information from the symptom analysis format can provide a clearer picture of the cause of the pain (see Chapter 3).

1. **Onset:** The nature of the onset of pain may suggest the cause of the problem. For example, rheumatoid symptoms begin gradually, whereas gout-related attacks are characterized by sudden onset that frequently awakens the client from sleep.
2. **Course since onset**
   a. **Precipitating events:** The client should be encouraged to try to recall those events that occurred *before* the onset of pain. Most individuals tend to forget minor injuries or unusual physical activity in the weeks before the pain began. For example, the client is unlikely to associate shoulder pain with recent home repair activities such as painting a large ceiling or to correlate symptoms and signs of infection in the preceding months with current joint pain.
   b. **Timing:** The time that pain occurs may also be diagnostic. The individual with osteoarthritis generally reports that the pain is worsened by increased use of the affected joint; therefore the affected person frequently has pain later in the day or when tired. The individual with rheumatoid arthritis generally reports that stiffness and pain occur early in the morning and notes some improvement after exercising the part.
3. **Location:** Note where the client feels pain as specifically as possible. A client frequently has difficulty in localizing the pain associated with joint disease. The client's description may involve large areas of the body (e.g., "my neck" [while moving the hand from the head to the thoracic vertebra], "my back," or "all down my arm"). This difficulty in localizing the pain may be related to whether the pain is deep or superficial and whether a nerve is involved. Trigger points—localized areas of hyperirritability that are tender when compressed—are helpful for diagnosis. When pressure is placed on a trigger point, it reproduces the client's symptoms.

   Describing the distribution of the pain will provide valuable information. Rheumatoid involvement is migratory (i.e., involving first one joint, which improves, then another). However, most infectious arthritis is confined to one joint. The joint involvement in rheumatoid arthritis tends to be symmetrical, whereas that of gout, psoriatic arthritis, and Reiter's syndrome tends to occur initially in one or two joints but becomes polyarticular in the later stages. Spondylitis is first detected in the spine and then spreads to peripheral joints (centrifugal spread), whereas rheumatoid arthritis starts peripherally in the hands and feet and then involves the large joints of the hips, shoulders, and spine in the later stages of the disease (centripetal spread).
   a. **Referred pain:** Ask the client to describe any referred pain. Individuals frequently feel spinal nerve root involvement in peripheral tissues. For instance, the client may experience lumbosacral nerve root irritation (sciatica) as pain in the thigh or the knee on the involved side. The area of referred pain corresponds with the segmental innervation of the structures by the dermatomes (see Figure 19-6).
4. **Quality:** Understanding the character of the pain may be helpful in determining its cause and in guiding the physical assessment of the involved joints. The quality of pain also differs according to the area affected. Nerve pain tends to be sharp and burning; vascular pain tends to be diffuse and aching; bone pain tends to be very localized, deep, and boring; muscle pain is dull, aching, and hard to localize (Magee, 1997). Dermatomal pain may be described with words associated with paresthesias, such as "prickling," "like an electric shock," "pins and needles," and "numbing." The client may describe pain of muscle origin as "pulled" or "charley horse." Joint pain descriptions may range along a spectrum from dull, aching, or stiff to excruciating and intolerable.
5. **Quantity:** Determine how much pain the client is experiencing. Use of a pain scale can help in determining the severity of the pain. This could be as simple as asking the client to rate the pain on a scale of 0 (no pain) to 10 (worst pain), or an actual pain measurement tool (see Figure 19-44) could be used. Be consistent in the method used so that the progression of the pain can be accurately monitored over time.
6. **Alleviating and aggravating factors:** Measures that alleviate or aggravate the pain can assist in your differential diagnosis of musculoskeletal pain. This information can be helpful in the differential diagnosis. Pain that decreases with rest usually suggests a mechanical problem that interferes with movement. Morning pain and stiffness that improve with activity suggest inflammation. For example, exercise alleviates pain in rheumatoid arthritis but worsens it in osteoarthritis. Conversely, rest alleviates pain in osteoarthritis but leads to stiffness and pain in rheumatoid arthritis.

> ■ HELPFUL HINT
>
> When evaluating the musculoskeletal system, it is helpful to consider joint, skeletal, and muscular problems and injuries separately.

Symptom Analysis

Joint Problems

1. **Onset:** specific date of first episode (or age when it occurred), sudden or gradual
2. **Course since onset:**
   Frequency: constant, episodic, periodic, occasional, change in pattern, similar episodes in the past
   Duration: length of episode, increasing or decreasing
   Timing: relationship of symptoms to specific events, time of day, or other symptoms
3. **Location:** which joint(s) affected
4. **Quality:** sharp, burning, aching, tearing, stiffness or limitation of movement, redness, increased warmth or swelling, locking, twinges, instability, or "giving way"
5. **Quantity:** number of joints involved, amount of pain (use pain scale)
6. **Setting:** occurring with certain activities (e.g., movements, sporting event, walking); at certain time of day; at work, home, recreational area
7. **Associated phenomena:** fever, weight loss, fatigue, malaise, rash, chronic diarrhea
8. **Alleviating and aggravating factors:** rest, specific movement, elevation, medications (e.g., diuretics), ice, heat, prolonged activity, injury, weather, specific foods, alcohol intake
9. **Underlying concern:** arthritis

Skeletal Problems

1. **Onset:** specific date of first episode (or age when it occurred), sudden or gradual
2. **Course since onset:**
   Frequency: change in pattern, similar episodes in the past
   Duration: length of episode, increasing or decreasing
   Timing: relationship of symptoms to specific events, time of day, or other symptoms
3. **Location:** which bone(s) affected, any radiation of pain (e.g., back pain with pain shooting down the leg)
4. **Quality:** pain associated with particular movement or weight bearing; localized tenderness, swelling, crepitus, limping, numbness, tingling or pressure; deformity or change in skeletal contour
5. **Quantity:** amount of pain (use pain scale)
6. **Setting:** occurred during sporting event, walking, at work, lifting, etc.
7. **Associated phenomena:** fever, weight loss, fatigue, malaise, past history of cancer, circulatory problems, numbness, tingling

8. **Alleviating and aggravating factors:** rest, movement (e.g., sudden or repetitive), elevation, medications, ice, heat, injury, stress, prolonged activity
9. **Underlying concern:** long-term disability or work limitations

Muscular Problems

1. **Onset:** specific date of first episode (or age when it occurred), sudden or gradual
2. **Course since onset:**
   Frequency: change in pattern, similar episodes in the past
   Duration: length of episode, increasing or decreasing
   Timing: relationship of symptoms to specific events, time of day, or other symptoms
3. **Location:** which muscle(s) affected, with specific movement (e.g., flexion, extension, etc.) or activity
4. **Quality:** localized or generalized pain, weakness, limitation of movement, paralysis, spasms, wasting, tremor, cramping, dull, aching
5. **Quantity:** amount of pain (use pain scale)
6. **Setting:** occurred during sport activity, walking, at work, etc.
7. **Associated phenomena:** fever, malaise
8. **Alleviating and aggravating factors:** rest, movement (e.g., sudden or repetitive), elevation, medications, ice, heat, injury, muscle contraction, stress, exercise
9. **Underlying concern:** long-term disability or work or athletic limitations

Musculoskeletal Injury

1. **Onset:** specific date of first episode (or age when it occurred); mechanism of injury: what happened—fall, direct trauma, overstretching, overuse; direction and magnitude of injuring force and how force was applied
2. **Course since onset:**
   Frequency: change in pattern, similar episodes in the past
   Duration: length of episode, increasing or decreasing
   Timing: relationship of symptoms to injury or specific events, time of day, or other symptoms
3. **Location:** specific areas affected
4. **Quality:** any noise with injury (popping, click, tearing); numbness; tingling; loss of sensation, strength, or mobility; warmth or coldness; swelling (immediate or gradual)
5. **Quantity:** amount of pain (use pain scale)
6. **Setting:** occurred during sporting event, walking, at work, etc.
7. **Associated phenomena:** loss of consciousness, other injuries
8. **Alleviating and aggravating factors:** rest, position of comfort, sudden or repetitive movement, stress, medications, heat and/or ice, exercise, home remedies
9. **Underlying concern:** limitation of functioning, long-term consequences

Preparation for Examination: Client and Environment

Thorough assessment of the musculoskeletal system requires appropriate exposure of the client. Have the ambulatory individual wear shorts or underwear, which will allow the extremities and the spine to be available for examination. Allow the female client to wear a bra or some other abbreviated form of chest cover. Make an effort to protect the client's sense of modesty, but recognize that you cannot accurately examine a fully clothed client.

For each examination, position the client in a way that allows for the greatest stabilization of the joints.

Technique for Examination and Expected Findings

The examination of neuromuscular coordination begins when you first meet and observe the client. Note normal body alignment and any obvious deformity. The examination continues as the client advances into the room, sits, rises from a sitting position, climbs onto the examining table, lies down, and rolls over. Note the client's speed, coordination, and strength of motion. In particular, note any clumsy, awkward, or involuntary movements and tremor or fasciculation. Assess the client's handshake to gain an estimate of muscle strength. Note the client's facial expression. Does he or she appear uncomfortable, apprehensive, deprived of sleep?

Explore musculoskeletal structure and function through inspection and palpation of the joints and muscles, assessment of active and passive ranges of motion, and tests for muscle strength.

Use the cephalocaudal (head-to-toe) organization for examination of the bones, joints, and muscles. This organization provides order and helps avoid omissions. Use side-to-side comparison of body parts as the basic criterion for

assessment. When injury or discomfort is involved, examine the unaffected side first.

The following discussion is organized differently from that in other chapters due to the nature of the musculoskeletal examination. First, general examination techniques for the musculoskeletal system are discussed, then components of the screening musculoskeletal examination are presented, followed by examination techniques for specific joints and muscles.

Inspection

General inspection of the musculoskeletal system includes a visual scanning for symmetry, contour, size, involuntary movement of the two sides of the body (tremors or fasciculations), gross deformities, areas of swelling or edema, and ecchymoses or other discoloration (Figure 18-10). Inspect the muscles for symmetry of size and contour. Measure asymmetry, noted as hypertrophy or atrophy, for verification.

Examine the posture, or stance, and body alignment from both in front of and behind the client. Note the structural relationships of the feet to the legs and the hips to the pelvis. For the upper extremities, compare the shoulder girdle and the upper trunk. Are the bony contours of the body symmetrical or is there an obvious deformity.

A deformity is an abnormality in appearance. **Varus** and **valgus** are terms used to describe an angular deviation from the normal structure of an extremity. The reference point is the midline of the body. In a varus deformity such as genu varum (bowleg) the angulation is away from the midline and the distal portion of the bone is displaced toward the midline (Figure 18-11). In a valgus deformity such as genu valgum (knock-knee) the angulation is toward the midline and the distal portion of the bone is displaced away from the midline (Figure 18-12). The name of the deformity is based on the joint involved.

Palpation

Palpate all joints, bones, and associated muscles. Palpate joints for the presence of tenderness, swelling, increased temperature, and crepitation. Gently palpate painful and tender joints, and always examine the pain-free side first. Pal-

---

Preparation for Examination

EQUIPMENT

Item	Purpose
Nonstretchable tape measure	To measure length of extremities and limb circumference
Goniometer	To measure joint range of motion

CLIENT AND ENVIRONMENT
1. Provide a warm room with adequate lighting.
2. Protect the client's sense of modesty while exposing as fully as possible the areas to be examined.
3. Explain each procedure before beginning to perform it.
4. Use short, clear instructions.
5. Arrange for extra examination time for older or debilitated clients.
6. Stabilize the joints by having the client sit or lie down.
7. Properly sequence the examination to minimize position changes from sitting to lying.
8. If there is pain, always examine the unaffected side first.

HELPFUL HINT

When palpating, note:
- Differences in tissue tension and thickness
- Abnormalities
- Temperature variation
- Pulses, tremors, fasciculations
- Dryness or excessive moisture
- Abnormal sensation
- Tenderness

Tenderness can be graded on a scale of I to IV:
I: Patient complains of pain
II: Patient complains of pain and winces
III: Patient winces and withdraws the joint
IV: Patient will not allow palpation of the joint

Data from Magee DJ: *Orthopedic physical assessment*, ed. 3, Philadelphia, 1997, WB Saunders.

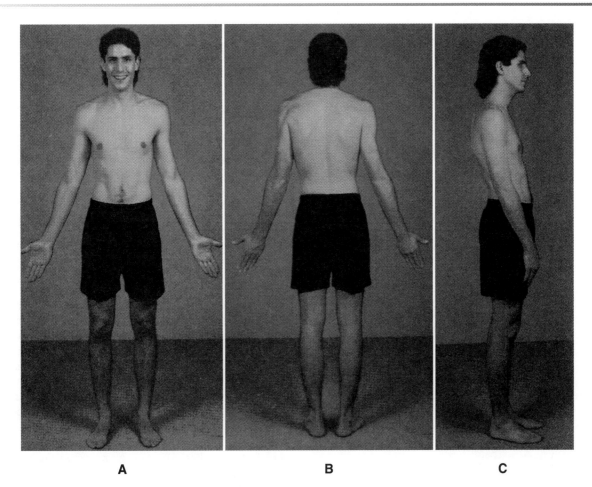

A   **B**   **C**

Figure 18-10   Inspection of overall body posture for symmetry of contour and size, gross deformities, swelling, and alignment of extremities. **A,** Anterior view. **B,** Posterior view. **C,** Lateral view.

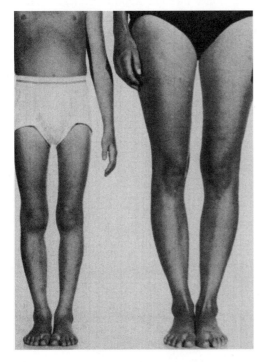

Figure 18-11   Varus deformity of the leg: bilateral genu varum (bowleg) in mother and son. (From Tachdijan MO: *Atlas of pediatric orthopedic surgery,* Philadelphia, 1994, WB Saunders.)

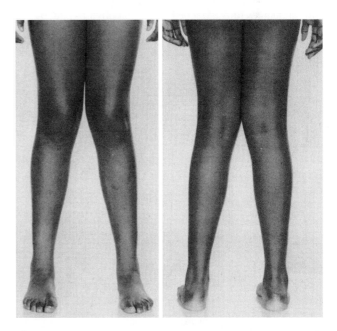

Figure 18-12   Valgus deformity of the leg: bilateral genu valgum (knock-knee) in an adolescent. (From Tachdijan MO: *Atlas of pediatric orthopedic surgery,* Philadelphia, 1994, WB Saunders.)

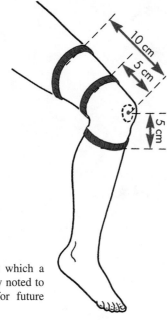

Figure 18-13 The sites at which a limb is measured are carefully noted to establish accurate location for future comparative measurements.

TABLE 18-1	**Anatomical Guideposts for Measuring Extremities**	
Area	From	To
Entire upper extremity	Tip of acromion process	Tip of middle finger
Upper arm	Tip of acromion process	Tip of olecranon process
Forearm	Tip of olecranon process	Styloid process of ulna
Entire lower extremity	Lower edge of antero-superior iliac spine	Tibial malleolus
Thigh	Lower edge of antero-superior iliac spine	Medial aspect of knee joint
Lower leg	Medial aspect of knee	Tibial malleolus

pate muscles to detect swelling, localized temperature changes, tone, and marked changes in shape. Note the consistency or tone of the muscle on palpation.

Measurement of Extremities

The musculoskeletal examination commonly includes measurement of the extremities for length and circumference. Take length measurements to verify the symmetry of two limbs or to determine whether the limbs are in the normal range. Take measurements with the client lying relaxed on a hard surface (examining table) with the pelvis level and the hips and knees fully extended and with both hips equally adducted. Apparent discrepancies in limb size are commonly a result of position.

The length of the upper extremity is the distance from the tip of the acromion process to the tip of the middle finger; the shoulder is adducted, and the other joints are at neutral zero (anatomical position: limb in extension). The length of the lower extremity is the distance from the lower edge of the anterosuperior iliac spine to the tibial malleolus (Table 18-1).

Measurement of Muscle Mass

Examine the muscles for gross hypertrophy or atrophy. Only in the markedly obese client are changes in muscle mass difficult to assess. The difference between the firm, hypertrophic muscle of the athlete and the limp, atrophic muscle of the paralytic is obvious both on inspection and on palpation. Although muscle size is largely a function of use or disuse of the muscle fibers, changes in the size of muscles may indicate disease. Malnutrition and lipodystrophy tend to reduce muscle size and markedly weaken the strength of contraction. Lack of neural input resulting from lesions of the spinal cord or the peripheral motor neuron may reduce muscle size by as much as 75% of the normal volume. Such a

decrease may occur over as short a time as 3 months. Measuring limbs at their maximal circumference may provide a baseline for comparison when swelling or atrophy is suspected on subsequent routine examinations.

Make sure that the limbs are in the same position and the muscles are in the same state of tension each time you take measurements. Several corresponding points may be measured above and below the patella and the olecranon process. To provide uniformity, some clinics routinely measure at 10 cm below and at points 10 and 20 cm above the middle patella. Regardless of the points you select, draw a small diagram showing the points measured to ensure consistency in future measures (Figure 18-13). Differences in symmetry or variations in limb size of less than 1 cm, noted at different times, are not significant (Figure 18-14). The dominant side is usually slightly larger than the nondominant side.

Measurement of Range of Joint Motion

A standardized method for measuring and recording joint motion has been published by the American Academy of Orthopaedic Surgeons (1965). This method describes the range of motion in degrees of deviation from a defined neutral zero point for each joint. The position of neutral zero is that of the extended extremity or the anatomical position.

Goniometry and arthrometry are terms that describe the measurement of joint motion. It is important to learn to use the **goniometer** to measure the range of motion and to communicate findings to other health team professionals.

The two arms of the goniometer are a protractor and a pointer that are joined at the zero point of the protractor (Figure 18-15). The hinge should provide sufficient friction so that the instrument remains in position when you pick it up to read it after placing it against the joint. You should be able to read the scale easily from a distance of 18 inches. Some goniometers have full-circle scales, whereas others have half-circle scales. For the sake of portability, the length of the arms is generally about 6 inches.

When you describe range of motion, differentiate whether it is active or passive motion. **Active range of mo-**

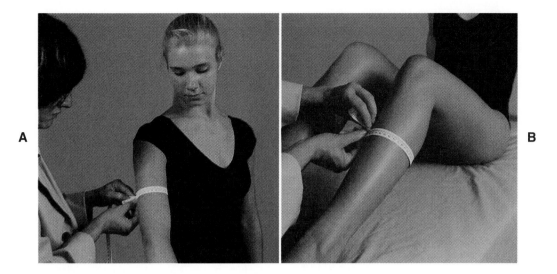

Figure 18-14 **A,** Measurement of upper midarm circumference. **B,** Measurement of midgastrocnemius circumference.

tion is when the client moves the joint. **Passive range of motion** is when you move the joint for the client. You should observe the client first in active motion and then, with the client relaxed, put the joints through passive range of motion. Measure any increase or limitation in range of motion with the goniometer. The normal ranges for active and passive motion should be the same.

Active Motion. Ask the client to move the joint through its full range. In normal (or full) active range of motion, joint movement is smooth and painless through its complete range and generally indicates the absence of any advanced lesion. Voluntary movement of the joints through their range of motion causes less muscle tension and joint compression than when the joints are moved against resistance, as in the strength tests. Therefore, assess active range of motion before testing muscle strength.

Passive Motion. Stabilize the client's joint with one hand while your other hand slowly moves the relaxed joint through the full range of its movement. When the range of motion is limited, examine further to determine whether (1) excess fluid is within the joint; (2) loose bodies, such as pieces of cartilage, are present in the joint; or (3) joint surface irregularity or contracture of the muscle, ligaments, or capsule exists. Moving the joint through the range of its motion may also reveal hypermobility of the joint. In such a situation, further examination should be directed toward differentiating among (1) a connective tissue disruption, such as the relaxation of the ligaments that occurs in Marfan's syndrome; (2) a ligamentous tear; and (3) an intra-articular fracture. An example of how this information might aid in diagnosis is when a joint can be flexed to a smaller angle with passive movement than with active flexion. Such a finding suggests a muscle problem rather than a problem within the joint.

Recording Range of Motion. Box 18-1 summarizes joint movements and the maximal expected angles of movement. Record limited joint movement from the angle of the

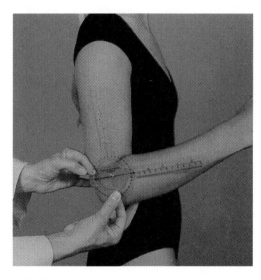

Figure 18-15 Use of a goniometer to measure range of motion of a joint.

starting position to the maximal angle reached during movement (e.g., from 20 to 50 degrees).

Screening Examination

The purpose of the screening musculoskeletal examination is to determine whether there is ease of function or functional impairment of the musculoskeletal system. This should be a part of the routine physical examination and need take only a few minutes.

The screening examination should include inspection, palpation, passive and active range of motion, muscle strength, and integrated function. This examination can be integrated into the regional examination. For example, assessing range of motion of the cervical spine is usually part of the head and neck examination. Box 18-2 describes com-

BOX 18-1

RECORDING RANGE OF MOTION IN DEGREES

CERVICAL SPINE

Flexion	45
Extension	50
Rotation (right)	70
Rotation (left)	70
Lateral bending (right)	40
Lateral bending (left)	40

SPINE

Forward flexion (C7 to S1 = 4 in)	70
Extension (standing)	30
Extension (lying)	20
Rotation (right)	45
Rotation (left)	45
Lateral bending (right)	35
Lateral bending (left)	35

SHOULDER

Forward flexion	180
Backward extension	60
Horizontal flexion	130-135
Horizontal extension	40
Abduction	180
Adduction	50
Internal rotation	90
External rotation	90

ELBOW

Flexion-extension	150
Hyperextension	0-15

FOREARM (ELBOW AND WRIST)

Pronation	80-90
Supination	80-90

WRIST

Extension	80
Flexion	70
Radial deviation	20
Ulnar deviation	30

THUMB

Abduction	50
Flexion—interphalangeal joint	80
Flexion—metacarpophalangeal joint	50
Flexion—carpometacarpal joint	15
Opposition to tip or base of little finger	

FINGERS

Flexion—distal interphalangeal joint	90
Flexion—proximal interphalangeal joint	100
Flexion—metacarpophalangeal joint	90
Extension—metacarpophalangeal joint	45
Hyperextension—distal interphalangeal joint	10
Abduction (measure from tips of fingers)	Varies
Adduction	Varies

HIP

Flexion (knees bent)	110-120
Extension	30
Abduction	45
Adduction	30
Internal rotation (hip and knee flexed)	40
External rotation (hip and knee flexed)	45

KNEE

Flexion-extension	135
Hyperextension	10

ANKLE

Dorsiflexion	20
Plantar flexion	50
Inversion hind foot (passive)	5
Eversion hind foot (passive)	5
Inversion	30
Eversion	20
Abduction forefoot (passive)	10
Adduction forefoot (passive)	20

GREAT TOE

Flexion—metatarsophalangeal joint	45
Extension—metatarsophalangeal joint	70
Flexion—interphalangeal joint (passive)	90

LATERAL FOUR TOES

Flexion—distal interphalangeal joint	60
Extension—distal interphalangeal joint	30
Flexion—proximal interphalangeal joint	35
Flexion—metatarsophalangeal joint	40
Extension—metatarsophalangeal joint	40
Abduction	Varies
Adduction	Varies

ponents of a screening musculoskeletal examination for sports participation for children and adolescents. It is presented in more detail in Table 26-19.

In the screening examination, assess joints through their active ranges of motion and describe the results as full range of motion. In joints that do not exhibit full range of motion, measure with the goniometer and record the results. Expect limitations in full range of motion in older individuals. If you note an abnormality or if the client has specific symptoms related to a specific bone, joint, or muscle group, then a more detailed examination of that area is required. General guidelines for the examination of bones, joints, and muscles are presented in the next section, followed by techniques for the examination of specific joints and muscles.

BOX 18-2

SCREENING MUSCULOSKELETAL EXAMINATION FOR CHILD AND ADOLESCENT SPORTS PARTICIPATION

- Observe posture and general muscle contour bilaterally
- Observe gait
- Ask patient to walk on tiptoes and heels
- Observe patient hop on each foot
- Ask patient to duck walk four steps with knees completely bent
- Inspect spine for curvature and lumbar extension, fingers touching toes with knees straight
- Palpate shoulder and clavicle for dislocation
- Check the following joints for range of motion: neck, shoulder, elbow, forearm, hands, fingers, and hips
- Test knee ligaments for drawer sign

From Seidel HM et al.: *Mosby's guide to physical examination,* ed. 4, St. Louis, 1999, Mosby.

Examination of Bones, Joints, and Muscles

Bones. Examine bones for deformities and tumors. Also examine bones for integrity by testing resistance to a deforming force. Palpate the bone to assess the presence of pain or tenderness. Tenderness of a bone may indicate tumor, inflammation, or the aftermath of trauma. Commonly, traumatic injuries are associated with damage to both bone and nerve. For example, paralysis of the ulnar and median nerves in the hand is often the result of a hand injury and may produce a clawlike posture of the hand.

Joints

Inspection and Palpation. Either make a systematic assessment of individual joints during the performance of the head-to-toe physical examination or examine all the joints at a preselected time during the examination. As with all bilateral structures, compare the paired joints, examining the unaffected side first.

The sequence for performing the examination of the joints is inspection, palpation, active range of motion, passive range of motion, and muscle strength testing. Use this sequence in a coordinated examination of each joint.

Begin the assessment with inspection of the joint for swelling, redness, deformity, subcutaneous nodules, or tumors. Let the presence of any observed abnormalities guide you in palpation. Palpate joints for the presence of pain with movement, tenderness, swelling, increased temperature, and crepitation. Palpate painful and tender joints lightly.

Give special consideration to the temporomandibular, sternoclavicular, manubriosternal, shoulder, elbow, wrist, hip, knee, and ankle joints.

Signs and Symptoms of Disorders. Pain, tenderness, swelling, partial or complete loss of mobility, stiffness, weakness, and fatigue are the signs and symptoms most commonly associated with disorders of the joints. Joint disease may be indicated by skin that feels warm, is red, has le-

sions, or is ulcerated. In psoriatic arthritis, skin lesions and pitting of the nails are involved in approximately 50% of cases. Pitting is the most commonly recognized change. Isolated pitting of a single nail may occur, or the pitting may be uniformly distributed across the nails.

Deformity. Deformities of the joint include absorption of tissues, flexion contracture, and bony overgrowth. Absorption may produce a flail joint, which makes the joint move erratically. Deformities result from scarring phenomena following inflammation and infection.

Swelling. The amount of swelling of the joint may range from difficult to detect to visually evident fluid within the joint (i.e., visible or palpable as a bulging of the joint capsule). Pressure on the sac at one point causes the fluid within it to shift and may lead to bulging at another site. The sac may vary from soft to tense, and the involvement may be symmetrical or unilateral. Often, the swelling is fusiform. Redness, warmth, swelling, and pain in a joint are the classic descriptors of an inflammatory process. The inflammation may be within the joint itself or in the soft tissue surrounding it. Swelling may also result from intra-articular effusion, synovial thickening, or bony overgrowth. In addition, swelling may result from the deposition of fat in the region adjacent to the joint. The synovial membrane is not palpable in normal joints. The palpation of a "boggy" or "doughy" consistency generally indicates a thickened or otherwise abnormal synovial membrane.

■ HELPFUL HINT

Possible causes of swelling:
Appears soon after injury → blood
Appears 8-24 hours after injury → synovial
Boggy, spongy feeling → synovial
Harder, tense feeling, warm → blood
Tough, dry → callus
Leathery, thickening → chronic problem
Soft, fluctuating → acute problem
Hard → bone
Thick, slow moving → pitting edema

Data from Magee DJ: *Orthopedic physical assessment*, ed. 3, Philadelphia, 1997, WB Saunders.

Tenderness. Injury and inflammatory processes cause joints to be tender. Arthritis, tendinitis, bursitis, and osteomyelitis are associated with tenderness in and around a joint. Therefore, it is important to attempt to determine which anatomical structure is tender.

Increased Temperature. Heat noted over a joint indicates inflammation and suggests rheumatoid or septic arthritis. Compare symmetrical joints for temperature when one joint is hot. Use the backs of the fingers when comparing temperature.

Redness. Vasodilation or inflammation occurs in the skin overlying a tender joint that is affected by septic arthritis and gouty arthritis.

Crepitation. Crepitation (crackling or grating sounds) produced by motion of the joint is caused by irregularities of the articulating surfaces. The coarseness of the surface may involve the cartilage or the bony capsule. Snapping (especially if its not painful) may be due to the movement of a tendon over a bony prominence.

Limitation of Range of Motion. The client may voluntarily limit the motion of a joint in response to pain. Spasm of the muscles involved in the movement of a joint may limit

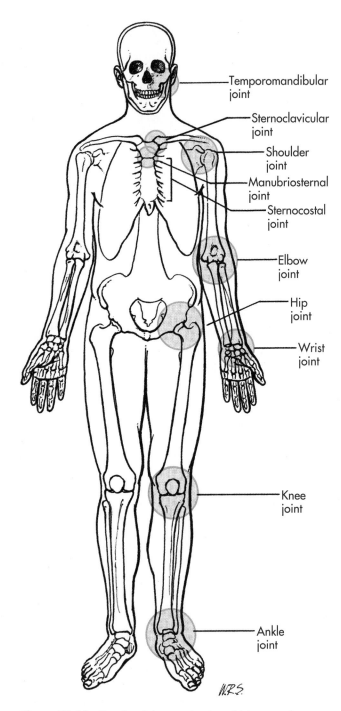

its motion. Mechanical obstruction to movement may accompany bony overgrowth and scar tissue. Limitation of motion in a joint is accompanied by weakness and atrophy of the muscles that are involved. Decreased range of motion occurs in joints in which there is inflammation of surrounding tissues, arthritis, fibrosis, or bony fixation (**ankylosis).**

Recording Joint Problems. To conveniently summarize the results of examination of the joints, circle the joint involved on a diagram (Figure 18-16) and briefly note any pathological condition.

Muscles. Examine muscles in symmetrical pairs (i.e., first one and then the other) for equivalence in size, contour, tone, and strength. Position the contralateral, matching muscle pairs uniformly while you examine them. Examine the muscles both at rest and in a state of contraction.

The assessment sequence is inspection, palpation, and testing of muscle strength. You may incorporate the examination of functional muscle groups into the examination of the joints.

Inspection and Palpation. Inspect the muscles for symmetry of size and contour. Measure asymmetry, noted as hypertrophy or atrophy, for verification. Use palpation to detect swelling, localized temperature changes, and marked changes in shape. Note the consistency of the muscle on palpation.

Muscle tone is the tension present in the resting muscle. You will also notice it in the slight resistance you feel when you passively move the relaxed limb. While palpating the muscle, be alert to **fasciculations,** which are involuntary contractions or twitching of groups of muscle fibers.

Ask the client to tell you of any sensations experienced while you feel the muscles and tendons. Then record the client's descriptions of pain or tenderness on palpation.

Tendon stretch reflexes, included as part of the neurological assessment discussed in Chapter 19, are generally altered in muscle disease, especially if the peripheral nerves are involved. For instance, the deep tendon reflexes are diminished in muscular dystrophy and polymyositis in proportion to the loss of muscle strength. A lengthened reflex cycle is characteristic of hypothyroidism, whereas a shortened period indicates the hypermetabolic state.

Recording Muscle Strength. Examiners commonly use the criteria in Table 18-2 for recording the grading of muscle strength.

Some examiners prefer to use simple descriptive words such as *paralysis, severe weakness, moderate weakness, minimum weakness,* and *normal.* Disability is considered to exist if (1) the muscle strength is less than grade 3, (2) external support may be required to make the involved part functional, (3) activity of the part cannot be achieved in a gravity field, and (4) external support is needed to perform movements. Muscle strength is expected to be greater in the dominant arm and leg. Movements should be coordinated and painless.

Perform a musculoskeletal screening test, unless you suspect a musculoskeletal problem. This will require a more indepth evaluation.

Screening Test for Muscle Strength. Muscle weakness in adults is generally mild and transitory. However, it may be

Figure 18-16 Results of the examination of joints may be summarized by circling on a diagram the joints involved and briefly noting the pathological condition.

the outcome of musculoskeletal, neurological, metabolic, or infectious problems. Therefore, an evaluation is necessary.

Although you can assess muscle strength throughout the full range of motion for each muscle or group of muscles, there are several simple screening tests that will allow you to find muscle or reflex abnormalities. One brief but effective approach is to observe the client carefully as he or she walks into the examining room, undresses, and gets on to the examination table. Watch for cues to neurological and motion deficit. This approach may also help you ascertain whether physical evidence can verify the chief complaint.

Table 18-3 gives an example of a formal screening examination. Place the client in the position that best allows movement through the full range. Apply resistance to the muscles. Muscle strength should be equal bilaterally. Grade the muscle contractions according to your judgment of the client's responses. The examination allows for a systematic testing of muscle groups from head to toe.

Specific Joints and Muscles

Temporomandibular Joint. The temporomandibular joint is the articulation between the mandible and the temporal bone (Figure 18-17). The joint is divided into two cavities as a fibrocartilaginous disk.

TABLE 18-2 Criteria for Grading and Recording Muscle Strength

Functional Level	Lovett Scale	Grade	Percent of Normal
No evidence of contractility	Zero (0)	0	0
Evidence of slight contractility	Trace (T)	1	10
Complete range of motion with gravity eliminated	Poor (P)	2	25
Complete range of motion with gravity	Fair (F)	3	50
Complete range of motion against gravity with some resistance	Good (G)	4	75
Complete range of motion against gravity with full resistance	Normal (N)	5	100

TABLE 18-3 Screening Test for Muscle Strength

Muscles Tested	Client Activity	Examiner Activity	Muscles Tested	Client Activity	Examiner Activity
Ocular musculature			Wrist musculature	Extend hand	Push to flex
Lids	Close eyes tightly	Attempt to resist closure		Flex hand	Push to extend
			Finger muscles	Extend fingers	Push dorsal surface of fingers
Yoke muscles	Track object in six cardinal positions			Flex fingers	Push ventral surface of fingers
Facial musculature	Blow out cheeks	Assess pressure in cheeks with fingertips		Spread fingers	Hold fingers together
	Place tongue in cheek	Assess pressure in cheek with fingertips	Hip musculature	In supine position raise extended leg	Push down on leg above knee
	Stick out tongue, move it to right and left	Observe strength and coordination of thrust and extension	Hamstring, gluteal, abductor, and adductor muscles of leg	Sit and perform alternate leg crossing	Push in opposite direction of crossing limb
Neck muscles	Extend head backward	Push head forward	Quadriceps	Extend leg	Push to flex leg
	Flex head forward	Push head backward	Hamstring	Bend knees to flex leg	Push to extend leg
	Rotate head in full circle	Observe mobility, coordination	Ankle and foot muscle	Bend foot up (dorsiflexion)	Push to plantar flexion
	Touch shoulders with head	Observe range of motion		Bend foot down (plantar flexion)	Push to dorsiflexion
Deltoid	Hold arms upward	Push down on arms	Antigravity muscles	Walk on toes	
Biceps	Flex arm	Pull to extend arm		Walk on heels	
Triceps	Extend arm	Push to flex arm			

INSPECTION AND PALPATION. Swelling appears as a tumescence over the joint, but it must be considerable to be visible. Palpate the joint by placing the fingertips anterior to the external meatus of the ear. In the normal joint there is a depression over the joint. Swelling may make this indentation difficult to feel. Palpate the jaw while the client moves it through its range of motion.

RANGE OF MOTION. To test range of motion, ask the client to do the following:

1. Open and close the mouth
2. Project the lower jaw (jutting of jaw)
3. Move the jaw from side to side (Figure 18-18)

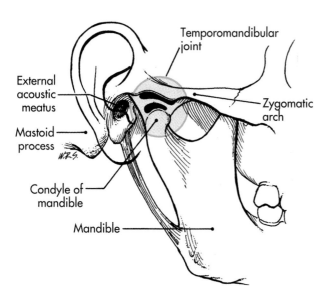

Figure 18-17 Temporomandibular joint. A fibrocartilaginous disk divides the articulation point into two synovial cavities. Note the proximity of this joint to the external acoustic meatus.

The normal range of distance between the upper and lower incisors is 3 to 6 cm. Measure lateral motion of the jaw when the client projects the jaw and moves it from side to side. Measure the distance that the midline of the lower lip deviates in each direction. The normal range of motion is 1 to 2 cm. Audible "clicks" on movement may be heard and are considered normal.

MUSCLE STRENGTH. To test muscle strength, ask the client to do the following:

1. Bite down hard while you palpate the masseter muscles.
2. Clench the teeth while you apply downward pressure on the chin.

These maneuvers also test the motor function of cranial nerve (CN) V.

Sternoclavicular Joint. The sternoclavicular joint is located at the juncture of the clavicle and the manubrium of the sternum. This joint is divided into two synovial cavities by a disk of cartilage and fibrous material. The joint is reinforced by a fibrous capsule and ligaments (Figure 18-19). The obtuse angle formed by the junction of the manubrium and the body of the sternum, called the angle of Louis, is used as a landmark for counting the ribs.

INSPECTION. Inspection of this joint is easy because little tissue overlies it. Swelling, redness, bony overgrowth, and dislocation are not difficult to see. Swelling of the joint appears as a smooth, round bulge. Although this joint is often overlooked, it is commonly involved in problems following surgery of the neck.

PALPATION. Palpate the joint with your fingertips. Movements of the shoulder depend on the normal function of this joint. Inflammation of the sternoclavicular joint may result in pain on movement of the shoulder girdle.

Cervical Spine. The cervical vertebrae are the most mobile of the spinal vertebrae. Flexion and extension occur between the skull and C1. Rotation occurs between C1 and C2.

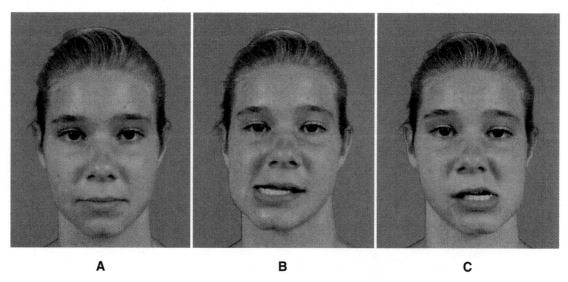

A   **B**   **C**

Figure 18-18 Lateral motion is determined by asking the client to move the lower jaw from side to side. The distance measured is the amount that the midline of the lower lip deviates in each direction. The midline of the stationary upper lip may be used as the baseline.

INSPECTION. Inspect the neck from both an anterior and a posterior position for deformities or abnormal posture. Note the alignment of the head with the shoulders. The cervical spine should be straight with the head erect. The normal spinal curvature should be concave in the cervical area.

PALPATION. Palpate the spinous processes of the cervical spine, including the trapezius, paravertebral, and sternocleidomastoid muscles. There should be symmetry in size, good tone, and no tenderness or muscle spasm.

RANGE OF MOTION. To evaluate range of motion, ask the client to do the following:

1. Touch the chin to the chest.
2. Extend the head backward as far as possible (Figure 18-20, A).
3. Bend the head laterally toward each shoulder (touch the ear to the shoulder without raising the shoulder) (Figure 18-20, B).
4. Rotate the head from side to side (pointing the chin toward each shoulder) (Figure 18-20, C).

MUSCLE STRENGTH. To evaluate muscle strength, ask the client to do the following:

1. Push the cheek against your hand (right and left sides). This maneuver also tests the motor function of CN XI (sternocleidomastoid muscle) (Figure 18-21, A).
2. Push the forehead against your hand (Figure 18-21, B).
3. Push the head back against your hand (Figure 18-21, C).

Shoulders. The shoulder joint is a ball-and-socket joint that is the articulation of the humerus and the glenoid fossa of the scapula (Figure 18-22). The joint is protected by the muscles and the ligaments. A fibrous capsule surrounds the joint completely. Overlying these structures is the subacromial bursa. The portion of the bursa that lies beneath the deltoid is called the subdeltoid bursa. The clavicle and the acromion process of the scapula are articulated by the acromioclavicular joint.

INSPECTION. Inspect the shoulders, including the muscles and the acromioclavicular joint, with the client standing with his or her back to you. Examine the contour and shape of the shoulders, and look for equality of shoulder height. Inspect the scapulae and related muscles. Anterior dislocation of the shoulder can be seen as a flattening of the lateral aspect of the shoulder. Joint swelling due to fluid collection may be visible only when the amount of fluid is moderate to large. Visible swelling generally appears over the anterior aspect of the shoulder.

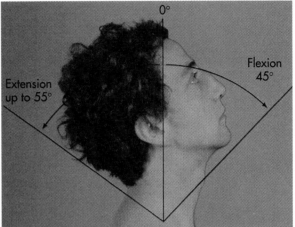

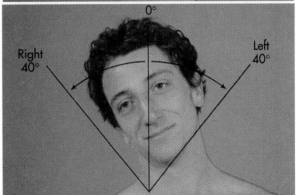

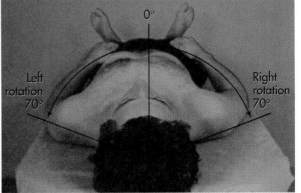

Figure 18-20 Range of motion of the cervical spine. **A,** Flexion and hyperextension. **B,** Lateral bending. **C,** Rotation.

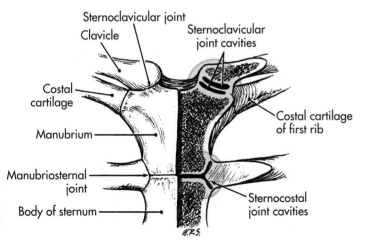

Figure 18-19 The sternoclavicular joint is divided into two synovial cavities. Movement of the shoulder girdle may cause pain when these joints are diseased. Manubriosternal joint examination is done largely by inspection and palpation, since these joints move minimally.

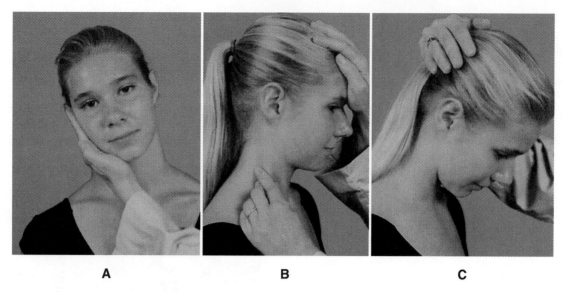

A **B** **C**

Figure 18–21 Examining the strength of the sternocleidomastoid and trapezius muscles. **A,** Rotation against resistance. **B,** Flexion with palpation of the sternocleidomastoid muscle. **C,** Extension against resistance.

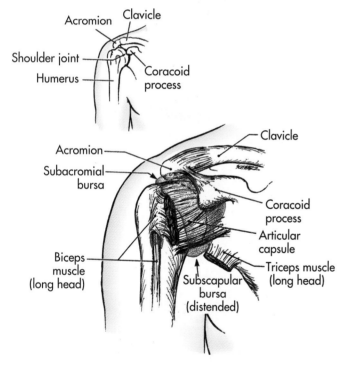

Figure 18–22 Shoulder joint.

PALPATION. Palpate the joint and the bursal sites. Sites to palpate include the acromion process, clavicle, scapulae, acromioclavicular joint, greater tubercle of the humerus, sternoclavicular joint, biceps groove, and area muscles. If you suspect neoplasia or infection, palpate the axilla for lymph nodes. Give special attention to the tendons of the teres minor and infraspinatus muscles (rotator cuff). Palpate these tendons for swelling, nodes, tears, and pain.

RANGE OF MOTION. To test for range of motion, ask the client to do the following (Figure 18-23):
1. Extend both arms forward (forward flexion).
2. Extend both arms backward (hyperextension).
3. Put the hands behind the back as if one were going to reach up to touch the shoulder blade (internal rotation).
4. Put the hands behind the head (external rotation).

MUSCLE STRENGTH. To test for muscle strength, ask the client to do the following:
1. Hold the arms upward while you try to push them down (deltoid muscles).
2. Extend the arms and then try to flex them while you try to pull them into extension (biceps muscle) (Figure 18-24).
3. Flex the arms and then extend them while you attempt to push them into a flexed position (triceps muscle) (Figure 18-25).
4. Shrug the shoulders while you try to push down on them (CN XI, trapezius muscle) (Figure 18-26).

Elbow. The elbow is the articulation of the humerus, the radius, and the ulna (Figure 18-27). The three articulating surfaces are enclosed in a single synovial cavity. The synovial membrane is generally palpable only on the posterior aspect of the joint. Radial and ulnar ligaments provide protection to the joint. The olecranon bursa is the largest bursa of the elbow, although several smaller bursae are present. Swelling and redness are easily visible over the posterior aspect of the elbow.

INSPECTION. Inspect the size and contour of the elbow in flexion and extension. Note deviations in the carrying angle of the arm while the arm is passively extended with the palm facing forward (Figure 18-28). The carrying angle is between 5 and 15 degrees in adults. Variations in the carrying angle are cubitus valgus (forearm farther outward than the arm) and cubitus varus (forearm carried more inwardly).

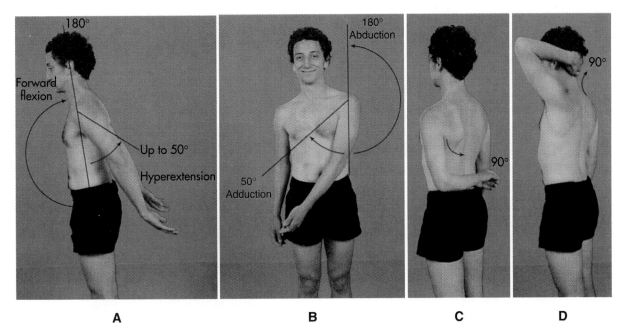

Figure 18-23   Range of motion of the shoulder. **A,** Forward flexion and hyperextension. **B,** Abduction and adduction. **C,** Internal rotation. **D,** External rotation.

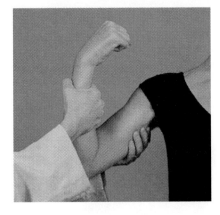

Figure 18-24   Assessment of biceps muscle strength. The client flexes her arm while the examiner attempts to pull the arm into extension.

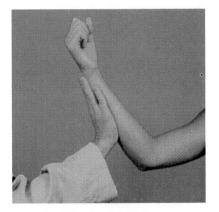

Figure 18-25   Assessment of triceps muscle strength. The client attempts to extend her arm while the examiner tries to push the arm into a flexed position.

These variations can be caused by acute injury, posttraumatic arthritis, or other forms of arthritis.

PALPATION.   With the client's arm flexed to approximately 70 degrees, palpate the elbow with the tips of the fingers while applying pressure on the opposite side of the joint with the thumb of the dominant hand. Support the arm with your other hand. Palpate the lateral and medial condyles, the olecranon process, and the grooves on either side of the olecranon process. Joint swelling is most often palpable in the medial groove (Figure 18-29).

RANGE OF MOTION.   To test range of motion (Figure 18-30), ask the client to do the following:

1. Bend and straighten the elbow.
2. Turn the hand face up (supination); face down (pronation).

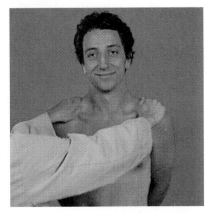

Figure 18-26   Assessment of trapezius muscle strength. The client shrugs his shoulders while the examiner attempts to push them down.

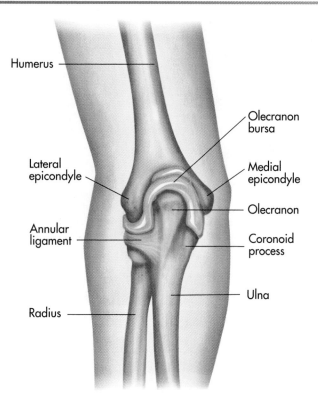

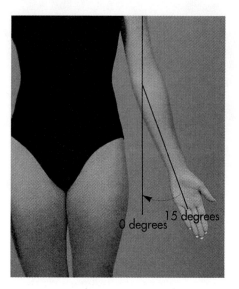

Figure 18-27   Elbow joint (left side, posterior view). (From Seidel HM et al.: *Mosby's guide to physical examination,* ed. 4, St. Louis, 1999, Mosby.)

Figure 18-28   The expected carrying angle of the arm is between 5 and 15 degrees in the adult.

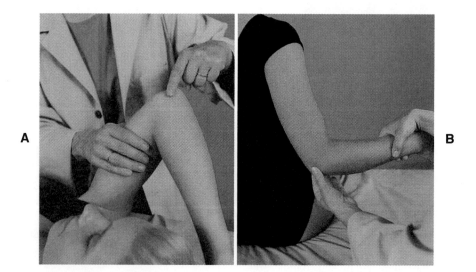

Figure 18-29   A, Examination of the extensor surface of the elbow joint with the client in the supine position. **B,** Examination of the extensor surface of the elbow joint with the client in the sitting position.

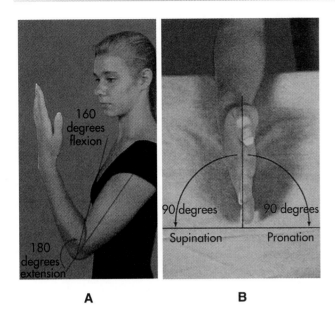

Figure 18-30 Range of motion of the elbow. **A,** Flexion and extension. **B,** Pronation and supination.

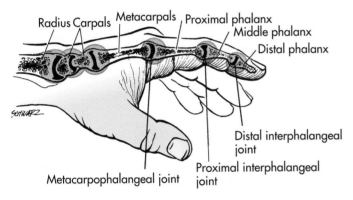

Figure 18-31 Joints articulating the bones of the wrist and hand.

MUSCLE STRENGTH. To test muscle strength, use the tests for the biceps and triceps muscles described in the section on shoulders.

Wrists, Hands, and Fingers. The wrist joint contains the points of articulation between the distal radius and the proximal portions of the following carpal bones: scaphoid (navicular), lunate, and triangular (Figure 18-31). An articular disk divides the radius from the ulnar bone and also separates the radius from the wrist joint. The wrist joint is protected by a fibrous capsule and ligaments. The joint is lined by synovial membrane.

INSPECTION. Inspect the wrist and the hands for position, contour, symmetry, smoothness, edema, atrophy or hypertrophy, and deformity. Swelling of the wrist joint most commonly appears on the dorsal surface distal to the ulnar tip. Swelling is easily visible over the dorsal surface of the hand because little tissue covers the joints.

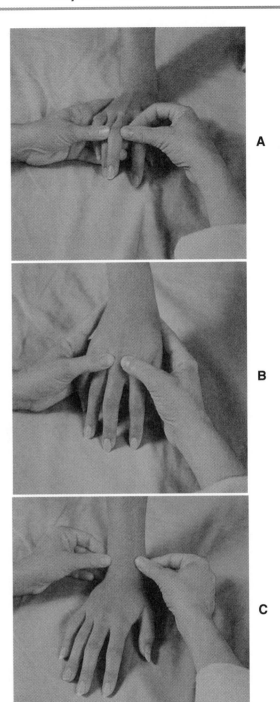

Figure 18-32 Palpation of joints of the hand and wrist. **A,** Interphalangeal joints. **B,** Metacarpophalangeal joints. **C,** Radiocarpal groove and wrist.

PALPATION. Use two hands for palpation of the wrist so that the thumbs and the index fingers are opposed on either side of the wrist. Apply enough pressure to outline bony and soft tissue structures. Palpate the joints between the carpal, metacarpal, and phalangeal bones. Use your thumbs and index fingers to palpate each of these joints (Figure 18-32).

RANGE OF MOTION.   To test range of motion of the hands and wrist (Figure 18-33), ask the client to do the following:

1. Spread the fingers apart and bring them back again.
2. Make a fist.
3. Touch the thumb to each fingertip and to the base of the little finger.
4. Bend the fingers up and down at the metacarpophalangeal joint.
5. Bend the hand up and down at the wrist.
6. With the palm facing down, turn the hand to the right (radial deviation) and to the left (ulnar deviation).

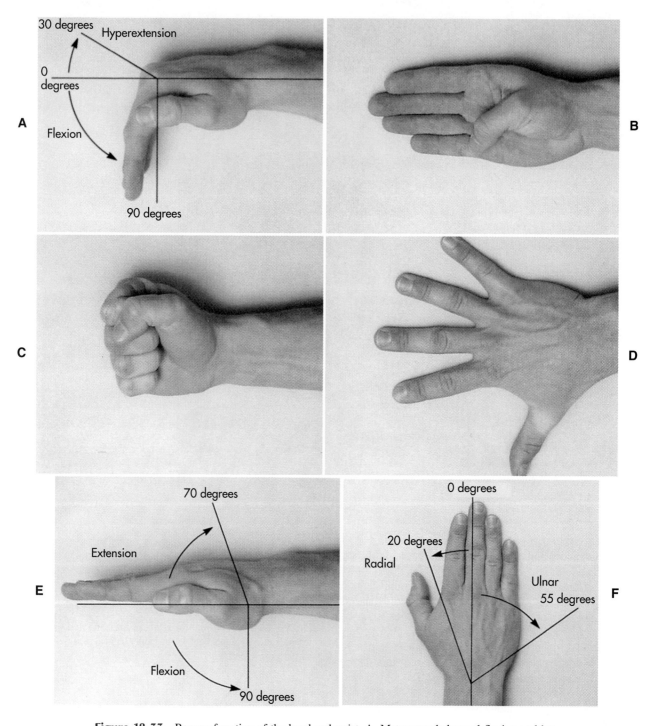

Figure 18-33   Range of motion of the hand and wrist. **A,** Metacarpophalangeal flexion and hyperextension. **B,** Finger flexion: the thumb to each fingertip and to the base of the little finger. **C,** Finger flexion: fist formation. **D,** Finger abduction. **E,** Flexion and hyperextension of the wrist. **F,** Radial and ulnar movement of the wrist. (From Seidel HM et al.: *Mosby's guide to physical examination,* ed. 4, St. Louis, 1999, Mosby.)

MUSCLE STRENGTH. To assess wrist strength, ask the client to do the following:

1. Maintain wrist flexion while you try to extend the wrist.
2. Try to extend the wrist as you try to flex it (Figure 18-34).

To assess grip strength, ask the client to squeeze your first two fingers as hard as he or she can (Figure 18-35). If you cross your fingers, you will not feel as much discomfort if the client is exceptionally strong.

To assess finger strength, ask the client to do the following:

1. Extend the fingers while you push down on the dorsal surface.
2. Flex the fingers while you push up on the ventral surface.
3. Spread the fingers as far apart as possible while you try to push them together (Figure 18-36).
4. Push the fingers as close together as possible while you try to pull them apart.

SPECIAL TESTS. Many tendons cross the wrist and hands to their insertions on the fingers. Thickening of the flexor tendon sheath of the median nerve (seen in carpal tunnel syndrome) is a common problem. It may lead to feelings of numbness, burning, and paresthesia along the distribution of the median nerve. The thickness of the sheath may be visible on the palmar surface of the wrist. Two tests may elicit these altered sensory phenomena. In the first of these tests, Phalen's test, the client is asked to maintain palmar flexion for 1 minute (Figure 18-37). The experience of numbness and paresthesia over the palmar surface of the hand and the first three fingers and part of the fourth is called Phalen's sign. The symptoms resolve quickly after the hand returns to the resting position. The second test, Tinel's test, consists of tapping over the median nerve (palmar aspect of wrist). The client's sensation of tingling or prickling is known as Tinel's sign (Figure 18-38).

Hips. The hip joint is the articulation of the **acetabulum** and the femur (Figure 18-39). It is a ball-and-socket joint that is protected by a fibrous capsule and ligaments. Three bursae reduce friction in the hip: (1) the trochanteric, between the posterolateral greater trochanter and the gluteus maximus; (2) the iliopectineal, between the anterior surface of the joint and the iliopsoas muscle; and (3) the ischiogluteal, situated over the ischial tuberosity.

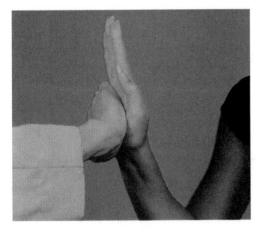

Figure 18-34 To assess wrist strength, the client attempts to extend her wrist while the examiner tries to flex it.

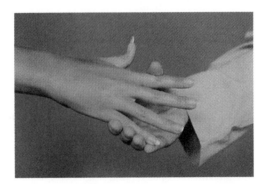

Figure 18-36 Assessment of finger strength.

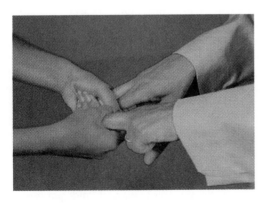

Figure 18-35 Assessment of grip strength.

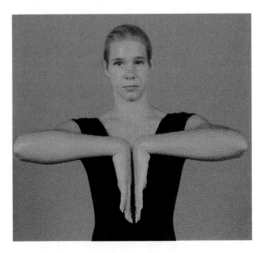

Figure 18-37 Phalen's test for carpal tunnel syndrome.

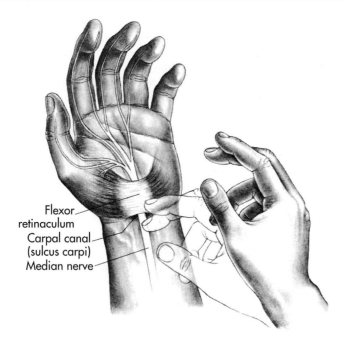

Figure 18-38   Elicitation of Tinel's sign. (From Seidel HM et al.: *Mosby's guide to physical examination,* ed. 4, St. Louis, 1999, Mosby.)

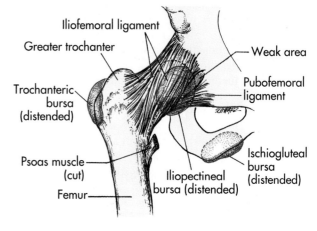

Figure 18-39   Hip joint.

INSPECTION.   Inspect the hips anteriorly and posteriorly while the client stands. Look for symmetry in the iliac crest height, size of the buttocks, and number and level of gluteal folds. Inspection of the hip joint includes an assessment of gait (see Chapter 9). A smooth and even gait indicates equal leg length and functional hip motion. Antalgic limp is characteristic of disease that produces pain in a hip joint; the body tilts toward the involved diseased hip in such a way that the weight of the body is directly over the hip. This limp decreases the need for abductor muscle movement and thus may alleviate muscle spasm. If the abductor muscles are weak (i.e., unable to support the pelvis), the unaffected hip may move downward in such a way that the weight is borne on that side. This condition is called Trendelenburg's limp.

PALPATION.   With the client supine, palpate the hips and the pelvis for stability, tenderness, or crepitus. The bursae are not palpable unless they are swollen. Swelling and tenderness are the diagnostic findings of pathological conditions of these structures.

RANGE OF MOTION.   To test range of motion of the hips (Figure 18-40), ask the client to do the following:

1. While supine:
   a. Raise the leg above the body with the knee extended.
   b. Bring the knee to the chest while keeping the other leg straight.
   c. Swing the leg laterally and medially while keeping the knee straight.
   d. Place the side of the foot on the opposite knee and move the flexed knee down toward the examining table (external rotation).

   e. Flex the knee and rotate the leg so that the flexed knee moves inward toward the opposite leg (internal rotation).
2. While either prone or standing, swing the straightened leg behind the body.

Muscle Strength.   To test muscle strength in the hips, place the client in a supine position. Then ask the client to do the following:

1. Raise the extended leg while you attempt to hold it down.
2. Push both legs against your hands while your hands are placed on the bed on either side of the client's knees.
3. Bring both legs together while your hands are placed on the bed between the client's knees.

To assess muscle strength in the hamstring, gluteal, abductor, and adductor muscles, ask the client to sit and perform alternate leg crossing (Figure 18-41).

Knee.   The knee joint is the articulation of the femur, the tibia, and the patella. The lining of the joint is a fibrous membrane. Synovial membrane covers the articular surface of the femur and the tibia with folds to the patella. The medial and lateral menisci are fibrocartilaginous disks with outside edges (**horns**) that are attached to the tibia and are continuous with the articular capsule. The medial convexity of the femur rotates with the inner portion of the meniscus that is attached to it. A spiral distortion of the menisci occurs on rotation, making these disks susceptible to rupture. The surfaces of the menisci have no synovial membrane. They are thought to aid the spread of synovial fluid, and this function may account for their existence. An anterior pouch in the

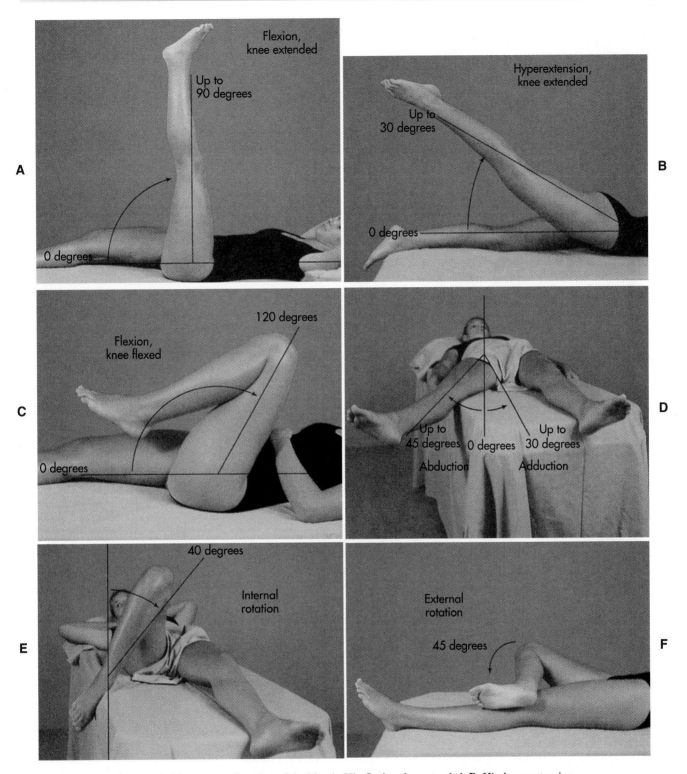

Figure 18-40 Range of motion of the hip. **A,** Hip flexion, leg extended. **B,** Hip hyperextension, knee extended. **C,** Hip flexion, knee flexed. **D,** Abduction. **E,** Internal rotation. **F,** External rotation.

knee joint that separates the patella and quadriceps tendon and muscle from the femur is called the suprapatellar pouch.

The bursae of the knee are numerous (Figure 18-42). On the anterior knee, the prepatellar bursa lies immediately in front of the patella. The superficial infrapatellar bursa lies anterior to the patellar ligament, and the deep infrapatellar bursa is behind the ligament. The bursae of the posterior knee include the two gastrocnemius bursae. One separates the lateral head of the gastrocnemius muscle from the articular capsule. The other divides the medial head of the gas-

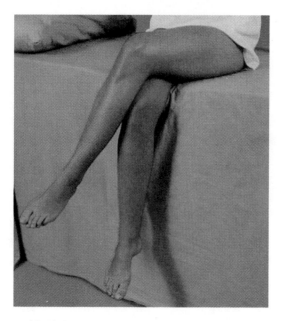

Figure 18-41 Alternate leg crossing for assessment of hamstring, gluteal, abductor, and adductor muscle strength.

trocnemius muscle from the articular capsule. In addition, a large bursa separates the medial head of the gastrocnemius muscle from the semimembranous muscle.

INSPECTION.   Inspect the knee with the client walking (to observe gait), sitting, and supine with knees extended. Be familiar with the normal contour of the knee because loss of contour may occur with swelling. The client may voluntarily maintain the knee at 15 to 20 degrees of flexion because the knee joint is at maximal capacity at this angle and thus pain is reduced. Swelling as a result of synovitis is most apparent at the suprapatellar pouch. Swelling caused by meniscal cysts appears at the lateral or the medial joint surface. Popliteal swelling is more obvious when the knee is extended. Swelling observed on the anterior aspect of the knee is called prepatellar bursitis or "housemaid's knee."

PALPATION.   Palpate the knee with the client in the sitting or supine position, whichever is more comfortable for the client. Apply downward pressure over the suprapatellar pouch to localize the synovial fluid in the lower portion of the articular cavity. Use the examining hand to palpate the lateral and medial joint surfaces with the fingers while using the thumb for stability (Figure 18-43).

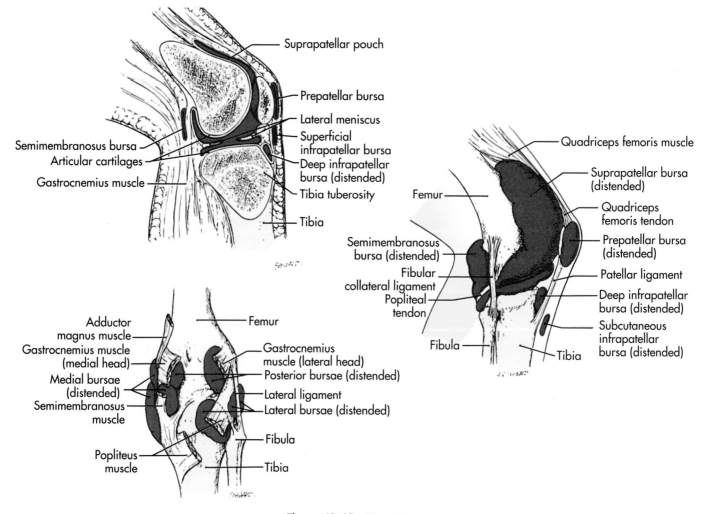

Figure 18-42 Knee joint.

In a second procedure for the examination of the knee, palpate the suprapatellar pouch with the thumb and the fingers of one hand while the other hand pushes the contents of the articular cavity upward. To do this, place your thumb on one side of the patella with the rest of your fingers on the other side to form an arch below the patella. Apply an inward and upward pressure to move any fluid upward into the suprapatellar bursa. Place the examining hand about 10 cm above the patella and move it gradually toward the patella. The following special tests involve palpating the knee to assess for swelling or fluid in the joint:

1. **Bulge sign.** A test for small effusions in the knee joint is called the bulge sign. Take the ball of your hand and firmly milk the medial aspect of the knee upward two to three times to displace fluid. Then press or tap behind the lateral margin of the knee (Figure 18-44). A positive bulge sign will show a swelling or bulge of fluid in the hollow area medial to the patella. The bulge sign is useful for assessing small effusions, but it may be absent in large effusions.

2. **Ballottement of the patella.** When considerable fluid is present in the suprapatellar pouch, ballottement of the patella may be possible (Figure 18-45). Ballottement involves applying downward pressure with one hand while pushing the patella backward against the femur with a finger of the opposite hand. Examine the popliteal region with the client in the prone position or while standing. Swelling of the joint in the popliteal

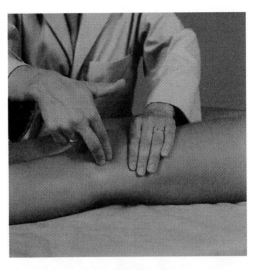

Figure 18-44 Testing for the bulge sign. After milking the medial aspect of the knee, the lateral side of the patella is tapped. The medial side is then observed for the presence of a bulge.

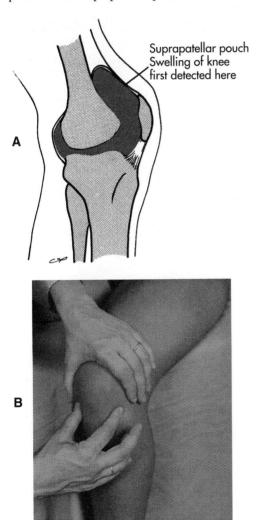

Figure 18-43 **A,** Knee effusion. **B,** Examination of the knee.

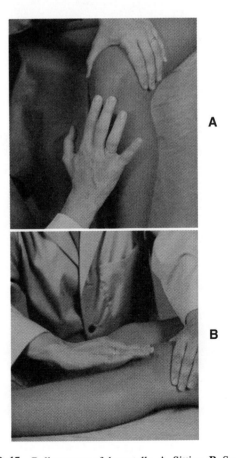

Figure 18-45 Ballottement of the patella. **A,** Sitting. **B,** Supine.

region, which is called **Baker's cyst**, is generally an extension of the articular cavity.

RANGE OF MOTION.   To test range of motion of the knee (Figure 18-46), ask the client to do the following:

1. Bend the knee.
2. Straighten and stretch the leg.

MUSCLE STRENGTH.   To test muscle strength in the knee, ask the client to do the following:

1. Extend the leg as you try to bend it (quadriceps muscle strength) (Figure 18-47).

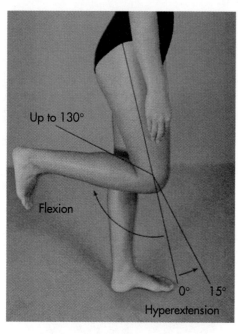

Figure 18-46   Range of motion of the knee: flexion and extension.

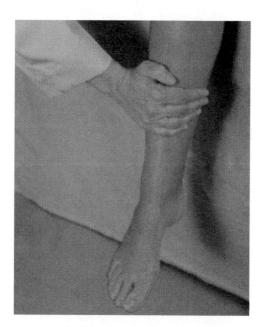

Figure 18-47   Assessment of quadriceps muscle strength. The client attempts to straighten the leg while the examiner tries to flex it.

2. Bend the knees as you try to straighten them (hamstring muscle strength) (Figure 18-48).

TESTS FOR LIGAMENT INJURY.   Sprains or tears of the ligaments are the most common injuries of the knee. In many sports, the knee is subjected to sudden strong forces. This makes knee injuries one of the most common types of athletic injury (Figure 18-49). Two sets of ligaments play a role in movement of the knee. They are the anterior and posterior cruciate ligaments and the medial and lateral collateral ligaments. The anterior cruciate ligament limits extension and rotation, whereas the posterior cruciate ligament stabilizes the femur against forward dislocation. The collateral ligaments prevent lateral and medial dislocation of the knee.

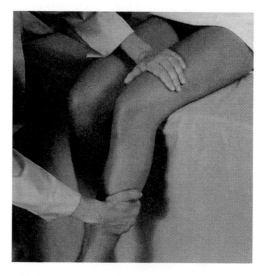

Figure 18-48   Assessment of hamstring muscle strength. The client flexes his knees while the examiner tries to straighten them.

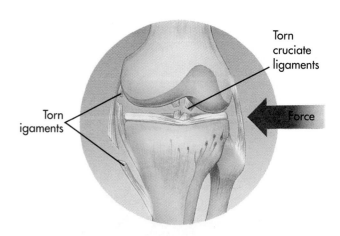

Figure 18-49   Knee injury. The knee is the largest and most vulnerable joint. Articular cartilages on the tibia as well as ligaments holding the tibia and femur together may be torn when the knee twists while bearing weight. (From Thibodeau GA, Patton KT: *Anatomy and physiology,* ed. 4, St. Louis, 1999, Mosby.)

Abnormal movements of the knee may indicate dislocation. You may be able to palpate the tears in the assessment of the knee.

To test the stability of the anterior and posterior cruciate ligaments, use the drawer test or the Lachman test (if you are assessing the anterior ligament).

1. **Drawer test**. For the drawer sign, have the client lie in a supine position with the knee flexed to 90 degrees and the foot flat on the examining table (Figure 18-50). Position yourself on the edge of the table so that you can stabilize the foot by sitting on the client's forefoot. Cup your hands around the tibia. To test the stability of the anterior cruciate

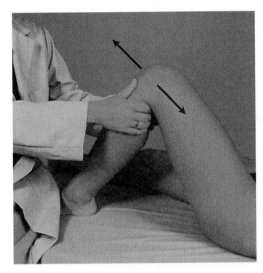

Figure 18-50 Examination of the knee with the drawer test for anterior and posterior stability.

ligament, pull the tibia toward you. If it slides forward from under the femur, the drawer test is positive and suggests a tear in the anterior ligament. To test the posterior cruciate ligament, push the tibia posteriorly. If it moves backward, the ligament is probably damaged. This test is usually performed in one continuous motion. Remember, first test the unaffected knee, then the affected knee, and compare findings.

2. **Lachman test**. The Lachman test is thought to be a better indicator of injury to the anterior cruciate ligament (Magee, 1997). Have the client lie in a supine position with the involved leg beside you. Place the client's knee between full extension and 30 degrees of flexion (close to the functional position of the knee). Stabilize the femur with one hand while you move the proximal aspect of the tibia forward with the other hand (Figure 18-51). If there is a soft or "mushy" feel and the infrapatellar slope disappears when the tibia is moved forward on the femur, the Lachman test is positive. This sign indicates damage to the anterior cruciate ligament, especially the posterolateral band. Remember, first test the unaffected knee, then the affected knee, and compare findings.

TESTS FOR MENISCUS DAMAGE. Indications of pathological conditions of the meniscus include (1) pain or tenderness on the lateral surfaces of the knee joint; (2) popping, snapping, or grating sounds with movement; and (3) inability to fully extend the knee ("locking"). The medial meniscus is more often injured than is the lateral. The two tests commonly used to aid in the diagnosis of a torn meniscus are the Apley test and the McMurray test.

1. **Apley test**. Attempt to elicit Apley's sign (Figure 18-52) in the client you suspect of having a

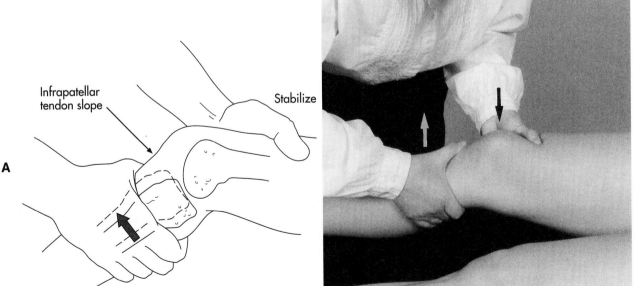

Figure 18-51 Hand position for the classic Lachman test (**A** and **B**). From Magee DJ: *Orthopedic physical assessment,* ed. 3, Philadelphia, 1997, WB Saunders.)

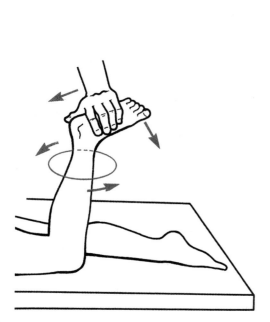

Figure 18-52 Elicitation of Apley's sign with compression.

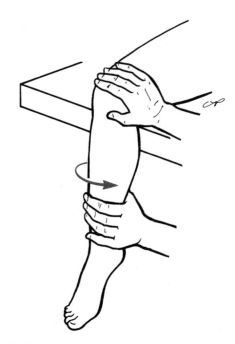

Figure 18-53 Elicitation of McMurray's sign to test the lateral meniscus.

loose object in the knee joint or one who has given a history of knee joint locking. Have the client assume the prone position with the suspected knee flexed to 90 degrees. Exert downward pressure on the foot so that the tibia is firmly opposed to the femur. Rotate the leg externally and internally. Locking of the knee, pain with the maneuver, or the sound of clicks is a positive sign and may indicate that a loose body, such as torn cartilage, is trapped in the articulation. Clicks or popping sounds are generated as the object escapes. Repeat the maneuver, applying traction to the leg while rotating the tibia internally and externally (distraction) rather than downward pressure (compression) on the foot. If the pain is worse when rotation plus compression is used, there is probably a meniscus injury. Pain that is worse when rotation plus distraction is used is probably ligamentous.

2. **McMurray test.** When the client states that he or she "feels something in the knee joint" or complains that "sometimes it just won't bend," attempt to elicit McMurray's sign (Figure 18-53). Perform this test with the client in the sitting position with the knee flexed to 90 degrees or in the supine position. Have the client internally rotate the leg while you slowly extend it with one hand. Use the other hand to provide resistance at the medial aspect of the knee. This maneuver tests the medial meniscus. Extension of the knee may not be possible (positive sign) if a loose body impedes its movement. Repeat the procedure by using external rotation and applying resistance to the lateral aspect of the knee. This maneuver tests the lateral meniscus.

Ankles and Feet. The ankle joint is the articulation of the tibia, the fibula, and the talus (Figure 18-54). The capsule is lined with synovia. The ankle joint is protected by ligaments on the medial and lateral surfaces but not on the anterior or posterior surfaces. The joint between the talus and the calcaneus bones is called the talocalcaneal, or subtalar, joint. The forward extension of the joint cavity is the articulation of the talus and the navicular bones. Articular capsules lined with synovial membrane separate the remainder of the tarsal, metatarsal, and phalangeal bones of the foot.

INSPECTION. Inspect the ankle and the foot with the client standing, walking, and sitting (not bearing weight). To best evaluate for swelling, examine the dorsal aspect of the foot because there is less tissue over the bone. Hallux valgus is a lateral deformity of the great toe in which it may lie above or below the second toe. The metatarsophalangeal joint is distorted in such a way that the first metatarsal bone is angled medially. A callus or bursal distention generally occurs at the joint (Figure 18-55, *A*). Hammer toe is a result of hyperextension of the metatarsophalangeal joint and flexion of the proximal phalangeal joint (Figure 18-55, *B*).

PALPATION. Palpate the anterior aspect of the ankle joint with your thumbs to assess for bogginess, swelling, or tenderness. Palpate the Achilles tendon for tenderness and nodules (Figure 18-56). Palpate the metatarsal and phalangeal joints with the fingers on the anterior surface and the thumb on the sole of the foot. Note any tenderness.

RANGE OF MOTION. To test range of motion of the ankle and foot (Figure 18-57), ask the client to do the following:

1. Point the foot up toward the ceiling.
2. Point the foot down toward the floor.

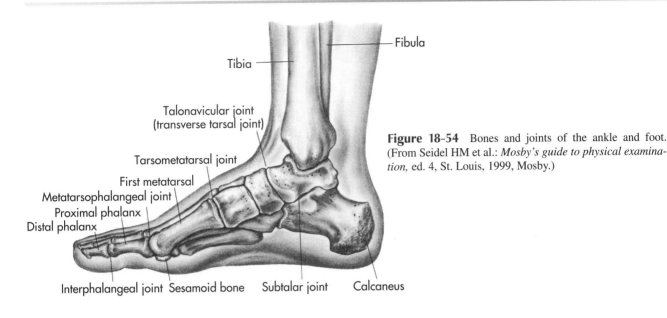

Figure 18-54 Bones and joints of the ankle and foot. (From Seidel HM et al.: *Mosby's guide to physical examination,* ed. 4, St. Louis, 1999, Mosby.)

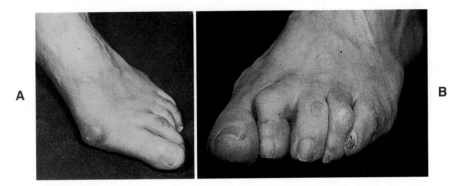

Figure 18-55 **A,** Hallux valgus with bunion. **B,** Hammer toes. (Courtesy Charles W. Bradley, DPM, California College of Pediatric Medicine. From Seidel HM et al.: *Mosby's guide to physical examination,* ed. 4, St. Louis, 1999, Mosby.)

3. With the foot bent at the ankle, point the medial side of the foot toward the floor (eversion) and repeat with the lateral side (inversion).
4. Rotate the ankle to turn the foot away from and then toward the other foot.

MUSCLE STRENGTH. To test muscle strength in the ankle and foot, ask the client to do the following:

1. Flex the foot upward against your hand.
2. Push the foot down against your hand (Figure 18-58).

Thoracic and Lumbar Spine

INSPECTION. Inspect the shape of the spine and its structural relationship to the shoulder girdle, thorax, and pelvis. The normal spinal curvatures are concave at the cervical area, convex at the thoracic area, and concave at the lumbar area. Note any differences in heights of the shoulders and the iliac crests. Unusual heights of the iliac crests suggest uneven leg lengths. Variations in spinal curvature may indicate a structural problem.

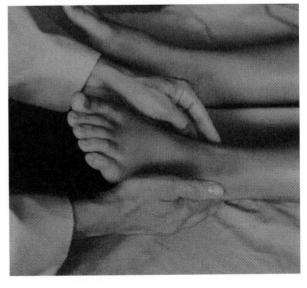

Figure 18-56 Examination of the ankle joint.

Scoliosis is a deformity of the spine that appears as a lateral deviation (Figure 18-59). This angling of the spine produces a downward slant of the thoracic cage on the affected side and an upward tilt of the pelvis on the contralateral side. A rotary deformity of the rib cage also occurs. The ribs protrude posteriorly on the convex side of the spine. A hump or "razorback" may be visible. The protrusion may become more obvious when the client bends over.

Scoliosis Assessment. To assess for scoliosis, ask the client to stand with the feet approximately 6 inches apart and bend over slowly to touch the toes. Stand behind the client and observe the movement of the spine as the client bends and comes back to an upright position (Figure 18-60). This maneuver provides a "skyline" view of the spine. Structural scoliosis, which is caused by vertebral rotation, tends to become more prominent as the client bends forward. Functional scoliosis, which compensates for structural abnormalities other than those associated with the vertebral column, disappears when the client bends forward. Also note symmetry of the muscles, movement, protrusions, or sharp angulation.

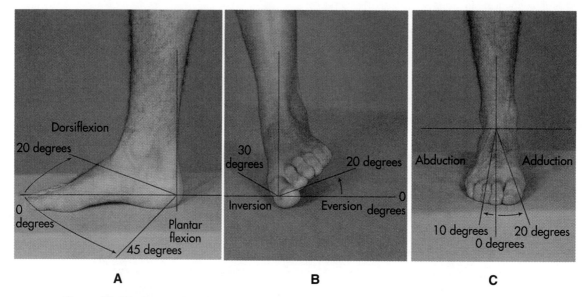

Figure 18-57 Range of motion of the ankle and foot. **A,** Dorsiflexion and plantar flexion. **B,** Inversion and eversion. **C,** Abduction and adduction.

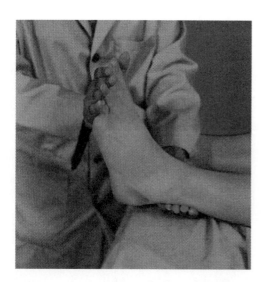

Figure 18-58 Testing muscle strength in the ankle and foot.

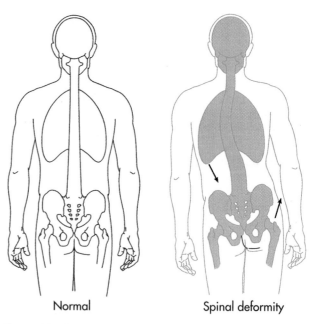

Figure 18-59 Deformity of the spine. Scoliosis is a lateral deviation of the spine. *Arrows* indicate the direction of the thoracic and pelvic tilt.

Kyphosis (humpback) is a flexion deformity (Figure 18-61, *B*). When the angle of the defect is sharp, the apex is called a gibbus.

Lordosis (swayback) is an extension deviation of the spine, commonly in the lumbar area (Figure 18-61, *B*).

PALPATION. Palpate the spinal processes as the client bends over to touch the toes (Figure 18-62). Palpate paravertebral muscles for symmetry, tenderness, and spasm. You may want to percuss for tenderness over the spinous process.

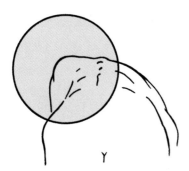

Figure 18-60 Rotary deformity of scoliosis produces a humpback or "razorback" deformity. This deviation is best demonstrated by asking the client to bend at the waist.

RANGE OF MOTION. To assess range of motion of the spine (Figure 18-63), ask the client to do the following:
1. Bend back as far as possible (hyperextend the spine).
2. Bend to the right and left side as far as possible (lateral bending). You may need to stabilize the client's pelvis.
3. Turn to the right and left in a circular motion (while you stabilize the pelvis).
4. Slowly bend forward at the waist and try to touch the toes (while you watch from behind the client and observe for signs of scoliosis).

ASSESSMENT OF GAIT. Evaluate gait in both phases—stance and swing—for rhythm and smoothness (Figure 18-64; see also Figure 9-3 and additional discussion in Chapter 9).

Stance is considered to consist of five phases: (1) initial contact—the weight loading or weight acceptance period of the stance leg—both feet are in contact with the floor so there is double support and the heel contacts the floor; (2) loading response—single support in which one leg carries the body weight while the other leg goes through the swing phase; (3) midstance—single support—here the body weight is transferred from the heel to the ball of the foot; (4) terminal stance—the heel leaves the ground as the stance leg unloads the body weight to the opposite limb—both feet are in contact so double support occurs; and (5) preswing—preparation for the leg swing phase. During the single support phases (2 and 3), the stance leg must be able to support the weight of the

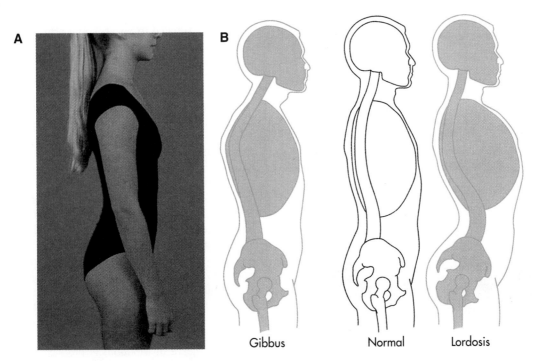

Gibbus   Normal   Lordosis

Figure 18-61 **A,** Normal curvature of the spine. **B,** Kyphosis—a flexion deformity of the spine—and lordosis—an extension deformity of the spine.

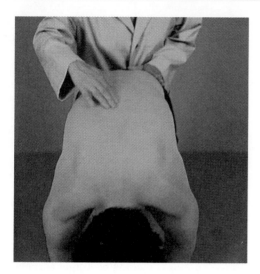

Figure 18-62   Palpation of the spinal processes as the client bends over.

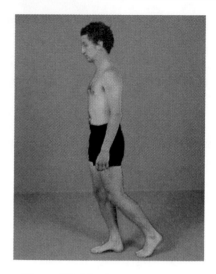

Figure 18-64   Assessment of gait.

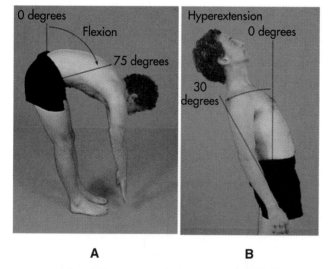

A   B

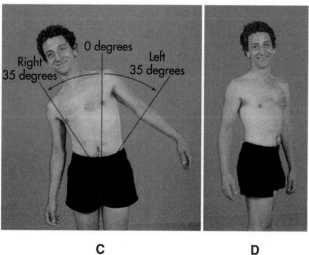

C   D

Figure 18-63   Range of motion of the thoracic and lumbar spine. **A,** Flexion. **B,** Hyperextension. **C,** Lateral bending. **D,** Rotation of the upper trunk.

body and balance on one leg. In addition, lateral hip stability is needed to maintain balance (Magee, 1997).

The swing phase occurs when the foot is moving forward and is not weight bearing. It consists of three processes: (1) initial swing (acceleration)—the foot is lifted off the floor; (2) midswing—the lifted foot travels ahead of the weight-bearing foot; and (3) terminal swing (deceleration)—the swinging foot slows in preparation for the initial contact with the floor (heel strike).

To describe the client's gait, include phase (conformity), cadence (symmetry, regular rhythm), stride length (symmetry, length of swing), trunk posture (related to phases), pelvic posture (related to phases), and arm swing (symmetry, length of swing).

If pain is present, describe it in relation to the phases of gait.

To assess gait, ask the client to walk naturally for a short distance so that you can observe the gait (if you have not already done so). Then ask the client to take a few steps on the toes and a few steps on the heels.

Special Maneuvers

STRAIGHT LEG-RAISING TEST.   The straight leg-raising test, which is also known as Lasègue's test (Figure 18-65), is used to test for sciatic nerve root irritation or a herniated lumbar disk at the L4, L5, and S1 levels. Perform the test for clients who complain of low back pain or pain that radiates down the leg. Have the client lie on the back on a firm surface with the leg and thigh as relaxed as possible. Slowly raise the foot, keeping the knee straight until the client complains of pain or tightness in the back or back of the leg. Lower the leg slightly until there is no pain or tightness and then dorsiflex the foot. A positive test includes the following responses: (1) pain (which extends down the back into the leg in the sciatic nerve distribution) is produced before 40 degrees is reached (80 to 90 degrees is normal hip flexion; pain after 70 degrees is probably joint pain; Figure18-66); (2) dorsiflexion aggravates the pain; and (3) pain relief occurs with

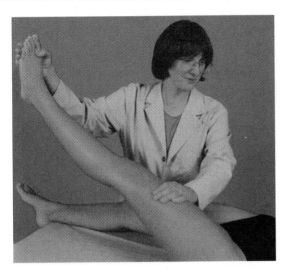

Figure 18-65 Straight leg-raising test.

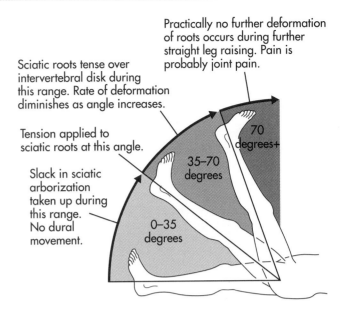

Practically no further deformation of roots occurs during further straight leg raising. Pain is probably joint pain.

Sciatic roots tense over intervertebral disk during this range. Rate of deformation diminishes as angle increases.

Tension applied to sciatic roots at this angle.

Slack in sciatic arborization taken up during this range. No dural movement.

70 degrees+

35–70 degrees

0–35 degrees

Figure 18-66 Observations on straight-leg raising with special reference to nerve root adhesions. (Adapted from, by permission of the publisher, *CJS* 9(1):44-48, 1966. ©Canadian Medical Association.)

flexion of the knee. Pain induced in this manner is caused by pressure on the dorsal roots of the lumbosacral nerves and is characteristic of a herniated disk. Repeat this maneuver with the other leg and compare the results. Nerve root irritation is suggested by pain in the lumbar area, hip, or posterior leg or by muscle spasm. If one leg is raised and pain is felt in the opposite side, then a large herniated **disk** is likely.

Thomas Test. The Thomas test evaluates flexion contractures of the hip. With the client in the supine position, ask the client to pull one knee up toward the chest as far as possible (Figure 18-67, *A*). In the individual with normal hip function, when the hip is flexed, the opposite leg remains flat on the examination table. For the individual with an immobile hip, the opposite hip and leg flex in response to flexion of the leg. Approximate the extent of the flexion contracture by noting the degree of flexion of the opposite leg (the angle between the client's leg and the table; Figure 18-67, *B*).

VARIATIONS FROM HEALTH

Osteoarthritis

Osteoarthritis is a degenerative joint disease characterized by a progressive loss of articular cartilage and formation of new bone at the joint surfaces and subchondral area. It occurs primarily in people older than 50 years, and the onset of signs and symptoms is insidious (see also Risk Factors box, p. 422.

Bony overgrowths that feel like hard, nontender nodules, 2 to 3 mm or larger in size, commonly occur in the fingers (Figure 18-68). When located in the distal interphalangeal joints, they are called Heberden nodes (nodules). When located in the proximal interphalangeal joints, they are called Bouchard nodes. Bony spurs, particularly in the knees, are also typical of osteoarthritis. Most symptoms are related to weight bearing and are relieved by rest.

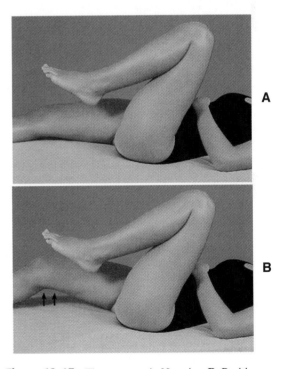

A

B

Figure 18-67 Thomas test. **A,** Negative. **B,** Positive.

Rheumatoid Arthritis

Rheumatoid arthritis is a chronic, systemic, inflammatory disorder that affects individuals of all ages, although its onset is most common in the 30s and 40s. It affects symmetrical joints. Deformities are related to inflammatory destruction of the joint with marginal bone erosion. Systemic complaints include fatigue and malaise in addition to joint pain. Joint inflammation is common, with marked edema,

Examination Step-by-Step

1. Observe the client for gait, ease of movement, ability to change positions, and signs of discomfort as the client enters the room and interacts during the examination.
2. Observe body alignment and stature with the client standing erect (front, back, and side). Note any deformities, spinal curvatures, atrophied or hypertrophied limbs, or age-related variations in posture and body size.
3. With the client sitting on the examination table, proceed with the examination.

HEAD

1. Inspect for musculature for facial symmetry of skinfolds, muscles, and wrinkles.
2. Palpate the temporomandibular joint while the client opens and closes the mouth.
3. To test range of motion, ask the client to:
   a. Open and close the mouth.
   b. Project the lower jaw.
   c. Move the jaw from side to side.
4. To test muscle strength, ask the client to:
   a. Bite down hard while you palpate the masseter muscles (CN V).
   b. Clench the teeth while you apply downward pressure on the chin.

CERVICAL SPINE

1. Inspect the neck for alignment and symmetry of skinfolds and muscles.
2. Palpate the cervical spine.
3. To evaluate range of motion, ask the client to:
   a. Touch the chin to the chest.
   b. Extend the head backward as far as possible.
   c. Bend the head laterally to each shoulder (touch the ear to the shoulder without raising the shoulder).
   d. Rotate the head from side to side (pointing the chin toward each shoulder).
4. To evaluate muscle strength, ask the client to:
   a. Push the cheek against your hand (right and left sides) (CN XI).
   b. Push the forehead against your hand.
   c. Push the head back against your hand.

SHOULDERS

1. Inspect the shoulders, including the muscles and the acromioclavicular joint, for contour and equality.
2. Palpate the shoulders and the bursal sites.

3. To test for range of motion, ask the client to:
   a. Extend both arms forward (forward flexion).
   b. Extend both arms backward (hyperextension).
   c. Put your hands behind your back as if you were going to reach up to touch your shoulder blade (internal rotation).
   d. Put your hands behind your head (external rotation).
4. To test for muscle strength, ask the client to:
   a. Hold the arms upward while you try to push them down (deltoid muscles).
   b. Extend the arms and then try to flex them while you try to pull them into extension (biceps muscle).
   c. Flex the arms and then try to extend them while you attempt to push them into a flexed position (triceps and muscle).
   d. Shrug the shoulders while you try to push down on them (trapezius muscle, CN XI).

ELBOWS

1. Inspect the elbows in both flexed and extended positions for carrying angle and contour.
2. Palpate the extensor surface of the ulna for nodules, the olecranon process and grooves, and the lateral epicondyles of the humerus for tenderness.
3. To test range of motion, ask the client to:
   a. Bend and straighten the elbow.
   b. Turn the hand face up (supination) and face down (pronation).

HANDS AND WRISTS

1. Inspect the dorsal and palmar surfaces of the hands for position, shape, contour, and number and completeness of digits. Inspect the wrists.
2. Palpate the hand and wrist joints.
3. To test range of motion of the hands and wrist, ask the client to:
   a. Spread the fingers apart and bring them back again.
   b. Make a fist.
   c. Touch the thumb to each fingertip and to the base of the little finger.
   d. Bend the fingers up and down at the metacarpophalangeal joint.
   e. Bend the hand up and down at the wrist.
   f. With the palm facing down, turn the hand to the right and to the left.

Examination Step-by-Step—cont'd

4. To test strength in the muscles of the hands and wrist, ask the client to:
   a. Maintain wrist flexion while you try to extend the wrist.
   b. Try to extend the wrist as you try to flex it.
   c. Squeeze your first two fingers as hard as he or she can.
   d. Extend the fingers while you push down on the dorsal surface.
   e. Flex the fingers while you push up on the ventral surface.
   f. Spread the fingers apart while you try to push them together.
   g. Push the fingers together while you try to pull them apart.

HIPS

1. Inspect the hips for symmetry in iliac crest height and level of gluteal folds.
2. Palpate the hips and the pelvis for stability, tenderness, and crepitus.
3. To test range of motion of the hips, ask the client (while supine) to:
   a. Raise the leg above the body with the knee extended.
   b. Bring the knee to the chest while keeping the other leg straight.
   c. Swing the leg laterally and medially while keeping the knee straight.
   d. Place the side of the foot on the opposite knee and move the flexed knee down toward the examination table (external rotation).
   e. Flex the knee and rotate the leg so that the flexed knee moves inward toward the opposite leg (internal rotation).
4. Ask the client (while either prone or standing) to swing the straightened leg behind the body.
5. To test muscle strength in the hips, ask the client (while supine) to:
   a. Raise the extended leg while you attempt to hold it down.
   b. Push both legs against your hands while your hands are placed on the bed on either side of the client's knees.
   c. Bring both legs together while your hands are placed on the bed between the client's knees.
8. To assess muscle strength in the hamstring, gluteal, abductor, and adductor muscles, ask the client to sit and perform alternate leg crossing.

KNEES

1. Inspect the knees for natural concavities and swelling.
2. Palpate the joint space and the popliteal space.

3. To test range of motion of the knee, ask the client to:
   a. Bend the knee.
   b. Straighten and stretch the leg.
4. To test muscle strength in the knee, ask the client to:
   a. Extend the leg as you try to bend it (quadriceps muscle strength).
   b. Bend the knees as you try to straighten them (hamstring muscle strength).

ANKLES AND FEET

1. Inspect the ankles and the feet during weight bearing and nonweight bearing for position, size, contour, and number of toes.
2. Palpate the ankle joint, Achilles tendon, and metatarsophalangeal joints.
3. To test range of motion of the ankle and foot, ask the client to:
   a. Point the foot up toward the ceiling.
   b. Point the foot down toward the floor.
   c. With the foot bent at the ankle, point the medial side of the foot toward the floor (inversion) and repeat with the lateral side (eversion).
   d. Rotate the ankle in order to turn the foot away from and then toward the other foot.
4. To test muscle strength in the ankle and foot, ask the client to:
   a. Flex the foot upward against your hand.
   b. Push the foot down against your hand.

THORACIC AND LUMBAR SPINE

1. Inspect the spine for alignment.
2. Palpate the spinous processes and the paravertebral muscles for tenderness and spasm.
3. To assess range of motion of the spine, ask the client to:
   a. Bend back as far as possible (hyperextend the spine).
   b. Bend to the right and to the left side as far as possible (lateral bending; you may need to stabilize the client's pelvis).
   c. Turn to the right and to the left in a circular motion (while you stabilize the pelvis).
   d. Slowly bend forward at the waist and try to touch the toes and then return to an upright position (watch from behind the client, take a "skyline view" of the spine, and observe for signs of scoliosis).

tenderness, pain, and limitation of movement. Stiffness early in the day is common. On palpation, joints will feel "boggy." Common deformities related to rheumatoid arthritis are ulnar drift, which is an ulnar deviation of the fingers caused by weakening of the capsuloligamentous structures and stretching of the extensor tendons (Figure 18-69, *A*); swan-neck deformity, which consists of flexion of the metacarpophalangeal and distal interphalangeal joints with hyperextension of the proximal interphalangeal joint (Figure 18-69, *B*); and boutonnière deformity, which is hyperextension of the metacarpophalangeal and distal interphalangeal joints with flexion of the proximal interphalangeal joint of the fingers

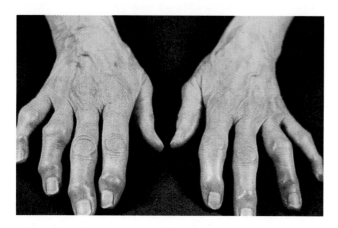

Figure 18-68 Degenerative joint disease. Heberden nodes at the distal interphalangeal joints and Bouchard nodes at the proximal interphalangeal joints. (Reprinted from the Clinical Slide Collection of the Rheumatic Diseases, copyright 1991, 1995, 1997. Used by permission of the American College of Rheumatology.)

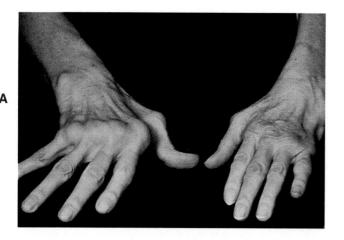

A

Figure 18-69 Deformities of the hand secondary to rheumatoid arthritis. **A,** Ulnar deviation and subluxation of metacarpophalangeal joints. **B,** Swan-neck deformities. **C,** Boutonnière deformity. (Reprinted from the Clinical Slide Collection of the Rheumatic Diseases, copyright 1991, 1995, 1997. Used by permission of the American College of Rheumatology.)

(Figure 18-69, *C*). Boutonnière deformity is the result of a tendon rupture and is also commonly seen after trauma.

Gout

Gout is a crystal-induced arthritis related to abnormalities in purine metabolism that result in prolonged hyperuricemia and subsequent deposition of uric acid crystals in the joint space. It can be caused by an overproduction of uric acid or an interference in uric acid excretion. It most commonly occurs in men older than 40 years. Joint involvement is usually monarticular. Classically, the proximal phalanx of the great toe is the joint affected. However, joints of the foot, ankle, and knee may also be affected. Pain is typically constant and severe (often called "exquisite") during an acute attack and is characterized by marked erythema, swelling, warmth, and tenderness (Figure 18-70, *A*). **Tophi**, hard, painless urate crystal deposits, may also occur on the ears and in the joints (Figure 18-70, *B*).

Osteoporosis

Osteoporosis is a systemic condition in which a decrease in bone mass occurs because bone resorption exceeds bone deposition. The bones become fragile, and fractures may occur even with minor trauma or during routine activities. The hips, vertebrae, and wrists are the most common fracture sites. Osteoporosis is most common in women (4:1, women/men). A decrease in calcium intake, decrease in estrogen production in women (menopause), lack of weight-bearing activities and exercise, and sedentary lifestyle are among the contributing factors (see the Risk Factors box on p. 422).

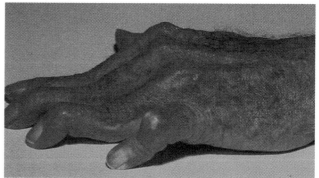

B

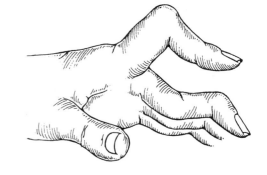

C

Muscle Weakness

The client who has difficulty in walking up steps or getting up from a sitting position or the client who is able to rise only by pushing off with the hands and arms or by pulling up by grasping some nearby furniture may have a problem involving the shoulder or hip girdle musculature. Further tests are necessary to ascertain the presence of muscular dystrophy, myasthenia gravis, parkinsonism, or polymyositis.

Myasthenia gravis should be strongly suspected if the following are true: (1) the client who has difficulty rising can rise easily after being instructed to sit back and relax for a few minutes; (2) the client is a woman in her 20s or a man in his 50s or 60s; (3) muscle atrophy is not present; and (4) the client has ptosis or extraocular muscle weakness resulting in diplopia.

Polymyositis is a progressive inflammatory disease that occurs in children and adults. It involves progressive symmetrical weakness of the limb girdles, neck, and pharynx. The client who has polymyositis may have pain; muscle atrophy; or a rash, particularly around the eyelids, and low-grade fever.

Parkinsonism may be the underlying cause when the aging client has difficulty rising from a chair. This impression is substantiated if the client says stiffness is a problem. In such a case, it is important to be alert for signs of flexion posture, slow and intermittent movement, frequent tremor, masked facies, or movement of several joint units at one time because these signs are also characteristic of Parkinson's disease.

The client who complains of intermittent bouts of muscle weakness requires methodical and careful investigation for ischemic attacks; disorders of glucose metabolism (diabetes); anemia; and serum electrolyte disturbances, particularly of potassium or calcium ion concentrations.

Transient ischemic attacks may cause a focal episode of motor dysfunction related to vascular disease, such as arteriosclerosis or essential hypertension. Listening for bruits over the neck vessels in the elderly client with muscle weakness is particularly important, since these bruits might strengthen the impression of vascular disease.

Clinical correlation of signs of muscle weakness and disease entities has shown that each neuromuscular disease has a general predilection for a particular group of muscles. A given pattern of weakness, then, suggests the possibility of a certain disease and excludes others. An example lies in the adage that peripheral muscle involvement in the extremities is of muscular origin, whereas distal disease is of neuropathic origin. Further explanation of the correlation of assessment data with underlying disease processes is presented in Table 18-4.

Hypokalemia

Since the ratio of the concentrations of potassium ions of the intracellular environment to the extracellular fluid determines the rate of cell firing, a deficit of this ion is accomplished by disorders of structure and function in muscular and neural tissues. Both skeletal and smooth muscles are affected by hypokalemia. The client complains of varying degrees of weakness and lassitude. Extreme hypokalemia may be accompanied by muscular paralysis. Some other signs that will help confirm hypokalemia as the cause of muscle weakness are abnormalities in motor and secretory activities of the gastrointestinal tract, changes in electrocardiograms, and dilute urine. Some of the conditions known to be correlated with a deficiency of potassium are diarrhea; excessive losses in the urine resulting from the use of chlorothiazide, mercurial diuretics, or steroid hormones; Cushing's syndrome; and primary aldosteronism.

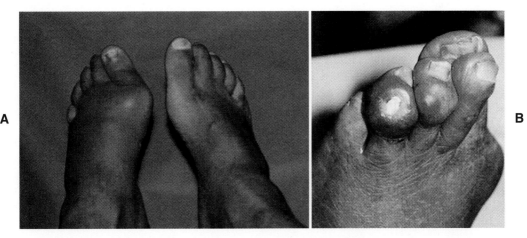

Figure 18-70 **A,** Inflammatory response of acute gout with swelling and inflammation of the first metatarsophalangeal joint left foot. **B,** Tophi due to chronic gout with ulceration over the distal interphalangeal joint of the fourth toe. (From Swartz MH: *Textbook of physical diagnosis: history and examination,* ed. 3, Philadelphia, 1998, WB Saunders.)

Involuntary Contraction of Skeletal Muscles

Fasciculations

Fasciculations are the visible, spontaneous contractions of a number of muscle fibers supplied by a single motor nerve filament. Visible dimpling or twitching may occur, although there is usually insufficient power generated to move the joint.

Fasciculations that occur during muscular contraction (twitching) are associated with conditions of irritability that result in poorly coordinated contraction of small and large motor units. Benign fasciculation occurs in the normal individual and is characterized by normal muscle strength and size. Rarely, myokymia, a rippling appearance of the muscle occasioned by numerous fasciculations, is noted in a normal individual.

Fascicular twitches noted during rest in a client with exaggerated muscular weakness and atrophy are characteristic of a peripheral motor neuron disorder. Generalized fascicular twitching that occurs in a progressive, wavelike pattern over an entire muscle and progresses to complete paralysis is characteristic of certain types of poisoning (organic phosphate) and of poliomyelitis.

TABLE 18-4	Topographical Patterns of Muscle Palsy	
Muscle Weakness or Paralysis	**Signs**	**Possible Cause**
Ocular	Diplopia Ptosis Strabismus	Myasthenia gravis Thyroid disease Ocular dystrophy and botulism
Bifacial	Inability to smile Inability to expose teeth Inability to close eyes	Myasthenia gravis Facioscapulohumeral dystrophy Guillain-Barré syndrome
Bulbar	Dysphonia Dysarthria Dysphagia Hanging-jaw facial weakness (may or may not be present)	Myasthenia gravis Myotonic dystrophy Botulism Diphtheria Poliomyelitis Early polymyositis
Cervical	Inability to lift head from pillow (hanging-head syndrome) Weakness of posterior neck muscles	Polymyositis Dermatomyositis Progressive muscular dystrophy
Bibrachial	Weakness, atrophy, and fasciculations of hands, arms, and shoulders (hanging-arm syndrome)	Amyotrophic lateral sclerosis
Bicrural	Lower leg weakness Floppy feet Inability to walk on heels and toes	Diabetic polyneuropathy
Limb-girdle	Inability to raise arms Inability to rise from sitting position Difficulty in climbing stairs without use of arms Waddling gait	Polymyositis Dermatomyositis Progressive muscular dystrophy
Distal limb	Footdrop with steppage gain Weakness of all leg muscles Wristdrop—weakness of handgrips ("claw hand"; later sign)	Familial polyneuropathy
Generalized or universal	Limb and cranial muscle weakness (acute in onset and periodic) Slow onset and progressive paralysis Atrophy Fasciculations of limb and trunk muscles No sensory loss Paralysis developing over several days Mild degree of generalized weakness	Electrolyte imbalance Hypokalemia Hypocalcemia Hypomagnesemia Motor system disease Guillain-Barré syndrome Glycogen storage diseases Vitamin D deficiency
Single muscles or groups of muscles	Inability to contract affected muscles	Thyrotoxic myopathy (almost always neuropathic)

Muscle Cramps and Spasm

Muscular spasm, or tremor (Table 18-5), may occur at rest or with movement and may be noted in the normal individual with metabolic and electrolyte alterations. Cramping is a common complaint following excessive sweating and with hyponatremia, hypocalcemia, hypomagnesemia, and hyperuricemia. Diseases that magnify these alterations are correlated with the presence of muscle spasm. A continuous spasm that is heightened by attempts to move the affected muscles occurs in tetanus and following the bite of the black widow spider. Paravertebral muscle spasm is often responsible for low back pain.

Muscle cramp commonly occurs after a day of vigorous exercise. As the feet cool, a sudden movement may trigger a strong contraction of the foot and leg. The musculature is visible, and the muscle feels hard on palpation. The spasm will cease in response to stretch of the fibers. In the case of the gastrocnemius muscle, the stretch can be achieved by dorsiflexion of the foot. Occasionally massage is helpful in relaxing the spasm.

Fasciculations commonly appear before and after the cramp. They are further evidence of the hyperexcitability of the neuromuscular unit. Muscle spasms occur more frequently when the client is dehydrated or sweating and in the pregnant client.

The cause of the pain associated with muscle cramp has not been determined, but some believe it is due to increased metabolic needs of the hyperactive muscles and the collection of the metabolic waste products, such as lactic acid, within the muscle.

Tetany

Hypocalcemia and hypomagnesemia may cause the involuntary spasms of skeletal muscle that resemble cramping. The calcium deficit causes depolarization of the distal segments of the motor nerve. Furthermore, a change occurs within the muscle fibers themselves, since nerve section or block does not prevent these tetanic contractions. Tetanic cramps can be elicited by percussing the motor nerve leading to a muscle group at frequencies of 15 to 20 per second. **Chvostek's sign** is the spasm of the facial muscles produced by tapping over the facial nerve near its foramen of exit. The instability of the neuromuscular unit is heightened by hyperventilation (alkalosis) and hypoxia (ischemia). Tetany in its mildest form affects the distal musculature in the form of carpopedal spasm, but it may involve all the muscles of the body, except those of the eye.

Myalgia

"I hurt all over" is commonly the chief complaint of the client with diffuse muscle pain that accompanies many types of systemic infection (e.g., influenza, measles, rheumatic fever, brucellosis, dengue fever, or salmonellosis). Soreness and aching are other descriptions given for this type of involvement. Little is known of the cause of myalgia.

Fibromyositis is inflammation of the fibrous tissue in muscle, fascia, and nerves. The client may complain of pain and tenderness in a muscle after exposure to cold, dampness, or minor trauma. Firm, tender zones, occasionally several centimeters in diameter, may be found on palpation. Palpation, active contraction, or passive stretching increases the pain.

Intense pain localized to a smaller group of muscles may be a result of epidemic myalgia, also called pleurodynia, "painful neck," or "devil's grip." Intense pain at the beginning of neurological involvement may occur in herpes zoster. The segmental pattern of the intense pain of herpes zoster is caused by the inflammation of spinal nerves and dorsal root ganglia that occurs 3 to 4 days before the skin eruption.

The initial symptoms of rheumatoid arthritis may be diffuse muscular soreness and aching, which may antedate the joint involvement by weeks or months. The muscles are tender, and the client describes the pain as occurring not at the time of activity but hours later. An increased sedimentation rate or a positive latex fixation test may support the conclusion of rheumatoid involvement.

TABLE 18-5 Tremor Classification

Cause	Type and Rate of Movement	Description
Anxiety	Fine, rapid, 10 to 12/sec	Irregular, variable Increased by attempts to move part; decreased by relaxation of part
Parkinsonism	Fine, regular, or coarse, 2 to 5/sec	Occurs at rest May be inhibited by movement Involves flexion of finger and thumb "pill rolling" Accompanied by rigidity, "cogwheel" phenomena, bradykinesia
Cerebellar tremor	Variable rate	Evident only on movement (most prominent on finger-to-nose test) Dysmetria (seen when client is asked to pat rapidly; pats are of unequal force and do not all arrive at same point)
Essential or senile	Coarse, 3 to 7/sec	Involves the jaw, sometimes the tongue, and sometimes the entire head
Metabolic		Disappears on complete relaxation or in response to alcohol Variable Client is obviously ill; if illness is a result of hepatic failure, client will have other signs such as palpable liver, spider nevi

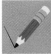

Sample Documentation and Diagnoses

FOCUSED HEALTH HISTORY (SUBJECTIVE DATA)

Ms. L, a 50-year-old executive secretary, complains of swelling and burning in both hands on and off for the past 2 weeks. States, "My hands hurt and the swelling is so bad in the morning, I can hardly type." States joints in hands feel warm, swollen, and tender. Pain and stiffness are worse in the morning, lasting about 1 to 2 hours. Improves over the course of the day. Has noticed increased fatigue, especially in the afternoon. Takes ibuprofen 600 mg for pain as needed. States has been in good health; no recent illnesses or change in weight. Denies any chronic illnesses or family history of arthritis. Is single and lives with her sister, who is in good health.

FOCUSED PHYSICAL EXAMINATION (OBJECTIVE DATA)

General appearance: 50-year-old Caucasian female who grimaces when hands are touched, tends to pull away, and guards both hands.

Extremities: Normal range of motion (ROM) in shoulders, elbows, hips, and knees; ROM of wrists is diminished—10 degrees radial, 25 degrees ulnar. Hands warm to touch; veins engorged with spindle-shaped swelling of the proximal interphalangeal (PIP) joints, third digits bilaterally. Ulnar deviation of metacarpophalangeal (MCP) joints noted. Tinel's and Phalen's tests negative.

Laboratory values: Erythrocyte sedimentation rate (ESR) elevated—25 mm/hr; white blood count mildly elevated with normal differential; red blood cell count slightly decreased (normocytic anemia); rheumatoid factor—positive.

DIAGNOSES

HEALTH PROBLEM

Probable rheumatoid arthritis; needs further evaluation

NURSING DIAGNOSES

Acute Pain Related to Inflammatory Process

Defining Characteristics

- Subjective communication of pain
- Self-focusing
- Guarding behavior
- Grimaces in pain

NURSING DIAGNOSES

Activity Intolerance Related to Anemia and Disease State

Defining Characteristics

- Verbal reports of fatigue and weakness especially in early afternoon
- Verbal reports of loss of energy

NURSING DIAGNOSES

Impaired Physical Mobility Related to Joint and Systemic Involvement

Defining Characteristics

- Limited range of motion of hands
- Decreased muscle strength and control of hands and wrist
- Impaired coordination of hands

Critical Thinking Questions

Review the Sample Documentation and Diagnoses box to answer questions 1 and 2.

1. What other history information would be helpful to obtain?
2. What history examination findings would you expect if Ms. L had osteoarthritis?
3. What physical examination findings are distinctive for rheumatoid arthritis?

4. What physical findings would you expect to see in the following problems: osteoarthritis, gout, and carpal tunnel syndrome?
5. Describe how you would assess active and passive range of motion (ROM). Discuss the implication of physical examination finding of differences between a joint's active and passive ROM.

Answers are available on the MERLIN website (www.harcourthealth.com/MERLIN/Barkauskas/). And be sure to check the website regularly for additional learning activities!

Remember to check out the Online Study Guide!
www.harcourthealth.com/MERLIN/Barkauskas/

Neurological System, Including Mental Status

Learning Objectives

On successful study of this chapter and completion of related learning experiences, the learner will be able to:
- Describe the anatomy and physiology of the central and peripheral neurological system.
- Identify six major areas of neurological assessment.

- Demonstrate and provide rationale for specific examination techniques for the neurological system.
- Explain the purposes for conducting a mental status examination.

Outline

Purpose of Examination

The purpose of the neurological examination is to determine (a) the presence of nervous system malfunction; (b) the location, type, and extent of nervous system lesions; and (c) the presence of healthy nervous system functioning for rehabilitation.

The neurological system integrates all the functions of the body. It controls cognitive and voluntary behavioral processes, as well as subconscious and involuntary body functions. The major functions of the neurological system are reception (sensory), integration, and adaptation. The nervous system receives stimuli from the environment, adjusts body functions to the environment, and effects changes to ensure homeokinesis, or survival.

PURPOSE OF MENTAL STATUS EXAMINATION

The mental status examination is an integral part of the neurological examination. In the context of the total health assessment, this appraisal begins with the initial contact with the client. Most examiners make assessments of mental status while obtaining the client's history and perform special tests of cognitive function afterward. The purpose of the mental status examination is to assess the client's current emotional and mental capacity and functioning. The mental status examination provides a baseline for a client's psychological state and specific information that helps to establish a nursing diagnosis. The examination includes a description of the client's:

- General appearance
- Behavior
- Mood or affect
- Characteristics of speech
- Orientation
- Thought processes
- Insight and judgment
- Memory and learning
- Perceptions and attitudes

The examiner focuses on assessing the client's ability to interact with the environment. Responses elicited during a single interview are only samples of the individual's thoughts and feelings. Fears regarding illness, family responsibilities, attitudes of others, and financial worries are some factors that can alter a client's feelings and behaviors. Considering the effects of prescription and illicit drugs on the client's mental processes and behaviors is important.

For the purpose of facilitating learning of this complex system, this chapter is organized with the physical assessment portion of the neurological examination presented first, followed by techniques for examination of mental status. This organization, however, is not the usual order for conducting the assessment; in practice, the mental status examination begins when the practitioner first encounters the client and continues throughout the examination (see Chapter 2).

ANATOMY AND PHYSIOLOGY

All components of the neurological system are highly interconnected and integrated in function. Maturation of the nervous system continues throughout childhood until early adolescence. For instructional purposes, the nervous system is divided into two major parts: (1) the central nervous system, which consists of (a) the brain and (b) spinal cord, and (2) the peripheral nervous system, which is composed of (a) 12 pairs of cranial nerves, (b) 31 pairs of spinal nerves, and (c) the autonomic nervous system. The autonomic nervous system is divided into the sympathetic (thoracolumbar) and parasympathetic (craniosacral) nervous systems. The autonomic nervous system is considered part of the peripheral nervous system because in most parts of the body innervated by these systems, their structures appear together.

Central Nervous System

Brain

The brain is made up of gray and white matter. Gray matter contains cell bodies, and white matter includes myelinated nerve fibers. The brain consists of the cerebrum, the largest part of the brain, which is composed of two hemispheres; the brainstem (midbrain, pons, and medulla): the diencephalon (thalmus, hypothalmus, epithalmus, and subthalmus); and the cerebellum (Figure 19-1). The left side of the brain controls language, whereas the right side is the nonverbal, or perceptual, hemisphere. Ninety percent of the population has a dominant left hemisphere, and these individuals are right-handed. The cerebral functions interact with the reticular activating system, located in the upper brainstem and diencephalon, to control conscious movement, thought, and perception. The major cerebellar functions influence mechanisms of equilibrium, muscle tone, and coordinated movement, such as control of gait (Figure 19-2).

Approximately 20% of the oxygen consumed by the body is used to provide energy to the brain. Since the brain depends totally on glucose for metabolism, a lack of oxygen for 2 to 5 minutes can result in irreversible brain damage. The circle of Willis, located at the base of the brain, is an arterial communication between the right and the left cerebral circulation. Its function is to equalize blood flow to various parts of the brain. Superficial and deep veins drain into the system of sinuses of the dura mater, which empties into the internal jugular vein.

Spinal Cord

A cross section of the spinal cord reveals H-shaped gray matter surrounded by white matter. The gray matter is made up of cell bodies, axons, and dendrites. The gray matter also

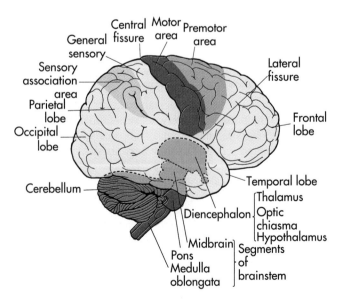

Figure 19-1 Lateral view of the brain. (Modified from Smith CG: *Serial dissections of the human brain*, Baltimore, 1981, Urban & Schwarzenberg.)

contains posterior (dorsal) and anterior (ventral) horns. The actual shape and extent of the white and gray matter vary at different levels of the cord. Figure 19-3 shows a cross section of the spinal cord, with a labeling scheme of laminae (layers) from I to X, as described by Rexed, to show the major longitudinal columns. The columns are identified according to similarity in appearance and function. For example, lamina V receives dorsal root afferent fibers from sensory fibers, such as those that transmit pain, temperature, and light touch (spinothalamic tract).

Motor and Sensory Pathways

Neurons that transmit impulses can be motor, sensory, or mixed. Motor neurons, or **efferent neurons**, carry impulses away from the central nervous system to effectors, located in muscles, organs, and glands. Sensory neurons, or **afferent neurons**, carry impulses to the central nervous system from receptors. General sensory afferent fibers involve sensation such as pain and light touch.

The dorsal nerve roots carry afferent (sensory) impulses from receptors to the dorsal root ganglia, in which cell bodies of the sensory nerves are located, to the spinal cord. Ventral roots carry efferent (motor) impulses from the spinal cord to the body.

In the spinal cord, descending tracts (pyramidal and extrapyramidal) carry efferent (motor) impulses away from the brain. Ascending tracts (dorsal columns or spinothalamic tract) carry afferent (sensory) impulses to the brain.

Sensory (Ascending) Pathways. Sensory impulses travel from the receptors through afferent fibers in the peripheral nerve, through the dorsal root, and to the spinal cord. Various types of receptors are stimulated by pain and temperature, position and movement, or visceral sensations of fullness or cramping. In the spinal cord, sensory impulses travel via two major pathways to higher levels of the nervous system: (a) the posterior columns and (b) the spinothalamic

tract. The lateral spinothalamic tract contains sensory fibers that transmit the sensations of pain and temperature. Fibers in the posterior columns transmit stimuli involved with position; vibration; light touch; and manipulation with digits, such as stereognosis and graphesthesia (see Figure 19-3).

Motor (Descending) Pathways

Pyramidal System. The pyramidal system (corticospinal tracts) consists of neurons of spinal cord white matter arranged in long columns, or fiber tracts, lateral to the gray matter. The majority of these columns cross to the contralateral side (desuccate) at the level of the medulla. Those that do not cross in the medulla continue as the anterior corticospinal tract and cross over at the cervical or thoracic level of the cord. The **pyramidal tract** uniquely transmits stimuli concerned with voluntary movements and temporal (time) and spatial (e.g., perceiving change over time) qualities (Figure 19-4).

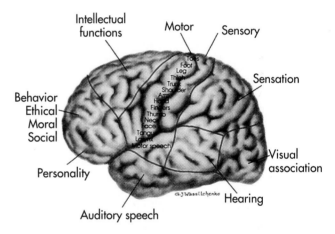

Figure 19-2 Functional subdivisions of the cerebral cortex.

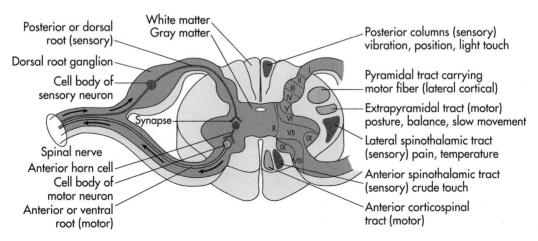

Figure 19-3 Cross section of the spinal cord. Spinal nerve roots and their neurons appear on the left side. Spinal nerve tracts appear in the white matter on the right side. All tracts and nerves are bilateral. (Adapted from Watson C: *Basic human neuroanatomy: an introductory atlas,* ed. 5, Boston, 1995, Little, Brown.)

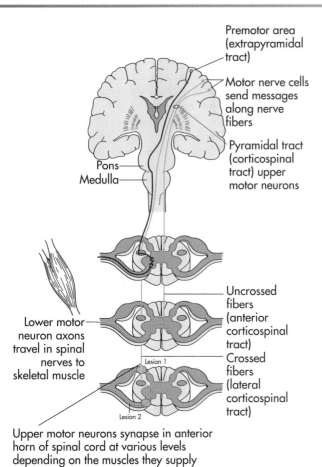

Figure 19-4 Major motor pathways between the cerebral cortex and lower motor neurons in the spinal cord. Lesion 1: Upper motor neuron with motor damage on the contralateral side. Lesion 2: Lower motor neuron with motor damage on the ipsilateral side.

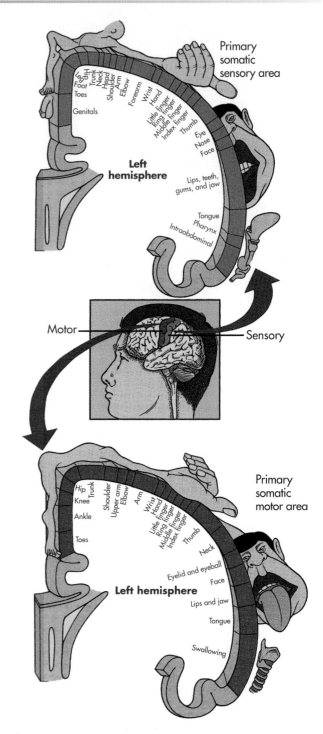

Figure 19-5 Representation of specific body parts in the motor strip of the frontal lobe. (From Thibodeau GA, Patton KT: *Anatomy and physiology*, ed. 4, St. Louis, 1999, Mosby.)

Upper and Lower Motor Neurons. A model of a two-neuron chain is used here to simplify understanding of the basic structure of the pyramidal tract. The chain begins in the motor area of the cerebral cortex, located anterior to the central sulcus. The size of the cortical area correlates with the degree of skilled function carried out by a particular body part (Figure 19-5). Note that the face and hands cover the largest areas. This neural chain travels to skeletal muscle and is contained in one of the many ascending and descending pathways in the spinal cord.

The **upper motor neuron** cell bodies are located in the cerebral cortex, and their axons cross over to the opposite side (contralateral) at the level of the medulla to synapse with the lower motor neuron cell body in the cranial nerve motor nuclei or the anterior horn of the spinal cord (see Figure 19-4). The axon of the **lower motor neuron** becomes the peripheral nerve. Because upper motor neurons affect motor activity only through the lower motor neurons, the latter are referred to as the final common pathway.

Damage to a lower motor neuron will cause motor impairment on the same (ipsilateral) side of the body, whereas

damage to an upper motor neuron leads to motor impairment on the contralateral side. For example, the facial nerve (cranial nerve [CN] VII) is a lower motor neuron. Damage to the motor portion of the right facial nerve results in impaired movement of the right side of the face. However, if a stroke damages the right upper motor neuron that synapses with the right facial nerve, the result would be impaired mo-

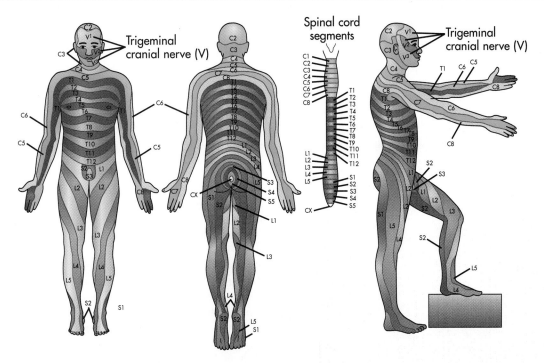

Figure 19-6 Dermatomes of the body. Each dorsal (sensory) spinal root innervates one dermatome. The first cervical nerve usually has no cutaneous distribution. The trigeminal nerve (CN V) supplies most of the general somatic sensory innervation to the anterior part of the head. (From Thibodeau GA, Patton KT: *Anatomy and physiology,* ed. 4, St. Louis, 1999, Mosby.)

tor function of the left side of the face, primarily its lower portion.

Extrapyramidal System. The **extrapyramidal system** is more complex than other motor pathways. It includes all the motor neurons originating in the motor cortex and the cerebellum outside the pyramidal tracts, and to the sensory (spinothalamic) tracts. The extrapyramidal tract integrates input from many sources and modifies the motor impulses of the pyramidal system, especially those needed to maintain posture, balance, and slow movement. Since the sensory tracts are located close to the corticospinal tracts in the spinal cord, it is common for both sensory and motor deficits to occur with spinal cord damage.

Peripheral Nervous System

Spinal Nerves

Each spinal cord nerve segment communicates with specific parts of the body through 31 pairs of spinal nerves, both afferent and efferent, at that level (eight cervical, 12 thoracic, five lumbar, five sacral, and one coccygeal). Each nerve is designated by a letter and a number to indicate its location. For example, C8 is the eighth cervical nerve. Each spinal nerve has a dorsal root, which carries afferent (sensory) impulses to the cord, and a ventral root, which carries efferent (motor) impulses away from the cord. Sensory fibers (dorsal root) from a single spinal nerve that serve a particular skin surface are collectively called a **dermatome** (Figure 19-6). Because of considerable overlap between adjacent der-

---

BOX 19-1

FIVE COMPONENTS OF A REFLEX ARC

1. Sensory (afferent) peripheral nerve
2. Intact interneuron (synapse) in the spinal cord
3. Motor (efferent) peripheral nerve
4. Intact neuromuscular junction (synapse in the muscle)
5. Competent muscle

---

matome areas, sensory loss results only if a number of dermatomes are damaged.

Reflex Arc

Reflexes are part of the motor system. They control automatic responses to stimuli at the level of the spinal cord (segmental response), freeing the cortex from involvement in most muscle movements that occur in the body. Reflexes provide rapid responses, such as withdrawal from painful stimuli. The simplest reflex arc is monosynaptic, in which the sensory fiber interacts directly with the motor neuron (Figure 19-7). See Box 19-1 for the five components of a reflex arc.

Skeletal muscles contract when they are stretched by contraction of the antagonistic muscle, the pull of gravity, or external manipulation. The muscles also contract when their tendons are stretched. Deep tendon reflexes (DTRs), or muscle stretch reflexes, are segmental responses elicited by striking a tendon with a reflex hammer. This stimulus stretches the neuromuscular spindles of the muscle group.

Figure 19-7 illustrates the deep tendon reflex, with the patellar tendon reflex used as an example. The patellar tendon of the quadriceps muscle is attached to the tibia. Tapping this tendon with a reflex hammer causes the muscle to be stretched, activating the muscle spindles and thereby the femoral (primary afferent) nerve, to the spinal cord. In the spinal cord the sensory neurons synapse with the alpha motor nerve in the cord segment (L3 and L4). The efferent

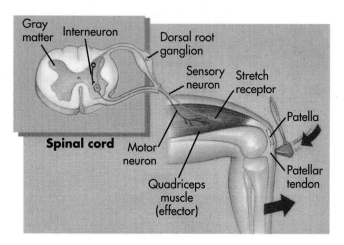

Figure 19-7 Deep tendon (stretch) reflex (knee-jerk or patellar tendon reflex). *Inset* shows afferent fibers from the muscle spindle and tendon organs, and efferent fibers to the muscle and spindle. Note that the patellar tendon of the extensor muscle attaches to the tibia below the knee. (From Thibodeau GA, Patton KT: *Anatomy and physiology,* ed. 4, St. Louis, 1999, Mosby.)

fibers carry impulses back to the muscle, resulting in contraction of the quadriceps muscle and extension of the leg. Dysfunction of the tendon reflex, therefore, could result from problems in the thigh muscle, the femoral nerve, or the segment of the spinal cord being tested.

Superficial Reflexes. Superficial reflexes are reactions that can be elicited by stroking the skin or muscle. Examples of these reflexes include the abdominal reflex, which tests spinal cord levels T8 through T12 (see Figure 17-31); the cremasteric reflex, observed in males (T12-L2) when stroking of the skin of the inner upper thigh results in testicular movement on the same side; and the plantar reflex (L4-L5, S1-S2), elicited by firmly stroking the lateral surface of the sole of the foot to stimulate plantar flexion of the toes.

Cranial Nerves

Twelve pairs of cranial nerves emerge from the brain or brainstem. Cranial nerves consist of fibers that have sensory (afferent) and motor (efferent) functions, as well as special sensory afferent functions such as vision, hearing, and equilibrium. Cranial nerves also contain special visceral efferent nerve fibers for voluntary motor function; special visceral afferent fibers carry visceral sensation, such as taste and smell (Figure 19-8).

CN I—Olfactory Nerve. The olfactory nerve is sensory for smell. The peripheral neurons of the olfactory nerve penetrate the nasal mucosa in the roof of the nose, the upper septum, and the medial wall of the superior nasal concha. Unless the individual sniffs or inspires deeply, most of the inspired air does not contact the olfactory epithelium; during normal respiration, inspired air does not rise that high in the nares (see Figure 13-5).

CN II—Optic Nerve. The optic nerve, sensory for sight, is described in Chapter 12 (see the discussions of ex-

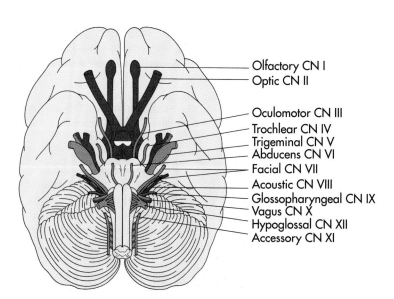

Figure 19-8 Diagram of the base of the brain showing the entrance or exit of the cranial nerves.

amination of visual acuity, visual fields, retinal fields, and the optic disc).

CN III—Oculomotor Nerve; CN IV—Trochlear Nerve; CN VI—Abducens Nerve. The oculomotor, trochlear, and abducens nerves, which control movement of the eyeball, elevation of the eyelid, and pupillary constriction, are always tested together. These cranial nerves are also described in Chapter 12 (note the sections on neuromuscular and extraocular muscle function and tests of eye movement).

CN V—Trigeminal Nerve. The trigeminal nerve is the motor to the muscles of mastication and sensory to the cornea; mucosa of the nose and mouth; and skin of the face and forehead in perceiving touch, temperature, and pain. The sensory fibers are contained in one of the three divisions of the nerve: ophthalmic, maxillary, or mandibular (Figure 19-9).

CN VII—Facial Nerve. The facial nerve is motor to the facial muscles and sensory to taste on the anterior two thirds of the tongue. Visceral sensation from the salivary glands and mucosa of the mouth and pharynx are also conducted by CN VII. In addition, the facial nerve carries parasympathetic fibers that stimulate secretion of the salivary glands; the lacrimal glands; and the mucosa of the nose, palate, and nasopharynx.

CN VIII—Acoustic Nerve. The acoustic nerve is composed of two divisions: the cochlear and the vestibular.

Cochlear Division. The cochlear division is sensory for hearing. Tests for cochlear function are described in Chapter 13.

Vestibular Division. Tests for vestibular functions, or **equilibrium**, are not routine in the physical examination. One method used to test vestibular function by producing changes in the flow of endolymph is the caloric test. In the caloric test, the examiner irrigates the client's ear with ice water; a normal reaction includes nausea, dizziness, and nystagmus.

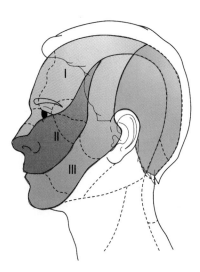

Figure 19-9 Cutaneous (sensory) fields of the head and upper part of the neck. The cutaneous fields of the three branches of the trigeminal nerve are identified as I, ophthalmic; II, maxillary; and III, mandibular.

CN IX—Glossopharyngeal Nerve; CN X—Vagus Nerve. The glossopharyngeal and vagus nerves are closely related both anatomically and physiologically, and they are tested as a unit. The glossopharyngeal nerve contains sensory and motor fibers. The sensory component is taste on the posterior third of the tongue and sensation from the tonsillar and pharyngeal mucosa. CN IX also has sensory fibers for the carotid sinus and body. The motor function of this nerve innervates the pharynx and parotid glands to control swallowing, gagging, and salivation.

The vagus nerve is sensory for the external ear and pharynx. It functions as a motor nerve to the soft palate, pharynx, larynx, and esophagus. CN X provides parasympathetic control to smooth and cardiac muscle and abdominal organs.

CN XI—Spinal Accessory Nerve. The spinal accessory nerve supplies the sternocleidomastoid and trapezius muscles with motor innervation.

CN XII—Hypoglossal Nerve. The hypoglossal nerve provides motor fibers to the muscles of the tongue, making possible articulation of lingual speech sounds and swallowing.

Autonomic Nervous System

The function of the autonomic nervous system is to maintain a stable internal environment for the body. The sympathetic nervous system, also called the thoracolumbar division, is activated during stress and brings about widespread responses, such as increased heart rate, vasodilation in skeletal muscle, reduction in gastric secretions, and dilation of bronchioles. These "fight or flight" responses enable us to be physically prepared to handle potential danger. Sympathetic (thoracolumbar) preganglionic fibers emerge from T1 to L2 levels of the spinal column.

The parasympathetic system, also called the craniosacral division, is associated with conservation; restoration; and maintenance of normal body functions, such as decreasing the heart rate and increasing gastrointestinal motility. Parasympathetic (craniosacral) preganglionic fibers emerge from the cranial nerves (III, VI, IX, X) and S1 through S4 segments of the spinal cord. A mnemonic device used to remember cranial nerves is: *On Old Olympus Towering Top A Finn And German Viewed Some Hops.*

EXAMINATION OF THE NEUROLOGICAL SYSTEM

Focused Health History

Clues to areas of abnormality may be evident during the client's history, such as orientation, speech, and ability to interact with the examiner. The presence of certain symptoms in a client who appears normal may indicate neurological problems (see Box 19-2 for major areas of the neurological examination). If any symptom is present, it is important to obtain further information about onset, course since onset (duration, intensity, frequency), location, quality, quantity, setting, associated phenomena, aggravating and alleviating factors, and the client's concerns (see Chapter 2).

Present Health/Illness Status

1. Presence of numbness, tingling, or loss of feeling
2. Difficulty with speaking, vision, or hearing
3. Any physical disability
4. Medications, including prescriptions, over-the-counter, and herbal preparations
5. Problems with coordination or balance
6. Change in behavior, memory, ability to communicate
7. Shakiness or tremors of the hands or legs
8. Presence of anxiety or depression
9. Recent changes in self, such as alterations in sleep habits, changes in sexual activity, unexplained weight gain or loss, difficulty in performing usual daily activities
10. Use of alcohol or other mind-altering drugs
11. Exposures to chemical agents, fumes, toxic substances

Family History

1. Headaches, stroke
2. Neurological conditions, such as Tay Sachs, Huntington's disease, muscular dystrophy
3. Mental illness, depression

Past Health History

1. Seizures, fainting, or dizziness
2. Headaches
3. Head injury, nerve injury, or major trauma
4. Neurosurgery
5. Mental illness, depression, anxiety, post-traumatic stress disorder
6. Stroke

Symptom Analysis

Hand Tremor or Shaking

1. **Onset:** sudden or gradual, recent occurrence or long-standing problem
2. **Course since onset:** frequency, timing to specific events, situations, duration
3. **Location:** unilateral or bilateral
4. **Quality:** specific characteristics of tremors such as fine movements, gross movements
5. **Quantity:** degree of impairment with usual activities

BOX 19-2

MAJOR AREAS OF NEUROLOGICAL EXAMINATION

1. Mental status (performed first during the interview, but in this chapter discussed after the other areas of examination)
2. Cranial nerves
3. Proprioception and cerebellar function
4. Motor function (see Chapter 18: Musculoskeletal System)
5. Sensory function
6. Deep tendon reflexes

6. **Setting:** environmental effects of home, work, stressful situations
7. **Associated phenomena:** change in sensory perceptions, weakness, lack of coordination
8. **Alleviating and aggravating factors:** effects of temperature, medications, rest, unintentional movements, anxiety
9. **Underlying concern:** interference with activities of daily living

Depression

(See also Box 27-3 on p. 678.)

1. **Onset:** gradual and progressive or sudden; review relationship to major life events/changes
2. **Course since onset:** change in symptoms
3. **Quality:** depressed mood, diminished interest or pleasure, unable to concentrate, thoughts of suicide, guilt, worthlessness
4. **Quantity:** degree of interference with work, family, sleep, activity, eating
5. **Setting:** environmental or situational effects on symptoms
6. **Associated phenomena:** weight loss or gain, lack of energy, social isolation, loss of memory, sleep disturbance, agitation
7. **Alleviating and aggravating factors:** effects of medications, alcohol and other drugs, counseling, social and family relationships, exercise
8. **Underlying concern:** suicidal thoughts, impaired social and physical functioning, a lack of motivation and hope

 Preparation for Examination

EQUIPMENT

Item	Purpose
Cottonball, disposable safety pin	Light touch, pain sensation, and localization
Tongue blade	Tongue strength, gag reflex
Tuning fork (512 cps)	Vibration sense
Ophthalmoscope	Optic nerve, pupil constriction
Reflex hammer	Deep tendon reflexes
Pencil and paper	Fine coordinated movements
Printed material	Reading and comprehension
Optional:	
Test tubes for cold and warm water	Temperature sensation
Aromatic substances	Olfaction
Sweet, sour substances	Taste
Calipers	Two-point discrimination

CLIENT AND ENVIRONMENT

Client clothed in loose-fitting gown over underwear
Quiet private room
Comfortable chairs
Examination table

Head Injury

1. **Onset:** describe the exact nature or mechanism of injury
2. **Course since onset:** any change in symptoms, especially change in level of consciousness, neurological changes, confusion
3. **Location:** describe precise extent and location of injury or trauma
4. **Quality:** mechanism of injury (e.g., blunt or open trauma, piercing trauma [was the client wearing a helmet when he or she fell off the bicycle?])
5. **Quantity:** severity of symptoms, Glasgow coma scale if loss of consciousness occurs and duration of unconsciousness
6. **Setting:** environmental exposures, such as traffic, heights; use of protective gear, padding, seat belts
7. **Associated phenomena:** nausea, vomiting, loss of memory, confusion, loss of hearing or vision, discharge from nose or ears
8. **Alleviating and aggravating factors:** effects of self-treatment, rest, activity
9. **Underlying concern:** permanent brain damage with loss of physical and cognitive function

Preparation for Examination: Client and Environment

A comprehensive physical examination often precedes a neurological examination, or the neurological examination can be integrated into the general physical examination. The neurological examination begins as soon as you, the examiner, and the client are introduced. Begin to form an overall impression and continue to make general observations before focusing on problem areas. Conduct the interview and examination in a quiet, private room without interruption. Perform the mental status examination with both you and the client comfortably seated. Conduct the remainder of the neurological examination with the client seated on the edge of the examination table or standing. Ask the client to remove shoes, socks, and outer clothing that covers the extremities. Give the client a loose-fitting gown to wear.

Technique for Examination and Expected Findings

Cranial Nerves

Table 19-1 summarizes the cranial nerves, including their functions, structures innervated, tests, and normal findings.

> **■ HELPFUL HINT**
>
> Be cautious about interpretating results whenever a client does not do something you have instructed. It may be simply a misunderstanding of directions and not a neurological defect. An isolated abnormal finding is very difficult to interpret.

CN I (Olfactory). Do not test CN I during a screening examination unless the history suggests a problem. Before testing the olfactory nerve, examine the nares for any signs of obstruction. Ask the client, with eyes closed, to sniff fa-

TABLE 19-1 **The Cranial Nerves**

Nerve	Function	Structure Innervated	Test	Normal Findings
I Olfactory	Sensory Smell	Olfactory epithelium in nasal cavity	Apply simple odors to one nostril at a time	Correct identification of odor
II Optic	Sensory Vision	Retina of eye	Visual acuity using Snellen chart Visual fields using a confrontation test Ophthalmoscopic examination	Correct identification of letters No visual fields defects Normal fundus
III Oculo motor	Motor Upward, downward, medial eye movement	Superior, medial, inferior rectus, inferior oblique, and levator palpebrae superior muscles	Flash light in one eye at a time EOM: Ask client to follow an object while you move it to left, then up and down left of midline; to right, then up and down right of midline	Direct and consensual light reflex Both eyes follow object in parallel
	Lid elevation Pupil constriction		Observe lids	Palpebral fissures equal Pupils constrict

TABLE 19-1	**The Cranial Nerves—cont'd**

Nerve	Function	Structure Innervated	Test	Normal Findings
IV Trochlear	Motor			
	Downward, medial eye movement	Superior oblique muscle	EOM	Same as EOM of CN III
V Trigeminal	Sensory			
	Face	Skin and mucosa of face and head via oph-thalmic, maxillary, and mandibular divisions	Test tactile and pain sensation of all three divisions	Normal sensory perception from entire face
	Scalp			
	Nasal mucosa			
	Buccal mucosa			
	Jaw muscles			
	Motor			
	Masseter muscle		Feel two masseter muscles as client bites down	Equal contraction of masseters and no deviation of mandible
	Temporal muscle			
	Digastric muscle		Corneal reflex	Blinking of eye
VI Abducens	Motor			
	Lateral eye movement	Lateral rectus muscle	EOM	Same as EOM of CN III
VII Facial	Sensory			
	External ear			
	Taste: anterior two thirds of tongue	Taste buds of anterior two thirds of tongue	Apply small amount of sugar or salt to ante-rior two thirds of tongue	Correct identifi-cation of substance
	Deep facial	Lacrimal, sublingual, and submandibular glands; other minor glands and mucosal surfaces		
	Motor			
	Facial movement	Facial, stapedius, stylo-hyoid, and posterior digastric muscles	Ask client to wrinkle forehead, close eyes, show teeth, whistle	Normal execution of movements
	Scalp muscle			
	Auricular muscle			
	Stylohyoid muscle	Middle ear		
	Digastric posterior belly	External ear		
	Parasympathetic			
	Salivation: submaxil-lary glands, sublin-gual glands			
	Lacrimation: lacrimal glands			
	Mucous membrane			
	Nasopharynx			
VIII Acoustic	Sensory			
	Cochlear: hearing	Spiral organ of cochlea	Hearing acuity using a watch or a whisper	Normal and bilat-erally symmet-rical hearing
			Rinne test (tuning fork on mastoid process)	Air conduction greater than bone conduction
			Weber test (tuning fork on center of forehead)	Heard in both ears equally
			Otoscopic examination	Normal tympanic membrane
	Vestibular: equilibrium	Ampullae of semicircu-lar ducts and maculae of saccule and utricle	Romberg test*	Able to maintain balance with eye closed

*Also a test of proprioception sense.

TABLE 19-1 **The Cranial Nerves—cont'd**

Nerve	Function	Structure Innervated	Test	Normal Findings
IX Glossopharyngeal	**Sensory** External ear Taste: posterior third of tongue Carotid: reflexes, baroreceptors and chemoreceptors, sinus, body	Taste buds of posterior third of tongue Parotid gland Pharynx (gag reflex), carotid sinus, posterior third of tongue, auditory tube, and middle ear Stylopharyngeus muscle External ear	Caloric	Nystagmus
	Motor Pharynx: gag reflex, swallowing, pharyngeal muscles Parotid gland: salivation		Touch pharynx with cotton applicator	Gag reflex Able to swallow
X Vagus	**Sensory** External ear Pharynx	External ear Carotid and aortic bodies; muscles of soft palate, pharynx, larynx, and esophagus	Listen to person talk	Lack of hoarseness
	Motor Swallowing, gag reflex Pronation Cardiac slowing Bronchoconstriction Gastric secretion Peristalsis	Epiglottis	Ask person to say "ah"	Both sides of soft palate contract and uvula remains in midline
	Parasympathetic Thoracic and abdominal viscera Aortic arch Chemoreceptors Baroreceptors	Smooth and cardiac muscles and glands of thoracic and abdominal organs through transverse colon		
XI Spinal Accessory	**Motor** Swallowing pharyngeal muscles Turning of head: sternocleidomastoid muscles Elevation of shoulders: trapezius muscles	Larynx and pharynx (with CN X)	Ask client to turn head to each side and shrug shoulders while you resist the movements	Strong contractions of sternocleidomastoid and trapezius muscles
XII Hypoglossal	**Motor** Muscles that move tongue: hypoglossus, genioglossus, styloglossus	Extrinsic and intrinsic muscles of tongue	Ask client to protrude tongue fully Move client's tongue side to side against resistance with tongue blade	Tongue protrudes in midline Good tongue strength

miliar odors, such as coffee, vinegar, or chocolate. Test each naris separately (Figure 19-10).

CN II (Optic). Test for visual acuity. See Chapter 12 for specific examination techniques.

CN III (Aculomotor), IV (Trochlear), VI (Abducens) (Extraocular Movements). See Chapter 12 for specific examination techniques.

CN V (Trigeminal). With the client's eyes closed, test for the presence of several types of sensation, comparing both sides and testing areas innervated by the three branches of the trigeminal nerve (Figure 19-11). Check whether the client perceives sensation equally on both sides. Test the corneal reflex only on an unconscious client by touching a wisp of cotton lightly to the cornea and observing a blink response. Test for light touch by using a wisp of cotton and asking the client to localize where the sensation is perceived. By alternating the sharp and dull ends of a safety pin, test for pain sensation; discard the safety pin after use. The sharp and smooth edges of a broken tongue blade can also be used. Test each branch on both sides of the face with a pain (sharp) stimulus. Testing for temperature sensation is not routine, since pain and temperature are both carried by the lateral spinothalamic tract.

Test muscles of mastication and the motor functions of the trigeminal nerve by palpating the masseter muscles (Figure 19-12) and the temporal muscles (Figure 19-13) while asking the client to bite down hard. Test jaw strength against resistance by applying downward pressure on the chin while asking the client to resist opening the mouth.

CN VII (Facial). Inspect the client's face for symmetrical movement when he or she looks at the ceiling, wrinkles the forehead, frowns, smiles, puffs out cheeks, and raises the eyebrows (Figure 19-14). Ask the client to close the eyes, first lightly and then tightly, while you try to open them. In infants, evaluate the facial muscles during crying. Evaluate tone and note any atrophy and fasciculations, or twitching, of a muscle group.

Testing for taste, salivation, and lacrimation is generally not part of the routine physical examination. When it is appropriate to test taste sensation, use an applicator to apply salty or sweet solutions to the anterior of each side of the tongue. Use a different applicator for each substance, and allow the client a sip of water between tests to avoid mixing tastes. Have the client leave the tongue protruded until he or she identifies the taste. To avoid spreading the test substance over the tongue, give the client a card with the words salty, sweet, sour, and bitter (the vagus nerve innervates sour and bitter taste on the posterior tongue) and ask the client to point to the one that best describes the solution on the tongue (Figure 19-15). Record the number of correct responses.

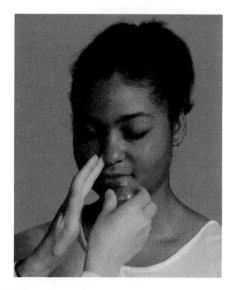

Figure 19-10 Testing for the ability to smell. The examiner asks the client to sniff while placing a test tube containing the test substance beneath the nostril. The examiner holds the other nostril closed.

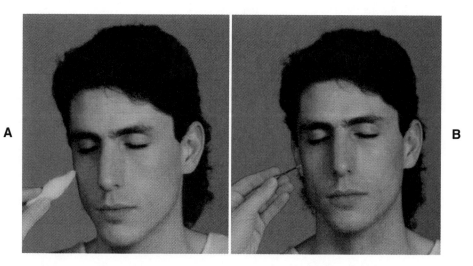

Figure 19-11 Testing for light touch (**A**) and pain (**B**) sensation. The examiner applies a wisp of cotton just firmly enough to stimulate the sensory nerve endings. To test for superficial pain, the examiner uses the sharp point of a safety pin, alternating with the dull end of the pin.

CN VIII (Acoustic). See Chapter 13.

CN IX (Glossopharyngeal) and X (Vagus). Testing of CN IX and CN X focuses on the musculature of the palate, pharynx, and larynx. Inspect the soft palate for symmetry. Identify the uvula and record any deviation from the midline. Test the gag reflex by touching the posterior wall of the pharynx with an applicator or a tongue blade; check for elevation of the palate and contraction of the pharyngeal muscles.

Note that the vagus nerve is functioning normally if the client can swallow and speak clearly without hoarseness.

Ask the client to say "ah," and note whether the palate rises symmetrically (see Chapter 13).

CN XI (Spinal Accessory). To test the spinal accessory nerve, evaluate the symmetry, size, and strength of the muscles. Ask the client to turn the head to one side against the resistance of your hand while you palpate the opposite sternocleidomastoid muscle (Figure 19-16).

To assess the trapezius muscles, ask the client to shrug the shoulders while you exert downward pressure. Evaluate the muscles for strength and symmetry (Figure 19-17).

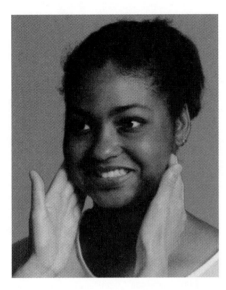

Figure 19-12 Palpation of the masseter muscles for size, strength, and symmetry to test CN V (trigeminal nerve).

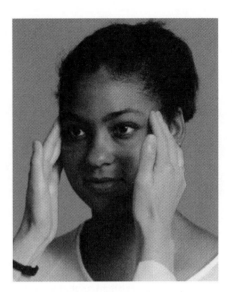

Figure 19-13 Palpation of the temporal muscles for size, shape, and symmetry to test CN V (trigeminal nerve).

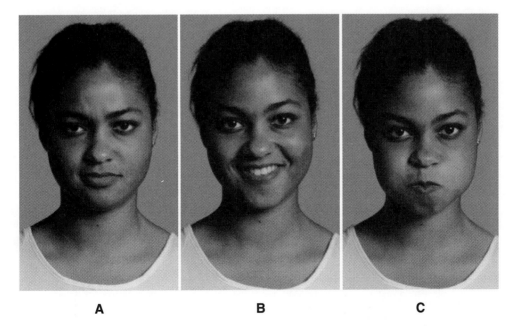

A   **B**   **C**

Figure 19-14 Testing motor function of CN VII (facial nerve). The examiner inspects the client's ability to frown **(A)**, smile **(B)**, and puff out the cheeks **(C)**.

CN XII (Hypoglossal). Inspect the tongue for size (atrophy), symmetry, and fasciculations. Ask the client to stick out the tongue as far as possible. Note the client's ability to stick the tongue straight out and the strength of the movement against lateral resistance produced with a tongue blade. Test the client's muscle strength by asking him or her to push out the cheek with the tongue while you push against it from the outside (Figure 19-18).

Proprioception and Cerebellar Function

The proprioceptive system of the nervous system maintains posture, balance, and coordination. The neural structures involved in proprioception are the posterior columns of the spinal cord, the cerebellum, and the vestibular apparatus. The posterior columns of the spinal cord carry stimuli from the proprioceptors in tendons and joints in addition to fibers for touch and two-point discrimination. Lesions affecting

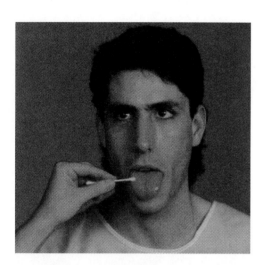

Figure 19-15 Testing for taste sensation (CN VII [facial nerve] and CN IX [glossopharyngeal nerve]). The examiner applies salty or sweet solutions to the anterior two thirds of the tongue and sour or bitter solutions to the posterior one third of the tongue. The right and left sides of the tongue are tested while the client's tongue is projected.

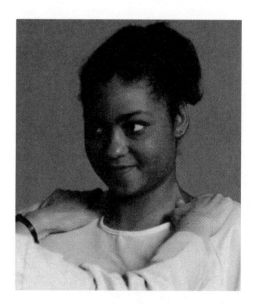

Figure 19-17 To test CN XI (spinal accessory nerve) and trapezius muscle strength, the client shrugs the shoulders against the resistance of the examiner's hands.

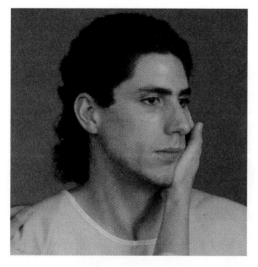

Figure 19-16 Assessing the symmetry, size, and strength of the sternocleidomastoid muscle in testing CN XI (spinal accessory nerve). The client is asked to turn the head to one side against the resistance of the examiner's hand. The contralateral sternocleidomastoid muscle will stand out as it contracts. The examiner palpates the visible muscle to assess tension.

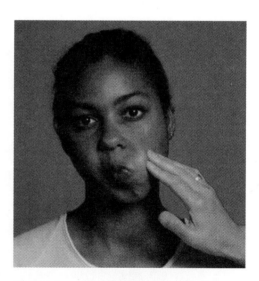

Figure 19-18 Assessing the strength of the tongue. The examiner asks the client to push against the inner surface of the cheek with as much strength as possible. The examiner palpates the external surface of the cheek simultaneously.

the posterior column impair muscle and position sense. The cerebellum integrates muscle contractions to maintain posture. Lesions affecting the cerebellum impair balance and coordination.

The vestibular system is concerned with correcting movements. Vestibular disease is characterized by vertigo, nausea, and vomiting. **Vertigo** is the illusion of a revolving movement of the individual or the environment. Nausea and

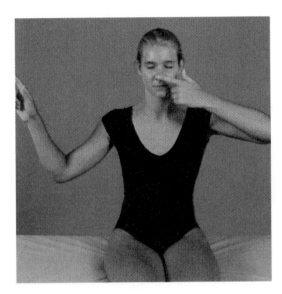

Figure 19-19 Testing cerebellar function. The client attempts to alternately touch the nose with the index finger of each hand, repeating the motion with increasing speed.

vomiting frequently accompany this condition. The following examination techniques are used to assess proprioception and cerebellar functions.

Finger-To-Nose Movements. Ask the client to touch his or her nose with the index finger of one hand and then the other, first with the eyes open and then with the eyes closed (Figure 19-19). A normal finding is the ability to accurately target the nose.

Finger-Nose-Finger Movements. Ask the client, with the eyes open, to touch his or her nose and then your finger at a distance of approximately 45 cm. Have the client increase the speed as you move your finger (Figure 19-20). Test each hand separately. Note the speed and accuracy of movement.

Rapid Alternating Movements. Ask the client to pat his or her knees with the palms of the hands followed by the backs of the hands at an ever-increasing rate (Figure 19-21). Then have the client perform thumb-to-finger opposition by touching each finger of one hand to the thumb of the same hand as rapidly as possible (Figure 19-22).

Heel to Shin. Ask the client to run the heel of each foot down the opposite shin (Figure 19-23).

Romberg Test. Ask the client to stand with the feet together, first with the eyes open and then with the eyes closed for about 15 seconds (Figure 19-24). Slight swaying is normal. Stand close enough to the client to prevent falling.

Coordination. Ask the client to walk naturally, then in a heel-to-toe fashion (Figure 19-25), and then to stand on each foot (Figure 19-26). If the client does this without difficulty, ask him or her to hop on one foot and then the other (Figure 19-27), and to do a deep knee bend (Figure 19-28).

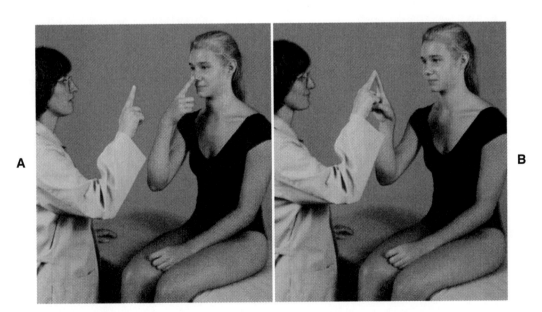

A   B

Figure 19-20 Testing cerebellar function. The client attempts to move the finger from the nose (**A**) to the examiner's finger (**B**) rapidly. The examiner's index finger is about 18 inches from the client's eye and moves the position of the finger target.

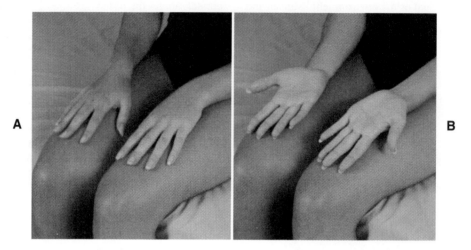

Figure 19-21   Testing cerebellar function: pronation (**A**) and supination (**B**) of the hands with progressively more rapid movement.

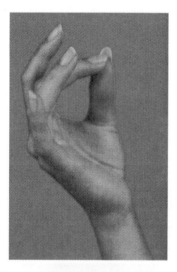

Figure 19-22   Testing cerebellar function. The examiner instructs the client to touch each finger to the thumb as rapidly as possible.

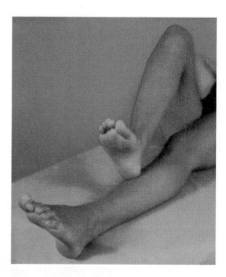

Figure 19-23   Testing cerebellar function. The examiner asks the client to run the heel of each foot down the opposite shin.

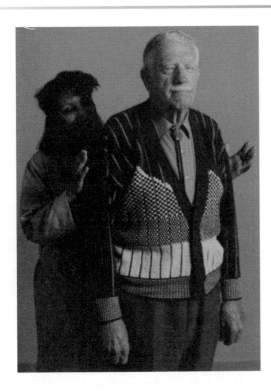

Figure 19-24 Testing the proprioceptive system. Romberg test: the client should be able to stand with the eyes closed and the feet together without swaying for approximately 5 seconds.

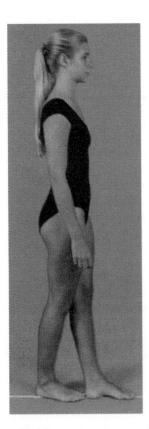

Figure 19-25 Testing the proprioceptive system. The client attempts to walk a straight line, placing heel to toe.

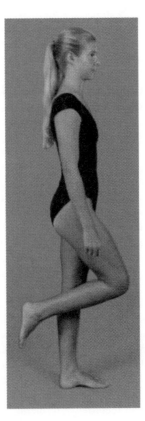

Figure 19-26 Testing the proprioceptive system. The client attempts to stand on one foot and then the other.

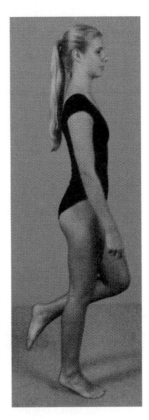

Figure 19-27 Testing the proprioceptive system. The client attempts to hop in place on one foot and then the other.

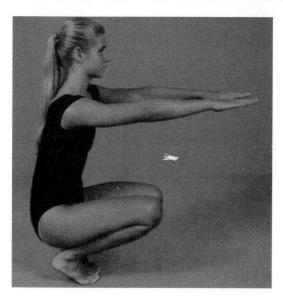

Figure 19-28   Testing the proprioceptive system. The client attempts a knee bend without support.

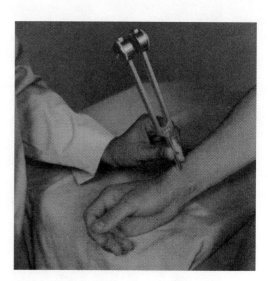

Figure 19-29   Testing sensitivity to vibration. The examiner applies the base of a vibrating tuning fork to a bony prominence, such as the wrist.

Since shoes can interfere with balance, have the client perform these tests without shoes.

Sensory Function

Although evaluating sensation over the entire skin surface is not necessary, stimuli should be applied strategically to test the dermatomes and the major peripheral nerves. A minimal number of test sites includes areas on the forehead, cheek, hand, and foot. In the screening examination, assume the nerve to be intact if sensation is normal at its most distal area. When there is evidence of dysfunction, localize the site of the dysfunction and map the boundaries. Sketch the region involved and describe the sensory change.

Variation in sensitivity of skin areas is normal. Use a stronger stimulus over the back, the buttocks, and areas where the skin is heavily cornified. Establish symmetry of sensation by checking first one spot and then the same area on the opposite side of the body.

Instruct the client to close the eyes during evaluation of sensory modalities. A client who is able to see the stimulus applied may be influenced by visual cues rather than responding to the specific sensory modality being tested.

■ HELPFUL HINT

Ensure that both you and the client are rested, because fatigue may result in errors. Otherwise you may interpret inattention or low motivation as a sensory loss. Also, to avoid predictability, vary the testing sites and the timing in applying the stimulus.

The following terms are useful in describing and recording sensory dysfunction:

Anesthesia: Absence of normal sensation.
Hyperesthesia: Extreme sensitivity of one of the body's senses.

Hypoesthesia: Abnormal weakness of sensation in response to sensory stimulation.
Paresthesia: Any subjective sensation, experienced as numbness, tingling, or a "pins and needles" feeling.

Light Touch Sensation.   Light touch and pain are mediated by different nerve endings. Sensory fibers for light touch enter the spinal cord and travel upward in the anterior spinothalamic tracts to the thalamus. Both anterior spinothalamic tracts must suffer destruction before transmission of light touch is lost.

Test light touch by contacting the skin with a wisp of cotton (see Figure 19-11, *A*). Does the client feel the touch of a wisp of cotton? Instruct the client to say "yes" or "now" when the touch is felt. If desired, combine this test with localization (a higher cortical function) by asking the client to state where he or she is touched. Compare each side of the body. Record areas of anesthesia or hyperesthesia.

Pain and Temperature Sensation.   Pain and temperature fibers both travel in the lateral spinothalamic tract. A screening examination does not include temperature assessment unless pain sensation is abnormal. To test temperature sensation, roll tubes filled with warm and cold water against the client's skin over dermatome areas. (First test the stimuli on your own skin to avoid burning the client and to provide a comparison.) Ask the client to say "hot," "cold," or "can't tell."

Evaluate the sensory perception of superficial pain by using the sharp and dull points of a safety pin or wooden tongue blade (see Figure 19-11, *B*). Compare each side of the body in the same locations as you test tactile sensation. Instruct the client to say "sharp" or "dull" when touched. Remember that each area examined must be touched with a sharp stimulus because dull touch simply validates light touch perception.

Vibration Sensation.   The normal client can perceive vibration as a buzzing or tingling sensation when a bony

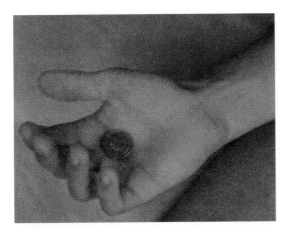

Figure 19-30   Testing for stereognosis. The normal client can identify a familiar object (coin, key) by touching and manipulating it.

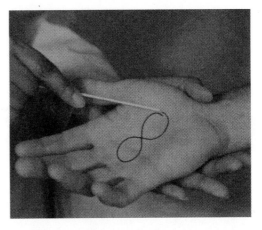

Figure 19-31   Testing for graphesthesia. The normal client can identify a number or letter written on the palm.

prominence, such as the wrist, elbow, or ankle, touches the base of a vibrating tuning fork. With the client's eyes closed, test vibratory sensation by applying the vibrating tuning fork to the wrists, elbows, knees, and ankles (Figure 19-29). Ask the client to say "yes" or "now" (1) when first feeling the vibrations and (2) when the vibrations stop. Dampen the vibrations of the tuning fork to move along more rapidly. Compare sensitivity from side to side and proximal to distal parts of the extremities. Apply the tuning fork to the most distal point of the extremity, since normal vibratory perception, or intactness of posterior columns, decreases from a proximal to a distal point.

In the older client vibratory sensation is diminished, particularly in the extremities.

Tactile Discrimination.   Tactile discrimination requires interpretation by the cerebral cortex. Three types of tactile discrimination are tested: (1) stereognosis, (2) two-point discrimination, and (3) extinction.

Stereognosis is the ability to recognize objects by touching and manipulating them. Test stereognosis with universally familiar objects, such as a key, safety pin, or coin (Figure 19-30). Test **graphesthesia** by asking the client to identify letters or numbers written on each palm with a blunt point. (Figure 19-31).

Two-point discrimination is the ability to sense whether one or two areas of the skin are being stimulated by pressure. There is considerable variability of perceptual ability over the different parts of the body. The following are minimal distances between the two points of the calipers at which the normal adult can sense simultaneous stimulation:

Tongue: 1 mm
Fingertips: 2.8 mm
Palms of hands: 8 to 12 mm
Chest, forearms: 40 mm
Back: 40 to 70 mm
Upper arms, thighs: 75 mm

To test two-point discrimination, apply disposable pins or a paperclip bent into a U shape to the skin simultaneously. Ask the client whether he or she feels one or two pinpricks (Figure 19-32).

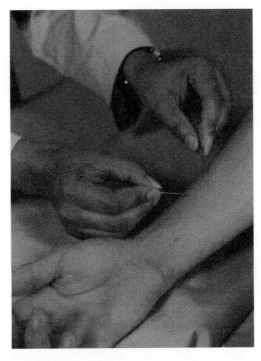

Figure 19-32   Testing for two-point discrimination. Disposable pins or paper clips bent into a U shape can be used.

To test for **extinction**, touch the skin on the same areas on both sides of the body. Failure to perceive touch on one side is called the extinction phenomenon. Normally, sensation is perceived on both sides.

Position Sense.   Position sense (**kinesthetic sensation**) is facilitated by proprioceptive receptors in the muscles, tendons, and joints. Perception of the position, orientation, and motion of limbs and body parts is obtained from kinesthetic sensations.

With the client's eyes closed and the joint in a neutral position, and with your fingers placed on each side of the client's digit (finger or toe), slightly move the position of the client's digit. Be careful not to touch other digits during this maneuver. Ask the client to describe how the position of the finger changes. Always move the digit to a neutral position before moving it again (Figure 19-33).

Reflexes

Deep Tendon Reflexes. Assess deep tendon reflexes to obtain information about the function of the reflex arcs and the spinal cord segments (Table 19-2). Elicit deep tendon reflexes by stretching (tapping) a tendon with a reflex hammer (Figure 19-34). Reflexes are graded using a 0-to-4 scale (Box 19-3).

BOX 19-3

GRADING DEEP TENDON REFLEXES

0	No response
1+	Low normal, slightly diminished response
2+	Normal
3+	More brisk than normal, not necessarily indicative of disease
4+	Brisk, hyperactive, clonus of tendon associated with disease

Record the symmetry of the reflex from one side of the body to the other. A succinct method of recording the reflex findings is the stick-figure representation (Figure 19-35). To obtain the best muscle contraction, test when the muscle is slightly stretched before the tendon is stretched (tapped with the reflex hammer).

Reinforcement is done to enhance a reflex. Ask the client to isometrically tense muscles not directly involved in the reflex arc being tested. For example, ask the client to clench the fists or to lock the fingers together and pull the hands apart (Figure 19-36) as you assess lower extremity reflexes. To reinforce the reflex arcs of the upper extremities, ask the client to clench the jaw or to tense the quadriceps. Document that reinforcement was used to elicit the deep tendon reflex.

Biceps Reflex (Figure 19-37). To check the biceps reflex, have the client flex the arm at the elbow. Place your

■ HELPFUL HINT

Compare reflexes bilaterally for symmetry, degree and speed of response, and recovery to original position. To accurately compare reflexes, make sure that each limb is in the same position.

TABLE 19-2 Reflexes Commonly Tested in the Physical Examination and Segmental Levels of the Central Nervous System Involved

Deep Tendon Reflexes	Segmental Level	Superficial Reflexes	Segmental Level
Biceps	C5, 6	Pharyngeal (gag)	Medulla
Triceps	C6, 7, 8	Abdominal (upper)	T7, 8, 9
Brachioradialis	C5, 6	Abdominal (lower)	T12; L1
Patellar	L2, 3, 4	Cremasteric	L1, 2, 3
Ankle (Achilles)	S1, 2	Gluteal	L4, 5
		Plantar	L4, 5; S1, 2

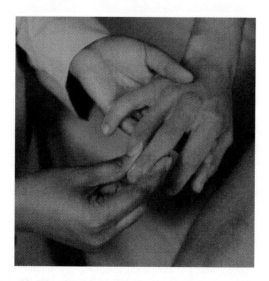

Figure 19-33 Testing for position sense. With the client's eyes closed, the examiner slightly changes the position of a digit up or down. The client describes how the position was changed.

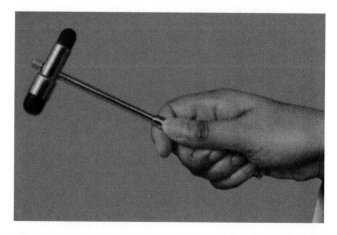

Figure 19-34 The examiner holds the reflex, or percussion, hammer in the dominant hand between the thumb and index finger and uses a striking motion to assess the deep tendon reflex.

thumb firmly over the biceps tendon to augment the tendon stretch. The thumb is struck with the reflex hammer and the response is flexion of the arm at the elbow.

Triceps Reflex (Figure 19-38). Tap the triceps tendon (above the olecranon process) with the reflex hammer. The normal response is extension of the elbow. Begin with the client's arm flexed at the elbow and resting in the client's lap. Alternatively, you can start with the client's arm flexed at the elbow and abducted while you hold it in position. The latter position sometimes allows for better viewing of the normal response of extension of the elbow.

Brachioradialis Reflex (Figure 19-39). To test the brachioradialis reflex, begin with the client's arm in a relaxed position. Strike the styloid process of the radius with the ham-

mer while palpating the tendon 3 to 5 cm above the wrist. The expected response is flexion of the elbow and pronation of the forearm. The fingers of the hand may also flex.

Patellar Reflex (Figure 19-40). For this test, the client's legs should be hanging freely over the side of the bed or chair, or the client should be resting in a supine position. Palpate the muscle above the patella with one hand while striking the tendon with the reflex hammer directly below the patella. The response is extension or kicking of the leg as the quadriceps muscle contracts.

Ankle (or Achilles) Reflex (Figure 19-41). Hold the client's foot in a slightly dorsiflexed position with one hand and strike the Achilles tendon with the reflex hammer. The response is plantar flexion of the foot.

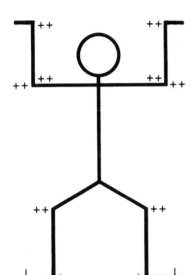

Figure 19-35 Stick-figure drawing for recording reflexes usually tested in the screening examination. Responses are coded from zero to "++++," with "++" values considered normal.

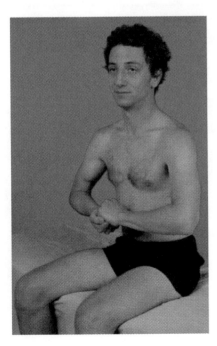

Figure 19-36 Reinforcement maneuver for deep tendon reflexes.

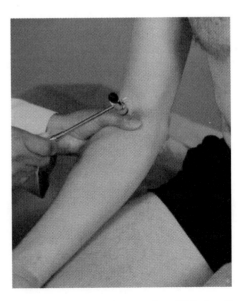

Figure 19-37 Eliciting the biceps reflex. With the client's arm flexed, the examiner places the thumb over the biceps tendon and strikes the thumb with the reflex hammer.

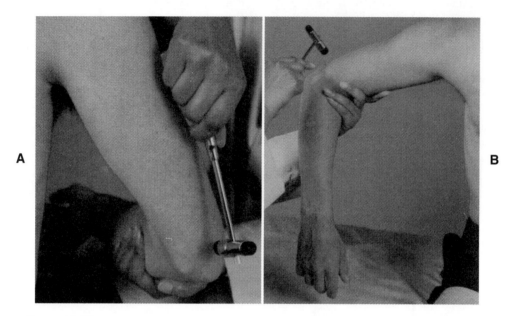

Figure 19-38 Eliciting the triceps reflex. **A,** With the arm flexed at the elbow, the examiner taps the triceps tendon. **B,** The examiner holds the flexed arm in position. The normal response is straightening or extension of the arm.

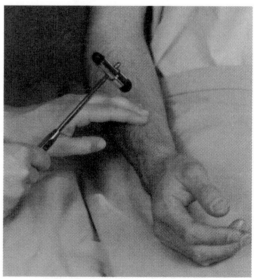

Figure 19-39 Eliciting the brachioradialis reflex. The normal response is flexion of the arm at the elbow, pronation of the wrist, or slight flexion of the fingers.

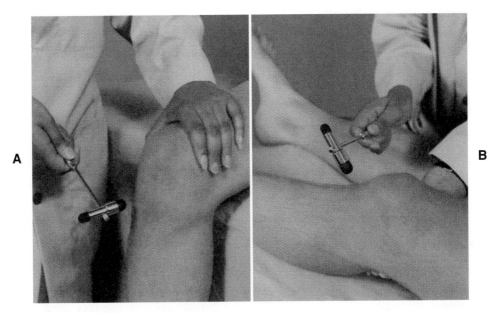

Figure 19-40 Eliciting the patellar reflex. With the client's legs hanging freely **(A)** or with the client in a supine position **(B),** the examiner strikes the tendon below the patella. The normal response is extension of the leg.

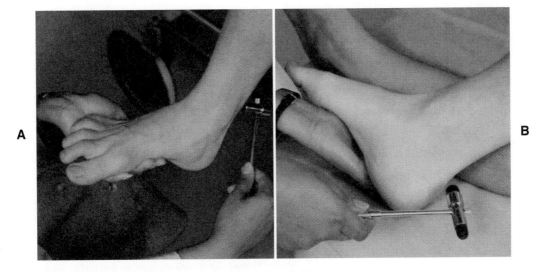

Figure 19-41 Eliciting the ankle reflex. **A,** Sitting. **B,** Lying down. The examiner strikes the Achilles tendon with the reflex hammer while holding the foot in a slightly dorsiflexed position. The normal response is plantar flexion of the foot.

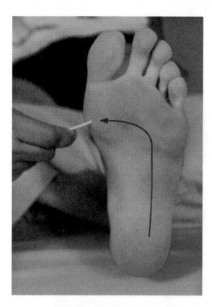

Figure 19-42   Eliciting the plantar reflex. The examiner applies a hard object along the lateral surface of the sole, starting at the heel and moving along the ball of the foot, ending beneath the great toe.

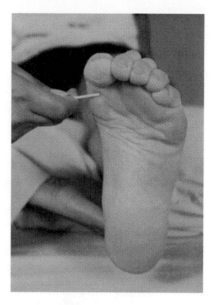

Figure 19-43   The normal response to plantar stimulation: flexion of all the toes.

Superficial Reflexes.   Superficial, or cutaneous, reflexes are obtained by stimulating the skin.

Plantar Reflexes (Figure 19-42).   Plantar reflexes are superficial reactions. Use a sharp stimulus to elicit the reflex. Apply the stimulus to the lateral border of the client's sole, starting at the heel and continuing across the ball of the foot and ending beneath the great toe. The response is flexion of the toes (Figure 19-43). Extension or dorsiflexion of the great toe and fanning of the others, which is abnormal, is called the Babinski response. Before a child can walk, fanning and extension of the toes are the normal response.

Abdominal Reflexes.   The abdominal reflexes are described in Chapter 17.

Cremasteric Reflex.   Stimulate the male client's inner thigh with a sharp object, such as the stick end of an applicator. The expected response is retraction (elevation) of the scrotum on the same side that the cremaster muscle contracts.

Gluteal Reflex.   Spread the client's buttocks and stimulate the perianal area. The response is contraction of the anal sphincter.

EXAMINATION OF MENTAL STATUS

Focused Health History

Assessment of mental status includes interviewing and observing. During the interview, make an overall assessment of whether the client is cooperative, friendly, or hostile. Obtain information about the client's educational and physical development; occupation; economic status; relationships; responsibilities felt toward family, work, or school; stressors (actual or perceived); goals (attainable and unrealistic); and support systems (individuals and affiliations).

Use therapeutic communication skills discussed in Chapter 2. Focus on obtaining data about symptoms, including how the client views these symptoms and how disruptive they are to the client and others. Compare and contrast your observations with the client's perceptions. Document a client's behaviors and words accurately; succinctly; and in measurable, descriptive terms. Use short, direct quotes only when doing so clarifies the situation:

- Not measurable: Client was very agitated during the interview.
- Measurable: During the 15-minute interview, client paced the room, bit her fingernails, and stated 4 to 5 times, "I'm really nervous today."

Preparation for Examination: Client and Environment

Equipment needed to conduct a mental status examination includes a pencil, paper, and reading material. The setting should be quiet and should provide privacy. Communication barriers related to age or culture can often be bridged through the use of qualified interpreters, friends, or family members. When information is obtained from sources other than the client, the examiner must understand the relationship of these individuals to the client and record who is the source of information.

General Appearance

Carefully observe the client's general physical appearance, grooming, manner of dress, facial expression, and body posture as a measure of mental function. Do not focus too early on obvious abnormalities, since the subtle clues may be missed.

TABLE 19-3	Level of Consciousness (Responsiveness)
Level	**Behaviors**
Consciousness	Appropriate response (rate and quality) to external stimuli; oriented to time, place, and person
Confusion	Inappropriate response to stimuli and decreased attention span and memory; reactions to simple commands
Lethargy (hypersomnia)	Drowsiness or increased sleep time; can be aroused; responds appropriately; may fall asleep again immediately
Delirium	Confusion, disorder perception, and decreased attention span; motor and sensory excitement; inappropriate reactions to stimuli; marked anxiety
Coma	Loss or lowering of consciousness
Stage I (stupor)	Arousable for short periods to verbal, visual, or painful stimuli; simple motor and verbal response to stimuli; slow responses; corneal and pupillary reflexes sluggish; deep tendon and superficial reflexes unaffected; pathological reflexes may be obtained
Stage II (light coma)	Simple motor and verbal (moaning) response to painful stimuli; mass motor movement or flexion (avoidance) response
Stage III (deep coma)	Decerebrate posturing to painful stimuli (extension of body and limbs and pronation of arms)
Stage IV	Flaccid muscles; pupillary reflex absent; apneic; on ventilator; superficial and some deep tendon reflexes present
Brain death	Two electroencephalographic (EEG) tracings 24 hours apart indicate absence of brain waves; cerebral function absent for 24 hours; failure of cerebral perfusion; expert opinion rules out hypothermia or drug toxicity (NOTE: All these behaviors must be present.)
Syncope	Temporary loss of consciousness (partial or complete) associated with increased rate of respiration, tachycardia, pallor, perspiration, and coolness of skin
Fugue state	Dysfunction of consciousness (hours or days) in which the individual carries on purposeful activity that he or she does not remember afterward
Amnesia	Memory loss over time or for specific subjects; individual affected responds appropriately to external stimuli

Grooming and Manner of Dress.   Observe the client's clothing to determine its appropriateness to time, place, age, and lifestyle. Grooming of hair and nails and general cleanliness should be noted. A disheveled appearance in someone who was previously well groomed is especially significant.

Posture.   Posture is important in providing clues to the client's feelings. The client who walks slowly into the room, barely lifting the feet, and who slumps in the chair while avoiding the examiner's glance may be showing signs of depression.

Coordination.   Assess general coordination of movement by observing the client's gait (see Chapter 9). To evaluate the complex coordination, give the client simple phrases to write and simple geometric figures to draw.

Behavior

Level of Consciousness.   Consciousness is awareness of one's thoughts and feelings and of the environment. The levels of consciousness (responsiveness) are generally described according to the behavior exhibited by the individual. Table 19-3 includes a useful categorization of the levels of consciousness. Response to pain may be the only indication of sensory stimulation. Stimuli used to assess response to pain include pinching of skin; pricking with a pin; pressure over supraorbital notches; or squeezing muscle masses or tendons, particularly the calf muscle. The client may respond by extension of limbs, facial grimacing, or withdrawal. Flexion responses are considered withdrawal responses and

therefore purposeful. Nonpurposeful responses are mass reactions or extension of limbs. If the client is alert and responsive, level of consciousness need not be assessed further. However, if the client appears drowsy or stuporous, a more complete assessment of level of consciousness is indicated.

Mood or Affect.   Affect is the observable manifestation of the internally experienced emotion or feeling state. In general, it is possible to estimate the client's emotional status or affective state from verbal and nonverbal behaviors. Affects may be described as labile if moods rapidly and abruptly shift. Observe the appropriateness and degree of affect to a given idea, as well as the range of affect.

To understand the client's perspective and to bring out the feelings of clients who resist offering information spontaneously, try the interview protocol described in Box 19-4.

Characteristics of Speech.   Evaluate the client's comprehension of and ability to use the spoken language. The client's manner of speech may offer clues about his or her thought processes. The mentally healthy individual answers questions frankly. Responses to your questions and instructions give valuable information about the client's comprehension and willingness to cooperate. Note failure to answer a question, other evasive replies, and unwarranted criticism of you as the examiner. Speech is especially difficult to evaluate when the client and examiner speak different languages.

Facial Expression.   Facial expression should be consistent with and appropriate to the topic. In some Southeast Asian cultures, direct eye contact is avoided, especially by

BOX 19-4

INTERVIEW PROTOCOL

How would you describe the problem that has brought you
    here?
What do you think is causing your problem?
Why do you think it happened to you?
Why do you think it started when it did?
How have your spirits been lately?
How do you feel life has been treating you?
Have you told anyone else about your feelings or problems?
Have you ever considered hurting yourself? If yes: Did you
    follow through and actually harm yourself? If yes: How
    did you do it?
Do you have any plans to harm yourself now? If yes: What
    are your plans?
Do you think about dying? If yes: How often?

Cultural Considerations
Behavior Variations

In many Asian cultures, an open display of one's distress is
not considered appropriate behavior.

women, since the examiner is considered to hold a position
of respect. In many cultures, acceptable expression of emotion varies greatly between males and females.

Cognitive Functions

Assess the client's orientation, attention, memory, use of
language, and intellectual skills. The Mini–Mental State
Examination (MMSE) is a practical 11-question instrument
used to assess orientation, memory, concentration, calculation, and language abilities (see discussion of Screening
Tests and Procedures).

   Orientation.   Assess orientation from the client's
awareness of person, place, and time. The following questions can help in obtaining this information:
PERSON:
   • What is your name? Address? Telephone number?
   • Who am I?
   • What is my job?
PLACE:
   • Tell me where you are. What is the name of this
     place?
   • What is the name of the town you are in?
   • Who brought you here?
TIME:
   • What day (month, year) is it?
   Record the degree of disorientation. Time is the orientation most commonly disordered in clients with mental disease. A disturbance of place orientation may accompany organic mental disorders or schizophrenia. An individual may
not be oriented to person in the aftermath of cerebral trauma
or seizures.

   Attention Span.   An appraisal of the individual's attention span includes the client's ability to maintain interest and
to concentrate. Attention span is one of the first mental functions to become affected in individuals who are fatigued,
anxious, or chemically impaired.

   Memory.   Memory is a general cerebral function. Impairment of memory occurs in both neurological and psy-

chiatric disorders. Some general questions that may help to
elicit a memory disorder are as follows:
   • Have you noticed any loss of memory?
   • Do you remember those things that happened years
     ago best or those that happened today or yesterday?
   Immediate Memory.   Immediate memory is verbalized
remembering immediately after presentation. Test immediate memory by digit recall. Two sample tests follow.
   To test your memory skills, I'd like you to repeat four series of numbers after me:
   7, 4
   9, 6, 5, 3
   8, 9, 4, 1, 5
   3, 8, 7, 4, 1, 6
   I will say some numbers. You say them backward. For instance, I say 8, 2; you say 2, 8:
   3, 8
   7, 2, 0
   5, 9, 2, 7
   The average individual can generally repeat five to seven
digits forward and four to six digits backward.
   Recent Memory.   Recent memory is verbalized after
several minutes to 1 hour. Examples of questions and exercises for assessing recent memory are as follows:
   • What were you doing before you came here today?
   • What time did you get up today?
   • What did you eat for breakfast today?
   Remote Memory.   Remote memory is verbalized after
hours, days, or years. At the beginning of the interview, give
the client three to five unrelated words to remember. Other
examples of questions for assessing remote memory are as
follows:
   • Where were you born?
   • Tell me the name of the high school you attended.
   • What was your mother's maiden name?
   In testing for memory, do not ask questions for which the
answers cannot be verified. Memory loss in organic dementia may involve disorders for immediate and recent events;
however, affected individuals may be able to recall events
from childhood with accuracy.
   Intellectual Functioning
   Abstraction Ability.   To assess abstraction ability, ask
the client to give the meaning of familiar proverbs, such as
the following:
   • A bird in the hand is worth two in the bush.
   • People who live in glass houses shouldn't throw
     stones.
   • Don't count your chickens before they hatch.
   • A rolling stone gathers no moss.

■ HELPFUL HINT

Interpretation of abstraction ability must take into consideration a client's cultural orientation, age, and educational level. Some proverbs may be culturally bound or more familiar to clients of a certain age group.

Ability to Learn (Comprehension).   The ability to learn includes abilities in perception, retention, association (interpretation), and recent memory. Give the client an address or a sentence that is not familiar and ask him or her to remember the content verbatim. For example:

Listen to me carefully. I am going to give you an address that I want you to remember. Later, I will ask you to repeat it for me: Apartment 13, Dover Hill Building.

Computation.   The following exercise is useful in assessing the client's computational abilities:

Ask the client to subtract 7 from 100. Have the client continue subtracting 7 from the resulting remainder for several more calculations.

The client is expected to be able to complete the computation in $1\frac{1}{2}$ minutes with fewer than four errors. Computation skills may be impaired by fatigue, depression, or anxiety.

Ability to Read.   Use a copy of a current newspaper to determine the client's reading skills. Be certain that the client is wearing corrective lenses if they are needed for reading. Impairment of the ability to read is called **dyslexia**.

General Knowledge.   Assessment of general knowledge may include an estimate of what the client has learned in school and his or her awareness of current events. Match inquiries to the educational, sociocultural, and life experiences of the client. Ask questions about presidents, capitals of countries, names of oceans, or current events in newspaper headlines.

Insight and Judgment.   Insight is the client's understanding of and beliefs about the cause and nature of his or her illness. Simple questions such as "Why did you decide to come here [name of health care facility] at this time?" allow clients to explain in their own words their comprehension of their health status. An example of an interview protocol designed to elicit information about the client's mental representation or beliefs about his or her health or illness follows:

• When did you first notice the problem?
• What do you think this problem does to you?
• How severe do you think this problem is?
• What do you feel is causing the problem?
• Have you noticed any troubling symptoms or feelings?
• What do you think is the best treatment for this problem?

Judgment is a skill necessary for evaluation, assessment, and decision making, particularly in those situations in which two or more experiences are related to one another. The individual who is able to evaluate a situation and deter-

mine the appropriate reaction(s) is said to have good judgment or reasoning ability. Assess judgment through the client's expressed attitudes to his or her social, physical, occupational, and domestic status and plans for the future.

Judgment may be impaired in highly charged emotional states, mental retardation, organic mental disorder, schizophrenia, effects of drugs and alcohol, and anxiety. Two examples of questions that elicit judgment skills follow:

• What would you do if you were in a theater when fire broke out?
• What would you do if you found a stamped, addressed envelope?

Thought Processes.   Verbal and nonverbal expressions are used to assess the client's ability to think logically and coherently.

Screening Tests and Procedures

Mini–Mental State Examination

Using the Mini–Mental State Examination (MMSE) (Box 19-5), ask the client the 11 questions in the order listed. The total possible score is 30. The test takes about 10 minutes to administer to a client with normal mental status functioning. Educational and culture can influence a client's performance. Generally a score of 20 to 24 suggests mild impairment; a score of 16 to 19, moderate impairment; and a score of 15 or less, severe deficit. Further diagnostic testing is needed before a definitive diagnosis of dementia can be made.

Pain Assessment Scale

A systematic assessment of pain intensity and pain management uses a pain rating scale (Figure 19-44). The client is asked to rate pain from 0 (no pain) to 10 (worst pain). Ratings of 3 to 5 are considered mild pain; ratings of 5 to 7 are considered moderate pain; and ratings greater than 7 are considered severe pain. For children, happy and sad faces are used to make the pain rating.

Glasgow Coma Scale

The Glasgow Coma Scale is an assessment tool that rates level of consciousness by assigning a numerical score to three behavioral evaluations: eye opening, verbal response, and motor response. The score is the sum of these ratings (Table 19-4). A person with normal consciousness would obtain a score of 15. Common postures found in nonresponsive clients are decorticate, decerebrate, and flaccid.

Special Tests

Data from standardized psychological tests to assess brain damage are more reliable than behavioral observations, although both examine the same functions, such as the speed of response, level of comprehension, and use of language. Neuropsychological testing assesses visual memory and psychomotor skills in depth by using a wide range of standardized tests. Testing is performed by a skilled clinician specifically trained to administer and interpret these tests.

BOX 19-5

MINI-MENTAL STATE EXAMINATION

MAXIMUM SCORE	SCORE	
		ORIENTATION
5	( )	What is the (year) (season) (date) (month)?
5	( )	Where are we: (state) (country) (town) (hospital) (floor)
		REGISTRATION
3	( )	Name 3 objects: 1 second to say each. Then ask the patient all 3 after you have said them. Give 1 point for each correct answer. Then repeat them until he learns all 3. Count trials and record. Trials
		ATTENTION AND CALCULATION
5	( )	Serial 7's. 1 point for each correct. Stop after 5 answers. Alternatively, spell "world" backwards.
		RECALL
3	( )	Ask for the 3 objects repeated above. Give 1 point for each correct.
		LANGUAGE
9	( )	Name a pencil, and watch (2 points) Repeat the following "No ifs, ands or buts." (1 point) Follow a 3-stage command: *"Take a paper in your right hand, fold it in half, and put it on the floor"* (3 points) Read and obey the following: Close Your Eyes (1 point) Write a sentence (1 point) Copy design (1 point)
30	( )	Total score ASSESS level of consciousness along a continuum _____
		Alert Drowsy Stupor Coma

BOX 19-5

MINI-MENTAL STATE EXAMINATION—cont'd

INSTRUCTIONS FOR ADMINISTRATION OF MINI-MENTAL STATE EXAMINATION

ORIENTATION

(1) Ask for the date. Then ask specifically for parts omitted (e.g., "Can you also tell me what season it is?"). One point for each correct.

(2) Ask in turn "Can you tell me the name of this hospital?" (e.g., town, country). One point for each correct.

REGISTRATION

Ask the patient if you may test his memory. Then say the names of 3 unrelated objects, clearly and slowly, about 1 second for each. After you have said all 3, ask him to repeat them. This first repetition determines his score (0-3) but keep saying them until he can repeat all 3, up to 6 trials. If he does not eventually learn all 3, recall cannot be meaningfully tested.

ATTENTION AND CALCULATION

Ask the patient to begin with 100 and count backwards by 7. Stop after 5 subtractions (93, 86, 79, 72, 65).
Score the total number of correct answers.
If the patient cannot or will not perform this task, ask him to spell the word "world" backwards. The score is the number of letters in correct order, e.g., dlrow = 5, dlorw = 3.

RECALL

Ask the patient if he can recall the 3 words you previously asked him to remember. Score 0-3.

LANGUAGE

Naming: Show the patient a wristwatch and ask him what it is. Repeat for pencil. Score 0-2.
Repetition: Ask the patient to repeat the sentence after you. Allow only one trial. Score 0-1.
3-Stage command: Give the patient a piece of plain blank paper and repeat the command. Score 1 point for each part correctly executed.
Reading: On a blank piece of paper print the sentence "Close your eyes," in letters large enough for the patient to see clearly. Ask him to read it and do what it says. Score 1 point only if he actually closes his eyes.
Writing: Give the patient a blank piece of paper and ask him to write a sentence for you. Do not dictate a sentence, it is to be written spontaneously. It must contain a subject and verb and be sensible. Correct grammar and punctuation are not necessary.
Copying: On a clean piece of paper, draw intersecting pentagons, each side about 1 in, and ask him to copy it exactly as it is. All 10 angles must be present and 2 must intersect to score 1 point. Tremor and rotation are ignored.
Estimate the patient's level of sensorium along a continuum, from alert on the left to coma on the right.

INITIAL PAIN ASSESSMENT TOOL   Date _____

Client's Name _____   Age _____
Diagnosis _____   Physician _____
                                             Nurse _____

I. LOCATION: Client or nurse marks drawing.

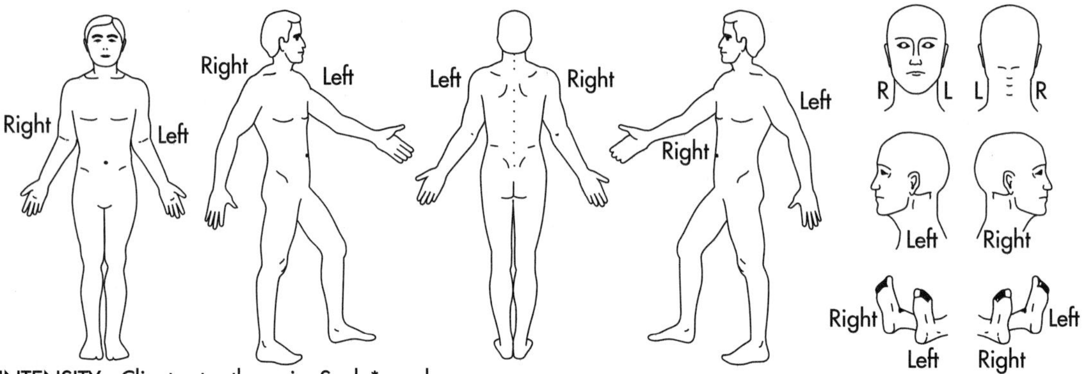

II. INTENSITY: Client rates the pain. Scale* used _____
    Present: _____
    Worst pain gets: _____
    Best pain gets: _____
    Acceptable level of pain: _____
III. QUALITY: (Use client's own words, e.g., prick, ache, burn, throb, pull, sharp) _____
    _____
IV. ONSET, DURATION VARIATIONS, RHYTHMS: _____
    _____
V. MANNER OF EXPRESSING PAIN: _____
    _____
VI. WHAT RELIEVES THE PAIN? _____
    _____
VII. WHAT CAUSES OR INCREASES THE PAIN? _____
    _____
VIII. EFFECTS OF PAIN: (Note decreased function, decreased quality of life) _____
    Accompanying symptoms (e.g., nausea) _____
    Sleep _____
    Appetite _____
    Physical activity _____
    Relationship with others (e.g., irritability) _____
    Emotions (e.g., anger, suicidal, crying) _____
    Concentration _____
    Other _____
IX. OTHER COMMENTS: _____
    _____

```
0  1  2  3  4  5  6  7  8  9  10
|__|__|__|__|__|__|__|__|__|__|
No                          Worst
pain                       possible
                            pain
```

FACES Pain Rating Scale:

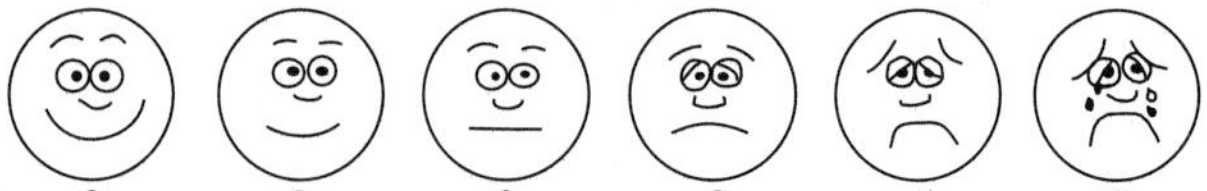

0 No hurt	1 Hurts little bit	2 Hurts little more	3 Hurts even more	4 Hurts whole lot	5 Hurts worst
Alternate coding 0	2	4	6	8	10

*Pain rating scales: 0-10 Visual Analog Scale *(left)* and FACES Pain Rating Scale *(right)*.

Figure 19-44   Pain assessment form. (Modified from McCaffery M, Pasero C: *Pain: clinical manual*, ed. 2, St. Louis, 1999, Mosby. Wong/Baker FACES Pain Rating Scale is from Wong DL, Hess FS.: *Wong & Whaley's clinical manual of pediatric nursing*, ed. 5, St. Louis, 2000, Mosby, Table 4-6, p. 316. Copyrighted by Mosby. Reprinted by permission.)

| TABLE 19-4 | Glasgow Coma Scale |

Best eye-opening response	Spontaneously	4
	To verbal command	3
	To pain	2
	No response	1
Best verbal response	Oriented, converses	5
	Disoriented, converses	4
	Inappropriate words	3
	Incomprehensible sounds	2
	No response	1
Best motor response	Obeys	6
To verbal command	Localizes pain	5
To painful stimulus	Flexion-withdrawal	4
	Flexion-decorticate	3
	Extension-decerebrate	2
	No response	1
	TOTAL	(3-15)

Decorticate: Rigid flexion; upper arms held tightly to sides of body; elbows, wrists, and fingers flexed; feet are plantar flexed, legs extended and internally rotated; may have fine tremors or intense stiffness

Decerebrate: Rigid extension; arms fully extended; forearms pronated; wrists and fingers flexed; jaws clenched; neck extended; back may be arched; feet plantar flexed; may occur spontaneously, intermittently, or in response to a stimulus

Modified from Chipps E, Clanin N, Campbell V: *Neurologic disorders,* St. Louis, 1992, Mosby.
From Wilson SF, Giddens JF: *Health assessment for nursing practice,* ed. 2, St. Louis, 2001, Mosby.

| TABLE 19-5 | Deep Tendon Reflex and Muscle Changes in Upper and Lower Motor Neuron Lesions |

Lesion	Common Cause	Characteristics
Upper motor neuron lesion (corticospinal tract)	Cerebral vascular occlusion	Hyperreflexia
	Cerebral neoplasm	Paralysis of voluntary movement
Spasticity (usually includes damage to parallel pathways)	Trauma	Babinski's sign present
		Minimal muscle atrophy
Lower motor neuron lesion (anterior horn cell, somatic motor part of cranial nerves)	Poliomyelitis	Muscle weakness
	Neoplasm	Paralysis
	Trauma	Muscle atrophy
		Hyporeflexia or absent reflexes
		Fasciculations

VARIATIONS FROM HEALTH

Variations in Sensory Function

Anosmia is the loss of the sense of smell. **Hyposmia** is an impaired sense of smell. In hyposmia, flavor perception is also impaired, since it is a synthesis of smell, taste, and perceptions from stimulation of end organs in the mouth and pharynx. The individual with CN I (olfactory) involvement may complain only of loss of the sense of taste.

Ageusia is the loss of taste or the lack of ability to discriminate sweet, sour, salty, and bitter tastes.

Shingles **(herpes zoster),** a very painful condition, is caused by the herpes varicella-zoster virus, the same virus that causes chickenpox. The virus may remain dormant in the dorsal root ganglia of some spinal nerves. With increasing age, the immune system is not as effective in keeping the virus inactive, and the reactivated virus causes shingles. Shingles appears on the skin as a painful papulovesicular rash that follows the course of peripheral, and sometimes cranial, nerves (see Figure 10-6). No specific treatment is available, and these lesions may ulcerate and keratinize. Neuralgia or anesthesia may remain after the rash disappears.

Variations in Motor Function

Multiple sclerosis (MS) is a demyelinating disease that involves deterioration of myelin sheaths of neurons in the central nervous system. Without the myelin, nerve impulses become short-circuited and do not reach their intended destinations. Evidence exists that this is an autoimmune disease triggered by a virus.

Symptoms of MS first appear between the ages of 20 and 40 years. The disease may progress rapidly or slowly. Symptoms vary but may include muscle weakness or paralysis, partial loss of sensation, visual changes, loss of bowel and bladder control, and loss of spinal cord reflexes. Some individuals experience remissions, when symptoms disappear for an unpredictable period of time. No cure exists for MS at present.

Table 19-5 summarizes the causes and characteristics of upper and lower motor neuron lesions. Bell's palsy is a facial nerve palsy of acute onset and unknown cause. Evidence of this lower motor neuron disorder, which results in paralysis of an entire side of the face, is the closing of only one eye when the client attempts to close both eyes. When

Examination Step-by-Step

There is no one method for conducting the neurological examination. Each examiner may develop his or her own method. If abnormalities are found, a more complete examination of that area is necessary. The order below is a logical one for performing the complete mental status and neurological examination.

1. During the interview, assess cerebral function:
   a. Observe appearance and behavior for appropriateness to the situation.
   b. Assess mental status for orientation to person, place, and time; attention span; and calculation.
   c. Assess recent and remote memory and abstract reasoning.
   d. Assess emotional status, observing affect, mood, thought content, and expression of ideas.
   e. Assess communication skills; ability to express oneself and to listen; clarity of expression.
2. With the client standing:
   a. Observe gait.
   b. Assess Romberg's sign (standing with feet slightly apart, eyes closed).
   c. Observe heel-to-toe walking (tandem gait, toe-walking, heel-walking).
   d. Test standing on one foot, then the other; hopping on each foot.
   e. Assess deep knee bend (optional).
3. With the client sitting, examine the following regions in a head-to-toe direction.

HEAD AND FACE

1. Observe facial symmetry (CN VII).
2. Have the client frown, smile, puff cheeks, close eyes tightly, and resist the examiner opening eyes.
3. Ask the client, with eyes closed, to indicate when and where he or she is touched with a cotton wisp on three areas of the face innervated by CN V.
4. Ask the client, with eyes closed, to indicate "sharp" or "dull" sensation when touched with a pin on three areas of the face innervated by CN V.

EYES

1. Observe symmetry of the lids, palpebral fissures (CN III).
2. Observe symmetry of the pupillary light reflex and pupil response (direct and consensual) to light and accommodation (CN III).
3. Test extraocular movements (CN III, IV, VI) for six fields of gaze.
4. Assess visual acuity using the Snellen chart (CN II).

5. Test visual fields by confrontation, having the client indicate when the examiner's fingers come into peripheral vision in eight visual fields (CN II).
6. Use an ophthalmoscope to examine CN II.

EARS

1. Test hearing acuity using Weber and Rinne tests (CN VIII).

NOSE

1. Test smell (CN I) (not done in screening examination).

MOUTH AND THROAT

1. Observe symmetrical rise of the soft palate with "ah" swallow (CN IX and X).
2. Assess jaw strength and symmetry (CN V).
3. Assess tongue strength (CN XII).
4. Test taste sensations (CN VII and IX) (not done in screening examination).

NECK

1. Test trapezius and sternocleidomastoid strength (CN XI).

OTHER

1. Assess cerebellar function and proprioception:
   a. Observe rapid alternating movements (upper and lower extremities).
   b. Perform finger-to-nose test.
   c. Perform finger-to-thumb test.
   d. Perform heel-down-shin test.
2. Test sensory function with the client's eyes closed:
   a. Assess light touch and pain on each extremity from distal to proximal.
   b. Test position sense.
   c. Check vibration sense.
   d. Test stereognosis (not done in screening examination).
   e. Test graphesthesia (not done in screening examination).
   f. Assess two-point discrimination (not done in screening examination).
3. Assess deep tendon reflexes.
   a. Test biceps reflex.
   b. Assess brachioradialis reflex.
   c. Test triceps reflex.
   d. Assess patellar reflex.
   e. Assess ankle jerk reflex.
   f. Assess plantar reflex.
4. Not tested in a screening examination:
   a. Extinction
   b. Reflexes: Corneal, abdominal, cremasteric, gluteal

the client tries to raise the eyebrows, the eyebrow on the affected side does not rise and the forehead does not wrinkle. The client may exhibit overflow of tears or be unable to hold fluids orally because of a sagging mouth.

Neck trauma is the most common cause of dysfunction of the spinal accessory nerve (CN XI). **Torticollis** is a condition of intermittent or constant contraction of the sternocleidomastoid muscle in which the head is flexed forward and the chin is rotated away from the affected side.

A cerebrovascular accident (CVA), or stroke, is damage to a blood vessel in the brain that results in lack of oxygen to that part of the brain. Either a blood clot (thrombosis) or hemorrhage, often from the rupture of an aneurysm, causes the interruption in circulation. The symptoms depend on the part of the brain affected. The onset of symptoms may be slow if a clot formation decreases blood flow before complete occlusion occurs. In the case of a ruptured aneurysm, however, the onset may be sudden. Recovery from a CVA

BOX 19-6

COMPARISON OF DISORDERS OF THE CEREBELLUM, POSTERIOR COLUMNS, AND VESTIBULAR APPARATUS

CEREBELLAR DYSFUNCTION

Ataxia present with eyes opened or closed
Clumsiness
Poor coordination
Tremor
Hypotonia
Nystagmus

POSTERIOR COLUMN DYSFUNCTION

Ataxia made worse with eyes closed
Positive Romberg's sign (swaying with eyes closed)
Inability to recognize limb position
Loss of two-point discrimination
Astereognosis
Loss of vibratory sense

VESTIBULAR APPARATUS DYSFUNCTION

Nystagmus
Nausea
Vomiting
Ataxia present with eyes opened and closed

depends largely on its location and the extent of damage and promptness of treatment. In many individuals, especially those who begin rehabilitation early, the brain is able to establish new pathways to compensate for damaged areas.

Lesions of the Dominant Cerebral Hemisphere

Aphasia, the inability to comprehend or use language symbols, is caused by a lesion in the cerebral hemisphere dominant for speech. The most common cerebral pathological condition associated with aphasia is vascular disease. Data show that 95% of persons who are right-handed and have a language deficit have lesions of the left cerebral hemisphere, whereas 70% of left-handed individuals with language impairment also have a lesion of the left cerebral hemisphere.

If the motor cortex for speech is involved, the person can understand written and spoken words but cannot contract the muscles used for speech to form words properly. Damage to the interpretation area of the cortex for speech results in the inability to comprehend the meaning of spoken words. Aphasia often accompanies **agnosia**, the inability to recognize once-familiar objects.

Lesions of the Nondominant Cerebral Hemisphere

A disturbance in the ability to perform a purposeful act when comprehension is intact is termed **apraxia**. For example, if given a fork, the client may be unable to use it to eat, or the client may be unable to dress or button a shirt.

Variations in Cerebellar Function

The client with cerebellar disease has difficulty with rapid patting and supination-pronation alterations. The problem involves both smooth control of muscles and the starting and stopping of motion. Clumsiness of movement and irregular timing are characteristic of affected individuals (Box 19-6).

Dyssynergia (impairment of muscle coordination or of the ability to perform movements smoothly) is loss of cerebellar function and results in intention tremor, or **hypotonia**.

Abnormalities of muscle tone, gait, speech, and nystagmus in lateral gaze may also indicate cerebellar dysfunction. Disturbances in the timing of movements may also be evident.

Ataxia is the impairment of position sense.

The client with a cerebellar gait walks with a wide base; the trunk and head are held rigidly; the legs bend at the hips; arm movements are not coordinated with the stride; and the client lurches and reels, frequently falling.

The client with cerebellar speech has slow, hesitant, or dysarthric verbalization.

Pathological Reflexes

Reflexes may be altered in pathophysiological changes involving the sensory pathways from the tendons and muscles or the motor component.

Babinski Response

The Babinski response is dorsiflexion of the great toe and fanning of the other toes. Lesions of the pyramidal tract or motor nerves may be present in the client with a Babinski response. A positive Babinski response is present in newborns and disappears by 24 months (see Figure 26-63).

Grasp Reflex

The **grasp reflex**, while present in individuals with widespread brain damage, is normal in infants younger than 4 months of age (Figure 19-45). To test the grasp reflex, place your index and middle fingers in the client's palm, entering between the client's thumb and the index finger. Gently withdraw your fingers, pulling them across the skin of the client's palm. A positive response consists of the client's grasping of your fingers.

Lesions of the Corticospinal Tract

Clients with lesions of the corticospinal tract perform fine movements of the hands, such as picking up coins or pencils, slowly. Also, they are able to perform thumb-to-finger opposition less rapidly.

Signs of Meningeal Irritation

Meningeal irritation most commonly results from infection or intracranial hemorrhages. Nuchal rigidity (stiff neck) is a common sign of meningitis and may be demonstrated by flexing the cervical spine, which produces discomfort in the posterior neck. In addition, the client cannot touch the chin to the chest.

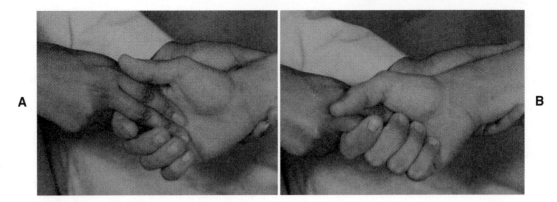

Figure 19-45 Eliciting the grasp reflex. **A,** The examiner places the index and middle fingers in the client's palm and gently withdraws them. **B,** A positive response consists of the client's grasping the examiner's fingers.

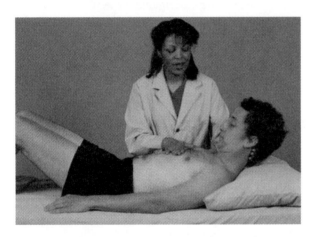

Figure 19-46 Eliciting Brudzinski's sign. With meningeal irritation, pain is elicited when the head is flexed.

Brudzinski's sign (Figure 19-46) is elicited with the client supine. Lift the client's head toward the sternum. The person with meningeal irritation will resist the movement and may flex the hips and knees. The movement is commonly accompanied by pain in the spine.

Variations in Mental Status

Confabulation is an attempt by the client to "fill in the gaps" with fabricated answers when he or she is unable to remember.

A client who rapidly skips from one complete idea to another without any relationship to the preceding idea may be manifesting **flight of ideas**.

It is important to carefully observe the client's affect to see whether it is congruent with the individual's verbal content. For example, a client who expresses little or no emotion while verbalizing the desire for self-harm or harm to others is demonstrating an incongruence between affect and verbal content.

Organic Brain Syndromes

Organic brain syndrome describes a symptom complex that causes an impairment of orientation, memory, or regulation of emotions. Affective symptoms, delusions, hallucinations, and obsessions may also be present. An acute brain syndrome (**delirium**) is one of short duration that is usually reversible. A chronic brain syndrome (**dementia**) is long-standing and often progressive in nature, with a less favorable prognosis.

Alzheimer's disease is a progressive, incurable form of mental deterioration that usually affects the elderly. Although the cause is not known, certain environmental factors bring out a genetic predisposition to this disease. Symptoms include confusion, forgetfulness, and loss of ability to execute simple tasks. As the disease progresses, a total loss of memory occurs. On autopsy the cerebral cortex shows structural changes, including increased fibrous tissue.

Affective (Mood) Disorders

The client with an affective disorder runs the gamut from depression to exaggerated euphoria, or mania. The highs and lows show little correlation with the person's life situation.

A **bipolar disorder** is diagnosed when mania is present or is indicated by the health history, whether or not depression occurs. Depression that occurs in the absence of mania is known as major unipolar depression.

Schizophrenic Disorders

Hallucinations and delusions are the diagnostic signposts of schizophrenia. **Delusions** are false beliefs that are improbable in nature. Hallucinations are visual perceptions for which no external stimuli can be ascertained. Hallucinations may be suspected in the person who appears preoccupied.

Anxiety

The client who demonstrates symptoms of severe anxiety has recurrent periods of abrupt-onset anxiety that end without intervention. The client complains of fright without a known object. The autonomic nervous system is activated, possibly resulting in such signs and symptoms as palpitations, breathlessness, dizziness, feeling of impending doom, headache, fatigue, nausea and vomiting, and diarrhea.

Phobia

Phobia is a highly disturbing, recurring, and unrealistic fear that may relate to any situation or object.

Sample Documentation and Diagnoses

FOCUSED HEALTH HISTORY (SUBJECTIVE DATA)

Mr. Z's chief complaint is that he feels too tired to get up in the morning. His wife died 3 months ago after a short illness. Since then, he reports feeling sad and lonely most of the time. Reports sleeping 2 to 3 hours per night and is tired all day. Reports a 10 lb weight gain in the past 2 months, which he attributes to increased intake of "junk" food, drinking 4 to 6 cans of beer per evening, and reduced physical activity. Says he sits home alone most of the time and has no close friends. Works on an assembly line and reports no job absences or injuries in the last 5 years but has been late for work five times in the past 2 weeks. Denies any history of mental illness, suicidal thoughts, or serious depression. Reports no sensory, motor, or coordination changes.

FOCUSED PHYSICAL EXAMINATION (OBJECTIVE DATA)

Mental status: Appears well-groomed; appropriate dress; slightly slumped posture. Gazed at the floor through most of the interview. Responds to questions appropriately. Oriented, alert, and cooperative throughout examination. Recent and remote memory intact.

Cranial nerves: Vision 20/30 both eyes with glasses (CN II); extraocular movement intact (CN III, IV, VI); jaw strength good (CN V); able to frown and smile (CN VII); correctly identifies whispered voice (CN VIII); swallows without difficulty (CN IX); palate rises symmetrically (CN X); able to turn head and shrug shoulders against resistance (CN XI); tongue midline (CN XII).

Cerebellar: Finger-to-nose, heel-to-shin, alternating movements done easily but slowly; Romberg negative; able to stand on each foot, hop, do knee bends, and heel-to-toe walk.

Face and extremities sensitive to light touch, localization, and pain; vibration and position sense intact.

DTRs: Bilaterally symmetrical, 1+, plantar reflex present.

DIAGNOSES

HEALTH PROBLEM

Situational depression since death of spouse

NURSING DIAGNOSIS

Ineffective Coping Related to Death of Spouse

Defining Characteristics

- Presence of life stress
- Inability to meet role expectations
- Alteration in societal participation
- Excess food intake, alcohol consumption
- Digestive, bowel, appetite disturbance; chronic fatigue or sleep pattern disturbance diagnoses

Critical Thinking Questions

Review the Sample Documentation and Diagnoses box to answer questions 1 and 2.

1. What aspects of the history were indicators of depression?
2. What additional information, if any, would you have obtained?
3. How would you modify the neurological assessment if the client to be examined was in a coma?
4. How would you modify the health history in a client who appears confused?
5. What health promotion activities would reduce the risk of unintentional head trauma or spinal cord trauma?

Answers are available on the MERLIN website (www.harcourthealth.com/MERLIN/Barkauskas/). And be sure to check the website regularly for additional learning activities!

Male Genitalia and Inguinal Area

Learning Objectives

On successful study of this chapter and completion of related learning experiences, the learner will be able to:
- Describe the anatomy and physiology of the male genitalia and inguinal region throughout the lifespan.
- Outline the history pertinent to the assessment of the male genitalia and inguinal region.
- Explain the related rationale for and demonstrate assessment of the male genitalia and inguinal region, including inspection and palpation techniques.

- Recognize abnormalities and common deviations of the male genital and inguinal region.
- Describe diagnostic techniques used to assess scrotal abnormalities and related causative factors.
- Compare the characteristics of inguinal and femoral hernias.

Outline

Purpose of Examination

The purpose of the examination of the male genitalia is to assess the health of the male genital organs. The examination also provides an opportunity for teaching the client about genital area self-examination.

The purpose of the inguinal area assessment for hernias is to determine the presence of inguinal and femoral hernias. This examination is addressed in conjunction with the male genital examination because most kinds of hernias are more common in males than in females. However, the inguinal area discussion pertains to the physical examination of both sexes.

ANATOMY AND PHYSIOLOGY OF MALE GENITALIA

The male genitalia include the penis, scrotum, testes, epididymides, vas deferens, seminal vesicles, and prostate (Figure 20-1).

Three columns of erectile tissue bound together by heavy fibrous tissue form the cylindrical shaft of the penis. The dorsolateral columns are called the corpora cavernosa. The ventromedial column, which contains the urethra, is called the corpus spongiosum. Distally the penis terminates in a cone-shaped entity called the **glans** penis. The glans penis is formed by an extension and expansion of the corpus spongiosum penis, which fits over the blunt ends of the corpora cavernosa penis. The corona is the prominence formed where the glans joins the shaft. The urethra traverses the corpus spongiosum, and the external urethral orifice is a slit-like opening located slightly ventrally on the tip of the glans.

The skin of the penis is thin, hairless, darker than the other skin on a person's body, and only loosely connected to the internal parts of the organ. At the area of the corona, the skin forms a free fold, called the **prepuce**, or foreskin. When allowed to remain, this flap covers the glans to a variable extent. Often the prepuce is surgically removed through circumcision (Figure 20-2).

The penis serves as the terminal excretory organ for urine and, with erection, as the means of ejaculating sperm. The physiological process of erection occurs when the two corpora cavernosa become engorged with approximately 20 to 50 ml of blood through decreased venous outflow and increased arterial dilation. Orgasm is a major pleasurable sensation accompanying emission of secretions from the epididymides, vas deferens, seminal vesicles, prostate, and penis.

The scrotum is a deeply pigmented cutaneous pouch that contains the testes and parts of the spermatic cords (Figure 20-3). An outer layer of thin, rugous skin overlying

a tight muscle layer (cremaster muscle) forms this sac. The left side of the scrotum is often lower than the right side because the left spermatic cord is usually longer. Internally, the scrotum is divided into halves by a septum; each half contains a testis and its epididymis and part of the spermatic cord. The testes are ovoid and are suspended vertically, slightly forward; they lean slightly laterally in the scrotum. The mediolateral surfaces are flattened. Each testis is approximately 4 to 5 cm long, 3 cm wide, and 2 cm thick.

The testes produce both spermatozoa and testosterone. The epididymides serve as receptacles for storage, maturation, and transmission of sperm. The vas deferens serves as a mechanism of transit from each epididymis to the seminal vesicles. The prostate produces the bulk of ejaculatory fluid. The dartos muscle of the scrotum controls the temperature of the testes by adjusting the distance of the scrotum, and consequently the testes, from the body. Spermatogenesis requires temperatures below 37° C (98.6° F). Therefore the scrotum appears low in hot weather and high in cold weather.

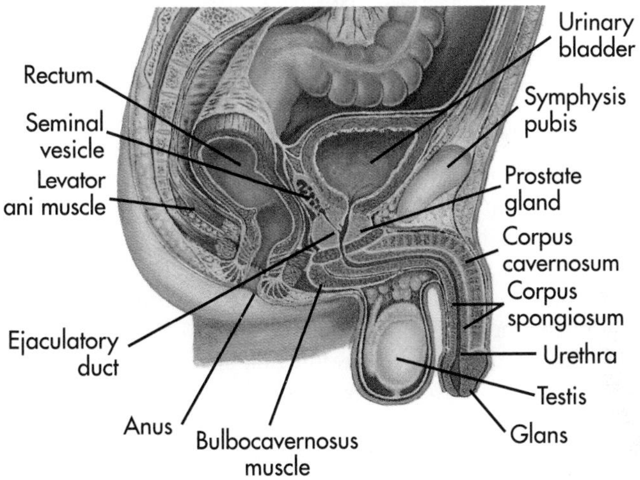

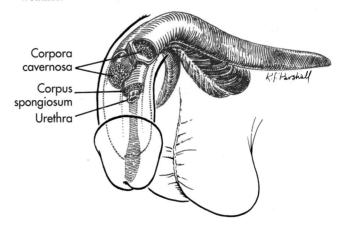

Figure 20-2   Circumcised penis.

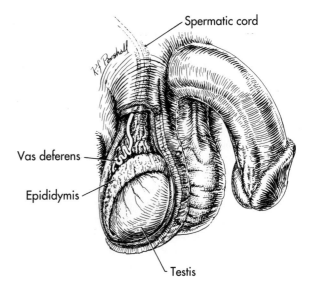

Figure 20-3   Scrotum and scrotal contents.

Figure 20-1   Male genitalia. (From Thibodeau GA, Patton KT: *Anatomy and physiology*, ed. 4, St. Louis, 1999, Mosby.)

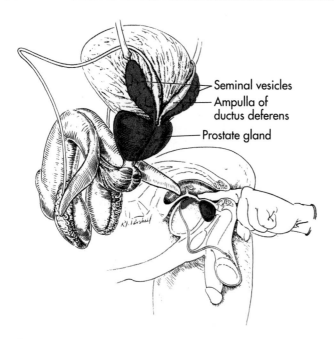

Figure 20-4   Prostate gland and seminal vesicles. Prostate examination.

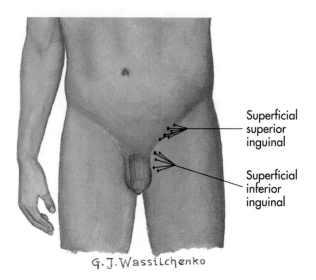

Figure 20-5   Inguinal lymph nodes. (From Seidel HM et al.: *Mosby's guide to physical examination*, ed. 4, St. Louis, 1999, Mosby.)

The epididymis is a comma-shaped structure that is curved over the posterolateral surface and upper end of the testis. It creates a visual bulge on the posterolateral surface of the testis. The ductus deferens (vas deferens) begins at the tail of the epididymis, ascends the spermatic cord, travels through the inguinal canal, and eventually descends over the fundus of the bladder (see Figure 20-1).

The prostate, a slightly conical gland, lies under the bladder, surrounds the urethra, and measures approximately 4 cm at its base (or uppermost) part, 3 cm vertically, and 2 cm in its anteroposterior diameter. The prostate gland is roughly the size and shape of a chestnut. It has three lobes: left and right lateral lobes and a median lobe. These lobes are not well demarcated from one another. The median lobe is the part of the prostate that projects inward from the upper posterior area toward the urethra. Enlargement of this lobe causes urinary obstruction in benign prostatic hypertrophy.

The posterior surface of the prostate lies in close contact with the rectal wall and is the only portion of the gland that is accessible to examination. Its posterior surface is slightly convex. A shallow median furrow divides all except the upper portions of the posterior surface into right and left lateral lobes.

The seminal vesicles are a pair of convoluted pouches, 5 to 10 cm long, that lie along the lower posterior surface of the bladder, anterior to the rectum (Figure 20-4).

The two groups of superficial nodes in the inguinal area are the superior and inferior inguinal nodes (Figure 20-5). These nodes receive most of the lymph drainage from the legs. The superior inguinal nodes lie somewhat horizontally along the inguinal ligament. They receive drainage from the abdominal wall below the umbilicus, the external genitalia (excluding the testes), the anal canal, the gluteal area, and

the inferior inguinal nodes. The inferior group lies somewhat vertically below the junction of the saphenous and femoral veins. This is a group of large lymph nodes that receives lymph from the superficial regions of the leg and foot. Lymph from the penile and scrotal surfaces drains to the inguinal nodes, but lymphatic drainage from the testes is deep into the abdomen.

EXAMINATION OF MALE GENITALIA
Focused Health History

The health history of the male reproductive system is integrated with the urinary system history and the sexual history. The client may need some explanation about the reasons for the exploration of the sexual history and reassurance that such information is important in assessing overall health.

Present Health/Illness Status

1. Patterns of urination: color of urine, frequency of urination
2. Changes in urination: frequency, urgency, amount of voidings, nocturia, dysuria, polyuria, color of urine, blood in urine, straining, difficulty in starting stream, incontinence
3. Satisfaction with sexual functioning
4. Use of contraceptives and safer sexual practices
5. Problems with sexual functioning: pain, difficulty in obtaining or maintaining an erection, premature ejaculation (for any positive responses, investigate frequency and characteristics associated with intercourse, partners, medications, and use of alcohol)

Risk Factors
Male Cancers

TESTICULAR CANCER

Age 20 to 35
History of undescended testes, groin hernia, or testicular swelling with mumps
Family history of testicular cancer
Caucasian
History of maternal use of oral contraceptives or diethylstilbestrol during pregnancy
History of maternal abdominal or pelvic x-ray examination during pregnancy
Higher social class
Never married or married late

PROSTATE CANCER

African-American
Age older than 50 years
Alcohol use
Diet high in animal fat
Family history of prostate cancer
Occupational exposure (e.g., cadmium, fertilizer, exhaust fumes)
Prostate specific antigen (PSA) level >4 ng/ml
Residence in the United States

SEXUALLY TRANSMITTED DISEASES

Multiple sexual partners
Intercourse with person(s) having multiple partners
Failure to use condoms with occasional partners

6. Pattern of scrotal self-examination
7. Penile discharge: color, amount, odor, associated symptoms, treatment, diagnoses
8. Penile lesions: appearance, associated symptoms, treatment, diagnoses
9. Scrotal and groin masses, swelling, tenderness, pain, treatment, diagnoses
10. Enlargements or hernias in the inguinal area: intermittent or constant, association with activity involving straining, groin pain, use of truss or similar device

Past Health History

1. Urinary tract infections, kidney disease, kidney stones, flank pain, prostate problems, undescended testicles
2. Reproductive history: number of children and current health
3. Sexually transmitted diseases or contacts
4. Reproductive system or hernia surgery
5. Trauma to genitourinary system

Family Health History

1. Cancer of prostate or testes
2. Infertility problems
3. Mother's use of hormones during pregnancy or exposure to radiation during pregnancy

Associated Conditions

1. Diabetes
2. Exposure to mumps after puberty

Personal and Social History

1. Alcohol use
2. Tobacco use
3. Drug use
4. Sexual partners: gender, total number, number in the past 6 months, and their health
5. Work and environmental exposures

Symptom Analysis

Urethral Discharge

1. **Onset:** gradual or sudden
2. **Course since onset:** changes in symptomatology
3. **Location:** more prominent at certain times of day or with different activities
4. **Quality:** color, consistency
5. **Quantity:** amount in specific measures (e.g., teaspoons or size of stain on underwear)
6. **Setting:** changes in sexual partners or practices
7. **Associated phenomena:** dysuria, painful ejaculation, fever, changes in urination, pruritus, arthritis, rashes
8. **Alleviating and aggravating factors:** trauma, exposure to sexually transmitted diseases, medications, efforts to treat and results of efforts
9. **Underlying concern:** sexually transmitted diseases

Scrotal Masses

1. **Onset:** exact date of onset, relationship to other illnesses (e.g., mumps)
2. **Course since onset:** changes in size or other characteristics
3. **Location:** exact location
4. **Quality:** surface characteristics, consistency, mobility, borders, tenderness
5. **Quantity:** size in centimeters
6. **Setting:** relationship to trauma
7. **Associated phenomena:** edema, obesity, recent infection, pain, fever, penile discharge
8. **Alleviating and aggravating factors:** changes with position, lifting, medications, efforts to treat and effects of efforts
9. **Underlying concern:** cancer

Erectile Dysfunction

1. **Onset:** onset and pattern of the problem
2. **Course since onset:** intermittent or consistent decrease in functioning
3. **Location:** relationship to variations in pattern of intercourse
4. **Quality:** inability to achieve erection, sustain erection, maintain complete erection, or ejaculate
5. **Quantity:** frequency of dysfunction
6. **Setting:** changes with setting of sexual intercourse or partners, stressors

Preparation for Examination

EQUIPMENT

Item	Purpose
Disposable latex gloves	To protect examiner from infection
Flashlight	To transilluminate scrotal mass
Material to make slide or culture per local protocols	To obtain specimen in case of abnormal discharge

CLIENT AND ENVIRONMENT

Client	Explain purpose and procedures
	Uncovered from the waist down
	Lying and standing for various parts
Environment	Warm
	Private

7. **Associated phenomena:** emotional problems, systematic disease, decreased libido, trauma, recent surgery, chronic illnesses (e.g., diabetes)
8. **Alleviating and aggravating factors:** medications, surgery, alcohol, drugs, changes in diet
9. **Underlying concern:** quality of sexual relations

Lesion on the Penis

1. **Onset:** date of onset
2. **Course since onset:** changes since onset, increase or decrease in size or characteristics
3. **Location:** exact location
4. **Quality:** color, appearance, surface characteristics, discharge (purulent or bleeding)
5. **Quantity:** number, size, extent of spread on skin surface, amount of associated pain
6. **Setting:** changes in sexual partners, travel
7. **Associated phenomena:** fever, malaise, enlarged lymph nodes, pain, headaches, pruritus, associated diagnoses, stress, immunosuppression, rash
8. **Alleviating and aggravating factors:** medications, lifestyle changes, sexual behavior, efforts to treat and results of efforts
9. **Underlying concern:** sexually transmitted disease

Preparation for Examination: Client and Environment

Both the client and the practitioner usually perceive the examination of the genital organs as being different from the examination of other body parts. Characteristically, the genital and rectal examinations are the last portions of the physical assessment. The practitioner precedes the examination with a thorough history of the urinary system and a history of sexual functioning. The examiner should generally take the sexual history during the history-taking portion of the assessment while the client is dressed.

In preparation for the physical assessment, advise the client of its purpose and the procedures involved in the examination. Assemble the needed equipment.

The client may be lying down (with the examiner standing) or standing (with the examiner sitting or standing for various portions of the examination). Trousers and shorts should be removed. Put on rubber gloves before initiating the examination, and wear them throughout the examination.

Technique for Examination and Expected Findings

Inspection of the Genital Area and Penis

The techniques of inspection and palpation are used to examine the male genitalia. Inspection and palpation are done consecutively for each portion of the genitalia. After the inguinal and genital areas have been exposed, inspect the skin, hair, and gross appearance of the penis and scrotum (Figure 20-6). General examination of the skin and hair is discussed in Chapter 10. Assess the size of the penis and the secondary sex characteristics in relationship to the client's age, general development, and sexual development.

The onset of the appearance of adult sexual characteristics is extremely variable. Pubic hair appears and the testes enlarge between the ages of 12 and 16 years. Penile enlargement and the onset of seminal emission normally occur between the ages of 13 and 17 years. Table 20-1 con-

TABLE 20-1   Developmental Changes in Appearance of the Male Genital Organs

Developmental Stage	Pubic Hair	Appearance	
		Penis	Testes and Scrotum
Stage 1 Sexual maturity	None except for fine body hair such as on abdomen	Size proportional to body size as in childhood	Size proportional to body size as in childhood
Stage 2 Sexual maturity	Sparse, long, slightly pigmented, thin at base of penis	Slight enlargement	Enlargement of testes and scrotum; reddened pigmentation; texture more prominent
Stage 3 Sexual maturity	Darkens, becomes more coarse and curly; growth extends over symphysis	Elongation	Enlargement continues
Stage 4 Sexual maturity	Continues to darken, thicken, and become coarser and more curly; growth extends laterally, superiorly, and inferiorly	Breadth and length increase; glans develops	Enlargement continues; skin pigmentation darkens
Stage 5 Sexual maturity	Adult distribution and appearance; growth extends to inner thighs, umbilicus, and anus and is abundant	Adult appearance	Adult appearance
Stage 6 Elderly clients	Sparse and gray	Decrease in size	Testes hang low in scrotum; scrotum appears pendulous

Illustrations modified from Tanner JM: *Growth at adolescence,* ed. 2, Oxford, 1962, Blackwell Scientific Publications.

tains a summary of developmental changes in the male genital system. See also Chapter 26 for a discussion of pediatric assessment.

Genital hair is coarser than scalp hair. It is similar in color and appearance to axillary and chest hair. In the adult male, pubic hair will be abundant in the pubic region and will extend in a diamond pattern, narrowing upward toward the umbilicus. The penis is hairless, and the scrotum may have a sparse distribution of hairs.

An ambulatory, cooperative client can assist in the examination by handling the penis and scrotum during inspection. The examiner must do all the handling for the debilitated client. It is important to examine all the surfaces, including the posterior surfaces, of the male genitalia.

The color of the penis ranges from pink to light brown in Caucasians and from light brown to dark brown in African-Americans. A prominent dorsal vein is often noted. Observe the entire penis for lesions, nodules, swelling, inflammation, and discharge. Then observe the glans and the urethral meatus for lesions and inflammation (Figure 20-7). If the client is uncircumcised, ask him to retract the prepuce from the glans, and carefully examine the glans and foreskin. If the uncircumcised client has retracted the foreskin for examination of the glans, remind him to return the foreskin to its usual position after the glans has been inspected.

If any discharge is present, obtain a smear and culture for gonorrhea and possibly chlamydial infection (see Chapter 21 for a discussion of procedures for obtaining smears and cul-

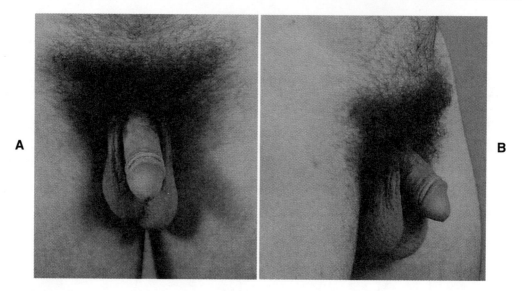

Figure 20-6 Normal appearance of the male genitalia. **A,** Frontal view. **B,** Lateral view. (NOTE: The left testis is lower than the right because of the length of the spermatic cord.)

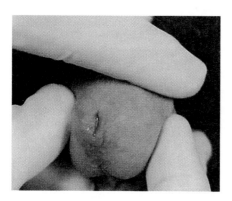

Figure 20-7 Usual position and appearance of the urethral meatus.

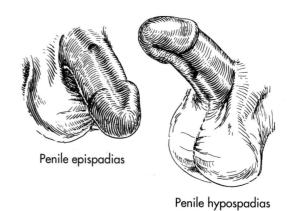

Penile epispadias

Penile hypospadias

Figure 20-8 Hypospadias, a malpositioning of the urethral meatus.

tures). If the client has reported a discharge but none is present, request him to strip the penis from the base to the urethra. If a discharge is then present, make a culture. The procedure for stripping the penis is as follows:

1. Grasp the base of the penis with the thumb and fingers, with the thumb at the front and the fingers behind.
2. While applying a moderate amount of consistent pressure, move the thumb and the fingers slowly from the base to the tip of the penis.

The urethral meatus should appear pink and slit-like and should be positioned rather centrally on the glans. When the distal urethral ostium occurs on the ventral corona or at a more proximal and ventral site on the penis or perineum, the condition is called **hypospadias** (Figure 20-8). **Epispadias** is a similar malpositioning of the urethral meatus in the dorsal area.

When hypospadias or epispadias is noted, describe the location of the urethral meatus as precisely as possible. Hy-

pospadias is classified as being glandular, penile, penoscrotal, or perineal. Epispadias is classified as being glandular, penile, or complete. Glandular refers to a location somewhere between the normal position and the junction of the glans with the body of the penis. Penile refers to a location on the penile shaft. Penoscrotal hypospadias indicates a positioning of the meatus along the anterior margin of the scrotum. Perineal hypospadias indicates a urethral orifice located on the perineum. Epispadias is described as complete when the urethral orifice is located anterior to and off the penis.

The prepuce, if present, should be easily retractable from the glans and returnable to its original position. **Phimosis** exists when retraction cannot occur (Figure 20-9). This condition presents problems with cleanliness and prevents observation of the glans and interior surfaces of the prepuce. If the foreskin has been partially retracted but has impinged on the penis so that it cannot be returned to its usual position, the condition is called **paraphimosis**.

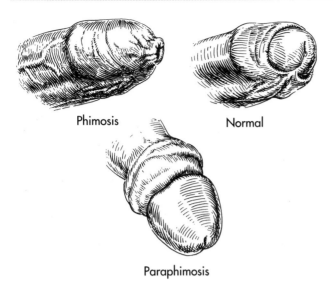

Phimosis   Normal

Paraphimosis

Figure 20-9   Phimosis, normal retraction of the prepuce, and paraphimosis.

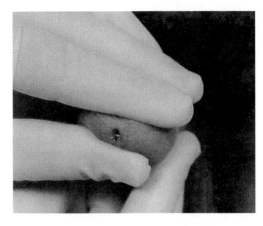

Figure 20-10   Compression of the glans to open the urethral meatus.

Palpation of the Penis

Carefully palpate the penile shaft with the thumb and the first two fingers of the examining hand. The penis should feel smooth and semi-firm. The overlying skin appears slightly wrinkled and feels somewhat movable over the underlying structures. Note any swelling, nodules, and induration as possible abnormal findings. Occasionally hard, nontender subcutaneous plaques are palpated on the dorsomedial surface. The client with this condition, called **Peyronie's disease**, may report penile bending with erection and painful intercourse.

Either compress the tip of the glans yourself or ask the client to compress the glans anteroposteriorly (Figure 20-10). This maneuver opens the distal end of the urethra for inspection. Observe for evidence of inflammation or lesions.

Inspection of the Scrotum

Instruct the client to hold the penis out of the way, and observe the general size, superficial appearance, and symmetry of the scrotum (Figure 20-11). The scrotum normally appears asymmetrical because the left testis is generally lower than the right testis. Also, the tone of the dartos muscle determines the size and position of the scrotum; this muscle contracts when the area is cold and relaxes when the area is warm. In advanced age, the dartos muscle is somewhat atonic, and the scrotum may appear pendulous.

The scrotal skin is more darkly pigmented than that of the rest of the body. To observe the scrotal skin, spread its rugated surface. Also, remember to inspect the posterior and posterolateral and anterior and anterolateral skin areas. A common abnormality, occurring as a single lesion or as multiple lesions, is that of **sebaceous cysts**. These are firm, yellow to white, nontender cutaneous lesions measuring up to 1 cm in diameter.

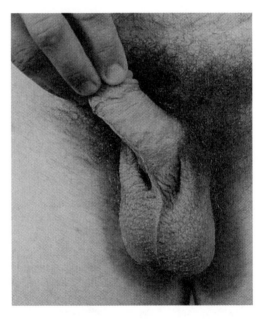

Figure 20-11   Normal appearance of the scrotum in the adult.

Palpation of the Scrotum

Before palpating the scrotum, assure the client that you will do this gently. The skin of the scrotum is not especially sensitive, but the contents are very sensitive. Palpate the contents of each half of the scrotal sac (Figure 20-12). Both testes should be present in the scrotum at birth. If they are not present, determine their location by retracing their course of descent back into the abdomen.

Palpate both testes with the thumb and index finger. Determine their consistency, size, shape, and response to mild

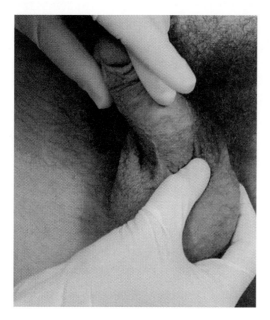

Figure 20-12   Palpation of the scrotal contents.

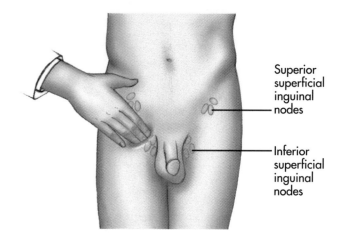

Superior superficial inguinal nodes

Inferior superficial inguinal nodes

Figure 20-13   Palpation of the inguinal lymph nodes.

pressure. The testes should be smooth, homogeneous in consistency, regular, equal in size, freely movable, and slightly sensitive to mild compression. If possible, palpate both testes simultaneously to allow for comparison between them.

Next, palpate each epididymis. The epididymides are located in the posterolateral area of the testes in 93% of the male population. In approximately 7%, the epididymides lie in the anterolateral or anterior areas. Palpate them and note their size, shape, consistency, and tenderness. To palpate the epididymides, pick up the scrotum just beneath the testes, using the thumb, first finger, and middle finger of each hand. Bring the fingers together under the testes. Next, move the fingers back several millimeters until the base of the testes is felt. Just under and behind the testes, you should feel the epididymides as tubular structures that collapse when gently compressed. Become accustomed to differentiating the consistencies of the testes and the epididymides and where each begins and ends. The epididymides should feel smooth, discrete, larger in their superior areas, and nontender.

Then palpate each of the spermatic cords by bilaterally grasping each between the thumb and index finger, starting at the base of the epididymis and continuing to the inguinal canal. The vas deferens feels similar to a smooth cord and is movable. The arteries, veins, lymph vessels, and nerves feel like indefinite threads along the side of the vas.

If swelling, irregularity, or nodularity is noted in the scrotum, an attempt should be made to transilluminate the focus area by darkening the room and placing a lighted flashlight behind the scrotal contents. **Transillumination** is noted by a red glow. On transillumination, the normal scrotum and epididymis will appear as dark masses with regular borders. Small areas of transilluminated space appear around the testes, with a larger transilluminated space appearing superior to the testes. The amount of transilluminated space su-

perior to the testes is dependent on the amount of scrotal relaxation. Because of concern about the transmission of disease, a disposable flashlight or a flashlight with a disposable plastic cover should be used. Serous fluid will transilluminate; tissue and blood will not and will appear dark.

The scrotum can be edematous, and palpation may produce pitting. Edema of the scrotum can occur in any condition that causes edema in the lower trunk (e.g., cardiovascular disease).

Palpation of the Regional Lymph Nodes

The lymph nodes of the inguinal areas may be assessed as part of the hernia examination or as part of the abdominal examination. Two sets of lymph nodes are assessed: superior inguinal and inferior inguinal (Figure 20-13).

The client can be lying down or standing for examination of the inguinal nodes. Flex the client's leg at the knee to relax the muscles of the inguinal area. Abduct the leg slightly; you may see a shallow, hollow space. Begin your palpation here, lightly at first, and then more deeply. Palpate from the anterosuperior iliac spine to the pubic tubercle. Do not confuse Poupart's ligament with enlarged lymph nodes. Enlarged lymph nodes will be close to the surface and fairly easy to feel. See Figure 20-13 for an illustration of lymph node palpation areas.

Palpation of the Prostate

With an ambulatory client, executing the rectal and prostate examination is done most satisfactorily with the client standing, hips flexed, toes pointed toward each other, and upper body resting on the examining table. This position flattens the buttocks, deters gluteal contraction, and makes the anus and rectum more accessible to evaluation. A debilitated client may be examined in the left lateral or lithotomy position. If

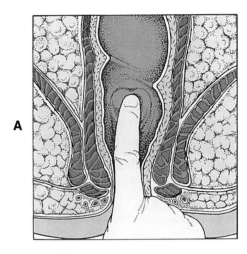

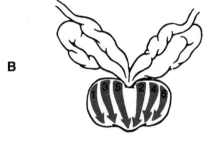

Figure 20-14 Palpation of the prostate. **A,** Position of the examiner's finger. **B,** Prostatic massage. *Arrows* indicate the areas of the prostate that are massaged and the sequence and direction of the massage.

the left lateral position is used, remind the client to flex his right knee and hip and to have his buttocks close to the edge of the examining table. The general procedure for the anal and rectal examination is described in Chapter 22. Perform the general rectal examination first. Then palpate the prostate gland and seminal vesicles with the pad of the index finger (Figure 20-14, *A*).

Visualize the prostate anatomy, its lobes, and its size in relationship to the bladder and the external anal sphincter. A common mistake of beginning practitioners is to palpate too deeply and mistake the base of the bladder for the prostate. Be sure to palpate the entire, accessible surface of the prostate. The prostate gland is located on the anterior rectal wall but should not be protruding into the rectal lumen.

■ HELPFUL HINT

In prostate examination, consider the following questions about the prostate:
• Surface: Smooth or nodular?
• Consistency: Rubbery, hard, boggy, soft, or fluctuant?
• Shape: Rounded or flat?
• Size: Normal, enlarged, or atrophied?
• Sensitivity: Tender or not?
• Movability: Movable or fixed?

Examination Step-by-Step

1. Inspect the condition of the skin and hair in the pubic region.
2. Inspect the pubic hair distribution. Assess the consistency of findings with the client's age.
3. Inspect the penis:
   a. Ask the client to retract the foreskin (if present).
   b. Inspect the glans for inflammation.
   c. Check the condition and position of the urethral meatus.
   d. Assess the skin for color, lesions, and swelling.
   e. Check the underside of the penis
4. Palpate the inguinal areas for nodes.
5. Palpate the penis:
   a. Compress the glans and check for inflammation or discharge.
   b. Examine the shaft of the penis for tenderness or induration (anterior and posterior surfaces).
   c. Strip the urethra for discharge (if symptomatic).
6. Inspect the scrotum:
   a. The client holds the penis out of the way.
   b. Inspect the skin and surface for color, symmetry, and swelling.
7. Palpate the scrotum:
   a. Spread the rugae to examine the surface for consistency, size, tenderness, and masses.
   b. Examine each spermatic cord for consistency, size, tenderness, and masses.
   c. Palpate the testes.
   d. Palpate the epididymides.
   e. Transilluminate any masses present.
8. Palpate the prostate gland (in conjunction with the rectal examination):
   a. Assess for extension into the lumen, surface characteristics, size, consistency, tenderness, and mobility.

Prostatic enlargement, or protrusion of the prostate gland into the rectal lumen, is commonly described in the following grades:
• Grade I: Encroaches less than 1 cm into the rectal lumen
• Grade II: Encroaches 1 to 2 cm into the rectal lumen
• Grade III: Encroaches 2 to 3 cm into the rectal lumen
• Grade IV: Encroaches more than 3 cm into the rectal lumen

The gland should be approximately 3 cm long, approximately 4 cm across at its base, symmetrical, movable, and of a rubbery (like a pencil eraser) consistency. Its median sulcus normally can be felt. The lateral margins of the prostate gland should be discrete, and a moderate degree of mobility can be noted when the tip of the index finger is hooked over the upper border of the gland and the gland is pulled down gently.

The proximal portions of the seminal vesicles can sometimes be palpated as corrugated structures above the lateral to the midpoint of the gland. Normally, they are too soft to

Additional Diagnostic Studies

Diagnostic Studies That *May* Be Indicated	Explanation of Test
Prostate-Specific Antigen (PSA)	PSA is a glycoprotein specific to the prostate but not to prostate cancer. It is normally produced by prostatic tissue. PSA is often elevated in men with prostate cancer. The American Cancer Society recommends annual PSA testing for all men over age 50, and for African-American men and men with a positive family history for prostatic cancer. A major limitation of the test is its poor specificity; abnormal results are often due to benign conditions. PSA findings under 4 ng/ml are considered normal. Results over 10 ng/ml are considered high. Between 4 ng/ml and 10 ng/ml, the results are considered borderline.
Fine-needle biopsy	Recommended when the PSA level is high
Transrectal or transurethral ultrasound	Recommended when the rectal examination findings are abnormal, but the PSA levels are borderline and a biopsy may be indicated. Helps to identify areas of the prostate most appropriate for biopsy.

From Woolf SH, Jonas S, Lawrence RS: *Health promotion and disease prevention in clinical practice,* Baltimore, 1996, Williams & Wilkins.

be palpated. Attempt to examine all available surfaces of the prostate gland and the entire area of the seminal vesicles. Significant abnormalities of the prostate gland or seminal vesicles include protrusion into the rectal lumen; hard, nodular areas; bogginess; tenderness; and asymmetry.

If infection is suspected, the prostate gland can be massaged centrally from its lateral edges to force secretions into the urethra (Figure 20-14, *B).* Stroke the prostate from its distal to proximal areas, with the order of strokes indicated in the illustration. Secretions at the urethral opening can be examined and cultured. It is important to massage all areas of the prostate accessible for palpation.

Screening Tests and Procedures

The U.S. Preventive Services Task Force (1996, p. 580) recommendation about screening for testicular cancer is as follows:

> There is insufficient evidence to recommend for or against routine screening of asymptomatic men in the general population for testicular cancer by physician examination or patient self-examination. Recommendations to discuss screening options with select high-risk patients may be made on other grounds.

Because this recommendation is somewhat ambiguous and since the self-examination is easily and quickly done during a bath or a shower, consider teaching it to every client and recommending that it be done monthly on some target date.

The U.S. Preventive Services Task Force (1996, p. 581) recommendation about screening for prostate cancer is as follows:

> Routine screening for prostate cancer with digital examinations, serum tumor markers (e.g., prostate specific antigen), or transrectal ultrasound is not recommended.

Table 20-2 presents information about the use of additional diagnostic studies that may be indicated if prostatic cancer is suspected.

VARIATIONS FROM HEALTH

Penis

Among the more common penile lesions are syphilitic chancre, condylomata acuminata, the vesicles of genital herpes, and cancer. See Figure 20-15 for illustrations of these various lesions. The syphilitic chancre is the primary lesion of syphilis. It begins as a single papule that eventually erodes into an oval or round red ulcer with an indurated base that discharges serous material. It is usually painless.

Condylomata acuminata are wart-appearing growths. They are caused by human papillomavirus and may be seen occurring singly or in multiple cauliflower-like patches on the penis and throughout the genital area. They can be transmitted to a partner via sexual intercourse.

Herpes lesions appear as painful clusters of superficial vesicles.

Carcinoma of the penis occurs most commonly on the glans and the inner lip of the prepuce. It may appear dry and scaly, ulcerated, or nodular. It is usually painless.

Scrotum

The common abnormalities of the scrotum are described and illustrated in Table 20-3. All scrotal masses should be described by their placement, size, shape, consistency, and tenderness and by whether they transilluminate.

Prostate

A hard single or multiple lesion on a firm and fixed prostate gland may indicate cancer. The initial lesion of carcinoma is commonly on the posterior lobe and can often be easily identified during the rectal examination. A soft, symmetrical, boggy, nontender prostate gland may indicate benign prostatic hypertrophy, a condition very common in men older than 50 years. In the later stages of this condition, the median sulcus may be obliterated. A boggy, fluctuant, or tender prostate gland may indicate acute or chronic **prostatitis**.

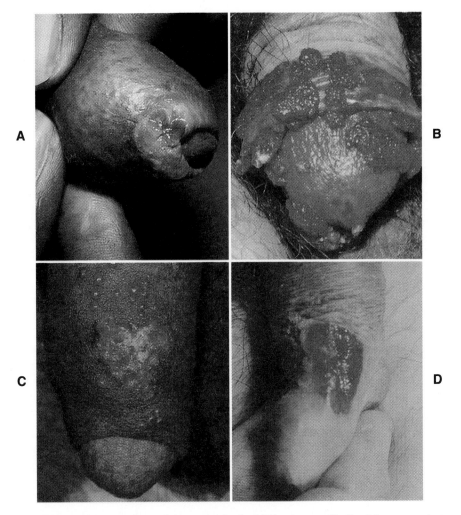

Figure 20-15   Various lesions of the penis. **A,** Syphilitic chancre. **B,** Condyloma acuminatum.
C, Genital herpes. **D,** Cancer of the penis.

TABLE 20-3	**Description of Scrotal Abnormalities**	
Abnormality	**Definition/Causation**	**History (Hₓ) and Physical Examination (PE) Findings**
Epididymal mass or nodularity 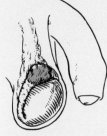	May be result of benign or malignant neoplasms, syphilis, or tuberculosis	(Hₓ) Usually painless (PE) Nodules are not tender; in tuberculosis lesions, vas deferens often feels beaded
Epididymitis 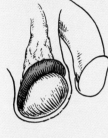	Inflammation of epididymis, usually resulting from *Escherichia coli*, *Neisseria gonorrhoeae*, or *Mycobacterium tuberculosis* organisms*	(Hₓ) Sudden onset of pain and rapid swelling in the scrotum; somewhat relieved by elevation; fever (PE) Red, swollen scrotum; spermatic cord often thickened and indurated; extreme pain with palpation; epididymis enlarged with overlying skin thick and edematous; pain relieved by elevation
Hydrocele 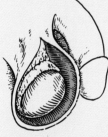	Accumulation of serous fluid between visceral and parietal layers of tunica vaginalis	(Hₓ) Painless; may be feeling of weight or bulk in scrotum (PE) Transilluminates; large, nontender, cystic mass; fingers can get above mass
Scrotal hernia 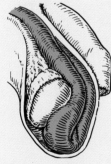	Hernia within scrotum; usually due to an indirect inguinal hernia	(Hₓ) History of swelling; pain with straining (PE) Enlarged scrotum; may reduce when supine; does not transilluminate; soft, mushy mass; bowel sounds auscultated; fingers cannot get above mass

TABLE 20-3   Description of Scrotal Abnormalities—cont'd

Abnormality	Definition/Causation	History (Hₓ) and Physical Examination (PE) Findings
Spermatocele 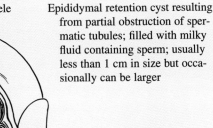	Epididymal retention cyst resulting from partial obstruction of spermatic tubules; filled with milky fluid containing sperm; usually less than 1 cm in size but occasionally can be larger	(Hₓ) Painless (PE) Transilluminates; round mass, feels like a third testis—round and freely movable; painless
Testicular tumor 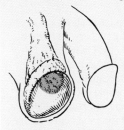	Multiple causes; most occur between the ages of 18 to 35	(Hₓ) Usually not painful (PE) Firm nodule, harder in consistency than normal testis; hydroceles may develop as result of a tumor; if testis cannot be palpated, fluid may need to be aspirated so that testis can be accurately evaluated
Torsion of spermatic cord 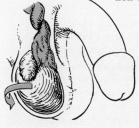	Axial rotation or volvulus of spermatic cord, resulting in infarction of testicle	(Hₓ) History of extreme pain of sudden onset and tenderness of testis; may also have lower abdominal pain, nausea, and vomiting; usually no fever (PE) Elevated mass in scrotum; pain not relieved by further elevation; more common in childhood or adolescence; followed by hyperemic swelling and hydrocele; cord is thick, swollen, and tender; cremasteric reflex is absent on affected side
Varicocele	Abnormal dilation and tortuosity of veins of pampiniform plexus; often described as "bag of worms" in scrotum	(Hₓ) Complaints of dragging sensation or dull pain in scrotal area (PE) Most often noted on left side; collapses when scrotum is elevated and increases when scrotum is dependent; more commonly present on left side; usually appears at puberty; feels like soft bag of worms

TEACHING SELF-ASSESSMENT

Genital self-examination is a means of early identification of scrotal cancer and sexually transmitted diseases. This examination shoud be taught to boys by age 15 and to all men who do not do already perform it.

At the initiation of the teaching, assess the male client's level of knowledge about genital self-examination, reinforce the importance of a monthly self-examination, and provide instruction for the examination. Accompany the examination with pictures of the anatomy of the male genitalia.

Teaching Self-Assessment

1. Regular monthly self-examination of your testicles and male organs is important because:
   a. Cancer of the testes is one of the most curable forms of cancer when detected early. The cure rate is approximately 90%.
   b. Cancer of the testes can affect males of any age but is most common between ages 15 and 35. It is much more likely in men whose testicles descended after infancy or never descended at all.
   c. Men can have normal sexual relations after being treated for cancer of the testicle.
   d. You may uncover some other problems, which if treated early, will prevent more serious problems and transmission to others.
   e. The examination only takes a minute.
2. Do the self-examination during or following a shower or warm bath, when the testes are relaxed, descended, and accessible for palpation.
3. Examine the penis for lesions and discharge:
   a. Inspect the head of the penis—retract the foreskin (if present).
   b. Examine the entire shaft.
   c. Inspect the urethral meatus for discharge (Figure 20-16, *A*).
4. Examine the skin and pubic hair for lesions and parasites.
5. Examine the scrotum and its contents:
   a. Use the thumbs and the index and middle fingers for examination, with the thumbs placed on the top and the fingers

on the underside of the scrotum (Figure 20-16, *B*). First, spread out the scrotal skin and examine the entire scrotum and the adjacent skin areas and note any rashes, sores, or bumps.
   b. Then, gently roll the contents of the scrotum between your thumbs and fingers. The normal testicle is about 1.5 to 2 inches long. It feels smooth, rubbery, and firm but not hard. It feels like a hard-boiled egg. On its back surface and top lies the epididymis, which feels like a ridge running up the backside of the testicle. The epididymis is the storage tube found behind each testicle. Each should feel soft and spongy and sometimes slightly tender. The spermatic cords extend from the bottom of the epididymides and up into the pelvis. The cords are made up of muscle fibers, blood vessels, and the vas deferens. The fibers and vessels will feel spongy, and the vas deferens feel like smooth, firm tubes, similar to a rod of cooked spaghetti.
   c. The examination should be painless unless the pressure is too hard or some problem exists. A small amount of tenderness may be noticed during the palpation of the testes and the epididymides; this is normal. *Any lump or change in texture, whether painful or not, should be reported to and assessed by a health care provider as soon as possible.*
6. After a few self-examinations you will become very familiar with the feel of your male organs. Any changes will leap out at you. Report anything new to your health care provider.

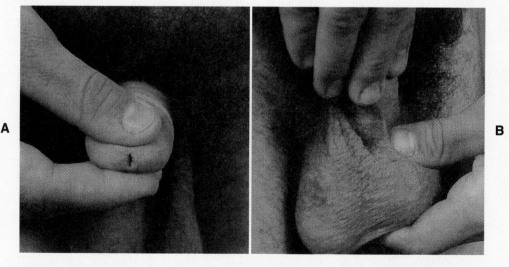

Figure 20-16   Male genital self-examination. **A,** Examination of the urethral meatus. **B,** Scrotal assessment.

ASSESSMENT OF INGUINAL AREA FOR HERNIAS

Anatomy of Hernias

The inguinal ligament (**Poupart's ligament**) extends from the anterosuperior spine of the ilium to the pubic tubercle. The inguinal canal is a flattened tunnel between two layers of abdominal muscle, measuring approximately 4 to 6 cm in the adult. Its internal ring is located 1 to 2 cm above the midpoint of the inguinal ligament. The spermatic cord traverses this internal ring, passes through the canal, exits the canal at its external (subcutaneous) ring, and then moves up and over the inguinal ligament and into the scrotum (Figure 20-17).

Hesselbach's triangle is the region superior to the inguinal canal, medial to the inferior epigastric artery, and lateral to the margin of the rectus muscle.

The femoral canal is a potential space for a femoral hernia just inferior to the inguinal ligament and 3 cm medial and parallel to the femoral artery. When the examiner's right hand is placed on the client's right anterior thigh with the index finger over the femoral artery, the femoral canal will be under the examiner's ring finger.

The three main types of pelvic area **hernias** are shown in Figure 20-18. Groin hernias arising above the abdominocrural crease are call inguinal hernias. Inguinal hernias may be classified as indirect, direct, or both. When both are present, the presentation is termed pantaloon hernia. The direct inguinal hernia emerges directly from behind and through the external inguinal ring. In the indirect inguinal hernia, the hernial sac enters the internal inguinal canal, and its tip is located somewhere in the inguinal canal or beyond the canal. In men, indirect inguinal hernias may descend into the scrotum.

The femoral hernias are found below the abdominocrural crease and result in the protrusion of abdominal contents through the femoral ring. The hernia emerges through the femoral ring, the femoral canal, and the fossa ovalis. The characteristics of the three main types of hernias are compared in Table 20-4.

EXAMINATION OF INGUINAL AREA

Focused Health History

Present Health/Illness Status

1. Pain or swelling in the groin

Past Health History

1. Surgery to the inguinal area
2. Infections in the legs or abdomen

Family Health History

1. Hernias

Symptom Analysis

Pain or Swelling in the Groin

1. Enlargement, swelling, or lump in the inguinal area
   a. **Onset:** time of onset and symptoms accompanying onset
   b. **Course since onset:** timing and nature of symptom appearance, pattern of symptoms since first appearance, changes in size of bulge
   c. **Location:** exact location of the enlargement
   d. **Quality:** appearance, reducibility, size, surface characteristics, type of accompanying tenderness or pain (e.g., dragging or heavy feeling)
   e. **Quantity:** size and changes in size
   f. **Setting:** changes with posture or specific activity, relationship to work or other labor

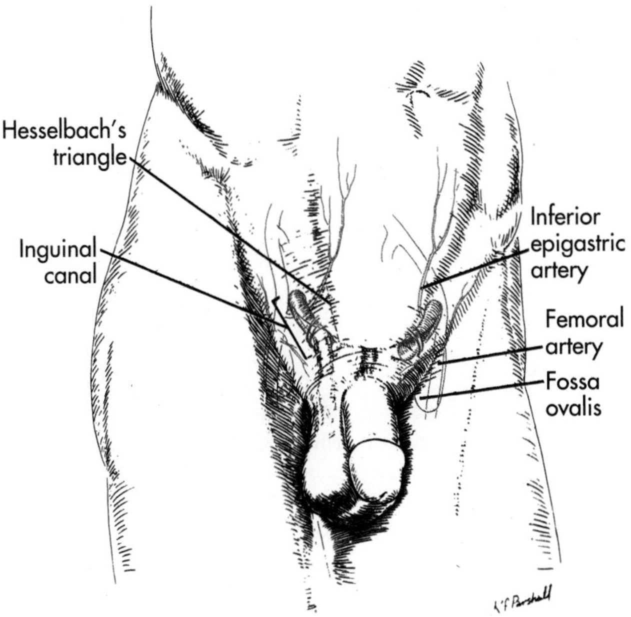

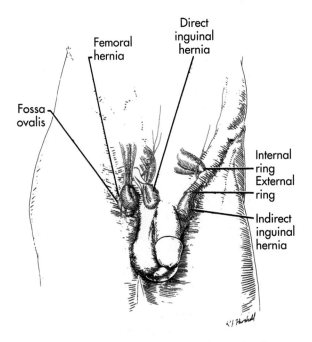

Figure 20-17 Superficial anatomy of the anterior pelvic area.

Figure 20-18 Three common pelvic area hernias.

TABLE 20-4	Comparison of Inguinal and Femoral Hernias		
	Inguinal Hernia		
	Indirect	**Direct**	**Femoral Hernia**
Course	Sac emerges through internal inguinal ring, lateral to inferior epigastric artery; can remain in canal, exit external ring, or pass into scrotum	Sac emerges directly from behind and through external inguinal ring; located in region of Hesselbach's triangle	Sac emerges through femoral ring, femoral canal, and fossa ovalis; observed medial to femoral artery
Incidence	More common in infants younger than 1 year and in young men 16 to 20 years; more common in men than in women at a ratio of approximately 4:1; 60% of all hernias	Most often observed in men older than 40 years; rarer than indirect hernia; accounts for 30% of hernias in males and 1.5% of hernias in females	Less common than inguinal hernias; seldom seen in children; more common in women; 4% of all hernias
Cause	Congenital or acquired	Congenital weakness exacerbated by (1) lifting, (2) atrophy of abdominal muscles, (3) ascites, (4) chronic cough, or (5) obesity	Acquired; may be caused by (1) stooping frequently, (2) increased abdominal pressure, (3) loss of muscle substance
Clinical symptoms and signs	Soft swelling in region of internal inguinal ring—swelling increases when client stands or strains, is sometimes reduced when client reclines; pain during straining	Abdominal bulge in area of Hesselbach's triangle, usually in area of internal ring; usually painless; easily reduced when client reclines; rarely enters scrotum	Right side more commonly affected; pain may be severe; strangulation frequent; sac may extend into scrotum, into labium, or along saphenous vein

Preparation for Examination

EQUIPMENT

Item	Purpose
Rubber gloves	Protect examiner from infection

CLIENT AND ENVIRONMENT

Client	Uncovered from the waist
	Preferably standing
Environment	Warm
	Private

g. **Associated phenomena:** presence of pain, tenderness, redness, changes in appearance of overlying skin
h. **Alleviating and aggravating factors:** medications, use of supportive devices, association with lifting or straining
i. **Underlying concern:** surgery

Preparation for Examination: Client and Environment

If a client has an inguinal or groin area hernia, he or she will probably complain of a swelling or bulging in that area, especially during abdominal straining. However, as part of the routine physical examination, all clients should be screened for inguinal and femoral hernias, even if they do not complain of groin swelling.

No special equipment is needed for the examination. The examiner should wear rubber gloves.

Technique for Examination and Expected Findings

Inspection and palpation are the techniques used for assessment of the inguinal area. Whenever possible, perform the examination for hernias with the client standing. However, if the client is debilitated or especially tense, perform the examination while he or she is lying down on a flat surface.

First, expose the areas of inguinal and femoral hernias and observe them with the client at rest and while the client holds his or her breath and exerts abdominal pressure by pushing the diaphragm into the abdomen. Straining is preferred to coughing because a more sustained pressure is elicited. Sometimes the impulse of coughing can be confused with the impulse of a hernia. Often, small hernias in women and children are more easily observed than felt because of the lack of fatty tissue in the area.

Palpate for a direct inguinal hernia by placing two fingers over each external inguinal ring and instructing the client to bear down. The presence of a hernia will produce a palpable bulge in the area.

To determine the presence of an indirect inguinal hernia, ask the client to flex the ipsilateral knee slightly while you attempt to direct your index or little finger into the path of the inguinal canal. When the finger has traversed as far as possi-

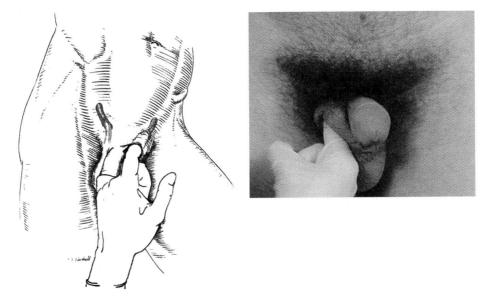

Figure 20-19 Examination of a male client for an indirect inguinal hernia.

Examination Step-by-Step

1. Inspect the inguinal area for bulges at rest and with straining.
2. Palpate the inguinal canals for a direct hernia—bilaterally at rest and with straining.
3. Palpate the inguinal canals for an indirect hernia—bilaterally at rest and with straining.
4. Palpate the femoral areas at rest and with straining.
5. Palpate the superior and inferior lymph nodes.

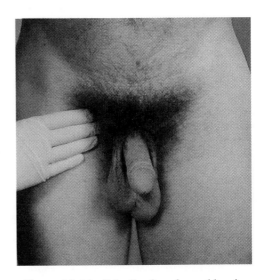

Figure 20-20 Palpation for a femoral hernia.

ble, ask the client to strain. A hernia will be felt as a mass of tissue meeting the finger and then withdrawing. To examine the client's left side, use the index or little finger of the left hand with the palm side out. For the client's right side, use the right hand. In women, the canal is narrow, and the finger cannot be inserted far, if at all. In men, the finger invaginates scrotal skin into the inguinal canal (Figure 20-19).

In both men and women, each fossa ovalis area is palpated while the client is straining (Figure 20-20). The femoral hernia will be felt as a soft tumor at the fossa, below the inguinal ligament and lateral to the pubic tubercle.

Occasionally the client may complain of the symptoms of hernia although none can be palpated. In such cases a load test is suggested. The client lifts a heavy object while the inguinal area is observed. A previously unobserved bulge may become prominent.

Sample Documentation and Diagnoses

FOCUSED HEALTH HISTORY (SUBJECTIVE DATA)

Mr. C, an 18-year-old college freshman, has come to the university health service complaining of pain on urination. Feels he needs to void every hour but produces only a small amount of urine. Has noted thick, white penile discharge for about 4 days—small, whitish yellow, dime-sized stains on his underwear. Denies fever; back, flank, or abdominal pain, or genital rash. No known allergies. No history of previous genitourinary disease. No prior history of sexually transmitted disease (STD). Had a recent episode of unprotected sexual intercourse about 10 days before examination. Is concerned that he has an STD and is avoiding all sexual activity.

FOCUSED PHYSICAL EXAMINATION (OBJECTIVE DATA)

Vital signs: BP 120/72, pulse 82, respirations 16, temperature 37.5° C (99.5° F)

Physical examination: Pubic hair pattern in adult male distribution. Skin clear of lesions. Circumcised penis with no lesions. Meatus red with a small amount of discharge apparent on tip. Testes and epididymides not tender and without masses or swelling. Inguinal and femoral canal areas without bulging or masses. Tenderness elicited in areas of superior inguinal lymph nodes, but no discrete lymph nodes palpated.

DIAGNOSES

HEALTH PROBLEM

Genitourinary infection

NURSING DIAGNOSES

Ineffective Sexuality Patterns Related to Effects of Infection and Pain

Defining Characteristics

- Decreased ability to have sexual intercourse due to genital pain
- Penile discharge
- Concern about unprotected sexual encounter

Anxiety Related to Threat to and/or Changes in Sexual Health Status

Defining Characteristics

- Uncertainty of health status
- Voiced worry over whether he has STD

Urinary Retention Related to Infection of Unknown Origin

Defining Characteristics

- Small, frequent voiding
- Sensation of bladder fullness

Critical Thinking Questions

Review the Sample Documentation and Diagnoses box to answer these questions.

1. Would you approach the history and physical examination differently, depending on whether Mr. C. indicated he had intercourse with a male or a female?

2. If he also had a painless nodule on his right testes, what additional historical information would you collect?

3. If the client were 50 years old and married, what additional historical information would you collect?

Answers are available on the MERLIN website (www.harcourthealth.com/MERLIN/Barkauskas/). And be sure to check the website regularly for additional learning activities!

Remember to check out the Online Study Guide!
www.harcourthealth.com/MERLIN/Barkauskas/

Chapter **21**

Female Genitalia

Learning Objectives

On successful study of this chapter and completion of related learning experiences, the learner will be able to:
- Describe the anatomy and physiology of the female reproductive system.
- Outline the history relevant to assessment of the female reproductive system.
- Explain the rationale for and demonstrate assessment of the female genitalia, including client positioning, inspection, speculum procedures, and palpation techniques.
- Recognize anatomical findings of bimanual vaginal and rectovaginal examinations.
- Recognize the common appearance of the vulva, vagina, and cervix.
- Describe procedures used to collect smears and cultures.

Outline

Purpose of Examination

The purpose of the screening examination of the female genitalia is to assess the health of the female reproductive system and to screen for various sexually transmitted diseases (STDs) and cervical cancer. The regional examination of the female genital system consists of (1) the abdominal examination, (2) inspection of the external genitalia, (3) palpation of the external genitalia, (4) the speculum examination, (5) specimen collection, (6) the bimanual vaginal examination, and (7) the rectovaginal examination. The examination of the inguinal area for hernias and nodes (see Chapter 20) and the assessment of the anus and rectum (see Chapter 22) are integrated into the examination of the genitalia.

ANATOMY AND PHYSIOLOGY

External Genitalia

The external female genitalia are termed the vulva or pudendum (Figure 21-1). A pad of fat called the mons pubis or mons veneris covers the symphysis pubis. In the postpubertal female, a patch of coarse, curly hair that extends to the lower abdomen covers the mons. The abdominal portion of the female escutcheon is flat and forms the base of an inverted triangle of hair.

The labia majora are two bilobate folds of adipose tissue extending from the mons to the perineum. After puberty, their outer surfaces are covered with hair and their inner surfaces are smooth and hairless. The labia minora are two folds of skin that are thinner and darker than the labia majora. The labia minora lie within the labia majora and extend from the clitoris to the fourchette. Anteriorly, each labium minus divides into a medial and a lateral part. The lateral parts join posteriorly to form the prepuce of the clitoris, and the medial parts join anterior to the clitoris to form the frenulum of the clitoris. The clitoris is composed of erectile tissue, homologous to the corpus cavernosum of the penis. Its body is normally about 2.5 cm long; the length of its visible portion is 2 cm or less.

The vestibule is the boat-shaped anatomical region between the labia minora. It contains the urethral and vaginal orifices. The urethral orifice is located approximately 2.5 cm posterior and inferior to the clitoris and is visualized as an irregular, vertical slit or an inverted V. The vaginal orifice, or **introitus**, lies immediately behind and inferior to the ure-thral orifice and can be observed as a thin vertical slit or as a large orifice with irregular skin edges, depending on the condition of the hymen. The hymen is a membranous, annular, or crescentic fold at the vaginal opening. When it is not perforated, it is usually a continuous membrane but on occasion may be cribriform. After perforation, small rounded fragments of hymen attach to the introital margins; these are called hymenal caruncles.

The ducts of two types of glands open on the vulva. Skene's glands are multiple, tiny organs located in the paraurethral area. They secrete a fluid that lubricates the vaginal vestibule during sexual intercourse. Their ducts, numbering approximately 6 to 31, lie inside and just outside of the urethral orifice and are usually not visible. When the urethral orifice is visualized as the center of a clock, these ducts open laterally and slightly posterior to the urethral orifice in approximately the 5 and 7 o'clock positions. Bartholin's glands are small, ovoid organs located lateral and slightly posterior to the vaginal orifice. During sexual excitement, these glands secrete mucus, which lubricates the introitus and promotes sperm motility and viability. Their ducts are approximately 2 cm long and open in the groove between the labia minora and the hymen in approximately the 5 and 7 o'clock positions relative to the introitus. These ducts are also usually not visible.

The perineum consists of the tissues between the introitus and the anus.

The pelvic floor consists of a group of muscles attached to points on the bony pelvis (Figure 21-2). These muscles form a suspended sling that assists in holding the pelvic con-

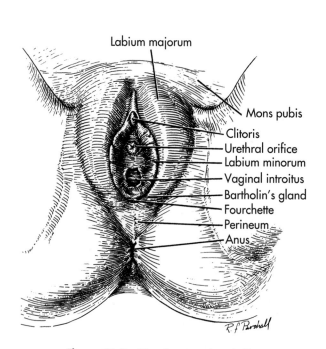

Figure 21-1 Female external genitalia.

Labium majorum
Mons pubis
Clitoris
Urethral orifice
Labium minorum
Vaginal introitus
Bartholin's gland
Fourchette
Perineum
Anus

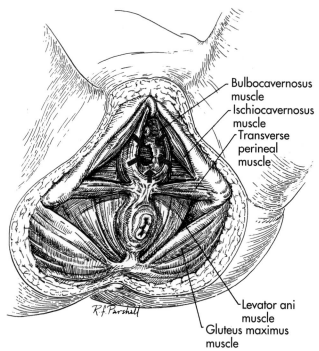

Figure 21-2 Muscles of the pelvic floor. *Arrows* illustrate the direction of contraction of the bulbocavernosus muscle.

Bulbocavernosus muscle
Ischiocavernosus muscle
Transverse perineal muscle
Levator ani muscle
Gluteus maximus muscle

tents in place. The muscles are pierced by the urethral, vaginal, and rectal orifices and function both passively as a pelvic support and actively in voluntary contraction of the vaginal and anal orifices.

Internal Genitalia

Figures 21-3 and 21-4 display the internal genitalia. The vagina is a pink, transversely **rugated**, collapsed tube that in the adult is approximately 9 cm long posteriorly and 6 to 7 cm long anteriorly. It inclines posteriorly at approximately a 45-degree angle with the vertical plane of the body. The vagina is highly dilatable, especially in its superior portion and anteroposterior dimension. When collapsed, it is roughly H-shaped in transverse section. Superiorly and usually anteriorly, the uterine cervix pierces the vagina. The recess between the portion of the vagina adjacent to the cervix and the cervix is called the vaginal **fornix**. Although it is actually a continuous circle, the fornix is anatomically divided into anterior, posterior, and lateral fornices.

The uterus is an inverted, pear-shaped, muscular organ that is flattened anteroposteriorly. It is usually found inclined forward 45 degrees from the vertical plane of the erect body and is approximately 5.5 to 8 cm long, 3.5 to 4 cm wide, and 2 to 2.5 cm thick in clients who have never been pregnant (i.e., nulligravidous clients). The uterus of a client who has borne and delivered a viable offspring (i.e., a parous client) may be normally enlarged an additional 2 to 3 cm in any of the three dimensions. The uterus is divided into two main parts: the body and the cervix. The body in turn is

composed of three parts: the fundus, the prominence above the insertion of the fallopian tubes; the body, or main portion, of the uterus; and the isthmus, the constricted lower portion of the uterus, which is adjacent to the cervix. The cervix extends from the isthmus into the vagina.

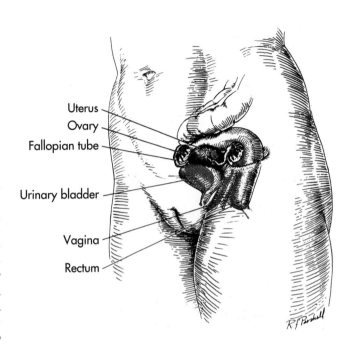

Figure 21-3   Internal female genitalia.

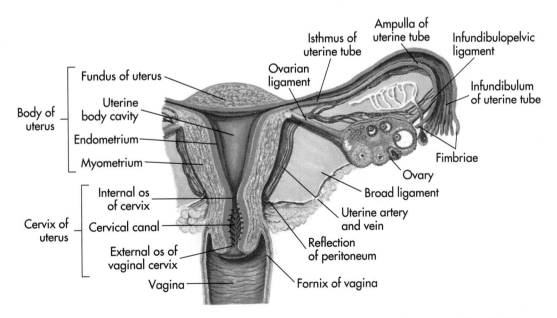

Figure 21-4   Cross-sectional view of internal female genitalia and pelvic contents. (From Seidel HM et al.: *Mosby's guide to physical examination,* ed. 4, St. Louis, 1999, Mosby.)

The uterine cavity communicates with the vagina through an **ostium**, the cervical os. The os is a small, depressed, regular, circular opening in clients who have not delivered an infant (i.e., nulliparous women). In women who have delivered children vaginally, the os is enlarged and irregularly shaped. The position of the uterus is not fixed; it is a relatively movable organ. The uterus may be anteverted, anteflexed, retroverted, or retroflexed in position; or it may be in midposition. (See Table 21-2 later in this chapter for illustrations of these positions.) Most commonly, in an adult with an empty bladder the uterus is usually anteverted and slightly anteflexed in position.

The ovaries are a pair of oval organs; each is approximately 3 cm long, 2 cm wide, and 1 cm thick. They are usually located near the lateral pelvic wall, at the level of the anterosuperior iliac spine. The two fallopian tubes insert in the upper portion of the uterus, are supported loosely by the broad ligament, and run laterally to the ovaries. Each tube is approximately 10 cm long.

The uterus, ovaries, and tubes are supported by four pairs of ligaments: the cardinal, uterosacral, round, and broad ligaments (Figure 21-5).

The rectouterine pouch, or Douglas' cul-de-sac, is a deep recess formed by the peritoneum as it passes over the intestinal surface of the rectum posterior to the uterus. It is the lowest point in the abdominal cavity.

The two groups of superficial nodes in the inguinal area are the superior and inferior inguinal nodes (see Chapter 20 for discussion of position and examination of the inguinal nodes). These nodes receive most of the lymph drainage from the legs. The superior inguinal nodes lie somewhat horizontally along the inguinal ligament. They receive drainage from the abdominal wall below the umbilicus, the external genitalia, the anal canal, the vulva and lower one third of the vagina, the gluteal area, and the inferior inguinal nodes. Lymph from around the internal female genitalia drains into deeper nodes, which are not accessible to palpa-

tion. The inferior group lies somewhat vertically below the junction of the saphenous and femoral veins. These large lymph nodes receive lymph from the superficial regions of the leg and foot.

EXAMINATION

Focused Health History

Present Health/Illness Status

The reproductive health history is fairly extensive. For a follow-up encounter in a health care system, much of the historical information will probably be on the record, and the focus of the interval history will be on the presenting health need or problem. The gynecological and obstetrical regional

Risk Factors
Female Cancers

CERVICAL CANCER

Age: between 40 and 55 years
History: cervical dysplasias, condylomata acuminata lesions, herpes infection, exposure to diethylstilbestrol, smoking, HIV positive
First coitus: early age
Sex partners: multiple or partner with multiple partners
Pregnancies: multiple
Low socioeconomic status

ENDOMETRIAL CANCER

Age: postmenopausal
Menarche: early
Menopause: late
Parity: low or infertility
Body weight: obese
History: hypertension, diabetes, endometrial hyperplasia, liver disease, pelvic irradiation, polycystic ovary syndrome, other cancers
Estrogen: history of replacement
Family history: endometrial, breast, or colon cancer
Personal history: middle to upper socioeconomic status

OVARIAN CANCER

Age: risk increases with age
History: ovarian dysfunction, anovulatory cycles, early menarche, late menopause, treatment for infertility, spontaneous abortions, cancer of breast or endometrium, irradiation of pelvic organs, endometriosis
Family history: ovarian or breast cancer
Environment: exposure to talc or asbestos
Diet high in animal fat

VULVAR CANCER

Age: risk increases with age
History: chronic vulvar inflammatory disorders, lower genital track neoplasia, diabetes, HIV infection
Cigarette smoking
Obesity
Environmental factors: exposure to environmental carcinogens

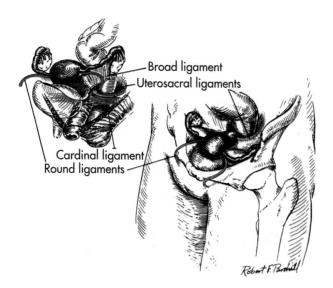

Robert F. Baraball

Figure 21-5 Ligaments of the internal female genitalia.

history for a new adult client will be, out of necessity, somewhat lengthy (see the following outline). Throughout the health history interview, record the following data about symptoms or problems: (1) onset (specific date, sudden or gradual), (2) course since onset, (3) location, (4) quality, (5) quantity, (6) setting, (7) associated phenomena, (8) alleviating and aggravating factors, and (9) the client's underlying concern.

A. Menstrual history
1. Age menses initiated (**menarche**)
2. Date of first day of last menstrual period (LMP)
3. Date of last normal menstrual period (LNMP) (NOTE: This date may be the same as or different from the LMP. Discrepancies may be clinically significant)
4. Pattern: frequency (days), duration (days), and amount of bleeding (in total number of tampons and/or pads used totally or per day); presence and size of clots (e.g., size of a quarter)
5. Associated symptoms premenstrually or during menses (**dysmenorrhea**): headaches, edema, pain, cramping, distention, weight gain, irritability, mood swings, breast tenderness, effect on activities of daily living, breast engorgement
   a. Frequency of dysmenorrhea—every cycle or other pattern
   b. Timing in the menstrual cycle
   c. Disability assessment
   d. Measures used for relief and effectiveness
6. Intermenstrual bleeding or spotting
7. Changes in cycle: **metrorrhagia, oligomenorrhea**
8. If menopausal—age at onset of symptoms, changing menstrual pattern, mood changes, hot flashes, irregular vaginal bleeding, emotional concerns, hormone replacement therapy

B. Self-care
1. Menstrual hygiene—especially length of time tampons are left intravaginally
2. Pattern of douching (including solution used, strength of solution, and frequency)
3. Use of feminine hygiene products
4. Type of material in underpants and pantyhose worn (e.g., cotton versus synthetic materials)
5. Habits of wearing tight clothing, especially pants and pantyhose
6. Planning for pregnancy, if applicable
7. Use of protection against sexually transmitted diseases
8. Date and results of last Papanicolaou (Pap) smear, any abnormalities on previous Pap smears

C. Medications: contraceptive, hormonal, or other prescribed for management of reproductive system problems
1. Name
2. Dosage
3. Purpose
4. Frequency
5. Duration
6. Side effects
7. Adherence

D. Past health history
1. Past gynecological diagnoses, procedures, and surgeries
2. Pregnancies: dates, duration of gestations, complications, condition of infants if live births, and other relevant outcomes (including abortions [spontaneous, elective, therapeutic] and ectopic pregnancies) (see Chapter 25 for a complete discussion of the obstetrical history)
3. Sexually transmitted diseases: diagnoses and treatment
   a. Gonorrhea
   b. Herpes simplex virus (HSV)
   c. Vaginitis
   d. Human immunodeficiency virus (HIV)
   e. Syphilis
   f. Human papillomavirus (HPV)
4. Infertility: length of time pregnancy attempted, pattern of sexual activity, knowledge of fertile period; abnormalities of the genital system, stress, nutrition, chemical substances, diagnosis and treatment, partner issues
5. Sexual abuse
6. Diabetes
7. Hypertension
8. Genitourinary problems
9. Cancer
10. Eating disorders

E. Family history
1. Reproductive problems
2. Cancer
3. Diabetes
4. Mother's use of hormones during pregnancy
5. Mother's age of menarche and menopause

F. Personal and social history
1. Sexual history
   a. Sexual preference
   b. Date of first intercourse
   c. Pattern of sexual encounters, including safe sex practices
   d. Number of partners
   e. Health of partners
   f. Number and health of partners' partners
   g. Satisfaction with intercourse
   h. Current sexual activity—satisfaction with partner and opportunities for intercourse
   i. Contraception used
2. Satisfaction with family and other significant relationships

Symptom Analysis

Abdominal/Pelvic Pain

1. **Onset:** date and time of onset, sudden or gradual
2. **Course since onset:** frequency, duration, and relationship to menstrual cycle; pattern of recurrence

3. **Location:** specific location of pain, radiation, relationship to exercise or other activity
4. **Quality:** sharp, dull, aching, burning, knifelike, throbbing, drawing
5. **Quantity:** response to pain, severity
6. **Setting:** relationship to a particular setting, intercourse in a particular position, or new partner
7. **Associated phenomena:** relationship to menstrual cycle, vaginal discharge or bleeding, gastrointestinal symptoms, abdominal distention or tenderness, pelvic fullness, malaise, fever, nausea, vomiting, constipation
8. **Alleviating and aggravating factors:** exercise, sexual activity, relationship to body functions and activities, previous medical care for the problem, medications, self-care methods and their results
9. **Underlying concern:** cancer, sexually transmitted diseases

Abnormal Bleeding

1. **Onset:** date and time of onset, sudden or gradual
2. **Course since onset:** frequency, duration, and relationship to menstrual cycle; pattern of occurrence
3. **Location:** relationship to activity, time of day
4. **Quality:** color—pink, red, dark red, brown; other characteristics—thin, thick, watery, mixed with mucus; if clots, how many and how large; odor
5. **Quantity:** what size of stain on underwear per a specific time period, or saturation of how many pads and tampons in a specific time period
6. **Setting:** relationship to exercise, recent injury, time of day
7. **Associated phenomena:** use of intrauterine contraceptive device (IUD), changes in regular menstrual flow, pain, cramping, abdominal distention, pelvic fullness, change in bowel habits, weight loss or gain
8. **Alleviating and aggravating factors:** stress, anxiety, weight loss or gain, obesity, sexual intercourse, medications
9. **Underlying concern:** pregnancy, cancer if menopausal

Vaginal Discharge

1. **Onset:** date of onset, previous similar problems
2. **Course since onset:** changes in discharge over time, relationship to menstrual cycle, sexual activity, exercise
3. **Quality:** color—white, yellow-green, gray, other consistency—thin, curdlike, purulent; odor—"fishy," foul
4. **Quantity:** amount, number of pads or tampons used or underwear changes
5. **Setting:** relationship to place or activity
6. **Associated phenomena:** vulvar itching, vaginal itching, rash, pain with intercourse, **dysuria**, abdominal pain, pelvic fullness, discharge in partner, change in partners, sexual practices, fever
7. **Alleviating and aggravating factors:** relationship to douching, nylon underwear or tight pants, use of an-

tibiotics, pregnancy, new brands of tampons or hygiene products, self-care attempts and results, diabetes
8. **Underlying concern:** sexually transmitted disease

Burning or Pain on Urination

1. **Onset:** exact date, sudden or gradual,
2. **Course since onset:** frequency; last episode; relationship of problems to changes in sexual intercourse frequency, technique, or partner; timing of discomfort in urination stream (e.g., beginning of voiding, midstream, or at the end of the voiding). patterns of recurrence
3. **Location:** location of any related discomfort
4. **Quality:** color of urine, consistency of urine, presence of blood or other matter, clarity, odor
5. **Quantity:** amount of each voiding
6. **Setting:** relationship to changes in daily schedule, travel, sexual practices
7. **Associated phenomena:** fever, chills, flank pain, urgency, frequency, dysuria, **hematuria**, vaginal bleeding or discharge, abdominal distention, pelvic fullness, flank pain, edema
8. **Alleviating and aggravating factors:** douches, traumatic sex, delay of urination, medications, past treatment, diet, attempts at self-treatment and the results
9. **Underlying concern:** urinary tract infection

Preparation for Examination: Client and Environment

Most female clients perceive the examination of their reproductive organs as being different from the examination of other body parts. Past admonitions of "do not touch" and "keep it covered" have created a population of anatomically unaware and sometimes inappropriately "modest" women who are often unnecessarily difficult to examine. This is particularly true of older women and members of certain ethnic groups. Most practitioners believe that they can obtain a great amount of information about a female client by examining the genital area and performing screening tests.

One cause of the female client's tenseness during an examination of the genital area may be fear of discovery of sexual activity. During the history, investigate areas of anatomical and physiological function and dysfunction. The review of systems on all clients should include a sexual history. (See Chapters 2 and 3 on interviewing and history taking for information about approaching clients about sensitive subjects and the structure of the history.) If you have skillfully accomplished this portion of the history and if the client has been cooperative, she should not be apprehensive about the possible discovery of sexual "secrets." Reassure the client about confidentiality if you note tenseness as you begin the examination.

During the taking of the history and the physical examination, be alert to any signs of abuse. During the history the patient may seem emotionally distraught and evasive and avoid eye contact. The concerns identified do not coincide with the degree of anxiety presented. She may appear guarded during the early parts of the physical examination. Signs may include bruising on the face, arms, legs, trunk, and the genital area. Tears in the vaginal and rectum also may indicate abuse.

Other causes of tenseness during the pelvic examination include fear of discovery of disease and the memory of previous, uncomfortable pelvic examinations. Many clients are not knowledgeable regarding the anatomy of the pelvic area. Determine the client's need for basic information regarding the structure of the genital organs and provide this instruction before the pelvic examination, along with a demonstration of the instruments and an explanation of the procedure. Show the speculum to the client and demonstrate the mechanism used to open and close it. Advise the client about the clicking sounds normally made by a speculum as it is opened and closed. A relatively short amount of time taken to inform and orient all female clients at their first examinations provides long-term benefits in preventing anxiety and increasing cooperation.

Most clients find it difficult to engage in lengthy conversations while in a lithotomy position. They do appreciate explanations and reassurances from examiners but prefer not to have to respond to questions until they are again upright and at eye level with the examiner. Questioning a client extensively during the pelvic examination is apt to make her tense.

Environmental conditions are also important in enhancing cooperation during examination of the genital area. The environment and the client should be warm. The examining area should be private and safe from unexpected intrusion. The room, the examiner's hands, and all materials touching the client should be warm.

Preparation for Examination

EQUIPMENT

Item	Purpose
Disposable latex gloves	To protect examiner and client from transfer of infectious organisms
Specula of various sizes	Inspection of internal genitalia
Long, sterile cotton-tipped swabs	To cleanse internal genitalia To obtain specimens for examination
Cotton balls	To cleanse tissues
Sponge forceps	To insert cotton or gauze to cleanse tissues
Lubricant* (water soluble)	To facilitate insertion of speculum and fingers for examination
Cytology fixative	To fix Papanicolaou (Pap) smear
Ayre spatulas	To obtain cell samples for Pap smear
Cervical brushes	To obtain endocervical specimens for Pap smears
Culture media	Inoculation of specimens from cervical and vaginal areas
Glass slides	For Pap smears and for preparing a sample of vaginal discharge for examination
Normal saline	To prepare discharge on slides to assess for presence of specific organisms
Potassium hydroxide	To prepare discharge on slides to assess for presence of specific organisms
pH tape	To test pH of vagina
Acetic acid	To test for human papillomavirus
Floor examination light	For visualization of internal structures
Hand mirror	To enable client to visualize internal genitalia

CLIENT

Explain the procedure, demonstrate equipment, and respond to questions

Have the client empty her bladder right before the examination.

Assist the client in assuming the lithotomy position.

1. Instruct the client to lie down on the examination table and help her to put her heels into the stirrups and to stabilize them. Some clients are more comfortable leaving on their shoes and/or socks. Also, padding the stirrups with a soft fabric is a helpful hint to increase comfort for the heels and feet.
2. Retract the end of the table if it is still extended.
3. Help the client to bring her buttocks to the very bottom edge of the table. Gently guide the client or advise her to feel and aim for the end of the table herself. Reassure her that she will not fall off the end of the table.
4. Redrape the client so that the knees and symphysis pubis are covered. Depress the drape between the knees so you can see the client's face for responses during the examination.
5. Reposition the upper torso so that the head and shoulders are slightly elevated to increase client comfort and assist relaxation of abdominal muscles.

ENVIRONMENT

Warm

Well lit with additional light available to assist the visualization of internal genitalia

Private

EXAMINER

Gloved throughout the examination

Standing and sitting (on a wheeled stool) between the client's legs during various parts of the examination

Monitoring the client's face throughout examination

---

*An amount of lubricant, sufficient for the examination, should be placed on a piece of paper or gauze. The examiner should avoid handling the tube of lubricant during the examination, since it might become contaminated during handling and become a mechanism of infection transmission. Also, single-use tubes of lubricant are available.

Clients should be advised not to douche or use vaginal medications or other inserts during the 24 hours preceding the pelvic examination and should be reminded to empty their bladders immediately before the examination.

Materials needed for the examination should be assembled and readily available before the client is put in the lithotomy position.

Some clients have difficulty assuming the **lithotomy position**, especially moving their buttocks sufficiently downward to the edge of the table. The practitioner can assist the

<table><tr><td>■ HELPFUL HINT</td></tr></table>

Teaching the client a relaxation technique often makes an examination shorter in length and, in the case of a very tense client, possible at all.

One successful relaxation technique is described in the following. Instruct the client to:
• Place her hands on her chest at about the level of the diaphragm.
• Breathe deeply and slowly through her mouth.
• Concentrate on the rhythm of breathing.
• Relax all body muscles with each exhalation.

The tense client is apt to hold her breath and tighten. Even the coached client may forget and hold her breath. A gentle reminder, advising her to keep breathing, usually enables the client to maintain relaxation. This technique is particularly helpful in the adolescent or virginal client, whose introitus may be especially small.

An additional relaxation, or, more specifically, distraction technique, is the placement of a sign or mobile above the examining table. Some clients appreciate having something to look at, and their attention is constructively diverted from the examiner's activities.

Sometimes clients can not differentiate tenseness versus relaxation of the perineum. Teaching Kegel contractions (i.e., voluntary contraction of the perineum) can sometimes be helpful in assisting clients to differentiate tenseness from relaxation.

client by asking the client to raise her buttocks (while the client is lying on the table with her heels in the stirrups) and by guiding the client's buttocks downward from a position at the client's side or from a position at the foot of the table. Clients usually feel more comfortable wearing shoes and/or socks when their feet are in the stirrups, rather than supporting their weight with their bare heels against the hard, cold metal of the stirrups.

The client and the examiner assume several positions for the examination. For the abdominal examination, the client is lying supine on the examination table and the examiner is facing the client's right side. For inspection and palpation of the external genitalia and the speculum examination, the client is in the lithotomy position (Figure 21-6) and the examiner is seated on a stool, facing the client's genitalia. For the bimanual examination and the rectovaginal examination, the client remains in the lithotomy position, and the examiner is standing.

The abdominal examination is discussed in Chapter 17 on assessment of the abdomen. The examination of the female genital system should be preceded by a thorough examination of the abdomen.

Always wear gloves on both hands for the genital area examination. If infection is suspected, double gloves may provide additional protection for the examiner. Also, double gloving facilitates changing of gloves between the vaginal examination and the rectovaginal examination. The top pair can be shed right before the rectovaginal examination. However in the case of infection or suspected infection, the examiner may want to double glove throughout the examination. Since items in the examination room may need to be handled during the examination (e.g., the lamp that needs to be adjusted or the container of cytology fixative for Pap smear), be careful about contamination of such items. Develop a routine that will prevent contamination, and have gloves readily available in case of need to change gloves during the examination.

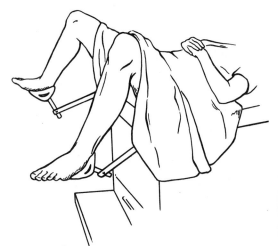
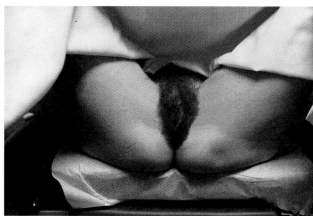

Figure 21-6 Lithotomy position for the female genital examination. (Photo from Seidel HM et al.: *Mosby's guide to physical examination,* ed. 4, St. Louis, 1999, Mosby.)

Technique for Examination and Expected Findings

Palpation of Regional Lymph Nodes

See Box 21-1 for general tips about conducting the examination. The lymph nodes of the inguinal areas are best assessed in the female client at the end of the abdominal examination. Two sets of lymph nodes are assessed: superior inguinal and inferior inguinal. (See Chapter 20 for discussion regarding examination of regional lymph nodes.)

The client must be lying down for the examination of the inguinal nodes. Flex the client's leg at the knee to relax the muscles of the inguinal area. Abduct the leg slightly; you may see a shallow, hollow space in the inguinal area. Begin your palpation here, lightly at first, and then more deeply. Palpate from the anterosuperior iliac spine to the pubic tubercle. Do not confuse Poupart's ligament with enlarged lymph nodes, which will be close to the surface and fairly easy to feel.

Inspection of the External Genitalia

With the client in the lithotomy position, sit on a stool, facing the external genitalia. Ask the client to relax and spread her knees apart. First, observe the skin and hair distribution.

Adult female hair distribution should be approximately shaped as an inverse triangle. Some abdominal hair is normal and may be hereditary. Male (diamond-shaped) hair distribution patterns in women are abnormal.

In the adolescent client, assess sexual maturity by observing breast growth and pubic hair growth. Table 21-1 outlines and illustrates sexual maturity ratings for the appearance of the female genitalia. When documenting your physical findings it is important to note the Tanner staging of breast and pubic hair development. (See Chapter 26 for additional information about the Tanner stages of sexual development.) Along with changes in quality and quantity of pubic hair, the following occur:

1. Increase in prominence of the labia majora
2. Enlargement of the labia minora
3. Increase in size of the clitoris
4. Increase in elasticity of vaginal tissue
5. Enlargement of the vagina and ovaries

Skin and Hair. Although the client knows she will be touched, she may startle when the fingers are placed on the genitalia at the initiation of the palpation. To enable the client to accommodate to the touching, touch her first on the inner thigh with the back of a hand before touching any part

BOX 21-1

TIPS FOR THE PELVIC EXAMINATION

Have everything you may need set up and within reach before the pelvic examination

Elevate the head of the examination table: Elevating the head of the examination table to about 30 degrees from the horizontal (1) allows eye contact and facilitates communication between the examiner and the client, (2) allows the practitioner to observe the client for responses to the examination, and (3) relaxes the abdominal muscles.

Position the examination lamp. The lamp is best positioned in front of the examiner's chest, a few inches below the chin, level with the perineum, but about 30 inches from it. This placement allows for maximum visibility for the examiner. Do not touch the lamp during the examination to avoid cross contamination.

Pace the examination. Speed is important, but it is important not to be abrupt or too fast to obtain the needed information.

Do not unnecessarily manipulate the speculum once it is inserted. Once inserted and locked into position, in most cases, a speculum will generally stay in place without being held.

Develop skill in performing a bimanual examination. Pelvic structures are caught and palpated between the abdominal and vaginal examining hands. With the abdominal hand, apply pressure with the flat of the fingers.

PROBLEM-SOLVING

Inability To Insert the Speculum Because of Client Discomfort

Try a Pederson speculum. Insert the speculum after asking the client to perform Kegel contractions followed by a Valsalva maneuver.

Inability To Insert Speculum Because of Vaginal Dryness

Use water on speculum or lubricant if specimens are not to be collected.

Failure To Find the Cervix on Insertion of the Speculum

This problem is usually caused by the speculum not being inserted far enough. Close the speculum and insert deeper. Other maneuvers include changing the angle of the speculum and moving the speculum from side to side. If the vaginal tissues are especially flaccid, use a larger speculum. Sometimes palpating the cervix before speculum insertion can assist in location with the speculum. The glove will prevent prolapse of the vaginal wall into the center of the open speculum.

Vaginal Walls Impede Visualizing Cervix

Use a larger speculum or retractor. Apply a glove, with fingertips cut off, over the speculum.

Inability To View Cervix Because of Extreme Posterior Position

Use a large, extra-long speculum; instruct client to bear down; raise hips on small pillow.

TABLE 21-1   Developmental Changes in the General Appearance of Female Genitalia

Developmental Stage	Description	Developmental Stage	Description
Stage 1 sexual maturity (preadolescence)	No pubic hair, except for fine body hair	Stage 4 sexual maturity	Texture and curl of pubic hair as in adult but not as thick and not spread over thighs (usually seen between ages 13 and 14)
Stage 2 sexual maturity	Sparse growth of long, slightly pigmented, fine pubic hair; growth is slightly curly and located along labia (usually seen between ages 11 and 12)	Stage 5 sexual maturity	Adult appearance in quality and quantity of pubic hair, which is spread onto inner aspect of upper thighs
Stage 3 sexual maturity	Pubic hair becomes darker, curlier, and spreads over symphysis (usually seen between ages 12 and 13)	Elderly	Pubic hair is thin, sparse, brittle, and gray

of the genitalia. Tell the client you will be placing your hand against her thigh. Then place it gently, but firmly there. This helps relax the client and enables the examiner to assess the degree of relaxation.

Inspect the total skin area for lesions and parasites. Use the gloved fingers of one hand (usually the thumb and index finger) to spread the hair and labia so that all skin surfaces can be adequately visualized. The skin should be the same color as the remainder of the body or slightly darker. The hair is normally coarse in texture and somewhat curly to very curly. Sebaceous cysts are often seen on the labia.

Labia.   The labia are flat in childhood, plump during adulthood, and atrophic in old age. Estrogen influences fat deposition, which causes a round, full appearance of the labia. The labia majora of the nulliparous client will be in close approximation, covering the labia minora and the vestibule area. After a vaginal delivery, the labia may appear slightly shriveled and gaping. Regardless of general appearance, the labia should appear reasonably symmetrical. The mucous membranes are normally dark pink and moist. The skin of the vulvar area is a slightly darker pigment than the skin of the rest of the body.

Clitoris.   Examine the clitoris for size, and examine the adjacent area for lesions. The visible portion of the clitoris should not exceed 2 cm in length and 1 cm in width. The area of the clitoris particularly is a common site for chancres of syphilis in the younger client and for cancerous lesions in the older client.

Urethral Orifice.   The urethral orifice appears slit-like, stellate, or as an inverted V and is of the same color as the membranes surrounding it. The openings of the paraurethral (Skene's) glands are not usually visible. Erythema or a polyp located in this area or a discharge from the urethra or gland ducts is abnormal.

Glandular Areas.   Observe the area of Bartholin's glands and their ducts for tenderness, swelling, erythema, duct enlargement, or discharge. The presence of any of these conditions is abnormal.

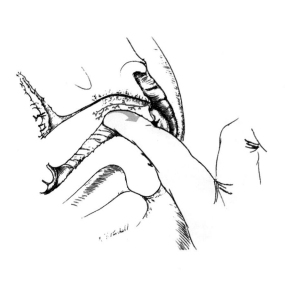

Figure 21-7 Palpation of Skene's glands.

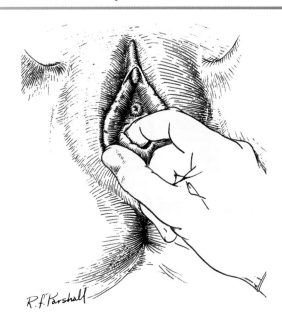

Figure 21-8 Palpation of Bartholin's glands.

Perineum. Inspect the perineum for lesions and evidence of an episiotomy and its healing. Also inspect the anal orifice at this time (see also Chapter 22).

Palpation of the External Genitalia

Labia. Use one hand to spread the labia open while the other hand is used to palpate the labia majora and labia minora. The labia should feel soft, and the texture should be homogeneous. Palpate any areas of observed abnormality below the skin surface to determine size, shape, consistency, movability, and tenderness.

Glands. Insert approximately half the index finger of the palpating hand into the vagina. First, gently milk the urethra and area of Skene's duct openings from about the level of 4 cm on the anterior vaginal wall down to the orifice (Figure 21-7). This procedure should not normally cause pain or discharge. If a discharge is present, a specimen is obtained with a swab and placed in sterile saline or a transporting fluid per local laboratory instructions and then transported to the appropriate laboratory. Then rotate the hand without removing the finger and palpate the area of Bartholin's glands and their ducts for swelling or tenderness (Figure 21-8). Palpate this area using the intravaginal finger and the thumb of that same hand on the external surface. Normally, Bartholin's glands are not palpable.

Perineum and Musculature of the Vaginal Introitus. While the finger is in the vagina, perform several maneuvers to assess the integrity of the pelvic musculature. Palpate the perineal area between the finger inside the vagina and the thumb of that same hand. In the nulliparous client, the perineum is felt as a firm, muscular body. After an episiotomy has healed, the perineum feels thinner and more rigid because of scarring. If this area is very thin and if the palpating fingers can almost approximate, the client may be experiencing bowel or sexual problems.

Ask the client to constrict her vaginal orifice around the examiner's finger while placed in the vagina. A nulliparous client will demonstrate a high degree of tone; a multiparous client, less tone.

Presence of Cystocele, Rectocele, Enterocele, and Uterine Prolapse. Place the index and middle fingers in the vagina, spread them laterally, and ask the client to push down against them. The presence of urinary stress incontinence, cystocele, rectocele, enterocele, or uterine prolapse can be observed if present. **Cystocele** is the prolapse into the vagina of the anterior vaginal wall and the bladder. Clinically, a pouching would be seen on the anterior wall as the client strains. **Rectocele** is the prolapse into the vagina of the posterior vaginal wall and the rectum. Clinically, a pouching would be seen on the posterior wall as the client strains. **Enterocele** is a hernia of the pouch of Douglas into the vagina. Clinically, a bulge would be seen emerging from the posterior fornix. If this is observed, the client should be additionally examined by assessing the effect of straining (1) during the speculum examination with the inserted speculum, half-opened and three fourths of its length into the vagina and (2) during the bimanual examination with the intravaginal fingers in the posterior fornix.

There are three degrees of uterine prolapse. In first-degree prolapse, the cervix appears at the introitus when the client strains. In second-degree prolapse, the cervix is outside the introitus when the client strains. In third-degree prolapse, the whole uterus is outside the introitus, and the vagina is essentially turned inside out when the client strains.

Inspection of the Internal Genitalia—Speculum Examination

You will have obtained clues regarding the most appropriate type and size of speculum to use in the speculum examination through the history and inspection of the external

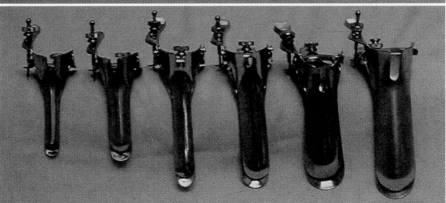

Figure 21-9 Vaginal specula. From left to right: **A,** Short-billed pediatric, pediatric, small Pederson, Pederson, small Graves, large Graves, plastic Graves. **B,** Short-billed pediatric, pediatric, small Pederson, Pederson, small Graves, large Graves. (From Seidel HM et al.: *Mosby's guide to physical examination,* ed. 4, St. Louis, 1999, Mosby.)

BOX 21-2

ABOUT SPECULA

A vaginal speculum consists of two blades, a handle, and some mechanism to open the distal end of the blades. There are two basic types: reusable metal and disposable plastic.

Metal and plastic specula operate somewhat differently, although both have (1) levers that, when depressed, open the distal ends of the blades; (2) mechanisms that allow for separation of the proximal ends of the blades; and (3) locking mechanisms. Metal specula have two positioning devices: depression of the lever opens the distal end of the blades, and fixing the screw on the lever locks the blades open at that point. In addition, the opening at the proximal end (and consequently the distal end) of the blades can be widened and locked wide by loosening and then lifting a plate attached to both the handle of the speculum and the upper blade.

The distal and proximal blade-opening mechanisms are connected in the plastic speculum. As the plastic lever is depressed in the plastic speculum, the distal end of the blades open. If the lever is fully depressed and then pushed upward on the handle, the proximal ends of the blades also widen. The lever fixes automatically into grooves on the handle of the speculum. The clicking sound of the plastic speculum is loud, sharp, and sometimes perceived as alarming to some clients, who think the speculum is breaking inside of them. Anticipatory warning about the sound of the plastic mechanism is advised. Plastic speculums also tend to get locked into position and are sometimes hard to release.

Because each type of speculum operates somewhat differently, the beginning examiner should practice with the mechanisms before using with clients.

genitalia. The two basic types of speculum shapes are the Graves speculum and the Pederson speculum (Figure 21-9 and Box 21-2). The Graves speculum is one of the most commonly used in examination of the adult female client. It is available in lengths varying from 3.5 to 5 inches (9 to 12.5 cm) and in widths from 0.75 to 1.5 inches (2 to 4 cm). The Pederson speculum is both narrower and flatter than the Graves speculum and is used with virgins, nulliparous clients, or clients whose vaginal orifices have contracted postmenopausally.

Warm a metal speculum before insertion. An effective way to do this is to run warm water over it. The warm water also assists in lubricating both the metal and plastic speculums and should be used as the method of lubrication if cultures and smears are to be taken. Gel lubricant is bacteriostatic and also distorts cells on Pap smears. Therefore do not use lubricant if cultures or smears are to be obtained.

Use the following procedure for speculum insertion:
1. Place the index and middle fingers of one hand about 2 cm into the vagina.
2. Spread the fingers and exert pressure toward the posterior vaginal wall. Advise the client that she will feel intravaginal pressure and ask her to relax the muscles you are pushing against.
3. Hold the speculum in the opposite hand with the blades between the index and middle fingers.
4. Ask the client to bear down. This maneuver helps to open the vaginal orifice and relax perineal muscles.
5. Insert the speculum blades obliquely along the top of the intravaginal fingers, taking advantage of the H configuration of the relaxed vagina (Figure 21-10, *A*).

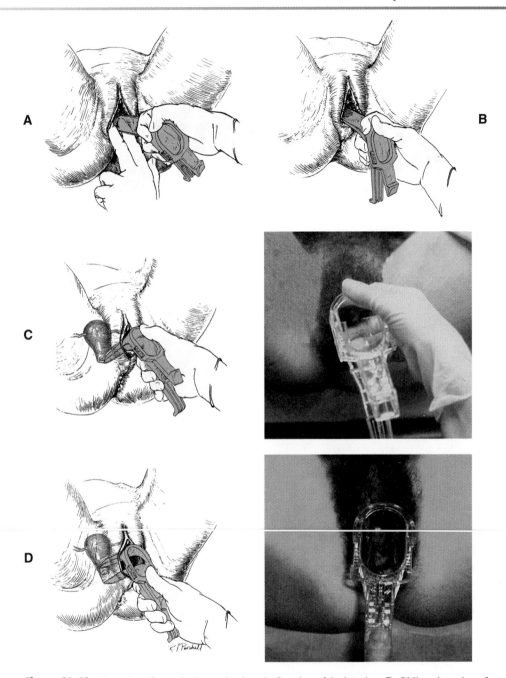

Figure 21-10   Procedure for vaginal examination. **A,** Opening of the introitus. **B,** Oblique insertion of the speculum. **C,** Final insertion of the speculum. **D,** Opening of the speculum blades. (**C** and **D** photos from Seidel HM et al.: *Mosby's guide to physical examination,* ed. 4, St. Louis, 1999, Mosby.)

6. Continue to insert the speculum at a plane parallel to the examining table until the end of the speculum has reached the tips of the fingers in the vagina. Then withdraw the intravaginal fingers (Figure 21-10, *B*).

7. Rotate the speculum to a transverse position, and alter the plane in adaptation to the plane of the vagina, approximately one of a 45-degree angle with the examining table (Figure 21-10, *C*). Insert the speculum until it touches the end of the vagina.

8. Depress the lever of the speculum; this opens the blades and allows visualization. Ideally, the cervix is seen between the blades (Figure 21-10, *D*). Some-

times, however, especially for the beginning examiner, it is not. In such cases the speculum is either anterior (usually the situation) or posterior to the cervix. If this occurs, withdraw the speculum halfway and redirect it into a different plane. Be careful not to pinch the patient, because the blades can catch tissue between them as they are being closed and rotated.

9. After the entire cervix is in view, fix the depressed lever in an open position.

If the client is tense and is resisting insertion of the speculum, do not withdraw the speculum but stop the insertion, leaving the speculum in its position. Remind the client

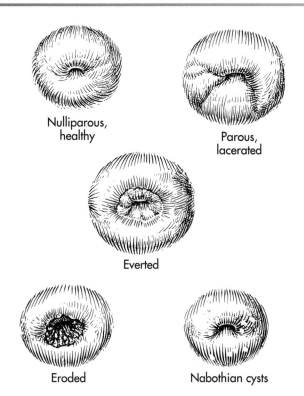

Nulliparous,
healthy

Parous,
lacerated

Everted

Eroded

Nabothian cysts

Figure 21-11   Common appearances and lesions of the cervix.

to use relaxation techniques, and continue the examination when relaxation has occurred.

Cervix.   Observe the cervix for color, position, size, projection into the vaginal vault, shape, general symmetry, surface characteristics, discharge, and shape of the os.

Color.   The normal color of the cervix is pink. The cervix is normally pale after menopause and cyanotic in pregnancy. Cyanosis can occur with any condition that causes systemic hypoxia or regional venous congestion. Hyperemia may indicate inflammation. An additional cause of pallor is anemia.

Position.   The position of the cervix is related to the position of the uterus. The cervix is usually midline and extends approximately 2 cm into the vagina. A cervix projecting more deeply than 3 cm into the vaginal vault may indicate uterine prolapse. A cervix situated on a lateral vaginal wall may indicate tumor or adhesion of a superior structure.

Size.   The cervix of women of childbearing age is usually 2 to 3 cm in diameter. A cervix larger than 4 cm in diameter is hypertrophied, and the presence of inflammation or tumor should be considered.

Surface Characteristics.   The cervix should look smooth and firm. Lesions and polyps are commonly seen on the cervix and require more than visual assessment to determine whether a pathological condition exists. Any irregularity or nodularity of the cervical surface should be considered possibly abnormal (Figure 21-11). One relatively benign condition is the presence of **nabothian** cysts, which appear as smooth, round, small (less than 1 cm in diameter), yellow or grayish white lesions. Nabothian cysts are caused by obstruction of the cervical gland ducts.

When the **squamocolumnar junction** is on the ectocervix, the columnar epithelium will appear as a red, relatively sym-

metrical circle around the os. This condition is called **eversion** or **ectropion**. It may be a normal variation of the placement of the squamocolumnar junction, or it may be caused by the separation by speculum blades of a cervix with an external os that has been altered and enlarged by childbirth. Erosions appear similar to eversions but are usually irregular, rough, and friable. Erosions commonly indicate pathological conditions and require further assessment and treatment. Because of the occasional presence of the squamocolumnar junction on the ectocervix and its visual similarity to erosions and other lesions, the differential assessment of a normal cervix from an abnormal cervix using inspection alone is impossible.

Diffuse punctuate hemorrhages, colloquially referred to as "strawberry spots," are occasionally observed in association with trichomonal infections.

Discharge.   The character of the normal cervical mucus varies in the menstrual cycle. Normal discharge is always odorless and nonirritating. Its color and consistency may vary from clear to white and from thin to thick and stringy. Colored, malodorous, or purulent discharges exuding from the os or present in the area of the cervix are probably abnormal.

Shape of the Os.   The cervical os of the nulliparous client is small and evenly round. The cervical os of a parous client who has had a vaginal delivery shows the effects of the stretching and laceration of childbirth and is irregular in shape.

Many clients have not seen their cervices. The client should be asked whether she wishes to see her cervix. This visualization can easily be accomplished through the use of a hand mirror.

After inspecting the cervix, obtain the Pap smear, culture for gonorrhea, and hanging drop specimen if indicated. The procedures for these are described at the end of this chapter.

Vagina.   Next, inspect the vagina. This step is done during speculum insertion, while the speculum is open and during its removal. Note the color and condition of the vaginal mucosa and the color, odor, consistency, and appearance of vaginal secretions. Pallor, cyanosis, and hyperemia may be present for the same reasons as described for the cervix. Leukoplakia may also occur on vaginal mucosa.

As with cervical discharge, vaginal discharge is normally odorless, nonirritating, thin or mucoid, and clear or cloudy. Also, the presence of some whitish, creamy material (**leukorrhea**) is normal. Describe any other vaginal discharge according to its color, odor, consistency, amount, and appearance.

After the inspection of the vagina, slowly withdraw the speculum. As it is withdrawn, loosen the nut, or catch, and control the lever again with the thumb. Slowly close the blades as they are withdrawn, and carefully rotate the speculum so that all areas of vaginal tissue are inspected. As the blades are closed, be careful to prevent pinching of tissue or the catching of hairs between the blades.

Inspect the speculum for odors and either discard it (plastic) or place it in a soaking solution (metal).

Palpation of the Internal Genitalia—Bimanual Vaginal Examination

The purpose of the bimanual examination is the palpation of the pelvic contents between the examiner's two hands (Figures 21-12 and 21-13): one in the vagina and the other on the lower

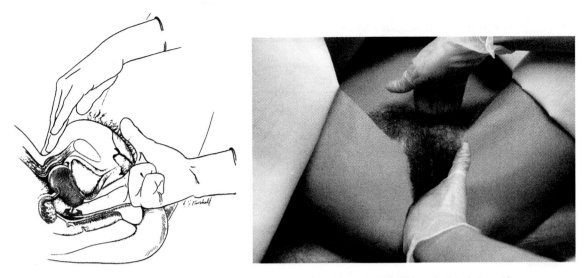

Figure 21-12 Bimanual palpation of the uterus. (Photo from Seidel HM et al.: *Mosby's guide to physical examination,* ed. 4, St. Louis, 1999, Mosby.)

abdomen. Examiners vary in their preference of the placement of the dominant, more sensitive hand. The beginning examiner should attempt alternating hands for examinations and then decide on a routine that is most workable individually.

The client remains in the lithotomy position. Stand between the client's legs. The vaginal examining hand assumes the obstetric position: index and middle fingers extended and together, thumb abducted, and fourth and little fingers folded on the palm of the hand. Lubricate the vaginal examining fingers. Spread the labia with the thumb and index finger of the opposite hand. Insert the lubricated fingers into the vagina with the palmar surface of the hand directed toward the anterior vaginal wall. Always palpate with the palmar surface of the fingers rather than with the less sensitive tips or backs. In the case of a young or old client with a small and narrow vagina, the examination may be performed with one intravaginal finger.

The other hand is placed on the abdomen and used to press the abdominal and pelvic contents toward the intravaginal hand. If the glove on this hand has been soiled by excessive discharge during the external genital inspection or speculum insertion, the glove on this hand should be changed before the bimanual vaginal examination.

Movement of both the intravaginal and abdominal hands should be slow and firm. To palpate adequately, the client must be relaxed. If the client becomes tense, stop the procedure and help the client relax; however, leave the examining hands in position.

Locate the cervix and assess it for size, contour, surface characteristics, consistency, position, patency of the os, and mobility. Use the palmar surfaces of both fingers to completely palpate the cervix and fornices. Gently place a fingertip into the external os to assess its patency. Determine on which vaginal wall the cervix is placed and whether the cervix is approximately midline. Place the fingers in the lateral fornices, and move (wag) the cervix back and forth between the fingers for 1 to 2 cm in each direction to assess for cervical motion tenderness. The cervix and uterus should be

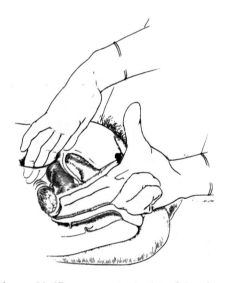

Figure 21-13 Bimanual palpation of the adnexa.

freely movable and should move without tenderness. An immobile or tender cervix and uterus are abnormal.

The surface of the cervix normally feels smooth. Nabothian cysts, tumors, or lesions will make it feel somewhat nodular or irregular. The consistency of the cervix is firm and slightly resilient and feels analogous to the tip of the nose. The cervix softens in pregnancy and hardens with tumors. The cervix is normally located on the anterior wall in the midline or on the posterior wall. A laterally displaced cervix may indicate tumor or adhesion. The external os in the nonpregnant client should admit a finger for about 0.5 cm. It should be open and firm. A stenosed external os is abnormal.

Assess the position, size, shape, surface characteristics, consistency, position, mobility, and tenderness of the uterine body and fundus. First, determine the position of the uterus because techniques used to assess the uterine body and fundus will vary with the uterine position in the client (Table 21-2). The uterus is in one of the three basic posi-

TABLE 21-2	**Findings in Bimanual Vaginal and Rectovaginal Examinations**

	Bimanual	
Position of Uterus	**Position of Cervix**	**Fundus Body of Uterus**
Anteverted	Anterior vaginal wall	Palpable by one hand on abdomen and fingers of other hand in vagina
Midposition	Apex of vagina	May not be palpable
Retroverted	Posterior vaginal wall	May not be palpable

TABLE 21-2 **Findings in Bimanual Vaginal and Rectovaginal Examinations—cont'd**

	Rectovaginal	
Anterior and Posterior Parts of Uterus	**Cervix**	**Body and Fundus**
Palpable as uterus is rotated even more anteriorly	Palpable through rectovaginal septum	May not be palpable by fingers in rectum
May not be palpable	Posterior portion felt through rectovaginal septum	May not be palpable
Posterior portion may be palpable by fingers in posterior fornix	May not be palpable by fingers in rectum	Body easily palpable by fingers in rectum; fundus may not be palpable

Continued

TABLE 21-2	Findings in Bimanual Vaginal and Rectovaginal Examinations—cont'd		
		Bimanual	
Position of Uterus	**Position of Cervix**	**Fundus Body of Uterus**	
Anteflexed	Anterior vaginal wall or apex	Easily palpable; angulation of isthmus may be felt in anterior fornix	
Retroflexed	Anterior vaginal wall or apex	May not be palpable	

tions: anteversion, midposition, or retroversion. Version in this context indicates deflection—specifically the relationship of the long axis of the uterus to the long axis of the body. If the axis of the uterus is deflected anteriorly, the uterus is said to be anteverted; if the uterus is deflected posteriorly, the uterus is said to be retroverted; and if the long axis of the uterus is roughly parallel to that of the total body, the uterus is in midposition. When the long axis of the uterus is not straight but is bent on itself, the uterus is said to be flexed. Thus the anteverted or retroverted uterus can be flexed, or bent on itself, to produce two additional variations of position: anteflexion and retroflexion.

The position of the cervix provides clues of the uterine position. A cervix on the anterior wall may indicate an antepositioned or retroflexed uterus; a centrally located cervix probably indicates a uterus in midposition; and a cervix on the posterior vaginal wall suggests a retroverted uterus.

Because approximately 85% of uteri are in anteposition (i.e., anteverted or anteflexed), first attempt palpation of the uterus anteriorly. Place the intravaginal fingers in the anterior fornix. Place the hand on the abdomen flat on the midline and in a position approximately halfway between the symphysis pubis and the umbilicus. This hand acts as a resistance against which the intravaginal fingers palpate the pelvic organs. In thin women the uterus can also be palpated with the abdominal hand. With the fingers in the anterior fornix, gently lift the tissues against the hand on the abdomen. If the uterus is in anteposition, it will be palpated between the hands. If the uterus is not palpated anteriorly, place the fingers in the posterior fornix and again raise them forward toward the hand on the abdomen. If the uterus is in retroversion, only the isthmus will be felt between the hands, and the corpus may be felt with the backs of the intravaginal fingers.

TABLE 21-2	**Findings in Bimanual Vaginal and Rectovaginal Examinations—cont'd**	
	Rectovaginal	
Anterior and Posterior Parts of Uterus	Cervix	**Body and Fundus**
Easily palpable	Same as anteverted	Same as anteverted
Not palpable	Palpable through rectovaginal septum	Angulation palpable; body and fundus easily palpable

Palpation of the body and fundus of the retroverted uterus is more difficult than palpation of the antepositioned uterus. In some cases the vaginal fingers can rotate the uterine fundus forward or upright by a combination of pressure in the posterior and lateral fornices combined with trapping of the fundus by the abdominal hand. If this cannot be done, palpate as much of the uterine surface as possible, and attempt a more thorough examination of the fundus during the rectovaginal examination.

Palpate the anterior, lateral, and posterior surfaces of the uterus by maneuvering its position and by "walking up" its surface with the intravaginal fingers.

Develop a mental image of the uterus as you perform the various assessments and maneuvers. In most cases you will not be able to palpate the uterus as a whole, but will develop impressions from the various maneuvers. The uterus should be pear shaped and approximately 5.5 to 8 cm long in the nonpregnant adult female. The contour should feel smooth and rounded, and the walls should be firm and smooth in all areas. When the uterus is moved between examining hands, it should be movable in its anteroposterior plane and the movement should not be painful to the client.

After palpating the uterus, examine the adnexal areas. The adnexal areas are the structures and spaces surrounding the uterus, including the fallopian tubes and ovaries. The structures in these areas are of a size, consistency, and position that they may not be specifically palpated. If you have appropriately examined the area and no masses larger than the normal-size ovaries are identified, assume that no masses are present.

Palpate each of the adnexal areas, left and right. Place the index and middle fingers of the intravaginal hand in one of the lateral fornices; place the hand on the abdomen on the ipsilateral iliac crest; and bring the hands together, moving in an inferior and medial direction, allowing the tissues lying between the two hands to slip between them (see Figure 21-13). The hand on the abdomen acts as resistance, and the intravaginal hand palpates the organs between the hands.

In premenopausal adult women the ovaries are felt about half of the time. If normal ovaries are palpated, they are smooth, firm, slightly flattened, ovoid, and no larger than 4 to 6 cm in their largest dimension. Ovaries of prepubertal girls or postmenopausal women are normally smaller than 4 cm in their largest dimension. The ovaries are sensitive to touch but are not tender. They are highly movable and will easily slip between the palpating hands. Normal fallopian tubes are not palpable. One clue to an ectopic pregnancy is the presence of arterial pulses in the adnexal areas.

Cordlike structures that are sometimes palpable in the adnexal area are round ligaments.

Rectovaginal Examination

The rectovaginal examination is uncomfortable for most women. However, because it enables examination not possible through the vaginal examination alone, it is recommended in all complete pelvic examinations. The rectovaginal examination allows for greater depth (approximately 2 cm higher) than the vaginal examination alone and enables assessment of the posterior portion of the uterus and pelvic cavity. Because the examination is uncomfortable, prepare the client for it by instruction regarding its purpose and anticipatory guidance about the possible feeling of urgency for bowel movement.

After completing the vaginal examination, withdraw the intravaginal hand, change the glove on the internal examining hand to prevent the possible transfer of infection from the vagina into the rectum, and lubricate the index and middle fingers. Advise the client that the next procedure is the last part of the pelvic examination and remind her to cooperate by relaxing the muscles. Next, ask the client to bear down. Then, place the index finger into the vagina in the

posterior fornix of the cervix, and place the middle finger into the rectum. (See Chapter 22 for a detailed explanation of the method for inserting the examining finger into the rectum.) Both fingers are inserted as far as possible. Place the other hand above the symphysis, as for the vaginal examination, and depress the abdominal hand to bring the pelvic contents into closer proximity to the fingers in the vagina and the rectum. During this maneuver the rectal finger should be able to palpate the posterior portion of the uterus.

The uterine position is confirmed by the rectal examination. If the uterus is retroverted, the finger in the rectum now palpates its body and fundus. In addition, the adnexal areas are reassessed. The procedure is the same as that described with the vaginal examination (Figure 21-14).

Palpate the areas of the rectovaginal septum and cul-de-sac. The rectovaginal septum should be palpated as a firm, thin, smooth, pliable structure. The posterior cul-de-sac is a blind pouch in the caudal peritoneum between the uterus and the rectum. Sometimes abnormal masses and normal ovaries are discovered in the cul-de-sac. Uterosacral ligaments may be palpable.

Complete the rectal examination (see Chapter 22), and help the client sit up when the examination is finished.

Because of the amount of lubricant used in the examination, the client may feel somewhat sticky. Provide her with disposable materials to clean herself and allow her to dress partially or completely (if the physical examination is completed). Often the pelvic and rectal examinations are the very last portions of the physical assessment, and complete dressing occurs before consultation about findings.

Special Maneuvers (Box 21-3)

Examination of Clients Who Are Unable To Assume the Lithotomy Position. The lithotomy position is optimal for a pelvic examination. However, it may be difficult for a very ill or debilitated client to assume and maintain the lithotomy

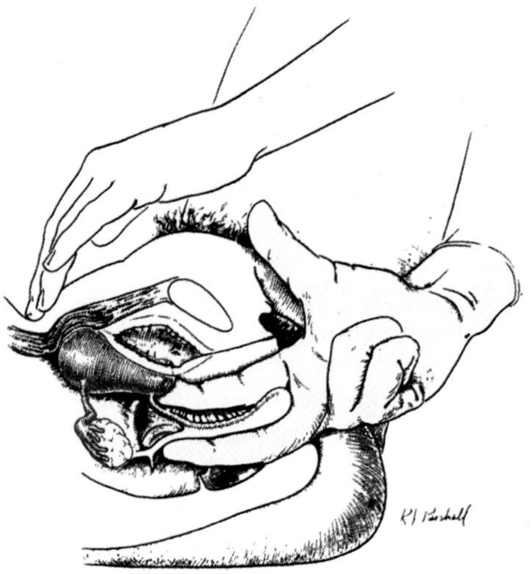

Figure 21-14 Rectovaginal palpation.

BOX 21-3

EXAMINATION OF A CLIENT WHO HAS HAD A HYSTERECTOMY

Determine as many details of the procedure as possible, especially the extent of the procedure.

On speculum examination the cervix will be absent. An identifiable suture line will be present. Take a Pap smear at the suture line with the blunt end of the spatula. Label the Pap smear requisition form with the fact of the hysterectomy.

The vaginal walls may appear as they would after menopause without replacement therapy—decrease in rugae and secretions.

In bimanual palpation the uterus will obviously not be present, but the adnexal areas should be palpated as in the usual examination.

All existing pelvic and lower organs will appear more prominent.

position. An alternative position for the female genital examination is a left lateral or Sims' position (Figure 21-15). The client's buttocks should be as close to the edge of the examining table as safety allows. Position the right leg on top of or over the left leg, and bend and abduct it. Stand behind the client. All the examination procedures described previously in this chapter can be performed with the client in this position.

Screening Tests and Procedures

The following recommendations are from the U.S. Preventive Services Task Force (1996).

Cervical Cancer.   Regular Pap tests are recommended for all women who are or have been sexually active. Testing should begin at the age when the woman initiates intercourse or around age 18 for women who are not sexually active. Pap tests are performed at an interval of 1 to 3 years, depending on the presence of risk factors, history, and clinical findings. Pap smears can be discontinued at age 65 if the previous pattern of Pap smear findings has been normal and no risk factors are present.

Healthy People 2010 (2000) has established the following national goals for Pap screening:

- Increase to 97% the percentage of women age 18 and older who have ever received a Pap test.
- Increase to 90% the percentage of women age 18 and older who received a Pap test within the preceding 3 years.
- Increase the proportion of sexually active females age 25 years and younger who are screened annually for genital chlamydia infections.
- Increase the proportion of all sexually transmitted disease clients who are being treated for bacterial STDs (chlamydia, gonorrhea, and syphilis) and who are offered provider referral services for their sex partners.

Chlamydial Infection.   Routine testing for *Chlamydia trachomatis* is recommended for the following groups of clients:

1. Asymptomatic persons who attend clinics for sexually transmitted diseases

2. Persons having specific risk factors for chlamydial infection: younger than 20 years of age, multiple sexual partners, or sexual partner with multiple sexual contacts
3. Recent sexual partners of persons with positive cultures
4. Pregnant women in the high-risk group at the first prenatal visit and at later visits if the risk for infection is high

Gonorrhea.   Routine cultures for *Neisseria gonorrhea* (similar to *C. trachomatis*) are recommended for the following groups:

1. Asymptomatic persons in high-risk groups: prostitutes, persons with multiple sexual partners
2. Persons who have had sexual contact with a person diagnosed with gonorrhea
3. Persons with a history of repeated episodes of gonorrhea
4. Pregnant women at the first prenatal visit and at a later visit if the risk for infection is high

Cervical Pap Smear

The Pap smear is taken to detect neoplastic cells in cervical and vaginal secretions. Normal and abnormal cervical and endometrial cells are shed onto the cervix and into the vagina and intermix with the normal secretions. The Pap smear is very accurate (95%) in detecting cervical cancer but only moderately effective in detecting endometrial cancer. Box 21-4 contains additional information about Pap smears.

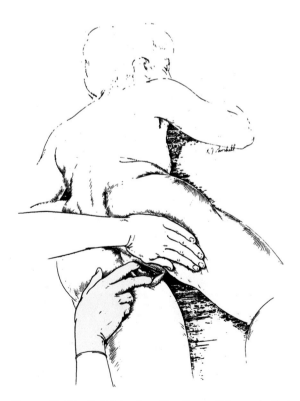

Figure 21-15 Left lateral position for genital examination.

✓	**Risk Factors**
	Abnormal Pap Smear

Early onset of sexual activity (before age 18)
Multiple sexual partners
Sexual partner with multiple sex partners (>3)
Smoking
History of illicit drug use
History of genital condylomata (HIV)
Sexual partner with genital condylomata (HIV)
History of sexually transmitted diseases
History of abnormal Pap smears
Diethylstilbestrol exposure in utero

BOX 21-4

ABOUT PAP SMEARS

CLIENT PREPARATION

Advise the client to avoid douching, using vaginal medications or other topical inserts, or tub baths for 48 hours before the procedure to avoid irritating the cervix.

Defer if menstrual flow or infection present.

Do not use lubricating jelly on the speculum.

Advise the client to avoid vaginal intercourse for 24 hours before the procedure.

Advise the client that a mild pinching may be momentarily felt as the endocervical sample and scrapings are taken.

Advise the client that a small amount of spotting may be noticed after the procedure.

FINDINGS

A report that indicates the presence of endocervical cells along with squamous cells or squamous metaplasia indicates an adequate sample.

CLASSIFICATION SYSTEM

Results are reported as classes or in cervical intraepithelial neoplasia (CIN) levels.

CLASS (CIN) SYSTEM

Class 1, or normal: no abnormal cells are present

Class 2, or atypia: atypical cells are present, but no evidence of malignancy

Class 3, or low-grade squamous intraepithelial lesion (SIL): mild dysplasia; cytological findings suggestive but not conclusive of malignancy; requires immediate follow-up

Class 4, or high-grade SIL: carcinoma in situ; cytological findings strongly suggestive of malignancy

Class 5, or invasive carcinoma: cytological changes are conclusive of malignancy.

CIN SYSTEM

CIN 1: mild and mild-to-moderate dysplasia (classes 2 and 3)

CIN 2: Moderate and moderate-to-severe dysplasia (class 3)

CIN 3: Severe dysplasia and carcinoma in situ (classes 4 and 5)

BETHESDA SYSTEM (NATIONAL CANCER INSTITUTE WORKSHOP, 1991)

The Bethesda system is a newer method that provides more extensive analysis of the specimen than earlier systems. This system is being recommended by national authorities. The components of this system are:

1. Adequacy of the specimen
2. General categorization of findings
3. Descriptive diagnoses
    a. Benign cellular changes
       I. Infection
       II. Reactive changes
    b. Epithelial cell abnormalities
       I. Squamous cell
       II. Glandular cell
    c. Other malignant neoplasms

Important

Secretions must be fixed before they dry. Drying will distort the cells and make interpretation difficult.

Pap smear findings do not constitute a definitive diagnosis of cancer or other disease. However, they can indicate the need for further assessment.

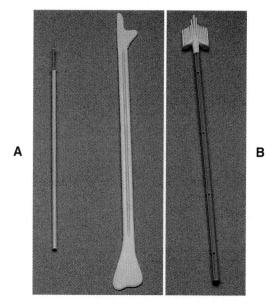

Figure 21-16 Implements used to obtain a Pap smear. **A,** Cytobrush and Ayre spatula. **B,** Cervex-brush. (**A** courtesy MEDSCAND (USA.), Inc., Hollywood, Fla. **B** courtesy UNIMAR, division of Cooper Surgical, Inc., Shelton, Conn.)

The client is in the lithotomy position, and the speculum has been inserted (only warm water should be used to lubricate the speculum). All materials listed earlier in the chapter are assembled. (Be sure the slides are clearly labeled with the client's identifying information.)

If a cervical mucous plug is present, remove it with a cotton ball held with forceps or a long cotton-tipped swab. Laboratories vary regarding the areas from which cell samples are to be obtained, the mixing of cells from two or more areas using a slide for each area or one slide for all specimen areas, and the fixing of cells. One procedure is described here. However, variations are acceptable, and the practitioner should consult with the cytopathologist reading the smears for locally recommended procedures. The following paragraphs describe methods for obtaining samples from the **ectocervix**, the **endocervix**, and the vaginal pool in that order. In the presented procedure three slides are used. The implements used to collect the Pap smear are displayed in Figure 21-16.

Ectocervical Specimen. Figure 21-17 illustrates the procedure for an ectocervical cervical specimen.

1. Insert the larger humped end of an Ayre spatula into the cervical os so that the cervix fits comfortably into the groove created by the two humps. With

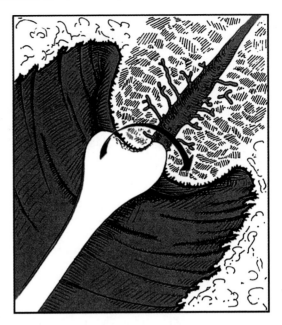

Figure 21-17 Cervical specimen taken using an Ayre spatula.

moderate pressure rotate the spatula 360 degrees, scraping the entire cervical surface and the squamo-columnar junction.

2. Spread the material from both sides of the spatula on a slide marked "cervix."
3. Fix the slide immediately by spraying it.

Endocervical Specimen

1. Insert a cylindrical-type brush into the cervical os until only the bristles closest to the handle are seen, and then rotate the brush 360 degrees in one direction (clockwise or counterclockwise).
2. Remove the brush and immediately rotate the entire surface of the brush onto a slide in the direction opposite to the one used to collect the specimen.
3. Avoid leaving a thick area of the specimen on the labeled slide.
4. Fix the slide immediately by spraying it with a fixative.

Vaginal Pool Smear Specimen

1. With the paddle or handle end of the Ayre spatula, scrape the area of the posterior cervical fornix.
2. Spread the material on the spatula in the area marked "vaginal pool."
3. Fix the slide immediately by spraying it or immersing it in a fixative solution.

New products (e.g., Cervex-brush) enable the simultaneous taking of ectocervical and endocervical specimens. These brushes are constructed with a bristle area, which is inserted into the cervix. Adjacent to the brush areas is a set of lateral bristles that rests along the ectocervix. After it is inserted, the brush is rotated three times to the left and then three times to the right while gentle pressure is applied. It is then withdrawn. The specimen from one side of the brush is placed on a slide; the brush is rotated and the specimen from the other side is applied in the same area of the slide. The specimen is immediately sprayed with a fixative.

New products are being developed to improve the accuracy of Pap smears, especially false negatives, which often result from sampling error. One of the technologies that is changing the way samples are collected is thin-layer technology. The actual sample is collected as previously described, but rather than smearing the cytological sample directly onto a microscope slide, the method suspends the sample cells in a fixative solution, disperses them, and then selectively collects them on a filter. Finally the cells are transferred to a microscope slide for cytological evaluation. Use of this method reduces the artifacts and reduces clumping of cells on the slides.

Gonorrheal Culture (Box 21-5)

Cultures for gonorrheal infection are performed on men and women at risk for the infection. In addition, all pregnant women should be screened for gonorrhea because of possible fetal complications. Cervical cultures are done for women, urethral cultures for men, and rectal and throat cultures for persons engaged in rectal or oral sex.

The female client is in the lithotomy position with a speculum inserted. The male client is in a supine position or sitting on the edge of the examination table with feet braced against the wall to prevent possible falling if vasovagal syncope occurs with the introduction of the specimen-collecting swab into the urethra.

1. In the female client obtain a specimen from the endocervical canal with a sterile cotton applicator. Insert a sterile cotton-tipped applicator approximately 0.5 cm into the cervical os. Rotate it 360 degrees and leave it in 30 seconds to ensure saturation (Figure 21-18). Ask the male client to milk the penis (see Chapter 20) and obtain a culture of the discharge from the urethral meatus. Then insert a sterile swab into the anterior meatus to collect discharge.
2. Inoculate a special culture plate or place the specimen in a special culture container as soon as possible, following local laboratory instructions.
3. If a Thayer-Martin culture plate is used, have the medium at room temperature; roll the swab in a large Z pattern on the culture plate; simultaneously rotate the swab as it is creating the Z so that all swab surfaces will be inoculated (Figure 21-19). Incubate the culture plate within 15 minutes of its in-

oculation in a warm, anaerobic environment. Place the culture plate, medium side up, in a candle jar, light the candle, tightly secure the cover of the jar, and leave the jar in a warm area until specimens can be placed in an incubator. In some clinics the inoculation is immediately cross-streaked with a sterile wire loop. Usually, however, this step is done in the laboratory, not in the examining room.

4. If another type of culture medium is used, follow instructions for specimen collection and handling.

Anal Culture. Figure 21-20 illustrates the procedure for an anal culture:

1. Insert a sterile cotton-tipped applicator into the anal canal for about 2 cm. Rotate the applicator 360 degrees and move it from side to side. Leave it in for 10 to 30 seconds to allow for absorption of secretion and organisms. If the swab contains feces, discard it and take another specimen.

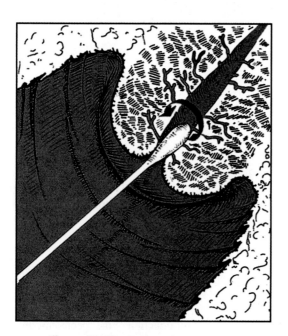

Figure 21-18   Endocervical specimen.

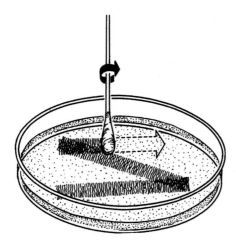

Figure 21-19   Inoculation of the Thayer-Martin culture.

2. Inoculate the culture plate and incubate it as described previously, using a separate culture plate labeled by source of specimen, or use transport medium per local laboratory instructions.

Oropharyngeal Culture

1. Obtain a specimen of secretion from the oropharynx with a sterile swab.

2. Inoculate the medium and incubate as described for endocervical specimens.

Chlamydial Culture

C. trachomatis is an organism that causes chlamydia, a common sexually transmitted disease. Detection is important because the organism causes trachoma, an eye disease resulting in the most common form of preventable blindness. Obtain vaginal and urethral specimens using a special Dacron swab. Wooden, cotton-tipped applicators may interfere with test results. Take the specimen as described earlier for gonorrhea cultures. Special culture material is inoculated with the specimen per instruction in the kit or by the laboratory. In males *Chlamydia* cultures are obtained by collecting clean-catch urine specimens.

Acetic Acid Wash

To screen for HPV, the causative agent for genital warts, perform the acetic acid wash test. After cervical and vaginal specimens have been taken, swab the cervix with a cotton–tipped applicator soaked in 5% acetic acid. Normally there is no change in the cervix. In the presence of the virus, a rapid blanching with jagged borders is observed.

The wet mount is a very commonly used, simple microscopic procedure that assists in the assessment of vaginal infections. It is indicated when there is vaginal discharge, vaginal or vulvar pruritus, vaginal or vulvar pain, or malodorous vaginal secretions.

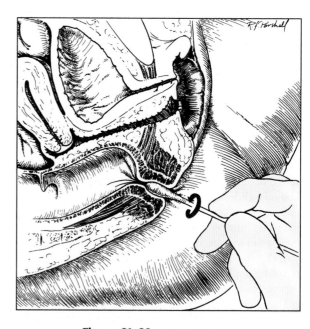

Figure 21-20   Anal specimen.

Various vaginal conditions are associated with the pH status of the vagina. Normally, the vaginal pH is 4. Changes in pH are noted with the following conditions: (1) candidiasis—pH 4 to 5; (2) bacterial vaginosis—pH greater than 4.5; and (3) trichomoniasis—pH 5.5 to 6.6.

Test for pH. To test for vaginal pH, touch a piece of pH-testing tape to vaginal secretions collected in the speculum blade after it is removed. Compare the color changes with the color codes on the outside of the pH tape container.

■ HELPFUL HINT

In preparing and examining wet mounts:
- If both saline and potassium hydroxide (KOH) slides are prepared, view the saline specimen first to allow time for the KOH to lyse cells.
- Trichomonads sometimes appear most mobile on a slide without a cover slip.
- Observe the slides with the ×10 objective and the light low.
- Start observing with the objective as close to the slide as possible.
- Use the coarse and fine focus knobs to improve visualization.
- First observe for squamous cells to estimate their number.
- Then switch to high power (×40) and increase the light if necessary.
- Look for bacteria, white blood cells, clue cells, trichomonads, and evidence of *Candida*. Vaginitis may have more than one cause, so do not stop examining the slide when one organism is found.
- When examining the KOH slide, start with low power. If hyphae are noted, confirm the impression under high power.

Modified from Hawkins JW, Roberto-Nichols DM, Stanley-Haney JL: *Protocols for nurse practitioners in gynecologic settings,* ed. 5, New York, 1995, Tiresias Press.

Wet Mounts. The interpretation of wet mount preparations in the context of data obtained from the history and physical assessment is presented in Table 21-3. The following is the procedure for obtaining vaginal specimens for the testing of the presence of *Trichomonas vaginalis, Candida albicans,* or bacterial vaginosis (also known as *Gardnerella* or *Haemophilus vaginalis*):

1. Obtain a specimen of vaginal secretions directly from the vagina or from material in the inferior speculum blade. For *T. vaginalis,* mix the secretions with a drop of normal saline solution on a glass slide. For *C. albicans,* mix the secretions with a drop of 10% potassium hydroxide (KOH) solution on a slide. For bacterial vaginosis, the secretions are mixed with a 10% potassium hydroxide solution.

2. Place a glass cover slip on the slides. Observe the slides under a microscope. Normally, all slides should have fewer than 10 white blood cells per field and be free of protozoa and yeast forms.

3. If bacterial vaginosis is suspected, perform a "whiff" test as the slide is being prepared with the KOH. If *G. vaginalis* is present, an unpleasant, "fishy" odor will be noted after the drop of KOH is added.

4. On the KOH slide, if the specimen is positive for *C. albicans,* hyphae and spores will be seen. If the specimen is positive for bacterial vaginosis, characteristic "clue cells" will be seen.

5. Immediately observe the saline slide under a microscope (Figure 21-21). If the specimen is positive for *T. vaginalis,* trichomonads will be seen on the saline slide. These are single-cell flagellates somewhat larger than a white blood cell (WBC), but smaller than a vaginal squamous epithelial cell.

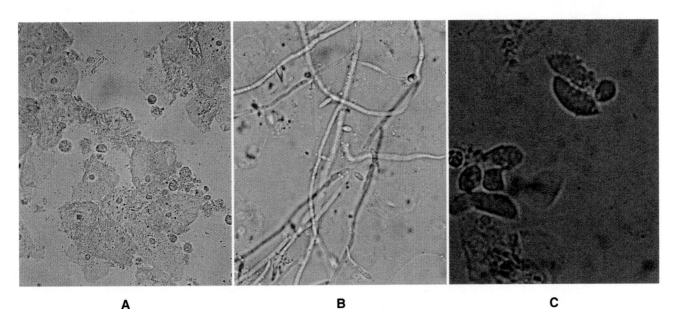

A   B   C

Figure 21-21 Microscopic appearance of vaginal microorganisms. **A,** Bacterial vaginosis: "clue cells." **B,** *Candida* vulvovaginitis: "budding, branching hyphae." **C,** Trichomoniasis: "motile trichomonads." (From Zitelli BJ, Davis HW: *Atlas of pediatric physical diagnosis,* ed. 3, St. Louis, 1997, Mosby.)

TABLE 21-3   **Comparisons Among Commonly Observed Vaginal Conditions**

	Normal	(Monitiasis) Candidiasis	Bacterial Vaginosis	Trichomoniasis	Chlamydia Infection	Gonorrhea	Atrophic Changes
Symptoms	None	Intense pruritus, burning	Pruritus, burning Constant wet feeling	Pruritus	Often no symptoms; mimics gonorrhea Sometimes urinary frequency, dysuria, or vaginal discharge	Variable; the majority of cases are asymptomatic Dysuria, abnormal uterine bleeding Abscesses Partner with STDs Variable	Vaginal and vulvar dryness, itching, burning Dyspareunia
Examination	Small amount of clear mucus Pink membranes	Thick, white, curdy discharge Vulva and vagina edematous	Profuse, thin, gray-white, malodorous discharge	Frothy, yellow-green discharge, worse during menstruation Vulva edematous Vagina red, with raised papules creating a "strawberry" appearance	Yellow or green mucopurulent discharge Friable cervix Cervical motion tenderness	May have no apparent findings or inflammation of vagina and cervix	Pale mucosa with friable areas that bleed easily
Odor	None	Yeast smell	Fishy or musty	Usually malodorous	No characteristic	None	No characteristic
Erythema	None	Present	Usually not present	Present	Variable	Variable	Variable
pH	3.5-4.1	4.0-5.0	>4.5	5.0-7.0	<4.5	<4.5	>4.5
Saline smear	Rare WBCs, large gram-positive rods, squamous epithelial cells	Budding filaments, spores, pseudohyphae	Clue cells	Many WBCs, trichomonads	No characteristic findings	No characteristic findings	Many WBCs, parabasal and intermediate cells, scarce superficial cells Folded, clumped epithelial cells
KOH preparation	No characteristic findings	Budding filaments, spores, pseudohyphae	Fishy odor with application of KOH	No characteristic findings	No characteristic findings	No characteristic findings	No characteristic findings

WBCs, White blood cells; *KOH*, potassium hydroxide.

Examination Step-by-Step

1. Palpate inguinal lymph nodes.
2. Inspect the external genitalia. Place your hand on the inner thigh to prepare the client for being touched.
   a. Skin color, condition, integrity
   b. Hair characteristics and distribution
   c. Labia majora: symmetry, color, inflammation, lesions
   d. Clitoris: size
   e. Labia minora
   f. Urethral opening: discharge, inflammation
   g. Vaginal opening: size, condition
   h. Perineum: condition, inflammation, lesions
   i. Anus
3. Palpate the external genitalia.
   a. Labia
   b. Skene's glands
   c. Bartholin's glands
4. Assess support of the pelvic musculature.
   a. Palpate the perineum.
   b. Test the vaginal introitus musculature.
   c. Assess for rectocele, cystocele, enterocele, and uterine prolapse.
5. Perform the speculum examination.
   a. Insert the speculum.
   b. Inspect the cervix and os for color, position, size, surface characteristics, discharge, and shape.
   c. Obtain specimens for cervical and vaginal smears and cultures if needed.
   d. Inspect the vaginal wall for color, surface characteristics, and discharge while withdrawing the speculum.
6. Perform bimanual palpation.
   a. Vaginal wall: smoothness, lesions
   b. Cervix and fornices: size, shape, position, mobility, patency of os, surface characteristics, tenderness
   c. Uterus: location, size, position, shape, mobility, tenderness
   d. Ovaries: size, shape, consistency, tenderness
   e. Adnexal areas: masses, tenderness
   f. Cul-de-sac: masses, tenderness
7. Perform rectovaginal palpation.
   a. Anus
   b. Rectovaginal septum: thickness, tone, nodules
   c. Rectum: masses, tone
   d. Uterus and adnexa
   e. Cul-de-sac

VARIATIONS FROM HEALTH

Skin and Labia

Common abnormalities of the skin and labia include parasites, skin lesions of all types, areas of leukoplakia, varicosities, hyperpigmentation, erythema, depigmentation, and swelling.

Parasites: Excoriations and erythematous areas are noted on the skin. Lice appear as dark spots on the skin, and their eggs (nits) are adherent to the pubic hair near the roots.

Skin lesions: Commonly seen skin lesions are those of HSV, appearing as small, shallow vesicles with surrounding erythema, and condylomata acuminata, which are the result of HPV infection and appear in single or multiple, cauliflower-like patches. HPV is a major risk factor for cervical cancer. Approximately 80% of cervical cancers show evidence of HPV.

Leukoplakia: This appears as white, adherent patches on the skin; it may be likened to spots of dried white paint. Leukoplakia is considered a precancerous lesion and requires further evaluation.

Vaginal Discharges

Vaginal discharges may result from various conditions of the uterus, cervix, and vagina. Causes include fungal, protozoal, viral, bacterial, spirochetal, and parasitic infections; benign and malignant neoplasms; chemical irritations; foreign bodies; fistulas; or poor hygiene. Full discussion of the various causes of discharges is beyond the scope of this text. However, clinical signs and symptoms accompanying common vaginal infections producing discharges are described (see Table 21-3) as follows:

Candida albicans

C. albicans is a fungus that causes approximately 20% of vaginal infections. Common symptoms of candidiasis are vulvovaginal itching; vulvar redness and swelling; and thick, white, curdlike (similar to cottage cheese) discharge. On examination the vulva and the vagina are commonly erythematous and edematous; curdlike white discharge may be present in labial folds and in the vagina; and the vagina and cervix may appear edematous and covered with adherent, thrushlike patches.

Bacterial Vaginosis

This is a bacterial vaginitis caused by *Gardnerella vaginalis* that is thought to account for 50% to 60% of vaginal infections. Clients complain of increased, watery, gray, malodorous vaginal discharge. Findings characteristic of the physical examination include little to no vulvar edema and a thin, creamy, gray-white, malodorous discharge covering the vagina and cervix.

Trichomonas vaginalis

This infection is caused by trichomonads, parasitic protozoans having motile flagella. Clients complain of watery, bubbly, profuse, yellowish-green, malodorous discharge, which is generally most severe immediately after menses. On physical examination, the vulva may appear erythematous, and a yellow-green, foul-smelling discharge is present at the introitus and in the vagina. In addition, the vagina may be erythematous and may have red, raised papules and petechiae.

Sample Documentation and Diagnoses

FOCUSED HEALTH HISTORY (SUBJECTIVE DATA)

Mrs. E, a 55-year-old female, is in for her annual gynecological examination. States that she has been feeling pressure "down there" all the time for the past 2 months. Feels as if she has to urinate all the time and dribbles urine frequently when she coughs, laughs, or sneezes. Has not had intercourse with her husband for 3 months because she is concerned she will urinate. Has been wearing pads to absorb urine leakage since about 6 months ago. Wears one pad during the day and one at night—they have been about half saturated when changed. Menarche was at age 14; cycle was regular every 30 days, with moderate to heavy flow for 5 days. Last menstrual period (LMP) was 5 years ago. Gravida 3/ para 3/ no abortions. Has had gynecological examinations yearly. Last Pap was 1 year ago, class I. No history of kidney disease. Had several bladder infections during her pregnancies and in early menopause, but no bladder infections for at least 10 years. Is not on hormone replacement therapy.

FOCUSED PHYSICAL EXAMINATION (OBJECTIVE DATA)

Female hair distribution. No masses; lesions; or swelling on labia, around clitoris, or perineum. Small amount of redness around urethral orifice. No discharge. No swelling or tenderness around Bartholin's glands. Old episiotomy scar on perineum.

Very weak vaginal musculature when asked to squeeze muscles around finger positioned in vagina. Anterior vaginal wall bulges, and a drop of urine escapes from urethral orifice when asked to push down.

Vaginal mucosa and cervix pale. Few secretions in vagina. No lesions noted.

No pain or tenderness with vaginal examination. Uterus anteverted, small, and firm without masses. No pain on moving cervix. Ovaries not palpated. No adnexal masses.

No lesions, tenderness, or pain noted on rectovaginal examination. No hemorrhoids or masses in anus or lower rectum.

DIAGNOSES

HEALTH PROBLEMS

Stress incontinence
Bladder prolapse

NURSING DIAGNOSES

Stress Urinary Incontinence Related to Prolapsed Bladder

Defining Characteristics

- Dribbling with increased abdominal pressure
- Urinary frequency
- Urinary urgency
- Poor vaginal musculature
- Bladder prolapse on examination

Sexual Dysfunction Related to Altered Body Structure and/or Function

Defining Characteristics

- Verbalization of fear of sex due to incontinence
- Embarrassed about stress incontinence

Ineffective Sexuality Patterns Related to Altered Body Structure and/or Function

Defining Characteristic

- Verbalization of fear due to incontinence

Teaching Self-Assessment

The teaching of genital self-examination may be indicated for clients in the following situations:

1. Clients using barrier or intrauterine contraceptive devices. The clients need to check the placement of devices.
2. Clients who have recurring vaginal infections.
3. Clients at risk for sexually transmitted diseases.
4. Clients who are starting to use tampons for the first time and may need to check whether one is removed before the new one is inserted.

The teaching session is initiated with a thorough presentation of the anatomy of the female genitalia and the normal appearance and feel of organs, structures, and discharge.

The following steps are recommended in teaching self-examination:

1. Find a comfortable position that will allow for viewing of the external genitalia with a mirror. A source of light from a nearby lamp is often necessary—positions can include sitting on the bed with knees bent, standing beside the toilet with one foot resting on the lid, or sitting in the bathtub or on the edge of a toilet seat.

2. Inspect the condition of the hair and skin over the genitalia. Spread the hairs and inspect all the surfaces of the labia. Look for bumps, sores, warts, and blisters.
3. Spread the labia and look at the clitoris for bumps, blisters, sores, and warts.
4. Look at the urethral opening and the area of Bartholin's glands for swelling or redness.
5. Insert a finger into the vagina, feel the consistency of normal tissue, and get used to the plane of the vagina.
6. Insert a finger deep into the vagina and locate the cervix. Feel the os and then feel the entire surface by circling it with the finger.
7. Look carefully at the type of discharge that is on the finger when it is taken out.

Some women's self-help groups teach self-examination by vaginal speculum. This is not recommended because of the difficulty of this maneuver on oneself and because professional judgment is needed for adequate assessment.

Critical Thinking Questions

Review the Sample Documentation and Diagnoses box to answer these questions.

1. Describe the components of a complete sexual history for a client suspected of having a sexually transmitted disease.

2. In the case of Mrs. E, which of the symptoms and physical findings are consistent with menopause?
3. What areas of self-care assessment are important in understanding Mrs. E's situation?

Answers are available on the MERLIN website (www.harcourthealth.com/MERLIN/Barkauskas/). And be sure to check the website regularly for additional learning activities!

Remember to check out the Online Study Guide!
www.harcourthealth.com/MERLIN/Barkauskas/

Anus and Rectosigmoid Region

Learning Objectives

On successful study of this chapter and completion of related learning experiences, the learner will be able to:
- Describe the anatomy and physiology of the rectosigmoid region.
- Outline the history relevant to rectosigmoid examination.
- Describe the expected appearance and characteristics of the anal and rectal structures accessible to examination.
- Explain the related rationale for and demonstrate assessment of the anus and rectum, including inspection and palpation techniques.
- Integrate the anal and rectal examination into the examination of the male and female reproductive tracts.
- Describe the assessment of stool characteristics and related pathological conditions.
- Describe procedures used to detect rectosigmoid pathology.
- Identify possible pathological conditions of the rectosigmoid region.

Outline

Purpose of Examination

The purposes of the rectal examination include assessment of anorectal status, the accessible pelvic viscera, the male prostate gland and seminal vesicles, and additional assessment of the female genitalia. The methods used to carry out this examination are inspection and palpation.

The rectal examination is an important component of every comprehensive physical examination. This type of examination is also indicated whenever the client is at risk for problems of the anorectal region or complains of symptoms that may indicate a problem or dysfunction of the region.

Because of the nature of the rectal examination, it is usually done at the end of the physical examination, which allows the client to clean himself or herself and dress on completion.

ANATOMY AND PHYSIOLOGY

The terminal gastrointestinal tract, which is called the rectosigmoid region, includes the anus, the rectum, and the caudal portion of the sigmoid colon.

Anus

The anal canal is the final segment of the colon. It is 2.5 to 4 cm long and opens into the perineum (Figure 22-1). The anal canal slants forward in a general line toward the umbilicus and forms a right angle with the rectum. The tract is surrounded by the external and internal sphincters, which keep it closed except when flatus and feces are passed. These sphincters are arranged in concentric layers. The striated external muscular ring is under voluntary control, whereas the internal smooth-muscle sphincter is under autonomic control. The internal sphincter is innervated from the pelvic plexus. Sympathetic stimulation contracts the sphincter; parasympathetic stimulation relaxes it. The anal canal, unlike the adjacent rectum, contains numerous somatic sensory nerves. Thus sensation in the canal is very keen.

The stratified squamous epithelial lining of the anus is visible to inspection because it extends beyond the sphincters, where it merges with the skin. Pigmentation and the presence of hair characterize this junction. Internally, the anal canal is lined by columns of mucosal tissue, which extend from the rectum and terminate in papillae. These anal columns, called the columns of Morgagni, fuse to form the anorectal junction. The spaces between these columns are called crypts.

The anal columns are invested with cross channels of **anastomosing** veins, which form mucosal folds known as anal valves. These anastomosing veins form a ring termed the zona hemorrhoidalis. When dilated, these veins are called internal hemorrhoids. The lower section of the anal canal contains a venous plexus, which has only a minor connection with the zona hemorrhoidalis and drains downward into the inferior rectal veins. Varicosed veins of this plexus are known as external hemorrhoids. Thus internal hemorrhoids occur superior to the pectinate line and are characterized by the moist, red epithelium of the rectum. External hemorrhoids are located inferior to the pectinate line and have the squamous epithelium of the anal canal or skin as their surface tissue.

Rectum

The rectum is the part of the gastrointestinal tract that is superior to the anal canal. Approximately 12 cm long, the rectum is lined with columnar epithelium. Superiorly the rectum has its origin at the third sacral vertebra and is continuous with the sigmoid colon. Its distal end dilates to form the rectal **ampulla**, which contains flatus and feces. Four semilunar transverse folds, the valves of Houston, extend across half the circumference of the rectal lumen. The purpose of these valves is not clear. They may serve to support feces while allowing flatus to pass.

Other Structures

The sigmoid colon has its origin at the iliac flexure of the descending colon and terminates in the rectum. Approximately 40 cm long, it is accessible to examination with the sigmoidoscope. Flexible fiberoptic instruments have made possible inspection of the mucosal surfaces of the entire sigmoid colon and of the other portions of the colon.

Other structures palpable during the rectal examination include the prostate, the structures of the female reproduc-

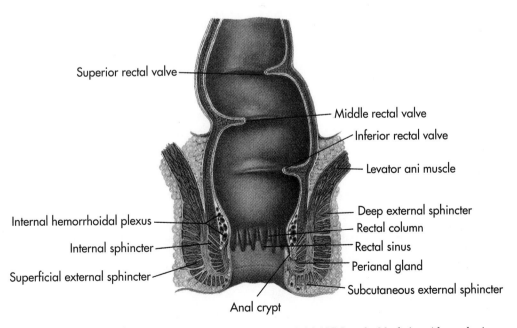

Figure 22-1 Anatomy of the anus and rectum. (From Seidel HM et al.: *Mosby's guide to physical examination,* ed. 4, St. Louis, 1999, Mosby.)

tive tract, and the inferior part of the abdominal cavity. The examination of the prostate is discussed in Chapter 20, and the female genital examination is discussed in Chapter 21. The lowest portion of the abdominal cavity, the peritoneal reflection, is palpable during the rectal examination. In males this area is termed the rectovesicular pouch and in females is termed the rectouterine pouch. This area extends down to within about 5.5 cm of the anal opening.

EXAMINATION

Focused Health History

In practice, the history of the anus and rectum is integrated into that of the gastrointestinal system. The regional history outlined here focuses on the distal portion of the gastrointestinal system. A regional history of the entire abdominal area is required for an adequate history of the anus and rectum. (See Chapter 17 for a discussion of history for the abdominal area.)

Present Health/Illness Status

1. Diet
   a. Intake of fiber and fluids
   b. Presence of lactose intolerance
2. Bowel habits
   a. Frequency of bowel movements
   b. Color of stools, odor
   c. Consistency of stools
   d. Changes in bowel patterns
   e. Any unusual signs or symptoms associated with defecation, such as mucus or blood
   f. Use of laxatives and enemas
   g. Pain with defecation
3. Rest and activity patterns
4. Medications: focus on medications intended to treat bowel problems and on those with intestinal tract side effects, such as iron
5. Date of last digital rectal examination, screening for fecal occult blood, and internal visualization procedures (e.g., colonoscopy or sigmoidoscopy)
6. Presence of risk factors for colorectal problems

Risk Factors
Anorectal Problems

Age greater than 50 years
Anal sexual practices
Travel to countries where parasitic and tropical diseases are common
Diabetes
Cardiac conditions
History of inflammatory bowel disease
Low-fiber, high-fat diet
Malignancies
Family history of cancer, Crohn's disease, ulcerative colitis

Past Health History and Associated Medical Conditions

1. Past history of anorectal problems, including prostate problems, hemorrhoids, anal fissure
2. Surgeries in region, including traumatic deliveries and episiotomy extensions
3. Trauma to rectum or perineal area
4. Neurological disorders
5. Cancer
6. Travel to countries or areas where exposure to parasitic diseases could have occurred
7. Diabetes
8. History of pelvic irradiation
9. Use of laxatives
10. Immobility

Family Health History

1. Family history of cancer or polyps in rectum or gastrointestinal tract
2. Crohn's disease
3. Ulcerative colitis
4. Bleeding disorders

Personal and Social History

1. Sexual practices, especially those involving the anus
2. Work environment—excessive sitting or lack of exercise
3. Sources of stress
4. Nutrition, especially fluids, fiber

Symptom Analysis

Bowel Movement Pattern Changes

1. **Onset:** specific date; sudden or gradual; association with diet, illness, stress, travel, other events
2. **Course since onset:** changes in daily pattern, frequency of bowel movements
3. **Location:** effect of change of location
4. **Quality:** type of stool—color, consistency, presence of matter other than feces such as mucus and blood, odor, explosiveness of movements
5. **Quantity:** amount and size of stool with each bowel movement, number of movements per day
6. **Setting:** differential patterns in various settings
7. **Associated phenomena:** incontinence, pain, fever, flatus, abdominal distention, nausea, vomiting, distention, cramping, diarrhea, constipation, straining or discomfort with defecation
8. **Alleviating and aggravating factors:** corrective measures taken and results; dietary changes; triggers that precipitate problem, such as dairy products
9. **Underlying concern:** fear of bowel cancer

Rectal Pain

1. **Onset:** specific date; sudden or gradual; association with diet, illness, changes in daily pattern, stress, travel, other events
2. **Course since onset:** frequency of pain, timing with defecation or straining of stool, relationship

to body position or activity, duration of episodes of pain
3. **Location:** specific location and radiation
4. **Quality:** acute, sharp, tearing, burning, throbbing, nagging
5. **Quantity:** amount of pain, effect on activities of daily living
6. **Setting:** differences by setting or activity
7. **Associated phenomena:** flatus, nausea, vomiting, diarrhea, constipation, distention, cramping, colic, pain, itching, burning, stinging, discharge; presence of blood, mucus, or other unusual substance in or on stool; swelling in anal region
8. **Alleviating and aggravating factors:** corrective measures taken and results; association with body position—sitting, standing, walking, lying down; medications; dissociation with bowel movements
9. **Underlying concern:** rectal abscess, cancer

Rectal Bleeding

1. **Onset:** specific date; sudden or gradual; association with defecation, diet, illness, changes in daily pattern, stress, travel, other events
2. **Course since onset:** relationship to defecation and changes in stool and bowel habits
3. **Location:** blood on or in stool
4. **Quality:** color of blood—bright red, dark red, or red-black; type of stool—color, consistency, presence of matter other than feces, odor
5. **Quantity:** amount—blood on tissue, spotting in toilet, active bleeding, or massive bleeding; frequency of bleeding episodes
6. **Setting:** relationship to a particular setting or activity
7. **Associated phenomena:** constipation, flatus, nausea, vomiting, distention, cramping, pain, weight loss, abdominal distention
8. **Alleviating and aggravating factors:** corrective measures taken and results, medications
9. **Underlying concern:** cancer, hemorrhoids

Stool Incontinence

1. **Onset:** specific date; sudden or gradual; association with diet, illness, changes in daily pattern, stress, travel, other events; relationship to anal intercourse
2. **Course since onset:** frequency of incontinent bowel movements, timing, duration
3. **Quality:** type of stool—color, consistency, presence of matter other than feces, presence of blood, odor
4. **Quantity:** amount
5. **Associated phenomena:** diarrhea, constipation, rectal prolapse, hemorrhoids, flatus, pain, nausea, vomiting, distention, cramping
6. **Setting:** relationship to a particular setting or activity
7. **Alleviating and aggravating factors:** diagnosis of impaction, cognitive impairment, neurological disorders; corrective measures taken and results; history of previous anal surgery, obstetric injury, anorectal

trauma, radiation-induced nerve or muscle injury, neurological disorders
8. **Underlying concern:** food poisoning, embarrassment

Constipation (Etiological Factors)

1. **Onset:** specific date; sudden or gradual; association with diet or fluid intake, illness, changes in daily pattern, stress, travel, other events
2. **Course since onset:** frequency of bowel movements
3. **Quality:** type of stool—color, consistency, presence of matter other than feces, odor, caliber of stool
4. **Quantity:** amount of stool with movements
5. **Associated phenomena:** bowel habits, flatus, nausea, vomiting, distention, cramping, pain, blood, mucus, straining with defecation, decreased appetite, colic, psychiatric or neurological disorders
6. **Setting:** relationship to a particular setting or activity, diet or specific foods
7. **Aggravating and alleviating factors:** dietary changes, motility disorders, structural abnormalities of the large bowel or anus, neurological disorders or injuries, endocrine disorders, medications taken, corrective measures taken and results, immobility, fluid intake
8. **Underlying concern:** pain, effect on activities of daily living

Preparation for Examination: Client and Environment

Most clients experience a significant amount of embarrassment and apprehension about the rectal examination. They may be concerned about the cleanliness of the area, the exploration of troubling symptoms, or pain. These fears can

Preparation for Examination

EQUIPMENT

Item	Purpose
Water-soluble lubricant	To enable more comfortable digital insertion and examination
Disposable gloves	To protect examiner's hands from feces and infection
Penlight	To observe skin of anus
Material for testing stool	To determine presence of occult blood
Anoscope	To visualize the rectum

CLIENT AND ENVIRONMENT

1. Provide a warm, private room with adequate lighting.
2. Explain examination.
3. Teach relaxation.
4. Reassure about sensations.
5. Position comfortably.
6. Drape adequately.

cause spasms of the anal sphincters and buttocks, which can make the examination unnecessarily uncomfortable. The following interventions can be used to alleviate anxiety and facilitate client cooperation so that a thorough and comfortable examination can be performed:

1. Teach the client relaxation techniques. Remind the client to continue slow, deep breathing during the examination. Breathing through an open mouth prevents Valsalva maneuvers.

2. Advise the client that unusual sensations may occur during the examination, especially the feeling that defecation is imminent; reassure the client that defecation is unlikely. Tell the client that sometimes flatus is passed during the examination and that this should not be a cause for embarrassment. Remind clients that they may feel an urge to void when the prostate is palpated.

3. If the client has fecal incontinence, protect the client and the examination area with appropriate padding.

4. Proceed with the examination in a sympathetic but confident manner.

5. Maintain gentleness in approach, avoiding undue force and allowing time for relaxation but not withdrawing the examining hand until the examination has been completed. However, if the client experiences extreme pain that persists, discontinue the examination.

6. Drape the client to avoid unnecessary exposure of the genitalia.

Technique for Examination and Expected Findings

Examine the client in one of the following positions, as shown in Figure 22-2 (also see Chapter 8):

1. *Left lateral or Sims' position.* The client lies on the left side with the superior thigh and knee flexed, bringing the knee close to the chest. The client's trunk should lie obliquely across the tabletop so

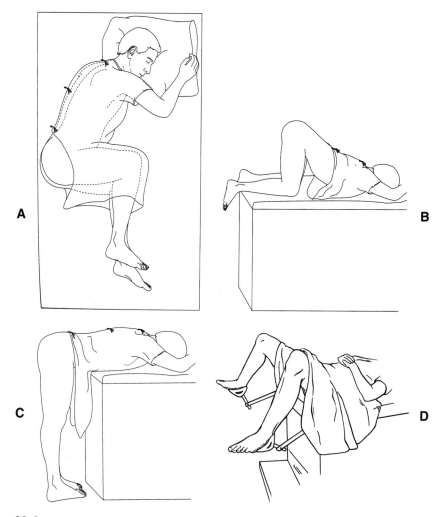

Figure 22-2 Positions for rectal examination. **A,** Left lateral or Sims' position. **B,** Knee-chest position. **C,** Standing position. **D,** Lithotomy position. (Squatting position is not shown because it is infrequently used.)

that the head rests on a pillow near the opposite edge. The hips should be flexed to an angle slightly less than 90 degrees, with the lower leg placed close to the opposite side of the table and parallel to its edge. The right side of the body should be displaced slightly forward. In this position the rectal ampulla is pushed down and posteriorly and thus is advantageously aligned for the detection of rectal masses. However, the upper rectum and the pelvic structure tend to fall away in this position. This examination position is good for bed-bound clients, for males, and for females who are not receiving a pelvic examination during this assessment.

2. *Knee-chest position.* The client kneels on the examining table with the shoulders and head in contact with the examining table. The knees are positioned more widely apart than the hips. The angle at the hip is 75 to 80 degrees. The prostate gland is best assessed with the client in this position. However, this position is uncomfortable and embarrassing for many clients.

3. *Standing position.* The client stands over the examining table with the hips flexed and the trunk resting on the table. Toes should be pointing in. This position is commonly used for examination of the prostate gland.

4. *Lithotomy position.* This position is used with female clients for a screening rectal examination following a pelvic examination. The client is supine with knees flexed and feet elevated and supported in stirrups.

5. *Squatting position.* The client squats on a firm, flat surface with the examiner behind the client. Rectal prolapse frequently can be noted when the client is in this position, and some lesions of the rectosigmoid region and pelvis can be felt especially well in this position. For all rectal examinations, the examiner should wear gloves on both hands throughout the entire procedure. Thorough hand washing after degloving is recommended.

Inspection

The manner in which the client sits throughout the history may provide some evidence of discomfort in the anal region. A client who continuously changes position during the examination may be having some anal discomfort.

Inspect the sacrococcygeal area for a pilonidal cyst or sinus. Normally, this area appears smooth and the overlying skin is healthy. Inspect the pilonidal area (at the tip of the coccyx) for dimples, sinus openings, or signs of inflammation. Also, palpate the pilonidal area at this time for tenderness, induration, or swelling.

The skin over a pilonidal sinus may have abundant hair growth. The accumulation of secretions within the sinus often leads to infection, which is generally accompanied by foul-smelling discharge and local tenderness.

Next, examine the skin of the entire perineal area for lesions and inflammation.

Spread the buttocks carefully with both hands to examine the anus and the tissue immediately surrounding it. The tissue surrounding the anal opening is more pigmented and coarser than the adjacent skin and is moist and hairless. The anal opening should remain closed and without discharge or leakage. Visually assess the perianal region for any lesions. **Skin tags**, scars, inflammation, perirectal abscesses, fissures, external hemorrhoids, fistula openings, condylomata acuminata (human papillomavirus), tumors, and rectal prolapse may be observed through this inspection.

After the initial inspection, ask the client to strain downward, as though defecating, and inspect the anus during straining. With this maneuver, it is possible to identify rectal prolapse, polyps, or internal hemorrhoids. Describe any abnormal findings in terms of clock position, with the 12 o'clock position being the apex of the anus (point closest to the symphysis pubis).

Palpation

Spread the buttocks with the nondominant hand. If the sphincter tightens, instruct the client to relax and reassure the client. Then, when the sphincter has relaxed, continue the examination. Occasionally painful lesions or bleeding may prevent completion of the examination unless a local analgesic agent is administered.

Lubricate the pad of the gloved index finger of the hand to be used for palpation. Instruct the client to strain downward against this finger. Then gently place the lubricated index finger of the examining hand against the anal opening. Exert firm pressure until the rectal sphincter begins to yield; then slowly insert the finger into the anal canal in the direction of the umbilicus as the sphincter relaxes (Figure 22-3). Note the tone of the anal canal at rest, which should be good. Then ask the client to tighten the sphincter around the examining finger to provide a measurement of muscle strength of the anal sphincter with contraction. Hypertonicity of the external sphincter may occur with anxious voluntary or involuntary contraction or as a result of an anal fissure or other local pathological condition. A relaxed or hypotonic sphincter is seen occasionally after rectal surgery, or it may be caused by a neurological deficiency.

The anal canal is short. The distance from the anal verge to the anorectal junction is less than 3 cm, which is roughly equivalent to the distance from the fingertip to the interphalangeal joint. Palpate the subcutaneous portion of the external sphincter on the inner aspect of the anal verge. Rotate the palpating finger to examine the entire muscular ring. A palpable indentation marks the intersphincteric line. Palpate the deep external sphincter through the lower part of the internal sphincter, which it surrounds. Bidigital palpation of the sphincter area, using the index finger and the thumb, yields more information than would be obtained by probing with the index finger alone. For bidigital palpation, press the thumb of the examining hand against the perianal tissue and move the examining index finger toward it. This technique is useful for detecting a perianal abscess and for palpating the bulbourethral (Cowper's) glands.

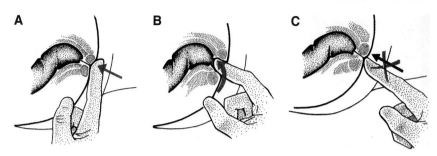

Figure 22-3 **A,** Digital pressure is applied against the anal verge until the external sphincter is felt to yield. **B,** The gloved, lubricated finger is slowly flexed and introduced in the direction of the umbilicus. **C,** Avoid this incorrect approach at a right angle to the sphincter (causes discomfort for the client and does not promote relaxation). NOTE: Illustrations are for a female in the lithotomy position. (Modified from Dunphy JE, Botsford TW: *Physical examination of the surgical patient: an introduction to clinical surgery,* ed. 4, Philadelphia, 1975, WB Saunders.)

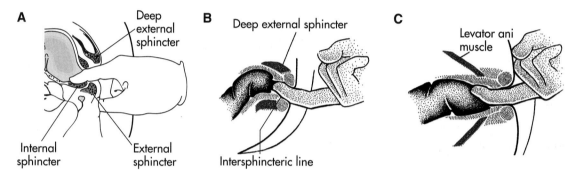

Figure 22-4 The subcutaneous portion of the external sphincter is palpated between the thumb and index finder (**A**), followed by digital exploration of the deep external sphincter (**B**). **C,** Palpation of the levator ani muscle. (NOTE: The technique for **A** is illustrated with a male leaning across the examination table. **B** and **C** are for a female in the lithotomy position. Techniques need to be slightly modified for examination of clients in other positions. Examination principles and sequences remain the same.) (Modified from Dunphy JE, Botsford TW: *Physical examination of the surgical patient: an introduction to clinical surgery,* ed. 4, Philadelphia, 1975, WB Saunders.)

Next assess the levator ani muscle; palpate laterally and posteriorly the area where the muscle is attached to the rectal wall on one side and then the other (Figure 22-4). Palpate the mucosa of the anal canal for tumors and polyps. Palpate the coccyx to determine its mobility and sensitivity. To assess muscular structures and the coccyx, perform bimanual examination with the index finger and the thumb.

Next insert the finger deeper into the canal to palpate the rectum. The posterior wall of the rectum follows the curve of the coccyx and the sacrum and feels smooth to the palpating finger. The examining finger is able to palpate the rectal canal a distance of 6 to 10 cm. To palpate the lateral walls of the rectum, rotate the index finger along the sides of the rectum. The ischial spines and the sacrotuberous ligaments can be identified through palpation. Rectal valves may be misinterpreted as protruding intrarectal masses, especially when they are well developed.

Because the prostate gland is situated anterior to the rectum, palpation through the mucosa of the anterior wall of the rectum allows for assessment of the size, shape, tenderness, surface characteristics, mobility, and consistency of the prostate gland. Ask the client to bear down so that an other-wise unreachable mass may be pushed downward into the range of the examining finger.

The prostate gland has a normal diameter of approximately 4 cm at its widest part. The palpating finger is used to identify the smooth lateral lobes separated by a central groove. The prostate, which is approximately 3 cm long, should protrude about 1 cm into the rectum, should feel rubbery and smooth, and should be slightly movable. The prostate should be nontender to palpation. (Ask the client specifically to report any tenderness to touch.) Note the presence of nodules. (A complete discussion of the prostate examination is included in the discussion of the assessment of the male genitalia in Chapter 20.)

The normal cervix can be felt as a small, round mass through the anterior wall of the rectum. In addition, a vaginal tampon or a retroverted uterus can be palpated through the rectal wall and mistaken for an abnormal mass. (See Chapter 21 for a complete discussion of the assessment of the female genitalia.)

At the termination of the examination, assist the client to a more comfortable position and offer the client tissues to remove any lubricant remaining around the anal opening.

TABLE 22-1   Assessment of Stool Characteristics

Description of Stool	Possible Explanation
Yellow or green	Severe diarrhea, sterilization of bowel by antibiotics, diet high in chlorophyll-rich vegetables, and use of the drug calomel
Light tan, gray	Absence of bile pigments, as may be found in blockage of common bile duct, pancreatic insufficiency, obstructive jaundice, and diets high in milk or fat and low in meat
Black, tarry	Bleeding into upper gastrointestinal tract, ingestion of iron compounds or bismuth preparations, and high proportions of meat in diet
Red	Bleeding from lower gastrointestinal tract; some foods such as beets
Translucent mucus on stool	Spastic constipation, nucleus colitis, emotional disturbance, and excessive straining
Bloody mucus	Neoplasm or inflammation of rectal canal
Mucus with pus and blood	Ulcerative colitis, bacillary dysentery, ulcerating cancer of colon, and acute diverticulitis
Fat in stool	Malabsorption syndromes, enteritis and pancreatic diseases, surgical removal of a section of intestine, steatorrhea, and chronic pancreatic disease
Blood-stained mucus in liquid feces	Amebiasis
Intermittent pencil-like stools	Spasmodic contraction in rectum
Persistent pencil-like stools	Permanent stenosis from scarring or other obstruction
Pipe stem and ribbon stools	Lower rectal stricture, anxiety and tension

Screening Tests and Procedures

Examination of Stool

After the examining finger has been withdrawn, examine the nature of any feces clinging to the glove (Table 22-1). Note the presence of pus or blood. Next, test a small quantity of the feces for the presence of occult blood using the instructions on commercially prepared kits for such testing. Fecal occult blood testing (FOBT) is a principal screening test for the early detection of colorectal cancers.

Two types of tests are commonly used for detecting fecal occult blood: guaiac-impregnated cards and other carriers that detect the peroxidase-like activity of hemoglobin (e.g., Hemoccult), and quantitative tests based on the conversion of heme to fluorescent porphyrins (e.g., HemoQuant). The guaiac-based tests are particularly sensitive to dietary factors.

Various factors other than bowel disease may contribute to occult blood in the stools. For example, the following factors might contribute to a positive test:

1. Bleeding gums following a dental procedure or resulting from another reason
2. Ingestion of red meat within 3 days of the test
3. Ingestion of fish, turnips, and horseradish within 3 days
4. Drugs that cause gastrointestinal bleeding, such as anticoagulants, aspirin, colchicine, iron preparations, nonsteroidal antiarthritics, and steroids
5. Other substances that might cause false-positive results for various reasons, such as oxidizing drugs, rauwolfia derivatives, and vitamin C
6. Lesions of the gastrointestinal tract

A single positive test result does not necessarily confirm the presence of gastrointestinal bleeding. A positive result is an indication to repeat the test at least three times while the client follows a meatless, high-residue diet. If the screening test is positive, the client is retested after 48 to 72 hours. Instruct the client to refrain from eating meat, poultry, fish,

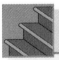

Examination Step-by-Step

INSPECTION

1. Spread the client's buttocks.
2. Observe the sacrococcygeal area.
3. Observe the perianal region for inflammation, lesions, hemorrhoids, and fissures.
4. Ask the client to bear down to determine presence of prolapse.

PALPATION

1. Lubricate the examining finger.
2. Insert the finger into the anus.
3. Place the pad of the finger gently along the anal verge.
4. Feel the sphincter tense and then relax. When the sphincter has relaxed, flex the tip of the finger and slowly insert it into the anal canal in the direction of the umbilicus.
5. Rotate the finger and palpate the entire muscular ring.
6. Assess tone by asking the client to contract the muscles.
7. Assess the perianal tissue and muscular structures through bidigital palpation.
8. Assess the accessible rectal wall.
9. Men: Palpate the prostate gland and the seminal vesicles on the anterior wall. Women: Perform the rectovaginal examination.

ASSESSMENT OF STOOL

1. Withdraw the examining finger.
2. Examine the feces on the gloved finger.
3. Test the stool for occult blood.

turnips, and horseradish during 3 days before testing. In addition, the client may need to temporarily discontinue the use of the following substances: iron preparations, oxidizing drugs, rauwolfia derivatives, indomethacin, colchicine, salicylates, phenylbutazone, oxybutazone, bismuth compounds, steroids, and ascorbic acid, and any drug that may cause gastrointestinal bleeding.

Screening for colorectal cancer is done through fecal occult blood testing and sigmoidoscopy. However, current screening recommendations vary.

Healthy People 2010 (U.S. Department of Health and Human Services, 2000) has established the goal of reducing

---

BOX 22-1

OTHER INVESTIGATIVE TECHNIQUES

ANOSCOPY

Use of an anoscope provides for a more complete examination of the anal canal and the internal hemorrhoidal zone than is possible through palpation alone.

PROCTOSCOPY

Use of a proctoscope provides visualization of the anus and the lower rectum. Approximately 9 to 15 cm of the lower intestinal tract can be visualized. The warmed and lubricated instrument is passed with the obturator for its full length. The obturator is removed, and the proctoscope is removed slowly while the examiner observes for ulcers, inflammation, strictures, or the cause of a palpable mass. Biopsy may be performed through the tube.

SIGMOIDOSCOPY

A sigmoidoscope allows for visual examination of the upper portion of the rectum, an area that cannot be felt with the examining finger, and also allows direct visualization of the lower 24 to 60 cm (flexible sigmoidoscope) of the gastrointestinal tract. This examination is particularly important since half of all carcinomas occur in the rectum and colon. The early detection of polyps and malignant lesions may result in early and successful treatment of an otherwise fatal disease.

COLONOSCOPY

Colonoscopy techniques allow the entire colon (from anus to cecum) to be visualized. Biopsy specimens can be taken through the colonoscope, and bleeding sites can be cauterized.

MANOMETRY

This technique measures intraluminal pressure by a balloon probe attached to a catheter that is connected to a pressure transducer and a polygraph.

SPHINCTER ELECTROMYOGRAPHY

Needle or surface electrodes are used to detect the contractile activity of striated muscle and to obtain separate recordings from the external sphincter and from the puborectalis muscle.

DEFECOGRAPHY AND BALLOON PROCTOGRAPHY

These radiological investigations are designed to image the rectum and the pelvic floor at rest and during contraction and defecation.

---

deaths from colon cancer to 13.9 per 100,000 persons from the 1998 baseline of 21.1. On behalf of achieving this objective the following objectives have been established:

- Increase to 50% the percentage of adults age 50 years and older who have received a fecal occult blood test within the preceding 2 years.
- Increase to 50% the percentage of adults age 50 and older who have ever received a sigmoidoscopy.

The U.S. Preventive Services Task Force (1996) recommends screening for colorectal cancer for all persons age 50 and older with FOBT or sigmoidoscopy, or both. There is insufficient evidence to determine which of these screening methods is preferable or whether the combination produces greater benefits than either test alone. There is also insufficient evidence to recommend for or against routine screening with digital rectal examination. FOBT is recommended on an annual basis, but there is insufficient evidence to recommend a schedule for sigmoidoscopy screening, although a frequency of every 3 to 5 years is common.

For persons with a family history of hereditary syndromes associated with a very high risk of colon cancer and those previously diagnosed with ulcerative colitis, high-risk adenomatous polyps, or colon cancer, regular endoscopic screening should be a part of routine diagnosis and screening.

The presence of a pathological condition detected by digital examination may be further explored by one of the procedures shown in Box 22-1.

VARIATIONS FROM HEALTH

Blood in the Stool

Bright red blood, in small or large amounts, may originate in the large intestine, the sigmoid colon, the rectum, or the anus. The stool is likely to be red-black if the bleeding is coming from the ascending colon. Colonic bleeding should be suspected when blood is mixed with the feces. Rectal bleeding is probably occurring when blood is observed on the surface of the stool. The presence of a good deal of blood in the stool may be associated with marked malodor.

A black, tarry stool (melena) may result from bleeding in the stomach or the small intestine; the blood is partially digested during its passage to the rectum. On the other hand, the black color may result from ingested iron compounds and bismuth preparations.

Abscesses

Abscesses of the lower gastrointestinal tract that can be identified by physical examination (Figure 22-5) include the following types:

1. Perirectal abscess: may be palpated as a tender mass adjacent to the anal canal. The increased temperature of the mass may be helpful in identifying the inflammatory process.
2. Ischiorectal abscess: may be palpated as a tender mass protruding into the lateral wall of the anal canal.

3. Supralevator ani muscle abscess: may be felt by the examining finger as a tender mass in the lateral rectal wall.

Anal Fissure

An anal fissure is a linear ulceration or laceration of the skin of the anus. Asking the client to bear down as though straining to evacuate stool may identify a thin tear of the superficial anal mucosa. Often a small amount of weeping can be noted around the tear. The fissure is most commonly found in the posterior midline of the anal mucosa (in more than 90% of affected patients) and less commonly in the anterior midline (Figure 22-6, *A* and *B*). An anal fissure usually results from trauma, such as that associated with the passage of a large, hard stool or with anal intercourse. The client may complain of local pain, itching, or bleeding. Pain generally accompanies the passage of stool, and blood may be observed on the stool or on the toilet tissue. The inspection finding may include a sentinel skin tag or ulcer through which the muscles of the internal sphincter may be visible at the base. Because the examination may be painful to the client, making relaxation of the anal muscle difficult, the use of a local anesthetic may be necessary.

Fecal Impaction

Fecal impaction is the accumulation and dehydration of fecal material in the rectum. When motility of the rectum is inhibited, the normal progression of feces does not occur and excessive amounts of water are reabsorbed through the bowel wall. The feces become hard and difficult to pass, and the accumulation may lead to complete obstruction. Fecal impaction is observed in individuals with chronic constipa-

tion and in those who have retained barium following gastrointestinal x-ray examination. The client complains of a sense of rectal fullness or urgency without ability to defecate to relieve the feeling. Frequent small liquid-to-loose stools may occur in incomplete obstruction. The dehydrated fecal mass is easily felt on palpation.

Fistula-in-Ano

Fistula-in-ano is an abnormal opening on the cutaneous surface near the anus. It usually results from a local crypt abscess but is also common in Crohn's disease. A tract from an anal fissure or infection that terminates in the perianal skin or other tissue is termed an anorectal fistula. This type of fistula usually originates from local crypt abscesses. The fistula is a chronically inflamed tube, made up of fibrous tissue surrounding granulation tissue that frequently can be palpated. The external opening is generally visible as a red elevation of granulation tissue. Local compression may result in the expression of serosanguineous or purulent drainage. Bidigital palpation is best accomplished with a finger in the anorectal

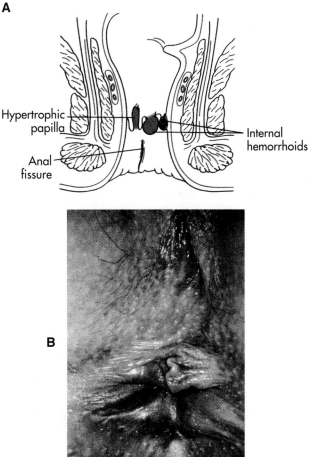

Hypertrophic papilla

Anal fissure

Internal hemorrhoids

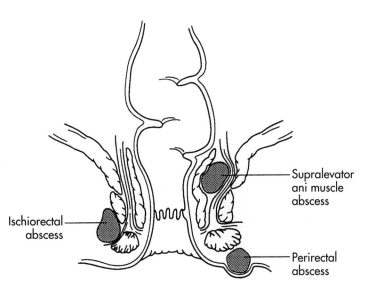

Figure 22-5 Common sites of abscess formation in the lower gastrointestinal tract.

Ischiorectal abscess

Supralevator ani muscle abscess

Perirectal abscess

Figure 22-6 **A,** Common problems of the anus and rectum. **B,** Actual appearance of lateral fissure. (**B** courtesy Gershon Efron, MD, Sinai Hospital of Baltimore.)

cavity that compresses the tissue against the thumb on the skin surface. The fistulous tract feels like an indurated cord.

The site from which drainage from an anal infection occurs can be identified by relating the location of the external opening of the fissure to the anus (Figure 22-7 and Table 22-2).

Hemorrhoids

Hemorrhoids are dilated, congested veins (Figure 22-8, *A* and *B*). Hemorrhoidal swelling is associated with increased hydrostatic pressure in the portal venous system. The pressure associated with hemorrhoids correlates positively with pregnancy, straining at stool, chronic liver disease, and sudden increases in intraabdominal pressure. Bowel habits also play a role: for example, hemorrhoids commonly occur with diarrhea, constipation, or incomplete bowel emptying. Local factors such as abscess or tumor may also contribute to venous stasis.

Hemorrhoidal skin tags are ragged, flaccid skin sacs located around the anus. They cover connective tissue sacs and are the locus of resolved external hemorrhoids. Clients de-

scribe these tags as painless. Internal hemorrhoids occur proximal to the pectinate line (see Figure 22-6), whereas external hemorrhoids are those that are seen distal to this boundary. External hemorrhoids are covered by skin or anal squamous tissue.

External hemorrhoids are often painful, particularly if an increase in stool mass stretches the skin. Because the mass is located near the sphincter muscles, spasm is not uncommon. External hemorrhoids often cause itching and bleeding on defecation. These dilated veins may not be apparent at rest; however, they may appear as bluish, swollen areas at the anal verge when thrombosed. A thrombosed hemorrhoid is one in which blood has clotted, both within and outside the vein.

Internal hemorrhoids generally do not cause pain unless thrombosis, infection, or erosion of overlying mucosal surfaces complicates them. Discomfort is increased if the hemorrhoids prolapse through the anal opening. Bleeding may occur from the internal hemorrhoids with or without defecation. **Proctoscopy** is generally necessary for their identification.

Fecal Incontinence

Loss of the voluntary ability to control defecation is called **incontinence**. It may range from the involuntary passage of

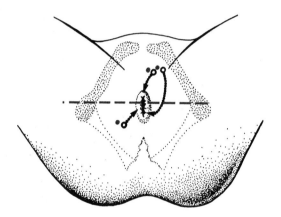

Figure 22-7 Salmon's law. Fissure location related to the aperture of the fistula. (Adapted from Dunphy JE, Botsford TW: *Physical examination of the surgical patient: an introduction to clinical surgery,* ed. 4, Philadelphia, 1975, WB Saunders.)

TABLE 22-2	Location of the Fistula Site Related to the External Opening	
	External Opening	**Location in Anus**
Goodsall's rule	Posterior to a line between ischial tuberosities	Posterior
	Radial from drainage site	Anterior
Salmon's law	Posterior to anus or more than 2.5 cm anterior or lateral	Posterior
	Anterior or less than 2.5 cm lateral	Anterior

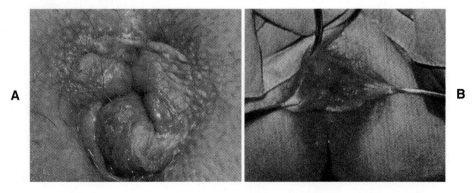

Figure 22-8 **A,** External hemorrhoids. **B,** Internal hemorrhoids. (**B** courtesy Gershon Efron, MD, Sinai Hospital of Baltimore.)

flatus to complete loss of sphincter tone. The loss of fecal gases or liquids may also occur in the presence of a normal sphincter in hyperdynamic bowel states.

Masses

The presence of a mass in the rectum deserves special attention because nearly half of the rectal masses discovered are malignant. However, most cancerous lesions are beyond the reach of the examiner's finger and require scoping to detect. The client commonly denies pain or other symptoms. Early lesions are felt as small elevations or nodules with a firm base. Ulceration of the center of the lesion results in a crater that may be palpated. An ulcerated carcinoma may be identified through palpation by its firm, nodular, rolled edge. If a lesion is palpated, describe its shape (annular or tubular), surface characteristics, borders, degree of fixation, and distance from the anus. The consistency of the malignant mass is often stony and hard, and the contour is irregular.

Pilonidal Cyst and Sinus

A pilonidal cyst is a hairy sac that develops in the sacral region of the skin. A pilonidal sinus is an abnormal channel that contains a tuft of hair and is most commonly situated over or close to the tip of the coccyx. Even though it is thought to be a congenital lesion, a pilonidal sinus is commonly first diagnosed between the ages of 15 and 30 years. It is located superficial to the coccyx, or lower sacrum. The sinus opening may look like a dimple, with another very small opening found in the midline. In other cases of pilonidal sinus, a cyst can be observed and palpated. In more advanced conditions, a sinus tract can be palpated. The affected area may become edematous, erythematous, and tender, and a tuft of hair may be observed. The ingrowth of the hairs is probably the cause of infection and cyst and fistula formation. These cysts and fistulas are generally removed surgically.

Pruritus Ani

Pruritus ani is a common chronic condition characterized by itching of the perianal skin. Excoriated, thickened, and pigmented skin may result from chronic inflammation associated with this condition. Itching and burning of the rectal area are most often traceable to pinworms in children and to fungal infections in adults. Clients with diabetes are particularly vulnerable to fungal infections. A dull, grayish pink color of the perianal skin is characteristic of fungal infections. The radiating folds of skin may appear enlarged, and the skin may be cracked or fissured. Pruritus ani that is characterized by dry and brittle skin is thought to be related to psychosomatic disease.

Rectal Polyps

Rectal polyps, which feel like soft nodules, are commonly encountered. They may be pedunculated (on a stalk) or sessile (irregularly moundlike, growing from a relatively broad base, and closely adherent to the mucosal wall). Because of their soft consistency, rectal polyps may be difficult or impossible to identify by palpation. Proctoscopy is usually necessary for identification, and a biopsy is performed to identify malignant lesions. A pedunculated rectal polyp occasionally prolapses through the anal ring.

Rectal Prolapse

Internal hemorrhoids are the most common type of tissue protrusion through the anal ring (Figure 22-9). The pink-colored mucosa is described as appearing like a doughnut or rosette. In the older client, however, protruding mucosa may herald eversion or prolapse of the rectum. Incomplete prolapse involves only mucosa, whereas complete rectal prolapse is also associated with the sphincters.

The client describes the prolapse of tissue through the anal ring as occurring with exercise or while straining at stool. Frequently, the client is able to push the mass back in with digital pressure. Inspection reveals a red, bulging mucosal mass protruding through the anal ring.

Rectal Tenesmus

Rectal **tenesmus** is painful straining at stool associated with spasm of the anal and rectal muscles. The chief complaint is a distressing feeling of urgency. The client should be questioned concerning the nature of the stool. A hard, dry stool indicates constipation. A bloody, diarrheal stool might indicate ulcerative colitis. When the client's stools are normally constituted, a rectal fissure may be the cause of tenesmus. The client with a perirectal inflammation, such as prostatitis or proctitis, may also experience tenesmus.

The client who complains of constant rectal pain should be examined carefully for thrombosed rectal hemorrhoids.

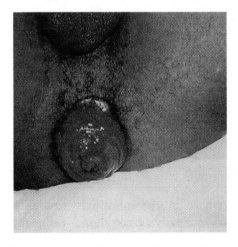

Figure 22-9 Prolapse of the rectum. (Courtesy Gershon Efron, MD, Sinai Hospital of Baltimore.)

Sample Documentation and Diagnoses

FOCUSED HEALTH HISTORY (SUBJECTIVE DATA)

Mrs. G, a 35-year-old married female, is complaining of burning and itching in the rectal area, especially after bowel movements, for about 2 months. Notes a small amount of blood on toilet tissue about once or twice a week after bowel movements. Over the past 2 months, bowel movements have not been regular (interval varies between 2× a day to once in 3 days). Stools are characteristically hard, and bowel movements are frequently painful. Has been taking a laxative (milk of magnesia) every 2 to 3 days for the past month. Denies abdominal pain; fecal incontinence; or a history of rectal infections, trauma, or surgeries. Has a history of hemorrhoids after her most recent pregnancy 3 years ago. Family history is negative for cancer and colon diseases. Three months ago started work outside of the home. Consequently, diet and activity patterns have changed. Eats fewer fruits and vegetables, drinks less water, and is less active.

FOCUSED PHYSICAL EXAMINATION (OBJECTIVE DATA)

Abdomen: Flat; bowel sounds normal and heard in all four quadrants. No organomegaly or tenderness on palpation. No masses.

Perianal area: Clean, no fissures or lesions.

Rectum and anus: Small, 1 × 1 cm, reddish blue, shiny mass visible at 5 o'clock position at anal opening. Tender on palpation. Two small skin tags at 3 and 9 o'clock positions.

Sphincter tone: Good.

Rectal walls: Smooth and without tenderness.

Stool: Brown and formed.

Hemoccult: Negative.

DIAGNOSES

HEALTH PROBLEM

Constipation; external hemorrhoid

NURSING DIAGNOSIS

Constipation Related to Low-Fiber Diet, Low Fluid Intake, and Inadequate Physical Activity

Defining Characteristics

- Frequency less than normal pattern
- Hard, formed stools; decreased quality
- Straining at stool
- Painful defecation

Critical Thinking Questions

Review the Sample Documentation and Diagnoses box to answer questions 1 and 2.

1. If Mrs. G's stool were light gray, what additional health issues would you consider?

2. If the client were a 23-year-old sexually active homosexual male, what factors could be contributing to painful defecation?

3. Describe the preparation for rectal examination of a 70-year-old male who has not had a physical examination for 20 years and who has symptoms of prostatic hypertrophy and a fear of cancer.

Answers are available on the MERLIN website (www.harcourthealth.com/MERLIN/Barkauskas/). And be sure to check the website regularly for additional learning activities!

Remember to check out the Online Study Guide!
www.harcourthealth.com/MERLIN/Barkauskas/

Integration of the Physical Assessment and Documentation

Learning Objectives

On successful study of this chapter and completion of related learning experiences, the learner will be able to:
- List the equipment and supplies needed for a complete physical examination.
- Prepare clients for a complete physical examination.

- Outline and perform procedures of a complete physical examination.
- Record findings from a complete physical examination.
- Describe guidelines to adapt the examination techniques that accommodate individual clients and client situations.

Outline

Performance of the Integrated Physical Examination

This chapter includes three sections: description of and outline for the performance of a comprehensive, integrated physical examination; description of the documentation of the comprehensive physical examination; and a worksheet for documenting a physical examination.

After practicing and acquiring proficiency in the performance of regional examinations, it is important to develop a systematic pattern for performing an integrated physical examination. In practice, practitioners perform both regional examinations, such as in acute care settings, and comprehensive multisystem examinations, such as in health maintenance programs.

In developing a personal routine for a complete examination, consider factors of efficiency and client comfort. The examiner who performs procedures systematically and efficiently conserves time and is less likely to forget a procedure or a part of the body than is the examiner who performs examinations haphazardly.

Clients who are ill or debilitated lose energy quickly. Follow a system of examination involving the fewest number of client position changes. This consideration for the client will enhance acceptability and decreases the number of examinations and portions of examinations deferred because of client intolerance.

The manner in which the examiner conducts the physical examination can enhance or compromise rapport developed during the history-taking interview. A disorganized examiner who leaves the room to obtain missing equipment, who changes positions several times in a short time period, or who has the client change positions frequently may lose the client's confidence. All of the equipment and supplies needed for the physical examination should be available in the room and within easy reach. See the boxes on p. 558 for a listing of equipment needed and hints about preparing the client and the environment for the examination.

The outline presented in this chapter under Technique for Examination is a suggested format for performing the comprehensive, integrated physical examination. It is intended as a guide for the beginning practitioner to use in

Preparation for Examination

EQUIPMENT

The equipment needed for a complete physical examination includes the following (the purposes and uses of all the listed items have been explained in the preceding chapters):

Cotton balls
Cotton-tipped swabs or applicator sticks
Drapes
Flashlights—both large with transilluminator and penlight
Gauze squares
Glass of water
Gloves—latex, disposable examination
Gowns
Marking pencil or pen
Materials for cover test
Materials to test pain and light touch sensation (pin, cotton ball)
Measuring tape
Nasal speculum (optional)
Odoriferous substances for cranial nerve I examination
Ophthalmoscope
Otoscope with pneumatic bulb insufflator
Printed material for near visual acuity and comprehension examination
Reflex (percussion) hammer
Ruler
Scale with height measurement attachment
Sharp and dull testing materials
Snellen eye chart (far vision acuity)
Sphygmomanometer with cuffs of various sizes
Stethoscope with diaphragm and bell heads
Substances for taste sensation evaluation (CN VII)
Thermometer
Tongue blades

Tuning forks (one 500-1000 cycles per second [CPS] for testing auditory function and one 100-400 CPS for testing vibratory sense)
Watch that records seconds

If a pelvic or a rectal examination is to be done, add the following equipment and supplies:

Lubricant (water soluble)
Materials to collect and prepare vaginal secretions or specimens for laboratory examination
Materials to examine fecal material for occult blood
Mirror
Vaginal specula of various sizes

CLIENT AND ENVIRONMENT

The physical examination should occur in a comfortable room that provides privacy, adequate lighting, and a reasonable amount of space for client and examiner movement. The recommended equipment for an examination room includes the following:

Desk with two chairs
Examination lamp
Examining table
Scale
Sink
Stand or counter to hold supplies
Stool

In preparation for the examination, the following procedures are recommended:

1. Check for availability of needed materials within easy reach.
2. Review examination procedure with client.
3. Have client empty bladder.
4. Have client undress and put on gown.

■ HELPFUL HINT

When performing the integrated physical examination:
• Warm hands and instruments.
• Keep fingernails short and smooth.
• Ensure a quiet, private setting.
• Adapt to the circumstances.
• Position the examining table away from a wall to enable maximum movement for yourself.
• Explain what you are doing and observing during the examination.
• Avoid vague or evaluative statements that the client may misunderstand.
• Advise the client of specific, possible uncomfortable and/or unusual sensations.
• Ask the client to tell you about unusual sensations or pain elicited during the examination.
• Expose the area to be examined fully to ensure a complete assessment, but drape all areas not being examined.

practice sessions. In actual client care situations, it may require adaptation because of the client's age or disability, examination protocols and priorities of the care agency, or examiner preference. The suggested format is designed to avoid excessive client and examiner movement. The approach integrates body systems into the examination of body regions.

Technique for Examination

The client enters the examination room, the examiner and the client greet each other, and the examiner observes the client (Figure 23-1).

Inspect General Appearance

1. Consistency of general appearance with age
2. Skin color
3. General state of nutrition
4. Posture

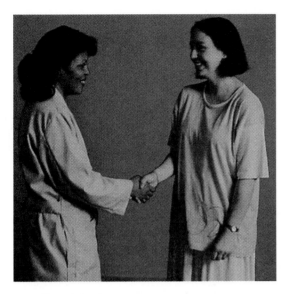

Figure 23-1 Examiner greeting the client.

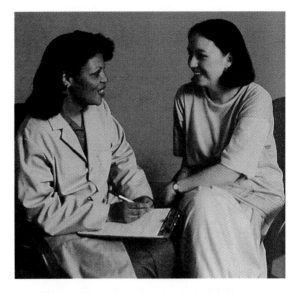

Figure 23-2 Interview for the health history.

5. Obvious physical deformities
6. Hygiene

Inspect Stature and Movement

1. Mobility
2. Symmetry
3. Posture
4. Body build
5. Gait

Inspect Demeanor

1. Facial expression
2. Composure
3. Speech
4. Orientation and mental status
5. Disposition
6. Eye contact

At this point in a comprehensive assessment, the examiner takes the health history (Figure 23-2).

Take Health History

The comprehensive health history is discussed in Chapter 3. The student is referred to that chapter for review as needed. Allow the client to remain in street clothes for the history-taking interview. Just before starting the physical examination, have the client change from street clothes into the examination gown.

The client is sitting on the bed or examining table and has put on an examination gown. The examiner is facing the client (Figure 23-3).

Take Measurements

1. Weight
2. Height

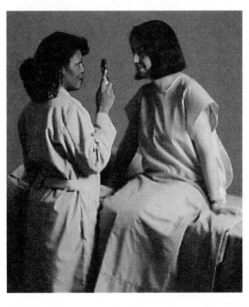

Figure 23-3 Client gowned and seated; examiner facing the client.

3. Temperature
4. Palpate pulses (radial and brachial)
5. Blood pressure (both arms sitting and standing)
6. Respiratory rate

Inspect and Palpate Upper Extremities

1. Examine skin (color, temperature, vascularity, lesions, hydration, turgor, texture, edema, masses), muscle mass, and skeletal configuration.
2. Examine nails (color and condition).

Examine Head

1. Inspect configuration of skull.
2. Inspect condition of skin, scalp, and hair (masses, parasites, lesions).
3. Inspect hair distribution.
4. Inspect face—appearance, expression, symmetry of structure and features, movements (cranial nerve [CN] VII).
5. Inspect head—size, shape, symmetry, extra movements.
6. Palpate skull, hair, and face (deformities, tenderness, lesions, texture, distribution, quantity).
7. Palpate and percuss paranasal (maxillary and frontal) sinus areas (tenderness). If sinuses tender, transilluminate.
8. Palpate temporomandibular joint (tenderness, crepitations).

Examine Eyes

1. Inspect eyebrows, eyelids, eyelashes, conjunctivae, corneas, sclerae, irides, pupils, and palpebral fissures.
2. Measure visual acuity (CN II).
3. Assess visual fields (CN II).
4. Determine alignment of eyes (perform cover test and corneal light reflex).
5. Test extraocular movements (CN III, CN IV, CN VI).
6. Palpate lacrimal sac.
7. Test pupillary responses (light and accommodation) (CN III).
8. The room should be darkened for the ophthalmoscopic examination. Perform ophthalmoscopic examination of lens, media, red reflex, disc vessels and retinal background (CN II).
9. Test corneal reflex (CN V, CN VII) if indicated.

Examine Ears

1. Inspect external ear (position, alignment, masses, lesions, tenderness).
2. Palpate external ear (masses, lesions, tenderness).

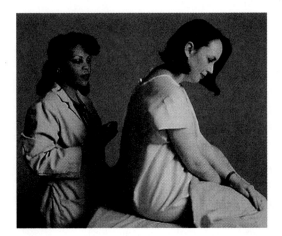

Figure 23-4 Client seated; examiner behind the client.

3. Perform otoscopic examination (inspect canals and tympanic membranes for color, position, landmarks, and integrity).
4. Determine auditory acuity (CN VIII).
5. Perform Weber and Rinne tests.

Examine Nose

1. Inspect alignment of septum and surface characteristics.
2. Determine patency of each nostril.
3. Test for olfaction (CN I) if indicated.
4. Using a speculum, inspect mucosa, septum, and turbinates (inflammation, allergy, lesions, epistaxis).

Examine Mouth and Pharynx

1. Using a penlight, inspect lips, total buccal mucosa, teeth, gums, tongue, sublingual area, roof of mouth, tonsillar area, and pharynx (as appropriate, for presence, condition, color, symmetry, surface characteristics, movement).
2. Palpate mouth with gloved hand if indicated.
3. Note mouth odor.
4. Test glossopharyngeal nerve (CN IX) and vagus nerve (CN X) ("ah" and gag reflex).
5. Test hypoglossal nerve (CN XII) (tongue movement).
6. Test taste (CN VII and CN IX) if indicated.

Complete Examination of Cranial Nerves

1. Test trigeminal nerve (CN V) (jaw clenching, lateral jaw movements, pain, and light touch to face).
2. Test facial nerve (CN VII). (Client smiles, raises eyebrows, shows teeth, puffs cheeks, keeps eyes closed against resistance.)
3. Test spinal accessory nerve (CN XI) (trapezius and sternocleidomastoid muscles).

Complete Examination of Head; Examination of Neck

1. Inspect surface characteristics and range of motion of the head and neck.
2. Palpate nodes (preauricular, postauricular, occipital, parotid, sublingual, submandibular, submental, anterior cervical, posterior superficial cervical, posterior cervical, internal jugular, supraclavicular, and intraclavicular nodes).
3. Palpate carotid arteries.
4. Palpate for position of trachea.
5. Observe thyroid area for swelling.
6. Palpate thyroid gland at rest and with swallowing (palpate anteriorly at this time; if a posterior approach is used, wait until position change when you are behind client).
7. Auscultate carotid arteries and thyroid gland for bruits.

The client is sitting on the bed or examining table, total chest uncovered if male, breasts covered if female (Figure 23-4). The examiner is standing behind the client.

Examine Back

1. Inspect skin
2. Inspect spine.

3. Palpate spine.
4. Palpate muscles and bones.
5. Palpate costovertebral area, asking client about tenderness.

Examine Lungs (Apices and Lateral and Posterior Areas)

NOTE: Apical, posterior, and lateral lung regions can usually be examined from a position behind the client.
1. Inspect respiration (depth, rhythm, pattern) and posterior and lateral thorax.
2. Palpate for thoracic expansion and tactile fremitus.
3. Percuss systematically.
4. Determine diaphragmatic excursion.
5. Auscultate systematically (breath sounds and adventitious sounds).
6. Auscultate for vocal resonance.

The client is sitting on the bed or examining table, with the gown off the shoulders and resting in the lap. The examiner is facing the client (Figure 23-5). Offer the female client a towel to cover areas of the chest not being examined while the gown is off the chest.

Examine Lungs (Anterior Areas)

1. Inspect skin and thoracic configuration.
2. Palpate external thorax for skin temperature and consistency, tenderness, and thoracic configuration.
3. Palpate for general assessment and tactile fremitus.
4. Percuss systematically.
5. Auscultate lungs systematically.
6. Auscultate for vocal resonance.

Examine Heart

NOTE: Additional examination in the supine position will be done later.

1. Inspect precordium (pulsations and heaving).
2. Palpate precordium (apical impulse, thrills, heaves, pulsations).
3. Ask the client to lean forward. Auscultate precordium (aortic area, pulmonic area, left sternal border, apical area).
4. Inspect jugular venous pulses and pressure.

Examine Breasts (Female Client and Male Client With Gynecomastia)

NOTE: All men should have a breast examination in the supine position.
1. Inspect breasts with client's arms and hands at the sides, above the head, and pressed into the hips, eliciting pectoral contraction for symmetry, mobility, dimpling.
2. Inspect breasts with client leaning forward.
3. If lesions are suspected or client is at risk for other reasons, palpate breasts in all four quadrants.
4. If client has large breasts, perform a bimanual examination.

Complete Palpation of Nodes in Upper Body and Upper Body ROM

1. Palpate axillary nodes (lateral axillary, posterior axillary, central axillary, anterior axillary, and apical axillary).
2. Palpate epitrochlear nodes.
3. Test ROM and strength of upper extremities.

The client is supine. The examiner is at the right side of the client (Figure 23-6).

Examine Breasts (Male and Female)

1. Position breasts for palpation.
2. Palpate breasts systematically in all four quadrants, areolar areas, and the tail of Spence.
3. Attempt to express secretion from the nipples.

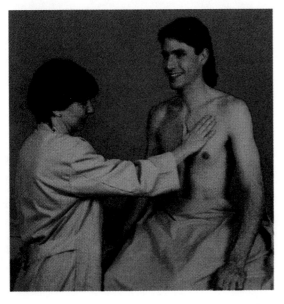

Figure 23-5 Client seated and disrobed to the waist; examiner facing the client.

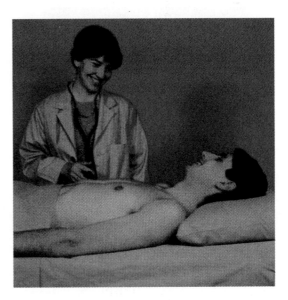

Figure 23-6 Client supine; examiner standing at the right side of the client.

Examine Heart

1. Inspect precordium (pulsations and heaves).
2. Palpate precordium (apical impulse, thrills, heaves, pulsations).
3. Auscultate apical rate and rhythm.
4. Auscultate precordium with both bell and diaphragm (supine and on left side in all major sound areas).
5. Inspect jugular venous pulses and pressure.
6. Measure supine blood pressure (both arms).

Examine Abdomen

1. Inspect abdomen at rest (skin characteristics, scars, contour, pulsations, movement, symmetry).
2. Inspect abdomen with client's head raised for integrity of abdominal musculature.
3. Auscultate bowel sounds, aorta, renal arteries, and femoral arteries.
4. Percuss abdomen in four quadrants.
5. Percuss and measure liver.
6. Percuss spleen.
7. Palpate all four quadrants lightly (tenderness, masses, organomegaly).
8. Palpate all four quadrants deeply (tenderness, masses, organomegaly).
9. Palpate liver, spleen, inguinal and femoral node and hernia areas, and femoral pulses.
10. Test abdominal reflexes.
11. Palpate inguinal areas for pulses, nodes, and hernias.

Examine Lower Extremities

1. Inspect skin (including between toes), presence of varicosities, hair distribution, muscle mass, symmetry, and skeletal configuration.
2. Palpate for temperature, texture, edema, popliteal pulses, posterior tibial pulses, and dorsal pedal pulses.

3. Test range of motion (toes, feet, ankles, knees, hips).
4. Test strength (toes, feet, ankles, knees, hips).
5. Test hips for stability.
6. Test sensation (pain, light touch, and vibration).
7. Test position sense.

The client is sitting on the bed or examining table. The examiner is standing in front of the client (Figure 23-7).

Assess Neural System

1. Elicit deep tendon reflexes (biceps, triceps, brachioradialis, patellar, and Achilles reflexes).
2. Test for plantar reflex bilaterally.
3. Test for coordination of upper and lower extremities (cerebellar function).
    a. Touch nose with rapidly alternating index fingers.
    b. Touch thumb with rapidly alternating fingers.
    c. With index finger, alternately touch own nose and examiner's rapidly moving finger.
    d. Run heel down tibia of opposite leg.
    e. Alternately and rapidly cross leg over knee.
    f. Perform figure eight in air with leg.
4. Test sensory function (face and extremities).
5. Test two-point discrimination—palms, thighs, back.
6. Test stereognosis, graphesthesia.
7. Test position sense in fingers and toes.
8. Test vibration sense in upper and lower extremities.

The client is standing. The examiner is standing next to and then behind the client (Figure 23-8).

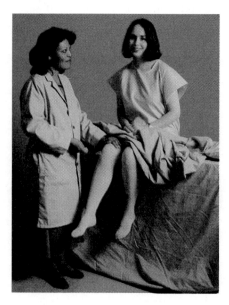

Figure 23-7 Client seated; examiner facing the client.

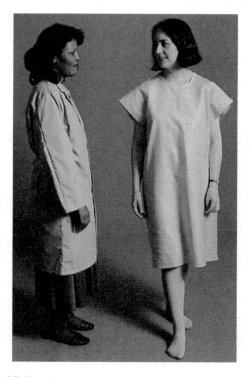

Figure 23-8 Client standing; examiner standing next to the client.

Examine Spine and Sacral Area

1. Inspect with client standing straight and then bending over for spinal deviation.
2. Test for range of motion—hyperextension, lateral bending, rotation of upper trunk.
3. Inspect sacrococcygeal and perianal areas.

Complete Assessment of Musculoskeletal and Neurological Systems

1. Inspect gait (tandem, heel walking, toe walking, usual).
2. Perform Romberg test.
3. With eyes closed, stand on one foot and then the other.
4. Hop in place on one foot and then the other.
5. Observe deep knee bends.

The male client is standing. The examiner is standing next to the client.

Male Genital Examination

1. Examine external genitalia.
   a. Inspect penis, urethral opening, pubic hair distribution, and scrotum.
   b. Palpate penis.
   c. Palpate scrotal contents.
2. Assess for presence of hernias.
   a. Observe for inguinal and femoral hernias at rest and with straining.
   b. Palpate bilaterally for femoral hernias.
   c. Palpate bilaterally for inguinal hernias.
3. Rectal examination
   NOTE: For this part of the examination, the client leans over the examination table, supporting the trunk with the forearms resting on the table.
   a. Inspect perianal area.
   b. Palpate rectum (sphincter tone and characteristics).
   c. Palpate prostate and seminal vesicles.
   d. Inspect characteristics of stool on gloved finger when removed.
   e. Examine for occult blood.

BOX 23-1

EXAMINATION OF THE BEDRIDDEN CLIENT

The regional and integrated examinations presented in this textbook are focused on clients who are able to sit and stand. For bedridden clients, the examination is adapted. A suggested sequence is (1) examination of the head, neck, anterior chest, and abdomen while the client is supine or supported in a sitting position on the bed; (2) examination of the back, posterior thorax, and skin while the client is rolled to the side; (3) completion of the examination with the client supine.

The female client is in the lithotomy position, genital area uncovered. The rest of the body is fully draped. The examiner is sitting, facing the genital area.

Female Genital Examination

1. Examine external genitalia.
   a. Inspect genitalia (pubic hair condition and distribution, labia, clitoris, urethral opening, perineum, perianal area, and anus).
   b. Palpate external genital area (labia, Bartholin's and Skene's glands).
2. Perform speculum examination (inspect vagina and cervix).
3. Obtain smears and cultures.
4. Perform bimanual vaginal examination (vagina, cervix, uterus, tubes, ovaries, muscle tone).
5. Perform bimanual rectovaginal examination (sphincter tone, rectovaginal septum, ligaments, uterus, tubes, ovaries, cul-de-sac).
6. Inspect appearance of feces on gloved finger when removed, and examine for occult blood.

Teaching Self-Assessment

While the client is still gowned, teach or review self-examinations appropriate to the situation (e.g., breast self-examination). Generally it is most effective to teach self-examinations during the corresponding portion of the practitioner's examination. However, there may be reasons to defer teaching until the end of the examination.

Completion of the Examination

When the examination and the teaching of self-examinations are completed, provide the client with disposable materials to clean areas where lubricant may remain. Then leave the examination room; allow the client privacy for dressing. Return to discuss findings and complete care.

Adapting the Physical Examination to Special Circumstances

See Box 23-1 for tips regarding adapting the physical examination to special circumstances.

DOCUMENTING THE PHYSICAL EXAMINATION (Box 23-2)

The record should describe what the examiner saw, heard, palpated, and percussed. Whenever appropriate, write the exact description. Avoid evaluations such as "normal," "good," or "poor," or use them judiciously. Too commonly, examiners describe a major system, such as the cardiovascular system, in one word, such as "normal." This description is limited because it does not indicate what components of that system were assessed or the examiner's parameters of normal. Pay

BOX 23-2

GUIDELINES FOR DOCUMENTING THE PHYSICAL EXAMINATION

1. Be specific.
2. Be concise.
3. Be complete.
4. Avoid using vague terms, such as "negative," "normal," or "good."
5. Specify parts of the examination omitted or deferred.
6. Use agreed-on and understood abbreviations.
7. Record exact size or placement of lesions—draw a picture or diagram.
8. Use illustrations when appropriate.

particular attention to fully describing systems about which the client has noted some problem. For example, if the client has ear pain, document specifically and completely all of the specific findings of the region and systems involved.

In documenting the physical examination, continuously attempt to achieve a balance between conciseness and comprehensiveness. To be concise, use outlines, phrases, and abbreviations. Sacrifice full sentences and write only essential words. Using a form for recording the physical examination is helpful. A form provides an outline into which data can be entered. Forms also serve as reminders for completeness, and they save time. If all members of a health care system

TABLE 23-1   Areas and Examples of Documentation for the Physical Examination

Area of Examination	Descriptions Usually Recorded	Descriptions Recorded in Detail If Abnormalities Are Present (Partial Listing Only)	Examples of Documentation

Vital signs	Temperature: oral, ear, axillary, or rectal
	Pulse
	Respiration
	Blood pressure: both arms in at least two positions (lying and sitting recommended)
	Weight (indicate whether client is clothed or unclothed)
	Height (without shoes)
		Blood pressure in standing position	T: 37° C (98.6° F) (oral)
			P: 76/min—strong and regular
			R: 16/min
			BP:
			    Lying: R, 110/70/60; L, 112/68/60
			    Sitting: R, 116/74/67; L, 120/76/65
			Wt: 170 lb, unclothed
			Ht: 5 ft, 3 in

General health	Appearance as relative to chronological age Apparent state of health Awareness Personal appearance Emotional status Nutritional status Affect Response Cooperation	Handshake Speech Respiratory difficulties Gross deformity Movements Unusual behavior	Slightly obese, alert, African-American male who looks younger than his stated age of 45; moves without difficulty; no gross abnormalities apparent; appears healthy and in no acute distress; is neatly dressed, responsive, and cooperative; responds appropriately; smiles frequently
Skin and mucous membranes	Color Edema Moisture Temperature Texture Turgor	Discharge Drainage Lesions: distribution, type, configuration Superficial vascularity Mobility Thickness	Skin: Uniformly brown in color; soft, warm, moist, elastic, of normal thickness; no edema or lesions Mucous membranes: Pink, moist, slightly pale
Nails	Color of beds Texture	Lesions Abnormalities in size or shape Presence of clubbing	Nailbeds pink; texture hard; no clubbing
Hair and scalp	Quantity Distribution Color Texture	Lesions Parasites	Hair: Normal male distribution; thick, curly; color black with graying at temples Scalp: Clean, no lesions
Cranium	Contour Tenderness	Lesions	Normocephalic, no tenderness

use the same forms systematically, they become extremely useful indexes for rapid information retrieval.

As recommended in the recording of the history (see Chapter 3), the beginning practitioner should record as many details as possible, including all findings from the examination. With increased skill and discrimination regarding the significance of findings, the practitioner will be able to weed out irrelevant information and consolidate significant data.

Table 23-1 is a guideline designed to assist the beginning recorder (see also Box 23-2). The first column in Table 23-1 indicates the body systems or regions that are examined. The second column contains a list of the areas of recording. These areas should be described for most clients. The third column is a partial list of areas to be recorded if abnormalities are suspected in the examination of that system. The fourth column contains examples of recording for each body system or area. The examples of recording do not relate to one client; therefore the fourth column should not be read as an example of the composite physical examination of one person. A sample worksheet for recording a physical examination can be found in Box 23-3 on pp. 570-574.

TABLE 23-1	Areas and Examples of Documentation for the Physical Examination—cont'd		
Area of Examination	**Descriptions Usually Recorded**	**Descriptions Recorded in Detail If Abnormalities Are Present (Partial Listing Only)**	**Examples of Documentation**
Face	Symmetry of movements Sinuses CN V CN VII	Tenderness Edema Lesions Parotid gland	Symmetrical at rest and with movement; jaw muscles strong, no crepitations or limitation in movement of temporomandibular joint; sinus areas not tender Sensory: Pain and light touch intact
Eyes	Visual acuity Visual fields Alignment of eyes Alignment of eyelids Movement of eyelids Conjunctiva Sclera Cornea Anterior chamber Iris Pupils: Size, shape, symmetry, reflexes (PERRLA may be used for "pupils, equally round, react to light and accommodation") Lens Lacrimal apparatus Ophthalmological examination (disc, vessels, retina, macular areas)	Eyebrows Tonometry Lesions Exophthalmos	Vision (distant with glasses): R, 20/40; L, 20/30; can read newspaper at 18 in; visual fields full Alignment: No deviation with cover test; light reflex equal; palpebral fissure normal Extraocular movements: Bilaterally intact; no nystagmus, ptosis, lid lag Conjunctiva: Clear, slightly injected around area of R inner canthus Sclera: White Cornea: Clear; arcus senilis, R eye Anterior chamber: not narrowed Iris: Blue, round Pupils: PERRLA Lens: Clear Funduscopic examination: Intact veins and arteries; disc round, margins well defined, color yellowish pink; macular areas visualized; no arteriolovenous (AV) nicking, hemorrhages, or exudates Lacrimal system: No swelling or discharge Corneal reflex: Present
Ears	Auricle Canal Otoscopic examination (color, presence of landmarks) Rinne and Weber tests	Position Discharge Pathological alterations present on otoscopic examination Lesions	Auricle: No lesions; canal free of cerumen and discharge Otoscopic examination: Drum intact; color pearly gray; land-

Continued

TABLE 23-1	Areas and Examples of Documentation for the Physical Examination—cont'd		
Area of Examination	Descriptions Usually Recorded	Descriptions Recorded in Detail If Abnormalities Are Present (Partial Listing Only)	Examples of Documentation
Ears—cont'd		Mastoid tenderness General tenderness	marks and light reflex in proper positions Hearing: Whispered voice heard in both ears at 3 ft Rinne and Weber tests heard equally in both ears, AC 2 × > BC or AC > BC 2:1
Nose	Patency of each nostril Turbinates and mucous membranes	External nose Olfaction Vestibule Transillumination of sinuses	Turbinates and membranes: Pink, moist, no discharge Nostrils patent Septum: Slightly deviated to R
Oral cavity	Buccal mucosa Gums Teeth (decayed, missing, filled) Floor of mouth Hard and soft palate Tonsillar areas Posterior pharyngeal wall Tongue position and movement	Breath odor Lips Lesions Laryngoscopic examination Palpation of mouth Parotid duct Taste	Membranes: Pink and moist, no lesions Gums: No edema or inflammation Teeth: In good repair Palate: Intact; moves symmetrically with phonation; gag reflex present Tonsils: Present, not enlarged Pharynx: Pink and clean Tongue: Strong, midline; moves symmetrically Taste: Able to differentiate sweet and sour
Neck	Movements: Rotation and lateral bend Symmetry Thyroid gland Tracheal position Glands and nodes	Postural alignment Tenderness Tone of muscles Lesions Masses	Full ROM; strong symmetrically; thyroid not palpable; trachea midline; no enlargement of head and neck regional nodes
Breasts and axillae	Axillary node Supraclavicular nodes Infraclavicular nodes Breasts: Inspection and palpation Nipples and areolar areas Discharge Masses	Retraction Dimpling	Breasts: Left breast slightly larger than right Surfaces smooth without dimpling or retraction No nodes palpable—axillary, infraclavicular, or supraclavicular; no masses, retraction, or discharge Nipples symmetrically positioned No masses or tenderness palpated
Chest and respiratory system	Shape of thorax Symmetry of thorax Respiratory movements Respiratory excursion Palpation: Tactile fremitus, tenderness, masses Percussion notes Diaphragmatic excursion and level Auscultation: Breath sounds, adventitious sounds	Deformity Use of accessory muscles of respiration Vocal resonance Egophony, bronchophony, whispered pectoriloquy	Thorax: AP diameter < lateral diameter; moves symmetrically at rest and with movements; excursion equal bilaterally; tactile fremitus equal bilaterally; no masses or tenderness; percussion tones resonant; diaphragmatic excursion 5 cm bilaterally vesicular breath sounds bilaterally; no adventitious sounds
Central cardiovascular system	Position in which heart was examined; lying, sitting, left lateral, recumbent Inspection: Bulging, depression, pulsation (precordial and juxtaprecordial) Palpation: Thrusts, heaves, thrills, friction rubs	Murmur or extra sound: Whether systolic or diastolic; intensity; pitch; quality; site of maximum transmission; effect of position, respiration, and exercise; radiation	Examined in sitting and lying positions; no abnormal pulsations or lifts observed; PMI in fifth ICS, slightly medial to the LMCL; no abnormal pulsations palpated Apical pulse: 72, regular; heart sounds; S^1 single sound; S^2 splits with inspiration; S^1 heard loudest at apex; S^2

TABLE 23-1	Areas and Examples of Documentation for the Physical Examination—cont'd		
Area of Examination	**Descriptions Usually Recorded**	**Descriptions Recorded in Detail If Abnormalities Are Present (Partial Listing Only)**	**Examples of Documentation**
Central cardiovascular system—cont'd	Apical impulse Auscultation: rate and rhythm, character of S_1, character of S_2, comparison of S_1 in aortic and pulmonic areas, comparison of S_1 and S_2 in major auscultatory areas, presence or absence of extra sounds—if present, description		heard loudest at base; no murmurs or other sounds
Arterial pulses	Radial pulse: Rate, rhythm; consistency and tenderness of arterial wall Amplitude and character of peripheral pulses: Superficial temporal, brachial, femoral, popliteal, posterior tibial, dorsal pedal Carotid pulses: Equality, amplitude, thrills, bruits	Any abnormality (analysis of type)	Radial pulse: Bilaterally equal, regular, strong; no tenderness or thickening of vessels; 76/min Peripheral pulses: Right Left Temporal 2+ 2+ Brachial 3+ 3+ Femoral 2+ 2+ Popliteal 0+ 0+ Posterior tibial Unable to palpate Dorsal pedal 1+ 1+ Carotid pulses: Equal, strong, no bruits
Venous pulses and pressures	Jugular venous pulsations, presence of waves a, c, and v Venous pressure: Distention present at 45 degrees	Hepatojugular reflex Analysis of jugular venous waves	Jugular venous distention, 5 cm with client at 45 degrees
Abdomen	Inspection: Scars, size, shape, symmetry, muscular development, bulging, movements Auscultation: Peristaltic sounds—present or absent; vascular bruits—present or absent Palpation Masses Tenderness (local, referred, rebound), tone of musculature Liver: Size, contour, character of edge, consistency, tenderness Kidney (indicate whether or not palpable) Costovertebral area: Tenderness Percussion: Liver size at MCL, spleen, masses	Diastasis Distention Mass or bulging (specific description) Palpable spleen: Size, surface contour, splenic notch, consistency, tenderness, mobility Palpable kidney: Location, size, shape, consistency Distention of urinary bladder Fluid wave Flank dullness Shifting dullness Aorta Gallbladder	Healed scar RLQ (appendectomy); slightly obese, protuberant; symmetrical, no bulging; bowel sounds present, no bruits; no abnormal movements; no masses; no tenderness; liver 11 cm in RMCL; no CVA tenderness; no organs palpated; muscle tone lax Area of midline diastasis: 6 cm × 2 cm inferior and superior to umbilicus 3 cm
Neural system	Orientation Intellectual performance Emotional status Insight Memory Cranial nerves Coordination Sensory: Touch, pain, position, vibration Babinski's sign Romberg test Reflexes	Thought content Speech Sensory: Hot, cold, two-point discrimination Stereognosis Involuntary movements	Alert, oriented ×3; mood appropriate and stable; remote and recent memory intact; serial calculations by subtracting 6 (starting with 100) accurate; insight normal; cranial nerves I-XII intact, examined and recorded in head and neck regions; all movement coordinated; able to perform rapid coordinated movements with upper and lower extremities

Continued

TABLE 23-1	Areas and Examples of Documentation for the Physical Examination—cont'd		
Area of Examination	**Descriptions Usually Recorded**	**Descriptions Recorded in Detail If Abnormalities Are Present (Partial Listing Only)**	**Examples of Documentation**
Neural system—cont'd			Deep tendon reflexes (0 to 4+) 0 = absent + (or 1+) = decreased ++ (or 2+) = normal +++ (or 3+) = hyperactive ++++ (or 4+) = clonus Sensory: Able to detect light touch, pain, and vibration to face, trunk, and extremities bilaterally and symmetrically; walks with coordination; able to maintain standing position with eyes closed
Extremities and musculoskeletal system	Both upper and lower extremities: General assessments—size, shape, mass, symmetry; hair distribution, color; temperature; edema; varicosities; tenderness; epitrochlear lymph nodes Bones and joints: Range of motion, tenderness, gait Muscles: Size, symmetry, strength, tone, tenderness, consistency Back: Posture; tenderness; movement—extension, lateral bend, rotation	Lesions Deformities Color and temperature: Changes on elevation and dependency Homans' sign Redness Heat Swelling Deformity Crepitations Contractures Muscle spasms Tenderness Atrophy Hypertrophy	Muscular development and mass normal for age; arms and legs symmetrical; skin warm, soft; male hair distribution on arms, legs, and feet; no edema, varicosities, or tenderness; no nodes palpated; joints nontender, not swollen; full ROM; good muscle tone, and strength equal bilaterally Back: full ROM; no tenderness or deformities

TABLE 23-1	Areas and Examples of Documentation for the Physical Examination—cont'd		
Area of Examination	**Descriptions Usually Recorded**	**Descriptions Recorded in Detail If Abnormalities Are Present (Partial Listing Only)**	**Examples of Documentation**
Anus and rectum	Anal area Skin Hemorrhoids Sphincter tone Rectum Tumors Stool color Occult blood	Lesions Fissures Pilonidal sinus Condition of perineal body Tenderness Proctoscopic examination	Skin clean, no lesions; sphincter tone good; no hemorrhoids or masses noted; stools brown, guaiac negative
Inguinal area	Hernia: Inguinal, femoral Nodes	Size, shape, consistency, tenderness, reducibility of hernia or nodes	Hernias not present; no enlargement of nodes noted
Male genitalia	Penis: Condition of prepuce, skin Scrotum: Size, skin, testes, epididymides, spermatic cords Prostate gland: Size, shape, symmetry, consistency, tenderness Seminal vesicles: Size, shape, consistency	Scars Lesions Structural alterations Masses Swelling Nodules	Penis: Circumcised, clean, no lesions Scrotum and contents: Normal size, no masses or tumors noted Prostate and inferior portions of seminal vesicles: Palpated; normal consistency; nontender Prostate: Not enlarged; rubbery; nontender Seminal vesicles: Not palpable
Female genitalia	External: Hair distribution; labia; Bartholin's glands, urethral meatus, Skene's glands (BUS); hymen; introitus Vaginal observation: Presence or absence of rectocele, urethrocele, cystocele; tissue; discharge (smears or cultures taken); cervix Bimanual examination: Cervix, uterus, adnexa Rectovaginal examination: Uterus, cul-de-sac, septum	Lesions Tumors Prolapses	Typical female hair distribution; no lesions or masses BUS: No tenderness, redness, or discharge Hymen: Present in caruncles Labia: Pink, no lesions Introital tone: Good; no prolapses; no scars; perineum thick Vagina: Pink; discharge—small amount, thin, clean, nonodorous Cervix: Pink, nulliparous, firm, not tender, movable, midline Uterus: Pear shaped, movable, normal size, firm, no masses Tubes: Not palpable Ovaries: Palpable, movable, not tender, approximately 2 ∞ 3 ∞ 2 cm; smooth surface, no lesions, firm consistency Rectovaginal septum: Thick and firm; no masses palpated in rectum or cul-de-sac

BOX 23-3

WORKSHEET FOR DOCUMENTING A PHYSICAL EXAMINATION

VITAL SIGNS

Temperature _____ Respiration _____ /min   BP   (L)   Arm   (R)

_____ Supine _____

_____ Sitting _____

_____ Standing _____

Height _____ ft _____ in   Weight _____ lb (with or without clothes [circle])

GENERAL INSPECTION

SKIN, HAIR, NAILS, MUCOUS MEMBRANES

HEAD

Scalp _____

Face _____

(CNs V, VII) _____

_____

Sinus areas _____

Nodes _____

Cranium _____

EYES

Visual acuity _____

Visual fields _____

Ocular movements (CNs III, IV, VI) _____

Convergence _____

Lids, lacrimal organs _____

Conjunctiva, sclera _____

Cornea (CN V) _____

Lens and media _____

Pupils: Pupillary reflexes (CN III) _____

        Light, direct and consensual _____

        Accommodation _____

Fundi (CN II) _____

EARS

External structures _____

Canal _____

BOX 23-3

WORKSHEET FOR DOCUMENTING A PHYSICAL EXAMINATION—cont'd

EARS—cont'd

Tympanic membranes and landmarks _____

Hearing (CN VIII) _____

NOSE

External structure _____

_____

Septum _____

Mucous membranes _____

Patency _____

Olfactory sense (CN I) _____

ORAL CAVITY

Lips _____

Buccal mucosa and ducts _____

Gums _____

Teeth _____

Palates and uvula (CNs IX, X) _____

Tonsillar areas _____

Tongue (CN XII) _____

Floor _____

Voice _____

Breath _____

Taste (CNs VII, IX) _____

NECK

General structure _____

_____

Trachea _____

Thyroid _____

Nodes _____

Muscles (CN XI) _____

BREASTS AND AREA NODES (AXILLARY, SUPRACLAVICULAR, INFRACLAVICULAR)

Inspection _____

Palpation _____

CHEST, RESPIRATORY SYSTEM

Chest shape _____

Type of respiration _____

Expansion _____

Fremitus _____

General palpation _____

Continued

BOX 23-3

WORKSHEET FOR DOCUMENTING A PHYSICAL EXAMINATION—cont'd

CHEST, RESPIRATORY SYSTEM—cont'd

Percussion _____

_____ Diaphragmatic excursion: (R) ___ cm (L) ___ cm

Breath sounds _____

_____

_____

Adventitious sounds _____

_____

CARDIOVASCULAR SYSTEM

Rate and rhythm: Radial (palpation) _____

Apical (auscultation) _____

Precordium: Inspection _____

   Palpation _____

   Auscultation _____

     S_1 _____

     S_2 _____

     Other sounds _____

      Murmur(s): Systolic _____

       Diastolic _____

Carotid arteries _____

Jugular venous distention _____

_____

Description of peripheral pulses

Brachial	Radial	Femoral	Popliteal	Dorsal pedal	Posterior tibial
R					
L					

ABDOMEN AND INGUINAL AREAS

Contour, tone _____

Scars, marks _____

Auscultation _____

_____

Liver _____ Span _____ cm at RMCL

Spleen _____

Kidneys _____ CVA tenderness _____

Bladder _____

Hernias _____

Masses _____

Palpation _____

_____

BOX 23-3

WORKSHEET FOR DOCUMENTING A PHYSICAL EXAMINATION—cont'd

ABDOMEN AND INGUINAL AREAS—cont'd

Percussion _____

Inguinal areas for hernias _____

Inguinal areas for nodes _____

GENITALIA

Female	**Male**
External _____	Penis _____
Glands _____	Scrotum _____
Vagina _____	Epididymides _____
Cervix _____	Testes _____
Uterus _____	

RECTAL EXAMINATION

Anus _____

Rectum _____

Prostate (male) _____

MUSCULOSKELETAL SYSTEM

Gait _____

Upper extremities _____

Lower extremities _____

Deformities _____

_____

Joint evaluation _____

_____

Muscle strength _____

_____

Muscle mass _____

Nodes _____

Range of motion _____

SPINE

Contour _____

Position _____

Motion _____

NERVOUS SYSTEM

Mental status _____

Language _____

Cranial nerves (summarize) _____

Motor: Coordination: Upper extremities _____

Lower extremities _____

Involuntary movements _____

Continued

BOX 23-3

WORKSHEET FOR DOCUMENTING A PHYSICAL EXAMINATION—cont'd

DEEP TENDON REFLEXES:

NOTE: +s denote finger jerks; brachioradialis, biceps, triceps reflexes; four-quadrant abdominal scratch reflexes; patellar Achilles reflexes; and plantar reflexes. Abdominal reflexes are recorded as 0 or +. Scale: 0-4 (++++); normal = 2 (++).

SENSORY

Light touch _____

Pain (pinprick) _____

Vibration _____

Position _____

❓ Critical Thinking Questions

1. How would you adapt the physical examination to a 25-year-old male with paraplegia?
2. How would you adapt the physical examination to a 75-year-old female with severe arthritis in her arm and leg joints?
3. How would you adapt the physical examination with a young male blind client?
4. How would you adapt the physical examination to a totally bed-bound client?
5. How would you prioritize the components of the physical examination for a healthy female population being served by a Pap smear screening clinic in which clients were scheduled every 20 minutes?

MERLIN   Answers are available on the MERLIN website (www.harcourthealth.com/MERLIN/Barkauskas/). And be sure to check the website regularly for additional learning activities!

Remember to check out the Online Study Guide!
www.harcourthealth.com/MERLIN/Barkauskas/

Clinical Reasoning In Determining Health Status

Learning Objectives

On successful study of this chapter and completion of related learning experiences, the learner will be able to:
• Apply the steps in gathering data to formulate a diagnosis.

• Describe the purposes of Nursing Interventions Classification and Nursing Outcomes Classification.
• Identify skills needed for evidence-based practice.

Outline

Purpose of Clinical Reasoning

The purpose of clinical reasoning is to apply knowledge gathered from the clinical evaluation of the client to complex decisions about the health status of the client and the treatment plan. Clinical reasoning, or clinical judgment, is the reasoning process used for health assessment information as the basis for further action.

DATA GATHERING PROCESS

The general health assessment provides the data, or information, needed to formulate a diagnosis and eventually a plan of treatment and evaluation. The data gathering process includes the following:

1. Data collection
2. Data validation
3. Data organization
4. Pattern identification

Data Collection

The general health assessment consists of data gathered from the first encounter with the client and during the health interview and physical examination. Laboratory data, if applicable, are also considered. In later follow-up with a client, the practitioner focuses the assessment by collecting data on a specific problem or concern.

Both history and physical examination data are collected using a system or framework. Dimensions of symptom analysis guide questions during a health history about a problem or symptom. A review of systems guides questions for a comprehensive review of a client's past and current health status. In the physical examination, the examiner can collect data using several organizing principles: head-to-toe, regional areas of the body (e.g., pelvic examination), or body systems (e.g., cardiovascular or neurological). Each of these methods provides a logical, organized framework for collecting physical assessment data. The practitioner's decision about which method to use is influenced by both needs and desires of the client. For example, if you see a client for a periodic health examination, use a head-to-toe approach. However, if a client who appears in acute distress stated she had just injured her hand, begin the assessment by focusing on the body region affected.

As you develop expertise as a practitioner, you will develop your own approach to data collection that is appropriate to the circumstances, such as the client's age, sex, emotional state, and acuity of the health problem or concern. Whatever approach is used, the examiner must think about the range of possibilities and be sensitive and open to the possible meaning of all signs and symptoms.

Data Validation

Validation is the process of making sure the data collected are accurate. Data obtained using an instrument with a measurement scale can be validated by repeating the measure. For example, if a weight on the clinic scale indicates a 10-pound weight loss since the last visit, you can repeat the weight to validate this measure. Verify information with the client by direct observation or interview. Preferably, validate information yourself, rather than relying on information obtained by others, especially if information involves subjective data open to interpretation. Strategies to validate data include the following:

1. Recheck your own data. Go back to an area of the physical examination to palpate or observe again.
2. Be sure other factors did not influence the accuracy of the data, such as while in a hurry to obtain a blood pressure, you used the wrong-size blood pressure cuff.
3. Always recheck information that is grossly abnormal. For example, repeat a blood pressure measurement of 200/110 mm Hg.
4. Ask someone, preferably more experienced, to collect the same data. If you hear a grade IV systolic heart murmur on physical examination, have another clinician also listen to the heart.
5. Recheck previous documentation to see whether abnormal findings were previously recorded.

Data Organization

Data are organized by clustering. The ability to do this efficiently depends on the examiner's knowledge and skill. Frameworks help to organize data and are discussed in more detail later in this chapter. The different chapters in this book present various frameworks for health assessment. For example, Chapter 16 presents a systems approach. Chapters 5 and 27 present a developmental approach that modifies the health history and physical examination for the client's age.

Pattern Identification

The examiner analyzes the data to determine whether gaps exist or whether more data are needed to make a diagnosis. For example, if a client states he has a loss of appetite, obtaining a weight is critical to determine whether weight loss has occurred. You would compare the current weight with previous weights to determine whether a pattern of weight change is evident. If no previous weights were recorded, you and the client would plan to obtain weight data at a designated frequency over the next month. You would then assess these data to detect any pattern of weight change.

DIAGNOSTIC REASONING PROCESS

Many investigators have studied how physicians diagnose illness. By comparison, few studies concern nursing decision-making. However, some of the research that has been done suggests that physicians and nurses use similar clinical reasoning processes. This conclusion seems reasonable, since researchers have suggested that both tradition and necessity require nurses to make both medical and nursing judgments.

The diagnostic reasoning process includes four major steps (Table 24-1).

Cue Recognition

In the first phase of diagnostic reasoning, the practitioner must recognize that a **cue** is significant in the context of the overall situation. A cue is a piece of information. It can consist of either subjective or objective data. For example, a subjective cue might be the client's statement, "I feel nervous." In contrast, an objective cue might be observing a client's hand tremor.

TABLE 24-1	**Stages of Diagnostic Reasoning**
Stage	**Example**
Cue recognition	Look at client's face—notice cyanosis as abnormal
Hypothesis formulation	Client is experiencing impaired gas exchange
Hypothesis testing	Arterial blood gas result: pH 7.32, P_{CO_2} 55 P_{O_2} 65. The client appears restless and confused. Weak cough effort.
Hypothesis evaluation	Do enough data exist to confirm the diagnosis of impaired gas exchange? If yes, then diagnosis is made. "Impaired gas exchange related to . . ."

Whether a cue is considered significant depends on the practitioner's ability to distinguish between normal and abnormal behavior, physical characteristics, and diagnostic findings. This ability, in turn, depends on the examiner's knowledge base and expertise. Even slight variations of normal findings may have a significance that is not at first obvious. A knowledgeable and experienced practitioner, for example, might note the slight pallor of a client's nailbeds and consider the diagnosis of anemia. In contrast, an inexperienced student might not notice the subtle change in nailbed color.

In summary, during the first phase of diagnostic reasoning, cue recognition, the practitioner receives thousands of pieces of information. Next, he or she begins to sort the data, keeping some pieces of information and ignoring others based on a working or tentative diagnosis. This process of sorting information is called clinical judgment. The remaining data or cues serve as a more efficient resource for the next step in the process: hypothesis formulation.

Hypothesis Formulation

During the second phase of diagnostic reasoning, the practitioner decides on possible explanations for the cues recognized in the previous step. This phase is often referred to as hypothesis formulation. **Inference** is the process of perceiving and interpreting a cue. The practitioner must be a critical observer to pick up all cues available. Before making any conclusions, the examiner first clusters or links the cues to determine any patterns. One cue, in isolation, is rarely enough to suggest a particular hypothesis or diagnosis. Rather, the presence of several cues that are usually or always associated with a specific problem helps indicate what other further information is necessary before a conclusion can be reached.

As in the first phase, a practitioner's knowledge and expertise strongly influence the diagnostic reasoning process and the interpretation and relative importance of the remaining cues. Often, the novice jumps to early and erroneous conclusions because he or she misinterprets cues, focuses on only one cue, or fails to eliminate irrelevant cues from the cues considered. As a practitioner gains knowledge and experience, he or she builds associations between cues and clinical situations. These associations enable the examiner to cluster cues into meaningful groups and formulate hypotheses.

The formulation of hypotheses or tentative conclusions helps focus further data collection efforts on a manageable group of possibilities. However, the practitioner must be careful not to limit further investigation to only one hypoth-

esis, since the likelihood of an accurate final diagnosis increases when several explanations are considered. The examiner must think about the more likely problems, since common problems occur with more frequency, while at the same time entertaining the probability that a rare problem might be presenting itself.

Hypothesis Testing

During the third stage of diagnostic reasoning, the practitioner focuses on gathering data to support or reject the previously generated hypotheses. This phase is called hypothesis testing. Examiners use many different data collection strategies during this stage. Tables 24-2 and 24-3 list methods of continued inquiry. One or more of these techniques may be appropriate for a given clinical situation. In addition, the practitioner may be more comfortable using some methods rather than others.

■ HELPFUL HINT

TO MINIMIZE BIAS IN HYPOTHESIS TESTING:
Don't maintain a narrow focus.
Don't jump to conclusions prematurely.
Do explore alternative explanations.
Do keep an open mind.
Do take your time.

Throughout the hypothesis testing phase, the practitioner needs to guard against having biases about hypotheses. Some of these biases may lead to prematurely accepting a possible explanation or prematurely rejecting an explanation (Table 24-4).

Hypothesis Evaluation

After the practitioner has investigated all reasonable explanations for the initial set of cues, he or she must evaluate each hypothesis in light of the new evidence collected and reach a final diagnosis or conclusion. Hypothesis evaluation requires synthesis of all data that have been collected, since information obtained to refute one hypothesis may support another. The practitioner might also find that the data suggest that more than one problem exists.

Careful recording of data collected is crucial. Failure to document data fully increases the chance that information

TABLE 24-2	**General Strategies for Hypothesis Testing**	
Approach	Explanation	Example
Cue based	Explore each aspect of initial cues until all facets are covered	Facial cyanosis—mucous membranes, ears, skin color
Hypothesis driven	Investigate the defining characteristics to confirm their presence or absence	Hypoxia? Hypercapnia? Restlessness? Confusion? Irritability? Inability to move secretions?
Systematic	Review body systems	Start with respiratory system, then move to cardiovascular system, etc
Hit or miss	No recognizable strategy	Ask client when last bowel movement took place

TABLE 24-3	**Hypothesis Testing Strategies Used by Experts**
Strategy	Explanation
Confirmation	Seek data to confirm hypothesis
Elimination	Eliminate hypothesis based on absence of key signs and symptoms (defining characteristics)
Discrimination	Investigate defining characteristics that separate diagnoses with similar signs and symptoms (i.e., look for those characteristics that are different)
Exploration	Consider investigation of diagnoses with similar manifestations

TABLE 24-4	**Biases Affecting Diagnosis**
Bias	Explanation
Frequency of occurrence	If the diagnosis being considered has been made frequently, it has a higher probability of being chosen.
Recency of experience	If the clinician has made the considered diagnosis in the recent past, the clinician may be more familiar with this diagnosis than with other related diagnoses.
Profoundness of memory	Vivid impressions of cases in which a certain diagnosis was made can influence the decision in favor of this diagnosis.

necessary to evaluate the hypothesis will be lost or forgotten. Missing data, in turn, can lead to erroneous conclusions. Chapter 23 contains an example of one form that can be used to record data during the assessment process.

During this phase of diagnostic reasoning, the practitioner determines which explanation has the most supporting data and chooses this hypothesis as the diagnosis. In some cases, however, the examiner can merely eliminate hypotheses until only the one with the highest probability remains.

INFORMATION CLASSIFICATION IN NURSING

The standardized nursing language for nursing diagnoses, the North American Nursing Diagnosis Association (NANDA) taxonomy, was introduced in Chapter 1. The clinical reasoning process described in this chapter culminates in the assignment of nursing diagnoses and other health diagnoses. These diagnoses serve as summary statements to specify the main health issues, which the practitioner will address with the client.

After the diagnoses are determined, the practitioner needs to consider what related and appropriate health outcomes are possible, given the clinical situation and the resources available. These outcomes will be the criteria against which the effectiveness of intervention will be evaluated. The Nursing Outcomes Classification (NOC) is another standardized nursing taxonomy, which can be used to evaluate the results of interventions. The NOC was first published in 1997 and was revised in 2000 (Johnson, Maas, and Moorhead, 2000). The NOC taxonomy is the culmination of an intensive scientific process to identify important outcomes sensitive to nursing interventions. The NOC contains 175 outcome labels. Each label is further specified by a set of indicators, which specify evidence for the attainment of the outcome.

For outcomes to be relevant, baseline assessment measurements are compared to similar measures during the care and the termination of care. Thus NOC measurements are also assessment measurements. To appreciate the close linkages between the history and physical examination and the NOC measures, the NOC measures have been classified according to the major headings of the health history and physical examination in Table 24-5.

TABLE 24-5	Analysis of the NOC by the Traditional Components of the History and Physical Examination

Assessment Component	NOC Outcomes	Assessment Component	NOC Outcomes

History

Development

Child adaptation to hospitalization
Child development: 2 months
Child development: 4 months
Child development: 6 months
Child development: 12 months
Child development: 2 years
Child development: 3 years
Child development: 4 years
Child development: 5 years
Child development: Middle childhood
  (6-11 years)
Child development: Adolescence
  (12-17 years)

General

Play participation
Rest
Sleep

Health behaviors

Adherence behavior
Compliance behavior
Health beliefs
Health beliefs: Perceived ability to perform
Health beliefs: Perceived control
Health beliefs: Perceived resources
Health beliefs: Perceived threat
Health orientation
Health promoting behavior
Health seeking behavior
Immunization behavior
Knowledge: Breastfeeding
Knowledge: Child safety
Knowledge: Contraceptive behavior
Knowledge: Diabetes management
Knowledge: Diet
Knowledge: Disease process
Knowledge: Energy conservation
Knowledge: Fertility promotion
Knowledge: Health behaviors
Knowledge: Health promotion
Knowledge: Health resources
Knowledge: Illness care
Knowledge: Infant care
Knowledge: Infection control
Knowledge: Labor and delivery
Knowledge: Maternal-child health
Knowledge: Medication
Knowledge: Personal safety
Knowledge: Postpartum
Knowledge: Preconception
Knowledge: Pregnancy
Knowledge: Prescribed activity

History—cont'd

Health behaviors— cont'd

Knowledge: Sexual functioning
Knowledge: Substance use control
Knowledge: Treatment procedure(s)
Knowledge: Treatment regimen
Pain control behavior
Prenatal health behavior
Risk control
Risk control: Alcohol use
Risk control: Cancer
Risk control: Cardiovascular health
Risk control: Drug use
Risk control: Hearing impairment
Risk control: Sexually transmitted diseases
Risk control: Tobacco use
Risk control: Unintended pregnancy
Risk control: Vision impairment
Risk detection
Safety behavior: Fall prevention
Safety behavior: Home physical environment
Safety behavior: Personal
Safety status: Falls occurrence
Safety status: Physical injury
Self-direction of care
Self-care: Non-parental medication
Self-care: Parenteral medication
Symptom control behavior

Nutrition

Breastfeeding establishment: Infant
Breastfeeding establishment: Maternal
Breastfeeding maintenance
Breastfeeding weaning
Nutritional status
Nutritional status: Biochemical measures
Nutritional status: Body mass
Nutritional status: Energy
Nutritional status: Food and fluid intake
Nutritional status: Nutrient intake
Weight control

Psychological system

Abusive behavior: Self-control
Acceptance: Health status
Aggression control
Anxiety control
Body image
Comfort level
Concentration
Coping
Decision-making
Depression control
Depression level
Dignified dying

Continued

TABLE 24-5	Analysis of the NOC by the Traditional Components of the History and Physical Examination—cont'd

Assessment Component	NOC Outcomes	Assessment Component	NOC Outcomes

History—cont'd

Psychological system—cont'd

Distorted thought control
Fear control
Grief resolution
Hope
Identity
Immobility consequences: Psycho-cognitive
Impulse control
Leisure participation
Loneliness
Mood equilibrium
Neglect recovery
Pain: Psychological response
Participation: Health care decisions
Psychological adjustment: Life change
Quality of life
Self-esteem
Self-mutilation restraint
Spiritual well-being
Substance addiction consequences
Suicide self-restraint
Symptom control behavior
Treatment behavior: Illness or injury
Well-being
Will to live

Sociological system

Abuse cessation
Abuse protection
Abuse recovery: Emotional
Abuse recovery: Financial
Abuse recovery: Sexual
Caregiver adaptation to patient institutionalization
Caregiver emotional health
Caregiver home care readiness
Caregiver lifestyle disruption
Caregiver-patient relationship
Caregiver performance: Direct care
Caregiver performance: Indirect care
Caregiver physical health
Caregivers stressors
Caregiver well-being
Caregiving endurance potential
Parent-infant attachment
Parenting
Parenting: Social safety
Role performance
Social interaction skills
Social involvement
Social support

Physical Examination

Cardiovascular system

Activity tolerance
Blood transfusion reaction control
Cardiac pump effectiveness
Circulation status
Coagulation status
Endurance
Energy conservation
Tissue perfusion: Abdominal organs
Tissue perfusion: Cardiac
Tissue perfusion: Cerebral
Tissue perfusion: Peripheral
Tissue perfusion: Pulmonary

Endocrine system

Blood glucose control

Functional status

Ambulation: Walking
Ambulation: Wheelchair
Self-care: Activities of daily living
Self-care: Bathing
Self-care: Dressing
Self-care: Eating
Self-care: Grooming
Self-care: Hygiene
Self-care: Instrumental activities of daily living
Self-care: Oral hygiene
Self-care: Toileting
Transfer performance

Gastrointestinal system

Bowel continence
Bowel elimination

General and skin

Abuse recovery: Physical
Body positioning: Self-initiated
Electrolyte and acid/base balance
Fluid balance
Growth
Hydration
Immobility consequences: Physiological
Infection status
Medication response
Pain: Disruptive effects
Pain level
Physical aging status
Psychomotor energy
Symptom severity
Thermoregulation
Tissue integrity: Skin and mucous membranes
Vital sign status

TABLE 24-5 Analysis of the NOC by the Traditional Components of the History and Physical Examination—cont'd

Assessment Component	NOC Outcomes	Assessment Component	NOC Outcomes
Physical Examination—cont'd		**Physical Examination—cont'd**	
General and skin—cont'd		*Reproductive—female and male*	
	Wound healing: Primary intention		Physical maturation: Female
	Wound healing: Secondary intention		Physical maturation: Male
Head, mouth, throat			Sexual functioning
	Oral health		Sexual identity: Acceptance
	Swallowing status		Symptom severity: Perimenopause
	Swallowing status: Esophageal phase		Symptom severity: Premenstrual syndrome
	Swallowing status: Oral phase	*Respiratory*	
	Swallowing status: Pharyngeal phase		Aspiration control
Immune system			Asthma control
	Immune hypersensitivity control		Respiratory status: Airway patency
	Immune states		Respiratory status: Gas exchange
Musculoskeletal system			Respiratory status: Ventilation
	Bone healing	*Sensory systems*	
	Joint movement: Active		Hearing compensation behavior
	Joint movement: Passive		Sensory function: Cutaneous
	Mobility level		Sensory function: Hearing
	Muscle function		Sensory function: Taste and smell
	Physical fitness		Sensory function: Vision
	Skeletal function		Vision compensation behavior
Neurological system		*Urinary system*	
	Neurological status: Central motor control		Urinary continence
	Balance		Urinary elimination
	Cognitive ability		Dialysis access integrity
	Cognitive orientation		Systemic toxin clearance: Dialysis
	Communication ability	**Additional Diagnoses, not Linked to the Individual Health History and Physical Examination**	
	Communication: Expressive ability		
	Communication: Receptive ability		
	Information processing	*Family*	
	Memory		Family coping
	Neurological status		Family environment: Internal
	Neurological status: Autonomic		Family functioning
	Neurological status: Central motor control		Family health status
	Neurological status: Consciousness		Family integrity
	Neurological status: Cranial sensory/motor function		Family normalization
	Neurological status: Spinal sensory/motor function		Family participation in professional care
	Sensory function: Proprioception	*Community*	
Pediatrics			Community competence
	Fetal status: Antepartum		Community health status
	Fetal status: Intrapartum		Community health: Immunity
	Newborn adaptation		Community risk control: Chronic disease
	Preterm infant organization		Community risk control: Communicable disease
	Thermoregulation: Neonate		Community risk control: Lead exposure
Pregnancy			
	Maternal status: Antepartum		
	Maternal status: Intrapartum		
	Maternal status: Postpartum		

From Johnson M, Maas ML, Moorhead S: *Nursing outcomes classification (NOC)*, ed. 2, St. Louis, 2000, Mosby.)

The linkages between the NANDA diagnoses and the outcome measures in the NOC have been proposed. For example, the outcomes suggested for two diagnoses, Bathing/Hygiene Self-Care Deficit and Dysfunctional Grieving are listed in the following:

NANDA Diagnoses	NOC Outcome Indicators
Bathing/Hygiene Self-Care Deficit	Self-Care: Activities of Daily Living
	Self-Care: Bathing
	Self-Care: Hygiene
	Self-Direction of Care
Dysfunctional Grieving	Concentration
	Coping
	Family Coping
	Grief Resolution
	Psychosocial Adjustment: Life Change
	Role Performance

The Nursing Interventions Classification (NIC) completes the set of taxonomies that can structure the clinical reasoning process. The NIC was first published in 1996 and revised in 1999 (McCloskey and Bulechek, 2000). It contains intervention labels, which are uniquely devised to describe nursing care. NIC is used to teach clinical decision-making, especially through the use of case studies that illustrate the relationship of nursing diagnoses and intervention to the client's signs and symptoms, history information, and existing health problems. NIC is useful in determining a client's needs and for providers to respond to these needs with a higher level of knowledge and critical thinking skills.

EVIDENCE-BASED PRACTICE

Evidence-based practice means integrating individual clinical experience with the best available evidence from systematic research. Evidence-based practice requires the practitioner to be engaged in life-long learning by doing the following:

1. Ask answerable questions.
2. Collect, with maximum efficiency, the best evidence to answer the question.
3. Critically evaluate the evidence for its truthfulness and usefulness.
4. Apply the results to clinical interventions.
5. Evaluate the outcomes of interventions.

The sources of scientific evidence are from randomized clinical trials, descriptive studies, case reports, and expert opinions. The randomized clinical trial is the best type of evidence to confirm cause-and-effect relationships.

Web-based sources such as the Cochrane Library are databases that have gathered the "best evidence" related to clinical problems. Access to Web-based data requires that the practitioner develop skills in health informatics—the application of computer technology to health care delivery. Practitioners will need to develop new skills in searching for and appraising information for a specific client in a specific clinical context.

In summary, developing expertise in clinical reasoning comes with the accumulation of knowledge and experience. It is a skill that develops with practice. Because human interaction and the specific environment influence judgment, practitioners must continuously ask themselves "Do I need more data?," "Is the diagnosis supported by sound rationale and literature?," and "Did I consider reasonable alternatives?"

? Critical Thinking Questions

1. Access MEDLINE, the Cochrane Library, or BestEvidence to answer the following question: What is the clinical research about how often an adult needs to engage in physical activity to experience health benefits?

2. Formulate a clinical question for which you will search the literature for research evidence.

 Answers are available on the MERLIN website (www.harcourthealth.com/MERLIN/Barkauskas/). And be sure to check the website regularly for additional learning activities!

Remember to check out the Online Study Guide!
www.harcourthealth.com/MERLIN/Barkauskas/

Chapter 25

Pregnant Clients

Learning Objectives

On successful study of this chapter and completion of related learning experiences, the learner will be able to:
- Describe the anatomical and physiological changes that occur in normal pregnancy.
- Outline the components of a reproductive history.
- Explain prenatal risk factors.
- Recognize physical signs of pregnancy associated with each stage of fetal development.
- Explain the rationale for and demonstrate prenatal assessment, including procedures essential to each prenatal visit.

- Delineate the usual findings of abdominal inspection, measurement, palpation, and auscultation, including:
  - Fundal characteristics
  - Fetal characteristics
  - Fetal heart tones and uterine souffle
- Delineate measurement techniques for the bony pelvis, including usual findings and common variations.

Outline

Purpose of Examination

This chapter focuses on the assessment of healthy pregnant women. It assumes and builds on knowledge of and skill in the physical examination of the adult client. The emphasis of this chapter is on the effects of the pregnant state on examination findings and the special techniques used to assess the health of the fetus and the client, as well as the woman's ability to deliver vaginally. To obtain complete information about the management of care for pregnant women, additional references are necessary.

PHYSICAL CHANGES IN PREGNANCY

A number of physical changes occur normally in pregnant women, many of which are noted in the physical assessment. The hormones produced by the fetal chorionic tissues and the placenta directly or indirectly initiate all the physiological changes of pregnancy. In early pregnancy the fetal trophoblast produces large amounts of human chorionic gonadotropic (HCG) hormone, which provides the basis for biological pregnancy testing. HCG is present in amounts detectable by immunological tests performed 8 to 10 days after conception.

Large amounts of estrogens and progesterone are produced during pregnancy. Estriol, an estrogen, is produced in large amounts during middle and late pregnancy. It is the basis for biological tests of placental and fetal well-being because a well-functioning placenta, a healthy fetus, and an intact fetal circulation are prerequisites for the continuous production of this hormone. The estrogens and progesterone maintain the decidua of pregnancy and cause the growth and hyperemia of the uterus, other pelvic organs, and the breasts.

Reproductive System Changes

Changes in the uterus include the development of the decidua, hypertrophy of muscle cells, increased vascularity, formation of the lower uterine segment, and softening of the cervix. During pregnancy the overall size of the uterus increases five to six times, its weight increases about 20 times, and its capacity increases from approximately 2 to 5000 ml.

Hormones supply the initial stimulus for uterine hypertrophy. During the first 6 to 8 weeks of pregnancy, the uterus will increase in size whether the pregnancy is uterine or extrauterine. In early pregnancy the uterus is only internally palpable. At approximately 10 to 12 weeks' gestation, the growing uterus is double its nonpregnant size and reaches the top of the symphysis, where it is palpable abdominally. The uterine fundus lies approximately halfway between the symphysis and the umbilicus at about 16 weeks' gestation and reaches the umbilicus at about 20 to 22 weeks' gestation. After 20 weeks' gestation, the average upward growth of the uterus is about 3.75 cm per month (1 cm per week). At approximately 36 weeks' gestation, the uterus reaches the xiphisternum. In the last month of pregnancy, the fundus of the uterus may drop several centimeters if the fetal head descends deep into the pelvis.

The position of the uterus changes during gestation. In early gestation an exaggerated anteflexion is common. As the uterus ascends into the abdomen, a slight dextrorotation develops. In early pregnancy the uterus changes from a flattened pear shape to a globular shape. The globular shape continues until approximately 20 to 24 weeks, when a definite ovoid shape develops and continues until delivery.

At approximately 6 to 8 weeks' gestation, the uterine isthmus becomes softened and easily compressible, and the cervix, on palpation, seems almost detached from the uterine fundus. At about 8 weeks' gestation, the entire uterus softens.

During pregnancy the uterus contracts intermittently. Painless contractions, called **Braxton Hicks** contractions, begin in early pregnancy and are first noted by the client and the examiner at about 24 weeks' gestation. These contractions can be stimulated by palpation of the uterus. If a contraction occurs during the abdominal examination, the examiner should wait until the contraction ends to continue palpation, and subsequently palpate more gently.

Three major changes occur in the cervix: (1) hypertrophy of the glands in the cervical canal, (2) softening of the cervix, and (3) bluish discoloration. These changes begin early in pregnancy—at about 6 weeks' gestation. Because of changes in the cervical epithelium, commonly a part of the squamous epithelium is replaced by an outward extension of the columnar epithelium, producing an observable cervical ectropion or eversion of the cervical canal. This condition usually persists throughout pregnancy but disappears soon after the delivery.

The increase in pelvic vascularity causes a bluish discoloration of the cervix, vagina, and vulva at about 6 to 8 weeks' gestation. In addition, the vaginal mucosa thickens, the connective tissue becomes less dense, and the muscular areas hypertrophy. These changes are reflected in palpatory findings of softening and relaxation. The hypertrophied glands secrete more mucus. The total vaginal discharge is increased and more acidic than normal.

Breast Changes

Breast changes begin at about week 8 of pregnancy, with enlargement of the breasts. Shortly afterward the nipples become larger and more erectile, the areolae become more darkly pigmented, and the sebaceous glands (Montgomery's tubercles) in the areolae hypertrophy. Sometimes an irregular secondary areola develops, extending from the primary areola. Hypertrophy of the breasts often causes a slight tenderness. In women with well-developed axillary breast tissue, the hypertrophy may produce symptomatic lumps in the axillae. Colostrum can be expressed from the breast at about week 24 of pregnancy. The colostrum appears clear and yellowish at first but becomes cloudy later.

Stretching of the skin on the breast may produce striae gravidarum, and increased vascular supply may visibly engorge superficial breast veins. See Figure 25-1 for illustrations of breast changes during pregnancy.

Abdominal Area and Gastrointestinal System Changes

The muscles of the abdominal wall stretch to accommodate the growing uterus, and the umbilicus becomes flattened or protrudes. The rapid stretching of abdominal skin may cause the formation of striae gravidarum, which appear pink or red during pregnancy and become silvery white after delivery. In the third trimester of pregnancy, the rectus abdominis muscles are under considerable stress, and their tone is diminished. A wide permanent separation of these muscles, called diastasis recti abdominis, may occur. This condition allows the abdominal contents to protrude slightly into the midline of the abdomen but requires no intervention.

In pregnancy peristaltic activity is reduced, resulting in decreased bowel sounds. Smooth muscle relaxation, or **atony**, contributes to a variety of changes in gastrointestinal function. These changes include a high incidence of pregnancy-associated nausea and vomiting, heartburn, and constipation. In addition, the increased regional blood flow to the pelvis and venous pressure contribute to hemorrhoids, a common source of discomfort in late pregnancy. Nausea and vomiting usually do not persist beyond the third month, but heartburn, constipation, and hemorrhoids are more characteristic and troublesome in late pregnancy.

Less frequently noted gastrointestinal symptoms include ptyalism, or excessive salivation, and pica, a craving for substances of little or no food value. Pica is often an expression of the folkways of some cultural groups. It becomes a concern when it interferes with good nutrition.

The enlarging uterus displaces the colon laterally, upwardly, and posteriorly. Since this displacement changes the anatomical situation of the appendix, signs of appendicitis during pregnancy may not be localized in **McBurney's point** of the right lower quadrant.

Skin, Mucous Membrane, Neck, and Hair Changes

The melanocytes in all parts of the skin are extremely active in pregnancy. There is a tendency toward generalized darkening of all skin, especially in skin that is hyperpigmented in the nonpregnant state. In some women a brownish-black pigmented streak may appear in the midline of the abdomen. This line of pigmentation is called the **linea nigra**. Some women develop a darkly pigmented configuration on the face that has been characteristically called the "mask of pregnancy," or **chloasma**. Scars and moles may also darken during pregnancy from the influence of melanocyte-stimulating hormone. Palmar erythema and spider nevi on the face and upper trunk also may accompany pregnancy.

Many pregnant women observe hypertrophy of the gums or **epulis**, resulting from hormonally induced, increased vascularity.

In more than 50% of prenatal clients, the thyroid gland is symmetrically enlarged as a result of hyperplasia of glandular tissue, new follicle formation, and increased vascularity.

The hair of pregnant women may straighten and change in oiliness. Some women experience hair loss, especially in the frontal and parietal areas. Occasionally, increases in facial and abdominal hair, resulting from increased androgen and corticotropic hormone, are noted.

Cardiovascular System Changes

Many changes, too numerous to discuss adequately here, occur in the maternal circulatory system during pregnancy. However, several major changes that alter the physical examination findings are summarized as follows.

Blood volume is increased up to 45%, and cardiac output is increased up to 30% in pregnancy, compared with the prepregnant state. Blood volume and cardiac output changes

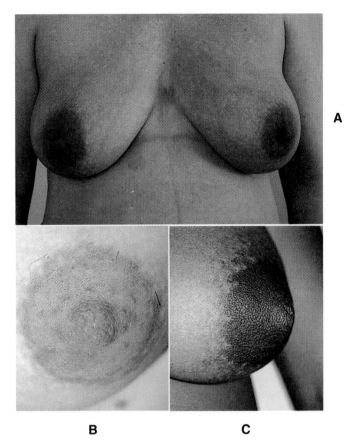

Figure 25-1 Breast changes in pregnancy. **A,** Note venous network, darkened areolae and nipples, and vascular spider. **B,** Increased pigmentation and the development of raised sebaceous glands known as Montgomery tubercles. **C,** Marked pigmentation in woman with dark skin. (**A** from Seidel HM et al.: *Mosby's guide to physical examination,* ed. 4, St. Louis, 1999, Mosby. **B** and **C** from Symonds EM, MacPherson MBA: *Color atlas of obstetrics and gynecology,* London, 1994, Mosby-Wolfe.)

contribute to auscultatory changes that are common in pregnancy. Heart sounds are accentuated, and a low-grade systolic murmur (usually grade II) is often noted.

As pregnancy advances, the heart is displaced upwardly and laterally. The apical impulse is displaced to a point 1 to 1.5 cm lateral of its location in the nonpregnant client. The pulse rate increases about 10 beats per minute from the prepregnancy rate, and palpitations may be noticed during pregnancy. The blood pressure is normally unchanged or may decrease in the second trimester. Several disorders in pregnancy may alter blood pressure. In some women, pregnancy induces hypertension, which abates after delivery. Also, increases in blood pressure accompany preeclampsia, a disorder observed in some pregnancies.

A progesterone-induced generalized relaxation of the smooth muscle, arteriolar dilation, and increased capacity of the vascular compartment occur. The systolic blood pressure remains the same or is slightly lower during midpregnancy. There is no change in the venous pressure in the upper body, but the venous pressure increases in the lower extremities when the client is supine, sitting, or standing because of the pressure of the gravid uterus. This situation predisposes the woman to varicosities of the legs and the vulva and to edema.

Respiratory System Changes

During pregnancy the tidal volume increases, and the respiratory rate increases slightly. Alveolar ventilation increases, and a more efficient exchange of lung gases occurs in the alveoli. Oxygen consumption rises by almost 20%, and plasma carbon dioxide content decreases.

As the uterus enlarges, it pushes the thoracic cage and diaphragm upward, and the thorax widens at the base. Physical assessment may reveal a change in respiration from abdominal to costal. In addition, dyspnea is a common complaint, especially in the last trimester, and deep respirations and sighing may be more frequent.

The tissue of the respiratory tract, sinuses, and nasopharynx manifests hyperemia and edema. This situation may contribute to engorgement of the turbinates, nasal stuffiness, and mouth breathing. Some women note increased nasal and sinus secretion and nosebleeds. Vocal cord edema may cause voice changes. Increased vascularity of the tympanic membranes and blockage of the eustachian tubes may contribute to decreased hearing, a sense of fullness in the ears, or earaches.

Musculoskeletal System Changes

The pelvic joints exhibit slight relaxation in pregnancy as a result of some unknown mechanism. This relaxation is maximal from about the seventh month onward. Because the gravid uterus has caused the pregnant client's weight to be thrust forward, the muscles of the spine are used to achieve a temporary new balance. The pregnant client throws her

| TABLE 25-1 | **Summary of the Physical Changes of Pregnancy** | | |

System or Region	Summary of Physiological and Physical Changes During Pregnancy	System or Region	Summary of Physiological and Physical Changes During Pregnancy
Skin and mucous membranes	Peripheral vascular vasodilation and increased numbers of capillaries result in increased blood flow, sweat, and sebaceous gland activity Increase in vascular spider veins and hemangiomas Thickening Fat is deposited in subdermal layers, especially on hips and buttocks Separations caused by stretching Increased pigmentation of face, nipples, areolae, axillae, and vulva Palmar erythema Linea nigra Chloasma (mask of pregnancy) Gum hypertrophy Ptyalism—excessive secretion of saliva	Respiratory system	Increase in thoracic transverse diameter of about 2 cm Rise in diaphragm up to 4 cm, compensated by increase in thoracic circumference of 5 to 7 cm Increase in costal angle to about 100 degrees Increase in tidal volume Dyspnea
Thyroid	Slight enlargement—may be palpable Increased vascularity with possible bruit Increased T_4 and T_3 levels Decreased T_3 uptake Unchanged thyroid function	Heart and blood vessels	Blood volume increases up to 45% Plasma volume increases 50% Splitting of S_1 and S_2 Loud S_1 S_3 may be heard Grade II systolic murmurs are commonly heard Diastolic murmurs are sometimes heard Increase in both thickness and mass of left ventricle Increase in stroke volume Cardiac output increases 30% Position of heart is shifted upward and to left Apex is rotated laterally—apex of heart is palpated more laterally than in nonpregnant state Vascular resistance decreases, and peripheral vasodilation occurs Varicose veins common in third trimester Increase in heart rate of 10 to 15 beats/min Blood pressure may drop in second trimester
Eyes	Mild corneal edema and thickening Fall in intraocular pressure Tears contain increase in lysozyme, resulting in blurred vision with contact lens wearing		
Ears, nose, and throat	Increased vascularity, resulting in symptoms of nasal stuffiness, decreased sense of smell, epistaxis, feeling of fullness in ears, and decreased hearing Increased vascularity and proliferation of gum tissue Laryngeal changes—hoarseness, voice changes, and cough		

shoulders back and straightens her head and neck. The lower vertebral column is hyperextended (Figure 25-2).

The musculoskeletal changes are often reflected in postural and gait changes, lower backache, and fatigue. Often the pregnant woman's gait is described as waddling, and her balance is less stable from about week 24 onward.

Urinary System Changes

A number of physiological changes occur during pregnancy, including a renal blood flow increased by as much as 50% and a glomerular filtration rate increased by up to 50% by the end of pregnancy. In addition, glucose reabsorption is decreased, resulting in glycosuria. The physical presence of the growing uterus causes displacement of the ureters and kidneys, especially on the right side. In the pelvis the growing uterus causes pressure on the bladder during the first and third trimesters, resulting in urinary frequency.

Neurological System Changes

The interrelatedness of the body systems during pregnancy, combined with the major physical changes, makes it difficult to isolate exclusively neurological system changes. Alterations that may be primarily neurological in origin include headaches and numbness and tingling of the hands. A summary of the physical changes that occur during pregnancy is provided in Table 25-1.

Endocrine System Changes

Increased oxygen consumption and fetal metabolic demands create an increase in the basic metabolic rate of 15% to 25%.

TABLE 25-1 Summary of the Physical Changes of Pregnancy—cont'd

System or Region	Summary of Physiological and Physical Changes During Pregnancy	System or Region	Summary of Physiological and Physical Changes During Pregnancy
Breasts and axillae	Sensations of fullness, tingling, and tenderness Enlarge two to three times nonpregnancy size Expansion of ductal system and secretory alveoli; on palpation, breasts feel coarsely nodular Increase in glandular tissues displaces connective tissue; breasts become softer and looser Areolae become more deeply pigmented, and diameter increases Nipples become more prominent, darker, and more erectile Veins engorge and become more visible Colostrum is secreted Striae may appear	Female genitalia	Uterine enlargement Softening of pelvic cartilage Strengthening of pelvic ligaments Pelvic congestion and edema Uterus, cervix, and isthmus soften; cervix appears blue Thickening of mucosa of vaginal walls and connective tissue Smooth muscle cells hypertrophy Increased length of vaginal walls Vaginal secretions increase and have acidic pH
Abdomen	Loss of abdominal muscle tone Striae may appear Rectus abdominis muscles may separate (diatasis recti) Gastric motility decreases, resulting in delayed emptying time Esophageal reflux Bowel sounds are diminished Constipation, nausea, and vomiting are common Displacement of appendix Tendency to hemorrhoid formation Enlargement caused by growing uterus and fetus Changes in bladder function and sensation Stool color may be green or black because of the use of supplementary iron	Anus and rectum	Decreased gastrointestinal tract tone and motility produce constipation Development of hemorrhoids is common
		Urinary system	Increased renal blood flow up to 50% in third trimester Increased glomerular filtration rate up to 50% Decreased resorption of glucose in renal tubules Displacement of ureters and kidneys Urinary frequency in first and third trimesters
		Musculoskeletal system	Increased mobility of sacroiliac, sacrococcygeal, and symphysis pubis joints Progressive lordosis in response to need to adjust to growing uterus
		Neurological system	Tension headaches Numbness and tingling of hands

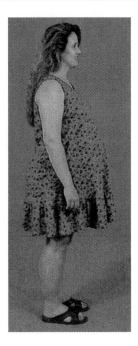

Figure 25-2   Posture of a pregnant woman.

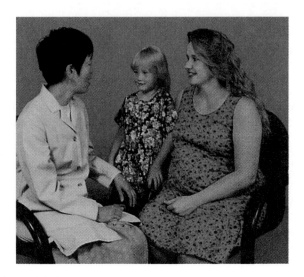

Figure 25-3   Interview with a pregnant woman and another family member.

This increase often causes feelings of warmth and heat intolerance.

A second endocrine system change is an increasing resistance to insulin as pregnancy progresses. This phenomena is related to the system's attempt to ensure sufficient glucose for fetal needs. Glycosuria may result when the renal tubules are unable to respond to increased amounts of glucose in the maternal circulatory system.

EXAMINATION

Prenatal Health History

A complete health history is an essential component of the initial visit for prenatal care (Figure 25-3). The structure of the health history is the same as that described for the adult client, with special attention given to the reproductive system and to the physical, social, and emotional readiness of the woman to incorporate a new child in her life.

The health history is important in pregnancy because information derived from it assists the practitioner in differentiating the client who is essentially healthy and expected to deliver a full-term, healthy baby from the high-risk expectant mother whose situation is likely to affect her own or her fetus' health negatively. High-risk clients are given special care in most health care systems. The early identification of risk factors and their effective management enable the prenatal care to result in maximal benefit for the mother, family, and infant.

The health history for the obstetrical client follows the same basic protocol as that presented for all adults in Chapter 3. However, in prenatal care the following areas of history taking should receive special and complete attention:

Biographical Information

1. Age
2. Race and/or ethnic background
3. Marital status and support network
4. Educational status

Past Obstetrical History

1. Gravidity and parity: A five-number code with the abbreviation **G-T-P-A-L** is often used to summarize gravity and parity information.

   G = **G**ravity: total number of pregnancies, including current one

   T = **T**otal number of full-term births

   P = Number of **P**reterm births (i.e., those between 21 and 37 weeks' gestation)

   A = Number of **A**bortions (i.e., those terminated at or before 20 weeks' gestation)

   L = Number of **L**iving children

   Thus, for example, the gravidity/parity 5-2-1-1-3 indicates the following: the client is pregnant for the fifth time; she has three living children, two of whom were delivered after full-term gestation and one of whom was premature; and she has had one abortion.

   Alternative methods of indicating parity include two-digit, three-digit, and four-digit codes.

   Two-digit codes: The first digit indicates gravidity, defined as the total number of pregnancies. The second digit represents parity, the number of live births (G-P). In the preceding example this code would be recorded as 5-3.

   Three-digit codes: The first digit indicates gravidity, the second digit represents parity, and the third digit indicates abortions (G-P-A).

Risk Factors
Prenatal Problems

The following factors have been associated with increased morbidity and mortality of mothers and infants. The examiner should take special note of these factors during the health history interview and its recording.

HABITS

Smoking
Alcohol consumption
Drug addiction

MATERNAL CHARACTERISTICS

Age—younger than 18 or older than 40
Poverty
Single status
Family disorganization
Conflict about pregnancy
Height less than 5 ft
Weight less than 100 lb
Inadequate diet
Low educational level

REPRODUCTIVE HISTORY

More than one previous abortion
Perinatal death
Infant weighing less than 2500 g
Infant weighing more than 400 g
Infant with isoimmunization or ABO incompatibility
Infant with major congenital or perinatal disease
Uterine anomaly
Myomas
Ovarian masses
Sexually transmitted infections

MEDICAL PROBLEMS

Anemia
Diabetes mellitus
Endocrine disorder
Heart disease
Hypertension
Pulmonary disease
Renal disease
Sickle cell disease

PRESENT PREGNANCY

Bleeding
Premature rupture of membranes
Anemia
No prenatal care
Preeclampsia or eclampsia
Hydramnios
Multiple pregnancy
Breech, transverse, or abnormal fetal position
Low or excessive weight gain
Hypertension (blood pressure greater than 140/90, a systolic increase of 30 mm Hg, or a diastolic increase of 15 mm Hg over baseline readings)
Abnormal fasting blood glucose level
Rh-negative sensitization
Exposure to teratogens
Viral infections
Sexually transmitted infections
Bacterial infections
Protozoal infections
Postmaturity

Four-digit codes: The first digit indicates gravidity, the second digit represents parity, the third digit indicates abortions, and the fourth digit represents the number of living children (G-P-A-L).

NOTE: The term nullipara describes a woman who has not given birth. The term includes women who are pregnant, but who have not yet given birth. This term is differentiated from the term nulligravida, which connotes a woman who has never been pregnant.

2. The following information is obtained for every past pregnancy:
   a. Date of delivery
   b. Duration of gestation
   c. Significant problems or complications of pregnancy, labor, and delivery
   d. Manner in which labor started, specifically whether labor was spontaneous or induced; if labor was induced, the reason for induction; if abortion, type (spontaneous [S] or induced [I])
   e. Length of labor
   f. Presentation of infant at delivery
   g. Type of delivery: vaginal or cesarean; if cesarean, the reason is noted
   h. Type of anesthesia used at delivery
   i. Condition of infant(s) at birth and sex and birth weight
   j. Postpartum problems, especially infection, hemorrhage, and thrombophlebitis
   k. Infant's problems—especially jaundice, respiratory distress, infection, and congenital anomalies
   l. Type of infant feeding
   m. Current health of child

Present Obstetrical History

1. Last normal menstrual period: An important task during the prenatal history is to estimate the expected date of confinement (EDC). Because the exact date of conception is unknown for the majority of prenatal clients, the EDC is calculated according to the first day of the last normal menstrual period (LNMP). The EDC is determined by counting backward 3 calendar months from the LNMP and adding 7 days (Nägele's rule). The year, of course, may change.

Example: If the LNMP were 10-15-97, the EDC would be 7-22-98.
Calculation: Tenth month − 3 months = the seventh month. The 15th day + 7 days = the 22nd day.

If the client has a history of irregular menses, the EDC can be more accurately estimated by physical examination than by using the LNMP. Critical events that aid in determination or validation of the EDC are the date of quickening (when the mother first notices fetal movement, usually at about 18 weeks) and the time at which the fetal heart tones can be auscultated (at 10 to 12 weeks for a Doppler instrument and at 16 to 20 weeks for a fetoscope). Because of the variation that characterizes these events, ultrasonic measurement of fetal size and growth is being used more commonly to date pregnancy and assess fetal growth, along with measurement of the progressive enlargement of the uterus.

2. Symptoms of pregnancy (e.g., breast tenderness, morning sickness, lower abdominal fullness)
3. Feelings about pregnancy, especially determination of whether pregnancy was planned or unplanned
4. Bleeding since LNMP
5. Date when fetal movements were first felt, if in second trimester
6. Fetal exposure to infections, radiation, and drugs (including oral contraceptives and spermicides)
7. Risk assessment

Current and Past Medical History and Gynecological History

1. Anemia
2. Bacterial and viral infections
3. Diabetes
4. Endocrine disorders
5. Heart disease
6. Hypertension
7. Sexually transmitted diseases
8. Urinary tract infections
9. Genital tract history, especially:
    a. Anomaly
    b. Cervical incompetence
    c. Myomas
    d. Ovarian mass
    e. Vaginal infections
    f. Surgery
    g. Abnormal Papanicolaou (Pap) test results
    h. Use of hormones (e.g., birth control pills)
    i. Menstrual history and functioning
    j. Endometriosis
10. Medication history: over-the-counter and prescribed drugs, including vitamins and folic acid
11. Current or past use of alcohol, tobacco, mood-altering drugs, or other nonprescribed drugs

Nutritional Assessment (see Chapter 6)

1. Prepregnant weight
2. Weight gain since conception
3. Dietary pattern—confirmation of ingestion of sufficient nutrients for the growing fetus; use of dietary supplements

Sexual History

1. Pattern of sexual activity
2. Satisfaction with sexuality and sexual activity
3. Partners: number and health
4. Contraception use and safe sex methods

Family and Partner Health History

Features of the family history that have special significance in pregnancy include diabetes, renal or hematological disorders, hypertension, multiple pregnancy, and congenital defects and retardation. It is important to know whether the primigravida's mother had preeclampsia or high blood pressure during pregnancies, especially if she convulsed.

During pregnancy the health of the baby's father assumes special importance as a component of the health history. The following factors about the health and health history of the baby's father are especially important:

1. Current health and relationship
2. Blood type and Rh factor
3. History of potential inherited disorders
4. Use of tobacco, alcohol, and illicit drugs
5. Risk factors for sexually transmitted diseases

Emotional, Psychological, and Developmental Status

Pregnancy is an important developmental event in a woman's life. The developmental tasks of pregnancy are: incorporation of the fetus; differentiation of the fetus and mother; and, eventually, separation from the fetus. These tasks roughly coincide with the three trimesters of pregnancy.

During the first trimester of pregnancy, the gravida is involved with the process of accepting the fetus as a fact and a part of her body. Most women initially experience some ambivalence about their pregnancy and a resultant increase in anxiety. Many body changes occur that cause increased somatic awareness and inward focus. Relationships with key persons, especially the child's father and the gravida's mother, become especially important. Unresolved feelings and conflicts undergo re-examination. Feelings of dependency and vulnerability occur and can be additional causes of anxiety.

In the second trimester the fetus develops a separate identity. The gravida has had some time to become accustomed to her body changes and often feels better physically because the nausea has ceased. The fetus's movements are an important event, confirming the presence of the fetus and reminding the woman of the independence of the fetal movements from her control. The woman begins to think about the infant and their future. Worries about the possibility of producing an abnormal infant are common.

In the last trimester the gravida prepares for her separation from the fetus and her entrance into a new relationship with the newborn. This time is occupied with preparatory activities, such as attending parents' classes and buying clothing and equipment for the newborn. Concerns about labor and delivery and the physical discomforts of late pregnancy contribute to the woman's readiness for separation from the fetus and her movement toward the tasks of parenthood.

Social, Economic, and Cultural Status

Because pregnancy and birth are important events in the development of any family and because the quality of the family affects the infant's health, the interviewer must assess the circumstances relating to the pregnancy and the family environment. In addition, all cultures view pregnancy and birth as significant events, and many have developed prescriptions and taboos around pregnancy. The following are several important areas of exploration in the social history across cultures:

1. Client's desire for, and feelings about, this pregnancy
2. Feelings of significant others regarding this pregnancy
3. Client's personal and culturally derived health beliefs about pregnancy
4. Client's knowledge regarding pregnancy and parenting
5. Amount of support and assistance provided by family and significant others (including father of child and children)
6. Economic burdens imposed on client or family by pregnancy
7. Condition of the family's physical and emotional environment
8. Presence or risk of physical or other abuse or other evidence of domestic violence

General Physical Examination

A complete physical examination should be performed on the first prenatal visit because (1) the examination may reveal problems that need special or immediate attention, and (2) initial data provide the baseline against which changes that occur later in pregnancy can be compared. The initial general physical examination of the prenatal client is the same as for other clients, except for special emphasis on the diagnosis of pregnancy, the assessment of pelvic adequacy, and the assessment of fetal growth and well-being.

Several signs unrelated to the reproductive system may be normally altered in pregnancy. Such alterations of physical findings are listed in Box 25-1.

Diagnosis of Pregnancy

The diagnosis of pregnancy takes into account both the history of subjective symptoms noticed by the client and the objective signs noted by the examiner. In addition, laboratory tests are especially helpful in confirming early pregnancy.

Traditionally the signs and symptoms of pregnancy have been categorized as (1) presumptive symptoms, (2) probable signs, and (3) positive signs. Presumptive symptoms are those concerns that the prenatal client identifies in the present illness and chief complaint parts of the history, as well as several additional general physical signs. They include the subjective data that may have led the client to seek confirmation of pregnancy. Presumptive symptoms include (1) absence of menses 10 or more days after the expected date of onset; (2) morning sickness, nausea, or appetite change; (3) frequent urination;

(4) soreness or a tingling sensation in the breasts; (5) Braxton Hicks contractions; (6) quickening; (7) abdominal enlargement; and (8) bluish discoloration of the vagina.

The following are probable signs of pregnancy: (1) progressive enlargement of the uterus; (2) softening of the cervix

BOX 25-1

PHYSICAL EXAMINATION FINDINGS ALTERED IN PREGNANCY

RESPIRATORY SYSTEM
Change in breathing from abdominal to costal
Shortening and widening at base of thoracic cage
Elevation of diaphragm
Increase in respiratory rate

CARDIOVASCULAR SYSTEM
Displacement of apical impulse laterally 1 to 1.5 cm
Grade 2 systolic murmur
Increase in pulse rate
Slight fall in blood pressure in second trimester

MUSCULOSKELETAL SYSTEM
Slight instability of pelvis
Alteration of standing posture and gait to compensate for gravid uterus

ABDOMINAL REGION
Contour changes because of gravid uterus
Striae gravidarum
Decrease in muscle tone
Linea nigra
Reduced peristaltic activity

SKIN AND MUCOUS MEMBRANES
Chloasma
Linea nigra
Hyperpigmentation of skin and bony prominences
Palmar erythema
Spider nevi on face and upper trunk
Striae gravidarum on breasts and abdomen
Gum hypertrophy

BREASTS
Enlargement
Large, erect nipples
Darkening of areolar pigment
Development of secondary areola
Hypertrophy of sebaceous glands in areola
Formation of colostrum
Tenderness on palpation
Striae gravidarum
Engorgement of superficial veins

OTHER ALTERATIONS
Straightening of hair
Loss of hair over frontal and parietal regions
Enlarged thyroid

Cultural Considerations
Cultural Influences in Pregnancy

CULTURE	CULTURAL PRESCRIPTIONS	CULTURAL RESTRICTIONS
African-Americans	Maternal relatives are primary advisors Geographia—eating of clay or earth Food cravings of food and nonfood substances	Avoid photography Bad luck to purchase clothing for unborn baby
Amish	Children perceived as a value—tendency to large families Perceive pregnancy as a normal life event	Avoid photography Want minimal intervention with birth
Appalachians	Eat well and take care of themselves Male fetuses are carried higher than female fetuses Childbearing and childbirth are natural processes	Picture taking can cause a stillbirth Reaching over one's head can cause cord to strangle the fetus Wearing opal can harm the baby Being frightened and eating strawberries and citrus fruit can cause birthmarks
Arab-Americans	High fertility A fetus carried high is a female and a fetus carried low is a male Cravings are indulged Excused from fasting May continue cigarette smoking and high caffeine ingestion Consume large quantities of olive oil	Tragedies can cause birthmarks
Chinese-Americans	Increase meat ingestion to strengthen the fetus Many women prefer a female practitioner	Avoid shellfish during the first trimester because it causes allergies Avoid iron as it may cause difficult delivery
Cuban-Americans	Eating coffee grounds cures morning sickness Eating a lot of fruit ensures a baby with a smooth complexion	Wearing necklaces during pregnancy causes the umbilical cord to be wrapped around the baby's neck
Egyptian-Americans	A family is not complete until there is a child Pregnancies occur early in a marriage Eating increases Cravings are indulged	
Filipino-Americans	Eat well Cravings should be satisfied—baby takes on some of the appearance of the craved food Lots of sleep at night Can demand attention, pampering from family Can indulge in laziness Women share advice with other women	Stay in a dependent position to avoid water retention Avoid sexual intercourse during the last 2 months of pregnancy Eating prunes, sweet foods, or squid Cautioned against taking any medications Stress and fear will harm the developing fetus
French Canadians	High fertility Fear of labor and delivery	Alcohol and tobacco discouraged Washing floors induces early labor
Greek-Americans	Tendency toward smaller families Children are important to a family Encouraged to eat large quantities of food—iron and protein are particularly important	Avoidance of funerals and viewing of deceased persons

From Giger JN, Davidhizar RE: *Transcultural nursing: assessment and intervention,* St. Louis, 1999, Mosby; and Purnell LD, Paulanka BJ: *Transcultural health care: a culturally competent approach,* Philadelphia, 1998, FA Davis.

at 4 to 6 weeks (Goodell's sign); (3) softening of the uterine isthmus at 6 to 8 weeks (Hegar's sign); (4) asymmetrical, soft enlargement of one uterine cornu at 7 to 8 weeks (Piskacek's sign); (5) bluish or cyanotic color of the cervix and upper vagina at 8 to 12 weeks (Chadwick's sign); (6) internal ballottement; (7) palpation of fetal parts; and (8) positive test results for HCG in the urine or serum. These signs are termed "probable" because clinical conditions other than pregnancy can cause any of them. However, if they occur together, a strong case can be made for pregnancy.

Cultural Considerations—cont'd
Cultural Influences in Pregnancy—cont'd

CULTURE	CULTURAL PRESCRIPTIONS	CULTURAL RESTRICTIONS
Haitian-Americans	Food: cornmeal, rice, beans, plantains, vegetables, red fruits	May not routinely seek prenatal care Dietary taboos: lima beans, tomatoes, black mushrooms, white beans, okra, lobster, fish, eggplant, black peppers milk, bananas
Iranians	Pregnancy is seen as desirable: a woman's prestige is elevated if she has a child Delivering the first child releases anxiety Cravings are seen as the fetus' need for certain foods Cravings must be satisfied Fruits and vegetables encouraged Sexual intercourse allowed until the last month Receives considerable support from the sixth month through the postpartum period Balance of hot and cold foods	Avoid fried foods and foods that causes gas Heavy work may cause a miscarriage
Irish-Americans	Eat a well-balanced diet	Should not reach over head as cord will wrap around fetus' neck Tragedies during pregnancy cause anomalies
Jewish-Americans	Children are a blessing Sterility is a curse The mother and her health are paramount	
Korean-Americans	Practice of Tai-kyo in which women are supposed to think only about good things in life and to maintain a calm attitude Eat perfect food	
Mexican-Americans	Pregnancy is natural and desirable May not value prenatal care Follow hot and cold theories of disease Sleep on their backs Engage in frequent intercourse to keep vaginal canal well lubricated for delivery Keep active to ensure a smaller baby and decrease the amount of amniotic fluid Wear some metal on their abdomens to prevent birth deformities	Walking in the moonlight causes deformities Avoid reaching over head to prevent cord from wrapping around fetus' neck
Navaho Indians	Do not seek prenatal care as pregnancy not considered an illness Twins are considered unfavorable	Reluctant to delivery in hospitals
Vietnamese-Americans	High fertility Prescriptive foods—noodles, sweets, sour foods, fruit Prescriptive foods vary by trimester Reduce food during the third trimester to produce an easier birth Prenatal care not a value Most comfortable with a female practitioner Maintenance of physical activity keeps the fetus moving and prevents edema, miscarriage, and premature delivery	Avoid fish, salty foods, and rice Avoid heavy lifting, strenuous work Raising the arms above the head causes the placenta to break Intercourse in late pregnancy cause infant respiration difficulty Cannot attend weddings or funerals Idleness causes prolonged labor and a large baby

The positive signs of pregnancy are those that prove the presence of a fetus: (1) documentation of a fetal heartbeat by auscultation, electrocardiogram, or Doppler instrument; (2) palpation of active fetal movements; and (3) radiological or ultrasonographic demonstration of fetal parts. Ultrasonographic techniques can demonstrate the presence of a gestational sac as early as 6 weeks' gestation. Doppler instruments can detect a fetal heartbeat as early as 10 to 12 weeks' gestation.

Currently clinical diagnosis of pregnancy is made by using laboratory tests in conjunction with the probable signs of pregnancy. Technology and marketing have made available reliable, low-cost home and in-clinic pregnancy tests that, in conjunction with clinical findings, can confirm the diagnosis of pregnancy early in the first trimester. The commonly used immunological pregnancy tests are the hemagglutination inhibition test and the latex agglutination test. These tests depend on an antigen-antibody reaction between HCG and an antiserum obtained from rabbits immunized against this antigen. These tests are available for use by both health professionals and laypersons and are very sensitive. Most commercial tests use standardized anti-HCG rabbit serum and dead cells or standardized latex particles coated with HCG. Anti-HCG serum is mixed first with a sample of the client's urine; then HCG-coated red blood cells or particles are added. The lack of agglutination is a positive test because urine that contains HCG has neutralized the HCG antibodies. If the urine sample contains no HCG, agglutination occurs, indicating a negative test for pregnancy.

Pregnancy tests based on the presence of HCG in the urine can be reliably performed from 2 days after the first day of a missed menses through 16 weeks' gestation. During this time the production of HCG is at its peak. Currently home pregnancy testing is widely available to women and is becoming a common method of self-assessment. Home pregnancy tests vary in accuracy and instructions. Although the techniques are relatively simple and straightforward, mistakes are possible, and a careful clinical assessment is always an important component of the diagnosis of pregnancy.

Several early clinical findings are used in conjunction with laboratory tests to diagnose pregnancy. In pregnancy a pelvic examination done approximately 6 to 8 weeks after the last normal menses shows uterine enlargement. The uterus first enlarges in the pelvis. By 12 weeks' gestation, the examiner can palpate the uterus abdominally just above the symphysis pubis. In addition to enlarging, the uterus becomes globular and then ovoid.

The uterus softens during pregnancy because of its increased vascularity. The isthmus of the uterus is the first part to soften. At about 6 to 8 weeks' gestation, the softened isthmus produces a dramatic palpatory finding. On palpation, the enlarged globular uterus feels almost detached from the cervix, which is still not completely softened, because the isthmus feels so indistinct (Figure 25-4). This phenomenon is called Hegar's sign. By 7 or 8 weeks' gestation, the cervix and the uterus can be easily flexed at their junction (McDonald's sign). Speculum examination shows cyanosis of the cervix as early as 6 to 8 weeks' gestation, a change that results from the increased vascularity in the area.

Often uterine enlargement does not progress symmetrically. Rather, the area of placental development enlarges more rapidly. This imbalance produces a palpatory asymmetrical enlargement of one uterine cornu, called Piskacek's sign (Figure 25-5).

The timetable for physical signs of pregnancy is presented in Table 25-2. This table also includes an outline of fetal development during pregnancy.

Technique for Examination and Expected Findings

Prenatal assessments include examination of both the mother and the developing fetus. After the initial assessment, examinations of the prenatal client are done at regular intervals. Re-examination schedules vary among health care services. However, a common schedule includes examinations done approximately every 3 to 4 weeks during the first 28 weeks of pregnancy, then every 2 to 3 weeks until 36 weeks and weekly thereafter.

Laboratory tests indicated during pregnancy are presented in Box 25-2.

Comfort of the client during the examination is especially important. Elevate the head of the examination table to prevent stress on the abdomen (Figure 25-6).

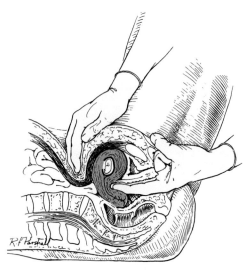

Figure 25-4 Hegar's sign: softening of the lower uterine segment.

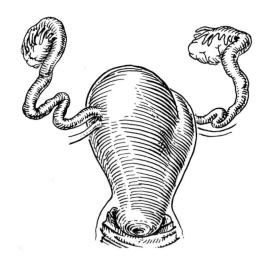

Figure 25-5 Piskacek's sign: asymmetrical enlargement of the uterine fundus.

At each prenatal revisit the examiner usually assesses the following:

1. Interval history
2. Weight gain
3. Blood pressure
4. Urine for glucose, albumin, and ketones
5. Legs for edema
6. Abdomen
   a. Determination of uterine growth through measurement of fundal height

TABLE 25-2 **Physical Signs of Pregnancy and Corresponding Stage of Fetal Development**

Sign	Approximate Gestation (Weeks Since Last Menses)		Fetal Development
Amenorrhea	2	0-4	Fertilization occurs
			Blastocyst implants
			Placental circulation established
			Organogenesis initiated
			Development of nervous system and vital organs initiated
			Anatomical structures and systems are in rudimentary form
			Size: 0.25 in by fourth week
Softening of cervix (Goodell's sign)	4-6		
Softening of cervicouterine junction (Ladin's sign)	5-6	5-8	All major organs in rudimentary form
			Fingers are present
Gestational sac may be noted by ultrasonography	6		Ears and eyes are formed
			Heart complete and functioning
Compressibility of lower uterine segment (Hegar's sign)	6-8		Development of muscles is initiated
			Size: 1.25 in by eighth week
Dilation of breast veins			
Pulsation of uterine arteries in lateral fornices (Oslander's sign)			
Flexing of fundus of cervix (McDonald's sign)			
Asymmetrical softening and enlarging of uterus (Piskacek's sign)			
Uterus changes from pear to globular shape			
Bluish coloration of vagina and cervix (Chadwick's sign)	8-12	9-12	Organs forming and growing
			Swallowing and sucking reflexes present
Detection of fetal heartbeat with a Doppler instrument	10-12		Body movements increase
			Size: 3 in, 0.5 ounces by 12th week
Uterus palpable just above symphysis pubis	12	13-16	Circulatory system established
			Size: 6 in, 4 ounces by 16th week
Ballottement of fetus possible by abdominal and vaginal examination	16		
Uterus palpable halfway between symphysis and umbilicus			
Fetal movements noted by mother (quickening)	16-20	17-20	Rapid growth
Pigment change may occur			Size: 8 in, 8 ounces by 20th week
Uterine fundus at lower border of umbilicus	20	21-24	Meconium present in intestines
Fetal heartbeat auscultated with fetoscope			Size: 11 in, 1-1.5 lb by 24th week
Fetus palpable	24		
Mother begins to notice Braxton Hicks contractions	24-26	25-28	Nervous system can control breathing and temperature
			Size: 12 in, 2-3 lb by 28th week
Uterus changes from globular to ovoid shape			
Fetus easily palpable, very mobile, and may be found in any lie, presentation, or position	28	29-32	Fat deposits under skin
			Size: 13 in, 3-5 lb by 32nd week
Uterus is approximately half the distance from umbilicus to xiphoid			
Fetus usually lies longitudinally with a vertex presentation	32	33-36	Primitive reflexes are present
			Size: 14 in, 5-6 lb by 36th week
Uterine fundus is approximately two thirds the distance between umbilicus and xiphoid			
Uterine fundus is just below xiphoid	34		
Vertex presentation may engage in pelvis	36-40	37-40	Less active because of crowding
			Size: 19-21 in, 6-8 lb by 40th week

BOX 25-2

LABORATORY TESTS

INITIAL PRENATAL ASSESSMENT

In addition to the appropriate tests for relevant risk factors, the following laboratory tests are characteristically included:

Blood type and antibody identification for D (Rh) incompatibility
Cervical smear for gonorrhea
Clean-catch urinalysis for glucose, albumin, and ketones and a microscopic examination
Clean-catch urine culture for asymptomatic bacteriuria
Complete blood count
General antibody screening test
Papanicolaou (Pap) smear
Rubella titer
Venereal Disease Research Laboratory (VDRL) test

TESTS DONE AS INDICATED FOR HIGH-RISK GROUPS

Antibody screening for *Toxoplasma gondii,* cytomegalovirus, herpes simplex virus, human immunodeficiency virus, and hepatitis B surface antigen
Genetic screening test

TESTS OFTEN DONE AT 24 TO 28 WEEKS' GESTATION

Cervical smear for *Chlamydia trachomatis*
Hemoglobin electrophoresis for all black women
Repeat antibody screening for women found to be negative for D antibodies
Repeat hemoglobin and hematocrit

Serum glucose screen and a mini-glucose tolerance test that consists of a fasting reading and a 1-hour glucose determination after a 50-g load
Tine test for purified protein derivative for tuberculosis

TESTS OFTEN REPEATED AT 32 TO 36 WEEKS' GESTATION

Cervical smear for gonorrhea
Hemoglobin and hematocrit
VDRL

SPECIAL SCREENING TESTS

Pregnant women with one or more of the following risk factors should be screened for diabetes: family history in parents or siblings; obesity high-risk ethnicity (American Indian, Hispanic, African American); history of glucose intolerance, hypertension, hyperlipidemia; history of gestational diabetes or macrosomia.

Screening ultrasonography can be used to assess gestational age, multiple gestation, and congenital anomalies in high-risk women or potentially high-risk situations. However, there is insufficient evidence to recommend for or against a single routine ultrasonographic scan in the second trimester in low-risk pregnant women. Routine third-trimester ultrasound examination of the fetus is not recommended (Woolfe, Jonas, and Lawrence, 1996). After a comprehensive review of the research on risk assessment in pregnancy, Andolsek and Kelton (2000) concluded that "studies of more than 15,000 low-risk pregnancies do not support the routine use of sonography for the diagnosis of fetal well-being or prediction of birth outcome" (p. 95).

---

b. Determination of fetal presentation and position (beginning at 28 weeks and continuing to full term)

c. Measurement of fetal heart rate

Interval History

At each visit it is important to ask the client about new symptoms and signs and to update information about any health problems or issues noted in the initial history. Sometimes flow sheets with common signs and symptoms are used to facilitate documentation. Commonly reviewed areas include the presence and character of fetal movements, vaginal discharge or bleeding, cramps, pelvic pressure, and signs and symptoms of urinary tract infection.

Weight Gain

At term the infant, uterine contents, and other changes in the body account for approximately 20 pounds of weight. Optimal weight gain during pregnancy, based on the lowest rate of complications and optimal birth weight of infants, is 24 to 27.5 pounds (a wider range is 20 to 30 pounds). High prepregnancy weight correlates significantly with an in-

creased risk of preeclampsia. Women with a low prepregnancy weight who gain little weight during pregnancy are more likely to have low-birth-weight infants (i.e., infants weighing 2500 g or less). Sudden weight gain, especially in the third trimester, usually indicates fluid retention, and this change should be evaluated in conjunction with maternal blood pressure. Apart from this transient cause of weight gain, many women tend to add to their body fat stores during pregnancy, and this weight gain may not be entirely lost after delivery. The gain in weight should occur gradually, averaging 1.5 to 2 pounds per month during the first 24 weeks and 0.5 to 1 pound a week during the remainder of the pregnancy.

Blood Pressure

Mean systolic blood pressure and mean diastolic blood pressure are essentially unchanged during pregnancy, except for a mild and transient decrease during the middle trimester in a normal pregnancy. However, hypertension contributes significantly to prenatal morbidity and mortality, and pregnancy-induced hypertension is a disease peculiar to pregnancy. This disorder typically develops after

Preparation for Examination

EQUIPMENT

In addition to all the equipment needed for a comprehensive physical examination that includes a pelvic examination, the following items are needed for the prenatal physical examination.

Item	Purpose
Measuring tape (50 cm or longer)	To assess growth of uterus
Doppler instrument or fetoscope	To auscultate fetal heart tones
Pelvimetric rulers	To measure various pelvic size dimensions

Client and the Environment

1. Provide a warm, private room.
2. Make sure that the client is adequately gowned and draped throughout the examination.
3. Help the client to assume various positions throughout the examination, as required by the assessment techniques.
4. Avoid allowing the client to lie on her back for extended periods because of the negative effects of the gravid uterus on the abdominal organs, the vessels, and the back. The most comfortable back-lying position is with the head elevated to about 45 degrees (Figure 25-6) and the knees slightly bent.

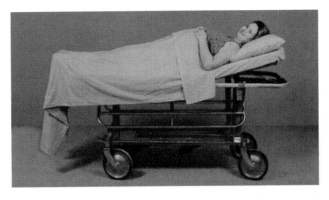

Figure 25-6 Elevation of the head and shoulders for a prenatal examination.

week 24 of pregnancy and is characterized by some combination of the following factors:

1. Systolic blood pressure of at least 140 mm Hg or a rise of 30 mm Hg or more above the usual level in two readings done 6 hours apart
2. Diastolic pressure of 90 mm Hg or more or a rise of 15 mm Hg above the usual level in two readings done 6 hours apart
3. Proteinuria
4. Edema of the face or hands
5. Excessive weight gain (more than 2.5 pounds per week)
6. Hyperreflexia

Assessment of Edema and Extremities

Ankle swelling and edema of the lower extremities occur in two thirds of women during late pregnancy. Women notice this swelling late in the day after they have been standing for some time. Sodium and water retention caused by steroid hormones, an increased hydrophilic property of intracellular connective tissue, and increased venous pressure in the lower extremities during pregnancy contribute to this edema. Assessment includes palpation of the ankles and pretibial areas to determine the extent of the edema and observation for hand, face, or generalized edema. Generalized edema may be manifested by pitting in the sacral area or by the appearance of a depression on the gravid abdomen from the rim of the fetoscope after it has been pressed against the abdomen to auscultate the fetal heart rate.

In addition to assessment for edema formation, examination of the legs includes inspection for varicose veins and dorsiflexion of the foot with the legs extended to check for Homans' sign and thrombophlebitis. In the presence of an elevated or a borderline elevated blood pressure, deep tendon reflexes should be assessed. Hyperreflexia and clonus, combined with other signs, may indicate pre-eclampsia.

Leg cramps during pregnancy may accompany extension of the foot and sudden shortening of leg muscles. This cramping may be caused by an elevation of serum phosphorus with a diet that includes a large quantity of milk.

Many discomforts and sensations in the legs result from compression of nerves caused by the pressure of the enlarging uterus. These include numbness in the lateral femoral area, resulting from compression of that nerve beneath the inguinal ligament. Medial thigh sensation may result from the compression of the obturator nerve against the side walls of the pelvis. Periodic numbness of the fingers occurs in at least 5% of gravidas. A brachial plexus traction syndrome apparently causes this from drooping shoulders. Drooping is associated with the increased weight of the breasts as pregnancy advances. Finger movement may be impaired by compression of the median nerve in the arm and hand, caused by physiological changes in the fascia, tendons, and connective tissue during pregnancy. This impairment, known as **carpal tunnel syndrome**, is characterized by a paroxysm of pain, numbness, tingling, or burning in the sides of the hands and fingers—particularly the thumb, second and third fingers, and the side of the fifth finger. (See Chapter 18.)

Abdominal Examination

As pregnancy progresses the uterus enlarges steadily. The height of the uterine fundus serves as a rough guide to fetal gestation and overall fetal growth. Figure 25-7 shows the expected fundal height at various gestational ages. At week 12 of pregnancy, the fundus is palpable just above the symphysis. At 16 weeks the fundus is approximately halfway between the symphysis and the umbilicus. At week 20 the fundus usually reaches the lower border of the umbilicus. After week 20 the uterus increases in height by approximately

3.75 cm per month (or about 1 cm per week) until weeks 34 to 36, when the fundus almost reaches the xiphoid. Then, in approximately 65% of gravidas, the fetal head drops further into the pelvis with "lightening." If this occurs, the fundal measurement at 36 weeks may be greater than that noted later in pregnancy. These benchmarks are averages, and it should be noted that the length of the torso and the position of the umbilicus are highly variable among clients. In prenatal assessment, the client serves as her own control for assessment of adequate progress of fundal growth.

Unless the fetal head drops into the pelvis, the fundal height between weeks 37 and 40 will stay approximately the same. During this period the fetus is growing, but the amount of amniotic fluid decreases.

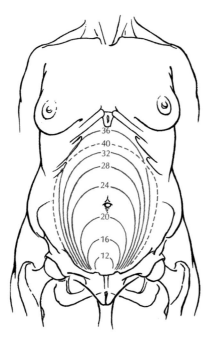

Figure 25-7 Approximate levels of the uterine fundus at various gestational points. Numbers indicate weeks of gestation.

The abdominal examination consists of the following components:

1. Inspection
2. Measurement of fundal height
3. Leopold's maneuvers for assessment of fetal position
   a. Fundal palpation
   b. Lateral palpation
   c. Pawlik's palpation
   d. Deep pelvic palpation
4. Auscultation

Inspection. In addition to the observations that are made during assessment of the abdomen (e.g., skin and scars), for the pregnant client the examiner observes the size and configuration of the enlarging uterus.

Normally the uterine size should relate to the estimated gestational age. Any discrepancy between observed size and estimated gestational age requires further exploration. A uterus larger than expected may indicate incorrect gestational age estimation, multiple pregnancy, or polyhydramnios. A smaller uterus may indicate a poorly growing fetus or miscalculation of gestational age.

Observation of the abdomen may provide the first clue to fetal presentation and position. An asymmetrical appearance or distention in width versus longitudinal enlargement may suggest a transverse or oblique fetal lie that palpation can verify. After approximately week 28, fetal movements may be seen.

Measurement of Fundal Height. Measurement of the height of the fundus provides a general assessment of the development of the pregnancy. Therefore such measurements should be taken at each prenatal visit. Before the fundal measurement is done, calculate the estimated gestational age based on the last normal menstrual period, and use the estimate of age as a benchmark against which fundal growth is assessed. Between 20 and 31 weeks' gestation, the fundal height in centimeters is approximately equal to the gestational age in weeks. In general, a 1 cm increase per week is a normal pattern.

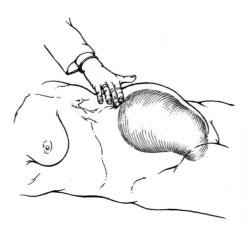

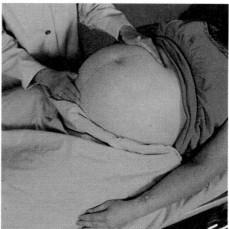

Figure 25-8 Palpation to determine the height of the uterine fundus.

The procedure for measuring the fundal height is as follows:

1. Determine the top of the fundus (Figure 25-8).
   a. Stand at the right side of the supine client, facing her head.
   b. Place your hands on each lateral side of the uterus midway between the symphysis and the fundus.
   c. Move the uterus from side to side between your hands with gentle pressure.
   d. Palpate up the sides of the uterus to the fundus, being sure to stay on the sides of the uterus.
   e. As you come near the fundus, your hands will come together, meeting at the top of the fundus.
2. Measure the distance to the fundal edge from the upper border of the symphysis with a measuring tape. Place the zero point of the tape at the top of the symphysis and measure the distance to the top of the fundus (Figure 25-9).

3. When the fundus is below the umbilicus, record the measurement in centimeters above the symphysis (preferable) or below the umbilicus. When the measurement is above the umbilicus, record the measurement in centimeters above the symphysis.

The measurement of fundal height is approximate, and estimates of fundal height measurement may vary 1 to 2 cm among examiners. However, measurement, if done consistently by one examiner or a team of examiners within a clinical situation, should provide an excellent picture of fetal growth with each visit. If fundal height is less than 4 cm less than expected, additional assessments of menstrual history or fetal status are indicated.

Leopold's Maneuvers for the Assessment of Fetal Position. Next, palpate the abdomen to determine fetal lie, presentation, position, attitude, engagement, and size.

The lie is the relationship of the long axis of the fetus to the long axis of the uterus. The lie can be longitudinal, oblique, or transverse (Figure 25-10).

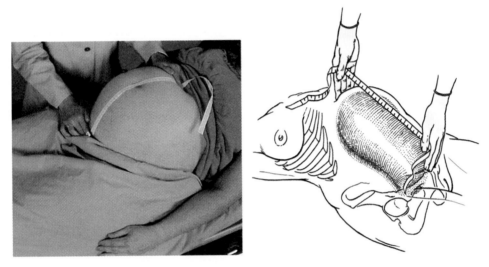

Figure 25-9 Measurement of fundal height.

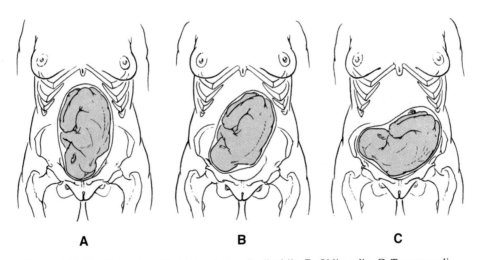

A   **B**   **C**

Figure 25-10 Examples of fetal lie. **A,** Longitudinal lie. **B,** Oblique lie. **C,** Transverse lie.

The presentation of the fetus is the fetal part that is most dependent. The presentation can be vertex, brow, face, shoulder, or breech (Figure 25-11).

The position is the relationship of a specified part of the fetal presentation, the denominator, to a particular part of the maternal pelvis (Figure 25-12). The denominator in a vertex presentation is the occiput *(O)*; in a breech presentation, it is the sacrum *(S)*; in a face presentation, it is the mentum (M), or chin; in a brow presentation, it is the frontum *(F)*; and in a transverse lie presentation, it is the scapula *(S)*. The posi-

tion is characteristically abbreviated according to the left or right of the pelvis, the denominator, and the pelvic part as follows:

Side of Pelvis	Denominator	Pelvic Part
L = Left	O = Occiput	A = Anterior
R = Right	S = Sacrum	P = Posterior
M = Mentum	T = Transverse	
F = Frontum		
S = Scapula		

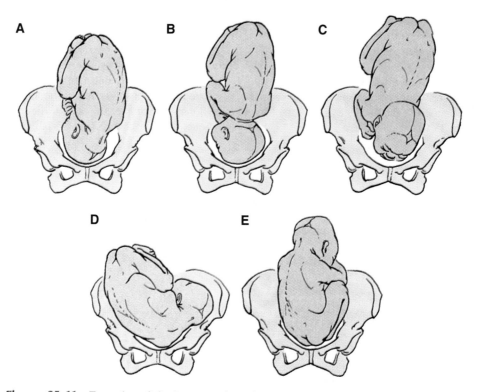

Figure 25-11   Examples of fetal presentation. **A,** Vertex. **B,** Brow. **C,** Face. **D,** Shoulder. **E,** Breech.

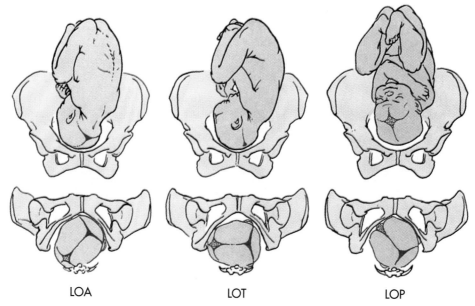

LOA   LOT   LOP

Figure 25-12   Examples of fetal position.

For example, if the occiput were presenting closest to the left anterior part of the pelvis, the fetal position would be LOA.

The fetal attitude is the relationship of the fetal head and limbs to its body (Figure 25-13). The fetus may be fully flexed, poorly flexed, or extended. When the fetus is fully flexed, the spine is flexed, the head is flexed on the chest, and the arms and legs are crossed over the chest and abdomen.

Engagement occurs when both the biparietal diameter and the suboccipitobregmatic diameter of the fetal head (the smallest anteroposterior diameter of the head when it is well flexed during labor) pass into the inlet of the pelvis (Figure 25-14). When this occurs, the fetal head can be felt at the level of the ischial spines on vaginal palpation.

Abdominal palpation determines fetal lie, presentation, position, attitude, engagement, and size. Systematically palpate the abdomen using Leopold's maneuvers in the four sequential steps as follows:
1. Fundal palpation
2. Lateral palpation
3. Pawlik's palpation
4. Deep pelvic palpation

Leopold's maneuvers are usually not especially productive until 26 to 28 weeks' gestation, when the fetus is large enough for its parts to be differentiated through abdominal and uterine structures.

For this examination the client is supine. Elevating the client's head and shoulders and bending the knees may assist in decreasing tension of the abdominal muscles and in making the examination more comfortable for the client.

■ **HELPFUL HINT**

In doing Leopold's maneuvers:
- Use the palmar surface of the fingers for palpating.
- Keep the fingers of the hand together.
- Apply firm, smooth, steady pressure as necessary to determine needed information.
- Avoid jabbing or poking movements.
- If uterine contraction occurs, wait for it to pass and then palpate less strongly.
- Have the client bend the knees to facilitate her comfort.
- Review findings with the client and teach her to recognize the fetal parts.

Fundal Palpation
1. Stand at the client's right side, facing her head.
2. Place the palmar surface of both hands on the uterine fundus to determine what part of the fetus is occupying the fundus (Figure 25-15).

Usually the buttocks of the fetus are in the fundus; they are felt as a soft, irregular, and slightly movable mass. The lower limbs are felt adjacent to the buttocks. If the head is in the fundus, it is felt as smooth, round, hard, and ballotable. The groove of the neck is felt between the trunk and the upper limbs. The head is freely movable in contrast to the buttocks, which can move only sideways and with the trunk.

Lateral Palpation (Figure 25-16)
1. While you are still facing the client's head, move both of your hands to either side of the uterus to determine the side on which the fetal back is located.
2. Support the fetus with one hand on one side while the other hand palpates the fetus on the other side.

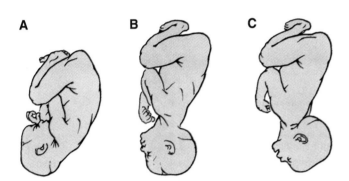

Figure 25-13 Fetal attitude. **A,** Fully flexed. **B,** Poorly flexed. **C,** Extended.

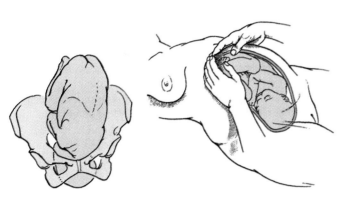

Figure 25-14 Engagement. Both the biparietal and suboccipitobregmatic diameters of the fetal head have passed into the inlet of the pelvis.

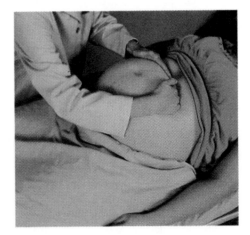

Figure 25-15 Palpation to determine the contents of the uterine fundus.

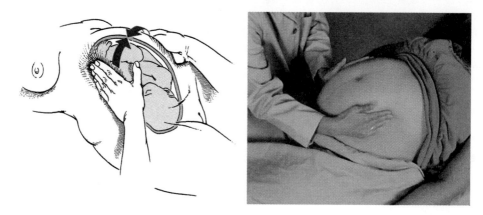

Figure 25-16   Palpation of the lateral uterine fundus to determine the position of the back and extremities of the fetus.

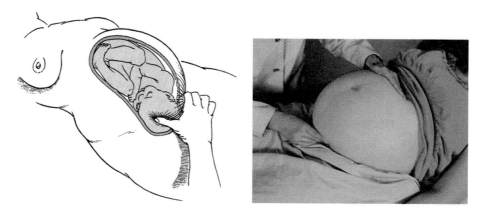

Figure 25-17   Pawlik's palpation to determine the fetal presenting part.

3. Then reverse the procedure to palpate each side of the uterus.

The fetal back is felt as a continuous, smooth, firm object, whereas the fetal limbs, or small parts, are felt as small, irregular, sometimes moving objects. On each side, palpate the flank to the midline, making special note of the edge of the fetal back as a landmark in determining the fetal position.

Pawlik's Palpation

1. Perform this procedure with the right hand only to determine what fetal part lies over the pelvic inlet. Place the right hand over the symphysis so that the fingers are on the left side of the uterus and the thumb is on the right side (Figure 25-17). The hand should be approximately around the fetal presenting part, usually the head.
2. Palpate the presenting part gently to determine its form and consistency.
3. Grasp and gently move the presenting part sideways back and forth between the thumb and fingers several times to determine its movability.

This palpation is done to confirm impressions about the presenting part and to determine whether the presenting part (usually the fetal head) is engaged. If the fetal head is movable above the symphysis, it is not engaged. If the head is not movable, it may be engaged. The only method of confirming engagement is pelvic examination to determine whether the biparietal diameter of the fetal head is level with the ischial spines.

Deep Pelvic Palpation

1. Change position (Figure 25-18). Remain on the client's right side but turn and face her feet.
2. Place a hand on each side of the uterus near the pelvic brim.
3. Ask the client to take a deep breath and to exhale slowly. As she does, allow your fingers to sink deeply above the pubic bones to palpate the presenting part and to determine the location of the cephalic prominence.

If the presenting part is the head, the location of the cephalic prominence (the forehead) helps determine the fetus's position and attitude. If the head is flexed, the occiput lies deeper in the pelvis, is flatter, and is less defined than the forehead, which is more prominent and on the same side as the small parts. If the head is not well flexed, the cephalic and occipital prominences are palpated at the same level, and the occipital part, on the same side as the back, may be more prominent.

Throughout these maneuvers, assess the congruence of the size of the fetus with the gestational age.

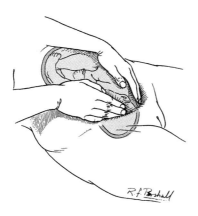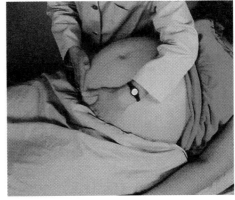

Figure 25-18 Deep pelvic palpation to determine the fetal attitude and descent.

Following is a series of questions that you, as the examiner, should mentally ask about each client during abdominal assessment and an indication of the procedures that assist in answering the questions.

Question	Source of Evidence To Answer Question
What is the fetal lie?	Abdominal inspection Lateral abdominal palpation
What is the fetal presentation?	Fundal palpation Pawlik's palpation Deep pelvic palpation
What is the fetal position?	Lateral palpation Deep pelvic palpation
What is the fetal attitude?	Deep pelvic palpation
Is the fetal growth congruent with gestational age?	Fundal height measurement All Leopold's maneuvers

Auscultation

The fetal heart rate is an indicator of fetal health status and requires monitoring throughout pregnancy. Auscultate the fetal heart rate with a special stethoscope called a fetoscope or a Doppler instrument. The Doppler instrument can be used to monitor the fetal heart rate after about 10 to 12 weeks' gestation as the fundus rises beyond the symphysis pubis. If you do not hear fetal heartbeats by Doppler monitoring after 12 to 14 weeks, re-evaluate the gestational age estimate or fetal status. With a fetoscope, the fetal heart rate can first be heard between 16 and 20 weeks' gestation.

Use of the fetoscope is demonstrated in Figure 25-19. The fetal heart rate is rapid and soft. Use of a fetoscope avoids noises produced by fingers on the stethoscope and takes advantage of the benefits of both air and bone conduction. The bell of an ordinary stethoscope can be used to auscultate fetal heart tones, but it is less effective than a fetoscope in transmitting fetal heartbeats, especially around 20 weeks.

The fetal heart rate is normally between 120 and 160 beats per minute, and the heartbeats resemble the sound of a watch's ticking heard through a pillow. These sounds are best heard through the fetal back. When the fetus is large enough for its position to be determined, place the bell of the fetoscope or the Doppler head on the fetus's posterior thorax. When the fetus is

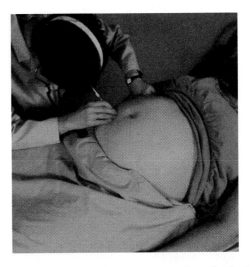

Figure 25-19 Use of a fetoscope to auscultate the fetal heart. NOTE: The hand on the bell of the fetoscope is used to adjust it. When the fetal heartbeats are actually being measured, the hand should be removed.

less than 20 weeks' gestation, the heart rate is often best heard at the midline, just above the pubic hairline.

Count the fetal heart rate for at least 15 seconds, and record it in number of beats per minute according to the location of maximal intensity (by the abdominal quadrant in which it is most prominent). The fetal heart rate is normally much faster than the maternal heart rate, and therefore it can usually be well differentiated from it. Moreover, the fetal and maternal heart rates are not synchronous. Differentiate the maternal rate by palpating the mother's pulse while auscultating the abdomen.

Sounds other than the maternal and fetal heart tones can be heard in the uterus. Blood rushing through the placenta is called uterine souffle. The uterine souffle is a soft, blowing sound that is synchronous with the maternal pulse. The intensity of the souffle has been interpreted as an indicator of uterine blood flow and placental function. A loud uterine souffle has been associated with high levels of urinary es-

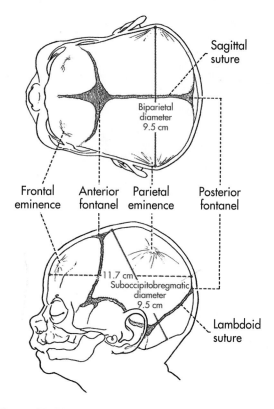

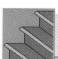

Figure 25-20 Various diameters of the fetal head at term.

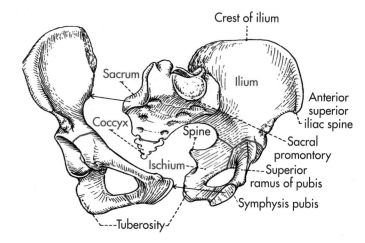

Figure 25-21 Bones of the pelvis.

Examination Step-by-Step

The following steps outline interval abdominal assessment for the pregnant client:
1. Measure fundal height.
2. Palpate the abdomen to determine fetal position using Leopold's maneuvers:
   a. Fundal palpation
   b. Lateral palpation
   c. Pawlik's palpation
   d. Deep pelvic palpation
3. Auscultate fetal heart tones

triol and a soft or absent souffle with lower estriol levels. Thus a soft or absent uterine souffle may indicate poor uterine blood flow and placental function, particularly in late pregnancy. Occasionally the blood flow in the umbilical artery can be auscultated. The sound is similar to a bruit and, as a rule, the rate is equal to the fetal heart tones. However, the sound does not have distinct heart sounds; rather it is similar to the uterine souffle.

Examination of the Bony Pelvis

The purpose of the examination of the bony pelvis is to determine whether the pelvic cavity is large enough to allow for passage of a full-term infant. Clinical pelvimetry is a gross estimate of the adequacy of the pelvis for delivery of a fetus. It is not uncommon for clients whose pelves have been assessed to be of borderline adequacy to deliver full-term infants vaginally. If the clinical assessment in early pregnancy indicates a possible inadequacy, the pelvis needs to be reassessed clinically and possibly by x-ray examination in late pregnancy and in relationship to the size of the infant at term. This examination is performed on the initial prenatal evaluation; it need not be repeated if the pelvis is of adequate size. However, if findings indicate that the pelvis is of borderline adequacy, or if you are unable to adequately perform the examination on the initial visit because of the client's tenseness and subsequent muscular contraction, repeat the examination at approximately 36 weeks' gestation. In the third trimester, the pelvic joints and ligaments relax,

and the client is more accustomed to examination. Thus you can more thoroughly and accurately accomplish examination of the bony pelvis at that time.

The examination of the bony pelvis is done not so much to diagnose the type of pelvis but to determine its configuration and size. Because the examiner does not have direct access to the bony structures and because the bones are covered with variable amounts of soft tissue, estimates are approximate. X-ray examination can provide precise bony pelvis measurements. However, x-rays are not needed or indicated for the vast majority of prenatal clients.

The assessment of the bony pelvis must be put in the perspective of the capacity necessary to accommodate a full-term fetus. When the head of a full-term fetus is well flexed, the two largest presenting diameters are the biparietal and the suboccipitobregmatic, each measuring approximately 9.5 cm (Figure 25-20).

The pelvis consists of four bones: the two innominate bones, the sacrum, and the coccyx. Each innominate bone consists of three bones that fuse after puberty. These three bones are the ilium, the ischium, and the pubis (Figure 25-21). The innominate bones form the anterior and lateral parts of the pelvis.

The sacrum and the coccyx constitute the posterior part of the pelvis. The sacrum is composed of five fused verte-

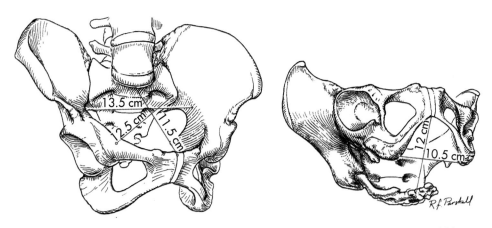

Figure 25-22 Planes of the pelvic inlet and midpelvis. (Measurements are averages within normal limits.)

brae. Its upper anterior part is called the sacral promontory, which forms the posterior margin of the pelvic brim. The coccyx is composed of three to five fused vertebrae and articulates with the sacrum.

The pelvis is divided by the brim into two parts: the false pelvis and the true pelvis. The false pelvis is the part above the brim and is of no obstetrical interest.

The brim and the area below it constitute the true pelvis. The true pelvis is divided into three parts: the inlet or brim, the midpelvis or cavity, and the outlet. The inlet is formed anteriorly by the upper margins of the pubic bones, laterally by the iliopectineal lines, and posteriorly by the anterior upper margin of the sacrum, the sacral promontory. The cavity is formed anteriorly by the posterior aspect of the symphysis pubis, laterally by the inner surfaces of the ischial and iliac bones, and posteriorly by the anterior surface of the sacrum. The outlet, which is diamond shaped, is formed anteriorly by the inferior rami of the pubic and ischial bones, laterally by the ischial tuberosities, and posteriorly by the inferior edge of the sacrum (if the coccyx is movable).

Each of the pelvic parts can be imagined as a series of planes: the plane of the brim (or pelvic inlet), the plane of the midpelvis, and the plane of the outlet. These planes are illustrated in Figure 25-22.

The plane of the inlet in an average female pelvis measures approximately 11 to 13 cm in the anteroposterior diameter and 13 to 14 cm in the transverse diameter. The anteroposterior diameter of the inlet, measured from the middle of the sacral promontory to the superior posterior margin of the symphysis pubis, is called the true conjugate and is an important obstetrical measurement. However, only radiographic methods can be used to directly assess this measurement. The true conjugate can be estimated by measuring the diagonal conjugate, which is the distance between the inferior border of the symphysis pubis and the sacral promontory. The diagonal conjugate is approximately 1 to 2 cm longer than the true conjugate, depending on the height and inclination of the symphysis. The clinical measurement of the diagonal conjugate, the most valuable single measurement of pelvic adequacy, is discussed later in this section.

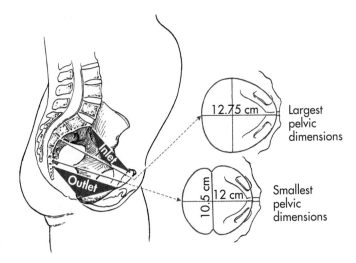

Figure 25-23 Pelvic outlet.

The midpelvis contains the planes of greatest and least pelvic dimensions. The plane of least pelvic dimensions is bounded by the junction of the fourth and fifth sacral vertebrae, the symphysis, and the ischial spines. The average dimensions of this plane are 12 cm (anteroposterior diameter) and 10.5 cm (transverse diameter). The transverse diameter is the distance between the ischial spines.

The pelvic outlet is composed of two triangular planes, having a common base in the most inferior part of the transverse diameter between the ischial tuberosities. The obstetrical anteroposterior diameter of the outlet is the distance between the inferior edge of the symphysis pubis and the edge of the sacrum (if the coccyx is movable). This measurement is usually 11.5 cm.

The transverse diameter of the outlet is the distance between the inner surfaces of the ischial tuberosities and usually measures approximately 11 cm (Figure 25-23).

Although there is a characteristic shape of the adult female pelvis that is different from the characteristic male pelvis, a female client may have any one of four types of human pelves, or a mixture of these types. In addition, the shape of the pelvis may have been distorted congenitally or by disease.

The four basic pelvic types, as originally classified by Caldwell, Maloy, and Swenson (1939), are (1) gynecoid, (2) android, (3) anthropoid, and (4) platypelloid.

The typical female pelvis is the gynecoid pelvis, which is found in approximately 40% to 50% of adult women. This pelvis is characterized by a rounded inlet, except for a slight projection of the sacral promontory; a deep posterior half made possible by a wide sacrosciatic notch and concave sacrum; and a wide anterior half made possible by a wide, subpubic angle.

The android pelvis is found in approximately 15% to 20% of adult women. This pelvic type is roughly wedge- or heart-shaped, with the transverse diameter of the inlet approxi-mately equal to the anteroposterior diameter but with the widest transverse diameter located closer to the sacrum. Other characteristics of the android pelvis include the following:

1. Narrow subpubic arch
2. Convergent side walls
3. Large, encroaching spines
4. Short sacrosciatic notch and sacrospinous ligament
5. Short interspinous diameter
6. Straight sacrum
7. Short intertuberous diameter

The anthropoid pelvis has an elongated anteroposterior diameter and is found in approximately 25% to 35% of women. It is characterized by the following:

1. Narrow subpubic arch
2. Prominent ischial spines

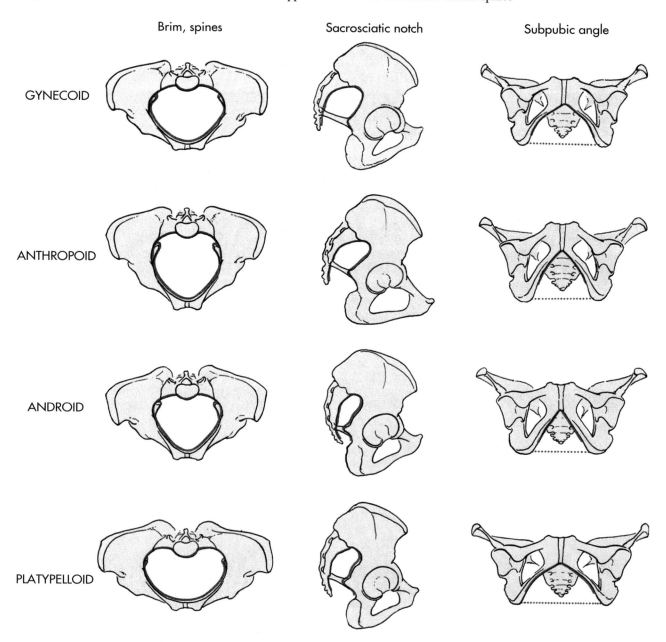

	Brim, spines	Sacrosciatic notch	Subpubic angle
GYNECOID			
ANTHROPOID			
ANDROID			
PLATYPELLOID			

Figure 25-24   Comparisons of various parts of the four basic pelvic types.

3. Wide sacrosciatic notch and long sacrospinous ligaments
4. Deeply curved sacrum

The platypelloid pelvis has a flattened anteroposterior dimension with a relative widening of the transverse diameter. This pelvic type is seen in approximately 5% of women. The platypelloid pelvis is characterized by the following:

1. Wide subpubic arch
2. Flat ischial spines
3. Wide sacrosciatic notch and long sacrospinous ligaments
4. Straight sacrum

The various dimensions of the four basic pelvic types are compared and contrasted in Figure 25-24. Pure pelvic types are unusual; most pelves are mixtures of two pelvic types, with the characteristics of one type predominating.

Because examination of the bony pelvis can be uncomfortable, perform it after the internal examination of the soft pelvic organs. In preparing the client, include an explanation of the procedure, the client's emptying of her bladder, and instructions on relaxation.

A standard procedure for the bony pelvis examination is recommended. Begin with examination of the anterior pelvis, proceed to lateral examination on one side, compare the initially examined side with the opposite side, and conclude with examination of the posterior and inferior parts.

The following bony pelvis parts and landmarks are especially important in examining the pelvis:

1. Subpubic arch
2. Symphysis pubis
3. Side walls
4. Ischial spines
5. Sacrosciatic notch
6. Sacrum
7. Coccyx
8. Sacral promontory
9. Ischial tuberosities

The following is a recommended procedure for assessment of the bony pelvis:

1. Palpate the width of the subpubic arch, and estimate its angle. Normally, both examining fingers should fit comfortably in the arch, which optimally forms an angle that measures slightly greater than a right angle (90-degree angle) (Figure 25-25).

2. Estimate the length and inclination of the symphysis pubis by sweeping the examining fingers under the symphysis (Figure 25-26). Also, palpate the retropubic curve of the forepelvis and envision its configuration. Measurement difficulties created by a large amount of soft tissue in the area and reliability with slope measurements preclude a precise estimation of the length and inclination of the symphysis. Essentially, you are screening for an unusually long or steeply inclined symphysis pubis and for an angular rather than a rounded forepelvis.

3. Examine the right or the left lateral pelvic area. First, palpate the side walls to determine whether they are straight, convergent, or divergent. Assess the splay of the side walls by following a line from the point of origin of the widest transverse diameter of the inlet downward to the inner aspect of the tuberosity. Another method for assessing the side walls is to place the examining fingers on the base of the ischial spine as a landmark and then to palpate above and below the landmark to determine the inclination.

4. Examine the ischial spine and the sacrospinous ligament on that same side. Assess the spines as being blunt, prominent, or encroaching. Outline the sacrosciatic notch with palpating fingers, if possible, and determine its width in centimeters or fingerbreadths. Often, tracing the entire notch is difficult, and the sacrospinous ligament is useful in estimating the width of the notch (Figure 25-27).

5. Examine the other side of the pelvis in the manner previously described to determine overall pelvic symmetry. Attempt to do this part of the examination with the palm of the hand up, rather than rotating the hand so that the palm is down.

6. Estimate the interspinous diameter by moving the examining fingers in a straight line from one spine across to the other (Figure 25-28). You may need to

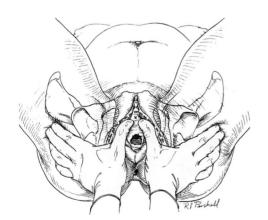

Figure 25-25 Method of estimating the angle of the subpubic arch.

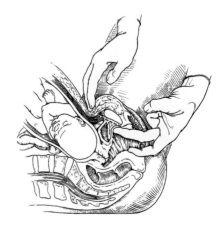

Figure 25-26 Estimation of the length and inclination of the symphysis pubis.

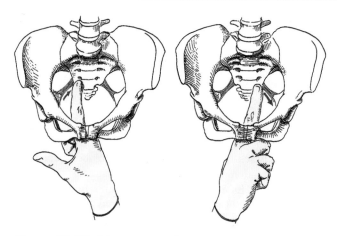

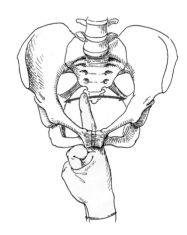

Figure 25-27 Measurement of the width of the sacrosciatic notch.

Figure 25-28 Measurement of the interspinous diameter.

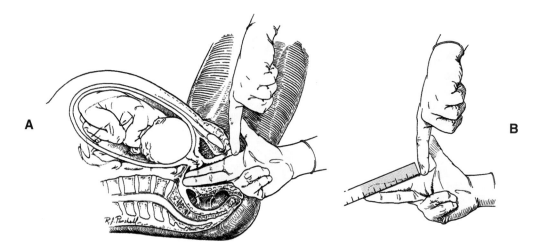

Figure 25-29 Measurement of the diagonal conjugate. **A,** Internal palpation. **B,** Use of a ruler to specify the estimation in centimeters.

pronate the hand for this estimation. Calculate the estimate in centimeters. The usual measurement is 10.5 cm.

7. Next examine the sacrum and the coccyx. Sweep the fingers down the sacrum, noting whether it is straight, curved, or hollow and whether its inclination is forward or backward. Examine the coccyx gently because it may be tender on movement. Gently press the coccyx backward to determine whether it is movable or fixed. Note its tilt as anterior or posterior.

8. Assess the diagonal conjugate last because this assessment can be uncomfortable for the client. A moderate amount of constant pressure is necessary to depress the perineum adequately. Exert pressure with your body rather than with the hand and forearm. Place your foot (the one on the same side as the examining hand) on a stool and the elbow of the examining arm on your thigh or hip. Then apply the needed pressure, controlling it with your body. For this examination, make sure that your fingers and wrist form a straight line with your forearm.

Locate the sacrum with the examining fingers, and with the middle finger "walk" up the sacrum until you reach the promontory or until you can no longer touch the sacrum. Mark the point where the client's symphysis touches your hand with the thumb of the opposite hand, and measure the distance in centimeters with a ruler (Figure 25-29). In obstetrical examining rooms, a ruler is often fixed to the wall for this measurement.

Often you will not reach the sacral promontory. Become familiar with the "reach" of your examining fingers and record the findings as greater than (>) the centimeters of this reach. Normally, the diagonal conjugate is >12.5 cm.

9. Withdraw the examining hand from the vagina, and measure the intertuberous diameter. Then, with both thumbs, externally trace the descending rami down to the tuberosities. Then make a fist and attempt to insert the fist between the tuberosities to measure the transverse diameter of an outlet (Figure 25-30). The intertuberous diameter is usually 10 to 11 cm.

TABLE 25-3   Recommendations of the U.S. Preventive Services Task Force for All Pregnant Women

Screening Recommendations	Other Recommendations
First Visit Screening Blood pressure Hemoglobin/hematocrit Hepatitis B surface antigen RPR or VDRL to screen for syphilis *Chlamydia* screen (<25 yr) Rubella serology or vaccination history D(Rh) typing, antibody screen Offer CVS (<13 wk) or amniocentesis (15-18 wk) (age >35) for detection of fetal abnormality Offer hemoglobinopathy screening Assess for problem or risk drinking Offer HIV screening Asymptomatic bacteriuria with urine culture (12-16 wk) **Follow-Up Visit Screening** Blood pressure Urine culture Offer multiple marker testing (15-18 wk) Offer serum α-fetoprotein (16-18 wk)	**Counseling** Tobacco cessation/effects of passive smoking Cease use of alcohol and other drugs Nutrition, including adequate calcium intake Encourage breast-feeding Use lap and shoulder belts Use infant safety car seats Sexually transmitted infection prevention **Chemoprophylaxis** Multivitamin with folic acid

Data from U. S. Preventive Services Task Force: *Guide to clinical preventive services: an assessment of the effectiveness of 169 interventions,* ed. 2, Baltimore, 1996, Williams & Wilkins.
CVS, Chorionic villus sampling (for this test, villus cells from the placenta are aspirated); *HIV,* human immunodeficiency virus; *RPR,* rapid plasma reagin; VDRL, Venereal Disease Research Laboratory.

Again, know the span of your own fist and estimate the intertuberous diameter accordingly.

In summary, the areas of bony pelvic examination and the assessment descriptors for these areas follow:

Sequence of Areas of Bony Pelvic

Examination	Assessment Descriptors
1. Subpubic arch	*Inclination:* Less than 90 degrees, more than 90 degrees
2. Side walls	*Direction:* Parallel, convergent, divergent
3. Ischial spines	*Size:* Small, average, large *Prominence:* Blunt, prominent, encroaching
4. Sacrosciatic	*Length:* Estimated width or length in notch; centimeters (usual length = 3 to 4 cm) sacrospinous ligament
5. Opposite	*Symmetry:* Symmetrical, asymmetrical pelvic side
6. Interspinous	*Length:* Estimated length in centimeters (usual length = diameter 10.5 cm)
7. Sacrum	*Shape:* Concave, straight, convex
8. Coccyx	*Position:* Straight, projects anteriorly, projects posteriorly *Movability:* Movable, fixed
9. Diagonal	*Length:* Actual length or length greater than the conjugate measurement that the examiner can reach (usual length = 12.5 cm)

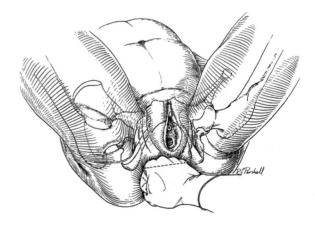

Figure 25-30   Use of a fist to estimate the intertuberous diameter.

10. Intertuberous	*Length:* Actual length in centimeters if Thom's pelvimeter diameter is used, or an estimated length using a closed fist (usual length is 10 to 11 cm)

Screening Tests and Procedures

General Recommendations

The recommendations of the U.S. Preventive Services Task Force (1996) and the American College of Obstetrics and Gynecologists are provided in Tables 25-3 and 25-4.

Teaching Self-Assessment

BREAST CARE

Wear a supportive bra that fits well.
Avoid nipple stimulation that would cause colostrum leakage.
Attend to any cracks or skin dryness immediately.

GASTROINTESTINAL HEALTH

For nausea: eat small, frequent meals; avoid spicy foods and
 fatty foods; get adequate rest; use antacids in moderation and
 with the permission of the health care provider.
For constipation: drink 8 to 10 glasses of water a day; increase
 fiber intake; exercise regularly.

URINARY TRACT HEALTH

Drink 8 to 10 glasses of water a day.
Avoid caffeinated beverages.
Void frequently and regularly.

MANAGING EDEMA

Elevate feet whenever possible.
Do not sit for more than 1 hour.
Take frequent short walks.
Wear supportive hose.

COMFORT

Lying on the left side with a pillow between the legs is usually
 the most comfortable position. This position also prevents
 supine hypotension.
Do low-intensity stretching exercises regularly.
Wear low-heeled, comfortable shoes.

TABLE 25-4	Recommendations of the U. S. Preventive Services Task Force for High-Risk Pregnant Women

Risk	Screening and Counseling Recommendations
High-risk sexual behavior	*Chlamydia* screening (first visit) Gonorrhea screening (first visit) HIV screening (first visit) HBsAg screening (third trimester) Repeat RPR/VDRL (third trimester)
Blood transfusion between 1978-1985	HIV screening (first visit)
Injection drug use	HIV screening (first visit) HBsAg (third trimester) Counseling to reduce infection risk
Unsensitized D-negative women	D(Rh) antibody testing (24-28 wk)
Risk factors for Down syndrome	Offer CVS (first trimester), amniocentesis (15-18 wk)
Prior pregnancy with neural tube defect	Folic acid 4 mg Offer amniocentesis (15-18 wk)

Data from U. S. Preventive Services Task Force: *Guide to clinical preventive services: an assessment of the effectiveness of 169 interventions,* ed. 2, Baltimore, 1996, Williams & Wilkins.
CVS, Chorionic villi sampling; *HBsAg,* hepatitis B surface antigen; *HIV,* human immunodeficiency virus,

Assessments Near Term

Two additional assessments of changes are done near the expected date of delivery: estimation of the length and dilation of the cervix and determination of the fetal station. Figure 25-31 illustrates a method of measuring the length of the cervix. Before 34 to 36 weeks' gestation, the cervix should maintain its usual length of 1.5 to 2 cm. During the last 4 weeks of gestation, the cervix shortens as the fetal head

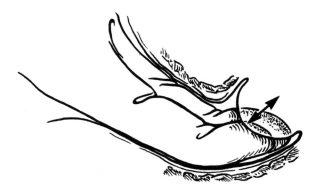

Figure 25-31 Measurement of cervical length. Use bidigital palpation to estimate the length of the cervix. Usual length before labor is 1.5 to 2 cm.

descends, and the internal cervical os softens and opens and is pulled upward and incorporated into the isthmus of the uterus. When the cervix shortens (effaces), it also begins to dilate. Cervical dilation is estimated by the diameter of the cervical os and is measured in centimeters—from 0 cm when closed to 10 cm when completely opened.

The degree of descent of the fetal presenting part, usually the head, is measured by the station. Station refers to the relationship of the presenting part to the plane of the ischial spines. If the lowest part of the presenting part is at the level of the spines, it is at station 0. Other stations of the fetal presenting part are the following:

Minus 3	At the pelvic inlet
Minus 2	One third of the distance from the inlet to the spines
Minus 1	Two thirds of the distance from the inlet to the spines
Station 0	At the level of the ischial spines
Plus 1	One third of the distance between the spines and the pelvic floor
Plus 2	Two thirds of the distance between the spines and the pelvic floor
Plus 3	At the pelvic floor

Sample Documentation and Diagnoses

FOCUSED HEALTH HISTORY (SUBJECTIVE DATA)

Mrs. A, a 24-year-old primigravid client, is in for a routine prenatal visit (estimated gestation of 20 weeks). Has been feeling better since last visit 1 month ago. Nausea and vomiting have ceased. Complains of mild pain in her breasts and a mild amount of lower abdominal and leg discomfort at night, which is alleviated by elevation of legs in the evening. Less urinary frequency than in early pregnancy, but gets up to void about two times each night. She and her husband are becoming more enthusiastic about the baby. Husband is assisting more around the home. Mrs A. plans to work until the baby is born and then take a 6- to 8-week postpartum leave. Fetal movements were first felt 3 weeks ago and are increasing in intensity. Occasional mild Braxton Hicks contractions noted. No vaginal bleeding or discharge. No other problems.

FOCUSED PHYSICAL EXAMINATION (OBJECTIVE DATA)

BP: 118/76.
Weight: 165 lb (prepregnant = 140 lb); 8 lb weight gain since last visit.
Urine: Negative for glucose, albumin, and ketones.
Extremities: No edema.
Breasts: Full; consistently glandular; no lesions palpated. Small amount of watery fluid expressed from both nipples.
Abdominal assessment: Fundus at umbilicus (consistent with estimated 20 weeks' gestation), measuring 19 cm. Fetal position uncertain because of small fetal size. Fetal heart tones heard in midline, regular at 158 beats/min.

DIAGNOSES

HEALTH PROBLEMS

Routine prenatal care

NURSING DIAGNOSES

Risk for Imbalanced Nutrition: More Than Body Requirements

Defining Characteristics
Weight 10% to 20% over ideal for height and frame
Weight gain of 25 lb in first 20 weeks of pregnancy

Acute Pain Related to Physical Body Changes During Pregnancy

Defining Characteristics
Pain in breasts
Pain in lower abdomen and legs

Disturbed Sleep Pattern Related to Frequent Urination at Night

Defining Characteristic
Interrupted sleep two times each night to void

Critical Thinking Questions

Review the Sample Documentation and Diagnoses box to answer questions 1 to 3.

1. This client asks about changes she should expect in herself and in the fetus during the next month. What would you tell her?
2. What weight in this client would you have expected between 16 and 20 weeks?
3. If this client were Mexican-American, what cultural issues might affect her response to prenatal care?
4. Your client is a recent immigrant from a country whose culture is not familiar to you. How would you assess the cultural influences on her pregnancy?
5. Describe the physical findings for a woman who is 12 weeks' pregnant.

 Answers are available on the MERLIN website (www.harcourthealth.com/MERLIN/Barkauskas/). And be sure to check the website regularly for additional learning activities!

Remember to check out the Online Study Guide!
www.harcourthealth.com/MERLIN/Barkauskas/

Chapter **26**

Pediatric Clients

Learning Objectives

On successful study of this chapter and completion of related learning experiences, the learner will be able to:
- Describe the usual schedule for well-child care.
- Perform a thorough pediatric health history that is appropriate for families with children during each developmental period (infants through adolescents).

- Identify strategies for obtaining history information from both the child and caregiver.
- Apply various strategies to address the emotional and developmental needs of both the child and the parents.
- Perform a comprehensive pediatric physical assessment, modifying it according to the differing needs of infants, young children, adolescents, and adults.

Outline

Purpose of Examination

To a large extent, pediatric care is health care aimed at promoting the health of the child and preventing illness and disability through early identification of problems, anticipatory guidance to help parents deal with physical and developmental issues before they become problems, and early and ongoing intervention for health care needs.

Ideally the practitioner performs the examination of the child over an extended time in a planned sequential pattern. The dynamic changes that occur throughout the child's normal growth and development require that the practitioner assess certain aspects carefully: increments in growth; changes in physiological function; and development of cognitive, social, and motor skills of the child during each examination.

The health of the child is determined by comparing the individual child's current growth achievements and parameters of health with those found in his or her previous examinations and with norms for children in the same age range. The practitioner should see the child frequently, usually every 2 to 3 months for well-child care during infancy, when growth changes are most rapid and dramatic. The practitioner should assess the older child at regular, but less frequent, intervals for well-child care.

To provide holistic care to the child, it is also important to consider the needs and concerns of the child's primary caretaker(s), usually the parents. The adults responsible for the child's care often have questions and concerns about the child's development and about their own ability to manage care. The practitioner needs to encourage them to express their concerns and to discuss their needs in addition to the needs of the child.

The examiner should have a sense of the parent as a person. What are the stresses and issues that the parents are dealing with? What impact do these factors have on their ability to parent? Parents who feel that their questions and concerns are being heard and that they are receiving support and respect will be better able to care for their children (Figure 26-1).

A part of each well-child assessment (and sick-child visit, if that is the only time that the family comes in for care, or if the potential for problems is apparent during an acute care visit) should address anticipatory guidance. Anticipatory guidance involves teaching parents what to expect in terms of their child's physical, cognitive, emotional, and social development. The goal of anticipatory guidance is to promote positive parent-child relationships and prevent the development of emotional and behavioral disturbances related to difficulties in parent-child interactions.

Commonly, problems develop because parents or caregivers are unaware that "problem" behaviors are in fact normal stage-specific behaviors related to development. Examples include the "stranger anxiety" demonstrated when a 9-month-old is picked up by his grandmother whom he sees infrequently and the "negativism" of the 2-year-old. Helping parents identify what is normal development versus abnormal or problem behavior can help parents feel more secure in their ability to respond to their children. For example, the 9-month-old will still cry when picked up by the "stranger," his grandmother, but his parents will be able to identify this reaction as a normal (although embarrassing) behavior rather than a reflection of being "spoiled" by his parents.

Anticipatory guidance also involves helping the parent identify and problem solve around problematic areas. Examples include talking with a parent about how to deal with

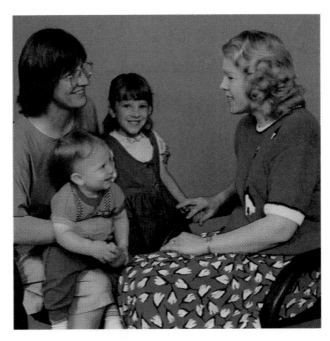

Figure 26-1 Attention to the concerns of both the parent and the child is an important component of the assessment.

negativism or temper tantrums and anticipating what to do if the child has a tantrum in the grocery store and helping parents who are planning to bring their 9-month-old child to a family reunion consider ways to introduce their child to relatives in a nonthreatening manner.

Anticipatory guidance can also be used to help new parents address potentially difficult issues before they become a source of family conflict. Common challenges parents face are differences in each parent's attitude toward discipline or differing expectations about the role each parent plays in child care activities.

Assessing the quality of the parent-child relationship is crucial. The practitioner should support positive interactions (Figure 26-2). Receiving recognition for their parenting skills is especially helpful for parents. The practitioner also should be alert to any signs of stress between the parent and the child. A mother who is concerned, anxious, or angry about a child's behavior or physical condition may actually be showing evidence of stress that can interfere with the mother-child relationship and ultimately with the child's development (Box 26-1 lists some parenting red flags). Identification of difficulties in the parent-child interaction allows the practitioner to initiate interventions to promote more positive interactions. This issue emphasizes the importance of considering needs of the parent or other adults caring for the child in addition to those of the child.

The practitioner should always demonstrate respect for both the child and the parent, be willing to listen to problems, and help in finding adequate solutions. Both the child and the parent will be aware of the practitioner's attitudes and will respond according to their impressions. In essence,

BOX 26-1

PARENTING RED FLAGS

MODERATE CONCERN

Disinclination to separate from child or prematurely hastening separation

Signs of despondency, apathy, or hostility

Fearful, dependent, apprehensive

Disinterested in or rejection of infant or child

Overly critical, mocking, and censuring of child; tendency to undermine child's confidence

Inconsistent in discipline or control; erratic in behavior

Very restrictive and overly moralistic environment

EXTREME CONCERN

Extreme depression and withdrawal; rejection of child

Intense hostility; aggression toward child

Uncontrollable fears, anxieties, guilt

Complete inability to function in family role

Severe moralistic prohibition of child's independent strivings

Domestic abuse or violence in the home

Self-destructive behaviors: alcohol or drug abuse

From Burns CE et al.: *Pediatric primary care: a handbook for nurse practitioners,* ed. 2, Philadelphia, 2000, WB Saunders.

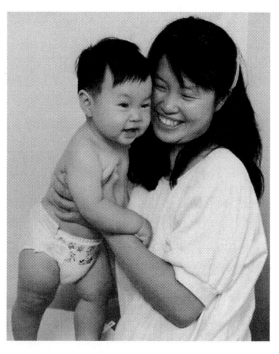

Figure 26-2 The quality of the parent-child interaction needs to be assessed, and positive attitudes should be supported.

it is important to be sensitive to the child as a growing, developing human being who is always changing.

This chapter discusses approaches to the child and the parent, as well as some techniques to obtain health information and to assess the child's health. In addition, it covers some of the physical differences between the child and the adult. Because it is not possible to include a survey of all the components of child development that are assessed, the reader is referred to the material on child developmental assessment in Chapter 5 and to standard pediatric texts for assistance in understanding the parameters of normal development and health of children.

GUIDELINES FOR HEALTH SUPERVISION

Much of the care given to children focuses on health promotion and the prevention of disease. The American Academy of Pediatrics (AAP) (1995) suggests the schedule of well-child care shown in Table 26-1 for the care of children who (1) are receiving competent parenting, (2) have no manifestations of any important health problems, and (3) are growing and developing in a satisfactory fashion. The following situations may warrant additional visits:

1. Firstborn or adopted children or those not with natural parents
2. Parents with a particular need for education and guidance
3. Families from a disadvantaged social or economic environment
4. Presence or possibility of perinatal disorders (e.g., prematurity, low birth weight, congenital defects, or familial diseases)
5. Children with acquired illness or previously identified diseases or problems

EXAMINATION

Pediatric History

The pediatric history provides the opportunity to interview both the child and the parent (or caregiver) to gather information about the child's health, development, relationships with others, and care. It also offers the opportunity for the child to become acquainted with the practitioner before being examined. The pediatric history is an adaptation of the model used for the adult history (see Chapter 3). It incorporates areas uniquely pertinent to the child, such as the history of the mother's health during the pregnancy, the history of birth and the neonatal period, and specific areas related to the child's psychosocial development (e.g., stage-related behaviors, school performance, peer relationships).

TABLE 26-1 Recommendations for Preventive Pediatric Health Care (RE9939)

Committee on Practice and Ambulatory Medicine

Each child and family is unique; therefore, these **Recommendations for Preventive Pediatric Health Care** are designed for the care of children who are receiving competent parenting, have no manifestations of any important health problems, and are growing and developing in satisfactory fashion. **Additional visits may become necessary** if circumstances suggest variations from normal.

These guidelines represent a consensus by the Committee on Practice and Ambulatory Medicine in consultation with national committees and sections of the American Academy of Pediatrics. The Committee emphasizes the great importance of **continuity of care** in comprehensive health supervision and the need to avoid **fragmentation of care.**

AGE[5]	Prenatal[1]	Newborn[2]	2–4d[3]	By 1 mo	2 mo	4 mo	6 mo	9 mo	12 mo	15 mo	18 mo	24 mo	3 y	4 y
				Infancy[4]						Early Childhood[4]				
HISTORY Initial/Interval	• ·	•	•	•	•	•	•	•	•	•	•	•	•	•
MEASUREMENTS Height and Weight		•	•	•	•	•	•	•	•	•	•	•	•	•
Head Circumference		•	•	•	•	•	•	•	•	•	•	•		
Blood Pressure													•	•
SENSORY SCREENING Vision	S	S	S	S	S	S	S	S	S	S	S	O[6]	O	
Hearing	O[7]	S	S	S	S	S	S	S	S	S	S	S	O	
DEVELOPMENTAL/ BEHAVIORAL ASSESSMENT[8]		•	•	•	•	•	•	•	•	•	•	•	•	•
PHYSICAL EXAMINATION[9]		•	•	•	•	•	•	•	•	•	•	•	•	•
PROCEDURES-GENERAL[10] Hereditary/Metabolic Screening[11]		←	•	→										
Immunization[12]		•	•	•	•	•	•	•	•	•	•	•	•	•
Hematocrit or Hemoglobin[13]								←	→	*	*	*	*	*
Urinalysis														
PROCEDURES-PATIENTS AT RISK Lead Screening[16]								*	→			*		
Tuberculin Test[17]										*	*	*	*	*
Cholesterol Screening[18]												*	*	*
STD Screening[19]														
Pelvic Exam[20]														
ANTICIPATORY GUIDANCE[21]	•	•	•	•	•	•	•	•	•	•	•	•	•	•
Injury Prevention[22]	•	•	•	•	•	•	•	•	•	•	•	•	•	•
Violence Prevention[23]	•	•	•	•	•	•	•	•	•	•	•	•	•	•
Sleep Positioning Counseling[24]	•	•	•	•	•	•								
Nutrition Counseling[25]	•	•	•	•	•	•	•	•	•	•	•	•	•	•
DENTAL REFERRAL[26]										←			•	

Used with permission of the American Academy of Pediatrics.

1. A prenatal visit is recommended for parents who are at high risk, for first-time parents, and for those who request a conference. The prenatal visit should include anticipatory guidance, pertinent medical history, and a discussion of benefits of breastfeeding and planned method of feeding per AAP statement "The Prenatal Visit" (1996).
2. Every infant should have a newborn evaluation after birth. Breastfeeding should be encouraged and instruction and support offered. Every breastfeeding infant should have an evaluation 48-72 hours after discharge from the hospital to include weight, formal breastfeeding evaluation, encouragement, and instruction as recommended in the AAP statement "Breastfeeding and the Use of Human Milk" (1997).
3. For newborns discharged in less than 48 hours after delivery per AAP statement "Hospital Stay for Healthy Term Newborns" (1995).
4. Developmental, psychosocial, and chronic disease issues for children and adolescents may require frequent counseling and treatment visits separate from preventive care visits.
5. If a child comes under care for the first time at any point on the schedule, or if any items are not accomplished at the suggested age, the schedule should be brought up to date at the earliest possible time.
6. If the patient is uncooperative, rescreen within 6 months.
7. All newborns should be screened per the AAP Task Force on Newborn and Infant Hearing statement, "Newborn and Infant Hearing Loss: Detection and Intervention" (1999).
8. By history and appropriate physical examination: if suspicious, by specific objective developmental testing. Parenting skills should be fostered at every visit.
9. At each visit, a complete physical examination is essential, with infant totally unclothed, older child undressed and suitably draped.
10. These may be modified, depending upon entry point into schedule and individual need.
11. Metabolic screening (e.g., thyroid, hemoglobinopathies, PKU, galactosemia) should be done according to state law.
12. Schedule(s) per the Committee on Infectious Diseases, published annually in the January edition of *Pediatrics*. Every visit should be an opportunity to update and complete a child's immunizations.
13. See AAP *Pediatric Nutrition Handbook* (1998) for a discussion of universal and selective screening options. Consider earlier screening for high-risk infants (e.g., premature infants and low birth weight infants). See also "Recommendations to Prevent and Control Iron Deficiency in the United States," *MMWR* 47 (RR-3):1-29,1998.
14. All menstruating adolescents should be screened annually.
15. Conduct dipstick urinalysis for leukocytes annually for sexually active male and female adolescents.
16. For children at risk of lead exposure consult the AAP statement "Screening for Elevated Blood Levels" (1998). Additionally, screening should be done in accordance with state law where applicable.
17. TB testing per recommendations of the Committee on Infectious Diseases, published in the current edition of *Red Book: Report of the Committee on Infectious Diseases.* Testing should be done upon recognition of high-risk factors.

Continued

TABLE 26-1 **Recommendations for Preventive Pediatric Health Care (RE9939)—cont'd**

	Middle Childhood[4]				Adolescence[4]										
AGE[5]	5 y	6 y	8 y	10 y	11 y	12 y	13 y	14 y	15 y	16 y	17 y	18 y	19 y	20 y	21 y
HISTORY Initial/Interval	•	•	•	•	•	•	•	•	•	•	•	•	•	•	•
MEASUREMENTS Height and Weight / Head Circumference / Blood Pressure	•	•	•	•	•	•	•	•	•	•	•	•	•	•	•
SENSORY SCREENING Vision	O	O	O	O	S	O	S	S	O	S	S	O	S	S	S
Hearing	O	O	O	O	S	O	S	S	O	S	S	O	S	S	S
DEVELOPMENTAL/ BEHAVIORAL ASSESSMENT[8]	•	•	•	•	•	•	•	•	•	•	•	•	•	•	•
PHYSICAL EXAMINATION[9]	•	•	•	•	•	•	•	•	•	•	•	•	•	•	•
PROCEDURES-GENERAL[10] Hereditary/Metabolic Screening[11]															
Immunization[12]	•	•	•	•	•	•	•	•	•	•	•	•	•	•	•
Hematocrit or Hemoglobin[13]	*				←—————————•[14]—————————————————→										
Urinalysis	•				←————————————————————•[15]——————————→										
PROCEDURES-PATIENTS AT RISK Lead Screening[16]															
Tuberculin Test[17]	*	*	*	*	*	*	*	*	*	*	*	*	*	*	*
Cholesterol Screening[18]	*	*	*	*	*	*	*	*	*	*	*	*	*	*	*
STD Screening[19]	*				*	*	*	*	*	*	*	*	*	*	*
Pelvic Exam[20]					*	*	*	*	*	*	*	* ←—*[20]—*→ *			
ANTICIPATORY GUIDANCE[21]	•	•	•	•	•	•	•	•	•	•	•	•	•	•	•
Injury Prevention[22]	•	•	•	•	•	•	•	•	•	•	•	•	•	•	•
Violence Prevention[23]	•	•	•	•	•	•	•	•	•	•	•	•	•	•	•
Sleep Positioning Counseling[24]	•	•	•	•											
Nutrition Counseling[25]	•	•	•	•	•	•	•	•	•	•	•	•	•	•	•
DENTAL REFERRAL[26]															

18. Cholesterol screening for high-risk patients per AAP statement "Cholesterol in Childhood" (1998). If family history cannot be ascertained and other risk factors are present, screening should be at the discretion of the physician.
19. All sexually active patients should be screened for sexually transmitted diseases (STDs).
20. All sexually active females should have a pelvic examination. A pelvic examination and routine Pap smear should be offered as part of preventive health maintenance between the ages of 18 and 21 years.
21. Age-appropriate discussion and counseling should be an integral part of each visit for care per the AAP *Guidelines for Health Supervision III* (1998).
22. From birth to age 12, refer to the AAP injury prevention program (TIPP*) as described in *A Guide to Safety Counseling in Office Practice* (1994).
23. Violence prevention and management for all patients per AAP Statement "The Role of the Pediatrician in Youth Violence Prevention in Clinical Practice and at the Community Level" (1999).
24. Parents and caregivers should be advised to place healthy infants on their backs when putting them to sleep. Side positioning is a reasonable alternative but carries a slightly higher risk of SIDS. Consult the AAP statement "Changing Concepts of Sudden Infant Death Syndrome: Implications for Infant Sleeping Environment and Sleep Position" (2000).
25. Age-appropriate nutrition counseling should be an integral part of each visit per the AAP *Handbook of Nutrition* (1998).
26. Earlier initial dental examinations may be appropriate for some children. Subsequent examinations as prescribed by dentist.

Key: • = To be performed   * = to be performed for patients at risk
S = subjective, by history   O = objective, by a standard testing method
←—•—→ = the range during which a service may be provided, with the dot indicating the preferred age.

American Academy of Pediatrics

NB: Special chemical, immunologic, and endocrine testing is usually carried out upon specific indications. Testing other than newborn (e.g., inborn errors of metabolism, sickle disease, etc.) is discretionary with the physician.

BOX 26-2

QUESTIONS FOR A HEALTH-BELIEFS HISTORY

What would you call this problem?
Why do you think your child has developed it?
What do you think caused it?
Why do you think it started when it did?
What do you think is happening inside the body?
What are the symptoms that make you know you know your child has this illness?
What are you most worried about with this illness?
What problems does this illness cause your child?
How do you treat it?
Is the treatment helpful?
What will happen if this problem is not treated?
What do you expect from the treatments?

From Dixon SD, Stein MT: *Encounters with children: pediatric behavior and development,* ed. 3, Philadelphia, 2000, WB Saunders.

Cultural differences and individual parental beliefs about childrearing and health influence the care of the infant and child and are revealed in the history of the child's care. The practitioner should respect these differences and make culturally sensitive decisions with regard to content and approaches in counseling. Box 26-2 lists some questions useful for obtaining information about the caregiver's cultural and health beliefs related to the child's situation.

The informant for the history may be a parent, a relative, a caretaker, and/or the child. Identify the informant and indicate the reliability of the information obtained. Commonly, the child, even the young child, participates in the interview and volunteers useful information. Indicate the information gained from the child as such in the history.

The comprehensive health history described in Chapter 3 is adapted for the pediatric client by making certain changes in format. The following developmental and nutritional data should be gathered before the review of systems, since these data are usually critical to the present health status of the infant or child:

1. Biographical information
2. Chief complaint or client's request for care
3. Present illness or health status
4. Past health history
5. Developmental data
6. Nutritional data
7. Family health history
8. Review of systems
   a. Physical systems
   b. Sociological system
   c. Psychological system
9. Anticipatory guidance

Biographical Information

The following information needs to be obtained in the biographical category. It is essentially the same as for the adult client, with the addition of the parents' information.

1. Full name
2. Address
3. Birth date
4. Sex
5. Race
6. Religion
7. Birthplace
8. Parents' names
9. Parents' marital status
10. Parents' ages
11. Source of referral
12. Usual source of health care
13. Source and reliability of information
14. Date of interview

Chief Complaint or Client's Request for Care

The chief complaint statement gives the reason for making the visit and should be recorded in the words of the informant. The informant could be the parent or the child. Elicit this information with a neutral question ("How may I help you today?"), since the visit may be for routine health care rather than for treatment of a health problem. The chief complaint statement for routine health care may be, "It is time for his checkup" or "It is time for his well-baby check."

When the visit is for a well-child examination, you may want to ask, "Before we begin the examination, are there any particular questions or concerns that you would like to discuss?" This question encourages the client, parent, or child to raise issues that may not be addressed in the health history format and reinforces the idea that their questions and concerns are important.

Present Health/Illness Status

The present illness or health status section incorporates the same categories of information obtained in the adult health history and includes a statement about the client's usual health; a description of the current concern, including the onset and chronological story; any relevant family history; any negative information; and a disability assessment. You may want to ask an open-ended question (e.g., "How has the baby been since you were last here?") to get a general picture of how things have been going (called an interval history). Also ask the parent the reason for seeking help at this time. Usually something significant has occurred that motivates the person to come for an evaluation. Physical changes in the child's condition, family stresses that make the problem more difficult to handle, or issues such as a similar problem in a friend or relative may have triggered the visit. Understanding these concerns will help in making your assessment of the situation and planning effective interventions.

Past Health History

The past health history of infants, young children, and any child with a possible developmental deficiency should include the following information:

1. Prenatal history
   a. Health of the mother while pregnant with this child
   b. Mother's feelings about the pregnancy

c. Amount of prenatal care and when initiated
d. History of complications (excessive weight gain; hypertension; vaginal bleeding; nausea and vomiting; urinary problems; or infections such as rubella, cytomegalovirus, or venereal disease)
e. Medications or drugs prescribed or used during the pregnancy
f. Use of alcohol, cigarettes, and other drugs (e.g., cocaine, heroin) during the pregnancy
g. Parity of the mother

2. Birth history
a. Date of birth
b. Hospital where child was born
c. Duration of the pregnancy
d. Nature and duration of the labor
e. Type of delivery
f. Use of sedation or anesthesia
g. Birth weight of the baby
h. State of the infant at birth and use of any special procedures
i. APGAR score and when it was measured (1 or 5 minutes), if known (Table 26-2)

3. Postnatal history
a. Any problems during the first days of life (including skin color, bleeding, seizures, respiratory distress, congenital anomalies or birth injuries, difficulty in sucking, rashes, or poor weight gain during the first days and weeks after birth)
b. Age of infant at discharge from hospital after birth

The past health history of *all* children includes the following information:

1. Past illnesses
a. Childhood illnesses (including communicable diseases such as chickenpox and rubeola)
b. Injuries/accidents
c. Hospitalizations
d. Operations
e. Other major illnesses
f. Frequency of infections

2. Allergies
a. Environmental
b. Food

c. Drug
d. Other

3. Immunizations, including booster inoculations (Figure 26-3). NOTE: Immunization schedules are updated several times a year as new immunizations are added and schedules are revised by the American Academy of Pediatrics (AAP) and the Centers for Disease Control and Prevention (CDC) Advisory Committee on Immunization Practices. The most current schedule is reported in the journal *Pediatrics* and in the CDC's *Morbidity and Mortality Weekly Reports*. This information may also be obtained from the AAP website at aap.org/policy, the CDC website at www.cdc.gov/nip, or the Immunization Action Coalition website www.immunize.org.

4. Habits
a. Sleep: Does child sleep through the night? Note naps, number of hours of sleep at night, bedtime routines
b. Elimination: Urination and bowel movements, toilet training, occurrence of accidents
c. Exercise: Types of activities, frequency, organized sports
d. Behavior patterns (e.g., fussiness, response to frustration, thumb-sucking, nail-biting) (e.g., What is your child like? Does he or she have a particularly fussy time during the day?)
e. Use of alcohol, tobacco, drugs, coffee, tea, colas
f. Discipline: Methods used, success, failure, concerns
g. Sexuality: Inquisitiveness about girl-boy differences and pregnancy; parental responses and sex education offered; concerns and questions parents/child may have about masturbation, menstruation, nocturnal emissions, development of secondary sex characteristics, dating, and sexual urges and activity

5. Medications taken regularly
a. By practitioner's prescription
b. By self-prescription (over-the-counter or use of prescription medications, use of herbal or alternative health care products)

TABLE 26-2   APGAR Scoring System for Newborns

Clinical sign	Assigned Score*		
	0	1	2
Heart rate	Absent	Slow (<100 beats/min)	>100 beats/min
Respiratory effort	Apnea	Slow and irregular	Immediate, strong
Muscle tone	Flaccid	Some flexion of arms and legs	Active movement
Reflex irritability†	No response	Grimace or cry	Crying vigorously
Color	Pale, blue	Body pink, extremities blue	Pink all over

*A score of 8 to 10 is excellent, 4 to 7 is guarded, and 0 to 3 is critical.
†Reaction when soft rubber catheter is inserted into the external nares.

Recommended Childhood Immunization Schedule
United States, January – December 2001

Vaccines[1] are listed under routinely recommended ages. ⬚Bars⬚ indicate range of recommended ages for immunization. Any dose not given at the recommended age should be given as a "catch-up" immunization at any subsequent visit when indicated and feasible. Ⓞvals indicate vaccines to be given if previously recommended doses were missed or given earlier than the recommended minimum age.

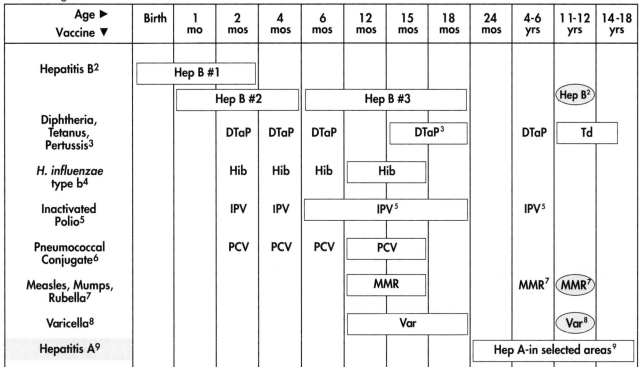

Age ▶ Vaccine ▼	Birth	1 mo	2 mos	4 mos	6 mos	12 mos	15 mos	18 mos	24 mos	4-6 yrs	11-12 yrs	14-18 yrs
Hepatitis B[2]	Hep B #1	Hep B #1	Hep B #2			Hep B #3					(Hep B[2])	
Diphtheria, Tetanus, Pertussis[3]			DTaP	DTaP	DTaP		DTaP[3]			DTaP	Td	
H. influenzae type b[4]			Hib	Hib	Hib	Hib						
Inactivated Polio[5]			IPV	IPV		IPV[5]				IPV[5]		
Pneumococcal Conjugate[6]			PCV	PCV	PCV	PCV						
Measles, Mumps, Rubella[7]						MMR				MMR[7]	(MMR[7])	
Varicella[8]						Var					(Var[8])	
Hepatitis A[9]									Hep A-in selected areas[9]			

Approved by the Advisory Committee on Immunization Practices (ACIP), the American Academy of Pediatrics (AAP), and the American Academy of Family Physicians (AAFP), website: http://www.aap.org/family/parents/immsch2001.pdf.

1. This schedule indicates the recommended ages for routine administration of currently licensed childhood vaccines, as of 11/1/00, for children through 18 years of age. Additional vaccines may be licensed and recommended during the year. Licensed combination vaccines may be used whenever any components of the combination are indicated and its other components are not contraindicated. Providers should consult the manufacturers' package inserts for detailed recommendations.

2. **Infants born to HBsAg-negative mothers** should receive the 1st dose of hepatitis B (Hep B) vaccine by age 2 months. The 2nd dose should be at least one month after the 1st dose. The 3rd dose should be administered at least 4 months after the 1st dose and at least 2 months after the 2nd dose, but not before 6 months of age for infants.

Infants born to HBsAg-positive mothers should receive hepatitis B vaccine and 0.5 mL hepatitis B immune globulin (HBIG) within 12 hours of birth at separate sites. The 2nd dose is recommended at 1-2 months of age and the 3rd dose at 6 months of age.

Infants born to mothers whose HBsAg status is unknown should receive hepatitis B vaccine within 12 hours of birth. Maternal blood should be drawn at the time of delivery to determine the mother's HBsAg status; if the HBsAg test is positive, the infant should receive HBIG as soon as possible (no later than 1 week of age).

All children and adolescents who have not been immunized against hepatitis B should begin the series during any visit. Special efforts should be made to immunize children who were born in or whose parents were born in areas of the world with moderate or high endemicity of hepatitis B virus infection.

3. The 4th dose of DTaP (diphtheria and tetanus toxoids and acellular pertussis vaccine) may be administered as early as 12 months of age, provided 6 months have elapsed since the 3rd dose and the child is unlikely to return at age 15-18 months. Td (tetanus and diphtheria toxoids) is recommended at 11-12 years of age if at least 5 years have elapsed since the last dose of DTP, DTaP or DT. Subsequent routine Td boosters are recommended every 10 years.

4. Three *Haemophilus influenzae* type b (Hib) conjugate vaccines are licensed for infant use. If PRP-OMP (PedvaxHIB® or ComVax® [Merck]) is administered at 2 and 4 months of age, a dose at 6 months is not required. Because clinical studies in infants have demonstrated that using some combination products may induce a lower immune response to the Hib vaccine component, DTaP/Hib combination products should not be used for primary immunization in infants at 2, 4 or 6 months of age, unless FDA-approved for these ages.

5. An all-IPV schedule is recommended for routine childhood polio vaccination in the United States. All children should receive four doses of IPV at 2 months, 4 months, 6-18 months, and 4-6 years of age. Oral polio vaccine (OPV) should be used only in selected circumstances. (See MMWR *Morb Mortal Wkly Rep* May 19,2000/49(RR-5);1-22).

6. The heptavalent conjugate pneumococcal vaccine (PCV) is recommended for all children 2-23 months of age. It also is recommended for certain children 24-59 months of age. (See MMWR *Morb Mortal Wkly Rep* Oct. 6, 2000/49(RR-9);1-35.)

7. The 2nd dose of measles, mumps, and rubella (MMR) vaccine is recommended routinely at 4-6 years of age but may be administered during any visit, provided at least 4 weeks have elapsed since receipt of the 1st dose and that both doses are administered beginning at or after 12 months of age. Those who have not previously received the second dose should complete the schedule by the 11-12 year old visit.

8. Varicella (Var) vaccine is recommended at any visit on or after the first birth-day for susceptible children, i.e., those who lack a reliable history of chickenpox (as judged by a health care provider) and who have not been immunized. Susceptible persons 13 years of age or older should receive 2 doses, given at least 4 weeks apart.

9. Hepatitis A (Hep A) is shaded to indicate its recommended use in selected states and/or regions, and for certain high risk groups; consult your local public health authority. (See MMWR *Morb Mortal Wkly Rep* Oct. 1, 1999/48(RR-12); 1-37.)

For additional information about the vaccines listed above, please visit the National Immunization Program Home Page at www.cdc.gov/nip or call the National Immunization Hotline at 800-232-2522 (English) or 800-232-0233 (Spanish).

Figure 26-3 The American Academy of Pediatrics' recommended childhood vaccination schedule— United States, January through December 2001.

TABLE 26-3 **Developmental Red Flags: Newborns and Infants**

Age	Physical Development (Autonomic Stability/ Rhythmicity/Sleep/ Temperament)	Psychosocial/ Emotional Skills	Cognitive and Visual Abilities	Language/ Hearing	Fine Motor (Feeding/Self-Care)	Gross Motor (Strength/ Coordination)
Newborn/ 1 mo	Lack of return to birth weight by 2-wk examination Poor coordination of suck/swallow Tachypnea/bradycardia with feedings Poor habituation to external stimuli	Diffuse nonverbal cues Poor state transitions Irritable	Doll's eyes No red light reflex Poor alert state	No startle to sound or sudden noises No quieting to voice High-pitched cry	Hands held fisted Absent or asymmetrical palmar grasp	Asymmetrical movements Hypertonia or hypotonia Asymmetrical primitive reflexes
3 mo	Less than 1-lb weight gain in 1 mo Head circumference increasing greater than 2 percentile lines on growth curve or showing no increase in size Continuing problems with poor suck/swallow Difficulty with regulation of sleep/wake cycle	Lack of social smile Withdrawn or depressed Lack of consistent, safe child care	No visual tracking Not able to fix on face or object	Does not turn to voice, rattle, or bell No sounds, coos, squeals	Hands fisted with oppositional thumb No hand to mouth activity	Asymmetrical movements Hypertonia or hypotonia No attempt to raise head when on stomach
6 mo	Less than double birth weight Head circumference showing no increase Continuation of poor feeding or sleep regulation Difficulty with self-calming	No smiles No response to play Solemn appearance	Not visually alert Does not reach for objects Does not look at caregiver	No babbling Does not respond to voice, bell, rattle, or loud noises even with startle	Does not reach for objects, hold rattle, hold hands together Does not grasp at clothes	Persistent primitive reflexes Does not attempt to sit with support Head lag with pull to sit Scissoring
9 mo	Parent control issues with feeding or sleep	Intense stranger anxiety or absent stranger anxiety Does not seek comfort from caregiver when stressed	Lack of visual awareness Lack of reaching out for toys Lack of toy exploration visually or orally	Lack of single or double sounds Lack of response to name or voice Does not respond to any words	No self-feeding No highchair sitting No solids Does not pick up toys with one hand	Does not sit even in tripod position No lateral prop reflex Asymmetrical crawl, handedness, or other movements
12 mo	Less than triple birth weight Losing more than 2 percentile lines on growth curve for weight, length, or head circumference Poor sleep/wake cycle Extreme inability to separate from parent	No response to game playing No response to reading or interactive activities Withdrawn or solemn	Not visually following activities in the environment	Inability to localize to sound Not imitating speech sounds Not using 2-3 words Does not point	Persistent mouthing Not attempting to feed self or hold cup Not able to hold toy in each hand or transfer objects	Not pulling self to stand Not moving around the environment to explore

From Burns CE et al.: *Pediatric primary care: a handbook for nurse practitioners*, ed. 2, Philadelphia, 2000, WB Saunders.

Developmental Data

The assessment of the development of the child is discussed in detail in Chapter 5. The history of the child's development is a component of that assessment and should provide clues that indicate when a more formal assessment is indicated. Box 5-5 in Chapter 5 summarizes normal child developmental milestones from 1 month to 5 years. Table 26-3 describes developmental findings for newborns and infants that indicate a need for close monitoring or more in-depth evaluation and/or referral.

The initial history should include the following information:
1. Age at which the young child attained specific developmental achievements:
   a. Held head erect
   b. Rolled over
   c. Sat alone
   d. Walked alone
   e. Said first words
   f. Used sentences
   g. Controlled feces
   h. Learned urinary continence
2. Current developmental performance. Assess developmental performance by asking specific questions related to expected abilities for the child's age range (see Box 5-5). You may want to ask a broad question (e.g., "What new things have you noticed your child doing since the last visit?") followed by a more specific question (e.g., "Has he rolled over yet?"). You may also determine development by the use of a screening tool such as the Denver Developmental Screening Test II (see Figure 5-1).
3. Any periods of slowed or decreased growth. Was this change in growth pattern evaluated? Were there any known or suspected causes for such growth or lack of growth (e.g., family stress, illness)? These questions can be asked either during the nutritional assessment or at this time.
4. Questions concerning developmentally appropriate activities (e.g., peer relationships, school achievement, dating) may be covered in the review of systems but are also appropriate to address here.

Nutritional Data

Questions regarding nutrition vary according to the child's age. More detailed and specific information may be obtained for the infant, who is growing rapidly, than for the older child.

Early Infancy (Birth to 6 Months)
1. Type of feeding (breast-feeding, brand of commercial formula, or home-prepared formula)
2. Frequency of feedings
3. Amount consumed with each feeding and during a 24-hour period: Be specific in terms of number of ounces per feeding, number and size of cans of formula used per day, type of formula and how formula is prepared (add water to concentrate versus ready to pour from can), and number of times and length of breast-feeding sessions per day

4. Any changes in feeding (e.g., from breast-feeding to bottle-feeding or addition of a supplementary bottle if breast-feeding, date of change, introduction of solids)
5. Any problems observed with feeding (e.g., colic or spitting up)
6. How long the mother plans to continue breast-feeding or bottle-feeding
7. Vitamin, iron, or fluoride supplements (including name of the preparation, when it was started, amount given, and method of administration)
8. Solid foods, including type (commercially prepared or home prepared), amount given, how they are given (by spoon or in bottle), and frequency
9. Water, including amount given, frequency offered, whether given plain or with a sweetener
10. Infant's appetite and reaction to eating

If the infant is receiving bottle-feedings, ask whether he or she is held for all feedings or whether the bottle is propped. The infant who goes to sleep with a bottle of milk or juice at bedtime or naptime, used in much the same way as a pacifier, is at risk for dental caries and destruction of the anterior maxillary teeth (referred to as "baby bottle syndrome," Figure 26-4). This practice also puts the child at risk for aspiration of fluids and middle ear infections.

The Breast-Fed Infant. If the infant is breast-feeding, obtain the following information about the mother:
1. How the mother feels she is doing with breast-feeding
2. Any questions or concerns about herself or the baby
3. Any problems with her breasts (e.g., discomfort, blisters, chafing, tenderness)
4. How the mother cares for her breasts
5. Mother's program of daily exercise, rest, diet, and fluid intake
6. Medications being taken (specify name, frequency, purpose, and effectiveness; see Table 26-4 for information on some drugs known to be excreted in

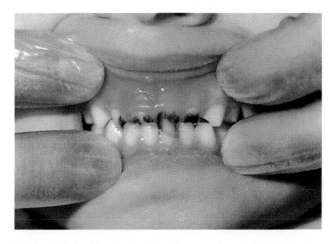

Figure 26-4 Nursing-bottle caries. Note extensive carious involvement of the maxillary primary incisors. (From Swartz M: *Textbook of physical diagnosis: history and examination,* ed. 3, St. Louis, 1998, Mosby.)

TABLE 26-4   Medications Affecting Breast-Feeding

Contraindicated Drugs	Drugs Requiring Temporary Cessation of Breast-Feeding	Drugs Whose Effect Is Unknown	Drugs Associated With Significant Effects
Bromocriptine Cocaine Cyclophosphamide Cyclosporine Doxorubicin Ergotamine Lithium Methotrexate Phencyclidine (PCP) Phenytoin	Radioactive compounds such as ^{64}Cu ^{67}Ga ^{111}I, ^{123}I, ^{125}I, ^{131}I Radioactive sodium ^{99m}Tc Need to stop breast-feeding for a minimum of 5 half lives of the drug	Antidepressants 　Amitriptyline 　Amoxapine 　Desipramine 　Dothiepin 　Doxepin 　Fluoxetine 　Fluvoxamine 　Imipramine 　Trazodone Antianxieties 　Diazepam 　Lorazepam 　Midazolam 　Prazepam 　Quazepam 　Temazepam Antipsychotics 　Chlorpromazine 　Chlorprothixene 　Haloperidol 　Mesoridazine 　Perphenazine Others 　Chloramphenicol 　Metoclopramide 　Metronidazole 　Tinidazole	5-Aminosalicylic acid Aspirin Clemastine Phenobarbital Primidone Sulfasalazine

From Burns CE et al.: *Pediatric primary care: a handbook for nurse practitioners,* ed. 2, Philadelphia, 2000, WB Saunders.

human milk and to have side effects in breast-fed infants)

7. Support mother receives from her spouse, family members, and/or friends
8. How long she plans to breast-feed and when (or if) she wants to introduce bottle-feeding
9. Whether the mother is using supplementary bottles and whether she is expressing breast milk or using formula; if she is using formula, what kind of formula; how is she storing breast milk; any problems with expressing milk
10. Need for any other information that the mother would like (e.g., resources, support groups, lactation consultation)

To determine whether the baby is getting enough breast milk, ask the mother:

1. How often the infant wets his or her diaper (should have at least eight wet diapers in a 24-hour period)
2. To describe the baby's bowel movements (often a large amount of soft yellow stool; frequency may vary from several times a day to every few days)

Later Infancy (6 to 12 Months). During this period the infant is beginning to vigorously manipulate his or her body and the environment. In addition to the questions outlined

for the period of early infancy, ask questions regarding the infant's developing skills:

1. Has the infant started using a cup, finger-feeding, or using a spoon?
2. Does the infant receive coarser foods such as junior foods or table foods?
   a. What foods does he or she like?
   b. Has there been any problem (diarrhea, rash) after eating any particular food?
   c. How often does the infant eat solids (meals and snacks) and how much is eaten?
3. How does the mother feel about the infant's developing independent feeding behaviors? What are her expectations of the child (e.g., child should not make a mess, should be able to use a spoon)?
4. Have there been any feeding problems?

Toddlerhood. During this stage the child's rapid growth rate slows. In addition, the child is experiencing an increased sense of independence and has the ability to feed himself or herself. This is a time when parents often become concerned about decreased food intake, and "battles" over feeding can develop. Therefore it is important to ask questions to determine the adequacy of food intake (recognizing that toddlers require smaller amounts of food than most parents realize) and the existence or signs of the development of feeding problems.

1. What does the child eat during a typical day?
   a. What foods does he or she like?
   b. Has there been any problem (diarrhea, rash) after eating any particular food?
   c. How often does the child eat meals and snacks? What are the amounts (e.g., tablespoonfuls, number of crackers)
   d. How does the child feed himself or herself (fingers, spoon, fork; holds cup; is still fed by parent)?
2. How do the parents feel about the toddler's feeding behaviors? What are their expectations of the child (e.g., should not make a mess; should be able to use a spoon, fork)?
3. Have there been any feeding problems?
   a. Have there been any "hunger strikes" (typical of an 18-month-old child)?
   b. Does the child go on "food jags" in which he or she will eat only one type of food?
   c. Is he or she a "picky eater"?
   d. Have there been many struggles for control over eating (parent trying to make the child eat), and how do these resolve?

Preschool Age, School Age, and Adolescence. The 24-hour recall method and the dietary history method are appropriate for obtaining information about the diet and eating habits of the child. In addition to general nutrition patterns, find out about the parents' attitudes toward eating and their response to any eating problems that might exist. Pay special attention to preadolescents' and adolescents' concerns about being "overweight." Assess for possible eating disorders and crash dieting. (Refer to the discussions of assessment of food intake, nutritional needs of children and adolescents, and clients with eating disorders in Chapter 6 for more details.)

Family Health History

The family medical history of the child is similar to the history obtained for the adult client (see Chapter 3). It includes the health and age of the grandparents, maternal and paternal aunts and uncles, parents, and siblings and the age at death and cause of death for deceased relatives. In addition, the pediatric family history should include information about miscarriages and stillbirths, congenital defects, and familial diseases.

Outline the family history information (an ideal way to present it is by drawing a family tree) to identify any illnesses or problems that may have implications for the child's future health and current health. The family tree, which is similar to the pedigree used in a genetic study, allows a study of the patterns of distribution of genetic traits in kindred people. When the information obtained in the family history reveals suspected genetic problems, refer the child and the parents to a specialist in genetics for diagnosis and counseling. Figure 26-5 illustrates a family tree for a pediatric client.

Review of Systems

The review of systems is essentially the same as that for the adult history (see Chapter 3), except for age-appropriate

modifications. The general format remains the same. Add the following review of system questions when taking the child's history.

Physical Systems

General. Recent and significant gain or loss of weight, failure to gain weight appropriate for age, or failure to increase in height.

Changes in Behavior. Variations from usual behavior such as increased crying, irritability, nervousness, withdrawal, or changes in sleep patterns. These questions are usually found under the review of the central nervous system in the adult history. However, behavior changes in children may represent the first symptoms of a problem in any physical system or may indicate psychosocial problems, including abuse and neglect.

Skin. Birthmarks, rashes, and acne.

Head. Injuries and headaches.

Eyes. Strabismus (crossed eyes), discharge, vision disturbance (behaviors that might be indicative of problems, such as sitting very close to the television, writing with the head near the desk, rubbing the eyes).

Ears. Ear infections, earaches, hearing loss (note loud speech, delayed speech, need to repeat questions), and previous hearing tests.

Nose. Has the child had a constant or frequent runny or stuffy nose (unilateral or bilateral); note the type of rhinorrhea.

Mouth and Throat. The age of eruption of teeth (comparison with siblings); the number of teeth at 1 year; loss of teeth; whether the child was born with a cleft lip or cleft palate; whether the child had thrush.

Neck and Nodes. Limitation of neck movement or enlarged nodes.

Breasts. In the newborn there may be breast enlargement secondary to maternal hormones that resolves spontaneously (but may be of concern to the parents).

Ask the preadolescent and the adolescent boy or girl whether he or she has noticed changes in the breasts. (Figure 26-6 describes the normal stages of breast development

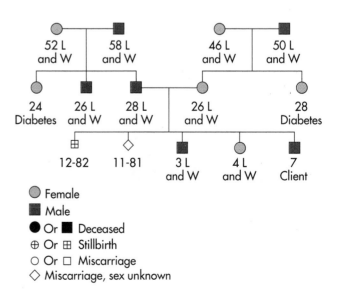

Figure 26-5 Family tree used in a pediatric history.

Stage		Breast development

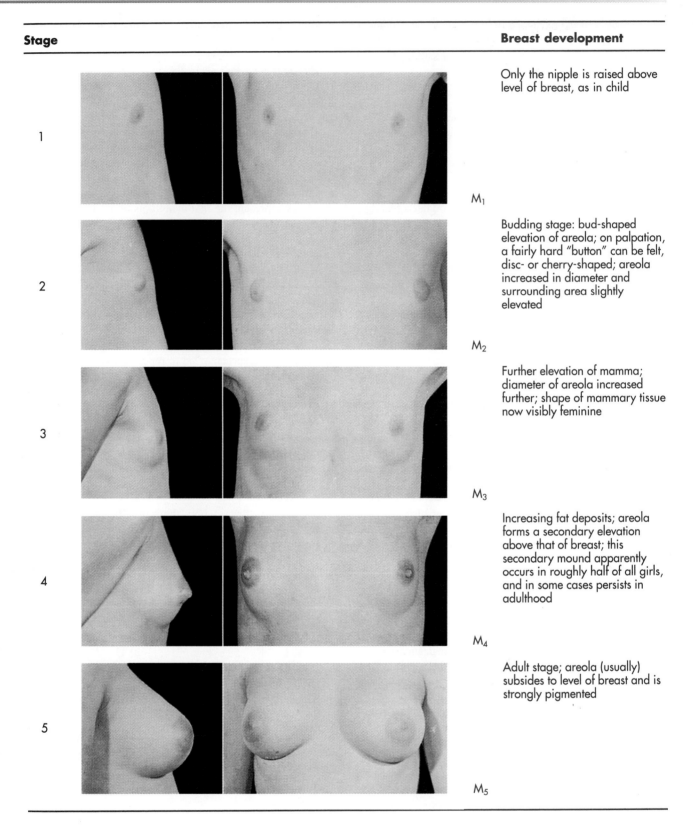

1 — M₁ : Only the nipple is raised above level of breast, as in child

2 — M₂ : Budding stage: bud-shaped elevation of areola; on palpation, a fairly hard "button" can be felt, disc- or cherry-shaped; areola increased in diameter and surrounding area slightly elevated

3 — M₃ : Further elevation of mamma; diameter of areola increased further; shape of mammary tissue now visibly feminine

4 — M₄ : Increasing fat deposits; areola forms a secondary elevation above that of breast; this secondary mound apparently occurs in roughly half of all girls, and in some cases persists in adulthood

5 — M₅ : Adult stage; areola (usually) subsides to level of breast and is strongly pigmented

Figure 26-6 Five stages of breast development in females. (Photographs from Van Wieringen JC: *Growth diagrams 1965 Netherlands second national survey on 0 to 24-year-olds*, Groningen, Netherlands, 1971, Wolters-Noordhoff; reprinted by permission of Kluwer Academic Publishers.)

in girls. Boys may experience some degree of transient gynecomastia during puberty.)

Inquire about individual concerns regarding breast development, such as comparisons made with peers or the unequal development of the breasts. This subject may be approached by acknowledging that such concerns are common at this age and stating that you would be happy to answer any questions the adolescent may have. For girls, teach self-breast examination once breast buds have begun to develop. (See also Chapter 14 for self-assessment tips.)

Respiratory System. Stridor, wheezing, episodes of croup, frequent colds, nighttime coughing, and reduced exercise tolerance. Does the child play as actively as other children or curtail strenuous exercise?

Cardiovascular System. Any history of heart murmur, and any evaluation and follow-up if a murmur is present; does the child experience fatigue on exertion, tire easily, turn blue?

Gastrointestinal System. Abdominal pain, constipation, diarrhea, change in continence, toilet training, and "accidents."

Genital System

MALE. Ask the preadolescent and adolescent male questions about the development of the secondary sex characteristics. (Figure 26-7 describes normal changes.) This discussion also provides an opportunity to teach about the normal changes that have occurred or are going to occur and to reassure the client that what he is experiencing is normal. Characteristics to ask about include the following:

- Appearance of hair on face and body
- Appearance of axillary hair
- Appearance of pubic hair
- Increase in size of testes
- Testicular self-examination (teach client) (See Chapter 20 for self-assessment tips.)

Ask about individual concerns regarding sexual development. An effective approach is to universalize concerns. For example, say: "Many boys your age have questions about…. What questions would you like me to answer?" Delete the question about impotence (from the adult history) until it is determined that the young man is sexually active.

FEMALE. Ask the preadolescent and adolescent female questions about the development of the secondary sex characteristics. (Figure 26-8 describes normal changes in girls.) This discussion also offers the chance to teach about the normal changes that have occurred or are going to occur and to reassure the client that what she is experiencing is normal. Characteristics to ask about include the following:

- Onset of menses (if menarche has occurred): determine whether periods are painful, how she felt about menarche (in addition to the routine adult menstrual history questions)
- Appearance of axillary hair
- Appearance of pubic hair

Ask about individual concerns regarding sexual development. Again, universalizing the question will make it more comfortable for the teenager to respond: "Many girls your age have questions about…." and "What questions would you like me to answer?"

Delete the questions (from the adult history) about obstetrical history until you determine that the girl is sexually active.

Delete the question about Papanicolaou (Pap) tests until the girl is 15 years old, unless you determine that (1) the girl younger than 15 years is sexually active or (2) was exposed to diethylstilbestrol (DES) before birth and has begun to menstruate.

BOTH SEXES. You should ask questions about sexual activity and sexually transmitted diseases once the child is about 10 years old. Explain the reason that the questions must be asked. Discuss "safer" sexual practices, contraception, and the option of abstinence, particularly if the client is sexually active.

Extremities and Musculoskeletal System. Ask about "growing pains," postural deformities or changes, changes in gait, and injuries to muscles or joints.

Central Nervous System. Ask about the child's ability to concentrate, hyperactivity, and headaches. Additional information about this system will be obtained in the developmental history and social history.

Sociological System

1. Relationship with family and significant others (can be done in the form of a family tree or genogram)
   a. Client's position in the family (birth order), natural child or adopted
   b. Person(s) with whom client lives
   c. Persons with whom client relates (Who is the primary caretaker? What are arrangements for baby-sitters or day care? Does the child have special friends?)
   d. Recent family crises or changes (include history of parental divorce, separation, or remarriage and birth or adoption of siblings)
2. Environment
   a. Home (Heated? Adequate hot water? Well or city water? Number of rooms, toilets, cooking facilities? Where does child play?)
   b. Neighborhood (safety issues, play areas, sense of community)
   c. Recent changes in environment
   d. To what degree are cultural and religious practices observed?
3. Occupational history (if appropriate)
   a. Jobs held
   b. Satisfaction with present and past employment
   c. Current place of employment
   d. Future goals concerning occupation, career, etc.
4. Economic status and resources
   a. Parents' occupations and sources of income
   b. Parents' perception of adequacy or inadequacy of income
   c. Arrangements for child care while parent(s) are at work: type of care (baby-sitter, child care center, relatives, after-school program), satisfaction with care, concerns about child care
   d. Effect of child's illness on parents' economic status; plans for care when child is sick if both parents work outside the home

Stage		Pubic hair	Penis	Scrotum
1	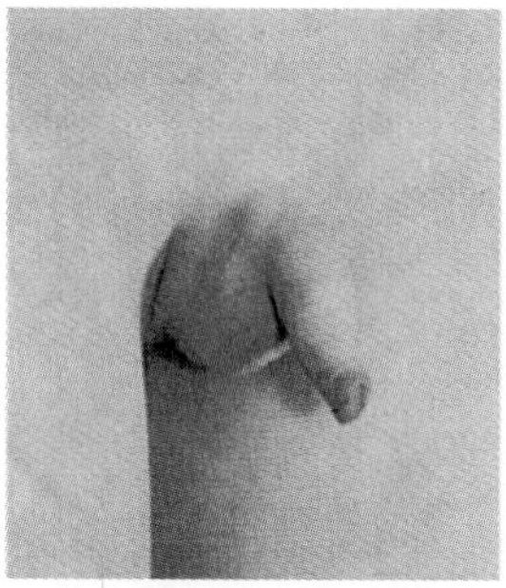	No pubic hair	Appears like smaller child's penis	Testes begins to enlarge, but scrotum remains small and undeveloped
2	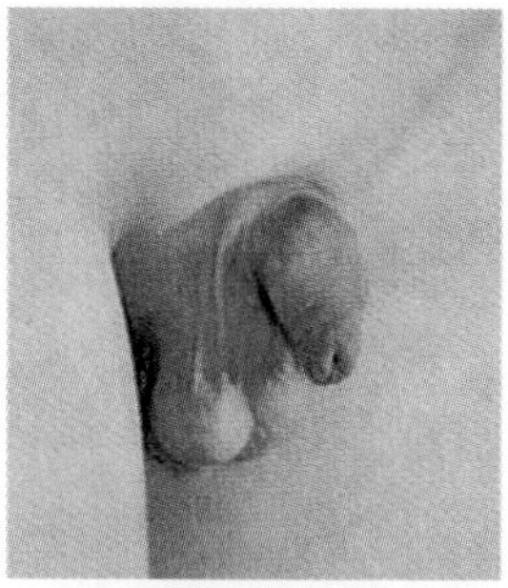	Pubic hair starting to develop; appears as straight, long, and downy texture	Little enlargement	Both testes and scrotum enlarge; scrotum begins to acquire darker skin tone and change in texture
3	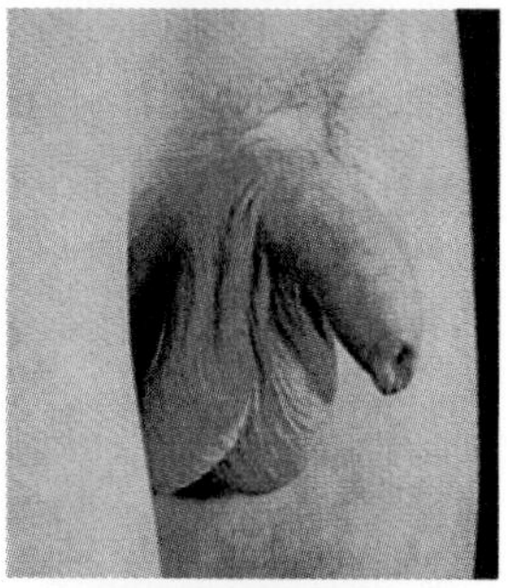	Increasing hair growth over entire pubic region; hair is dark, curly, and beginning to become coarse	Penis begins to enlarge; enlargement is more in length than in general size	Growth and skin texture continue to develop
4	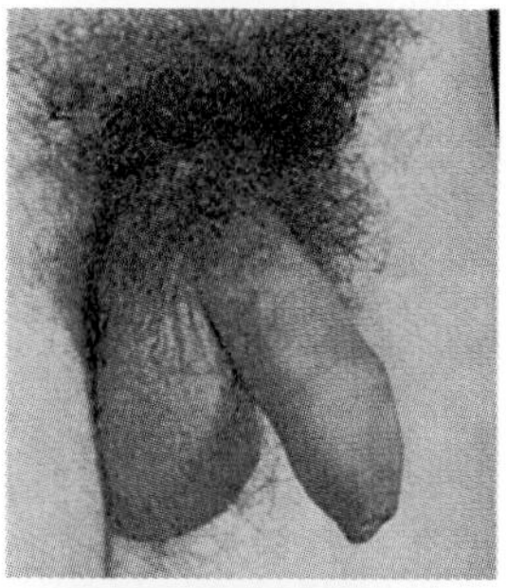	Hair is thick and coarse over entire pubic area	Penis grows in both length and diameter; glans also develops	Scrotum is like that of adult—darker tone and testes are almost adult size
5	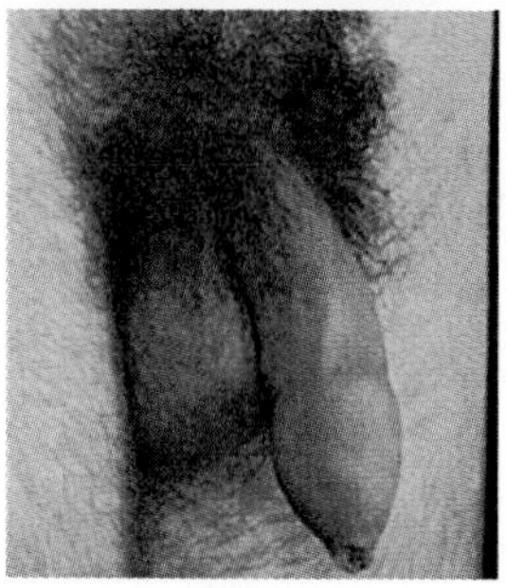	Mature pubic hair distribution, including on upper medial thighs	Adult appearance of penis	Full development and adult-appearing testes

Figure 26-7 Tanner's sex maturity development in males. (Photographs from Van Wieringen JC: *Growth diagrams 1965 Netherlands second national survey on 0- to 24-year-olds*, Groningen, Netherlands, 1971, Wolters-Noordhoff; reprinted by permission of Kluwer Academic Publishers.)

Stage		Pubic hair development
1	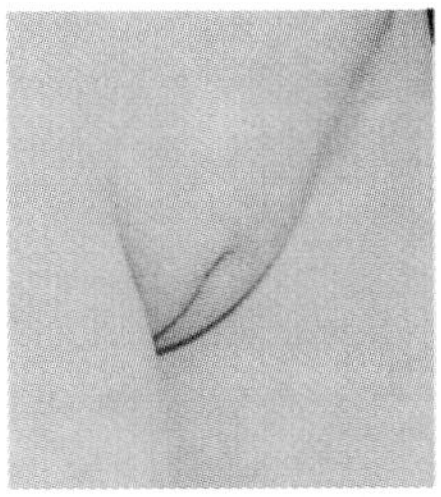	No growth of pubic hair
2	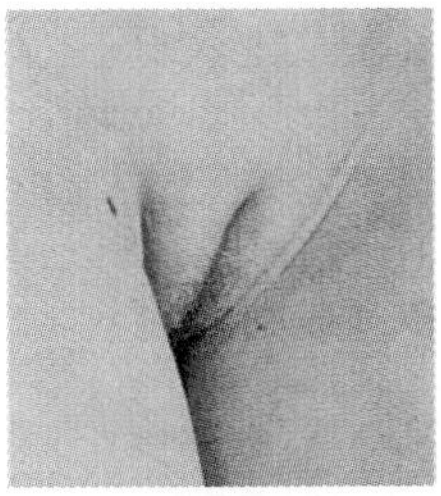	Initial, scarcely long, straight, downy and slightly pigmented pubic hair, especially along labia
3	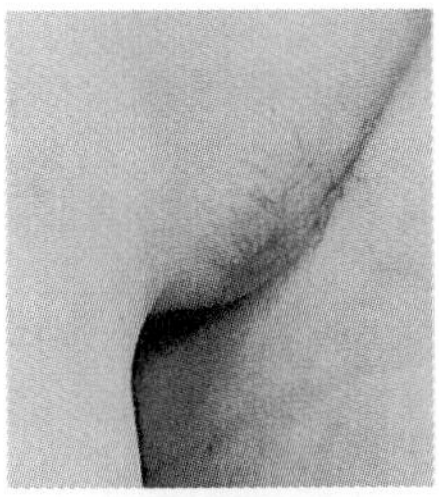	Pubic hair is darker, coarser, and curly, and spread sparsely over entire pubis in typical female triangle
4	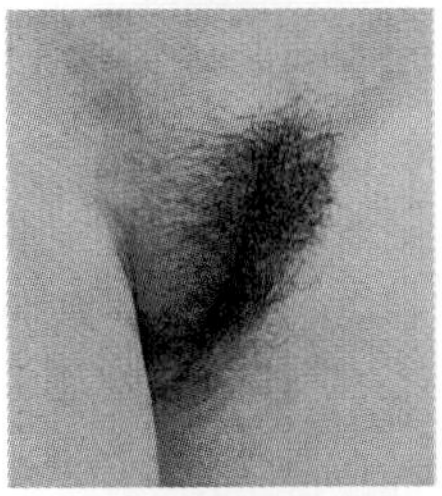	Pubic hair is denser, curly, and in an adult distribution, but less abundant and restricted to pubic area
5	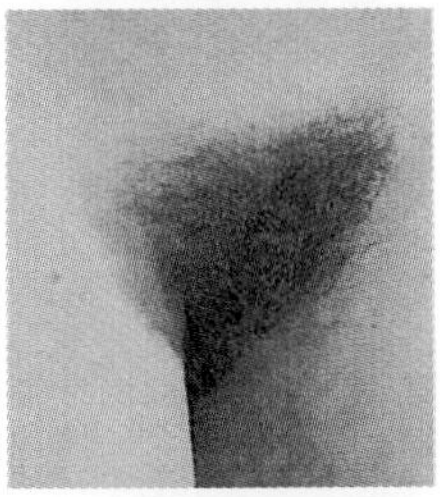	Pubic hair is adult in quantity, type, and pattern, with lateral spreading to inner aspect of thighs
6	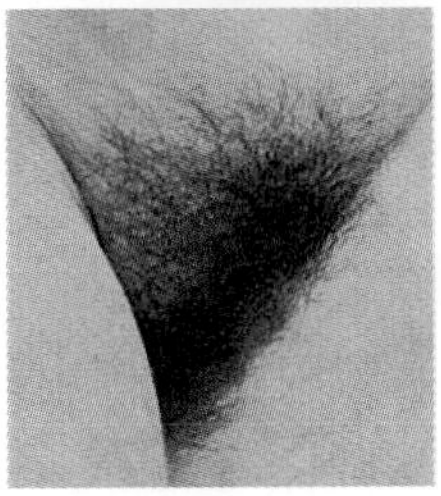	Further extension laterally, upward, or over the upper thighs (this stage may not occur in all women)

Figure 26-8 Tanner's sex maturity development in females. (Photographs from Van Wieringen JC: *Growth diagrams 1965 Netherlands second national survey on 0-24-year-olds*, Groningen, Netherlands, 1971, Wolters-Noordhoff; reprinted by permission of Kluwer Academic Publishers.)

5. Educational level (this area may also be covered in the developmental assessment section)
   a. Name of child's school
   b. Current grade level (Has child ever been held back or skipped a grade?)
   c. Judgment of intellect relative to age (parent may be asked to make this judgment by asking how this child performs compared with siblings or other children of the same age)
   d. Satisfaction with school, relationships with teacher and other students, safety in school, bullying, etc.
   e. Concerns about school performance
6. Daily profile (describe a typical day)
   a. Sleep, rest, activity patterns
   b. Social activities (play activities)
   c. Special weekend activities
   d. Recent changes in daily activities
   e. Parental concerns and management of any specific behavior, such as masturbation, thumb-sucking, nail-biting, temper tantrums, or bed-wetting
7. Patterns of health care
   a. Private physician, managed care, or community primary care agencies
   b. Dental care
   c. Preventive care
   d. Emergency care

Psychological System.   The outline for the psychological system review provided in Chapter 3 (and repeated here) is appropriate for use with the child and parent with the addition of information about the child's personality style. Include both the parent and the child in your assessment because it will be the parent who is primarily responsible for the child's care during the childhood years. The adolescent child will be more responsible for self-care but will continue to need direction and support from an informed, understanding parent.

You can describe personality in general terms such as outgoing or shy. One way of describing the child's personality that practitioners have found useful in working with families is to identify the child's behavioral or temperament style. Temperament refers to the way an individual deals with new situations and life in general. Chess and Thomas (1986) have identified nine temperament categories (Table 26-5) that can be combined to form three behavior profiles—the easy child, the difficult child, and the slow-to-warm-up child (Box 26-3). These patterns appear to exist over long periods and may affect the child's adjustment to a variety of childhood situations. Chess and Thomas emphasize that the style itself is not problematic; it is the degree of "fit" between the child's style and his or her environment, in particular the parents, that determines the degree of difficulty experienced. Interventions should be directed at helping parents to understand their child's style and to work with that style rather than against it (see suggestions in Box 26-3).

In assessment of the adolescent client (age 12 years and older), it is important to explore some additional areas, including depression and suicide potential, involvement with drugs and alcohol, and sexuality. Boxes 26-4 and 26-5 and Table 26-6 give suggestions for what to cover and how to get the most information in the adolescent interview.

Always inform teenage clients that the information they share will be kept confidential, unless they or someone else is in danger of physical harm. At the same time, encourage teens to talk with their parents about these issues.

1. Personality: How does the parent describe the child's general characteristics? What are his or her temperament characteristics (see Table 26-5 and Box 26-3)? How do these characteristics influence the child's interactions with family, friends, peers, teachers, etc.?
2. Cognitive abilities (for the child, this information may be included in the developmental assessment)
   a. Comprehension
   b. Learning patterns
   c. Memory

TABLE 26-5	**Characteristics of Temperament**

Temperament Characteristic	Description
Activity	What is the child's activity level? Is the child moving all the time he or she is awake, some of the time, or rarely?
Rhythmicity	How predictable is the child's sleep/wake pattern, feeding schedule, and elimination pattern?
Approach/withdrawal	What is the child's response when presented with something new such as a new toy, an experience, or new person? Does he or she immediately approach or turn away?
Adaptability	How quickly does the child get used to new things? Quickly or not at all?
Threshold of response	How much stimulation does the child require for calming? A quiet voice and touch or more intense, loud voice or firm grasp?
Intensity of reaction	Are the child's responses (crying or laughing) very subtle or extremely intense?
Quality of mood	Is the child's mood usually outgoing, happy, joyful, pleasant or unfriendly, withdrawn, or quiet?
Distractability	How easily is the child distracted from outside disturbance such as a phone ringing, TV, siblings?
Attention span and persistence	How long will the child continue to play with a particular toy or engage in a certain activity? Does this continue even when there are distractions?

From Burns CE et al.: *Pediatric primary care: a handbook for nurse practitioners,* ed. 2, Philadelphia, 2000, WB Saunders.

BOX 26-3

TEMPERAMENT STYLES AND PARENTING GUIDELINES

EASY CHILD (approximately 40% of the population)

Easygoing children are even tempered, regular, and predictable in their habits and have a positive approach to new stimuli. They are open and adaptable to change and display a mild to moderately intense mood that is typically positive.

Guidelines for Parents

- Adapts to almost any parenting approach and is easy to manage if expectations are clearly defined and consistent and not incongruent with what the child finds in the outside world.
- Seldom develops behavior problems. If behavior problems occur, it is because there is conflict between home-taught values and those of the outside world. Because of this child's easy adaptability, it is important not to initiate any practice or ritual that is undesirable to continue over time, as the child will quickly incorporate that practice into own living pattern.
- Spend separate time with this child who may be easily overlooked because is so "easy."
- Because this child is highly adaptable, may always do what others wish even if it is not in own best interest.
- Teach this child how to discriminate and develop own rules.
- Teach child caution since child is generally positive in approach and may not use caution when meeting strangers and thus get into dangerous situations.

SLOW-TO-WARM-UP CHILD (approximately 15% of the population)

Slow-to-warm-up children typically react negatively and with mild intensity to new stimuli and, unless pressured, adapt slowly with repeated contact. They respond with only mild but passive resistance to novelty or changes in routine. They are quite inactive and moody but show only moderate irregularity in functions.

Guidelines for parents

- Use a patient, relaxed, persevering approach. New situations or rules should be presented gradually but repeatedly without pressure. Because of some common elements in the traits in the difficult and slow-to-warm-up personality types, some management guidelines apply to both personality types.
- Refuse to compete with the child or demand strict adherence to every rule in the home. Such action only increases a negative display of behavior.
- Try not to explode at the child as fury only exaggerates inappropriate behavior.
- Clearly identify on a regular basis what behaviors will be accepted and what behaviors are unacceptable. The child also needs help in identifying what behaviors are contingent to the situation at hand. This clarification should occur at times when the child is not misbehaving because, if tense, the child may not hear the rules. Be consistent in en-

forcing established limits. A democratic approach is least overwhelming for this child; however, an autocratic approach may also work as long as it is not in the extreme.
- This child learns slowly, so much repetition of the rules is necessary.
- Build in daily successes for this child.
- Maintain established routines while child is mastering a rule or behavioral expectation.
- Key words to management: firmness, repeated exposure, consistent reinforcement, patience.

DIFFICULT CHILD (approximately 10% of the population)

Difficult children are highly active, irritable, and irregular in their habits. Negative withdrawal responses are typical, and they require a more structured environment. These children adapt slowly to new routines, people, or situations. Mood expressions are usually intense and primarily negative. They exhibit frequent periods of crying, and frustration often produces violent tantrums.

Guidelines for parents

- A firm, consistent approach that emphasizes the positive is most effective with this temperament style. Aspects of a child's temperament that may have undesirable consequences if allowed unrestricted expression should be controlled and limited in a calm but firm and consistent manner.
- Patience is essential. Parents need to exert an active effort to avoid negative parent-child relationships that may arise out of the child's constant stressful behaviors.
- Parents of this temperament style cope best if they take turns and give each other a daily chance to get away from the child. Certain activities may predictably cause negative behaviors, but it is important to persist in introducing the child to the situations or expectations so that the child can eventually learn control. Parents may wish to take turns handling the child during these experiences since it takes a great deal of energy.
- Provide gradual and repeated reinforcement, both positive and negative, for expected behaviors so that the child can internalize (problems in behavior usually arise from conflict between the child and almost any aspect of the environment, whether it be parents, new situations, or the world outside).
- Give a minimum number of rules at a time (one to three). The rules need to be straightforward and unencumbered by explanations or choices.
- Finally, provide constructive avenues for excess emotions and energy.

MIXED TEMPERAMENT CHILD (approximately 35% of the population)

Determine which of the other three personality types seems to predominate in this child and respond appropriately.

From Wong DL et al.: *Whaley and Wong's nursing care of infants and children,* ed. 6, St. Louis, 1999, Mosby; and Fox JA: *Primary health care of children,* St. Louis, 1997, Mosby.)

TABLE 26-6 **Opening Lines—Good and Bad**

Poor	Better	Reason
Home		
Tell me about mom and dad.	Where do you live, and who lives there with you?	Parent(s) may have died or left the home. Open-ended question enables one to collect "environmental" as well as personal history.
Education		
How are you doing in school?	What are you good at in school? What is hard for you? What grades do you get?	Poor questions can be answered "okay." Good questions ask for information about strengths and weaknesses and allow for quantification/objectification.
Activities		
Do you have any activities outside of school?	What do you do for fun? What things do you do with friends? What do you do with your free time?	Good questions are open-ended and allow patient to express himself.
Drugs		
Do you do drugs?	Many young people experiment with drugs, alcohol, or cigarettes. Have you or your friends ever tried them? What have you tried?	Good question is an expression of concern with specific follow-up. With younger teens, it is best to begin by asking about friends.
Sexuality		
Have you ever had sex? Tell me about your boyfriend/girlfriend.	Have you ever had a sexual relationship with anyone? Most young people become interested in sexual relationships at your age. Have you had any with boys, girls, or both? Tell me about your sex life.	What does the term "have sex" really mean to teenagers? Asking only about heterosexual relationships closes doors at once.

From Goldenring JM, Cohen E: Getting into adolescent heads, *Contemp Pediatr* 5:75-86, 1988.

BOX 26-4

SUICIDE RISK/DEPRESSION SCREENING

1. Sleep disorders (usually induction problems; also early/frequent waking or greatly increased sleep and complaints of increasing fatigue)
2. Appetite/eating behavior change
3. Feelings of "boredom"
4. Emotional outbursts and highly impulsive behavior
5. History of withdrawal/isolation
6. Hopeless/helpless feelings
7. History of past suicide attempts, depression, psychological counseling
8. History of suicide attempts, depression, or psychological problems in family or peers
9. History of drug/alcohol abuse, acting-out/crime, recent change in school performance
10. History of recurrent serious "accidents"
11. Psychosomatic symptomatology
12. Suicidal ideation (including significant current and past losses)
13. Decreased affect on interview, avoidance of eye contact—depression posturing
14. Preoccupation with death (clothing, music, media, art)

Modified from Goldenring JM, Cohen E: Getting into adolescent heads, *Contemp Pediatr* 5:75-86, 1988.

3. Response to illness and health
   a. Reaction to illness
   b. Coping patterns
   c. Value of health
   d. Use of well-child and health promotion services
4. Response to care
   a. Perceptions of the caregivers
   b. Compliance
5. Cultural implications for care
   a. Patterns of therapy
   b. Beliefs about child care and childrearing
   c. Patterns of illness response

Anticipatory Guidance

As noted earlier in the chapter, anticipatory guidance should be addressed at each visit. This area includes evaluating the parents' understanding of child development and education, upcoming developmental changes, and questions or issues of concern. The focus should be individualized to the family's needs. In addition, information about child safety (e.g., child-proofing the home; use of bicycle helmets, seatbelts; Figure 26-9) needs to be communicated. This information is most effective when it is offered just before a developmental change is about to occur. Boxes 26-6 and 26-7 provide guidelines for such information.

Anticipatory guidance information may be most easily integrated into other parts of the health history. For example,

BOX 26-5

THE HEADSS PSYCHOSOCIAL INTERVIEW FOR ADOLESCENTS

HOME

Who lives with client? Where?

Own room?

What are relationships like at home?

What do parents and relatives do for a living?

Ever institutionalized? Incarcerated?

Recent moves? Running away?

New people in home environment?

EDUCATION AND EMPLOYMENT

School/grade performance—any recent changes? Any dramatic past changes?

Favorite subjects—worst subjects? (Include grades.)

Any years repeated/classes failed?

Suspension, termination, dropping out?

Future education/employment plans/goals?

Any current or past employment?

Relations with teachers, employers—school/work attendance?

Recent change of schools—number of schools in last 4 years?

ACTIVITIES

With peers (What do you do for fun? Where and when?)

With family or clubs?

Sports—regular exercise?

Church attendance, clubs, projects?

Hobbies—other home activities?

Reading for fun—what?

TV—how much weekly—favorite shows?

Favorite music?

Does patient have care, use seat belts?

History of arrests—acting-out—crime?

DRUGS

Use by peers? Use by patient? (Include alcohol/tobacco.)

Use by family members? (Include alcohol/tobacco.)

Amounts, frequency, patterns of use/abuse, and car use while intoxicated?

Source—how paid for?

SEXUALITY

Orientation?

Degree and types of sexual experience and acts?

Number of partners?

Masturbation (Normalize.)

History of pregnancy/abortion?

Sexually transmitted diseases—knowledge and prevention?

Contraception? Frequency of use?

Comfort with sexual activity, enjoyment/pleasure obtained?

History of sexual/physical abuse

SUICIDE/DEPRESSION

Feelings about self—both positive and negative

History of depression or other mental health problems

Prior suicidal thoughts or attempts

Sleep problems—difficulty getting to sleep, early waking

Modified from Goldenring JM, Cohen E: Getting into adolescent heads, *Contemp Pediatr* 5:75-86, 1988; and Siberg G, Iannone R: *The Harriet Lane Handbook,* St. Louis, 2000, Mosby.

---

when you are getting information about the child's current developmental achievements, you can tell the parent what to look for over the next few months. For example, "Now that your baby has started to crawl, you can expect that he will start to explore new and potentially dangerous areas of your home." This approach can lead to a discussion of safety concerns that the parent will need to consider related to the child's mobility and ability to get into things (e.g., safety gates, plugs for electrical outlets, door/cupboard latches).

Preparation for Examination: Client and Environment

How you conduct the interview and physical examination will vary according to the child's age, development, and behavior and the type of setting in which the care is being provided and the purpose of the encounter. If you do not give consideration to the child's age and development, the examination is likely to be incomplete. If the child is fearful or fatigued, you will need to be more creative, patient, and selective (if possible) in performing the examination.

In carrying out a pediatric examination, keep in mind that each visit for health care is a learning experience for the

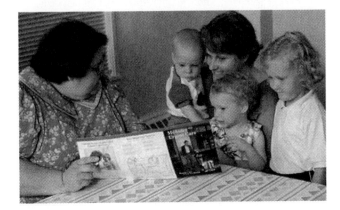

Figure 26-9 Anticipatory guidance needs to be addressed at each visit and should be individualized to the family's needs.

child and the parent(s). The experience may result in increased confidence in themselves and others, or it may produce feelings of failure and distrust toward the professionals who are caring for them. Thus it is important to provide opportunities to develop positive relationships during the visits for routine health care (Figure 26-10).

BOX 26-6

ANTICIPATORY GUIDANCE TOPICS

PRENATAL AND NEWBORN

Prenatal Visit

Health: Pregnancy course, worries, tobacco, alcohol, drug use, hospital and pediatric office procedures

Safety: Infant car seat, crib safety

Nutrition: Planned feeding method

Child care: Help after birth, later arrangements

Family: Changes in relationships (spouse, siblings), supports, stresses, return to work

Newborn Visits

Health: Jaundice, umbilical cord care, circumcision, other common problems, when to call the physician's office

Safety: Infant car seat, smoke detector, choking, keeping tap water temperature below 120° F

Nutrition: Feeding, normal weight loss, spitting, vitamin and fluoride supplements

Development/behavior: Individuality, "consolability," visual and auditory responsiveness

Child care: Importance of interaction, parenting books, support for primary caregiver

Family: Postpartum adjustments, fatigue, "blues," special time for siblings

FIRST YEAR

0 to 6 Months

Health: Immunizations, exposure to infections

Safety: Falls, aspiration of small objects or powder, entanglement in mobiles with long strings, curtain cords

Nutrition: Supplementation of breast milk or formula, introduction of solids, iron

Development/behavior: Crying/colic, irregular schedules (eating, sleeping, eliminating), responding to infant cues, reciprocity, interactive games, beginning eye-hand coordination

Child care: Responsive and affectionate care, caregiving schedule

Family: Return to work, the nurturing of all family relationships (spouse and sibling)

12 MONTHS

Safety: Locks for household poisons and medications, gates for stairs, ipecac, poison center telephone number; outlet safety covers; avoidance of dangling cords or tablecloths; safety devices for windows/screens, toddler car seat at 20 pounds; avoidance of toys with small detachable pieces; supervision of child in tub or near water

Nutrition: Need to discourage use of bottle as a pacifier or while in bed; offer cup and soft finger foods (with supervision); introduce new foods one at a time

Development/behavior: Attachment, basic trust versus mistrust, stranger awareness, night waking, separation anxiety, bedtime routine, transitional object

Child care: Prohibitions few but firm and consistent across caregiving settings; discipline defined as "learning" (not punishment)

Family: Spacing of children

SECOND YEAR

2 Years

Health: Immunizations

Safety: Climbing and falls common; need to supervise outdoor play; ensure safety caps on medicine bottles; note dangers of plastic bags, pan handles hanging over stove, and space heaters

Nutrition: Avoidance of feeding conflicts (decreased appetite common); period of self-feeding, weaning from breast or bottle; need to avoid sweet or salty snacks

Development/behavior: Autonomy versus shame/doubt, ambivalence (independence/dependence), tantrums, negativism, getting into everything, night fears, readiness for toilet training, self-comforting behaviors (thumb-sucking, masturbation), speech, imaginative play, no sharing in play, positive reinforcement for desired behavior

Child care: Freedom to explore in safe place; day care; home a safer place to vent frustrations; needs show of affection, language stimulation through reading and conversation

Family: Sibling relationships

From Foye HR: Anticipatory guidance. In Hoekelman R et al.: *Primary pediatric care,* ed. 3, St. Louis, 1997, Mosby.

Also, remember that any separation of the child from the parent may provoke anxiety in both parties and may increase their level of fear and distrust. Encourage parents to participate in the examination and support their young child. This participation may be done by holding the child during the examination or by soothing the child in other ways.

The older child may be able to participate more freely without the parent present. Most parents will recognize the older child's need to develop independence and encourage the child to participate alone. Finally, prepare the child and the parent for any new or painful procedures. An appreciation for the feelings of children and parents will make them more cooperative.

Developmental Approach to Examination

Conduct the physical examination of the child in an organized and systematic manner, taking into account differences between an adult and a pediatric examination. Perform distressing parts of the examination at the end if you believe that the child will be unable to cooperate. You can alter the order of the examination to accommodate the individual child's behavior (e.g., listening to the heart and lungs early in the examination before crying starts or becomes more vigorous). Similarly, you may begin the examination of a child with a body part that is least likely to interfere with developing a sense of trust and confidence (e.g., the hands or the eyes). Table 26-7 presents a summary of the

BOX 26-6

ANTICIPATORY GUIDANCE TOPICS—cont'd

PRESCHOOL

2 to 5 Years

Health: Toothbrushing, first dental visit

Safety: Need for close supervision near water or street; home safety factors include padding of sharp furniture corners, fire escape plan for home, and locking up power tools; should have car lap belt at 40 pounds and bike helmet; should know (a) name, address, and telephone number; (b) not to provoke dogs; and (c) to say "no" to strangers

Nutrition: Balanced diet; need to avoid sweet or salty snacks; child should participate in conversation at meals

Development/behavior: Initiative versus guilt; difficulty with impulse control and sharing; developing interest in peers, high activity level; speaking in sentences by age 3; speech mostly intelligible to stranger by age 3; reading books; curiosity about body parts; magical thinking; egocentrism

Child care: Need for daily special time with parent(s), bedtime routine; need to talk about day in day care, limit TV and watch with child, reprimand privately, answer questions factually and simply; adjustment to preschool, kindergarten readiness

Family: Chores, responsibilities

MIDDLE CHILDHOOD

5 to 10 Years

Health: Appropriate weight; regular exercise; somatic complaints (limb and abdominal pain, headaches); alcohol, tobacco, and drug use; sexual development; physician and child dealings (more direct)

Safety: Bike helmets and street safety; car seatbelts; swimming lessons; use of matches, firearms, and power tools; fire escape plan for home; saying "no" to strangers

Nutrition: Balanced diet, daily breakfast, limited sweet and salty snacks, moderate fatty foods

Development/behavior: Industry versus inferiority; need for successes, peer interactions, adequate sleep

School: School performance, homework, parent interest

Family: More time away but continuing need for family support, approval, affection, time together, and communication; family rules about bedtime, chores, and responsibilities; guidance in using money; parent(s) should encourage reading; limit TV watching and discuss programs seen together

Other activities: Organized sports, religious groups, other organizations, use of spare time

ADOLESCENCE

Discuss with Adolescent

Health: Alcohol, tobacco, and drug use; need for dental care, physical activity, immunizations

Safety: Bike and skateboard helmet and safety, car seatbelts, driving while intoxicated, water safety, hitchhiking, risk-taking

Nutrition: Balanced diet, appropriate weight, avoidance of junk foods

Sexuality: Physical changes, sex education, peer pressure for sexual activity, sense of responsibility for self and partner, OK to say no, prevention of pregnancy and sexually transmitted diseases, breast and testes self-examination

Development/relationships: Identify versus role confusion, family, peers, dating, independence, trying different roles

School: Academics, homework

Other activities: Sports, hobbies, organizations, jobs

Future plans: School, work, relationships with others

Discuss with Parent

Communication: Let adolescent participate in discussion and development of family rules; needs frequent praise and affection, time together, interest in adolescent's activities

Independence: Parent and child ambivalence about independence; expect periods of estrangement; promote self-responsibility and independence; still needs supervision

Role model: Actions speak louder than words—parents provide model for responsible, reasonable, and compassionate behavior

different approaches used for the physical examination at different developmental stages.

Infant. Usually, little difficulty is encountered in performing the physical examination of the infant in the first 6 months of life, since the infant has little fear of strangers. The parent or the examiner can distract the infant with repetitive vocal sounds and smiles. However, since the examination of the ears and mouth may cause distress, these areas should be saved for the end of the examination. Take advantage of the opportunities that are offered. If the infant is quiet or sleepy, start with the auscultation of the chest and do so while the caretaker is still holding the infant. If the infant is playful and active, start with the extremities and wait for a quieter moment to examine the chest.

During the last half of the first year of life, the infant experiences an increasing fear of strangers. In this situation, conduct the entire examination while the infant is held on the parent's lap (Figure 26-11). Even under the best of circumstances, creating an ideal situation may not be possible. The infant may remain resistant throughout the examination. If this happens, you need to be efficient in carrying out the examination in the least amount of time and with minimal restraint of the infant. The parent often experiences discomfort or embarrassment because of the infant's behavior and will need reassurance that the infant is behaving normally.

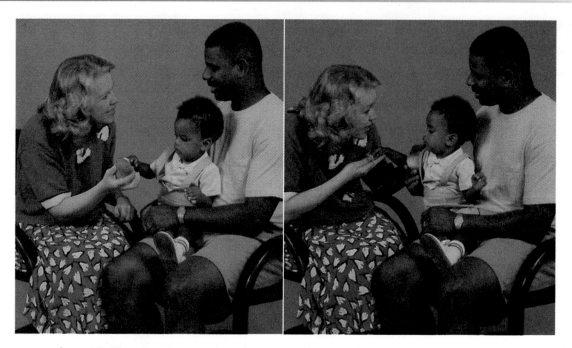

Figure 26-10   The physical examination can be a learning experience for both the parent and the child. It is important to listen to the parent's concerns and to assess the child's needs during the interview.

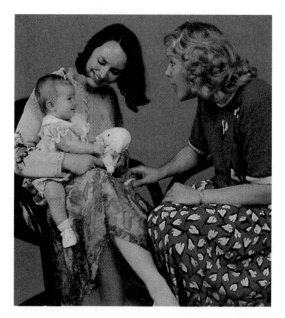

Figure 26-11   The interview is a time for the child to become familiar with the examiner, as well as a time to gather information.

The situation is ideal for helping the parent to understand normal development and the needs of the infant at this age.

Toddler.   The child from 1 to 3 years of age is a challenge to even the most experienced examiner. At this time the child is learning to use his or her body and to manipulate and experiment with all aspects of the environment. The child may see any restraint in the pursuit of desired activities as an interference, resulting in unhappiness or frustration for the child. At this age the child is experiencing a

---

BOX 26-7

**PERTINENT INFORMATION
FOR ANTICIPATORY GUIDANCE**

A. Information about the *child*
 1. Concerns—expressed by parent or child
 2. Health current status and follow-up of past problems
 3. Routine care—feeding, sleep, and elimination
 4. Development—evaluated by school performance or with standardized tests (e.g., Denver Developmental Screening Test, Early Language Milestone Scale)
 5. Behavior—temperament and interaction with family, peers, and others
B. Information about the *child's environment*
 1. Family composition (at home)
 2. Caregiving schedule—who and when
 3. Family stresses—e.g., work, finances, illness, death, move, marital, and other relationships
 4. Family supports—relatives, friends, organizations, maternal resources
 5. Stimulation in the home
 6. Stimulation/activities outside the home, e.g., preschool/school, peers, organizations
 7. Safety

From Foye HR: Anticipatory guidance. In Hoekelman R et al.: *Primary pediatric care,* ed. 3, St. Louis, 1997, Mosby.

---

good deal of pleasure from recently acquired skills such as walking and talking and is enjoying the new ability to manipulate objects such as doors and wastebaskets. Yet the child is still unsure of strangers and needs the parent's presence to feel safe.

TABLE 26-7	Age-Specific Approaches to Physical Examination During Childhood	
Position	**Sequence**	**Preparation**
Infant		
Before sits alone: supine or prone, preferably in parent's lap; before 4 to 6 months: can place on examining table After sits alone: use sitting in parent's lap whenever possible If on table, place with parent in full view	If quiet, auscultate heart, lungs, abdomen Record heart and respiratory rates Palpate and percuss same areas Proceed in usual head-to-toe direction Perform traumatic procedures last (eyes, ears, mouth [while crying]) Elicit reflexes as body part examined Elicit Moro reflex last	Completely undress if room temperature permits Leave diaper on male Gain cooperation with distraction, bright objects, rattles, talking Have older infants hold a small block in each hand; until voluntary release develops toward end of the first year, infants will be unable to grasp other objects (e.g., stethoscope, otoscope) Smile at infant; use soft, gentle voice Pacify with bottle of sugar water or feeding Enlist parent's aid for restraining to examine ears, mouth Avoid abrupt, jerky movements
Toddler		
Sitting or standing on/by parent Prone or supine in parent's lap	Inspect body area through play: "count fingers," "tickle toes" Use minimal physical contact initially Introduce equipment slowly Auscultate, percuss, palpate whenever quiet Perform traumatic procedures last (same as for infant)	Have parent remove outer clothing Remove underwear as body part examined Allow to inspect equipment; demonstrating use of equipment is usually ineffective If uncooperative, perform procedures quickly Use restraint when appropriate; request parent's assistance Talk about examination if cooperative; use short phrases Praise for cooperative behavior
Preschool Child		
Prefer standing or sitting Usually cooperative prone/supine Prefer parent's closeness	If cooperative, proceed in head-to-toe direction If uncooperative, proceed as with toddler	Request self-undressing Allow to wear underpants if shy Offer equipment for inspection; briefly demonstrate use Make up "story" about procedure: "I'm seeing how strong your muscles are" (blood pressure) Use paper-doll technique Give choices when possible Expect cooperation; use positive statements: "Open your mouth"
School-Age Child		
Prefer sitting Cooperative in most positions Younger child prefers parent's presence Older child may prefer privacy	Proceed in head-to-toe direction May examine genitalia last in older child Respect need for privacy	Request self-undressing Allow to wear underpants Give gown to wear Explain purpose of equipment and significance of procedure, such as otoscope to see eardrum, which is necessary for hearing Teach about body functioning and care
Adolescent		
Same as for school-age child Offer option of parent's presence	Same as for older school-age child	Allow to undress in private Give gown Expose only area to be examined Respect need for privacy Explain findings during examination: "Your muscles are firm and strong" Matter-of-factly comment about sexual development: "Your breasts are developing as they should be" Emphasize normalcy of development Examine genitalia as any other body part; may leave to end

From Wong DL et al.: *Whaley and Wong's nursing care of infants and children.* ed. 6, St. Louis, 1999, Mosby.

The 2- or 3-year-old child may be charming and cooperative or difficult to examine. Whichever the case, you will be required to make many modifications in the organization of the examination. You may examine the child in a standing position while you are seated or perform the examination with the child on the parent's lap. The child usually does not like to have all clothing removed at one time but will often cooperate if only one article of clothing is removed at a time while you carry out the examination. The child needs positive reinforcement for cooperative behaviors. He or she also needs the opportunity to handle and use the examining instruments (Figure 26-12). The child may enjoy doing so but may reject the offer if it is too fear-provoking. Despite the difficulties in examining the child of this age, the child's ability to relate more positively at each subsequent visit can be rewarding and profitable for the examiner.

Preschooler. At 3 or 4 years of age the child is usually able to understand and cooperate during the examination. He or she is anxious to please and is usually a delightful participant. At this stage the child has better control of feelings and behavior than the younger child does but may still lose control if fear is great. It is important to keep in mind the child's previous experiences with health care providers and the fears or problems associated with certain aspects of the examination (otoscopic examination in particular). The child should receive recognition for his or her efforts to participate so that the self-image will be enhanced. The child of this age especially enjoys trying out the examiner's equipment and will likely demonstrate this new learning in future play activities; this experience is a way to incorporate the role of the examiner and to master fears (Figure 26-13). The child may prefer to try the equipment on a doll or a stuffed animal. Examination techniques or procedures can also be demonstrated first on a doll or stuffed animal. Again, for some children it may be helpful to permit the child to remain on the caregiver's lap.

School-Age Child. You can approach the school-age child in much the same way that you approach the adult. At this stage the child is usually curious and interested and benefits from explanations of what you are going to do. This child wants to perform well and will usually cooperate. However, the child may have concerns about his or her body and may feel threatened by the examination, particularly if he or she has had past negative experiences. Encourage the child to ask questions. Respect the child's sense of modesty, and attempt to conduct the examination with as little exposure as possible.

Adolescent. The adolescent period is a challenging one for parents, the adolescent, and health care providers. Many physical, developmental, and emotional changes occur during this time (Table 26-8 and Figures 26-14 and 26-15). Adolescents are not easy to anticipate, since behaviors are not predictable at this stage. They may be angry and hostile or charming and self-confident. Adolescents are primarily concerned about themselves and have the egocentric belief that others are as preoccupied with their own behavior and appearance as they are. They are likely to anticipate the responses of other people based on self-beliefs, self-criticism, and self-admiration. Adolescents self-consciously play to an audience because they believe that their behaviors, thoughts, and appearance are important to many people. Despite this egocentric view, adolescents will be responsive to a nonjudgmental examiner who encourages relevant conversation. This type of dialogue may not happen during the first visit, but if the experience is worthwhile to him or her, the adolescent may reveal more of these concerns at a later visit.

If possible, the adolescent should be the primary informant for the interview. The parent also provides significant data, particularly about the adolescent's past health history, the family health history, and the family situation, but the adolescent's perspective is also important. This approach

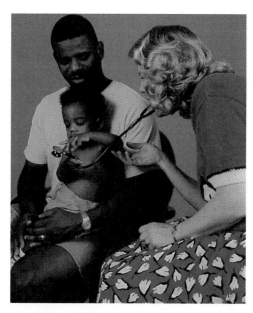

Figure 26-12 The toddler needs the opportunity to handle and use the examining instruments from the safety of the parent's lap.

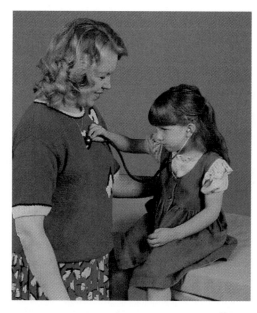

Figure 26-13 The preschool-age child enjoys trying out the examiner's equipment.

TABLE 26-8 **Adolescent Psychosocial and Pubertal Development**

Early Adolescence (11 to 14 Years)	Middle Adolescence (15 to 17 Years)	Late Adolescence (18 to 21 Years)
Cognitive Development		
Concrete thinking: Present oriented; appreciate immediate reactions to behavior but little sense of later consequences	*Early abstract thinking:* Inductive/deductive reasoning; understands later consequences; very self-absorbed, introspective; lots of daydreaming and fantasies	*Abstract thinking.* Adult ability to think abstractly; philosophical; intense idealism about love, religion, social problems
Social/Emotional Development		

Identity concerns:
  Concrete sense of morality and rule driven
  Preoccupation with physical image
  Moody
  Friendship with same-sex peers
  Experimentation is a common phenomenon
  Peer values do not replace parents
  May begin to experiment with mood or mind-altering substances
  May experiment/explore homosexual behavior
  May experiment/explore heterosexual behavior
	More comfortable with sexual identity; gay youth at risk for depression and suicide ideation, also sadness
	Moodiness continues
	Identity centers on "Who am I?"
	Strives toward autonomy
	Sensitive to social norms of peer group; conforms to perceived peer attitudes and behaviors
	Identifies with group or clique
	May develop relationship with single romantic partner
	Limited capacity for emotional intimacy
		Focuses on vocational and personal options
		Uses life experience to generate options and temper decision making
		Capacity for moral reasoning
		Able to formulate ethical principles
		Capacity for mature emotional intimacy in relationships
		Adult sense of self

School-Vocation		
Adjustment to middle school Need to be time efficient May see decrease in scholastic performance as demands increase Truancy may begin	Adjustment to senior high school Academic decisions Increased anxiety about academic performance, especially if college bound Safety in school; students carry weapons, may experience fear of physical harm	Decisions on whether to go to college, join workforce, or enter military Should be a time of choice and empowerment
Family		
Heightened need for privacy Ambivalence about emotional independence Opinionated Challenges family rules, values, behaviors Still needs continued supervision and limit setting that promote increasing autonomy in decision making Family members are important role models Potential for sexual abuse increases as adolescent emerges sexually and begins to challenge behavior	Increased individuation and autonomy Extremely opinionated and challenging Increased family conflict, especially over issues of control Spends less time with family Peer groups take on greater importance Parents may be frustrated; continued communication is important	Relationships more accepting and harmonious More adult-to-adult interactions Family feels sense of loss as adolescent independence increases or can experience freedom

Physical

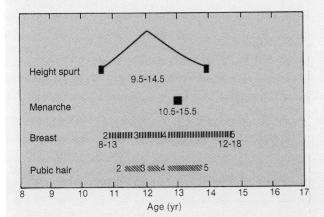

Figure 26-14 Approximate timing of developmental changes in girls. Numbers indicate stages of development. The range of ages during which some of the changes occur is indicated by inclusive numbers below them. (From Marshall WA, Tanner JM: *Arch Dis Child* 44:291, 1969.)

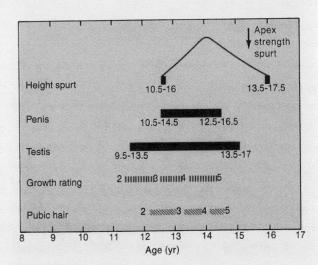

Figure 26-15 Approximate timing of developmental changes in boys. Numbers indicate stages of development. The range of ages during which some of the changes occur is indicated by inclusive numbers below them. (From Marshall WA, Tanner JM: *Arch Dis Child* 45:13, 1970.)

Modified from Levenberg P, Elster A, editors: *Guidelines for adolescent preventive services (GAPS): clinical evaluation and management handbook,* Chicago, 1995, American Medical Association.

supports the adolescent's sense of independence and can help in the development of rapport with the client.

Spend some time talking with the adolescent alone, in addition to talking with the parents (Figure 26-16). This approach allows the adolescent to discuss private concerns. In general, the physical examination of the adolescent should be performed without the parent present. At the beginning of the visit, explain to the client and the parent that the policy is to meet with the parent and the child together for the history to make it as complete as possible and then to speak with and examine the child age 12 or older alone. Explain that after the examination, you will again meet with the parent and the child to discuss your findings and plans and to answer any questions that the parent and the child may have. Most parents are not offended by this approach. If for cultural or individual reasons, it is not acceptable to the parent or the adolescent, conduct the history and examination with the family together.

Establishing a sense of confidentiality with the adolescent is important. Reassure the adolescent client that the information shared will remain between you and the client, unless he or she gives you permission to share it with the parents or others or unless a problem becomes a threat to the client or to others. If you obtain information that cannot be kept confidential because of the laws of a particular state or the rules of health care practice, you must inform the client of this matter. As mentioned earlier, this should be introduced at the beginning of the visit and then again should such need arise.

Since adolescent clients may be self-conscious and easily embarrassed, it is important to make sure that they wear a gown during the examination and that they are given complete privacy for dressing and undressing.

Technique for Examination and Expected Findings

The physical examination provides the opportunity to obtain objective information about the child. Although, in general, most of the information comes from the history, physical examination findings assume greater importance when the parents are poor historians and the child is too young to communicate.

The physical examination of the infant or child varies according to the primary purpose of the visit. Three types of examinations might be performed. The first is the screening of a healthy child. Such an examination is usually complete but does not go into great depth in regard to a particular organ system. The second is the evaluation of a chief complaint, in which a more intensive examination of a particular area (and related regions) may be in order. The third is the follow-up examination of a complaint or disease that has been under treatment in which the focus is usually one or two organ systems. Sometimes these three types of examinations are combined, particularly when it is the child's first visit and he or she is in need of a screening examination and a careful evaluation of the chief complaint.

Methods of Restraint

On some occasions the physical examination involves an uncooperative child. You may need to use one or more of a variety of safe child-restraint methods. Clinical experience and knowledge of the child's behavior during previous visits will aid in choosing a safe restraint method. When restraint is necessary, carry out the procedure as quickly as possible and without criticism of the child.

One of the most common methods for restraining the infant or young child when examining the ears, nose, and mouth is done with the aid of the parent or another adult. Place the child in the supine position with the arms extended, and have the assisting adult hold the arms alongside the head (Figure 26-17). For an older child who cannot cooperate, use the same method with a second adult holding the child's legs.

Another method for the older child is sometimes called the "hug." Have the child sit on the parent's lap with the legs to the side and one arm tucked under the parent's arm while the parent holds the child's other arm securely (Figure 26-18). Obtain greater immobility of the child by having the parent

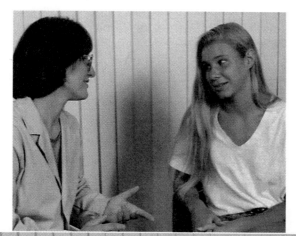

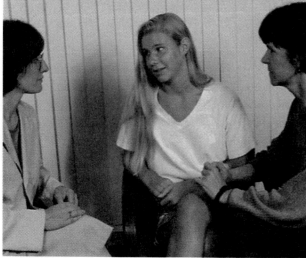

Figure 26-16 It is important to meet with the adolescent both alone and with the parent.

place the child's legs between his or her own (Figure 26-19). If the parent is uncomfortable about assisting with restraint, you may ask another adult to help. However, the child usually feels less threatened if the parent does the holding.

Measurements

Take measurements of the temperature, pulse rate, respiratory rate, blood pressure (for children older than 3 years), height, and weight as part of the physical examination of the child. In addition, note the measurements of the head circumference for the child who is younger than 3 years. Comparing the physical measurements of a child with those of other healthy children over time makes it possible to determine whether the child is progressing within normal parameters or whether significant deviations exist.

Assessment of Vital Signs

Temperature. The body areas commonly used for obtaining temperature measurements—the mouth, the axilla, the rectum, and the ear canal and tympanic membrane—and types of thermometers are discussed in detail earlier in the text (see Chapter 9) and are briefly reviewed here. The child's ability to cooperate and the health status determine the method selected.

Axillary Temperature. You can obtain an axillary temperature on any child. This method reduces the risk of injury and is less intrusive than rectal or oral reading. Use the axillary route, whenever possible, to obtain the newborn's temperature. This approach may also be preferable for toddlers and preschoolers.

Consider using the axillary temperature when the child objects to the rectal temperature and the oral temperature is not appropriate. Many practitioners recommend using the axillary method first and confirming an elevated temperature with a rectal or oral reading. Place the thermometer tip deep into the axilla and hold the arm close to the body for at least 5 minutes (a digital thermometer reading will be faster). Restrain the child by using the "hug" if necessary.

Oral Temperature. Generally reserve the oral temperature reading (with a glass thermometer) for children who are 5 to 6 years and older. Younger children may be able to use a digital thermometer. The child must be able to understand not to bite on the glass or digital thermometer and to keep the mouth closed during the procedure. Place the ther-

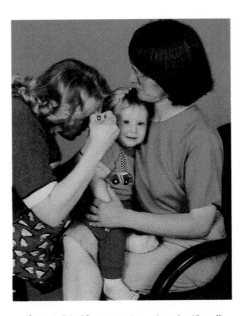

Figure 26-18 Restraint using the "hug."

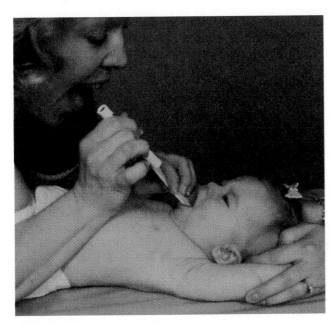

Figure 26-17 Restraint of the young child with the parent assisting.

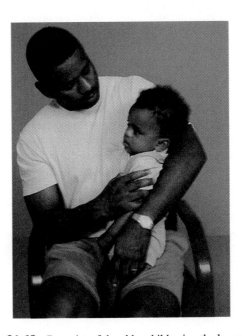

Figure 26-19 Restraint of the older child using the leg restraint.

mometer under the tongue for at least 5 minutes; it can take up to 7 minutes to reach the maximum temperature (for a glass thermometer [a digital thermometer will be much quicker]). Sometimes the child's health condition (e.g., mouth breathing or limited intellectual functioning) interferes with being able to use this method.

Tympanic Thermography. A more recent method for taking temperatures is tympanic thermography (see Chapter 9). The tympanic thermometer is placed in the ear canal and uses an infrared sensor to detect the temperature of blood flowing through the eardrum. For the most accurate results, make sure to straighten the ear canal by pulling on the pinna (see Figure 26-44). Take three measurements and record the highest one. The thermometer registers within 2 seconds. The ease and speed of this approach is making it the preferred method for use in many health care settings.

Rectal Temperature. Obtaining a rectal temperature has been a common practice during the first few years of a child's life. However, many now recommend using this method only when no other route can be used. The main drawbacks are the danger of perforation of the rectum in the newborn and young infant and the increased discomfort for the young child, who experiences this as an intrusive procedure. Do not use this method with children who cannot tolerate this kind of stimulus to the central nervous system (CNS), as is the case with some children who have epilepsy, or with children who are receiving chemotherapy that affects the gastrointestinal mucosa.

A safe restraint method for taking a rectal temperature of a young infant is to lay the child face down on the parent's lap or on a padded table. Have the adult place the left forearm firmly across the child's hip area so that the child cannot raise the buttocks off the adult's lap or the table. Use the thumb and forefinger of the nondominant hand to separate the buttocks, and gently insert the lubricated thermometer with the dominant hand. Do not insert the thermometer any farther than 1 inch (2.5 cm). Deeper insertion increases the risk of perforation, since the colon curves posteriorly at a depth of $1\frac{1}{4}$ inches (3 cm). The temperature registers within 3 to 4 minutes on a glass thermometer (a digital thermometer reading is much quicker).

The infant's rectum is quite short; therefore insert the thermometer only a short distance. Three considerations help to determine sufficient entry: noting that the column of mercury is rising steadily, inserting no more than 1 inch (2.5 cm), and observing a decrease in the child's effort to push against the thermometer. It is normal for the child to push against the thermometer as the rectal sphincter muscles contract in response to the stimulus. Wait until the sphincter relaxes before continuing to insert. Hold the thermometer firmly enough to keep the child from pushing it out. Use care to hold the thermometer firmly but not to push it in farther. Also, hold the child securely to prevent jerking and subsequently pushing the thermometer farther into the rectum.

Temperature regulation is less exact in children than in adults. The time of day and the child's activity level need to be considered when assessing temperature. Children may normally have elevated temperatures after vigorous play, af-

ter eating, later in the afternoon, or when excited (Barness, 1998). The rectal temperature is normally higher in infants and younger children, and the average temperature is greater than 37.2° C (99° F) until age 3 years. After age 3 the average temperature is similar to that of adults (98.6° F; 37° C).

When a temperature is being recorded, it is important to indicate the route of measurement (rectal, oral, axillary, tympanic). However, do not add or subtract degrees based on route, since there is disagreement as to how much variability in temperature exists. The increase in temperature with even a minor infection is usually greater in infants and young children than in adults. However, young infants with a severe infection may have a normal or subnormal temperature. Therefore it is also important to consider the child's general appearance (e.g., lethargic with decreased responsiveness versus happy and playful) to evaluate the significance of the child's body temperature.

Pulse and Respiration. Apprehension, crying, and physical activity, as well as the examination procedure itself, can alter a child's heart and respiratory rates. Thus, if possible, take these measurements while the child is at rest, either sleeping or lying quietly.

If the child has been active, delay taking the measurement until the child has relaxed for about 5 to 10 minutes. If you must measure the respiratory rate and the heart rate while the child is crying or agitated, note this information next to your recording of the rate.

Examine the child's pulse for rate, rhythm, quality, and amplitude, just as for an adult. Auscultation of the heart—measuring the apical pulse—is the most easily obtained pulse in a young infant. The average heart rate of the infant at birth is 140 beats per minute. At 2 years of age the child's heart rate has adjusted downward to 110. At 10 years the rate is 85, and by the time the child reaches age 18, the pulse may have decreased to 82. A child, usually an adolescent, who engages in exercise regularly, such as swimming laps, may exhibit a much slower rate (i.e., in the 60s).

Table 26-9 lists the normal ranges of heart rates for children. Heart rhythm in children is not always regular. Often the rate will change in relation to the respiratory cycle. The heart rate accelerates during inspiration because of the increase in pressure in the thoracic cavity and decreases during expiration. This phenomenon, which is called sinus arrhythmia, is considered normal in children.

Palpation of the brachial and femoral pulses is an essential step in the examination of the young infant. Irregularities often are the first signs of serious heart dysfunction. The amplitude and rhythm of the femoral pulse are expected to equal those of the brachial pulse. Absence or weakness of the femoral pulse indicates the possibility of coarctation of the aorta in the young infant. Table 26-10 compares some differences in amplitude, quality, and site and how they may relate to the differential diagnosis of heart disorders in children.

Obtain the respiratory rate by inspection or auscultation. In infants, respiratory movements are primarily diaphragmatic and are observed by abdominal movement. Since these movements are commonly irregular, you need to count them for a full minute for accuracy. The average range of

TABLE 26-9 Normal Ranges of Heart Rates for Children

Age	Rate (Beats/Min)		
	Resting (Awake)	Resting (Sleeping)	Exercise (Fever)
Newborn	100-180	80-160	Up to 220
1 week to 3 months	100-220	80-180	Up to 220
3 months to 2 years	80-150	70-120	Up to 200
2 years to 10 years	70-110	60-100	Up to 180
10 years to adult	55-90	50-90	Up to 180

Modified from Gillette PC: Dysrhythmias. In Adams FH, Emmanouilides GC, Riemenschneider TA, editors: *Moss' heart disease in infants, children, and adolescents,* ed. 4, Baltimore, 1989, Williams & Wilkins.

TABLE 26-10 Amplitude, Quality of Heart Rate, and Site as They Relate to Differential Diagnosis of Heart Dysfunction in Young Infants and Children

Amplitude, Quality, Site	Cardiac Dysfunction
Narrow, thready	Congestive heart failure
	Severe aortic stenosis
Bounding	Patent ductus arteriosus
	Aortic regurgitation
Pulsation in suprasternal notch	Aortic insufficiency
	Patent ductus arteriosus
	Coarctation of aorta
Palpable thrill in suprasternal notch	Aortic stenosis
	Valvular pulmonary stenosis
	Coarctation of aorta, occasionally patent ductus arteriosus

Data from Kempe CH et al.: *Current pediatric diagnosis and treatment,* ed. 9, Los Altos, Calif., 1987, Lange Medical Publications.

TABLE 26-11 Variations in Respiration with Age

Age	Rate/Min
Premature	40-90
Newborn	30-80
1 yr	20-40
2 yr	20-30
3 yr	20-30
5 yr	20-25
10 yr	17-22
15 yr	15-20
20 yr	15-20

Data from Lowrey GH: *Growth and development of children,* ed. 8, St. Louis, 1986, Mosby.

normal respirations is 30 to 80 per minute in the newborn period compared with 20 to 30 per minute in the 2-year-old. By 10 years of age the respiratory rate has adjusted to 17 to 22 per minute, and by age 20 it averages 15 to 20 per minute. Table 26-11 shows variations in respiration with age.

Blood Pressure. The levels of systolic and diastolic blood pressure gradually increase during childhood, and normally a considerable variation exists in a child's pressure. The systolic pressure of the child may be raised by crying, vigorous exercise, or anxiety. Therefore choose a time when the child is quiet and comfortable to obtain this measurement.

The National Task Force on Blood Pressure Control in Children recommends that children 3 years or older have their blood pressure measured annually as part of their regular health care. The child of this age is usually able to cooperate when you explain the procedure for obtaining a blood pressure measurement. Routinely measuring the blood pressure of the child younger than 3 years is unnecessary, unless there are indications of underlying problems such as renal or cardiac disease.

The most common method of measuring the blood pressure of the child is still auscultation with a mercury or aneroid sphygmomanometer. The selection of the cuff size and the method of measuring the blood pressure are described in detail in Figure 26-20.

The size of the cuff is important because a cuff that is too small causes falsely elevated values. Pediatric cuffs are available in several sizes for newborns, infants, and children. A pediatric stethoscope with a small diaphragm is also essential when measuring the blood pressure of a young child. The systolic pressure is recorded as the point at which the Korotkoff sounds are initially heard. The diastolic pressure is recorded as the point at which the fourth-phase Korotkoff

sound is heard, when the sound first becomes muffled. The fifth-phase Korotkoff sound is the disappearance of all sound. In young children the fourth and fifth sounds commonly occur simultaneously, and sometimes the Korotkoff sounds are heard all the way to zero.

The Doppler instrument, although relatively expensive, is useful with young infants and children. It measures systolic blood pressure, which is the first sound heard. Even though the Doppler device is useful for systolic measurement, it has not been found to be reliable for diastolic pressure measurement.

If a Doppler instrument is unavailable, you can use the flush method to approximate the mean blood pressure. (This method is rarely used, but it is helpful to know it for situations in which advanced technology is unavailable.) Elevate the extremity, with the uninflated cuff in place. Stroke or milk the arm from the hand to the elbow. Inflate the cuff to a point above the estimated systolic blood pressure. Slowly

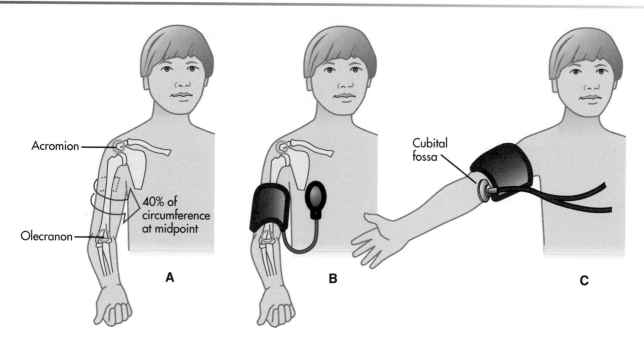

Figure 26-20 Determination of proper cuff size and blood pressure measurement in children. **A,** The cuff bladder width should be approximately 40% of the circumference of the arm, measured at a point midway between the olecranon and the acromion. **B,** The cuff bladder should cover 80% to 100% of the circumference of the arm. **C,** Blood pressure should be measured with the cubital fossa supported at the heart level. The stethoscope is placed over the brachial artery pulse, proximal and medial to the cubital fossa, below the bottom edge of the cuff. (Modified from National High Blood Pressure Education Program Working Group on Hypertension Control in Children and Adolescents: update on the 1987 Task Force Report on High Blood Pressure in Children and Adolescents, *Pediatrics* 98(4):649-658, 1996.)

■ **HELPFUL HINT**

When taking a child's blood pressure:
- The child should be seated. Take the measurement routinely in the right arm held at heart level.
- Do not press too hard with the stethoscope.
- If no pediatric cuff is available, use an adult cuff around the child's thigh and place the stethoscope over the popliteal area (behind knee) to hear Korotkoff sounds. This measurement averages about 10 mm Hg higher than blood pressure taken in the arm.
- Refer the child with abnormally high serial readings to a physician.
- Blood pressure readings between the 90th and 95th percentiles are high-normal and require further evaluation for risk factors for hypertension.
- Significant hypertension is blood pressure persistently between the 95th and 99th percentiles for age, height, and sex.

---

release the pressure. A sudden reddening or "flush" of the extremity (as compared with the other extremity) will occur at a point about halfway between the systolic and diastolic pressures.

The 1996 AAP Update on the 1987 Task Force Report on High Blood Pressure in Children and Adolescents found that body size, along with sex and age, must be considered to ac-

curately assess blood pressure in children and adolescents. Commonly, very tall children have been misclassified as hypertensive. When height was factored in, their blood pressures were found to be normal. Conversely, very short children, judged to be normotensive, may in fact have high-normal or elevated blood pressures. Based on a detailed review of epidemiological samples, the AAP (1996) developed new blood pressure tables adjusted for height, as well as age and sex (Tables 26-12 and 26-13).

To determine blood pressure status, obtain the height percentile from a standard growth chart; these can be found at the CDC website (www.cdc.gov/growthcharts/). Then compare the child's systolic and diastolic blood pressures with the numbers provided in the boys' or girls' table (as appropriate) for age and height percentiles. A normal blood pressure is less than the 90th percentile for height. If the child's systolic or diastolic blood pressure is at or more than the 95th percentile for height, repeated measurements are indicated to rule out hypertension. Blood pressure measurements between the 90th and 95th percentiles for height are considered high-normal and require additional observation and evaluation for risk factors for hypertension. A blood pressure measurement more than the 95th percentile on at least three occasions over a 6- to 12-month period (in the absence of symptoms) is required for a diagnosis of hypertension. Although early essential hypertension is not a common problem in children, elevated blood pressure in children of-

TABLE 26-12   Blood Pressure Levels for the 90th and 95th Percentiles of Blood Pressure for Girls Ages 1 to 17 Years by Percentiles of Height

Age (Yr)	Blood Pressure Percentile*	Systolic Blood Pressure by Percentile of Height (mm Hg)							Diastolic Blood Pressure by Percentile of Height (mm Hg)†						
		5%	10%	25%	50%	75%	90%	95%	5%	10%	25%	50%	75%	90%	95%
1	90th	97	98	99	100	102	103	104	53	53	53	54	55	56	56
	95th	101	102	103	104	105	107	107	57	57	57	58	59	60	60
2	90th	99	99	100	102	103	104	105	57	57	58	58	59	60	61
	95th	102	103	104	105	107	108	109	61	61	62	62	63	64	65
3	90th	100	100	102	103	104	105	106	61	61	61	62	63	63	64
	95th	104	104	105	107	108	109	110	65	65	65	66	67	67	68
4	90th	101	102	103	104	106	107	108	63	63	64	65	65	66	67
	95th	105	106	107	108	109	111	111	67	67	68	69	69	70	71
5	90th	103	103	104	106	107	108	109	65	66	66	67	68	68	69
	95th	107	107	108	110	111	112	113	69	70	70	71	72	72	73
6	90th	104	105	106	107	109	110	111	67	67	68	69	69	70	71
	95th	108	109	110	111	112	114	114	71	71	72	73	73	74	75
7	90th	106	107	108	109	110	112	112	69	69	69	70	71	72	72
	95th	110	110	112	113	114	115	116	73	73	73	74	75	76	76
8	90th	108	109	110	111	112	113	114	70	70	71	71	72	73	74
	95th	112	112	113	115	116	117	118	74	74	75	75	76	77	78
9	90th	110	110	112	113	114	115	116	71	72	72	73	74	74	75
	95th	114	114	115	117	118	119	120	75	76	76	77	78	78	79
10	90th	112	112	114	115	116	117	118	73	73	73	74	75	76	76
	95th	116	116	117	119	120	121	122	77	77	77	78	79	80	80
11	90th	114	114	116	117	118	119	120	74	74	75	75	76	77	77
	95th	118	118	119	121	122	123	124	78	78	79	79	80	81	81
12	90th	116	116	118	119	120	121	122	75	75	76	76	77	78	78
	95th	120	120	121	123	124	125	126	79	79	80	80	81	82	82
13	90th	118	118	119	121	122	123	124	76	76	77	78	78	79	80
	95th	121	122	123	125	126	127	128	80	80	81	82	82	83	84
14	90th	119	120	121	122	124	125	136	77	77	78	79	79	80	81
	95th	123	124	125	126	128	129	130	81	81	82	83	83	84	85
15	90th	121	121	122	124	125	126	127	78	78	79	79	80	81	82
	95th	124	125	126	128	129	130	131	82	82	83	83	84	85	86
16	90th	122	122	123	125	126	127	128	79	79	79	80	81	82	82
	95th	125	126	127	128	130	131	132	83	83	83	84	85	86	86
17	90th	122	123	124	125	126	128	128	79	79	79	80	81	82	82
	95th	126	126	127	129	130	131	132	83	83	83	84	85	86	86

From National High Blood Pressure Education Program Working Group on Hypertension Control in Children and Adolescents: update on the 1987 Task Force Report on High Blood Pressure in Children and Adolescents, *Pediatrics* 98(4):649-658, 1996.

*Blood pressure percentile was determined by a single reading.

†Height percentile was determined by standard growth curves.

ten correlates with hypertension in early adulthood (AAP, 1996). Monitoring blood pressure in children and promoting appropriate lifestyle interventions in those at risk may help to avoid long-term problems.

Growth Measurements

The routine measurement of growth is a screening procedure rather than a diagnostic procedure. Yet such measurement can provide clues to serious health problems. Growth is a continuous process that the practitioner must evaluate over time. Successive serial measurements plotted on a standardized growth chart provide objective information about the individual child's rate and pattern of growth in comparison with the general population. This information is useful in providing reassurance to parents and professionals regarding the child who is growing normally; in assessing the nutritional status of the child; in identifying the child who may have abnormalities that are affecting the various growth parameters, such as growth-hormone deficiency, inflammatory bowel disease, and cardiac and renal disorders; and in identifying children who are at risk for or are experiencing growth problems.

By far the most significant current growth problem in the United States is an increase in obesity in children and ado-

TABLE 26-13 Blood Pressure Levels for the 90th and 95th Percentiles of Blood Pressure for Boys Ages 1 to 17 Years by Percentiles of Height

Age (Yr)	Blood Pressure Percentile*	Systolic Blood Pressure by Percentile of Height (mm Hg)							Diastolic Blood Pressure by Percentile of Height (mm Hg)†						
		5%	10%	25%	50%	75%	90%	95%	5%	10%	25%	50%	75%	90%	95%
1	90th	94	95	97	98	100	102	102	50	51	52	53	54	54	55
	95th	98	99	101	102	104	106	106	55	55	56	57	58	59	59
2	90th	98	99	100	102	104	105	106	55	55	56	57	58	59	59
	95th	101	102	104	106	108	109	110	59	59	60	61	62	63	63
3	90th	100	101	103	105	107	108	109	59	59	60	61	62	63	63
	95th	104	105	107	109	111	112	113	63	63	64	65	66	67	67
4	90th	102	103	105	107	109	110	111	62	62	63	64	65	66	66
	95th	106	107	109	111	113	114	115	66	67	67	68	69	70	71
5	90th	104	105	106	108	110	112	112	65	65	66	67	68	69	69
	95th	108	109	110	112	114	115	116	69	70	70	71	72	73	74
6	90th	105	106	108	110	111	113	114	67	68	79	70	70	71	72
	95th	109	110	112	114	115	117	117	72	72	73	74	75	76	76
7	90th	106	107	109	111	113	114	115	69	70	71	72	72	73	74
	95th	110	111	113	115	116	118	119	74	74	75	76	77	78	78
8	90th	107	108	110	112	114	115	116	71	71	72	73	74	75	75
	95th	111	112	114	116	118	119	120	75	76	76	77	78	79	80
9	90th	109	110	112	113	115	117	117	72	73	73	74	75	76	77
	95th	113	114	116	117	119	121	121	76	77	78	79	80	80	81
10	90th	110	112	113	115	117	118	119	73	74	74	75	76	77	78
	95th	114	115	117	119	121	122	123	77	78	79	80	80	81	82
11	90th	112	113	115	117	119	120	121	74	74	75	76	77	78	78
	95th	116	117	119	121	123	124	125	78	79	79	80	81	82	83
12	90th	115	116	117	119	121	123	123	75	75	76	77	78	78	79
	95th	119	120	121	123	125	126	127	79	79	80	81	82	83	83
13	90th	117	118	120	122	124	125	126	75	76	77	78	79	80	
	95th	121	122	124	126	128	129	130	79	80	81	82	83	83	84
14	90th	120	121	123	125	126	128	128	76	76	77	78	79	80	80
	95th	124	125	127	128	130	132	132	80	81	81	82	83	84	85
15	90th	123	124	125	127	129	131	131	77	77	78	79	80	81	81
	95th	127	128	129	131	133	134	135	81	82	83	83	84	85	86
16	90th	125	126	128	130	132	133	134	79	79	80	81	82	82	83
	95th	129	130	132	134	136	137	138	83	83	84	85	86	87	87
17	90th	128	129	131	133	134	136	136	81	81	82	83	84	85	85
	95th	132	133	135	136	138	140	140	85	85	86	87	88	89	89

From National High Blood Pressure Education Program Working Group on Hypertension Control in Children and Adolescents: update on the 1987 Task Force Report on High Blood Pressure in Children and Adolescents, *Pediatrics* 98(4):649-658, 1996.

*Blood pressure percentile was determined by a single measurement.

†Height percentile was determined by standard growth curves.

lescents. The CDC (2000) noted that one in five children is at risk of being overweight and 10% of children are overweight or obese. In addition, they reported that the number of overweight children has doubled during the past 15 years and that 70% of overweight children ages 10 to 13 will become overweight and obese adults. Currently more than one half of all American adults are overweight. Research indicates that, in general, children are heavier today than in 1977, but height has remained virtually unchanged. This trend is associated with low levels of physical activity rather than increased food consumption (Barlow and Dietz, 1998). This trend highlights the importance of early intervention to prevent these problems and the need to monitor growth at every visit.

Three parameters of growth are routinely measured during each examination of the child younger than 3 years old: recumbent length, body weight, and head circumference. For the child older than 3 years, standing height and weight measurements are obtained. Assessment of body segments, skinfold thickness, bone age, and dentition may be useful for further study of body growth, but it is not usually included in the routine physical examination. These parameters are then plotted on growth charts, which provide a visual representation of the child's growth pattern.

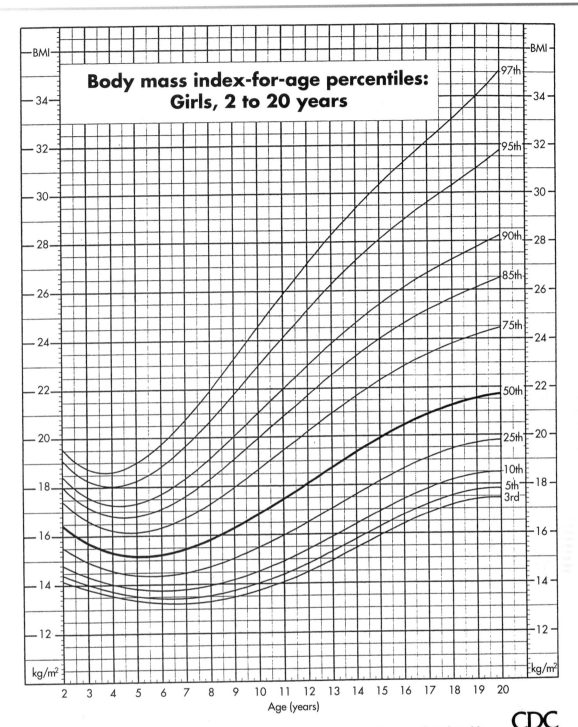

Figure 26-21 Body mass index-for-age percentiles: girls, 2 through 20 years. (Developed by the National Center for Health Statistics in collaboration with the National Center for Chronic Disease Prevention and Health Promotion [2000].)

Growth Charts. In June 2000 the CDC released revised growth charts based on new data and improved statistical procedures. The revised pediatric growth charts better reflect the current racial and ethnic diversity in the United States and include size and growth patterns of both breast-fed and formula-fed infants. In addition, 3rd and 97th percentiles were added to all the charts, and charts were extended to track the growth pattern of children and young people through age 20. The revised charts for children age 2 to 20 years include the body mass index (BMI) (Figure 26-21), which is believed to be a more sensitive measure of both risk for and actual overweight and underweight.

The BMI is a single number that evaluates an individual's weight status in relation to height to determine underweight and overweight. It has been used as the first indicator in assessing body fat and has been the most common method of tracking weight problems and obesity among adults (see Chapter 6). Studies have shown that children as young as age 2 years can demonstrate a risk for future weight problems if they have a high ratio of body fat and a family history of weight problems. It is hoped that use of the BMI will make it easier to assess the child's risk for obesity and result in earlier interventions to address this major public health concern.

The CDC's new charts are based on data gathered through the National Health and Nutrition Examination Survey (NHANES III), which are data from physical examinations on a cross-section of Americans from all over the country. Two groups of charts were developed from the data: the first for the age interval from birth to 36 months and the second for the interval from 2 to 18 years. The charts for infants (birth to 36 months) were developed separately for boys and girls and include graphs for head circumference, recumbent length by age, weight by age, and weight by length. The charts for children ages 2 to 18 years are in separate versions for boys and girls and include graphs for stature (standing height) by age, weight by age, and weight by stature of prepubescent children and BMI-for-age according to sex-specific charts. The standard growth charts are available on the CDC website (www.cdc.gov/growthcharts/). Figure 26-21 shows a BMI chart, the most recent addition to the standard growth charts.

The appropriate use of the charts requires that consistent measurement techniques be used at each point in time. For instance, do not record standing height or stature on the birth-to-36 months chart, since the infant will appear shorter than if the recumbent length were used. There can be a difference of up to 1 inch between recumbent and standing measures of the same child. Record standing height on the chart for 2- to-18-year-olds.

To interpret growth measurements, you need to take into account several factors. First, children whose weight and height fall between the 5th and 95th percentiles are likely to be growing normally. Evaluate and follow closely, however, those who fall below the 5th or above the 95th percentiles. Also follow closely the child who has a sudden increase or decrease in dimensions. Consider the size of the parents when looking at the child's growth pattern. If both parents are small or large, their children's growth likely will be similar. The overall pattern of growth is more important than any single measure.

The relationship between height and weight is also significant. Pay specific attention to children who have a disparity between these two measures. For example, a child whose height falls in the 75th percentile but whose weight falls in the 25th percentile needs more in-depth evaluation and monitoring. Other areas of concern are a child's failure to show expected increases in height and weight, particularly during peak growth periods such as infancy and adolescence, and sudden changes in height or weight from the child's growth curve (e.g., sudden increases or decreases).

Length or Height. Measure recumbent length (birth to 3 years) with the child in the supine position with the legs extended. To measure length, facilitate the procedure by having two people participate. The parent is usually available and interested in providing this assistance. If you use a measuring board, place the infant's head against the fixed headboard, and have the parent hold it in the midline while you gently push on the infant's knees until the legs are fully extended and both heels are firmly touching the movable footboard. If a measuring device is not available, follow the same procedure, placing the child on a paper-covered flat surface and marking the paper at the top of the child's head and at the bottom of the heels (Figure 26-22, *A*). Measure the distance between the two points (Figure 26-22, *B*).

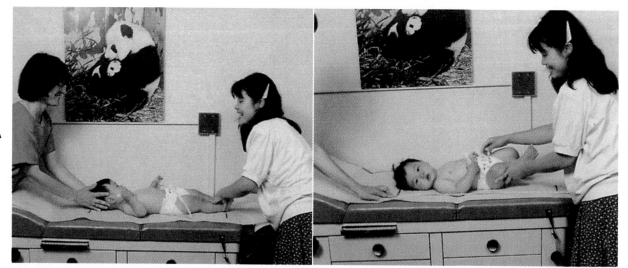

Figure 26-22 **A,** Measuring recumbent length with the parent's assistance. The child is placed on a paper-covered flat surface, and marks are made at the head and feet. **B,** The distance between the two marks is measured while the child relaxes.

Measure standing height or stature (2 to 18 years) with the youngster's shoes off. Ask the child to stand as tall as possible with heels on the ground and look straight ahead so that the top of the head is parallel with the ceiling. The feet should be together, and the shoulders, buttocks, and heels should be touching the wall without any flexion of the knees (Figure 26-23). Bring a block, squared at right angles against the wall, or a measuring board to the top of the child's head. When a measuring device is not available, you can make a mark on the wall at the top of the child's head and measure the distance from the floor.

Weight. To weigh the child, use an appropriately sized beam scale with nondetachable weights. Two scales are suggested: one for infants and small children, which measures weights to the nearest 0.5 ounce or 10 g, and one for older children and adults, which measures weights to the nearest 0.25 pound or 100 g. Before weighing the child, check the scale to determine whether it is balanced. Return the weights to the zero setting and make sure that the balance is resting in the middle.

When infant growth charts (birth to 36 months) are used, weigh the child naked on the infant scale (Figure 26-24). With the charts for older children (2 to 18 years), use the upright adult scale, ideally with the child dressed only in underpants or a light gown. Record what the child was wearing when the measurement was taken (e.g., in diaper, shoes removed; Figure 26-25).

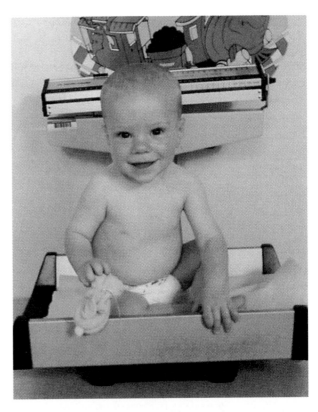

Figure 26-24 Weighing the young infant.

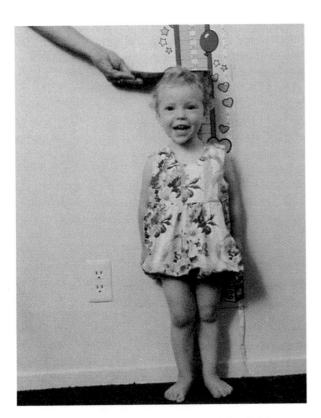

Figure 26-23 Measurement of standing height.

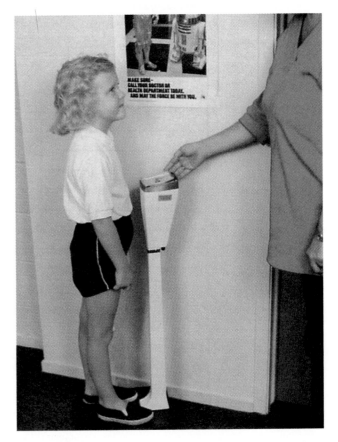

Figure 26-25 Weighing the older child. Ideally, the child would be dressed only in underwear or a light gown with shoes removed.

Head Circumference.   Measure the head circumference during each examination of children between birth and 36 months and in any child whose head size is questionable. Pass a nonstretchable tape measure over the most prominent part of the occiput and just above the supraor-

bital ridges (Figure 26-26). The average head circumference at birth is 35 cm (14 inches) and by age 2 has increased to 49 cm (19.2 inches). The head circumference is an important measure to obtain because it is related to intracranial volume and allows an estimation of the rate of growth of the brain. Plot sequential measurements on the appropriate growth chart. Check any discrepancy or deviation, with consideration given to the conditions of microcephaly and hydrocephaly.

Always measure the head circumference of the child who is suspected of having a neurological problem or a developmental delay, regardless of age.

Chest Circumference.   The measurement of the circumference of the chest at delivery and in early infancy has become significant in that it may indicate birth injury, congenital anomalies, or system dysfunction (e.g., cardiac enlargement). Otherwise, measuring the chest circumference on a regular basis beyond early infancy is unnecessary. Exceptions to this might include observed body disproportion or malformation of the thoracic cage. Measure the chest circumference of the child by placing a nonstretchable cloth tape measure at the level of the nipple, with the child in a supine position. Take the measurement midway between inspiration and expiration.

Growth curves of the body as a whole and of three types of tissue—lymphoid, neural, and genital—demonstrate the age ranges when children are expected to exhibit growth spurts (Figure 26-27).

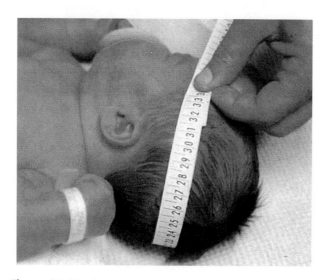

Figure 26-26   Appropriate placement of the measuring tape to obtain the head circumference. (From Seidel HM et al.: *Mosby's guide to physical examination,* ed. 4, St. Louis, 1999, Mosby.)

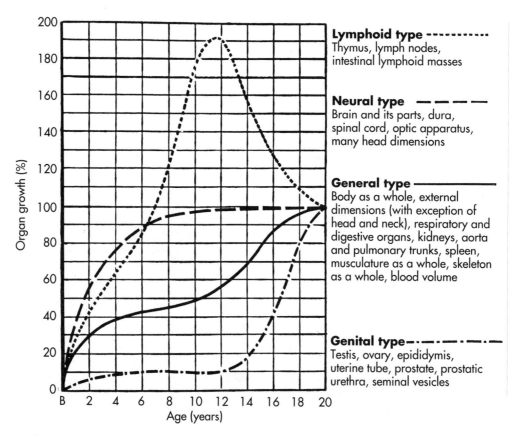

Figure 26-27   Differential organ growth curves. (From Harris JA et al.: *The measurement of man.* Minneapolis, 1930, University of Minnesota Press.)

Body Mass Index. The BMI is used differently with children than it is with adults (Kuczmarski et al., 2000). The interpretation of BMI depends on the child's age. As children grow, their body fatness changes over the years. In addition, girls and boys differ in their body fatness as they mature. The CDC (2000) recommends the following approaches to determine the BMI. First, obtain height and weight measurements and then do *one* of the following:

1. Look the BMI up on a table. The CDC provides the CDC Table for Calculated BMI Values for Selected Heights and Weights for Ages 2 to 20 Years at the CDC website (www.cdc.gov/growthcharts).
2. Access a website BMI calculator. The CDC Web BMI calculator can be found at the CDC website (www.cdc.gov/growthcharts).
3. Compute the BMI on a calculator using one of the following formulas:
   - English version:

     Weight in pounds ÷ Height in inches ÷ Height in inches × 703 = BMI. (*Example:* Joey weighs 33 pounds, 4 ounces and is 37⅝ inches tall. His BMI is 33.25 pounds divided by 37.625 inches, divided by 37.625 inches × 703 = 16.5.)

   - Metric version:

     Weight in kilograms ÷ [Height in meters]² = BMI

   or

     Weight in kilograms ÷ Height in meters ÷ Height in meters × 10,000 = BMI. (*Example:* Sharon weighs 16.9 kg and is 105.2 cm tall. Her BMI is 16.9 divided by 105.2 cm divided by 105.2 cm × 10,000 = 15.3.)

Using the CDC BMI-For-Age Growth Chart. Each of the CDC BMI-for-age charts contains a series of curved lines that indicate specific percentiles. The percentile curves show an expected pattern of growth—the BMI decreases during the preschool years, then increases into adulthood. In the United States, the BMI reaches its lowest point around 4 to 6 years of age. It then begins a gradual increase through adolescence and most of adulthood. The upward trend after the low point, or dip, in BMI percentile curves is called the "adiposity rebound." Children whose adiposity rebound begins at younger ages are more likely to have an increased BMI as an adult (CDC, 2000).

■ **HELPFUL HINT**

Proper documentation of height and weight onto growth charts is as important as proper assessment. Age- and sex-specific growth charts are readily available on the Internet (www.cdc.gov/growthcharts).

If a child is born prematurely, use the "corrected age" on growth charts and developmental assessments until the child is 2½ years old. To calculate corrected age, subtract the number of weeks the child was born prematurely from the child's chronological age. Example: One would expect a 15-month-old child born 6 weeks prematurely to be in the same growth and developmental range of normal as a 13½-month-old.

Plot the BMI-for-age by finding the child's age on the horizontal scale, then following a vertical line to the BMI.

To identify underweight and overweight children and adolescents, use the following cut-off points:
- Underweight BMI-for-age is less than the 5th percentile
- At risk of overweight BMI-for-age is greater than the 85th percentile
- Overweight BMI-for-age is greater than the 95th percentile

General Inspection

The general inspection of the child includes observations similar to those of the adult examination (see Chapter 9). These include changes in facies, posture, and body contour; hygiene; and changes in gait. Also keep in mind those physical and behavioral characteristics that are expected for the individual child at the present chronological age (Figure 26-28). Chapter 5 describes the normal physical and behavioral changes that occur during the child's development. Observations made about the child's development during the interview and examination may indicate the need for a more formal assessment.

Observe and describe the child's behavior during the visit. Is this a quiet, shy child or an active, restless child? Is this child comfortable during the visit, or anxious and afraid? Does the child respond to the parent or other adults in an appropriate way?

Each child is a unique being, and it is a challenge to observe and record a description of any child's behavior. Keep in mind that behavior observed during a visit for health care may not be typical for that child but may reflect stress or anxiety related to the visit or to some encounters just prior to the visit.

It is also important to assess and record your general impression of the child during a visit for an acute problem. The

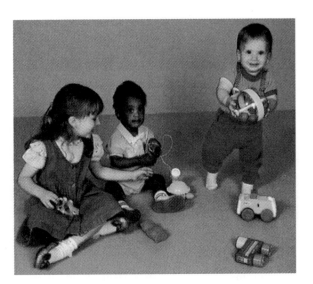

Figure 26-28 Observations of children at play in the waiting area, as well as during the examination, can provide helpful information about their behavioral styles and development.

child's general behavior can be an important clue to the severity of an illness. For example, a child with a fever of 104° F (40° C) but who is happy and playful may be less severely ill than an infant with a fever of 99.9° F (37.2° C) who is lethargic or highly irritable.

Skin, Hair, and Nails

Assess the skin for color, texture, temperature, moisture, turgor, and any rashes or lesions. Observe the hair for color, texture, quality, and distribution. Assess the nails for color, shape, texture, and quality.

The examination of the skin provides valuable information about the general health of the child and evidence of specific skin problems. Inspect and palpate the skin of the entire body at each examination. Since the normal condition of the skin changes with age, it is important to become familiar with those changes seen in children, as described in the following sections.

Newborns and Infants.   The skin of the newborn is soft and smooth and appears almost transparent. The superficial vessels are prominent, giving the skin its red color. Use natural daylight to assess for jaundice. A mild degree of jaundice is commonly present after the second or third day in normal infants. However, if the jaundice is severe or occurs within the first 24 hours, you should consider the presence of a serious problem.

Small papular patches, called nevus flammeus, may be present over the occiput, forehead, and upper eyelids in the newborn period; these patches usually disappear by the end of the first year of life. The nose and cheeks are commonly covered by small white papules called milia (Figure 26-29), caused by plugging of the sebaceous glands during the neonatal period. Both sweat and sebaceous glands are present in the newborn, but they do not function until the second month of life. Some desquamation is common during the first weeks and varies in individual babies.

Mongolian spots, which are blue or bluish brown, irregularly shaped, flat areas, occur in the sacral and buttocks areas of some infants, usually those who have darkly pigmented skin (Figure 26-30). These spots usually disappear by the end of the first year or by the second year, but occasionally they persist for a longer time.

A considerable amount of fine hair, called lanugo, covers the body of the newborn and is lost during the first weeks of life. The nails of the full-term newborn are well formed and firm, in contrast to those of the premature infant, which are imperfectly formed.

During the first year of life the proportion of subcutaneous fat continuously increases, and raw areas resulting from skin rubbing against skin are more prevalent in young, obese infants. This condition is called **intertrigo** (see Figure 10-27). During the second year of life, the proportion of subcutaneous fat decreases and intertrigo is less common.

Skin turgor is a good indicator of hydration status. Check skin turgor by grasping the skin on the abdomen between your thumb and index finger, releasing it, and observing how quickly it returns to its normal shape (Figure 26-31).

Children and Adolescents.   After the first year of life, the normal child shows little change in the skin until the onset of puberty, when considerable development of both sweat and sebaceous glands occurs. Associated with the development of the sebaceous glands is acne vulgaris, which is so common in its mildest forms that it is sometimes considered a normal physiological change. Early evidence of acne is the occasional comedo, or blackhead, on the nose and chin. At age 13 or 14 years, papules and small pustules may begin to appear (Figure 26-32). However, by age 16, many children will have recovered completely. Changes in the amount and distribution of hair also occur (see Figures 26-7 and 26-8). Hair growth becomes heavier; the appearance of pubic, axillary, and most of the more prominent body hair is influenced by sexual development during adolescence. (See Chapter 10; in particular, see Figures 10-15, *B* and *D,* 10-23 to 10-28, *B,* 10-33, *B,* 10-36, 10-38, and 10-39 for common dermatologi-

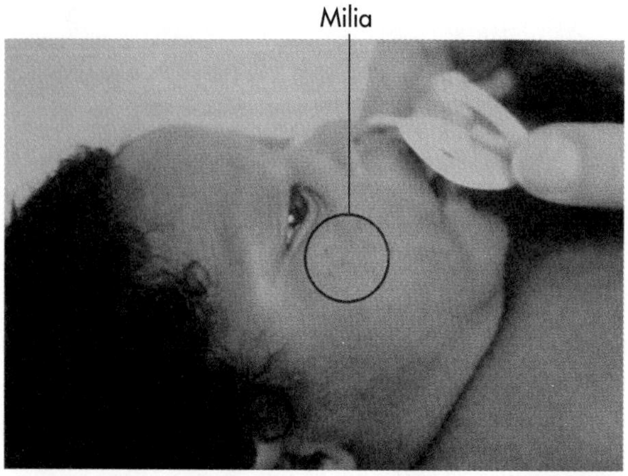

Milia

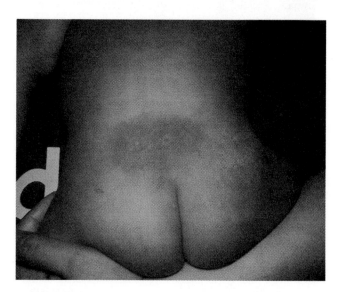

Figure 26-29   Milia in an infant. (From Seidel HM et al.: *Mosby's guide to physical examination,* ed 4, St. Louis, 1999, Mosby.)

Figure 26-30   Mongolian spot in the sacrococcygeal area, its most common location. (From Shah BR, Laude TA: *Atlas of pediatric clinical diagnosis,* Philadelphia, 2000, WB Saunders.)

cal conditions in children and adolescents.) Viral exanthems are also very common in childhood. It is helpful to be aware of these and get history information about associated phenomena related to or preceding the onset of a rash to determine the source of the rash.

Lymph Nodes

Inspect and palpate the lymph nodes for size, mobility, temperature, and tenderness.

Infants and Children.   Lymph nodes in children have the same distribution as those in adults, but the nodes are usually more prominent until puberty (Figure 26-33). The amount of lymphoid tissue is considerable at birth and increases steadily, peaking between ages 8 and 10 and gradually decreasing during adolescence (see Figure 26-27). Shotty, discrete, movable, small, nontender nodes are common in the normal healthy child in the occipital, postauricular, axillary chains (size less than 0.5 cm) and in the anterior and posterior cervical, parotid, submaxillary, sublingual, and inguinal areas (size less than 1 cm). These are particularly notable in school-age children. It is rare to find any palpable lymph nodes in the supraclavicular or epitrochlear areas.

Palpate lymph nodes as you would in the adult examination, assessing location, size, number, consistency, tenderness, mobility, and attachment to other structures. Lymph nodes that have grown rapidly, are "suspiciously" large (2 to 3 cm), tender, fixed to associated tissue, and relatively immobile require further investigation. As with adults, any palpable supraclavicular lymph nodes are of concern and require in-depth evaluation.

Examine lymph nodes during the examination of each part of the body.

Adolescents.   The examination is the same as for adults (see Chapter 11).

Head and Neck

Inspect the head for shape and symmetry. Palpate the fontanels in the infant and young child.

Newborns and Infants.   The shape of the newborn's head is often asymmetrical as a result of the molding that occurs during the passage through the birth canal. It may be a few days or weeks before the normal shape is restored. The newborn has a skull that molds easily because the bones of the cranium are not fused, which allows for some overlapping of the bones. Trauma may result in caput succedaneum or cephalhematoma (Figure 26-34). **Caput succedaneum** is an edematous swelling of the superficial tissues of the scalp manifested by a generalized soft swelling not bounded by suture lines. This condition is temporary and is usually resolved within the first few days of life. **Cephalhematoma** occurs as a result of bleeding into the periosteum and results in swelling that does not cross the suture line. Most cephalhematomas are absorbed within 2 weeks to 3 months. Flattening of the head often occurs in normal children, but it can also indicate problems such as mental retardation or rickets.

Palpate the sutures of the skull, which can usually be felt as ridges until the age of 6 months. Palpate the fontanels during each examination of the infant and young child to determine the size, shape, and presence of any tenseness or bulging. Normally, the posterior fontanel closes by 2 months of age and the anterior fontanel closes by the end of the second year (Figure 26-35). Tenseness or bulging of the fontanel is most easily detected when the child is in a sitting position and should be assessed when the child is quiet. Bulging may occur with increased intercranial pressure (or when the child is crying). The fontanel may be depressed when the infant is dehydrated or malnourished. Note early closure or delayed closure of the fontanel. Early closure can result from microcephaly and delayed closure from prolonged intracranial pressure.

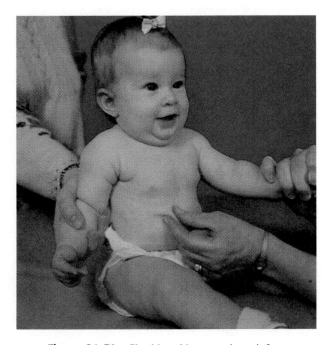

Figure 26-31   Checking skin turgor in an infant.

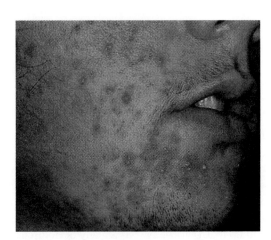

Figure 26-32   Acne in an adolescent. (From Habif TP: *Clinical dermatology: a color guide to diagnosis and therapy,* ed. 3, St. Louis, 1996, Mosby.)

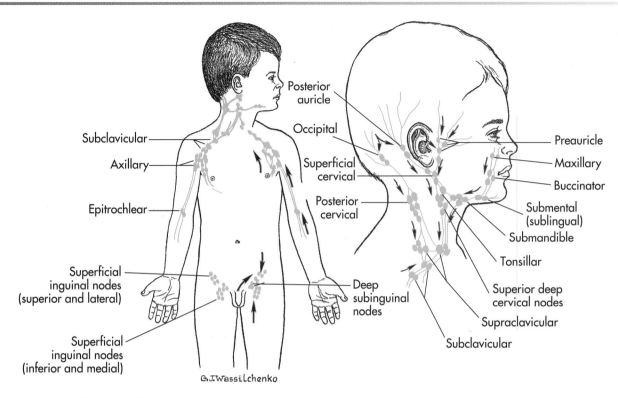

Figure 26-33 Location of superficial lymph nodes. *Arrows* indicate directional flow of lymph. (From Wong DL et al.: *Whaley and Wong's nursing care of infants and children,* ed. 6, St. Louis, 1999, Mosby.)

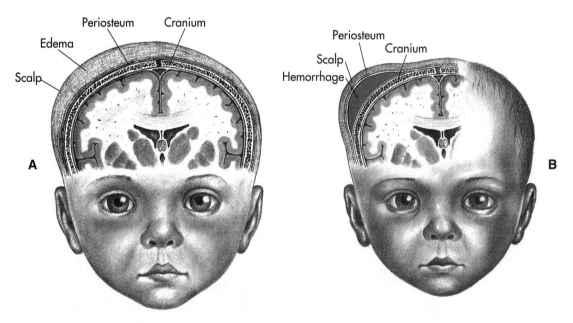

Figure 26-34 Common areas of scalp swelling in the newborn as a result of birth trauma. **A,** Caput succedaneum. **B,** Cephalhematoma. Note that the swelling does not cross the suture lines. (From Seidel HM et al.; *Mosby's guide to physical examination,* ed 4, 1999, St. Louis, Mosby.)

The importance of measuring the head circumference of the child up to 3 years of age has already been discussed.

Transillumination of the skull is a useful procedure in the initial examination of the infant and for any infant with an abnormal head size. Perform transillumination in a com-pletely darkened room with an ordinary flashlight equipped with a rubber adaptor. Place the light against the infant's head. If the cerebrum is absent or greatly thinned, as from increased intracranial pressure, the entire cranium lights up. Often, defects transilluminate in a more limited way. Aus-

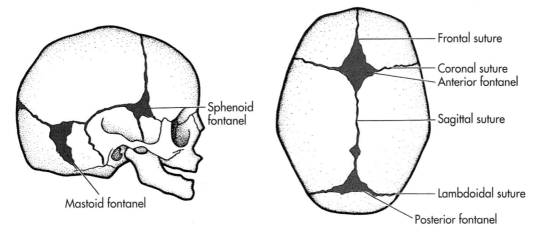

Figure 26-35   Skull bones of the infant, showing fontanels and sutures.

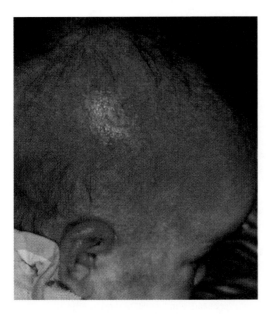

Figure 26-36   Seborrheic dermatitis of the scalp in an infant. (From Habif TP: *Clinical dermatology: a color guide to diagnosis and therapy,* ed. 3, St. Louis, 1996, Mosby.)

cultation of the skull may reveal bruits, which are commonly found in normal children up to 4 years of age. After the age of 4 years, bruits are evidence of problems such as aneurysms or increased intracranial pressure.

Inspect the young infant's scalp for evidence of crusting, which often results from a seborrheic dermatitis commonly called "cradle cap" (Figure 26-36).

Inspect the shape of the face. A facial paralysis is most easily observed when the child cries or smiles and the asymmetry is increased. An abnormal or unusual facies may indicate conditions or syndromes such as Down syndrome, a chromosomal abnormality (Figure 26-37, *A*), or fetal alcohol syndrome, a preventable cause of mental retardation related to alcohol consumption during pregnancy (Figure 26-37, *B*). Early recognition of these conditions can help initiate supportive interventions for the child and family.

Examine the neck with the child lying flat on the back. Note the size of the neck. The neck of the infant normally is short. It lengthens at about 3 or 4 years of age. Palpate the lymph nodes, thyroid glands, and trachea. Carefully palpate the sternocleidomastoid muscle. A mass on the lower third of the muscle may indicate a congenital torticollis. Palpate the clavicles for evidence of fracturing in the newborn.

Children and Adolescents. Percuss the frontal and maxillary sinuses by the direct method and palpate them in the child who is older than 2 or 3 years. Until that age, the sinuses are too small and poorly developed for percussion or palpation (Figure 26-38).

Palpate the submaxillary and sublingual glands in the same way as in the adult examination. Check for local swelling of the parotid gland by observing the child in the sitting position with the head raised and the neck extended and by noting any swelling below the angle of the jaw. You can feel the swollen parotid gland by palpating downward from the zygomatic arch. Unilateral or bilateral swelling of the parotid gland usually indicates mumps.

Inspect the size of the neck and associated structures. Palpate the trachea, thyroid gland, and lymph nodes as you would in an adult examination.

Finally, with the child lying flat on the back, determine neck mobility by lifting the child's head and turning it from side to side or bringing the chin forward to touch the chest. Any resistance to flexion may indicate meningeal irritation (see the section on the neurological examination for a more detailed description).

Eyes

Examination of the eyes is most easily accomplished when the child is able to cooperate. The school-age child can participate in the adult format for the eye examination (see Chapter 12). The infant and young child are much more of a challenge to the examiner.

Newborns and Infants. Visual function at birth is limited, but it improves as the structures develop. Vision can be tested grossly in the very young infant by noting the pupillary response to light. This is one of the most primitive visual functions and is normally found in the newborn. The blink reflex is also present in normal newborns and young infants. The infant will blink the eyes when a bright light is introduced. It is important to make sure that the infant has a full red reflex in each eye. A white reflex could indicate a cataract or retinoblastoma. It is often difficult to catch the young infant with his or her eyes open when you want to examine them. To facilitate the eye examination in the young infant, have the parent hold the infant upright securely against the parent's chest with the infant's face looking over the parent's shoulder. Movement to an upright position will often stimulate the infant to open his or her eyes.

At 5 or 6 weeks of age, the child should be able to fixate and give some evidence of following a bright toy or light.

When 3 or 4 months old, the infant begins to reach for objects at different distances. At 6 to 7 months of age, the infant can have a funduscopic examination, although it is not routinely performed at this early an age.

Test extraocular movements (EOMs) during the first weeks of life, as soon as the child is able to demonstrate following of movement. You can also at least partially examine the visual fields in infants and young children by having the child sit on the parent's lap with the head in the midline and one eye covered. As the light or bright object is brought into the visual field, the child will look at it or reach for it. In the older child, test EOMs as you would for an adult.

Inspect the outermost structures of the eyes in the same way as in the adult examination. In infants, look for evi-

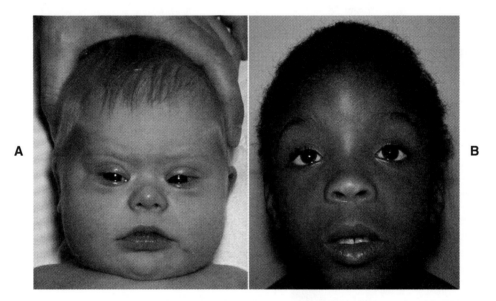

Figure 26-37 **A,** Down syndrome. Note depressed nasal bridge, epicanthal folds, mongoloid slant of eyes, low set ears, and large tongue. **B,** Fetal alcohol syndrome. Note the poorly formed philtrum; widespread eyes, with inner canthal folds and mild ptosis; hirsute forehead; short nose; and relatively thin upper lip. (From Zitelli BJ, Davis HW: *Atlas of pediatric physical diagnosis,* ed. 3, St. Louis, 1997, Mosby.)

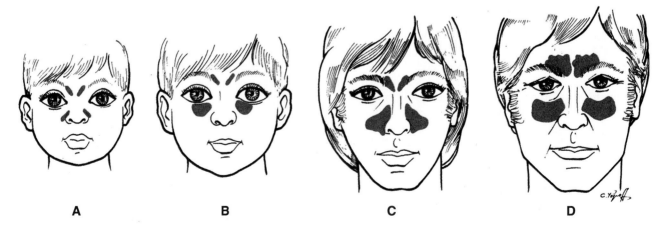

Figure 26-38 Development of the frontal and maxillary sinuses. **A,** Early infancy. **B,** Early childhood. **C,** Adolescence. **D,** Adulthood.

dence of nasolacrimal duct obstruction. Tears are not present at birth but are often produced by 4 months of age. The nasolacrimal duct is sometimes not patent until 1 year. This may cause a chronically tearing eye that may be clear or purulent. To confirm nasolacrimal duct obstruction, press over the nasolacrimal ducts. Mucoid or purulent discharge will confirm an obstruction.

Children and Adolescents. For children 3 to 6 years of age, a Snellen E chart can be used. Ask the child to hold the fingers in the same direction as the fingers of the E. You can also use Allen picture cards. The child identifies pictures, such as a tree, a telephone, a car, a house, and a teddy bear on an Allen card from a distance of 15 feet. Familiarizing the child with the procedure before testing may be helpful (Figure 26-39). The young child is normally farsighted and does not achieve visual acuity of 20/20 until the age of 7 years.

Tests for strabismus (squint, cross-eye), an imbalance of the extraocular muscles, are important because strabismus can lead to **amblyopia**, a type of blindness in the affected eye. Early recognition is essential to restore binocular vision, since the prognosis for a successful outcome for the child older than 6 years is poor. Occasional strabismus may occur in a young infant up to the age of 6 months as he or she attempts to focus on a close object. Fifty percent of all children with strabismus will manifest symptoms by age 1 year and 80% by 4 years (Fox, 1997).

An easy method for detecting strabismus is the corneal reflex test (or Hirschberg's test). Shine a bright light from a flashlight or ophthalmoscope directly into the eyes from about 16 inches (40.5 cm). In normal eyes the reflection of the light should fall symmetrically within each pupil. Any deviation warrants further evaluation.

Another more accurate test to assess muscle imbalance is the cover-uncover test (see Chapter 12). You can use this test in both younger and older children. Have the child focus on an object. Cover one eye with your hand, a card, or specially designed eyewear and observe the uncovered eye for movement (Figure 26-40, *A*). Then uncover the eye and observe the recently covered eye for movement (Figure 26-40, *B*). If movement is noticed in either or both eyes, strabismus is present.

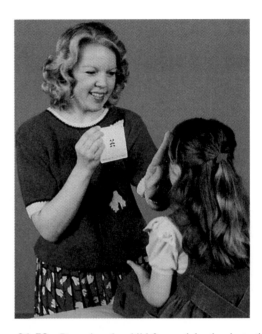

Figure 26-39 Preparing the child for participation in testing of visual acuity.

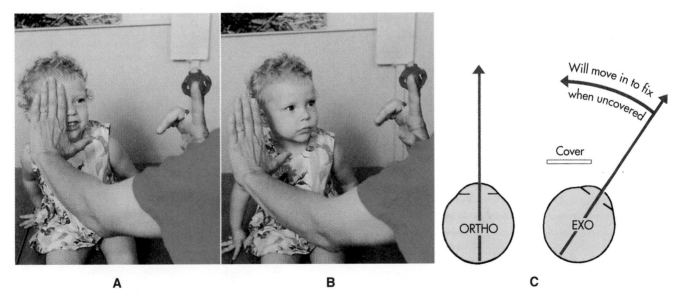

Figure 26-40 Cover-uncover test for strabismus. **A,** Have the child look at an object (preferably a brightly colored toy) and cover one eye. Observe the uncovered eye for movement. **B,** While the child is still focused on the object, uncover the eye and observe it for movement. **C,** Exophoria: as the eye is uncovered, it shifts to fixate on the object. (**C** from Prior JA, Silberstein JS, Stang JM: *Physical diagnosis: the history and examination of the patient,* ed. 6, St. Louis, 1981, Mosby.)

The type of strabismus is determined by the combination of movements. Repeat the test to examine the other eye. Transient strabismus is common during the first months of life. If it persists beyond 6 months of age, however, or becomes fixed at an earlier age, the child should be referred to an ophthalmologist.

The ophthalmoscopic examination depends on the child's ability to cooperate and the examiner's efficiency in observing as much as possible in a limited time. Attempts to restrain the child and force his or her eyes to remain open often prove unsuccessful. If possible, direct the child's attention toward an object or light while you approach without touching the child. The appearance of the red reflex alone is important information for ruling out opacities of the cornea and lens and cataracts. Attempt to use the ophthalmoscope to observe the red reflex at each examination of the infant and child, beginning in the first weeks of life.

Ears

Examination of the ears is often difficult; however, it is important because the immature structure of the young child's ears makes them more prone to infection. In the infant, the eustachian tube is shorter and wider than in the adult. It is also in a more horizontal position than in the adult, which makes it easier for pathogens to infect the middle ear.

■ HELPFUL HINT

Pneumotoscopy is an important technique to learn, especially when working with children. It involves gently blowing air into the ear canal (either with a rubber squeeze bulb or gently blowing or sucking with the end of the rubber tube in the examiner's mouth). The normal tympanic membrane will move in and out as positive and negative pressures are applied. In the presence of infection, there is fluid behind the tympanic membrane and therefore a decrease in mobility when pressure is applied.

Newborns, Infants, and Young Children. Inspect and palpate the external ear and the posterior mastoid areas for any obvious deformities. Note the position and size of the ears. Normally, the top of the ear is on a horizontal line with the inner and outer canthi of the eye (Figure 26-41). There is sometimes an association between "low set" ears and congenital anomalies such as renal agenesis.

Next use the otoscope. Make sure the otoscope has new batteries or is fully charged since a dim light will give a yellow tint. The ear examination becomes more difficult as the infant grows older. It is usually helpful to spend some time preparing the child by letting him or her see the light and by inserting the speculum gently for only a few seconds and then removing it to assure the child that the procedure does not hurt (Figure 26-42). When restraint is necessary, have the parent firmly hold the child (Figure 26-43).

Before inserting the otoscope, inspect the meatus for evidence of a foreign body or external otitis. In infancy and early childhood, the auditory canal is directed upward: pull the pinna of the ear down and back to aid in visualization (Figure 26-44). Hold the otoscope so that the hand holding it rests firmly on the head; the top of the speculum is inserted only $\frac{1}{4}$ or $\frac{1}{2}$ inch into the canal to avoid any unnecessary discomfort. For the older child, pull the pinna up and back to visualize the tympanic membrane (Figure 26-45).

Before you examine the tympanic membrane, carefully inspect the canal for evidence of furuncles, redness, or exudate. Inspect the tympanic membrane for color, light reflex, and the usual landmarks of the bony prominences of the middle ear. If you suspect that fluid or pus is present behind the tympanic membrane, you will need to check mobility of the tympanic membrane. This can be done with pneumotoscopy or a tympanogram.

Pneumotoscopy involves use of an otoscope with a speculum that has a hole through which a puff of air can be introduced by an attached bulb. The speculum must fit tightly in the canal to create a good seal. Air insufflation of the tympanic membrane allows the examiner to observe

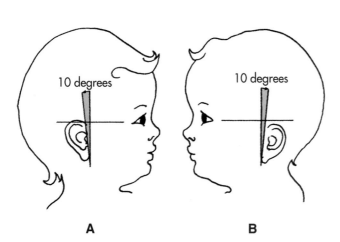

Figure 26–41 Ear alignment. **A,** Normal. **B,** Abnormal. (From Whaley LF, Wong DL: *Nursing care of infants and children,* ed. 4, St. Louis, 1991, Mosby.)

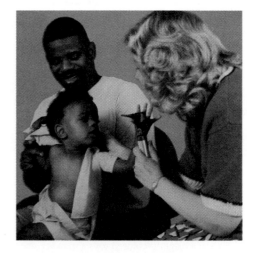

Figure 26–42 It is helpful to let the child see the speculum and examine it in preparation for the otoscopic examination.

tympanic membrane movement as both positive and negative pressures are gently applied to it (see also Chapter 13). This is especially helpful to differentiate a red tympanic membrane caused by crying (good mobility) to a red tympanic membrane caused by otitis (no mobility). A tympanogram uses sound rather than air to detect movement. Figure 26-46 shows common middle ear findings, including mobility. For additional examples of abnormal tympanic membranes, see Chapter 13.

If the canal is filled with cerumen, you may need to remove the cerumen by irrigation or curettage (see also Chapter 13). Water irrigation should be done with body temperature water and may be preferable to curettage, particularly with small children. Never irrigate if you suspect a perforation of the tympanic membrane. Removing the cerumen with a curette requires skill and experience. The procedure may cause pain and bleeding and may result in increased crying, which only exacerbates the redness of the mem-

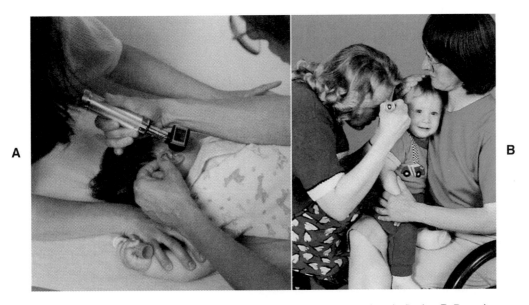

Figure 26-43 Positioning for restraining the child for an ear examination. **A,** Supine. **B,** Restraint using the "hug."

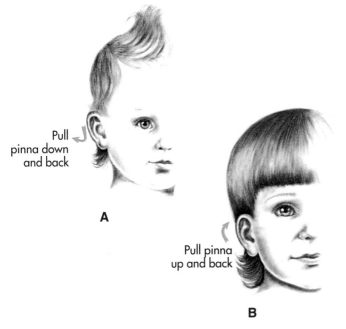

Figure 26-44 Straightening the ear canal in the infant (**A**) and in the child older than 3 years (**B**). (From Whaley LF, Wong DL: *Nursing care of infants and children,* ed. 4, St. Louis, 1991, Mosby.)

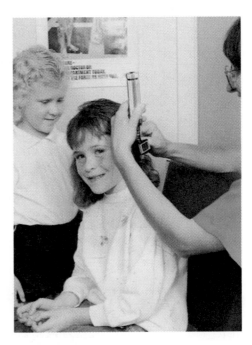

Figure 26-45 Examination of the ear in an older child.

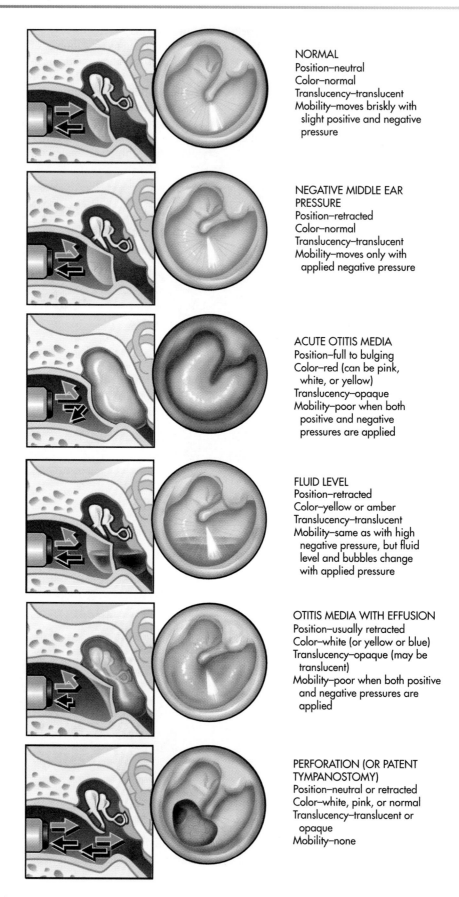

NORMAL
Position–neutral
Color–normal
Translucency–translucent
Mobility–moves briskly with
    slight positive and negative
    pressure

**NEGATIVE MIDDLE EAR
PRESSURE**
Position–retracted
Color–normal
Translucency–translucent
Mobility–moves only with
    applied negative pressure

ACUTE OTITIS MEDIA
Position–full to bulging
Color–red (can be pink,
    white, or yellow)
Translucency–opaque
Mobility–poor when both
    positive and negative
    pressures are applied

FLUID LEVEL
Position–retracted
Color–yellow or amber
Translucency–translucent
Mobility–same as with high
    negative pressure, but fluid
    level and bubbles change
    with applied pressure

OTITIS MEDIA WITH EFFUSION
Position–usually retracted
Color–white (or yellow or blue)
Translucency–opaque (may be
    translucent)
Mobility–poor when both positive
    and negative pressures are
    applied

**PERFORATION (OR PATENT
TYMPANOSTOMY)**
Position–neutral or retracted
Color–white, pink, or normal
Translucency–translucent or
    opaque
Mobility–none

Figure 26-46   Common conditions of the middle ear as assessed with the otoscope. (Modified from
Bluestone CD, Klein JO: *Otitis media in infants and children,* Philadelphia, 1988, WB Saunders.)

brane. Flexible plastic curettes are available and seem easier for many children to tolerate. Often cerumen that is not dry but fairly soft will move during the examination. Visualization of the membrane then becomes possible without the need for any special procedures to remove the cerumen. Avoid discomfort so that the child will not become conditioned to expect pain with future ear examinations.

In the infant, test hearing by asking an assistant to stand behind the child and make a noise, such as a hand slap, several inches away from the child's ear while you observe the child for an eye blink. This test is often inaccurate, since the child may be responding to air movement. In the young child, hearing can be grossly tested with the whispered voice. Stand behind the child, occlude one ear with your hand, and whisper the child's name. The child will usually turn when his or her name is heard. Repeat this step to test the other ear.

Older Children and Adolescents. The examination for the ears is similar to the adult examination (see Chapter 13). Continued emphasis should be placed on the auditory acuity, particularly in children who have had repeated ear infections. Audiometric testing should be performed on all school-age children.

Nose

Newborns and Infants. Infants are obligate nose breathers, so any nasal obstruction may cause respiratory distress. Simply clearing the nasal passages may resolve the problem.

Children and Adolescents. Purulent secretions are common with any nasal infection, including the common upper respiratory infection. Children with redness, discharge, and crusting on the cartilaginous outer edges of the nostrils may have a beta-hemolytic streptococcal infection. Watery nasal secretions may indicate foreign bodies, the common cold, or an allergy.

Inspect the nostrils. Note any unusual shape of the nose, flaring of the nostrils (which occurs with any type of respiratory distress), and the character and amount of discharge.

Look at the tip of the nose. A permanent transverse crease is commonly seen in allergy sufferers and is caused by the "allergic salute," which is when the individual uses the palm or forefinger to rub the nose upward and outward.

Examine the septum, turbinates, and vestibule by pushing the tip of the nose upward with the thumb of the nondominant hand and shining a light into the naris. A speculum is usually not necessary for adequate visualization, and it might cause the child to be apprehensive.

Mouth and Oropharynx

The mouth and oropharyngeal area can be examined last, since this examination often provokes fear in the child. However, it is helpful to some children to do this examination first. For example, the child who is anticipating discomfort may be relieved to have it accomplished and then can cooperate with the rest of the examination. Deciding on this approach requires knowledge about the individual child's behavior and responses. This information may be obtained during the history or in discussion with the parent.

The procedures are the same as in the adult examination. However, the young child will probably need to be restrained by the parent (Figure 26-47, *A*). The older child is usually able to cooperate (Figure 26-47, *B*). The examination findings are different from those of adults.

Newborns and Infants. In the young infant inspect and palpate the palate for a cleft. The palatal arch should be dome shaped with no clefts in either the hard or soft palate. A bifid uvula may indicate a submucous cleft palate (a cleft covered by membrane), which cannot be identified by inspection alone. Examine the palate by placing the finger inside the mouth with the fingerpad toward the roof, eliciting the sucking reflex. This soothes the infant and allows palpation of the palate for a cleft and evaluation of the infant's suck.

Inspect the pharynx. The buccal mucosa should be pink and moist. Check any white patches on the buccal mucosa and tongue for signs of thrush (candidiasis). Nonadherent

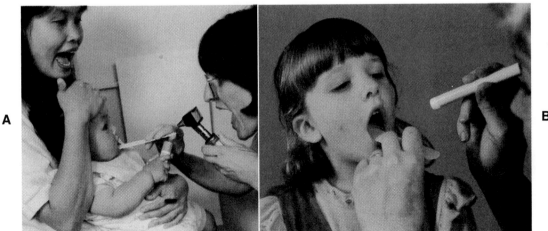

A   **B**

Figure 26-47 Positioning the child for examination of the mouth. **A,** The young child often requires restraint by the parent and encouragement from both the parent and the examiner. **B,** The older child is usually cooperative.

patches are usually due to milk deposits. Adherent patches suggest candidiasis.

Children and Adolescents. Inspect the teeth for number and for caries. The number of deciduous and permanent teeth and the pattern of eruption are determined by the child's age and development. There are 20 deciduous teeth, and their eruption is completed by the age of 2½ years. The first permanent molar and the lower incisor erupt at 6 years of age (Figure 26-48). Check the teeth for signs of decay. Baby-bottle caries due to the erosive effects of a nighttime bottle of juice or milk may be seen as multiple brown areas or caries on the upper and lower incisors (see Figure 26-4). Mottled or pitted teeth may be the result of excessive fluoride and tetracycline treatment during tooth development.

Inspect the pharynx. The buccal mucosa should be pink and moist. The tonsils are normally larger in children than in adults, and they usually extend beyond the palatine arch until the age of 11 or 12 years (Figure 26-49). Figures 13-28 and 13-29 provide examples of enlarged tonsils. Figure 13-30 shows the system for grading tonsillar enlargement.

Epiglottitis. Although currently less common a problem due to the advent of the Hib immunization, it is important to be aware of the signs and symptoms of epiglottitis, which is considered a *medical emergency.* Before routine immunization, epiglottitis was most often seen in children between the ages of 3 and 7 years. Symptoms of epiglottitis include an abrupt onset of severe sore throat, sudden high fever, croupy cough, apprehension, and a focus on breathing in a formerly active child. The classic presentation is of the child in a sitting position, leaning forward (tripoding), with his or her mouth open, tongue protruding, and drooling. Drooling is a particularly characteristic sign. These are indicators of impending airway obstruction. No one should examine the child's mouth until the child is in a setting where immediate intubation is possible (usually an operating room) because the examination may trigger a complete airway obstruction.

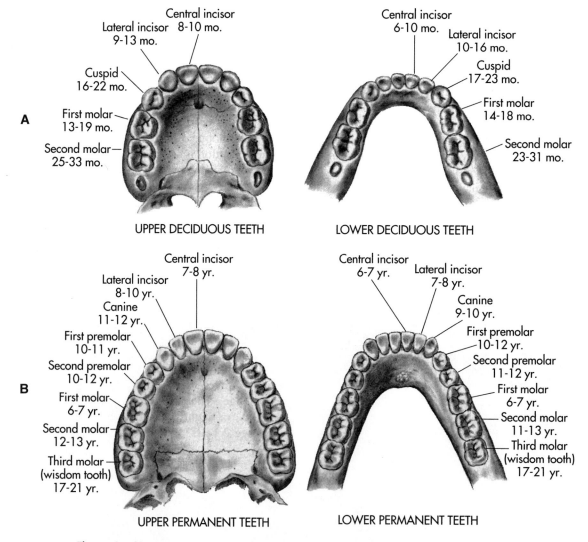

Figure 26-48   A, Dentition of deciduous teeth and their sequence of eruption. **B,** Dentition of permanent teeth and their sequence of eruption. (From Seidel HM et al.: *Mosby's guide to physical examination,* ed. 3, St. Louis, 1995, Mosby.)

A child with epiglottitis will have a markedly inflamed "cherry red" pharynx with copious secretions.

Chest

Begin the examination of the chest with an inspection of its general shape and circumference. Observe the respiratory rate while the infant or child is undisturbed. The resting respiratory rate varies considerably with age (see Table 26-10). Examination of the chest is the same as in adults (see Chapter 15). The findings vary with age.

Newborns, Infants, and Young Children. Inspect the chest. In infancy the chest is almost round; the anteroposterior diameter equals the transverse diameter (i.e., barrel chest). This shape changes as the child grows from preschool to school age. The chest circumference is normally the same as, or slightly less than, the head circumference until age 2 years.

Respiratory activity in infants and young children is abdominal and does not become primarily thoracic until age 7 years. Little intercostal motion is seen in healthy infants and young children. Therefore, if you observe intercostal motion in the young child (retractions), suspect respiratory distress. Other signs of distress are nasal flaring and a respiratory grunt.

Percuss the chest. In the newborn the chest is hyperresonant throughout. If necessary, you can perform palpation and evaluate for tactile fremitus while the child is crying. Perform percussion of the chest by using either the direct or the indirect method. The child's chest is normally more resonant than that of the adult.

Auscultation follows the same pattern as in the adult exam. Breath sounds will seem much louder because of the thinness of the chest wall and are almost all bronchovesicular (Figure 26-50). Often tracheal breath sounds are transmitted down to the chest. To avoid mistaking these for crackles, hold the stethoscope over the mouth and listen, then compare the sounds from the mouth with the lung sounds.

Older Children and Adolescents. The examination for the respiratory system is the same as the adult examination.

Heart

A quiet child and environment are necessary for accurate assessment of the heart (Figure 26-51). Therefore, if possible, make this the first part of the examination when the child is quiet and relaxed. The examination of the cardiovascular system as discussed in Chapter 16 for the adult applies to the examination of the child; however, some cardiac findings of normal children are not considered normal in adults.

Newborns, Infants, and Young Children. The pulse rate in children of different ages is discussed earlier in this chapter (see Table 26-8). The palpation of pulses in all the extremities is a part of the cardiovascular examination. The pulses in the lower extremities, especially the femoral pulses, are of special importance in children. Their absence or diminution may indicate coarctation of the aorta (see Table 26-9).

During infancy the position of the heart is more nearly horizontal and has a larger diameter in comparison with the total

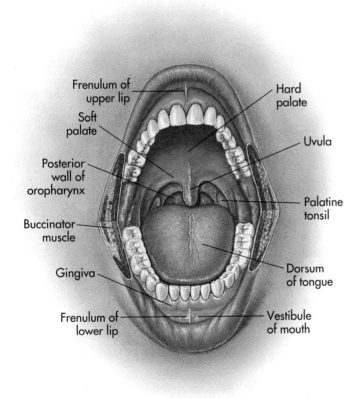

Figure 26-49 Anatomic structures of the oral cavity. (From Seidel HM et al.: *Mosby's guide to physical examination*, ed. 4, St. Louis, 1999, Mosby.)

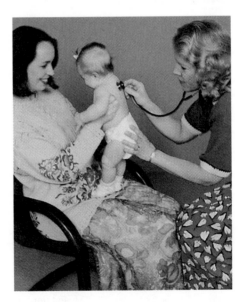

Figure 26-50 Examination of the lungs. The young child is more comfortable and cooperative on the parent's lap.

diameter of the chest than it does in the adult (Figure 26-52). The apex is one or two intercostal spaces above what is considered normal for the adult. Therefore the apical impulse in young children is normally felt in the fourth intercostal space immediately to the left of the midclavicular line. This location changes gradually, and by 7 years of age the apical impulse is normally found in the fifth intercostal space at the midclavicular line.

Sinus arrhythmia is a normal finding in infants and children. The degree of arrhythmia is less in the young infant and greatest in the adolescent. The heart sounds are louder because of the thinness of the chest wall. They are also of a higher pitch and shorter duration than those of the normal adult. A splitting of the second heart sound can be heard in the second left intercostal space in most infants and children. The physiological split normally widens with inspiration. A third heart sound is present in approximately one third of all children and is best heard at the apex.

Many children have murmurs without heart disease. The significance of a murmur may be difficult to determine. Innocent murmurs are characteristically systolic in timing; are grade 1 or 2 in intensity; have a soft, blowing quality; and are not transmitted to other areas. It is not always possible to determine whether the murmur is innocent or pathological by auscultation alone, although murmurs of grade 3 or louder usually indicate heart disease. A venous hum is commonly present in children. It is a continuous, low-pitched sound originating in the internal jugular vein that is heard either above or below the clavicles (see Figure 16-28). It is accentuated in the upright position and disappears when the child is lying down. Because it is not pathologically significant, a venous hum should be differentiated from a murmur. Table 26-14 summarizes the more common childhood murmurs and associated findings. Tables 16-9 and 16-10 provide a review of cardiac murmurs. Any murmur that is symptomatic (e.g., accompanied by chest pains or palpitations) requires further evaluation.

Abdomen

The abdomen is somewhat easier to examine in the child than in the adult because of the child's thinner abdominal

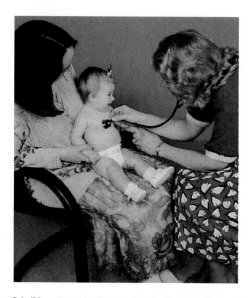

Figure 26-51 Auscultation of the heart requires a quiet child. Doing the examination on the parent's lap increases the child's comfort and cooperation.

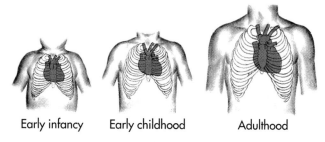

Early infancy   Early childhood   Adulthood

Figure 26-52 Position of the heart at various ages. (From Seidel HM et al.: *Mosby's guide to physical examination,* ed. 2, St. Louis, 1991, Mosby.)

TABLE 26-14	**Cardiovascular Murmurs of Childhood**				
Condition	**Cycle**	**Location**	**Radiation**	**Pitch**	**Other Signs**
Ventricular septal defect	Pansystolic	Left sternal border at the fourth or fifth intercostal space	Over the precordium, rarely to the axilla	High	Thrill at left lower sternal border
Mitral insufficiency	Pansystolic	Apex	Axilla	High	S_1 decreased S_3
Pulmonic stenosis	Systolic ejection	Left second or third intercostal space	Left shoulder	Medium	Widely split S_2 Right-sided S_4 Ejection click
Patent ductus arteriosus	Continuous	Left second intercostal space	Left clavicle	Medium	Machinery-like, harsh Thrill
Venous hum	Continuous	Medial third of clavicles, often on the right	First and second intercostal spaces	Low	Can be obliterated by pressure on the jugular veins

From Swartz MH: *Textbook of physical diagnosis: history and examination,* ed. 3, Philadelphia, 1998, WB Saunders.

wall. To gain the child's cooperation, several approaches may be helpful. For example, a baby bottle may calm the infant; the young child may be more comfortable and relaxed if examined while sitting on the parent's lap. Find the approaches that are most productive in particular situations (Figure 26-53).

Newborns and Infants. The order of the abdominal examination procedures for the infant and young child is the same as with the adult: inspection, auscultation, percussion, and then palpation.

In infants the abdomen is protuberant due to poor development of the abdominal muscles. Observe the umbilicus. It is normally closed and puckered. In the neonate, the umbilical stump dries within 1 week after birth, hardens and falls off usually by day 10 to 14, and skin covers the area by 3 to 4 weeks. Umbilical hernias are common in all infants up to age 2 and up to age 7 in African-American children (Figure 26-54). Diastasis of the rectus muscle, a separation of the rectus muscle with a visible bulge along the midline, is also a common finding. This usually disappears by early childhood as the abdominal muscles strengthen.

To facilitate palpation of the abdomen, flexing the infant's knees with one hand while palpating with the other will relax the infant's abdominal muscles. The liver is palpable 1 to 2 cm below the right costal margin in the first year of life. If it extends more than 2 cm below the costal margin, investigate further. The spleen is normally palpable 1 to 2 cm below the left costal margin in the first weeks of life. Note any increase in size. Any evidence of tenderness may indicate serious blood dyscrasias or other problems.

Children. The child's abdomen should appear slightly rounded, soft, and symmetrical. The abdomen is larger than the chest in children younger than 4 years old and appears pot-bellied in both the supine and sitting positions. The child up to 13 years old will have a pot belly in the standing position. This normal shape must be differentiated from true distention caused by enlargement of organs or the presence of

tumors, cysts, severe malnutrition, or ascites. A depressed abdomen may result from dehydration or malnutrition.

Abdominal movement should be synchronous with respirations. Respirations are largely abdominal in children up to 7 years of age. Any splinting or loss of movement may indicate peritonitis, appendicitis, or other acute problems. Also, observe the abdomen for peristaltic waves (indicating pyloric stenosis) or dilated veins (indicating liver disease).

Auscultate the abdomen in the same manner as described in the examination of the adult—before percussion and palpation. Listen for peristaltic sounds.

Percussion may be useful in obtaining the boundaries of the liver, spleen, and any tumors. Children may be intrigued by the percussion sounds, especially the gastric bubble. Having the child listen for the gastric bubble sound is one way to make the examination seem less threatening.

Palpate in the same way as in the examination of the adult, except for the modifications in approach and in the positions of the child. Light palpation enables you to determine the tenseness of the abdominal muscles, the presence of superficial masses, and the presence of tenderness. The child is often not able to pinpoint the area of tenderness, and only by watching the facial expressions can you determine the point of maximal tenderness.

Determine tissue turgor by grasping a few inches of skin and subcutaneous tissue over the abdomen, pulling it up, and

---

■ HELPFUL HINT

Many children become anxious or very ticklish during the abdominal part of the examination. To help the child relax, make sure he or she keeps the knees bent while lying on the back, and have the child keep a hand over yours as you palpate. You can also have the child's hand under your examining fingers during palpation.

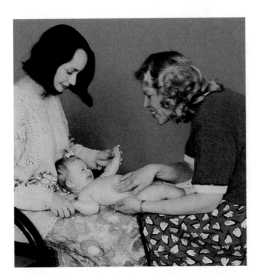

Figure 26-53 Examination of the abdomen in an infant.

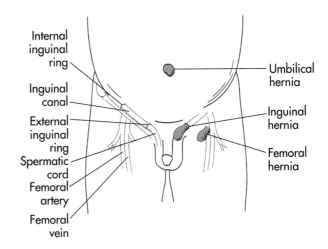

Figure 26-54 Location of hernias.

then quickly releasing it (see Figure 26-31). If the creases formed do not disappear immediately, dehydration is present.

Do deep palpation in all four quadrants by single-hand or bimanual methods. Palpate the inguinal and femoral regions for hernias, lymph nodes, and femoral pulses (see Figure 26-54).

Genitalia

The examination of the genitalia of both male and female children usually includes inspection and palpation.

As part of the genital examination, you need to consider the child's or the adolescent's stage of pubertal development. The Sexual Maturity Rating (SMR) scale developed by Tanner (1962) is composed of five classes, which are based on pubic hair and breast development in females (see Figures 26-6 and 26-8) and pubic hair and genitalia development in males (see Figure 26-7). This information is important for identifying abnormal puberty and also for reassuring the adolescent that he or she is normal. Record the SMR, or Tanner stage, at the initial visit and yearly thereafter.

Male Genitalia.   In the male child, two primary areas are examined: the penis and the scrotum. First examine the foreskin of the penis. The foreskin of the uncircumcised infant is normally tight for the first 2 or 3 months of life and does not retract easily. If the tightness persists beyond this period, it is called phimosis. Determine whether this condition causes any interference with urination. Do any retraction of the foreskin carefully, since the delicate membranes attached to the foreskin may be easily torn, resulting in adhesions.

Next examine the meatus to determine its position and the presence of any ulceration. The meatus is normally located at the tip of the shaft. An abnormal location of the meatus on the ventral surface is called hypospadias; an abnormal location on the dorsal surface is called **epispadias**.

Inspect the scrotum for evidence of enlargement. An enlarged scrotum may be indicative of a hernia or hydrocele.

Palpate the scrotum to determine whether the testes are descended (Figure 26-55).

Use your index finger to block the inguinal canal and gently push toward the scrotum. Use the finger and thumb of the opposite hand to palpate the scrotum and grasp the testes as they are pushed downward into the scrotum. In an infant, block each inguinal canal with the nondominant hand and palpate the testes as soon as the diaper is removed before the cold room air causes retraction. If you cannot easily palpate the testes in an older boy, have him sit in a chair with his legs apart, his heels on the seat of the chair, and his arms around his knees. This procedure interrupts the cremasteric reflex and creates pressure by flexing the abdomen and the thigh. You will feel the testes as a soft mass about 1 cm in diameter. The testes are considered descended if you can palpate them in the scrotum, regardless of whether there is subsequent retraction into the inguinal canal.

For the adolescent male, follow the same procedure as for the adult male. Remember, teaching about testicular self-examination is important since the risk for testicular cancer is greatest in 15- to 35-year-old males when hormonal activity is greatest and early detection is important for the prognosis (see Chapter 20 for more details).

Female Genitalia.   Inspect the genitalia of the female child by separating the labia majora with the thumb and the forefinger to expose the labia minora, urethral meatus, and vaginal orifice (Figure 26-56). Examine the young infant in a supine position on the mother's lap with the knees held in a flexed position and separated. Sit facing the mother and child. The older child can help by spreading back her labia with her hands (Figure 26-57).

Urethral discharges are pathological and indicate infection somewhere in the urinary tract. A bloody vaginal discharge during the first month of life (secondary to residual maternal hormones) is normal but not common. Purulent or mucoid vaginal discharge indicates infection or the presence of a foreign body.

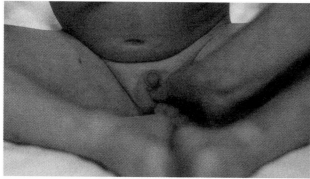
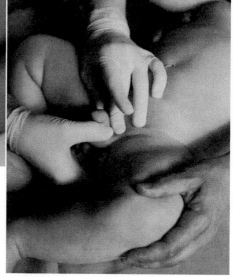

A

B

Figure 26-55   **A,** Preventing the cremasteric reflex by having the child sit in the "tailor" position. **B,** Palpation of the scrotum to determine whether the testes are descended, blocking the inguinal canal. (**A** From Wong DL et al.: *Whaley and Wong's nursing care of infants and children,* ed. 6, St. Louis, 1999, Mosby.)

Inspect the labia and the clitoris for any abnormality in size or for evidence of adhesion or infection. Inspect the vaginal area; usually it is not palpated. An imperforate hymen may be apparent if there is fluid behind it.

The vaginal examination is usually omitted for the child. If concerns or symptoms require such an examination, an experienced clinician or a gynecologist should examine the child. Vaginal examinations should be performed on the adolescent who is sexually active, has been sexually assaulted, is considering contraception, requests such an examination, or has indications of an infection or other pelvic disorder. The age at which the first pelvic examination is recommended varies, depending on the previously mentioned criteria, but between ages 16 and 18 years is commonly accepted.

Musculoskeletal System

Infants and Young Children. The skeleton of the infant and young child is made up largely of cartilaginous tissues, which account for the relative softness and malleability of the bones. It is also the reason that many defects identified early in life can be corrected with more ease than in later years.

Conduct much of the musculoskeletal examination while watching the child or while playing with the child. Since the infant or younger child is not able to understand directions, you can perform much of the examination by helping the child passively go through range-of-motion movements. An older child is able to follow directions, and you can complete a routine musculoskeletal examination.

Inspect the neck, extremities, hips, and spine for symmetry, increased or decreased mobility, and anatomical defects. Observe the gait by asking the child to walk back and forth.

In the child, the normal configuration of the legs is reached by age 6 years. Figure 26-58 shows the sequence of changes that normally occur between birth and age 6. The newborn at rest assumes the position maintained in utero,

and the feet are rarely straight. The feet are usually held in the varus (forefoot turned in) or valgus (forefoot turned out) position and simulate the clubfoot. To determine whether this is a true abnormality or a transient position, scratch the outside and inside borders of the foot. The normal foot will usually assume a right-angle position with the leg. If this is a fixed deformity, or if it is difficult to bring the foot to the neutral position, refer the infant for an orthopedic evaluation (Table 26-15 and Box 26-8).

Infants generally have bowlegs until 12 to 18 months. When they begin walking, their gait is wide based. Some children tend to evert their feet so that they bear weight on the inner aspects of the feet, and this is normal. The young child also has a fat pad under the arch of the foot and may appear flat-footed until about 3 to 4 years of age. The child's bowlegged appearance changes as the gait improves, and then the child becomes mildly knock-kneed (Figure 26-59).

Intoeing may result from metatarsus varus (forefoot turned in); medial tibial torsion, in which the entire foot turns in while the knee remains straight; or medial femoral torsion, in which the entire leg turns in with the foot and knee turned medially. A child who has intoeing as a result of a fixed deformity of the forefoot that cannot be corrected to neutral should be referred for orthopedic care. The problems of medial tibial torsion and medial femoral torsion are more cosmetic than functional and usually disappear by age 4 or 5 years.

Examine the hips for congenital dislocation or subluxation at every routine visit during the first year of life. In congenital dislocation, the head of the femur is found outside the acetabulum, and relocation may or may not be possible. Subluxation means that the capsule is lax enough to allow the femoral head to be displaced but not dislocated. Clinical signs of an abnormal hip may be asymmetry of the skinfolds, creases on the dorsal surfaces, and an apparent leg length inequality (Figure 26-60). However, these signs may not be apparent in the young infant who has a hip that is susceptible to dislocation rather than a dislocated hip.

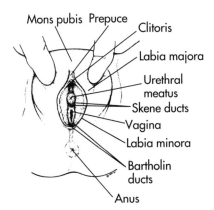

Figure 26-56 External structures of the genitalia in a prepubertal female. Labia are spread to reveal deeper structures. (From Whaley LF, Wong DL: *Nursing care of infants and children,* ed. 4, St. Louis, 1991, Mosby.)

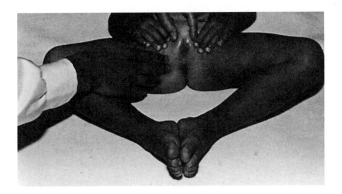

Figure 26-57 Position for examining the genitalia in a female child. (From Wong DL: *Whaley and Wong's nursing care of infants and children,* ed. 5, St. Louis, 1995, Mosby.)

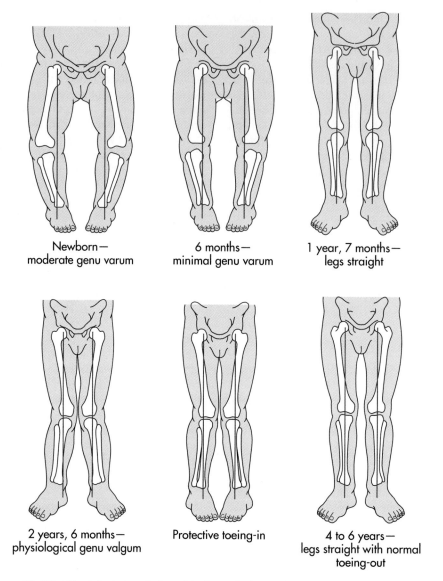

Newborn—
moderate genu varum

6 months—
minimal genu varum

1 year, 7 months—
legs straight

2 years, 6 months—
physiological genu valgum

Protective toeing-in

4 to 6 years—
legs straight with normal
toeing-out

Figure 26-58 Physiological evolution of the lower limb at various ages in infancy and childhood. (From Tachdjian MO: *Pediatric orthopedics,* Philadelphia, 1972, WB Saunders.)

TABLE 26-15	Four Primary Deformities of the Foot in Relation to the Position of the Heel, Forefoot, and/or Toes			
Primary Deformity	**Heel**	**Forefoot**		**Toes**
Varus	Inverted	Adducted inverted (sole in)		
Valgus	Everted	Abducted everted (sole out)		
Equinus	Plantar flexed			At level lower than heel
Calcaneus	Dorsiflexed			At level higher than heel
Combinations				
Equinovarus	Plantar flexed inverted	Adducted inverted (sole in)		At level lower than heel
Equinovalgus	Plantar flexed everted	Abducted everted (sole out)		At level lower than heel
Calcaneovarus	Dorsiflexed inverted	Adducted inverted (sole in)		At level higher than heel
Calcaneovalgus	Dorsiflexed everted	Abducted everted (sole out)		At level higher than heel

Data from Swanger R: *Common problems of toddlers and preschoolers,* lecture, 1972.

The examination of the hips is done with the infant in the supine position. Flex the infant's hips and knees, and then abduct the hips fully. In the newborn, each thigh should abduct to almost 90 degrees (Figure 26-60, *C*). Any limitation in the abduction of either or both hips may indicate dislocation.

To check the stability of the individual hip, place your middle finger over the greater trochanter (Figure 26-60, *D*) with your thumb placed medially. Adduct the thigh while still in the flexed position and apply pressure along the long axis of the femur in the direction of the posterior lip of the acetabulum. As dislocation occurs, you will feel the click of exit of the femur out of the acetabulum (Barlow's test). You will feel a similar click or "clunk" when you reverse the maneuver by abducting the hip and the head of the femur slips back into the joint (Ortolani's maneuver). When you feel lateral movement of the head of the femur without dislocation, the hip is subluxed. In the Barlow's test, each hip is evaluated separately. In the Ortolani test, the hips may be evaluated simultaneously.

Most dislocated hips in the newborn will relocate naturally. However, an unstable hip may become fixed in the dislocated position during the first weeks of life and the Ortolani maneuver cannot be done to replace the head. Dislocated hips can resolve spontaneously, but there is no way to be sure this will happen. Refer the infant suspected of having a dislocation to an orthopedist without delay, since treatment is far more effective at an early age.

Inspect and palpate the spine. Examine the young infant in a sitting position while bending the child forward on your hand. In the young infant and child, a tuft of hair or small dimple usually located toward the distal portion of the spine, but which may appear anywhere from the coccyx to the skull, may indicate underlying spina bifida or may be only a superficial anomaly. If a dimple is apparent, note its interior and depth. A dimple often indicates a dermoid cyst, which may become a site of infection. The young infant and child should be examined for congenital scoliosis, whereas the child age 10 years or older should be examined for idiopathic scoliosis.

Older Children and Adolescents.   In older children and adolescents, the method of musculoskeletal examination is the same as for the adult. All children should have a spinal examination during each health visit. Observe the shoulders for symmetry in the standing position (Figure 26-61). Ask the child to bend the shoulders forward with the arms hanging freely and the head down. In this position you can observe any prominence of one side of the rib cage. If a scoliosis is suspected, refer the child to an orthopedist.

The AAP has developed the 2-minute orthopedic screening examination, which includes 12 simple steps. The examination assesses musculoskeletal alignment; flexibility and proprioception; and loss of range of motion, function, or

BOX 26-8

ORTHOPEDIC DISORDERS COMMON TO VARIOUS AGE GROUPS OF CHILDREN

NEONATE
Oligohydramnios
  Compressed face
  Limb deformities
  Thoracic compression
  Lung hypoplasia
Prolonged breech position
Dislocation of hip
Deformations of knee
Hyperextension of knee
Dislocation of knee
Foot deformities
  Calcaneovalgus
  Metatarsus adductus
  Equinovarus
  Overlapping toes
Craniofacies
  Compressed face
    Molding of calvaria
    Mandibular asymmetry
  Torticollis
Dislocated hip(s)
Postural scoliosis

PRESCHOOLER
Postural-orthopedic abnormalities of foot
Abnormalities of toenail
Disorders of skin
Deviations in gait
Poor foot hygiene
Inadequate footgear

SCHOOL-AGE CHILD
Idiopathic adolescent scoliosis
Other types of scoliosis
Kyphosis
Lordosis
Alignment problems of lower extremity
Juvenile arthritis
Athletic injuries
  Unstable knee
  Upper extremity, elbow clean
  Epiphyseal injuries

YOUNG ADULT
Disabling low back pain
Osteoarthritis
Athletic injuries
  Jogging-related injuries

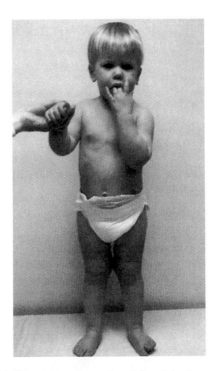

Figure 26-59 Genu valgum (knock-knee) in the young child. (From Seidel HM et al.: *Mosby's guide to physical examination,* ed. 4, St. Louis, 1999, Mosby.)

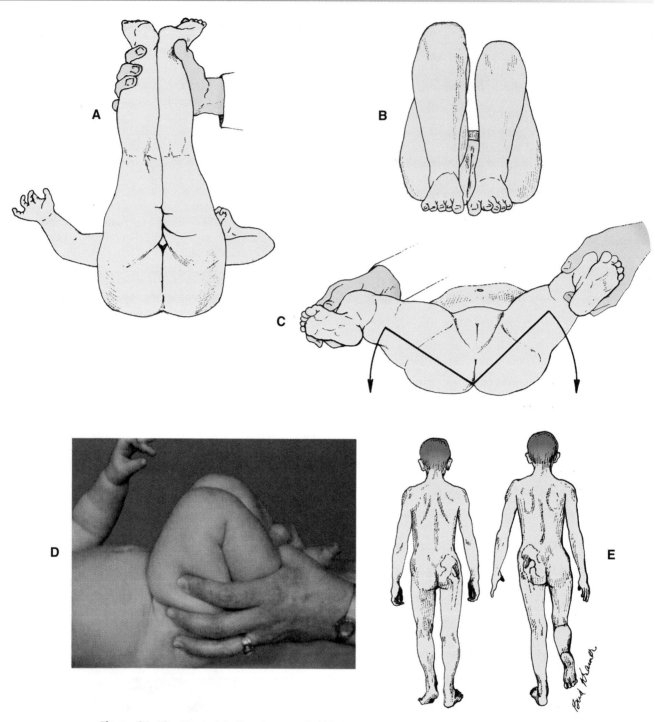

Figure 26-60 Physical findings in congenital hip location. **A,** Thigh fold asymmetry is often present in infants with unilateral hip dislocation. An extra fold can be seen on the abnormal side. The finding is not diagnostic, however. It may be found in normal infants and may be absent in children with hip dislocation or dislocatability. **B,** Leg length inequality is a sign of unilateral hip dislocation (Galeazzi's sign). It is not reliable in children with dislocatable but not dislocated hips or in children with bilateral dislocation. **C,** Limitation of hip abduction is often present in older infants with hip dislocation. Abduction of greater than 60 degrees is usually possible in infants. Restriction or asymmetry indicates the need for careful radiological examination. **D,** Adduction of the hips; note placement of fingers over the trochanter. **E,** Trendelenburg sign. In single-leg stance, the abductor muscles of the normal hip support the pelvis. Dislocation of the hip functionally shortens and weakens these muscles. When the child attempts to stand on the dislocated hip, the opposite side of the pelvis drops. When bilateral dislocation is present, a wide-based Trendelenburg limp will result. (**A** to **C** and **E** from Scoles P: *Pediatric orthopedics in clinical practice,* ed. 2, St. Louis, 1988, Mosby.)

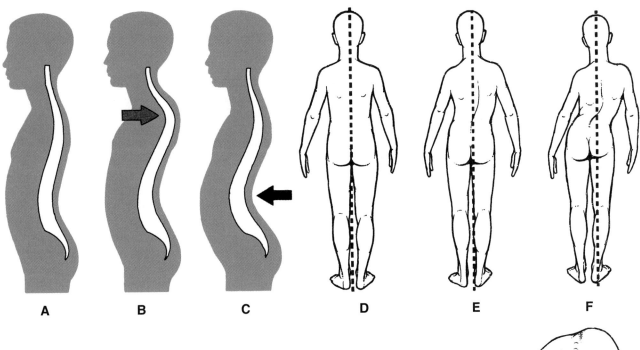

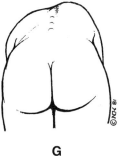

Figure 26-61   Defects of the spinal column. **A,** Normal spine. **B,** Kyphosis. **C,** Lordosis. **D,** Normal spine in balance. **E,** Mild scoliosis in balance. **F,** Severe scoliosis not in balance. **G,** Rib hump and flank asymmetry seen in flexion caused by rotary component.

TABLE 26-16   The 2-Minute Orthopedic Examination

Instructions	Observations
Stand facing examiner	Acromioclavicular joints, general habitus
Look at ceiling, floor, over both shoulders; touch ears to shoulders	Cervical spine motion
Shrug shoulders (examiner resists)	Trapezius strength
Abduct shoulders 90 degrees (examiner resists at 90 degrees)	Deltoid strength
Full external rotation of arms	Shoulder motion
Flex and extend elbows	Elbow motion
Arms at sides, elbows 90 degrees flexed; pronate and supinate wrists	Elbow and wrist motion
Spread fingers; make fist	Hand or finger motion and deformities
Tighten (contract) quadriceps; relax quadriceps	Symmetry and knee effusion; ankle effusion
"Duck walk" four steps (away from examiner with buttocks on heels)	Hip, knee, and ankle motion
Stand with back to examiner	Shoulder symmetry, scoliosis
Knees straight, touch toes	Scoliosis, hip motion, hamstring tightness
Raise up on toes, raise heels	Calf symmetry, leg strength

injury sequelae (Table 26-16). When problems are suspected refer the child for evaluation by an orthopedist.

Athletic injuries are becoming more common with the increase in organized sports activities for preadolescents and adolescents. The growing child is at risk for epiphyseal frac-

tures, since the epiphyseal plate is the weakest part of the long bones and has the least resistance to stress. Stress fractures of the tibia or the femur occur commonly, and the affected child complains of pain in the proximal region of the tibia or distal part of the femur. A painful knee may be caused by a dislocation of the patella. Another common cause of knee pain in young athletes is Osgood-Schlatter disease in which there is a partial avulsion of the tibial tubercle and painful swelling in the associated area. The history of the child's recent activities will give some indication of the kind of injury sustained.

Neurological System

The nervous system manifests dynamic growth and change from the newborn period through young childhood. Sensory and motor development proceeds with the increase in myelinization. Myelinization follows a cephalocaudal (head-to-toe) and proximodistal (head, neck, trunk, and extremities) pattern. Clinically, these changes become apparent as the infant achieves the expected developmental milestones (see Box 5-5 on p. 82).

Newborns, Infants, and Young Children. In children younger than 2 years old the neurological assessment is closely related to the increasing myelinization and maturation of the neural system. In this age group you can only estimate the degree of maturation rather than quantify it. You must adapt the formal neurological examination of the infant or child to the age of the individual. In infants and children, a complete neurological examination consists of assessment of the following: the cranial nerves and special senses, the motor system, coordination and cerebellar function, sensation, and both superficial and deep reflexes. In this age range, the primary mode of examination is one of observation and inspection, reinforced by palpation and passive manipulation.

Observe the child in the natural state and then with intentional stimulation such as a noise or a toy. Such observation is the best opportunity to determine how the child's overall function and behavior meet age-related norms. There are seven areas to assess: general appearance, symmetry of spontaneous movements, body positioning, posture, movement of extremities, presence of seizure activity, and responsiveness to the parents and the environment.

A good tool for assessing neurological status in an infant and young child is the Denver Developmental Screening Test (DDST-II) (described in Chapter 5 and shown in Figure 5-1). The DDST-II assesses gross and fine motor skills, language skills, and social skills as compared with other children of the same age. This is a screening tool that can provide clues to the child's neurological status. When deviations from the norm occur, the infant or child should be closely monitored and/or evaluated with more definitive measures.

Since the neurological system affects every other system, integrate the neurological examination with other parts of the physical examination. For example, changes in skin pigmentation, lesions, masses in the abdomen, abnormal size and shape of the head, gaps and protrusions in the spinal column, and limited range of motion can all reflect a disease, lesion, or injury to the nervous system.

Remember that a child is going through an intense period of development that is in part related to the increasing myelinization and maturation of the neural system. This means that meticulous observation of the child's developmental progress is important. Indicators of how well the

neurological system is functioning include characteristics such as the quality, pitch, loudness, and duration of a child's cry; the level of drowsiness; the degree of irritability; symmetry and smoothness of movement; and social, adaptive, language, and motor skills.

Assess for primitive reflexes in the newborn and young infant. The automatic infant reflexes that are normal at birth disappear at approximately 4 to 6 months of age, as voluntary control begins to develop. They include the Moro reflex, palmar grasp reflex, plantar grasp reflex, placing reflex, stepping reflex, asymmetric tonic neck reflex, sucking reflex, and rooting reflex. Table 26-17 describes several reflexes found in full-term infants. Figure 26-62 illustrates these reflexes. Table 26-18 includes descriptions of the sucking and rooting reflexes. A positive Babinski response (Figure 26-63) is normally present in the newborn and disappears by the age of 12 to 24 months or when the child begins to walk (Compare Figure 26-63 with Figure 19-43, an example of the negative Babinski in an adult). Ankle clonus may also be present in the newborn. Absence of these reflexes at birth may indicate a severe problem of the central nervous system. Persistence of these reflexes beyond age-appropriate norms usually indicates nervous system abnormality.

Cranial nerves in infants are not directly tested but are indirectly evaluated during the physical examination (see Table 26-18). Patellar tendon reflexes are present at birth. The Achilles and brachioradial tendon reflexes become testable at age 6 months. In infants, use the flat surface of a finger to briskly tap the tendon (rather than a reflex hammer).

Children. Examine the child age 2 years or older with the same methods used for an adult (see Chapter 19). Alter the conversation, directions, and developmental tasks to be more suitable to the child's interests and knowledge level.

In a child more specific examination is possible than with the infant. You can now include auditory testing, funduscopic examination, and stereognosis testing. Expand the assessment to observe the quantity and quality of spontaneous voluntary motor activity, the ease in performing voluntary movements, lateral dominance, spontaneous drawing, articulation of sounds, and language acquisition. Note the child's auditory discrimination, memory, reading, speech, and calculation skills. Also, assess the child for awareness of body parts, spatial orientation, and emotional lability. There are a number of "soft" neurological signs that can provide subtle clues to a neurological delay or deficit in the school-age child. Table 26-19 describes some of these findings and the age when their continued presence would be of concern.

Cranial nerves can be tested with modification of the adult format by making the tasks more of a game. Table 26-20 gives detailed information on techniques for evaluating cranial nerve function in young children.

When assessing movement, look for signs of generalized weakness as is seen in muscular dystrophy. Observe the child rising from a supine position to a standing position. A child with good muscle strength will be able to rise without using the arms for leverage. A child with generalized muscle weakness will demonstrate the Gowers' sign, which in-

TABLE 26-17	Primitive Reflexes Routinely Evaluated: Procedure for Examination, Expected Findings, Time of Appearance and Disappearance

Reflex (Appearance)	Procedure and Findings
Palmar grasp (birth)	Making sure the infant's head is in midline, touch the palm of the infant's hand from the ulnar side (opposite the thumb). Note the strong grasp of your finger. Sucking facilitates the grasp. It should be strongest between 1 and 2 months of age and disappear by 3 months (Figure 26-62, *A*).
Plantar grasp (birth)	Touch the plantar surface of the infant's feet at the base of the toes. The toes should curl downward. It should be strong up to 8 months of age (Figure 26-62, *B*).
Moro (birth)	With the infant supported in semisitting position, allow the head and trunk to drop back to a 30-degree angle. Observe symmetrical abduction and extension of the arms; fingers fan out, and thumb and index finger form a **C**. The arms then adduct in an embracing motion, followed by relaxed flexion. The legs may follow a similar pattern of response. The reflex diminishes in strength by 3 to 4 months and disappears by 6 months (Figure 26-62, *C*).
Placing (4 days of age)	Hold the infant upright under its arms next to the table or chair. Touch the dorsal side of the foot to the table or chair edge. Observe flexion of the hips and knees and lifting of the foot as if stepping up on the table. Age of disappearance varies (Figure 26-62, *D*).
Stepping (between birth and 8 weeks)	Hold the infant upright under the arms and allow the soles of the feet to touch the surface of the table. Observe for alternate flexion and extension of the legs, simulating walking. It disappears before voluntary walking (Figure 26-62, *E*).
Tonic neck or "fencing" (by 2 to 3 months)	With the infant lying supine and relaxed or sleeping, turn the head to one side so the jaw is over the shoulder. Observe for extension of the arm and leg on the side to which the head is turned and for flexion of the opposite arm and leg. Turn the infant's head to the other side, observing the reversal of the extremities' posture. This reflex diminishes at 3 to 4 months of age and disappears by 6 months. Be concerned if the infant never exhibits the reflex or seems locked in the fencing position. This reflex must disappear before the infant can roll over or bring its hand to its face (Figure 26-62, *F*).

Modified from Seidel HM et al.: *Mosby's guide to physical examination,* ed. 4, St. Louis, 1999, Mosby.

TABLE 26-18	Testing Procedures and Expected Behaviors for Indirect Cranial Nerve Evaluation in Newborns and Infants

Cranial Nerves	Procedures and Observations
CN II, III, IV, and VI	Optical blink reflex: shine a light at the infant's open eyes. Observe the quick closure of the eyes and dorsal flexion of the infant's head. No response may indicate poor light perception. Gazes intensely at close object or face. Focuses on and tracks an object with the eyes. Doll's eye maneuver: see CN VIII.
CN V	Rooting reflex: touch one corner of the infant's mouth. The infant should open the mouth and turn the head in the direction of stimulation. If the infant has been recently fed, minimal or no response is expected. Sucking reflex: place your finger in the infant's mouth, feeling the sucking action. The tongue should push up against your finger with a fairly good rate. Note the pressure, strength, and pattern of sucking.
CN VII	Observe the infant's facial expression when crying. Note the infant's ability to wrinkle the forehead and the symmetry of the smile.
CN VIII	Acoustic blink reflex: loudly clap your hands about 30 cm from the infant's head; avoid producing an air current. Note the blink in response to the sound. No response after 2-3 days of age may indicate hearing problems. Infant will habituate to repeated testing. Moves eyes in direction of sound. Freezes position with high-pitched sound. Doll's eye maneuver: hold the infant under the axilla in an upright position, head held steady, facing you. Rotate the infant first in one direction and then in the other. The infant's eyes should turn in the opposite direction of the head movement at exactly the same pace of the rotation. If the eyes do not move in the expected direction, suspect a vestibular problem or eye muscle paralysis.
CN IX and X	Swallowing and gag reflex.
CN XII	Coordinated sucking and swallowing ability. Pinch infant's nose: mouth will open and tip of tongue will rise in a midline position.

Modified from Thompson JM et al.: *Mosby's clinical nursing,* ed. 4, St. Louis, 1997, Mosby. In Seidel HM et al.: *Mosby's guide to physical examination,* ed. 4, St. Louis, 1999, Mosby.

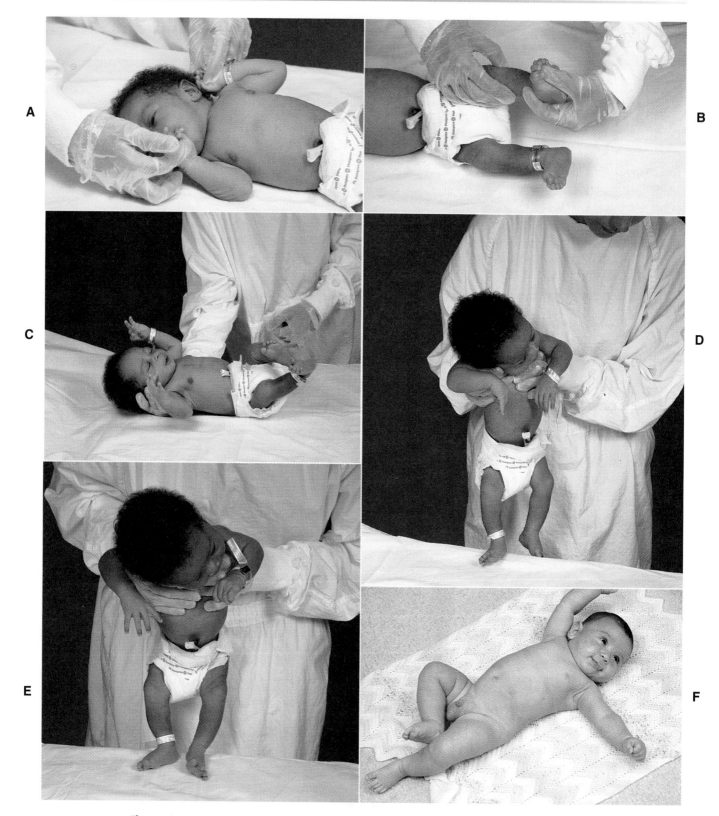

Figure 26-62   Elicitation of the primitive reflexes. Note: The preferred state for testing the primitive reflexes is "quiet alert," neither hungry nor drowsy. **A,** Palmar grasp. **B,** Plantar grasp. **C,** Moro reflex. **D,** Placing reflex. **E,** Stepping reflex. **F,** Asymmetric tonic neck reflex. (From Seidel HM et al.: *Mosby's guide to physical examination,* ed. 4, St. Louis, 1999, Mosby.)

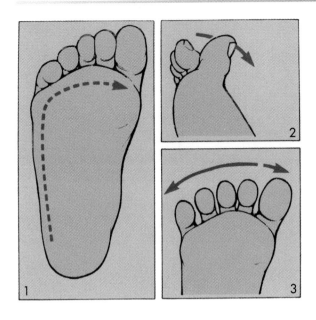

Figure 26-63 Babinski response. *1,* Direction of stroke; *2,* dorsiflexion of big toe; *3,* fanning of toes. (From Wong DL et al.: *Whaley and Wong's nursing care of infants and children,* ed. 6, St. Louis, 1999, Mosby.)

TABLE 26-19	Activities for Evaluating Neurologic Soft Signs in Children	
Activity	Soft Sign Findings	Latest Expected Age of Disappearance (Years)
Walking, running gait	Stiff-legged with a foot slapping quality, unusual posturing of the arms	3
Heel walking	Difficulty remaining on heels for a distance of 10 ft	7
Tip-toe walking	Difficulty remaining on toes for a distance of 10 ft	7
Tandem gait	Difficulty walking heel-to-toe, unusual posturing of arms	7
One-foot standing	Unable to remain standing on one foot longer than 5-10 sec	5
Hopping in place	Unable to rhythmically hop on each foot	6
Motor-stance	Difficulty maintaining stance (arms extended in front, feet together, and eyes closed), drifting of arms, mild writhing movements of hands or fingers	3
Visual tracking	Difficulty following object with eyes when keeping the head still; nystagmus	5
Rapid thumb-to-finger test	Rapid touching thumb to fingers in sequence is uncoordinated; unable to suppress mirror movements in contralateral hand	8
Rapid alternating movements of hands	Irregular speed and rhythm with pronation and supination of hands patting the knees	10
Finger-nose test	Unable to alternately touch examiner's finger and own nose consecutively	7
Right-left discrimination	Unable to identify right and left sides of own body	5
Two-point discrimination	Difficulty in localizing and discriminating when touched in one or two places	6
Graphesthesia	Unable to identify geometric shapes you draw in child's open hand	8
Stereognosis	Unable to identify common objects placed in own hand	5

From Seidel HM et al.: *Mosby's guide to physical examination,* ed. 4, St. Louis, 1999, Mosby.

volves rising from a sitting position by placing the hands on the legs, pushing the trunk up, and "climbing up himself" to reach a standing position (Figure 26-64).

Adolescents. The examination for older children and adolescents is the same as for the adult (Chapter 19).

Tests for Meningeal Irritation. Regardless of a child's age, if you suspect meningeal irritation during an illness episode, note the presence of the following: paradoxical irritability, Kernig's sign, and Brudzinski's sign. With para-

doxical irritability, the child is irritable (not easily comforted) when held by the parent, contrary to his or her usual behavior. To elicit Kernig's sign, have the child lie on the table, face up, with the leg bent at the knee. Attempt to extend the hip by raising the knee. If you encounter pain and resistance, the maneuver is positive for meningeal irritation. Obtain Brudzinski's sign by having the child lie supine on a table. Bend the neck gently. If the child's knees flex spontaneously, this sign is positive for meningeal irritation.

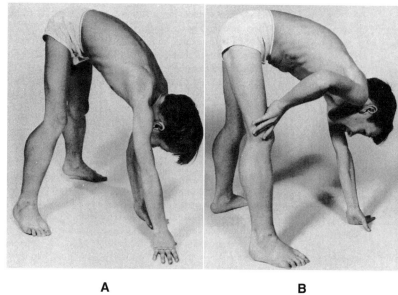

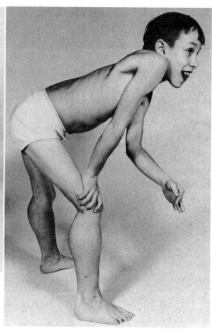

Figure 26-64 Gowers' sign of generalized muscle weakness. **A,** Maneuvers to position supported by both arms and legs. **B,** Pushes off floor to rest hand on knee. **C,** Then pushes self upright. (From Swaiman KF, Wright FS: *Pediatric neuromuscular diseases,* St. Louis, 1979, Mosby.)

TABLE 26-20	Cranial Nerve Examination Procedures for Young Children
Cranial Nerves	**Procedures and Observations**
CN II	If the child cooperates, the Snellen E or Picture Chart may be used to test vision. Visual fields may be tested, but the child may need the head immobilized.
CN III, IV, and VI	Have the child follow an object with the eyes, immobilizing the head if necessary. Attempt to move the object through the cardinal points of gaze.
CN V	Observe the child chewing a cookie or cracker, noting bilateral jaw strength. Touch the child's forehead and cheeks with cotton and watch the child bat it away.
CN VII	Observe the child's face when smiling, frowning, and crying. Ask the child to show the teeth. Demonstrate puffed cheeks and ask the child to imitate.
CN VIII	Observe the child turn to sounds such as bell or whisper. Whisper a commonly used word behind the child's back and have the child repeat the word. Perform audiometric testing.
CN IX and X	Elicit gag reflex.
CN XI and XII	Instruct older child to stick out the tongue and shrug the shoulders or raise the arms.

Modified from Bowers AC, Thompson JM: *Clinical manual of health assessment,* ed. 4, St. Louis, 1992, Mosby. In Seidel HM et al.: *Mosby's guide to physical examination,* ed. 4, St. Louis, 1999, Mosby.

• • •

The importance of conducting a comprehensive, holistic assessment of the child to promote physical, developmental, and psychosocial health as well as to prevent problems cannot be overemphasized. A thorough working knowledge of growth and development, combined with solid physical assessment skills and an appreciation of the need to include the family in the assessment process, will help the practitioner successfully assess pediatric clients and promote the health of children and their families (Figure 26-65).

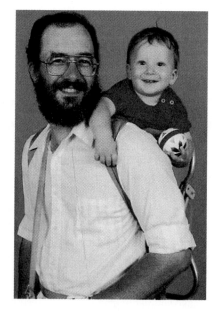

Figure 26-65 Assessment of both the child and family is important for promoting health.

Sample Documentation and Diagnoses

FOCUSED HEALTH HISTORY (SUBJECTIVE DATA)

Debbie, a 7-year-old Caucasian female, has been brought to the clinic by her mother because of a sore throat and fever for the past day. She has been in good health except for approximately four colds since her visit 1 year ago. She has no known allergies to any medications. Her mother states that Debbie has had a fever of up to 102.7° F oral; (39.3° C) since yesterday. The fever comes down with acetaminophen 320 mg taken every 4 to 6 hours. Her last dose of acetaminophen was about 3 hours ago. Debbie also complains of a sore throat. She has been drinking some liquids but eating little since she has had the fever and sore throat. Debbie denies any pain when bending her neck, abdominal pain, or pain with urination. Her mother states that Debbie is tired but alert and moderately active. She states that several of Debbie's classmates have strep throat and she is concerned that Debbie may also have strep throat. No one else in her family is sick.

Debbie is in the second grade of the urban elementary school. She states that she enjoys school but thinks her teacher is "too hard sometimes." Her mother says that all school reports are good and that Debbie has many friends in school and in the neighborhood and has recently started "sleeping over" with her girlfriends. Her mother states that everyone in the family is fine—no major stresses or life changes.

FOCUSED PHYSICAL EXAMINATION (OBJECTIVE DATA)

General appearance: Cooperative, pleasant, 7-year-old Caucasian female who appears flushed and feverish.
Temperature: 38.8° C (101.8° F) (tympanic membrane).
Eyes: Clear, no discharge or redness.
Ears: Tympanic membranes pearly with landmarks visible.
Nose: Pink mucosa; slight, clear discharge.
Mouth: Pink, no lesions.
Throat: Tonsils red, swollen 3+, white exudate bilaterally.
Neck: Enlarged and tender tonsillar nodes bilaterally.
Chest: Lungs clear; breath sounds clear anteriorly and posteriorly, resonant to percussion, no adventitious sounds.

DIAGNOSES
HEALTH PROBLEM
Pharyngitis: Possible Group A Streptococcal Infection

NURSING DIAGNOSES
Acute Pain Related to Inflammation of Throat

Defining Characteristics
• Tonsils red, swollen, enlarged
• Verbal expression of sore throat
• Decreased intake related to sore throat

Imbalanced Nutrition: Less Than Body Requirements Related to Sore Throat

Defining Characteristics
• Reported decreased food or drink intake
• Lack of interest in food
• Sore, inflamed throat

Critical Thinking Questions

Review the Sample Documentation and Diagnoses box to answer questions 1 and 2.
1. If Debbie's general appearance showed her to be extremely ill appearing, apprehensive, and leaning forward to breathe with her mouth open and excessively salivating, how would your physical examination differ?
2. Given the new information in question 1, what would you consider the probable cause of Debbie's pharyngitis?

3. You are conducting a routine well-child examination. Describe how you would adjust the sequencing of your examination for an infant, a toddler, a preschooler, a school-age child, and an adolescent.
4. Describe the new CDC recommendations for assessing growth in children from birth to 36 months and children ages 2 to 20 years. How do they differ from the previous approaches? In what ways are they useful or problematic?

Remember to check out the Online Study Guide!
www.harcourthealth.com/MERLIN/Barkauskas/

Aging Clients

Purpose of Examination

This chapter highlights areas of assessment that may differ in older adults. The health history and physical examination of the older client focus on the management of chronic illness, maximizing functional ability, and prolonging an independent and active life. Assessment is often done in an interdisciplinary team that may include physicians, advanced practice nurses, social workers, nutritionists, pharmacists, and physical and occupational therapists. The initial assessment of the older client will serve as a baseline from which to compare change over time.

DEMOGRAPHICS

The percentage of the American population older than age 65 tripled between 1900 and 1990. Since 1990, the 65-and-older population increased by 10%, and by 2000, approximately 13% of the entire population was older than 65 (Administration on Aging [AOA], 2001). By 2030, when the baby boom generation has aged, about 20% of the population will be older than 65. While the actual maximum lifespan has not increased (approximately 110 years), the number of older persons living into their 80s and 90s has increased. In 1997 older adults who reached the age of 65 could expect to live an average of 19 additional years for women and 15 years for men. The fastest growing segment of the American population is the group of individuals older than 85.

The majority of older adults live active, independent lives in the community. Retired from one career, older adults may embark on a second career or pursue a lifelong hobby on a full-time basis. For many older adults this is a time when energy, previously devoted to work and caring for family, is directed toward new and creative projects. Most older adults have one or more chronic health problems. The extent to which chronic problems cause illness and functional disability depends on the type and severity of the problem, co-existing problems, environmental factors such as financial and social resources, and the individual's perception of health and personal coping strategies.

Health care providers strive to help older adults maximize their functional abilities and quality of life. The most prevalent chronic physical problems in older adults are outlined in Box 27-1. About 15% of older adults have some problem with cognition that affects functioning.

BOX 27-1

MAJOR CHRONIC CONDITIONS IN OLDER ADULTS

Arthritis	Hypertension
Cataracts	Orthopedic impairments
Diabetes	Sinusitis
Hearing impairments	Varicose veins
Heart disease	Visual impairments

USE AND COST OF HEALTH CARE

Data prepared by the Administration on Aging (AoA) (2001) indicate that older individuals account for a disproportionate number of hospital stays and noninstitutionalized older adults also had more physician contacts than younger persons. Slightly more than 1% of the population age 65 to 74 years live in nursing homes, but by age 85, this percentage increases to almost 20%. Health care is expensive for older adults. Older adults averaged more than $2800 out-of-pocket medical expenses in 1997, almost twice the expense for those younger than 65. Although most older adults are eligible for Medicare insurance, Medicare does not pay for many of the key expenses incurred by older adults, such as medications, hearing aids, dental care, and routine vision care. For many older adults these expenditures are a financial burden. In 1998, 17% of those older than 65 were considered poor or near poor. Lack of financial resources can cause people to ration their medications, delay seeking care, or avoid care. This behavior may lead to worsening health conditions and lengthy, expensive hospital stays that might otherwise be avoided.

Nurses are likely to care for older clients in a variety of settings. And, since after age 65 there are 149 women for every 100 men, a majority of these clients are likely to be women.

EXAMINATION

Health History

Older adults are likely to have different types of problems than younger and middle-aged adults. This section discusses the presentation of conditions that are more likely to occur in older adults and significantly affect their daily function. These conditions are sometimes referred to as "geriatric syndromes" and include falls, incontinence, delirium, inappropriate medication use, mental status and mood impairment, functional impairment, and poor nutrition. Although these conditions are not diseases, they do place the client at risk for functional decline, morbidity, and mortality.

Altered Clinical Presentation

Diseases associated with "classic" symptoms in young and middle-aged adults may be associated with more general symptoms in later life. For example, a myocardial infarction in an older person may present with mental confusion, a fall, or nausea and vomiting, as opposed to crushing substernal pain radiating down the left arm commonly seen in younger patients. In addition, the presence of one condition may mask another. For example, a person with severe chronic obstructive lung disease may not be active enough to develop the symptoms of angina despite the presence of severe ischemic heart disease.

Concomitant Disease

Since multiple medical problems are common in older adults, an examination directed at one symptom may uncover more than one problem. When examining the client for a complaint of recurrent falls, the examiner may discover that the falls are related to hurrying to the bathroom to avoid an incontinence episode.

Accumulated Life History

Intelligence does not decline with age. Respect older adults for their knowledge, wisdom, and accumulated life experiences. Remember that the person has lived with his or her body a long time and may be able to detect subtle changes in health status better than the health professional. The older adult may have a long history of medical problems, and the interview may become lengthy. Whenever necessary, gently redirect the conversation to obtain the most pertinent history while at the same time avoiding giving the client the impression that offered information is not valued. To redirect the interview, say, "This is valuable information that I would like to hear about at some later point in time, but right now I need to focus on your problem of dizziness."

The following impairments are more commonly encountered in older adults. Awareness of these conditions will assist you in focusing questions on specific signs and symptoms that may indicate the presence of impairment.

Mental Status and Mood Impairment

Dementia. Dementia is a clinical syndrome characterized by a decline in memory and intellectual functioning that significantly interferes with work or social functioning (American Psychiatric Association, 1994). Several different diseases may cause dementia. The most common cause of dementia is Alzheimer's disease, in which neuron loss and a decrease in chemical transmitters occur in certain areas of the brain. Other causes of dementia include multiple strokes, alcohol abuse, Parkinson's disease, Huntington's disease, and acquired immunodeficiency disease. Box 27-2 lists the criteria from the *DSM-IV* required to make a diagnosis of dementia.

Older clients are more likely to have symptoms of dementia, since the prevalence of dementia increases with age. At age 65, about 1.5% of the population has dementia; this percentage increases to about 50% at 90 years.

The answers to the following questions may provide information about the client's mental status:

- Did the client come to the appointment alone or accompanied by someone?

BOX 27-2

DSM-IV DEMENTIA CRITERIA

A. Multiple cognitive deficits, including:
  1. Memory impairment
  2. One or more of the following:
    a. Aphasia
    b. Apraxia
    c. Agnosia
    d. Disturbance in executive function
B. No. 1 and No. 2 must significantly impair occupational or social functioning

BOX 27-3

DSM-IV MAJOR DEPRESSION CRITERIA

Presence of five or more of the following:
  1. Depressed mood
  2. Diminished interest or pleasure
  3. Weight loss or gain
  4. Insomnia or hypersomnia
  5. Psychomotor agitation or retardation
  6. Fatigue or loss of energy
  7. Feelings of worthlessness or guilt
  8. Diminished energy to think or concentrate
  9. Recurrent thoughts of death, suicidal ideation

• Is the client appropriately dressed?
• Is the client having difficulty answering questions?

Not all clients need a formal assessment of their mental status. If, however, the examiner suspects some impairment in mental status, such as memory loss, he or she can use a number of standardized assessment instruments to evaluate mental status. The Mini-Mental Status Examination (MMSE) (Folstein, Folstein, and McHugh, 1975) is a commonly used 30-item screening tool that assesses orientation, registration, attention and calculation, recall, and language (see Box 19-5). A score of 30 indicates optimal function. A score of 23 or less suggests some type of mental status impairment; however, dementia may be present even with a score greater than 23. If dementia is suspected, refer the client to a physician for a complete evaluation. No diagnosis is made or excluded solely on the basis of the MMSE score.

Depression.   Depression is the most common mood disorder in late life. The 1991 NIH Panel Development Conference on the Diagnosis and Treatment of Depression in Late Life defines depression as a syndrome that includes physiological, affective, and mental symptoms. Box 27-3 outlines the *DSM-IV* criteria for depression.

A 1997 update of the 1991 consensus statement suggests that depression may be underdiagnosed in older adults by health care providers who attribute depressive symptoms to the multiple problems associated with aging (Lebowitz et al., 1997). About 1% to 2% of community-dwelling older adults suffer from major depression, and about 13% to 27% suffer from subsyndromal depression. Subsyndromal depression occurs when an older adult has symptoms of depression that do not meet the *DSM-IV* criteria for major depression but which do cause the individual physical and/or functional disability (Lebowitz et al., 1997; Lyness et al., 1999). Subsyndromal depression is a relatively new concept, and research is ongoing to determine the best methods of treatment for this condition. Because some of the symptoms of depression, such as weight loss, sleep disturbances, and fatigue, may be associated with other conditions, depression may easily be missed in older adults. Simply asking the client, "Do you feel sad, blue, or depressed much of the time?" provides insight into the client's mood. Assessing for depression is an impor-

tant part of the health history for older adults, particularly for men because older Caucasian men are at the highest risk for suicide of any age group.

A number of questionnaires are available to assess for depressive symptoms. The Geriatric Depression Scale (GDS) (Yesavage et al., 1983) is a 30-item questionnaire designed specifically to screen for depression in the elderly. Table 27-1 is a 15-item shortened form of the original 30-item GDS. Similar to the MMSE, the GDS score does not diagnose or exclude depression. Refer a client who scores between 5 and 9 on the GDS-Short Form to a physician for further evaluation of possible depression. Also, if the history suggests depression even in the absence of a high GDS score, refer the client for further evaluation.

Delirium.   Delirium is an acute change in mental status and is diagnosed when a client has symptoms that meet the *DSM-IV* criteria outlined in Box 27-4.

Delirium usually occurs during an acute medical illness, and studies have reported that 5% to 35% of hospitalized elderly clients develop delirium during their hospitalization. Delirium may develop in a few hours, and the client, who previously was thinking clearly, suddenly becomes disoriented, restless, or lethargic and may hallucinate. This sudden impaired ability to think rationally may alternate with periods of clear thinking. Delirium is distinguished from dementia by its rapid onset. Delirium most often occurs in clients who had normal mental status before surgery or before developing an acute illness. Almost any acute disorder that affects brain function, such as hypoxia, fever, dysrhythmias, and anemia, can cause delirium. One of the major causes of delirium in the older adult is medications. While delirium is most prevalent in hospitals, acutely ill older clients may be brought into a clinic accompanied by family members who report sudden and dramatic changes in the older adult's mental status. Because delirium is often the first indication of an underlying acute problem, report acute changes in mental status.

Functional Impairment

The older client's ability to maintain independence depends on his or her ability to perform the skills to meet basic physical and daily life management needs or to secure these

TABLE 27-1	Geriatric Depression Scale (Short Form)		

Choose the Best Answer for How You Felt the Past Week.

1. Are you basically satisfied with your life?		Yes	No*
2. Have you dropped many of your activities and interests?		Yes*	No
3. Do you feel that your life is empty?		Yes*	No
4. Do you often get bored?		Yes*	No
5. Are you in good spirits most of the time?		Yes	No*
6. Are you afraid that something bad is going to happen to you?		Yes*	No
7. Do you feel happy most of the time?		Yes	No*
8. Do you often feel helpless?		Yes*	No
9. Do you prefer to stay at home, rather than going out and doing new things?		Yes*	No
10. Do you feel you have more problems with memory than most?		Yes*	No
11. Do you think it is wonderful to be alive now?		Yes	No*
12. Do you feel pretty worthless the way you are now?		Yes*	No
13. Do you feel full of energy?		Yes	No*
14. Do you feel that your situation is hopeless?		Yes*	No
15. Do you think that most people are better off than you are?		Yes*	No

From Sheikh JL, Yesavage JA: *Clin Gerontol* 5:165-173, 1986. In Ham RJ, Sloane PD: *Primary care geriatrics: a case-based approach,* ed. 3, St. Louis, 1997, Mosby.

Each answer indicated by * counts as one point. Scores between 5 and 9 suggest depression, scores above 9 generally indicate depression.

BOX 27-4

DSM-IV DELIRIUM CRITERIA

1. Reduced attention
2. Impaired sensorium
3. Fluctuating course
4. Disorganized thinking
5. Subacute onset

BOX 27-5

ACTIVITIES OF DAILY LIVING

Dressing	Bowel control
Transferring	Bladder control
Feeding	Walking
Bathing	Climbing stairs
Toileting	Grooming

BOX 27-6

INSTRUMENTAL ACTIVITIES OF DAILY LIVING

Telephoning	Shopping
Reading	Meal preparation
Leisure activities	Laundering
Medication management	Housekeeping
Money management	Home maintenance

needs through family or community resources. Basic physical skills are referred to as **activities of daily living (ADLs)**, and life management skills are called **instrumental activities of daily living (IADLs)** (see Boxes 27-5 and 27-6). One or more physical and psychological impairments can greatly affect the client's ability to perform ADLs or IADLs. Assess ADL and IADL function in the older client.

The most accurate assessment of ADL and IADL function is direct observation of the client performing each specific task. In the hospital, physical and occupational therapists often administer tests of ADL and IADL function in the rehabilitation department where clients can be observed performing these tasks. If unable to directly observe clients performing ADL or IADL tasks, ask clients whether they can perform the various ADL and IADL tasks alone or with assistance. If assistance is required, find out who provides the assistance and with what frequency. Ask the caregiver what ADL or IADL tasks the client can perform. In addition, simply observing the client entering the room, sitting in a chair, and undressing for the examination provides clues about several ADL functions. One quick and easy assessment of mobility is the timed get-up-and-go test (Podsiadlo and Richardson, 1991). Time the client getting up from a

chair, walking 10 feet, turning around, walking back to the chair, and sitting back down (Figure 27-1). Use a standard armchair with a seat height of about 20 inches. The time required to perform this test varies with clients; however, highly mobile, independent older adults can perform the test in about 10 seconds (Podsiadlo and Richardson, 1991). Detect changes over time by repeating this test at subsequent visits. The examiner can also observe the client's ability to function with assistive devices (Figure 27-2).

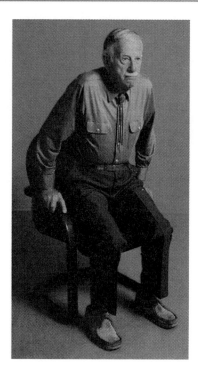

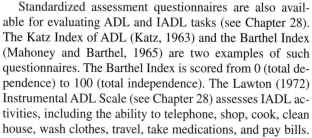

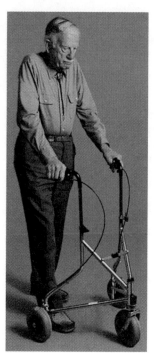

Figure 27-1 The timed "get-up-and-go" test measures the time it takes the client to rise from a chair, walk 10 feet, turn around, return to the chair, and sit down.

Figure 27-2 Many older clients use assistive devices, such as a Delta walker, to provide additional stability when ambulating.

Standardized assessment questionnaires are also available for evaluating ADL and IADL tasks (see Chapter 28). The Katz Index of ADL (Katz, 1963) and the Barthel Index (Mahoney and Barthel, 1965) are two examples of such questionnaires. The Barthel Index is scored from 0 (total dependence) to 100 (total independence). The Lawton (1972) Instrumental ADL Scale (see Chapter 28) assesses IADL activities, including the ability to telephone, shop, cook, clean house, wash clothes, travel, take medications, and pay bills.

Incontinence.   Between 15% and 35% of older adults living at home and up to 50% of nursing home residents have incontinence (Fantl et al., 1996). Incontinence is an involuntary loss of urine with or without warning. The incontinent older adult may experience physical, psychological, and financial burdens. For example, fear of an accident may lead to restriction of outside activities and contribute to social isolation. In response to the significant physical, psychological, and social problems associated with urinary incontinence, the U.S. Department of Health and Human Services Agency for Health Care Policy Research (now the Agency for Healthcare Research and Quality [AHRQ]) established practice guidelines for the management of urinary incontinence in 1992 and revised these guidelines in 1996.

Incontinence may be transient or established. Transient incontinence is acute in onset and is often related to a change in health status, such as a urinary tract infection, medications, stool impaction, delirium, polyuria, or restricted mobility. Often several of these factors are present during hospitalization, and it is not uncommon for older adults to develop incontinence when hospitalized.

Established incontinence occurs when leakage of urine persists after suspected causes (e.g., decreasing a dose of diuretic) have been treated. The AHCRQ guidelines describe categories of established urinary incontinence based on the type of incontinence symptoms. The most common categories are urge, stress, mixed, overflow, and functional incontinence (see Table 27-2). Urge incontinence is the most common cause of incontinence in older adults and may result from stroke, Parkinson's disease, dementia due to Alzheimer's disease, or it may be present in individuals without apparent neurological disease. Urge incontinence is characterized by little warning before voiding large amounts of urine. A client may state, "I just can't seem to get to the bathroom on time."

Stress incontinence is the second most common cause of incontinence in older women and is the result of bladder outlet incompetence. Stress incontinence causes involuntary loss of urine when abdominal pressure increases, such as when the woman coughs, laughs, lifts, or suddenly stands. Relaxation of the pelvic floor muscles allows the proximal portion of the urethra and bladder neck to be displaced into the urogenital diaphragm with increased abdominal pressure. The amount of urine lost may vary from a few drops to a large quantity.

Overflow incontinence is caused by overdistention of the bladder, with subsequent leakage of urine from the bladder. Overdistention of the bladder results from an underactive bladder muscle or obstruction to the outflow of urine from the bladder. One of the most common causes of overflow incontinence is prostate enlargement, resulting in urethral obstruction. Overflow incontinence due to obstruction from an

TABLE 27-2   Categories of Incontinence by Symptoms

Symptoms	Cause
Urge	
Urgency, little warning before voiding, usually large amounts of urine	Stroke, dementia, Parkinson's disease
Stress	
Involuntary loss of urine with increased abdominal pressure such as coughing, sneezing, lifting, or standing	Relaxation of pelvic floor muscles
Overflow	
Dribbling of urine from distended bladder or bladder contracts reflexively without warning, mixed urge and stress	Prostatic hypertrophy, diabetes, bladder nerve injury
Functional	
Urine leakage before getting to bathroom	Environmental or personal factors

enlarged prostate is the second most common type of incontinence in older men. This type of incontinence may present with constant dribbling.

Mixed incontinence is generally a combination of urge and stress incontinence.

Functional incontinence results from a variety of environmental and personal factors that impede getting to the bathroom before voiding occurs. Restricted mobility, bathroom location, and decreased manual dexterity or balance may cause incontinence in the absence of any urinary tract dysfunction or may exacerbate pre-existing incontinence.

Clients are often reluctant to volunteer information about incontinence symptoms. Some individuals have the mistaken belief that incontinence is a normal part of aging that must be tolerated. State the following to help the client relate incontinence symptoms, if present: "Some older people have a problem with leakage of urine at inappropriate times. This is not something that normally happens with aging and can be treated. Do you ever have problems with leakage of urine?" Asking the question in this way informs the client that other people have a similar problem, it is not normal, and it may be treatable. If a client is experiencing symptoms, ask about the frequency and amount of the incontinence, associated activities, medications, eating and drinking habits, and current management of the problem by the client. Instruct the client on how to complete a voiding diary. The diary is an account of the frequency and amount voided, incontinent episodes, and associated activities.

Falls.   Falls are a common occurrence in the older population. As many as one third of older adults who live at home fall each year. This increases to about 50% by age 80. Accidents are the sixth leading cause of death for individuals older than 65; falls are the leading type of accident in this age group. About 5% of falls result in a fracture, with the most common fracture sites being the humerus, wrist, pelvis, ankle, and hip.

Risk factors for falls include sensory impairment such as visual changes and proprioceptive and vestibular dysfunction; neurological disorders resulting in gait impairment or mental status impairment; musculoskeletal disorders affecting strength and mobility; cardiovascular conditions, particularly orthostatic hypotension; and medications. Situational factors such as acute illness or an unfamiliar environment may precipitate a fall in individuals with or without predisposing risk factors. Falls are sometimes nonspecific signs of acute illness. For example, a nursing home resident falls, and in the course of the assessment after the fall the nurse measures a temperature of 38.9° C (102° F), and a subsequent diagnosis of pneumonia is made.

Ask clients whether they have fallen in the past 6 months. Obtain a detailed history about any reported falls, including risk factors for falls, frequency of falls, activity at the time of the fall, a description of the environment in which the fall occurred, and any injuries associated with the fall. For clients who live alone, always ask whether they were able to get up from the fall or whether they had to wait for help. The physical examination for clients who report a fall should include a neurological, musculoskeletal, and cardiovascular examination to assess for visual, balance, and gait impairment; muscle weakness; dysrhythmias; and postural changes in blood pressure.

Inappropriate Medication Use

Older adults are the largest consumers of prescription medications and also purchase many nonprescription medications, vitamin and mineral supplements, and herbal preparations. Several factors place the older client at risk for the ingestion of inappropriate medication, including multiple diseases, multiple health care providers, nonprescription medication use, sharing medications, and rationing medications. Older adults who see several different physicians for different problems may accumulate multiple medications, some of which may potentiate or lessen the effect of others. Because of limited financial resources, the older adult may purchase only a portion of prescribed medications or may ration the medication, such as taking a pill once a day that is prescribed to be taken three times a day.

Dosage for some medications may be altered for older clients because of age-related changes in the responsiveness of receptor cells or the distribution, metabolism, and excretion of medications. Since variability exists among older clients, consider medication dosages on an individual basis.

Instruct the client to bring all prescribed and over-the-counter medications to the examination, whether the client is currently taking them or not (people often stockpile unused medications at home). Using the last refill date on the bottle and the dose schedule, calculate the number of pills that should remain. Compare this number with the actual number of pills remaining to determine whether the client is using the medication as ordered. Assess the number and type of medications in relation to the client's physical problems. Question the client about medications that do not seem to correspond with information obtained during the health history. For instance, a client might bring in a bottle of thyroid medication and fail to mention any thyroid problem. Conversely, the client may relate a diagnosis of hypertension and not have any antihypertensive medication. If you notice a discrepancy between the way in which a medication was prescribed and the way in which the client takes the medication, explore reasons for this discrepancy.

The greater the number of medications prescribed, the greater the likelihood that not all will be ingested. Clients may have difficulty opening the medication bottles, reading the labels, or remembering to take their medications. Advise clients that they can request easy-to-open pill bottles from their pharmacist. Suggest medication reminder boxes, which have compartments for both the days of the week and different times of the day. The client, a family member, or a community nurse can sort medications into these compartments. Discourage clients from sharing medications with family members and friends.

Poor Nutrition

Nutritional status depends on the amount and type of food in the diet. Calorie requirements decrease with age. This decrease is likely due to both the change in body composition with age and the change in activity level with age (Abbasi, 1998). As individuals age, the percentage of body fat increases and the percentage of muscle or lean body mass decreases. With a decrease in lean body mass there is a decrease in the basal metabolic rate (BMR) and a decreased need for calories. Activity level changes with age. Some older adults become less active due to chronic illness and mobility problems, and others become more active as they have increased time for recreational activities. An older adult who regularly engages in activities such as golf, swimming, or bicycling will need more calories than someone who is sedentary (see Chapter 6).

Since the older client may need fewer calories with increasing age, the type of food eaten is important to ensure adequate nutrient intake and to prevent poor nutritional status. The nutritional history should focus on both caloric needs and the types of food consumed. Inquire about where the client eats, how often meals are skipped, the usual intake, the facilities available for food preparation, the resources available to purchase food, and the ability to prepare food. Focus history questions on special dietary needs (e.g., is the client on a restricted sodium diet?); clinical symptoms such as sore mouth; difficulty with chewing or swallowing; history of fractures; mood; mental status; and medications.

A 3-day diet record provides a good indication of food consumption, and many computer programs are available to calculate the energy and nutrient intake based on this 3-day record. You can mail this record, along with instructions for use, to clients before their appointment. Specifically ask clients about calcium intake since most adults do not con-

sume the recommended daily requirement of 1200 mg calcium. Deficiency in calcium intake places older adults at risk for osteoporosis. Although both men and women can develop osteoporosis, the prevalence is higher in women.

Poor nutritional status, as defined by the 1991 Nutrition Screen Initiative (Dwyer, 1992), includes nutritional deficiencies, as well as dehydration, undernutrition, nutritional imbalances, obesity, and excesses such as alcohol abuse (see Chapter 6). The Nutrition Screen Initiative developed a plan for self-screening and professional nutritional screening for older adults. The client self-assessment screen is called the Checklist to DETERMINE Nutritional Health. The client is asked questions about the following nutritional risk factors:

- **D**isease, chronic or acute
- **E**ating habits
- **T**ooth loss
- **E**conomic hardship
- **R**educed social contact
- **M**ultiple medications or drugs
- **I**nvoluntary weight loss or gain
- **N**eeded assistance with self-care
- **E**ighty years of age or older

The purpose of this self-screening form is to encourage clients to examine their nutritional intake and to seek professional help if they appear to be at risk. If a client scores greater than 2 on this self-screen, additional nutritional screening is required.

Weight is a predictor of mortality in hospitalized older adults (Abassi, 1998). A body mass index (BMI) of less than 23 or more than 30 is associated with increased mortality in older adults (Abbasi, 1998). Height may be difficult to obtain in some older clients because of kyphosis, inability to stand, or inability to maintain balance. When the client cannot stand, estimate height by measuring the length from the bottom of the foot to the anterior knee with the ankle and knee at a 90-degree angle (see Table 6-8).

Compare current weight to usual body weight to determine whether the client has had a greater than 5% weight loss in the past 6 months.

Comprehensive Geriatric Assessment

It is apparent that the health assessment of the geriatric client may be complex and time-consuming. Older clients with multiple complex problems often benefit from a comprehensive geriatric assessment (CGA). Such an assessment by team members from a variety of disciplines may improve the accuracy of assessment, discharge planning and placement, and functional status.

In 1987 the National Institutes of Health convened a consensus conference on geriatric assessment. The convening group defined CGA as a multidisciplinary evaluation in which the multiple problems of older persons are uncovered, described, and explained, if possible, and in which the resources and strengths of the person are catalogued, the need for services is assessed, and a coordinated care plan is developed to focus interventions for the person's problems (*Geriatric Assessment Methods*, 1988). The various domains covered by CGA are physical, mental, social, economic, functional, and environmental status. More recently, several models of comprehensive geriatric assessment have emerged. A multidomain assessment requires considerable time since a core team consisting of at least a physician, nurse, and social worker all evaluate the client. Many geriatric assessment teams also include physical and occupational therapists, a pharmacist, and a nutritionist. Often, the members of the various disciplines use standardized screening questionnaires, such as those mentioned previously, as they perform their assessment of the client. Because a comprehensive geriatric assessment is time-consuming and costly, generally only frail, older clients with changing multiple physical and functional problems are targeted for this type of evaluation (Williams, 1998).

Preparation for Examination: Client and Environment

Examiner-Client Interaction

Older adults may be accompanied by a spouse, adult child, or other relative or friend. Note how the client walks into the examination room. Observe whether the client requires the assistance of another person or an ambulation assistance device, such as a cane or walker. An inability to get to the examination room independently may indicate some type of sensory, functional, or mental status impairment. If relatives accompany independent and competent older adults into the examination room, determine the client's wishes regarding the presence of these individuals in the examination room. If the client requests that a relative or friend remain in the room, pay careful attention to who is answering questions and spontaneously providing information. A relative answering questions for the client may indicate that the client has some type of cognitive impairment and cannot answer. Politely but firmly inform the relative or friend that the client should be allowed to answer the questions first and that any additional information the relative or friend can supply will be welcomed after the client speaks.

Ask whether the client needs help in getting undressed for the examination or in getting dressed after the examination. Clients may need extra time and assistance in getting on and off the examining table. For clients who cannot easily get up on the examination table, a part or all of the examination may be performed with the client in the chair. Some clients may tire quickly during the examination. If this occurs, adjust the sequence of the examination to include the most relevant assessments based on the presenting problem first.

Examples of age-related questions to include in the health history for an elderly client are listed in Box 27-7. During the interview, determine whether the client appears to have problems with memory, ambulation, and/or dressing. If the client has limitations in any of these areas, determine what assistance you will need to provide the client in undressing for the examination, getting on and off the examining table, and redressing. The procedure for performing the physical examination on the older adult is similar to that outlined in previous chapters for each body system. As with

BOX 27-7

QUESTIONS TO DETERMINE POTENTIAL AGE-RELATED IMPAIRMENTS

1. Do you ever have a problem with urine leaking?
2. Have you fallen in the past 6 months?
3. Do you often feel sad, blue, down in the dumps, or depressed?
4. Do you often travel places away from home alone?
5. Do you have enough money to purchase your medications?
6. Do you sometimes skip your medications?
7. Do you skip meals often?

all clients, make sure the examination room is quiet and the temperature is comfortable.

Auditory Impairment

The loss of auditory acuity is the most common sensory loss among aging individuals and may impede history taking. Face the client directly, since many people with a hearing impairment rely to some extent on lip-reading. Use simple, direct questions and avoid shouting. Shouting obscures the consonant sounds, sounds that are lost with hearing impairment in late life. Lowering the voice and speaking slightly louder may help. Amplification devices may assist in communication and are discussed later in this chapter.

Technique for Examination and Expected Findings

General Inspection

The physical changes that highlight the aging process are graying of the hair and wrinkling of the skin. Because of loss of connective tissue, body contours may appear sharper and hollows deeper, such as the orbits of the eyes and the axilla.

Skin

Age Changes. Heredity, changes in the connective and epithelial tissues, endocrine alterations, and vascular changes all influence aging changes of the skin. Excessive exposure to sun accelerates these changes. The skin epidermis decreases in thickness. The melanocytes lose some of their ability to protect the skin from ultraviolet light. With chronic sun exposure, some melanocytes may be destroyed, resulting in hypopigmentation, or white spots, on the skin. Sun exposure can also stimulate melanocytes to produce hyperpigmented areas called lentigines. **Lentigines** are flat, tan to brown macules and are usually located on sun-exposed surfaces. They may be as large as 1 or 2 cm.

The dermis decreases in thickness, and as a result, the skin takes on a thin, translucent appearance. Sun exposure changes the structure of the dermal layer and contributes to sagging and wrinkling of the skin. With thinning of the dermis, less support exists for capillary walls, and blood vessel walls dilate. Visible dilated vessels are called **telangiectasias**, or spider angiomas (see Figure 10-15, *C* and *E*). Skin capillaries are also more fragile. A bump to the skin can cause blood to leak through the capillaries into the dermis, resulting in bruising known as **senile purpura**. Ask the client how bruising occurred, since bruising may indicate a recent fall. A client unaware of bruising may have decreased sensory perception.

Subcutaneous fat decreases with age. Whereas sebaceous glands may increase in size, their ability to function decreases. This decrease in function, together with water loss from the skin, contributes to dry skin or xerosis, a common complaint in older clients.

Lesions. Various skin lesions are common with increasing age. **Seborrheic keratoses** are benign, raised, warty-type lesions usually located on the face, shoulders, and trunk. The borders are irregular, and the surface scaly. These lesions have a "pasted-on," greasy appearance. Early lesions may be yellowish to tan, with the color changing to dark brown or black over time. Although benign, some people request their removal for cosmetic purposes (see Figure 10-25).

Skin tags are soft, flesh-colored lesions and are attached to the skin by a stalk. They vary in size from a pinhead to a pea and are most commonly found on the vertical and lateral surfaces of the neck and the axillary area. Like seborrheic keratoses, these lesions have little clinical importance but may be removed if they are irritated by clothing or for cosmetic reasons.

Cherry angiomas are another type of benign skin lesion that occur with increased frequency in older adults. These lesions are caused by proliferation and dilation of the superficial capillaries of the skin. They are bright red, soft, and dome shaped with a diameter of 1 mm or greater (see Figure 10-15, *A*).

Actinic keratoses are pink to slightly red, dry lesions with indistinct borders. Rough adherent scales cover the lesions. These lesions occur over sun-exposed areas, such as the face, ears, and dorsal surfaces of the hands and arms. A small percentage of these actinic keratoses will transform into squamous cell skin cancers. Therefore these lesions are generally removed (see Figure 10-20).

Basal cell skin cancer is the most common of all cancers, and its occurrence increases with age. Look for lesions that are nodular with rolled borders, translucent, and pearly in appearance. Telangiectasias are common inside the nodule. These lesions, which may be ulcerating, are most often located on sun-exposed body surfaces (Figure 27-3). Basal cell skin cancer is locally invasive and destructive but does not metastasize. Several techniques are available to remove these lesions, depending on the patient and the size and location of the cancer.

Pressure sores, or decubitus ulcers, tend to occur more often in elderly persons who are bed-bound, wheelchair-bound, or sit in one place for long periods. Box 27-8 presents the Braden Scale for predicting pressure sore risk.

Hair and Nails. Hair growth and nail growth change with age. Scalp, axillary, and pubic hair thins and decreases. Eyebrow, nostril, and ear hair becomes coarser, and some older women develop an increase in facial hair. A loss of hair pigment contributes to graying of hair. Nail growth slows, and nails may yellow and lack luster. Some nails may become thin and split, whereas others, especially the toenails, may thicken.

Head and Neck

Eyes. The cells responsible for lubricating the conjunctiva decrease, and "dry eye syndrome," characterized by a scratchy sensation with chronic irritation, may develop. Observe for an arcus senilis, the accumulation of calcium and cholesterol salts at the limbus of the eye (see Figure 12-32). This appears as a grayish to gray-white arc or halo and has no association with elevated serum cholesterol or other systemic illness. The cornea tends to become hazy. Pupils decrease in size, react more slowly to light, and dilate more slowly in the dark. As a result, the older adult requires more time to adapt to a dark room. Restriction of upward movement of the pupil occurs with age, and the client may have to tip the head back farther to look up.

Lids. Loss of fat from the orbit of the eye causes a sunken appearance. A decrease in strength of the muscles allowing the lids to shut tightly may result in an ectropion (see Figure 12-27). This is the turning out of the lower lid, exposing the punctum of the lower lid. If this occurs, tears do not drain properly and the client may complain of excess tearing. The opposite condition, entropion, is a turning inward of the lower lid caused by muscle spasm. The eyelashes of the lower lid contact the conjunctiva and cornea. If chronic irritation occurs, surgical correction may be necessary. The muscles that hold the upper lid open may weaken, causing lid droop or ptosis. The lid droop may hamper vision and can be corrected with surgery. Tear production may decrease and contribute to complaints of dry eyes.

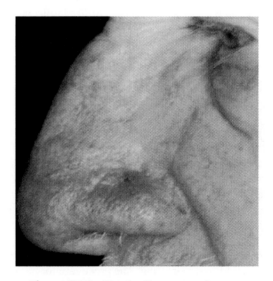

Figure 27-3 Basal cell cancer on the nose.

Vision. The ability to accommodate decreases progressively with age. This condition is called presbyopia and increases with frequency after age 40. Assess for presbyopia by checking near vision with a hand-held reading card or newspaper. The ophthalmoscopic examination may be more difficult because of the smaller pupil size. Look for mildly narrowed vessels, granular pigment in the macula, and a loss of bright macular and foveal reflexes. The fundus itself lacks luster and may appear more yellow.

Cataract, glaucoma, and **age-related macular degeneration (AMD)** are eye problems that occur more commonly in the older client. A cataract is an opacity in the lens that gradually impairs vision (see Figure 12-33). A client who complains about glare from headlights when driving a car at night may have a cataract. The most common type of glaucoma in the older adult is open-angle glaucoma. Measuring intraocular pressures on a regular basis helps to detect glaucoma early. AMD, a loss of central vision, is one of the leading causes of blindness in the elderly. Laser therapy is one method of treatment for AMD. Clients with AMD may also be referred to low-vision specialists for assessment of magnification aids.

Ears

Outer Ear. Aging changes begin to appear in the outer ear between ages 30 and 50. The skin becomes dry and less resilient, and connective tissue is lost. Pruritus may occur in the external auditory canal, leading to scratching. Remind clients not to use cotton-tip applicators to relieve itching. Hair growth may be visible along the periphery of the helix, antihelix, and tragus of the pinna. The hairs are coarse and wirelike. The pinna increases in both length and width, and the earlobes are elongated. There is a decrease in cerumen production, and this reduction correlates with an increased dryness in cerumen. This may contribute to the increased tendency toward cerumen impactions.

Middle Ear. Degenerative changes in the joints of the bones of the middle ear occur with increasing age. These changes, however, do not appear to have an appreciable effect on sound transmission.

Inner Ear. The specialized cells of the auditory pathways have a limited ability to regenerate. Approximately 24% of individuals between ages 65 and 74 and 39% of those older than 75 have hearing loss. A variety of genetic and environmental factors contribute to this age-related hearing loss, called **presbycusis**. Two common types of presbycusis are sensory and neural presbycusis. Sensory presbycusis is associated with degeneration of the organ of Corti and involves the inability to hear high-frequency sounds. Neural presbycusis is primarily a loss of speech discrimination. Neural presbycusis is associated with a decrease in the cochlear neurons while the organ of Corti remains functional.

A mild loss of speech frequency may pose little problem for the older person when listening to normal, clearly spoken conversation in a quiet room. In rooms with environmental noise, such as churches, restaurants, or movie theaters, a mild hearing loss may present greater hearing problems.

If you suspect hearing loss, check for and remove any cerumen impactions. If hearing problems persist, refer the client to an audiologist. Several aids are available for amplification of sound. The purpose of a hearing aid is to increase the intensity of the sound with as little distortion as possible. Several types of hearing aids are available: behind-the ear, eyeglass with aid, in-the-ear, in-the-canal, and body aids (Figure 27-4). The older adult may fear the social stigma associated with hearing aids. Successful adjustment to an aid depends largely on the client's motivation in wanting to use the aid.

Situation-specific assistive listening devices (ALDs) amplify speech for the hearing-impaired (Figure 27-5). An ALD is the size of a small transistor radio. A microphone is

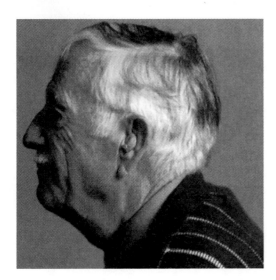

Figure 27-4 In-the-ear hearing aid.

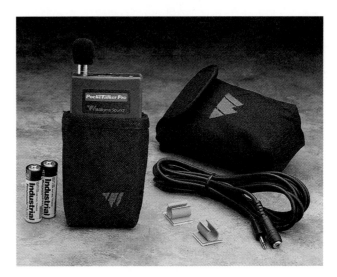

Figure 27-5 Assistive listening device. (Courtesy Williams Sound Corporation, Eden Prairie, Minn.)

BOX 27-8
BRADEN SCALE FOR PREDICTING PRESSURE SORE RISK

Patient's Name _____

Evaluator's Name _____

Date of Assessment _____

	1	2	3	4			
SENSORY PERCEPTION Ability to respond meaningfully to pressure-related discomfort	**1. Completely Limited** Unresponsive (does not moan, flinch, or grasp) to painful stimuli, due to diminished level of consciousness or sedation. *or* Limited ability to feel pain over most of body.	**2. Very Limited** Responds only to painful stimuli. Cannot communicate discomfort except by moaning or restlessness. *or* Has a sensory impairment which limits the ability to feel pain or discomfort over ½ of body.	**3. Slightly Limited** Responds to verbal commands, but cannot always communicate discomfort or the need to be turned. *or* Has some sensory impairment which limits ability to feel pain or discomfort in 1 or 2 extremities.	**4. No Impairment** Responds to verbal commands. Has no sensory deficit which would limit ability to feel or voice pain or discomfort.			
MOISTURE Degree to which skin is exposed to moisture	**1. Constantly Moist** Skin is kept moist almost constantly by perspiration, urine, etc. Dampness is detected every time patient is moved or turned.	**2. Very Moist** Skin is often, but not always moist. Linen must be changed at least once a shift.	**3. Occasionally Moist** Skin is occasionally moist, requiring an extra linen change approximately once a day.	**4. Rarely Moist** Skin is usually dry, linen only requires changing at routine intervals.			
ACTIVITY Degree of physical activity	**1. Bedfast** Confined to bed.	**2. Chairfast** Ability to walk severely limited or nonexistent. Cannot bear own weight and/or must be assisted into chair or wheelchair.	**3. Walks Occasionally** Walks occasionally during day, but for very short distances, with or without assistance. Spends majority of each shift in bed or chair	**4. Walks Frequently** Walks outside room at least twice a day and inside room at least once every two hours during waking hours.			
MOBILITY Ability to change and control body position	**1. Completely Immobile** Does not make even slight changes in body or extremity position without assistance.	**2. Very Limited** Makes occasional slight changes in body or extremity position but unable to make frequent or significant changes independently.	**3. Slightly Limited** Makes frequent though slight changes in body or extremity position independently.	**4. No Limitation** Makes major and frequent changes in position without assistance.			

	1. Very Poor	2. Probably Inadequate	3. Adequate	4. Excellent
NUTRITION *Usual* food intake pattern	Never eats a complete meal. Rarely eats more than ⅓ of any food offered. Eats 2 servings or less of protein (meat or dairy products) per day. Takes fluids poorly. Does not take a liquid dietary supplement. *or* Is NPO and/or maintained on clear liquids or IVs for more than 5 days.	Rarely eats a complete meal and generally eats only about ½ of any food offered. Protein intake includes only 3 servings of meat or dairy products per day. Occasionally will take a dietary supplement. *or* Receives less than optimum amount of liquid diet or tube feeding.	Eats over half of most meals. Eats a total of 4 servings of protein (meat, dairy products) per day. Occasionally will refuse a meal, but will usually take a supplement when offered. *or* Is on a tube feeding or TPN regimen which probably meets most of nutritional needs.	Eats most of every meal. Never refuses a meal. Usually eats a total of 4 or more servings of meat and dairy products. Occasionally eats between meals. Does not require supplementation.
FRICTION AND **SHEAR**	**1. Problem** Requires moderate to maximum assistance in moving. Complete lifting without sliding against sheets is impossible. Frequently slides down in bed or chair, requiring frequent repositioning with maximum assistance. Spasticity, contractures or agitation leads to almost constant friction.	**2. Potential Problem** Moves feebly or requires minimum assistance. During a move skin probably slides to some extent against sheets, chair, restraints, or other devices. Maintains relatively good position in chair or bed most of the time but occasionally slides down.	**3. No Apparent Problem** Moves in bed and in chair independently and has sufficient muscle strength to lift up completely during move. Maintains good position in bed or chair.	

© Copyright Barbara Braden and Nancy Bergstrom, 1988.
Total Score

placed near the sound source while the listener places earphones in the ears. Sound travels to the earphones via infrared, audio loop, FM radio, or direct audio input. The sound is enhanced, and extraneous noise is reduced. Many theaters, churches, and lecture halls have such devices. These devices may also be used in examination rooms or hospital rooms.

Nose.   Olfactory function decreases with age, and many older adults have a decreased ability to correctly identify odors. Although smell is not routinely assessed in the physical examination, question the client about altered smell since failure to detect the smell of smoke or gas can be life-threatening. In addition, a decreased sense of smell may contribute to decreased food intake.

Mouth.   The number of taste buds does not decline with aging. There is no age-related deterioration in the ability of healthy older adults to taste sweet, sour, salty, and bitter at usual concentrations. Older adults are retaining more of their teeth longer. When tooth loss occurs, it is due to two major causes: dental caries and periodontal disease. Periodontal disease is the major cause of tooth loss in the older adult. Dental caries in older adults tends to develop at the root or bottom of the tooth along the gum where gingival recession or periodontal disease causes exposure of the root surface.

Healthy adults do not have diminished saliva production. Decreased salivary function does, however, occur commonly as a side effect of medications with anticholinergic effects. Box 27-9 lists medications that commonly cause dry mouth, or **xerostomia**. The decreased salivary function causes the xerostomia. Xerostomia is also caused by irradiation of the salivary glands or salivary tumors. Observe for dry oral mucous membranes and dry tongue. Saliva has many functions, including antibacterial and antifungal activity, oral lubrication, buffering of bacteria-produced acids, mechanical cleansing, remineralization of teeth, and as an aid in mastication. Decreased saliva may contribute to caries formation. Instruct clients with xerostomia to brush their teeth after every meal and to avoid moistening their mouth with candy unless it is sugar-free. A variety of salivary lubricants are available to moisten the mouth in clients who have xerostomia.

The majority of oral cancers develop after age 40. Individuals with a history of tobacco and/or alcohol abuse are particularly at risk for developing an oral cancer. Carefully inspect the oral mucosa for red or white lesions. Remove any dentures during the examination, since poorly fitting dentures can cause trauma to the oral mucosa. In addition, oral candidiasis may be present on areas of the mucosa where the dentures rest.

Breasts

With increasing age the amount of fat in the breast increases as the glandular tissue atrophies. Breast consistency and shape change, and breasts are often described as pendulous (see Figure 14-5, *F*). The incidence of breast cancer in the United States increases with age; therefore the detection of a lump is significant and requires evaluation. Most recommendations suggest a mammogram every 2 years for women 40 to 49 years old, annually for women between ages 50 and 59, and every 2 years after age 60.

Respiratory System

Calcification occurs in the costochondral joints of the ribs, and the chest wall becomes less compliant. Skeletal changes in the spine may cause an increase in the anteroposterior diameter of the chest. If this occurs, breath sounds may be more difficult to hear during auscultation.

Cardiovascular System

Age-Related Changes.   Diseases of the cardiovascular system are common in the elderly and are the leading cause of death in this age group. Maximal heart rate decreases with age. Despite a decrease in heart rate, healthy older adults can maintain a normal cardiac output during exercise by increasing their stroke volume. Although healthy older adults maintain normal cardiac output, many older clients have cardiac disorders and decreased cardiac output and decreased activity tolerance.

Blood Pressure.   Isolated systolic hypertension and orthostatic hypotension are two problems commonly associated with changes in blood pressure in older adults.

Systolic blood pressure increases with age because of increased stiffness of the aorta and its branches. **Isolated systolic hypertension** occurs when the systolic blood pressure is greater than 160 mm Hg in the presence of a normal diastolic pressure. Isolated systolic hypertension occurs more frequently in older adults and is associated with an increased risk for strokes and fatal cardiovascular events. Research has shown that treating isolated systolic hypertension in older adults reduces the likelihood of strokes.

Postural, or orthostatic, hypotension occurs when the systolic blood pressure drops 20 mm Hg or more when the client goes from a lying or sitting position to a standing position. Baroreceptor sensitivity remains intact in healthy older adults and is not a likely cause of postural hypotension. One common cause of postural hypotension is medications, particularly antihypertensive medications, diuretics, and medications with anticholinergic effects.

In older clients, measure blood pressure in both arms with the client lying and standing, or sitting and standing.

BOX 27-9

CLASSES OF MEDICATIONS KNOWN TO CAUSE XEROSTOMIA

Anticholinergics	Antipsychotics
Antidepressants	Antispasmodics
Antihistamines	Decongestants
Antihypertensives	Diuretics
Antiparkinsonians	

Have the client lying or sitting at rest for at least 15 minutes before taking the initial blood pressure reading. Then have the client stand, and take the blood pressure immediately. If you record a drop in the standing blood pressure, retake the blood pressure again in 1 minute. A drop in blood pressure on rising places the older client at risk for light-headedness and falls. If these symptoms occur, refer the client to a physician for further evaluation. In addition, instruct the client to sit on the edge of the bed or chair for a couple of minutes before standing and have a firm object such as a heavy chair close by to use for support if needed.

Heart. Precordial palpation may be difficult in those elderly who have an increased anterorposterior diameter. Kyphosis, which often occurs in the older client, may cause a downward dislocation of the cardiac apex (see Figure 18-61, *B*).

With age, there is an increase in fibrosis and calcification of the aortic valve cusps, a condition called aortic sclerosis. The thickening of these valves, together with dilation of the aorta, may cause a systolic murmur. Aortic sclerosis is of little clinical significance unless the sclerosed valve progresses to aortic stenosis. The aortic sclerosis murmur is best heard at the right base. It is low in intensity and short in duration, and it peaks early in systole. The differential diagnosis of aortic stenosis versus aortic sclerosis is difficult and best made by an echocardiogram. A fourth heart sound (S_4) is common with increased age and is often heard along with an aortic sclerotic murmur. An S_4 in the older client is most likely a result of decreased ventricular compliance.

Abdomen

In some older clients the general loss of fibroconnective tissue and muscle wasting may make the abdominal wall slacker, thinner, and easier to palpate. In other clients, increased fat deposits around the abdomen may make palpation more difficult.

Reproductive System

Female Client. Cells of the reproductive tract and the breasts are estrogen dependent for growth and function. The decline of estrogen production starting at menopause is responsible for many changes in the tissues of older female clients (see Table 21-1).

The ovaries, uterus, and cervix decrease in size. The ovaries may not be palpable. The vagina narrows and shortens. The vaginal epithelium atrophies; the surface is thin, pale, fragile, and easily traumatized; and intercourse may be painful. The frequency of intercourse in older women depends on the availability of a partner, physical health, previous sexual activity, and desire. Table 27-3 lists changes in the phases of intercourse in the older woman. Vaginal estrogen creams often provide relief for painful symptoms associated with atrophic vaginitis. Observe for vaginal erosions, ulcerations, and adhesions.

Male Client. Testosterone declines in older males. This decline occurs later than the decline in estrogen in the female. Testes decrease in size and are less firm on palpation.

Sperm production either remains the same or decreases slightly, and sperm motility decreases. The prostate gland is enlarged, and secretion is impaired. The seminal fluid is reduced in amount and viscosity.

These changes do not necessarily mean a decrease in libido or a loss in the sense of satisfaction from intercourse. Most men older than 60 reported having intercourse one or two times a week. Table 27-4 lists changes in the phases of intercourse in the older man (see also Table 20-1).

Musculoskeletal System

With increasing age, thinning of the intervertebral discs and shortening or collapse of the intervertebral bodies result in loss of height. Changes in the spine also contribute to the development of kyphosis and an increase in anteroposterior diameter.

TABLE 27-3	Changes in the Four Phases of Intercourse in the Aging Female Client	
Phase	**Alteration**	
Excitement	Delay in production of vaginal secretion and lubrication	
Plateau	Reduction in vaginal length and width expansion	
	Decreased uterine elevation	
	Labia majora flaccid and do not elevate and flatten against perineum	
	Labia minora do not undergo sex color change from pink to burgundy or become congested	
	Clitoral size decreases after 60 years of age	
Orgasm	Shorter than in younger persons	
Resolution	Occurs more rapidly	

TABLE 27-4	Changes Observed in the Four Phases of Intercourse in the Aging Male Client	
Phase	**Alteration**	
Excitement	Slower increment in excitement	
	Sex flush less in duration and intensity	
	Diminished involuntary spasms	
	Increased time to obtain erection	
	Lessened testicular elevation and scrotal sac vasocongestion in erection	
Plateau	Longer duration	
	Increase in penile diameter due to less preejaculatory fluid emission	
Orgasm	Shorter duration	
	Fewer contractions in expulsion of semen bolus	
Resolution	Lasts 12 to 24 hours	
	Loss of erection may take only a few seconds	

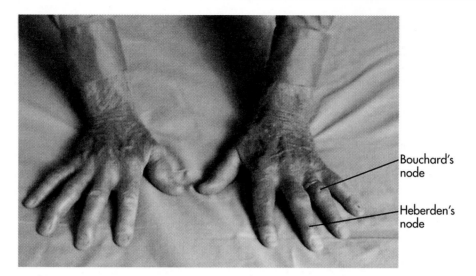

Bouchard's node

Heberden's node

Figure 27-6 Heberden's and Bouchard's nodes.

Muscle mass and strength decrease with age. You can easily see atrophy of muscle by observing the back of the hands where grooves are present between the bones.

Osteoarthritis is a common age-related condition involving joints throughout the body, particularly the spine, knees, hips, and fingers. Most clients older than 60 will have osteoarthritic changes in the spine. Accumulated injuries to the cartilage over time cause slow-but-progressive deterioration of the joint. With loss of cartilage, bony overgrowths protrude from the bone into the joint capsule. These overgrowths can cause angular deformities, pain, and limited mobility. In the spine, these overgrowths are called osteophytes. Bony enlargement of the dorsolateral and dorsomedial aspects of the distal and proximal joints of the fingers are called **Heberden's nodes** and Bouchard's nodes, respectively (Figure 27-6; see also Figure 18-68).

Nervous System

The assessment of mental status and cranial nerves has been discussed previously. Motor strength may decrease slightly with age. Investigate further any asymmetry of strength. Vibratory sensation decreases with age, especially in the feet and ankles. The posture may become stooped. Changes in gait, including a decreased stride length, anteroflexion of the upper torso, flexion of the arms and knees, and a diminished arm swing, may contribute to postural unsteadiness. Deep tendon reflexes remain intact in healthy elderly people, although they may be more difficult to elicit. In many older clients, ankle jerks may be diminished or absent.

SUMMARY

Demographic trends indicate a growing proportion of the population that will be older than 65 years. The examiner will need to identify normal age-related changes and those changes related to disease and adverse environmental and lifestyle factors to support the client in functioning at an optimal level of health.

Sample Documentation and Diagnoses

FOCUSED HEALTH HISTORY (SUBJECTIVE DATA)

Mrs. P, an 83-year-old female who lives alone, complains of dizziness when getting out of bed in the morning and occasionally later during the day when going from a sitting to a standing position. Describes the sensation as "the room spinning around." Yesterday morning she lost her balance getting out of bed and fell. Reports no injuries. Denies unsteadiness when she walks. One week ago her doctor prescribed a diuretic for high blood pressure. She has been taking the tablet once daily in the morning as prescribed.

FOCUSED PHYSICAL EXAMINATION (OBJECTIVE DATA)

Vital signs: BP—lying: 160/70 right arm, 156/72 left arm; immediate standing: 130/64 right arm, 132/62 left arm; 1-minute standing: 140/80 right arm; 146/78 left arm. Temperature 37.1° C (98.8° F) (oral).
General appearance: Well-groomed, frail-looking woman, appropriately dressed and able to provide history without hesitation.
Lungs: Breath sounds vesicular without crackles or wheezes.
Heart: Rate and rhythm regular without murmurs or extra sounds.
Extremities: Pulses 2 + /4 in all extremities. Muscle strength 3/5 bilaterally. Skin thin, intact, no edema or lesions present.
Neuro: Gait slow and slightly wide based. Rising from a chair after sitting 15 minutes caused light-headedness and slight swaying on rising.

DIAGNOSES

HEALTH PROBLEM

Orthostatic hypotension

NURSING DIAGNOSIS

Risk for Injury Related to Lightheadedness Secondary to Orthostatic Hypotension
Defining Characteristics
• Internal regulatory function—integrative dysfunction
• External—pharmaceutical agent (diuretic)

? Critical Thinking Questions

1. Mr. Smith is an 80-year-old retired English professor from whom you are obtaining a health history. What questions do you need to ask to identify conditions that more commonly occur in older adults?
2. As you obtain the health history, you notice that Mr. Smith is unable to answer certain questions about his daily functioning. How will you modify your assessment?
3. You proceed to the physical examination. What physical findings are normal changes with aging?

Answers are available on the MERLIN website (www.harcourthealth.com/MERLIN/Barkauskas/). And be sure to check the website regularly for additional learning activities!

Remember to check out the Online Study Guide!
www.harcourthealth.com/MERLIN/Barkauskas/

Clients With Functional Limitations

Learning Objectives

On successful study of this chapter and completion of related learning experiences, the learner will be able to:
- Describe the rationale for including functional assessment data in a health assessment.
- Define the terms, variables, and parameters used for functional assessment.

- Describe the content of functional assessment tools.
- Discuss the application of functional assessment tools.
- Adapt the physical examination to clients with functional disabilities.

Outline

Purpose of Examination

The various components of the physical examination and health history provide an indication of the health of a client's body systems and data about the relationship of the client with the environment. For most clients, the data also implicitly provide information about self-care and overall functional abilities. For special populations, however, including the elderly and clients with functional limitations, the usual components of the health assessment may be insufficient in providing adequate information regarding the client's capabilities and activities. This chapter presents and discusses several approaches to measuring functional status, guidelines to incorporate a functional assessment into the routine health assessment, and adaptation of the physical assessment to a disabled client.

Persons with disabilities are a major, new focus in the most recent Healthy People objectives (*U. S. Department of Health and Human Services, 2000*). The following national goals and objectives for persons with disabilities have been established:

• Promote the health of people with disabilities, prevent secondary conditions, and eliminate disparities between people with and without disabilities in the U.S. population.

• Include in the core of all relevant *Healthy People 2010* surveillance instruments a standardized set of questions that identify "people with disabilities."

• Reduce the proportion of children and adolescents with disabilities who are reported to be sad, unhappy, or depressed. The 2010 target is 17% from a 1998 baseline of 31%.

• Reduce the proportion of adults with disabilities who report feelings such as sadness, unhappiness, or depression that prevent them from being active. The 2010 target is 7% from a 1998 baseline of 28%.

• Increase the proportion of adults with disabilities who participate in social activities. The 2010 target is 100% from a 1998 baseline of 95.4%.

• Increase the proportion of adults with disabilities reporting sufficient emotional support. The 2010 target is 79% from a 1998 baseline of 70%.

• Increase the proportion of adults with disabilities reporting satisfaction with life. The target is 96% from a 1998 baseline of 87%.

• Reduce the number of people with disabilities in congregate care facilities, consistent with permanency planning principles, from approximately 93,000 persons at 1998 baseline to 47,000.

• Eliminate disparities in employment rates between working-age adults with and without disabilities. The target is 82% from a 1998 baseline of 52%.

• Increase the proportion of children and youth with disabilities who spend at least 80% of their time in regular education programs. The target is 60% from a 1998 baseline of 45%.

KEY TERMS AND DEFINITIONS

Several conceptual definitions are useful for understanding the discussion in this chapter and other literature in the area of functional assessment. The World Health Organization (WHO) (1980) developed the following definitions to standardize terminology and facilitate communication in this area.

An impairment is any loss or abnormality of psychological, physiological, or anatomical structure or function. An impairment is independent of its etiology and does not necessarily mean that a disease is still present. An example of an impairment is loss of a limb.

A disability is any restriction or lack of ability to perform an activity in the manner or within the range considered normal for a person of the same age and similar circumstances. A disability may be temporary or permanent and can occur in any component of human functioning. A disability is the functional consequence of an impairment. Different impairments may result in similar disabilities, and the same impairments do not necessarily result in similar disabilities. Not all impairments result in disability. An example of a disability is inability to climb stairs.

A handicap is a disadvantage for a given individual, resulting from impairment or a disability that limits or prevents the fulfillment of a role that is normal for that individual. A handicap is characterized by a difference between what an individual appears to be able to do and the expectations of the particular group of which he or she is a member. The state of being handicapped is strongly influenced by existing societal values. An example of a handicap is joblessness.

Functional status refers to the normal or characteristic performance of the individual. Functional status can be conceptualized into the following four categories:

1. Physical function: sensory-motor performance
2. Mental function: intellectual, cognitive, or reasoning capabilities of the individual
3. Emotional function: affect and effectiveness in coping psychologically with life stresses
4. Social function: performance of social roles or obligations

The following additional definitions are derived from legislative practice (NH Rev Stat Ann 464-A:2[VII], [XI] [1983]; cited in Nolan, 1984, p. 213).

Incapacity means a legal, not a medical, disability and shall be measured by functional limitations. It shall be construed to mean or refer to any person who has suffered, is suffering, or is likely to suffer substantial harm due to an inability to provide for his or her personal needs for food, clothing, shelter, health care, safety, or an inability to manage his or her property or financial affairs.

Functional limitations connote behavior or conditions in an individual that impair his or her ability to participate in and perform minimal activities of daily living that secure and maintain proper food, clothing, shelter, health care, or safety for himself or herself.

The following models by Granger, Seltzer, and Fishbein (1987), based on the work of Nagi (1975) and Wood (1975), provide insight into the relationships among some of the concepts related to functional limitations.

Nagi Model

Pathologic condition →	*Impairment* →	*Functional limitations* →	*Disability*
Interruption or interference with normal and processes efforts of the organism to regain a normal state	Anatomical, physiological, mental, or emotional abnormalities or loss	Limitation in performance at the level of the whole organism or person	Limitation in performance or socially defined roles and tasks within sociocultural and physical environments

Wood Model

Disease or disorder (Intrinsic)	→ Impairment (Exteriorized)	→ Disability (Objectified)	→ Handicap (Socialized)
The intrinsic pathology or anatomical disorder	Loss or abnormality of psychological, physiological structure or function at organ level	Restriction or lack of ability to perform an activity in a normal manner	Disadvantage due to impairment or disability that limits or prevents fulfillment of a normal role for that person

These models demonstrate several issues related to the culture of disabilities. Health care professionals often focus on factors on the left side of the models (i.e., the pathologies, diseases, and impairments). In contrast, persons with disabilities focus on the right side of the models (i.e., on the life decisions changes made in adaptation to the physical issues). Therefore, in addition to understanding the physical problems, the practitioner needs to assess the meaning of the functional limitation in the individual client's life.

TABLE 28-1	Recommendations for Communicating About Persons With Disabilities

Recommended Terminology	Terminology to Avoid
Persons who have disabilities	Disabled, crippled, handicapped persons The blind Epileptics
Person who uses a wheelchair, crutches, etc.	Confined to a wheelchair; has to use crutches, unable to walk without braces
Individual or person who has (name of problem)	Victim of Suffers from Afflicted with Burdened with Stricken Crippled Diseased Disabled Poor Unfortunate Tragic
Individual who has (describe what the person has accomplished)	Courageous Inspirational Heroic

Adapted from Curtis KA: Communicating with persons who have disabilities. Reprinted from Davis CM: *Patient practitioner interaction: an experiential manual for developing the art of health care,* ed. 3. Thorofare, NJ, 1998, SLACK, with permission from SLACK, Inc.

CULTURAL DIMENSION OF CARE TO PERSONS WITH DISABILITIES

Sometimes persons without major disabilities are unsure about how to address and label persons with disabilities. Too often persons with disabilities are described in ways that emphasize the disability and minimize the person or evoke pity. Table 28-1 contains recommendations for addressing persons with disabilities. The overall principle is to put the person, rather than the disability, first.

UNDERSTANDING THE CULTURAL CONTEXT OF DISABILITIES

Disabilities are perceived differently among cultures. In some cultures and during some phases of cultural development, some groups have perceived disabilities as shameful and have hidden a disabled family member. With the development of rehabilitation and occupational health services, the understanding of disabilities has increased across cultures. Assessing cultural beliefs and practices related to disability and rehabilitation is important in situations in which functional issues are involved.

INTEGRATING FUNCTIONAL ASSESSMENT INTO THE ROUTINE EXAMINATION

Functional Assessment Variables

Functional assessment can include a broad range of areas for examination. In practice, the examiner chooses assessment areas that are relevant to a particular client or client group. For example, basic and instrumental activities of daily living would be important for assessment of a residential geriatric population, whereas the examiner would choose other assessment parameters for a rehabilitation unit accepting transfers from intensive care units. The following is a list of general categories of functional assessment areas:

Basic Activities of Daily Living (ADLs)

Bathing
Dressing and undressing
Eating
Grooming and personal hygiene
Managing brace or prosthesis
Skin care
Toileting

Instrumental Activities of Daily Living (IADLs)

Cooking
Managing business affairs
Managing medications
Managing personal finances
Preparing balanced meals
Shopping
Using problem-solving skills
Capacity to work

Mobility

Ascending and descending stairs
Bed activities—turning, sitting, and shifting
Body movement
Capability of upper and lower extremities
Operating a wheelchair
Transferring—between bed and wheelchair, wheelchair and chair, or chair and toilet
Traveling
Walking on level surface
Ability to operate a motor vehicle

Medical Condition

Amount of medical care needed
Continence—bowels and bladder
Speech

Communication

Auditory comprehension
Language expression (gestural)
Language expression (verbal)
Reading
Writing (motor)
Written language expression

Senses

Hearing
Vision

Mental Capability

Ability to comprehend movies and books
Ability to manage travel instructions
Ability to play games and work on hobbies

Attention span
Awareness of current events
Communication
Judgment and reasoning
Memory
Memory of appointments and commemorations
Orientation
Reading
Understanding
Writing

Resources

Amount of assistance received from others
Significant others
Social interaction
Social support

Behavioral and Emotional Areas

Amount of supervision required
Cooperation
Depression
Presence of emotional or psychiatric disorders

General Assessment With Emphasis on Functional Status

You can perform the functional assessment at any time during the routine health assessment. If you are using a standardized tool, this assessment is probably most logical at the end of the history and before the examination. Findings may provide guidance for particular follow-up during the physical examination.

Cultural Considerations
Cultural Implications of Disabilities

CULTURAL GROUP	RESPONSE TO DISABILITIES
Appalachians	Handicapped persons readily accepted
	Disability is a natural and an inevitable part of the aging process
	Rehabilitation discouraged
Arab-Americans	Attitudes toward the disabled are generally negative and expectations with respect to education and rehabilitation are low
	Disabled often kept from public view
Chinese-Americans	Becoming more supportive of the disabled, although use of support services is rare
	Disabilities should be hidden
Egyptian-Americans	Disabilities are not hidden
	Public sympathy and acceptance for the disabled
	Families assume responsibility for the care of disabled members and do not expect public support services
	Actively seek health care assistance with disabilities
Filipino-Americans	Major concerns about hereditary diseases are associated with the selection of a marriage partner
	Care for disabled at home
French-Canadians	Physically disabled persons are protected from discrimination and abuse
	Large-scare adaptation of the environment to accommodate access for the disabled
Iranian-Americans	Up until 1980 disabled were hidden, and attitudes were negative; however, since that time, rehabilitation has been accepted
Vietnamese-Americans	Disabled persons are cared for by their families
	Some families are very secretive about disabled members

Data from Purnell LD, Paulanka BJ: *Transcultural health care: a culturally competent approach*, Philadelphia, 1998, FA Davis.

The functional assessment requires no equipment in addition to that used in a comprehensive examination; most of the approaches require only interview and observation. Be prepared, however, to verify responses to various questions as needed. For example, you may want to ask the client to demonstrate operation of a wheelchair or ability to climb stairs. The best location for functional assessment is often the client's own surroundings, where environmental adaptations enable a full range of independent activities (Figures 28-1 through 28-3). Table 28-2 outlines the major

TABLE 28-2   Functional Assessment Emphases in the History and Physical Examination

Areas of Assessment	Special Emphases	
History (see Chapter 3)		
Present illness	Determine how present illness interferes with client's ability to carry out self-care and work and to execute roles appropriate for age and social situation	
Past health history	Gain knowledge of abilities before incapacitating illness or situation to understand expectations and set rehabilitation goals	
Family health history	Note genetically transmitted disabling conditions	
Review of systems	Determine capabilities of the systems unaffected by the disability; these strengths will support rehabilitation	
	Complete a review of affected and likely-to-be-affected systems	
Social history	Describe in detail relationships and living arrangements and the adequacy of those relationships and living arrangements; for a hospitalized client after an unanticipated traumatic event, the accessibility of the living arrangements and the willingness of family and significant others to assist are important	
	Determine adequacy of income to support client and family	
	Obtain information about the social support available to the client, the issues created by the disability, and the coping strategies used within the family	
Employment history	Note the nature of the client's work and the client's ability to continue to manage that work or return to that work	
	Determine the meaning of work to the client; the client's perception of the current job; and, if applicable, the effect the loss of the job and work might mean	
Physical Examination		
Neurological evaluation (see Chapter 19)	Mental status	Atrophy
	Orientation to time, place, and person	Spontaneous muscle activity
	Memory	Mood
	Attention span	Insight
	Ability to perform calculations	Sensory status
	Abstract thinking	Reflexes
	Behavior	Vision
	Ability to follow commands	Hearing
	Judgment	Swallowing
	Motor system	Speech and language
Musculoskeletal, soft tissue, and joint evaluation (see Chapter 18)	Inspection—symmetry, postural attitudes, scars, edema, atrophy, masses, skin changes	
	Palpation—muscles, bones, joints for local and general spasm, masses, swelling, or tenderness	
	Measurement of active and passive range of motion with a goniometer	
	Joint stability	
	Muscle strength, tone, increase in spasticity or rigidity, hypotonia or flaccidity	
	Finger flexion	
	Gait and mobility—use of assistive devices, ability to transfer, demonstration of methods of mobility and transfer	
Cardiac status (see Chapter 16)	Complete assessment	
	Physical endurance or capacity	
Respiratory status (see Chapter 15)	Adequacy of ventilation	
	Ability to clear tracheobronchial secretions	
	Physical endurance or capacity	
	Psychological reaction to breathing difficulties	
Skin (see Chapter 10)	Condition of pressure areas—ischial, sacral, and trochanteric prominences	
Bladder function	If incontinence or retention, extensive urological evaluation	
	If intermittent self-catheterization or Foley used, review of technique	
Bowel function (see Chapter 17)	Review pattern and interventions used to achieve regular pattern	
Pain	Quality, location, temporal characteristics, provocative factors, alleviating factors	
	Incapacitation caused by pain	

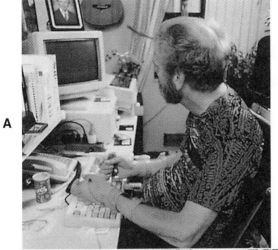

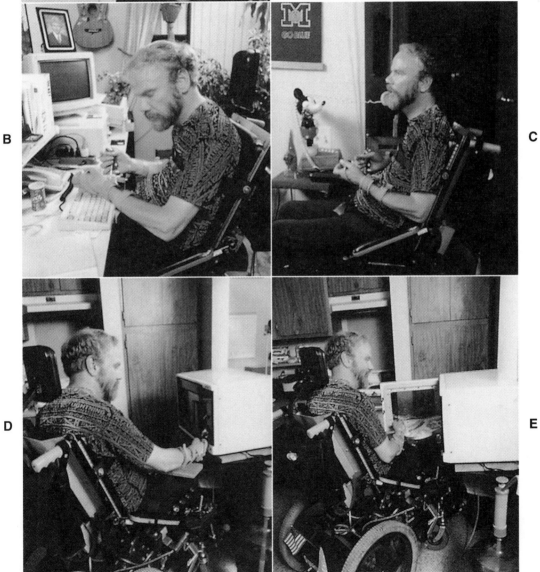

Figure 28-1 Assessing clients in their own surroundings allows for a full evaluation of the clients' capabilities. This man with quadriplegia is able to work and manage a number of activities of daily living quite independently in his home. **A** and **B,** Using a computer to work at home. **C,** Adapting a telephone to enable full use of this resource. **D** and **E,** Using a board to transfer frozen meals into and out of a microwave oven for independent food preparation.

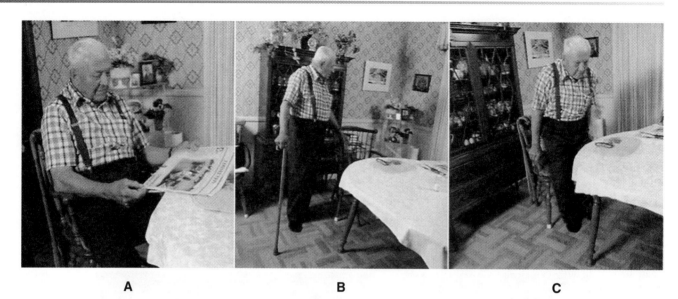

A **B** **C**

Figure 28-2 The elderly enjoy being able to sit in familiar surroundings and engage in activities that they have enjoyed all of their lives. **A,** This elderly man with a walking disability enjoys sitting at the kitchen table and reading the daily newspapers in several languages. **B,** He demonstrates his method of walking with the use of two canes. **C,** He demonstrates his method of lowering and lifting himself up from his chair.

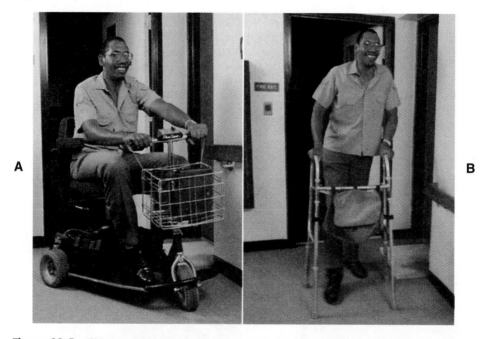

A **B**

Figure 28-3 This man with paraplegia works outside his home each day and engages in a number of other outside activities. **A,** He demonstrates use of a mobile chair designed for his needs. **B,** He demonstrates his mobility in getting around his apartment building with a walker.

components of the history and physical examination and identifies the areas in which an assessment, focused on functional status, would require special emphasis.

Adapting the Physical Assessment to the Client With Functional Limitations

The general components of physical assessment should be adapted to the client's disabilities. General principles include the following:

- Fully understand the nature of the disability before you begin the assessment.
- Enlist the client's recommendations for making the examination most comfortable.
- Determine what type of assistance is needed.
- Be gentle.
- Be patient.
- Use family members or other caregivers as needed, but involve the client as fully as the limits of physical ability, sensory abilities, and emotional capacities allow.

Many deaf clients read lips; speak slowly and enunciate each word clearly and in full view. Keep your face within visual contact of the client. Whenever possible, use a signer as an interpreter for clients who sign. When using a signer, be sure you look at the client when conversing rather than at the signer to establish and maintain rapport with the client.

In the case of a blind person, be creative about teaching with models or other three-dimensional aids, which can be felt by the client. Allow the client to manually examine the instruments to be used for the examination. Orient the client to the examination room. Be sure to keep explaining what you are doing and planning to do.

Adapting the Gynecological Examination

If the client is physically impaired from the waist down, the gynecological examination will require adaptation. Rather than using the standard gynecological position with the legs in stirrups, other positions can be used, including a side lying position or a diamond shaped position. For the side lying position, the client lies on her right side with the knees as close to her chest as possible. The speculum examination and the digital examination can be managed with the practitioner behind the client. For the diamond position, the woman lies on her back, with the knees bent, hips abducted, and the pads of the feet together. In either position, assistants may be needed to help the client assume and maintain the position.

FUNCTIONAL ASSESSMENT TOOLS

Choosing and Administering Functional Assessment Tools

In practice with a given client group, a practitioner may choose to use standardized tools for all clients or to integrate functional assessment questions and techniques into the routine health assessment as individual situations may indicate. Either method has advantages as well as disadvantages (Box 28-1). Because standardized tools are devised to yield comparable numerical scores, they are useful in situations in which information must be summarized for communication across systems and providers or when client, program, or other outcome evaluation is desired for care planning or discharge planning purposes. However, standardized tools often are not fully applicable across all groups and may include items not relevant for specific clients or client groups.

The examiner can integrate appropriate functional assessment parameters into the client's health assessment. Such integration can be effective if the examiner takes a highly individualized approach to the health history and physical examination and if sufficient time is available to add items. However, difficulty in obtaining reliable data in vulnerable populations may foster neglect in obtaining functional assessment information that could influence choice and scope of intervention.

Pinholt et al. (1987) compared the sensitivity and specificity of routine assessments and comprehensive functional assessment instruments. They found that physicians and nurses could identify severe impairments with routine approaches, but more prevalent and less prominent impairments were poorly recognized. The authors recommended the use of functional assessment instruments to detect moderate impairments, especially those remediable through early intervention.

If you choose to use standardized tools to measure functional assessment in a given population, first determine the variables of primary interest and then match those variables with items on extant tools. When examining potential screening and assessment tools, assess both the content of the items and the scope of measurement. For example, you may want to determine whether a certain functional disability exists or the extent to which the functions are enabled by human or mechanical assistance, or both.

Desirable characteristics of a functional assessment tool include the following:

1. *Applicability:* Appropriate for the client population.
2. *Continuity:* Applicable to the client population across phases of care.
3. *Ease in administration:* Can be administered by various types of health care professionals.
4. *Efficiency:* Balance between comprehensiveness and time required for administration.
5. *Reliability:* Demonstration of good test-retest and inter-rater reliability.
6. *Validity:* Findings consistent with other assessment data.
7. *Sensitivity:* Ability to differentiate differences among clients and changes in a given client during various stages of treatment.

BOX 28-1

ADVANTAGES AND DISADVANTAGES— TWO MAIN FUNCTIONAL ASSESSMENT APPROACHES

INTEGRATION INTO GENERAL ASSESSMENT
Advantages

Flexible
Individualized
Focus on variables of interest

Disadvantages

Can be incomplete
Lack of standardized terminology
Generally unsuitable for statistical analyses

STANDARDIZED TOOLS
Advantages

Objective
Explicit
Standardized

Disadvantages

May include irrelevant items
Issues of validity and reliability

Although numerous tools have been developed to measure functional status, this chapter presents only some of the extant tools based on their potential applicability to a health assessment framework. Criteria for selection included length of the tool; broad applicability to the elderly or the persons with disabilities; ability to complement the usual components of a history and physical examination; ease of administration; and published data about the tool's conceptual bases, validity, reliability, usability, and quality.

The functional assessment tools in this chapter generally are designed to be administered by health care professionals. Sometimes the care provider may request that the client or client caregiver administer the tools (e.g., after hospital discharge and between clinic visits). However, findings from various studies comparing client self-report with professional and caregiver assessments indicate that the type of rater may influence scores. McGinnis et al. (1986) compared the use of a modified Barthel Index by clients and health care professionals. Findings indicated that assessments were significantly different between groups, with providers rating clients higher in abilities than they rated themselves at a time immediately before discharge.

Rubenstein et al. (1984) compared the ratings of hospitalized elderly by various groups using three instruments: the Lawton Personal Self-Maintenance Scale (PSMS), the Instrumental Activities of Daily Living (IADL) Scale, and the Katz Activities of Daily Living (ADL) Scale. Comparisons of ratings by the clients themselves, the clients' nurses, and the clients' significant others revealed that the PSMS scores by clients were significantly higher than those of significant others, that the clients' IADL scores were significantly higher than scores by the nurses and significant others, and that client scores for the ADLs were significantly higher than the nurses' scores. The authors concluded that clients may overestimate their abilities and that significant others may underestimate clients' functional abilities as compared with professional nursing assessments.

Another issue regarding functional assessment is the relative reliability of various forms of client self-report. Spiegel, Hirshfield, and Spiegel (1985) observed that clients with arthritis were more willing to admit difficulties with self-care activities in a self-administered questionnaire than in a personal interview.

Thus take care in selecting the most relevant functional assessment tool for the client and client group, understand its limitations, and understand how its limitations may affect the responses of clients and others.

Specific Functional Assessment Tools

This section of the chapter presents a number of standardized functional assessment tools that may be useful with populations commonly seen in ambulatory and long–term-care settings. Numerous other tools exist; see DeLisa and Gans (1998) and Dittmar and Gresham (1997) for additional information about the tools presented in this chapter and for information about tools designed for special populations and for research applications.

Katz ADL Index (Revised Version 1976)

The original Katz ADL tool was among the earliest tools to standardize functional assessment. The Katz tool is a general measure of self-care and a very limited measure of mobility. It is probably most applicable with populations in which a level of disability is assumed or already established (e.g., elderly individuals with chronic illness). The tool is short and very easy to administer; therefore the examiner could easily include a version on a printed history form. Its scoring approaches allow for comparison of a given individual over time or compilation across client groups.

Both the original and revised versions focus on several basic activities of daily living and are very easy to administer and score (Katz et al., 1963; Katz and Akpom, 1976). The revised version of the Katz ADL Index (Table 28-3) measures self-care and mobility, specifically the following activities:

Bathing
Dressing
Toileting
Transferring
Continence
Feeding

The examiner rates each activity as 1 or 0, with 1 indicating performance of the activity without human help and 0 indicating performance of the activity with human assistance or that the activity is not performed at all. The scores form an ordinal scale, as noted on the top portion of Table 28-3.

The original Katz tool has been adapted for scoring using a Likert-type scale, with a scale range of 0 to 3 (0, complete independence; 1, use of a device; 2, use of human assistance; 3, complete dependence). No category exists for clients who use both a device and human assistance. The examiner adds the scores to obtain an overall score. A community-based version of the Katz tool adds items of walking and grooming but excludes continence. Brorsson and Asberg (1984) have judged the reliability and validity of the tool as good.

PULSES Profile

The PULSES Profile was developed by Moskowitz and McCann (1957) to assess the functional independence of chronically ill elderly persons. The PULSES instrument (Table 28-4) measures impairment, and the title of the tool is an acronym for its assessment components:

P—Physical condition
U—Upper limb functioning
L—Lower limb functioning
S—Sensory components
E—Excretory function
S—Support factors

The examiner scores each dimension using an ordinal scale from 1 to 4, with 1 representing essential intactness and 4 representing total dependence. The six categories are equally weighted, and the examiner sums the scores to produce a total score ranging from 6 to 24. Scores greater than 12 imply serious impairment, and scores greater than 16 usually reflect severe disability.

TABLE 28-3	Index of Independence in Activities of Daily Living: Scoring and Definitions

The index of Independence in Activities of Daily Living is based on an evaluation of the functional independence or dependence of clients in bathing, dressing, going to toilet, transferring, continence, and feeding. Specific definitions of functional independence and dependence appear below the index.

A—Independent in feeding, continence, transferring, going to toilet, dressing, and bathing
B—Independent in all but one of these functions
C—Independent in all but bathing and one additional function
D—Independent in all but bathing, dressing, and one additional function
E—Indepenent in all but bathing, dressing, going to toilet, and one additional function
F—Independent in all but bathing, dressing, going to toilet, transferring, and one additional function
G—Dependent in all six functions
Other—Dependent in at least two functions, but not classifiable as C, D, E, or F

Independence means without supervision, direction, or active personal assistance, except as specifically noted in the following paragraphs. This is based on actual status and not on ability. A client who refuses to perform a function is considered as not performing the function, even though he or she is deemed able.

Bathing (Sponge, Shower, or Tub)

Independent: Assistance only in bathing a single part (such as back or disabled extremity) or bathes self completely
Dependent: Assistance in bathing more than one part of body; assistance in getting in or out of tub or does not bathe self

Dressing

Independent: Gets clothes from closets and drawers; puts on clothes, outer garments, braces; manages fasteners; act of tying shoes is excluded
Dependent: Does not dress self or remains partly undressed

Going to Toilet

Independent: Gets to toilet; gets on and off toilet; arranges clothes; cleans organs of excretion (may manage own bedpan used at night only and may or may not be using mechanical supports)
Dependent: Uses bedpan or commode or receives assistance in getting to and using toilet

Transfer

Independent: Moves in and out of bed independently and moves in and out of chair independently (may or may not be using mechanical supports)
Dependent: Assistance in moving in or out of bed and/or chair; does not perform one or more transfers

Continence

Independent: Urination and defecation entirely self-controlled
Dependent: Partial or total incontinence in urination or defecation; partial or total control by enemas, catheters, or regulated use of urinals and/or bedpans

Feeding

Independent: Gets food from plate or its equivalent into mouth (precutting of meat and preparation of food, such as buttering bread, are excluded from evaluation)
Dependent: Assistance in act of feeding (see above); does not eat at all or parenteral feeding

Modified from Katz S et al.: The index of independence in activities of daily living, progress in development of the index of ADI, *Gerontologist* 10:23, 1970.

Several authors have reviewed the reliability and validity evidence for the scale (Jette, 1985; McDowell and Newell, 1996), and they have assessed it as acceptable.

The main limitations of the tool are the general focus on a broad array of categories and redundancy with items commonly measured in a routine history and physical examination. The instrument was designed for use in a rehabilitation setting and is probably most applicable in situations in which changes in levels of impairment are anticipated.

Barthel Index

The Barthel Index (BI) (Mahoney and Barthel, 1965; Granger, 1982) (Table 28-5) is a weighted index for assessing dependence in various areas of self-care, mobility, and continence. The original scale contains 10 items that the examiner scores with a weighted rating of 15, 10, 5, or 0, depending on the amount of help the client needs to perform the function. Total scores range from 0 (total dependence) to 100 (total independence) and are intended to indicate the amount of assistance a client requires. A score of 60 indicates the threshold

TABLE 28-4 **PULSES Profile**

	P Physical Condition	U Upper Extremities	L Lower Extremities	S Sensory Function	E Excretory Functions	S Social and Mental Status
	Cardiovascular, pulmonary, and other visceral disorders	Shoulder girdles, cervical and upper dorsal spine	Pelvis, lower dorsal and lumbosacral spine	Vision, hearing, and speech	Bowel and bladder	Emotional and psychiatric disorders
Normal	1 Health maintenance	1 Complete function	1 Complete function	1 Complete function	1 Continent	1 Compatible with age
Mild	2 Occasional medical supervision	2 No assistance required	2 Fully ambulatory despite some loss of function	2 No appreciable functional impairment	2 Occasional stress incontinence or nocturia	2 No supervision required
Moderately severe	3 Frequent medical supervision	3 Some assistance necessary	3 Limited ambulation	3 Appreciable bilateral loss or complete unilateral loss of vision or hearing Incomplete aphasia	3 Periodic incontinence or retention	3 Some supervision necessary
Severe	4 Total care Bed or chair confined	4 Nursing care	4 Confined to wheelchair or bed	4 Total blindness Total deafness Global aphasia or aphonia	4 Total incontinence or retention (including catheter and colostomy)	4 Complete care in psychiatric facility

Modified from Moskowtiz E: PULSES profile in retrospect, *Arch Phys Med Rehabil* 66:648, 1985; and Moskowitz E, McCann CB: Classification of disability in the chronically ill and aged, *J Chron Dis* 5:343, 1957 (reprinted with permission from Elsevier Science).

P. *Physical* condition, including diseases of the viscera (cardiovascular, pulmonary, gastrointestinal, urologic, and endocrine) and cerebral disorders that are not enumerated in the lettered categories below.
   1. No gross abnormalities, considering the age of the individual.
   2. Minor abnormalities not requiring frequent medical or nursing supervision.
   3. Moderately severe abnormalities requiring frequent medical or nursing supervision yet still permitting ambulation.
   4. Severe abnormalities requiring constant medical or nursing supervision confining individual to bed or wheelchair.
U. *Upper* extremities, including shoulder girdle, cervical and upper dorsal spine.
   1. No gross abnormalities, considering the age of the individual.
   2. Minor abnormalities with fairly good range of motion and function.
   3. Moderately severe abnormalities but permitting the performance of daily needs to a limited extent.
   4. Severe abnormalities requiring constant nursing care.
L. *Lower* extremities, including the pelvis, lower dorsal and lumbosacral spine.
   1. No gross abnormalities, considering the age of the individual.
   2. Minor abnormalities with a fairly good range of motion and function.
   3. Moderately severe abnormalities permitting limited ambulation.
   4. Severe abnormalities confining the individual to bed or wheelchair.
S. *Sensory* components relating to speech, vision, and hearing.
   1. No gross abnormalities, considering the age of the individual.
   2. Minor deviations insufficient to cause any appreciable functional impairment.
   3. Moderate deviations sufficient to cause appreciable functional impairment.
   4. Severe deviations causing complete loss of hearing, vision, or speech.
E. *Excretory* function (i.e., bowel and bladder control).
   1. Complete control.
   2. Occasional stress incontinence or nocturia.
   3. Periodic bowel and bladder incontinence or retention alternating with control.
   4. Total incontinence, either bowel or bladder.
S. *Mental and emotional status.*
   1. No deviations, considering the age of the individual.
   2. Minor deviations in mood, temperament, and personality not impairing environmental adjustment.
   3. Moderately severe variations requiring some supervision.
   4. Severe variations requiring complete supervision.

TABLE 28-5 Original Barthel Index

	With Help	Independent
1. Feeding (if food needs to be cut up = help)	5	10
2. Moving from wheelchair to bed and return (includes sitting up in bed)	5-10	15
3. Personal toilet (wash face, comb hair, shave, clean teeth)	0	5
4. Getting on and off toilet (handling clothes, wipe, flush)	5	10
5. Bathe self	0	5
6. Walking on level surface (or if unable to walk, propel a wheelchair)	10	15
	0*	5*
7. Ascend and descend stairs	5	10
8. Dressing (includes tying shoes, fastening fasteners)	5	10
9. Controlling bowels	5	10
10. Controlling bladder	5	10

From Mahoney FI, Barthel DW: Functional evaluation: the Barthel index, *Maryland State Med J* 14(2):61-65, 1965.

*Score only if unable to walk.

Instructions for scoring the Barthel Index (NOTE: A score of zero is given when the patient cannot meet the defined criterion):

1. Feeding
   10 = Independent. The patient can feed himself a meal from a tray or table when someone puts the food within his reach. He must put on an assistive device if this is needed, cut up the food, use salt and pepper, spread butter, etc. He must accomplish this in a reasonable time.
   5 = Some help is necessary (when cutting up food, etc., as listed above).
2. Moving from wheelchair to bed and return
   15 = Independent in all phases of this activity. Patient can safely approach the bed in his wheelchair, lock brakes, lift footrests, move safely to bed, lie down, come to a sitting position on the side of the bed, change the position of the wheelchair, if necessary, to transfer back into it safely, and return to the wheelchair.
   10 = Either some minimal help is needed in some step of this activity or the patient needs to be reminded or supervised for safety of one or more parts of this activity.
   5 = Patient can come to a sitting position without the help of a second person but needs to be lifted out of bed, or if he transfers with a great deal of help.
3. Doing personal toilet
   5 = Patient can wash hands and face, comb hair, clean teeth, and shave. He may use any kind of razor but must put in blade or plug in razor without help, as well as get it from drawer or cabinet. Female patients must put on own make-up, if used, but need not braid or style hair.
4. Getting on and off toilet
   10 = Patient is able to get on and off toilet, fasten and unfasten clothes, prevent soiling of clothes, and use toilet paper without help. He may use a wall bar or other stable object of support if needed. If it is necessary to use a bed pan instead of a toilet, he must be able to place it on a chair, empty it, and clean it.
   5 = Patient needs help because of imbalance or in handling clothes or in using toilet paper.
5. Bathing self
   5 = Patient may use a bathtub, a shower, or take a complete sponge bath. He must be able to do all the steps involved in whichever method is employed without another person being present.
6. Walking on a level surface
   15 = Patient can walk at least 50 yards without help or supervision. He may wear braces or prostheses and use crutches, canes, or a walkerette but not a rolling walker. He must be able to lock and unlock braces if used, assume the standing position and sit down, get the necessary mechanical aides into position for use, and dispose of them when he sits. (Putting on and taking off braces is scored under dressing.)
   10 = Patient needs help or supervision in any of the above but can walk at least 50 yards with a little help.
6a: Propelling a wheelchair
   5 = If a patient cannot ambulate but can propel a wheelchair independently. He must be able to go around corners, turn around, maneuver the chair to a table, bed, toilet, etc. He must be able to push a chair at least 50 yards. Do not score this item if the patient gets score for walking.
7. Ascending and descending stairs
   10 = Patient is able to go up and down a flight of stairs safely without help or supervision. He may and should use handrails, canes, or crutches when needed. He must be able to carry canes or crutches as he ascends or descends stairs.
   5 = Patient needs help with supervision of any one of the above items.
8. Dressing and undressing (Women need not be scored on use of a brassiere or girdle unless these are prescribed garments.)
   10 = Patient is able to put on and remove and fasten all clothing, and tie shoelaces (unless it is necessary to use adaptations for this). The activity includes putting on and removing and fastening corset or braces when these are prescribed. Such special clothing as suspenders, loafer shoes or dresses that open down the front may be used when necessary.
   5 = Patient needs help in putting on and removing or fastening any clothing. He must do at least half the work himself. He must accomplish this in a reasonable time.
9. Continence of bowels
   10 = Patient is able to control his bowels and have no accidents. He can use a suppository or take an enema when necessary (as for spinal cord injury patients who have had bowel training).
   5 = Patient needs help in using a suppository or taking an enema or has occasional accidents.
10. Controlling bladder
    10 = Patient is able to control his bladder day and night. Spinal cord injury patients who wear an external device and leg bag must put them on independently, clean and empty bag, and stay dry day and night.
    5 = Patient has occasional accidents or cannot wait for the bedpan or get to the toilet in time or needs help with an external device.

TABLE 28-6	Modified Barthel Index Scoring			
Independent		**Dependent**		
I Intact	II Limited	III Helper	IV Null	
10	5	0	0	Drink from cup/feed from dish
5	5	3	0	Dress upper body
5	5	2	0	Dress lower body
0	0	−2		Don brace or prosthesis
5	5	0	0	Grooming
4	4	0	0	Wash or bathe
10	10	5	0	Bladder continence
10	10	5	0	Bowel continence
4	4	2	0	Care of perineum/clothing at toilet
15	15	7	0	Transfer, chair
6	5	3	0	Transfer, toilet
1	1	0	0	Transfer, tub or shower
15	15	10	0	Walk on level 50 yards or more
10	10	5	0	Up and down stairs for one flight or more
15	5	0	0	Wheelchair/50 yards—only if not walking

Modified from the presentation of the Modified Barthel Index in Fortinsky RH, Granger CV, Seltzer GB: The use of functional assessment in understanding home care needs, *Med Care* 19:489, 1981.

between independence and dependence; a score of 40 or less indicates severe dependence; and a score of 20 or less reflects total dependence in self-care and mobility. Granger, Albrecht, and Hamilton (1979) reported the test-retest reliability and inter-rater agreements as 89% and 95%, respectively.

Fortinsky, Granger, and Seltzer (1981) modified the original BI (Table 28-6). The modified BI contains 15 items and the following changes: two items of dressing (i.e., upper and lower body) rather than one general item; additional items for use of brace or prosthesis, transfer to toilet, and transfer to tub or shower; and differentiation of items for walking and propelling a wheelchair.

Advantages of the BI include its widespread use, the clarity of scoring, and completeness of the set of items.

IADL Scale

The IADL Scale (Lawton, 1972) (Table 28-7) measures behaviors that are more cognitively and less directly physically oriented than the other self-care scales. The tool's eight items measure the client's ability to use a telephone, shop, prepare food, keep house, do laundry, use public transportation, take responsibility for one's medications, and handle finances. The examiner scores each item on a 3-, 4-, or 5-point scale that reflects the amount of assistance used or limitation in performing the activity.

The Instrumental ADL Scale expands the concept of self-care beyond specific and basic physical ability by measuring performance in the usual household maintenance activities. The examiner could use this scale with community-based

TABLE 28-7	Instrumental Activities of Daily Living Scale

A. Ability to use telephone
  1. Operates telephone on own initiative—e.g., looks up and dials numbers.
  2. Dials well-known numbers.
  3. Answers telephone but does not dial.
  4. Does not use telephone at all.
B. Shopping
  1. Takes care of all shopping needs independently.
  2. Shops independently for small purchases.
  3. Must be accompanied on any shopping trip.
  4. Completely unable to shop.
C. Food preparation
  1. Plans, prepares, and serves adequate meals independently.
  2. Prepares adequate meals if supplied with ingredients.
  3. Heats and serves prepared meals, or prepares meals but does not maintain adequate diet.
  4. Needs to have meals prepared and served.
D. Housekeeping
  1. Maintains house alone or with occasional assistance.
  2. Performs light daily tasks such as dishwashing, bedmaking.
  3. Performs light daily tasks but cannot maintain acceptable level of cleanliness.
  4. Needs help with all home maintenance tasks.
  5. Does not participate in any housekeeping tasks.

E. Laundry
  1. Does personal laundry completely.
  2. Launders small items—rinses socks, stockings, etc.
  3. All laundry must be done by others.
F. Mode of transportation
  1. Travels independently on public transportation or drives own car.
  2. Arranges own travel by taxi but does not otherwise use public transportation.
  3. Travels on public transportation when assisted or accompanied by another.
  4. Travel limited to taxi or automobile with assistance of another.
  5. Does not travel at all.
G. Responsibility for own medications
  1. Is responsible for taking medications in correct dosages at correct time.
  2. Takes responsibility if medications are prepared in advance in separate dosages.
  3. Is not capable of dispensing own medications.
H. Ability to handle finances
  1. Manages financial matters independently (budgets, writes checks, pays rent, bills, goes to bank), collects and keeps track of income.
  2. Manages day-to-day purchases but needs help with banking, major purchases, etc.
  3. Incapable of handling money.

Modified from Brody E, Lawton MP: Philadelphia Geriatric Center, 5301 Old York Road, Philadelphia, Pa 19141.

populations and individuals whose mobility is compromised or who are at risk of progressive debilitation (e.g., the frail elderly).

Physical Self-Maintenance Scale

The Physical Self-Maintenance Scale (PSMS) (also known as the Lawton and Brody Scale, 1969) (Table 28-8) includes six items of self-care and mobility that the examiner rates using a unique Guttman-type scale for each item. The six items are toileting (including continence), feeding, dressing, grooming, physical ambulation, and bathing. The examiner may use either of two scoring methods: a count of the number of items for which disability is noted or a severity scale summing the response codes for each item, resulting in a summary score ranging from 6 to 30.

This tool demonstrates good reliability and validity (McDowell and Newell, 1996). The scale is probably most applicable to homebound or institutionalized populations. Administration is easy and rapid.

Rapid Disability Rating Scale

The Rapid Disability Rating Scale–2 (Linn and Linn, 1982) (Table 28-9) is an 18-item global disability scale measuring assistance needed with activities of daily living; disability; and special problems according to the assistance required or degree of disability. Each item is briefly defined and has op-

tions of 4 scale points. The total scores range from 18 to 72, with higher values indicating greater disability.

The scale demonstrates high reliability in use (McDowell and Newell, 1996; Rothstein, 1985), and the initial results of validity examination are positive.

This tool contains several items that the examiner would include in the routine health assessment (e.g., hearing, sight, diet, and medication), and it may be most appropriate for screening situations.

Functional Status Rating System

The Functional Status Rating System (Forer, 1981) (Table 28-10) measures the amount of assistance needed in self-care and mobility and the amount of impairment in communication, psychosocial adjustment, and cognitive function. It is unusually comprehensive for a functional assessment tool, covering 30 items under five topics. Although the tool may in small part duplicate portions of the health assessment, most of the items measure new assessment factors.

The amount of currently available psychometric information about the tool is limited.

Functional Independence Measure and Functional Assessment Measures

A recent innovation in the field of rehabilitation is the proposal of a uniform, national data system for functional as-

TABLE 28-8   Physical Self-Maintenance Scale

A. Toilet
  1. Cares for self at toilet completely, no incontinence.
  2. Needs to be reminded, or needs help in cleaning self, or has rare (weekly at most) accidents.
  3. Soiling or wetting while asleep more than once a week.
  4. Soiling or wetting while awake more than once a week.
  5. No control of bowels or bladder.
B. Feeding
  1. Eats without assistance.
  2. Eats with minor assistance at mealtimes and/or with special preparation of food, or help in cleaning up after meals.
  3. Feeds self with moderate assistance and is untidy.
  4. Requires extensive assistance for all meals.
  5. Does not feed self at all and resists efforts of others to feed him.
C. Dressing
  1. Dresses, undresses, and selects clothes from own wardrobe.
  2. Dresses and undresses self, with minor assistance.
  3. Needs moderate assistance in dressing or selection of clothes.
  4. Needs major assistance in dressing but cooperates with efforts of others to help.
  5. Completely unable to dress self and resists efforts of others to help.
D. Grooming (neatness, hair, nails, hands, face, clothing)
  1. Always neatly dressed, well-groomed, without assistance.

  2. Grooms self adequately with occasional minor assistance (e.g., shaving).
  3. Needs moderate and regular assistance or supervision in grooming.
  4. Needs total grooming care, but can remain well-groomed after help from others.
  5. Actively negates all efforts of others to maintain grooming.
E. Physical ambulation
  1. Goes about grounds or city.
  2. Ambulates within residence or about one block distant.
  3. Ambulates with assistance of (check one)
      a ( ) another person, b ( ) railing,
      c ( ) cane, d ( ) walker, e ( ) wheelchair.
      1 ____ Gets in and out without help.
      2 ____ Needs help in getting in and out.
  4. Sits unsupported in chair or wheelchair, but cannot propel self without help.
  5. Bedridden more than half the time.
F. Bathing
  1. Bathes self (tub, shower, sponge bath) without help.
  2. Bathes self with help in getting in and out of tub.
  3. Washes face and hands only, but cannot bathe rest of body.
  4. Does not wash self but is cooperative with those who bathe him.
  5. Does not try to wash self and resists efforts to keep him clean.

Modified from the Physical Self-Maintenance scale in Lawton MP, Brody EM: Assessment of older people: self-maintaining and instrumental activities of daily living, *Gerontologist* 9:180, 1969.

TABLE 28-9	Rapid Disability Rating Scale–2

Directions: Rate what the person *does* to reflect current behavior. Circle one of the four choices for each item. Consider rating with any aids or prostheses normally used.

Assistance with Activities of Daily Living

Eating	None	A little	A lot	Spoon-feed: intravenous tube
Walking (with cane or walker if used)	None	A little	A lot	Does not walk
Mobility (going outside and getting about with wheelchair, etc., if used)	None	A little	A lot	Is housebound
Bathing (include getting supplies, supervising)	None	A little	A lot	Must be bathed
Dressing (include help in selecting clothes)	None	A little	A lot	Must be dressed
Toileting (include help with clothes, cleaning, or help with ostomy, catheter)	None	A little	A lot	Uses bedpan or unable to care for ostomy/catheter
Grooming (shaving for men, hairdressing for women, nails, teeth)	None	A little	A lot	Must be groomed
Adaptive tasks (managing money/ possessions; telephoning; buying newspaper, toilet articles, snacks)	None	A little	A lot	Cannot manage

Degree of Disability

Communication (expressing self)	None	A little	A lot	Does not communicate
Hearing (with aid if used)	None	A little	A lot	Does not seem to hear
Sight (with glasses, is used)	None	A little	A lot	Does not see
Diet (deviation from normal)	None	A little	A lot	Fed by intravenous tube
In bed during day (ordered or self-initiated)	None	A little (<3 hr)	A lot	Most/all of time
Incontinence (urine/feces, with catheter or prosthesis, if used)	None	Sometimes	Frequently (weekly +)	Does not control
Medication	None	Sometimes	Daily, taken orally	Daily: injection (+ oral if used)

Degree of Special Problems

Mental confusion	None	A little	A lot	Extreme
Uncooperativeness (combats efforts to help with care)	None	A little	A lot	Extreme
Depression	None	A little	A lot	Extreme

Modified from the presentation of the Rapid Disability Rating Scale–2 as published in Linn MW, Linn BS: The rapid disability rating scale–2, *J Am Geriatr Soc* 30:380, 1982. Reprinted by permission of Blackwell Science, Inc.

sessment. This standardized database would establish a uniform language and set of definitions for communicating disability and rehabilitation information. Toward this end, the major researchers in the field have developed the minimum data set for the field, the Functional Independence Measure (FIM) tool. The FIM tool measures 18 items in the categories of self-care, mobility, locomotion, communication, and social cognition. The 7-point rating scale is designed to assess the patient's level or degree of independence, the amount of assistance required, use of adaptive or assistive devices, and the percentage of a given task completed successfully. The FIM requires 15 to 20 minutes for administration and can be performed by a variety of health care professionals.

The staff of the Santa Clara Medical Center (California), has expanded the FIM to a 29-item scale, titled the Functional Assessment Measures (FAM). The expanded tool uses the same rating scheme and requires 20 to 25 minutes for administration. The summary rating scale for the FIM and the FAM is presented in Table 28-11. The 11 items added to the eighteen-item FIM tool components are identified by asterisks. Currently the FIM is one of the most commonly used functional assessment tools.

SUMMARY

Use of an organized functional assessment is recommended for all clients whose daily activities may be affected by impairments or disabilities; the elderly and the handicapped are the more obvious examples of such groups. The literature has shown that health care providers often do superficial assessments of this assessment area and may not appreciate

TABLE 28-10	**Functional Status Rating System**

Functional Status in Self-Care

A. *Eating/feeding:* Management of all aspects of setting up and eating food (including cutting of meat) with or without adaptive equipment.

B. *Personal hygiene:* Includes setup, oral care, washing face and hands with a washcloth, hair grooming, shaving, and makeup.

C. *Toileting:* Includes management of clothing and cleanliness.

D. *Bathing:* Includes entire body bathing (tub, shower, or bed bath).

E. *Bowel management:* Able to insert suppository and/or perform manual evacuation, aware of need to defecate, has sphincter muscle control.

F. *Bladder management:* Able to manage equipment necessary for bladder evacuation (may include intermittent catheterization).

G. *Skin management:* Performance of skin care program, regular inspection, prevention of pressure sores, rashes, or irritations.

H. *Bed activities:* Includes turning, coming to a sitting position, scooting, and maintenance of balance.

I. *Dressing:* Includes performance of total body dressing except tying shoes, with or without adaptive equipment (also includes application of orthosis and prosthesis).

Functional Status in Mobility

A. *Transfers:* Includes the management of all aspects of transfers to and from bed, mat, toilet, tub/shower, wheelchair, with or without adaptive equipment.

B. *Wheelchair skills:* Includes management of brakes, leg rests, maneuvering and propelling through and over doorway thresholds.

C. *Ambulation:* Includes coming to a standing position and walking short to moderate distances on level surfaces with or without equipment.

D. *Stairs and environmental surfaces:* Includes climbing stairs, curbs, ramps or environmental terrain.

E. *Community mobility:* Ability to manage transportation.

Functional Status in Communication

A. *Understanding spoken language*

B. *Reading comprehension*

C. *Language expression (non-speech/alternative methods):* Includes pointing, gestures, manual communication boards, electronic systems.

D. *Language expression (verbal):* Includes grammar, syntax, and appropriateness of language.

E. *Speech intelligibility*

F. *Written communication (motor)*

G. *Written language expression:* Includes spelling, vocabulary, punctuation, syntax, grammar, and completeness of written response.

Functional Status in Psychosocial Adjustment

A. *Emotional adjustment:* Includes frequency and severity of depression, anxiety, frustration, lability, unresponsiveness, agitation, interference with progress in therapies, motivation, ability to cope with and take responsibility for emotional behavior.

B. *Family/significant others/environment:* Includes frequency of chronic problems or conflicts in client's relationships, interference with progress in therapies, ability and willingness to provide for client's specific needs after discharge, and to promote client's recovery and independence.

C. *Adjustment to limitations:* Includes denial/awareness, acceptance of limitations, willingness to learn new ways of functioning, compensating, taking appropriate safety precautions, and realistic expectations for long-term recovery.

D. *Social adjustment:* Includes frequency and limitation of social contacts, responsiveness in one-to-one and group situations, appropriateness of behavior in relationships, and spontaneity of interactions.

Functional Status in Cognitive Function

A. *Attention span:* Includes distractability, level of alertness and responsiveness, ability to concentrate on a task, ability to follow directions, immediate recall as the structure, difficulty, and length of the task vary.

B. *Orientation*

C. *Judgment reasoning*

D. *Memory:* Includes short- and long-term.

E. *Problem-solving*

Summary of Rating Scales

Self-Care and Mobility Items

1.0 = Unable—totally dependent
1.5 = Maximum assistance of 1 or 2 people
2.0 = Moderate assistance
2.5 = Minimal assistance
3.0 = Standby assistance
3.5 = Supervised
4.0 = Independent

Communication, Psychosocial, and Cognitive Function Items

1.0 = Extremely severe
1.5 = Severe
2.0 = Moderately severe
2.5 = Moderate impairment
3.0 = Mild impairment
3.5 = Minimal impairment
4.0 = No impairment

Modified from S.K. Forer.

the client's capabilities or limitations. This lack of appreciation may cause inappropriate or insufficient treatment, lack of support, and neglect of problems that may be treatable.

The approaches and tools presented in this chapter have applicability across the range of settings and circumstances in which practitioners perform health assessments. Because the functional assessment is not a routine component of the health assessment, a standardized approach across practitioners does not exist for general populations. The practitioner is advised to explore the assessment options and to select and use, as indicated, the most applicable and useful approaches and tools.

| TABLE 28-11 | **Functional Assessment Measures Summary Worksheet** |

Rating Scale: 7 Complete independence (timely, safely)
6 Modified independence (extra time, device)
5 Supervision
4 Minimal assist (subject 75% of task)
3 Moderate assist (50%-74% of task)
2 Maximal assist (25%-49% of task)
1 Total assist (subject 25% of task)

Self-Care Items

1. Feeding　　　　　　　　　　　　　　　Adm ___ Goal ___ D/C ___ F/U ___
2. Grooming　　　　　　　　　　　　　　Adm ___ Goal ___ D/C ___ F/U ___
3. Bathing technique ____　　　　　　　Adm ___ Goal ___ D/C ___ F/U ___
4. Dressing upper body　　　　　　　　Adm ___ Goal ___ D/C ___ F/U ___
5. Dressing lower body　　　　　　　　Adm ___ Goal ___ D/C ___ F/U ___
6. Toileting　　　　　　　　　　　　　　Adm ___ Goal ___ D/C ___ F/U ___
7. Swallowing*　　　　　　　　　　　　Adm ___ Goal ___ D/C ___ F/U ___

Sphincter Control

8. Bladder management　　　　　　　　Adm ___ Goal ___ D/C ___ F/U ___
9. Bowel management　　　　　　　　　Adm ___ Goal ___ D/C ___ F/U ___

Mobility Items

Transfers Technique _____

10. Bed, chair, wheelchair　　　　　　Adm ___ Goal ___ D/C ___ F/U ___
11. Toilet　　　　　　　　　　　　　　　Adm ___ Goal ___ D/C ___ F/U ___
12. Tub or shower　　　　　　　　　　　Adm ___ Goal ___ D/C ___ F/U ___
13. Car transfers*　　　　　　　　　　　Adm ___ Goal ___ D/C ___ F/U ___

Locomotion

14. Walking/wheelchair　　　　　　　　Adm ___ Goal ___ D/C ___ F/U ___
15. Stairs　　　　　　　　　　　　　　　Adm ___ Goal ___ D/C ___ F/U ___
16. Community mobility*　　　　　　　　Adm ___ Goal ___ D/C ___ F/U ___

Communication Items

17. Comprehension　　　　　　　　　　Adm ___ Goal ___ D/C ___ F/U ___
18. Expression　　　　　　　　　　　　Adm ___ Goal ___ D/C ___ F/U ___
19. Reading*　　　　　　　　　　　　　Adm ___ Goal ___ D/C ___ F/U ___
20. Writing*　　　　　　　　　　　　　　Adm ___ Goal ___ D/C ___ F/U ___
21. Speech intelligibility*　　　　　　　Adm ___ Goal ___ D/C ___ F/U ___

Psychosocial Adjustment Items

22. Social interaction　　　　　　　　　Adm ___ Goal ___ D/C ___ F/U ___
23. Emotional adjustment*　　　　　　　Adm ___ Goal ___ D/C ___ F/U ___
24. Adjustment to limitations*　　　　　Adm ___ Goal ___ D/C ___ F/U ___
25. Vocational reentry*　　　　　　　　　　　　　　　　　D/C ___ F/U ___

Cognitive Function

26. Problem solving　　　　　　　　　　Adm ___ Goal ___ D/C ___ F/U ___
27. Memory　　　　　　　　　　　　　　Adm ___ Goal ___ D/C ___ F/U ___
28. Orientation*　　　　　　　　　　　　Adm ___ Goal ___ D/C ___ F/U ___
29. Attention*　　　　　　　　　　　　　Adm ___ Goal ___ D/C ___ F/U ___

The Functional Assessment Measures tool was developed by the staff of the Santa Clara Medical Center, Santa Clara, Calif. *D/C,* At discharge; *F/U,* at follow-up.
*Items added to the original FIM assessment tool. The FIM was developed by the Task Force for the Development of a Uniform Data System for Medical Rehabilitation, Department of Rehabilitative Medicine, Buffalo General Hospital, Buffalo, N.Y.

Sample Documentation and Diagnoses

FOCUSED HEALTH HISTORY (SUBJECTIVE DATA)

Mr. K, a 59-year-old plumber, who had a diagnosis of left hemiplegia and aphasia 6 days after he suffered a cerebrovascular accident, has just been transferred from the neurological intensive care unit onto the medical floor to stabilize his condition before transfer to the rehabilitation center. Because of Mr. K's speech dysfunction, his wife provided his history. Mr. K was admitted 6 days ago unconscious after he did not awaken to the alarm clock. He was noted to respond only to deep pain; his left arm and leg were limp. Two days later, he regained consciousness; was unable to move his left arm or leg; and was unable to speak clearly, swallow, or perform any activities of daily living (ADLs). Wife states client is unable to move his left arm or leg, speak clearly, swallow, or do his own ADLs. He owns his own business and was extremely active in his business and with family prior to his CVA. The couple has three adult children living outside of the home and a teenager, age 16, at home.

FOCUSED PHYSICAL EXAMINATION (OBJECTIVE DATA)

Mental status: Client is lying in bed; body slumps slightly to left; appears alert but has difficulty maintaining eye contact. Speech slow, requires much effort, and is garbled. Hard to determine whether appropriate. Seems to understand words spoken to him. Follows requests slowly but appropriately within limits of motor weakness. Some drooling.

Cranial nerves:

I:	Not tested.
II:	Acuity 20/20 in both eyes without correction, fields by confrontation—left homonymous hemianopia, fundi reveal intact vessels without exudate, clear disc margins.
III, IV, VI:	Extraocular movements (EOMs) intact; slight left-sided ptosis; no nystagmus; pupils equal, round, react to light and accommodation (PERRLA).
V:	Sensation intact to pinprick and light touch. Jaw strength weak on left.
VII:	Flat nasolabial fold on left; motor weakness on left lower face. Unable to wrinkle forehead bilaterally; unable to smile on left side.
VIII:	Hearing intact.
IX, X:	No swallowing or gag reflex present; uvula rises slightly to right on phonation.
XI:	Shoulder shrug; head movement weaker on left.
XII:	Tongue protrudes slightly to right; no tremors.

Cerebellar: Unable to move left hand or leg, unable to support weight. Spasticity in left arm and leg. Unable to stand and walk unassisted. Unable to perform finger-to-nose or heel-to-shin maneuver on left side. Right side intact but slow.

Sensory: Pinprick and light touch present but decreased on left arm and leg. Vibration intact. Position sense decreased on left, intact on right. Stereognosis intact.

Deep tendon reflexes (DTRs): Right side intact 1 + ; left side 0; Babinski present left side. Plantar reflex absent left side, intact on right side.

Functional Assessment Measure Score = 87 of a possible 203.

DIAGNOSES

HEALTH PROBLEM

Cerebrovascular accident with left hemiplagia

NURSING DIAGNOSES

Impaired Swallowing Related to Neuromuscular Impairment (Absent Gag Reflex)

Defining Characteristics

- Observed evidence of difficulty swallowing
- Observed coughing/choking when swallowing
- Assessed no gag or swallowing ability

Impaired Nutrition: Less than Body Requirements Related to Muscle Weakness (Mastication and Swallowing)

Defining Characteristics

- Inability to swallow
- No gag reflex
- Observed inadequate food intake

Risk for Impaired Skin Integrity Related to Prolonged Immobility

Defining Characteristics

- Physical immobility—cannot move left side
- Incontinence of both bladder and bowel—excretion on skin

Continued

Sample Documentation and Diagnoses—cont'd

Bowel Incontinence Related to Cognitive/Perceptual Impairment
Defining Characteristics
- Involuntary passage of stool
- Inability to communicate need (aphasia)

Total Urinary Incontinence Related to Cognitive/Perceptual Impairment
Defining Characteristics
- Lack of perineal or bladder filling awareness
- Unawareness of incontinence
- Inability to communicate need (aphasia)

Impaired Physical Mobility Related to Neuromuscular Impairment
Defining Characteristics
- Inability to purposefully move within the physical environment
- Decreased muscle strength
- Impaired coordination
- Level IV—is dependent and at this time does not participate in movement

Bathing/Hygiene, Dressing/Grooming, Feeding, and Toileting Self-Care Deficits Related to Neuromuscular Impairment
Defining Characteristics
- Inability to wash body or body parts
- Inability to obtain or get to water source
- Inability to regulate temperature or flow of water
- Impaired ability to put on or take off necessary items of clothing
- Impaired ability to obtain or replace articles of clothes, fasten clothing, and maintain appearance at a satisfactory level
- Level IV—is dependent and does not participate in self-care at this time

Disturbed Sensory Perception (Kinesthetic) Related to Neuromuscular Impairment
Defining Characteristics
- Measured change in sensory acuity
- Altered communication patterns
- Inability to sit or stand
- Motor incoordination

Unilateral Neglect Related to Neuromuscular Impairment, Inability to Move Left Side
Defining Characteristics
- Consistent inattention to stimuli on affected side
- Lack of positioning and/or safety precautions regarding left side
- Does not look toward affected side

Disturbed Body Image Related to Nonintegration of Change in Body Function and Limitations
Defining Characteristics
- Verbalized feelings of powerlessness in relation to body
- Depersonalization of part or loss by impersonal pronoun
- Refusal to verify actual change in body
- Change in ability to estimate spatial relationship of body to environment

Impaired Verbal Communication Related to Neuromuscular Impairment
Defining Characteristics
- Speaks or verbalizes with difficulty
- Difficulty forming words
- Difficulty expressing thoughts verbally

Critical Thinking Questions

Review the Sample Documentation and Diagnoses box to answer these questions.

1. Which of the functional assessment tools presented in this chapter would be useful in assessing Mr. K's rehabilitation progress?

2. How would you adapt the physical examination to clients with similar disabilities?

3. What additional information from the family would be helpful to obtain in this situation?

Answers are available on the MERLIN website (www.harcourthealth.com/MERLIN/Barkauskas/). And be sure to check the website regularly for additional learning activities!

Remember to check out the Online Study Guide!
www.harcourthealth.com/MERLIN/Barkauskas/

Glossary

abatement Decrease in intensity of a pain or other symptom.

abduction Movement away from the axial line (for a limb) or the median plane (for the digits).

acceptance Recognition of what is said without necessarily agreeing.

accommodation Process by which the refractive power of the lens of the eye is increased through contraction of the ciliary muscle, which causes increased thickness and curvature of the lens. The accommodation response of the pupils consists of convergence of the eyes and constriction of the pupils as the gaze shifts from a distant to a near point.

acculturation Process of adapting to a culture different from the one in which a person was encultured.

acetabulum The large, cup-shaped cavity at the juncture of the ilium, the ischium, and the pubis, in which the ball-shaped head of the femur articulates.

acini Small, saclike dilations found in various glands.

acoustic stethoscope Instrument used in mediate auscultation, consisting of two earpieces connected by means of flexible tubing to a diaphragm, which is placed on the client's skin.

actinic keratoses Pink to slightly red, dry, scaly lesions with indistinct borders and a malignant potential.

active listening Communication technique that involves concentration on what is said by blocking out environmental noise, distractions, and intrusive thoughts. Active listening conveys a nonverbal message to the speaker that what is being said is valued.

active range of motion Purposeful joint movement performed by the client without assistance from the examiner.

activities of daily living (ADLs) Basic physical needs of dressing, transferring, feeding, bathing, toileting, bowel and bladder control, walking, climbing stairs, and grooming.

acute Characterized by sharpness and severity; usually involves rapid onset and short duration.

adaptation Process by which the eye becomes more sensitive to either reduced or increased illumination.

adduction Movement toward the axial line (for a limb) or the median plane (for the digits).

adnexal Being next to or near another, related structure—the ovaries and fallopian tubes in the case of female genitalia.

adolescence The stage of life beginning at puberty and extending to adulthood.

affect Outwardly manifested emotional range attached to ideas. *Appropriate affect:* emotional tone in harmony with the accompanying idea, thought, or verbalization. *Blunted affect:* disturbance manifested by a severe reduction in the intensity of affect. *Flat affect:* absence or near absence of any signs of affective expression. *Inappropriate affect:* incongruence between the emotional feeling tone and the idea, thought, or speech accompanying it. *Labile affect:* rapid changes in the emotional feeling tone that are unrelated to external stimuli.

afferent neuron Any neuron that transmits nerve impulses from the periphery toward the central nervous system (sensory).

age-related macular degeneration (AMD) Degeneration of the macula leading to decreased central vision.

ageusia Loss of the sensation of taste or of the ability to discriminate sweet, sour, salty, and bitter tastes.

agnosia Inability to discriminate sensory stimuli. *Acoustic or auditory agnosia:* impaired ability to recognize familiar sounds. *Tactile agnosia:* impaired ability to recognize familiar objects by touch or feel. *Visual agnosia:* impaired ability to recognize familiar objects by sight. *Somatagnosia:* disturbance in recognition of body parts.

alopecia Partial or complete lack of hair resulting from normal aging, endocrine disorder, drug reactions, skin disease, and other causes.

alveoli Small, thin-walled sacs through which gas exchange takes place between alveolar air and pulmonary capillary blood.

amblyopia Reduced vision in an eye that appears structurally normal on ophthalmoscopic examination.

amenorrhea Absence of menstruation.

ampulla Rounded, saclike dilation of a duct, canal, or any tubular structure.

712

anastomosing Joining.

anesthesia Absence of normal sensation, especially sensitivity to pain, such as induced by an anesthetic substance or hypnosis or as occurs with traumatic or pathophysiological damage to nerve tissue.

aneurysm Localized dilation of an artery. Most prominent and significant in the aorta but also occurs in peripheral vessels.

angina pectoris Pain that is substernal and/or radiating to the left arm, neck, or jaw; frequently correlated with myocardial ischemia. May be accompanied by a feeling of suffocation or impending death. Attacks are often related to exertion, emotional stress, or exposure to intense cold.

anisocoria Condition in which the pupils of the two eyes are of unequal size.

ankylosis Rigidity and consolidation of a joint.

annulus Dense, fibrous ring surrounding the tympanic membrane.

anonychia Complete absence of the nail.

anorexia Loss of appetite.

anosmia Inability to smell.

anterior triangle Landmark on the neck formed by the edge of the mandible (superiorly), the sternocleidomastoid muscle (laterally), and the midline of the trachea (medially). Used to describe the location of physical findings.

anuria Absence of excretion of urine.

anxiety Motor tension, autonomic hyperactivity, apprehension, or hyperattentivenss.

aortic valve Heart valve separating the left ventricle from the aorta.

aphasia Dysfunction or loss of the ability to express thoughts by speech, writing, symbols, or signs. *Fluent aphasia:* ability to produce words but with frequent errors in the choice of appropriate words or in the creation of words. *Nonfluent aphasia:* inability to produce words, either in spoken or written form.

apical impulse Pulsation of the apex of the heart against the chest wall, normally at the fifth left intercostal space in the midclavicular line.

Apley's sign Pain, locking of the knee, or clicking evoked with rotation of a flexed knee. Positive sign is indicative of a loose object in the knee (cartilage) that occurs with a torn meniscus.

apnea Cessation of breathing in the end-expiratory position.

apraxia Impairment of the ability to carry out purposeful skilled acts despite an intact sensory and motor system, such as an inability to draw or construct forms of two or three dimensions.

aqueous humor Fluid secreted in the ciliary body, which is found in the anterior chamber of the eye.

arcus senilis Grayish to gray-white, opaque arc or halo surrounding the cornea; generally occurs in individuals older than 50 years.

areolae Pigmented areas surrounding the nipples. Their color varies from pink to brown.

arrhythmia Any deviation from the normal pace of the heart. Kinds of arrhythmias include atrial fibrillation, atrial flutter, heart block, premature atrial contraction, and sinus arrhythmia.

arterial insufficiency Inadequate supply of blood by way of the arteries to peripheral areas.

arterial pressure Force exerted by the blood against the arterial walls.

arteriosclerosis Common arterial disorder characterized by hardening, thickening, loss of elasticity, and calcification of arterial walls, resulting in a decreased blood supply, especially to the cerebrum and the lower extremities.

arteritis Inflammatory condition of the inner layers or the outer coat of one or more arteries.

arthralgia Any pain that affects a joint.

arthritis Inflammation of a joint.

ascites Abnormal accumulation of fluid containing large amounts of protein and electrolytes within the abdominal cavity.

asthma Paroxysmal dyspnea (wheezing) resulting from obstruction of the bronchi or spasm of smooth muscle.

astigmatism Condition involving irregularity of the spherical curve of the cornea in which light rays cannot be focused in a point on the retina.

ataxia Impairment of coordination of muscular activity.

atelectasis Incomplete expansion of a lung compromised since birth; collapse of the adult lung.

atherosclerosis Type of arteriosclerosis characterized by deposits (atheromas) of cholesterol, lipoid material, and lipophages in the walls of large arteries and arterioles. This condition usually occurs with aging and is often associated with obesity, hypertension, and diabetes.

atony (atonic) Weak; lacking normal tone.

atrioventricular (AV) block Impairment of impulse conduction from the atria to the ventricles that occurs at the AV node or the bundle of His (or its branches).

atrioventricular (AV) valves Valves in the heart through which blood flows from the atria to the ventricles. The left AV valve is the mitral valve. The right AV valve is the tricuspid valve.

atrium (*pl,* atria) One of the two upper chambers of the heart. The right atrium receives deoxygenated blood from the superior and inferior vena cavae. The left atrium receives oxygenated blood from the pulmonary veins.

atrophy Wasting; decrease in the size of a cell, tissue, organ, or body part.

auditory ossicles Series of three small bones (malleus, incus, stapes) that extend across the middle ear.

augmentation Technique used to reinforce expression of deep tendon reflexes. The individual isometrically tenses muscles not directly involved in the reflex arc.

auricle External ear; also called pinna.

auscultation Examination technique done by listening, usually through a stethoscope.

autonomic nervous system Part of the peripheral nervous system that regulates involuntary vital function, including the activity of the cardiac muscle, the smooth muscle, and the glands. It has two divisions: (1) the sympathetic nervous system accelerates heart rate, constricts blood vessels, and raises blood pressure; (2) the parasympathetic nervous system slows heart rate, increases intestinal peristalsis and gland activity, and relaxes sphincters.

axillary tail of Spence Anatomical projection of breast tissue into the axilla.

axon Cylindrical extension of a nerve cell that conducts impulses away from the neuron cell body.

Baker's cyst Swelling in the popliteal space resulting from herniation of the synovial membrane of the knee.

ballottement Palpation technique used to assess a floating object. Fluid-filled tissue is pushed toward the examiner's hand so that the object will float against the examiner's fingers.

basal cell skin cancer Nodular, translucent lesions with small blood vessels often seen inside the nodule.

behavior Any observable, recordable, and measurable move, response, or act (verbal or nonverbal) of an individual.

bigeminal, bigeminy Pattern of arrhythmia consisting of coupled or paired ventricular beats; alternating QRS complexes are ventricular premature depolarizations.

bigeminal pulse Abnormal pulse in which two beats in close succession are followed by a pause during which no pulse is felt.

bipolar disorder Affective or mood disorder characterized by periods of mania alternating with periods of depression, with normal mood intervals occurring between the two.

bitemporal hemianopsia Loss of vision in both temporal fields of vision.

blepharitis Inflammation of the eyelid margins.

body image A person's subjective concept of his or her physical appearance.

body language The conveyance of messages by movements or gestures of the body or limbs, facial expressions, and eye contact. Body posture may convey a variety of emotions, including anger, anxiety, boredom, attention, or indifference.

borborygmi Audible bowel sounds, generally caused by gas propulsion through the intestine.

bounding pulse Pulse that, on palpation, feels full and spring-like because of an increased thrust of cardiac contraction or an increased volume of circulating blood within the elastic structures of the vascular system.

bradycardia Circulatory condition in which the myocardium contracts steadily but at a rate of less than 50 beats per minute.

bradypnea Abnormally slow rate of breathing.

brain stem Portion of the brain that comprises the medulla oblongata, the pons, and the mesencephalon. It performs motor, sensory, and reflex functions and contains the corticospinal and the reticulospinal tracts. The 12 pairs of cranial nerves arise mainly from the brainstem.

Braxton Hicks contraction Irregular tightening of the uterus that begins in the first trimester and increases in frequency, duration, and intensity as the pregnancy advances.

bronchiectasis Chronic dilation of one or more bronchi.

bronchioles Small airways of the respiratory system extending from the bronchi into the lobes of the lungs.

bronchitis Inflammation of one or more bronchi; condition may be chronic or acute.

bronchophony Sound of the voice as heard with abnormally increased clarity and intensity through the stethoscope over the lung parenchyma in an area of consolidation.

bronchovesicular Related to breath sounds from bronchial tubes and alveoli.

bruit Murmur or blowing sound heard over the peripheral vessels, indicating increased flow or stenosis of the vessel.

bruxism Compulsive, unconscious grinding of the teeth, especially during sleep.

buccal Pertaining to the cheek.

buffalo hump Accumulation of fat on the back of the neck associated with the prolonged use of large doses of glucocorticoids or the hypersecretion of cortisol caused by Cushing's syndrome.

bursa Sac or saclike cavity filled with fluid and located in sites where friction would otherwise develop, such as in a joint or over a bony prominence.

bursitis Inflammation of a bursa.

caput succedaneum Localized pitting edema in the scalp of a newborn that may overlie the sutures of the skull.

caries Decay of the calcified protein of teeth.

carpal tunnel syndrome Entrapment of the median nerve in the carpal tunnel, resulting in paresthesia, pain, and muscle weakness.

caruncle Small, fleshy projection located at the inner canthus of the eye.

cataplexy Condition characterized by sudden muscular weakness and hypotonia, caused by emotions, such as anger, fear, or surprise; often associated with narcolepsy.

cataract Opacity in the lens that gradually impairs vision over time.

caudad Toward the tail or end of the body; away from the head.

central sleep apnea Form of sleep apnea resulting from a decreased respiratory center output. Characterized by cessation of both airflow and respiratory movements.

cephalad Toward the head; away from the tail or end.

cephalhematoma Swelling caused by subcutaneous bleeding and accumulation of blood in the scalp of a newborn; usually the result of birth trauma.

cerebellum Part of the brain located in the posterior cranial fossa behind the brainstem. Its functions are concerned with coordinating voluntary muscular activity.

cerebrum Largest part of the brain, consisting of the right and left cerebral hemispheres. Its many functions include movement, sensation, learning, and memory.

cerumen Earwax produced by the apocrine and sebaceous glands within the ear canal.

chalazion Sebaceous cyst on the eyelid that is formed by distention of a meibomian gland.

cherry angiomas Benign, bright red, small, dome-shaped skin lesion.

chief complaint or concern The major reason for seeking care stated in the client's own words.

chloasma Tan or brown pigmentation, particularly of the forehead, cheeks, and nose.

choana Funnel-shaped channel.

cholesterol Fat-soluble crystalline steroid alcohol found in animal fat, oil, and egg yolk. Increased levels of serum cholesterol may be associated with the pathogenesis of atherosclerosis.

chordae tendineae Strands of tendon attaching the atrioventricular valves to the papillary muscles at the heart.

chorionic Pertaining to the chorion, a fetal membrane composed of trophoblast that forms the fetal portion of the placenta.

choroid Thin, highly vascular membrane covering the posterior five sixths of the eye, located between the retina and the sclera.

chronic obstructive pulmonary disease General term for disease involving airway obstruction, such as chronic bronchitis, emphysema, or asthma.

Chvostek's sign Spasm of the facial muscle evoked by tapping branches of the facial nerve; may be caused by hypocalcemia or hypomagnesemia.

ciliary body Thickened part of the vascular tunic of the eye that joins the iris with the anterior portion of the choroid; produces aqueous humor and regulates its outflow.

ciliary movement Waving motion of the hairlike processes projecting from the epithelium of the respiratory tract.

circadian pattern (circadian rhythm) Cyclical pattern of period based on a 24-hour cycle, especially the repetition of certain physiological phenomena, such as sleeping and walking.

circumduction Circular movement.

cirrhosis Disease characterized by destruction of liver parenchyma. The affected liver is characterized by fibrous tissue and yellow-tan nodules.

claudication Weakness of the legs accompanied by cramplike pains in the calves, caused by poor circulation of the blood to the leg muscles. This condition is exacerbated by walking.

clubbing Proliferation of soft tissue of the terminal phalanges, generally associated with relative hypoxia of peripheral tissues, loss of the angle between the skin and the nail base, and sponginess of the nail base.

coarctation Tightening or compression of the walls of a vessel, producing a narrowed lumen.

cochlea Conical bony structure of the inner ear, perforated by numerous apertures for passage of the chochlear division of the acoustic nerve.

cognitive Pertaining to the mental processes of knowing, thinking, learning, and judging.

colic Acute abdominal pain associated with smooth muscle contraction of the gastrointestinal tract.

colitis Inflammation of the colon.

concha Body structure that is shell shaped, such as the cavity in the external ear that surrounds the external auditory meatus.

conduction Process in which heat is transferred from one substance to another because of a difference in temperature.

conductive hearing loss Diminished ability to hear caused by the inability of vibrations to travel to or through the inner ear to an intact auditory nerve.

condyloma (condylomata acuminata) Hyperkeratotic exophytic lesions of stratified squamous epithelium; these develop as small, elevated, soft nodules that enlarge and coalesce to become cauliflower-like excrescences.

confabulation Fabrication of facts or events in response to questions about situations that are not recalled because of memory impairment.

congenital Present at birth.

conjunctiva Mucous membrane that lines the inner surfaces of the eyelids and the anterior part of the sclera.

conjunctivitis Inflammation of the conjunctiva.

consensual reaction Constriction of the pupil of one eye when the other eye is being stimulated by light.

consolidation Process in which liquid or solid replacement of lung parenchyma as exudate from an inflammatory condition is amassed.

constipation Infrequent or difficult evacuation of feces; often associated with drying and hardening of the stool.

contour Surface outline or shape of the part being described.

contracting A contract is an oral or written agreement between the provider and client that makes explicit the expectations of each party.

contractures Abnormal, usually permanent condition of a joint, characterized by flexion and fixation and caused by atrophy and shortening of muscle fibers or loss of the normal elasticity of the skin.

convection Transfer of heat through a gas or liquid by the circulation of heated particles.

convergence Coordinated medial movement of the eyes in fixing on a near object.

Cooper's ligaments Suspensory ligaments of the breast.

cor pulmonale Right-sided heart hypertrophy and right ventricular failure resulting from pulmonary hypertension.

cornea Convex, transparent anterior part of the eye that makes up one sixth of the outermost tunic of the eye bulb.

cornu Any horn-shaped structure.

coronary artery disease Any one of the abnormal conditions that may affect the arteries of the heart and produce various pathological effects, especially the reduced flow of oxygen and nutrients to the myocardium.

corticotropic Of or pertaining to stimulation of the adrenal cortex.

crackles Discrete, noncontinuous sound resembling fine crackling, radio static, or hairs being rubbed together as heard through a stethoscope; generally produced by air bubbling through an exudate.

cramp Involuntary, painful skeletal muscle contraction.

crepitus (crepitation) Dry, crackling sounding (1) the lung, when air passes through abnormally accumulated moisture; (2) the joints, when dry synovial surfaces rub together, and (3) the skin, when air is present subdermally.

cretinism Disease caused by congenital lack of thyroid hormone; characterized by retarded physical and mental development, deafness, dystrophy of bones and soft tissue, and abnormally low concentrations of thyroid hormones.

cribriform Perforated, like a sieve.

crisis Sudden change in the course of a disease.

cryptorchidism Failure of one or both of the testicles to descend into the scrotum.

cue Something that is noted by using the five senses (taste, touch, smell, sight, and hearing). A cue can be either subjective data or objective data.

culture Complex, integrated system that includes knowledge, beliefs, skills, art, morals, law, customs, and any other acquired habits and capabilities of a group of people.

cupping Increased posterior curvature of the optic disc caused by the increased intraocular pressure of glaucoma, which gradually exerts pressure posteriorly against the optic disc.

cyanosis Dusky blue color of the skin and mucous membranes, seen especially in the lips and nail beds, caused by an excess of deoxygenated hemoglobin in the blood (saturation less than 75% to 85% or PaO_2 less than 50 mm Hg), or a structural defect in the hemoglobin molecule.

cystocele Herniation of the urinary bladder into the anterior vaginal wall.

dacryoadenitis Inflammation of the lacrimal gland.

dacryocystitis Inflammation of the lacrimal sac.

decidua Endometrium during pregnancy that is shed in the postpartum period.

defervescence The diminishing or disappearance of a fever.

defining characteristics Signs and symptoms that help to confirm a diagnosis.

delirium Clouded state of consciousness; reduction in clarity of awareness of the environment accompanied by a reduced capacity to shift, focus, and sustain attention to environmental stimuli.

delusion False belief that is improbable in nature; not influenced by contrary experience or related to the client's cultural and educational background.

dementia Loss of cognitive abilities of sufficient magnitude to interfere with social or occupational functioning. It involves impairment of memory, abstract thinking, or judgment or other disturbance of high cortical function.

dendrite Branching process that extends from the cell body of a neuron. Each neuron usually possesses several dendrites, which receive impulses that are conducted to the cell body.

depression Term used to define (1) a mood, (2) a syndrome, and (3) an illness. The mood of depression is described as dejection and lowering of functional activity; it is a normal experience that may be incurred in response to frustration and loss. The syndrome of depression includes a depressed mood in combination with one or more of the following symptoms: inability to concentrate, anorexia, weight loss, and suicidal ideas. The illness of depression is characterized by the syndrome of depression but lasts longer. Related functional impairment may include the inability to carry on daily activities, particularly work.

dermatome Area on the surface of a body innervated by afferent fibers from one spinal root.

detrusor Bladder muscle.

dextrocardia Rare condition in which the position of the heart is reversed and lies on the right side of the chest.

diagnostic Pertaining to the identification of a disease or condition by a scientific evaluation of physical signs, symptoms, history, laboratory tests, and procedures.

diarrhea Increased frequency and liquid content of fecal evacuation.

diastasis recti abdominis Separation of the two rectus muscles along the median line of the abdominal wall. May occur as a result of pregnancy or obesity.

diastolic (diastole) The force of blood against the arterial wall during the filling phase of the cardiac cycle, and the time between contractions of the atria or the ventricles during which the blood enters the relaxed chambers.

dicrotic match Interval between the two peaks of a dicrotic pulse.

dicrotic pulse Presence of two sphygmographic waves to one beat of the pulse.

diplopia Double vision; simultaneous perception of two images for a single object.

disease Abnormality of structure or function that has a single pathogenic mechanism and a predictable course.

disorientation Lack of awareness as to time, place, or person.

dorsiflexion Backward bending.

dullness Decreased resonance on percussion, such as percussion sound produced over the liver.

dysarthria Difficult, poorly articulated speech.

dyschezia Painful defecation.

dyscoria Abnormality in the shape of the pupil.

dyslexia Disturbance in understanding the written word; difficulty in reading.

dysmenorrhea Painful menstruation.

dyspareunia Difficult or painful sexual intercourse in women.

dyspepsia Impairment of the ability to digest food, especially discomfort after eating a meal.

dysphagia Difficult or painful swallowing.

dysplasia Disorder in the size, shape, or organization of adult cells; any abnormal development of tissues or organs.

dyspnea Difficult or labored respiration; shortness of breath.

dyssynergia Inability to perform movements smoothly or an impairment in muscle coordination.

dysuria Difficult or painful urination.

ecchymosis Discoloration of an area of the skin or mucous membranes caused by the extravasation of blood into the subcutaneous tissues as a result of trauma to the underlying blood vessels or fragility of the vessel walls.

ecogram Diagram that maps the network of significant others, including friends, neighbors, peers, and associates.

ectocervix The outside portion of the cervix.

ectomorph A person whose physique is characterized by slenderness, fragility, and predominance of structures derived from the ectoderm.

ectopic pregnancy Abnormal pregnancy in which the conceptus implants outside the uterine cavity.

ectropion Turning outward of the lower lid of the eye.

edema Abnormal increase in the quantity of interstitial fluid.

efferent neuron Any neuron that transmits nerve impulses from the central nervous system toward the periphery (motor).

egophony Voice sound of a nasal or bleating quality, as heard through a stethoscope; often defined by asking the client to say "ee," which sound like "ay" in an area of consolidation.

ejection click High-pitched clicking sound produced by the forceful opening of a diseased aortic or pulmonic valve, heard soon after the first heart sound.

embolism Sudden obstruction of an artery by a clot or other foreign substance. Symptoms vary with the degree of occlusion that the embolism causes, the character of the embolus, and the size, nature, and location of the occluded vessel.

embolus Foreign object, quantity of air or gas, bit of tissue or tumor, or piece of thrombus that circulates in the bloodstream until it becomes lodged in a vessel.

emphysema Condition involving entrapment of air within tissue, either interstitial or pulmonary. *Pulmonary emphysema,* or chronic obstructive pulmonary disease, results from permanent dilation of enlargement of the passages peripheral to the terminal bronchiole, which causes increased resistance to airflow. *Interstitial emphysema* is the presence of air in the subcutaneous tissue mediastinum or connective tissue of the lung resulting from air leakage through a damaged portion of the respiratory passages or alveoli; may result in swelling of tissue or a distinctive crackling sound called crepitation.

enculturation Process of acquiring one's cultural identity as it is transmitted by the previous generation.

endocardium Lining of the heart chambers.

endocervical Pertaining to the inside of the cervix.

endocervix Membrane lining the canal of the uterine cervix.

endolymph Fluid found in the membranous labyrinth of the internal ear.

endometriosis Presence of endometrial stroma and glands in ectopic locations, such as the ovaries, pelvic peritoneum, or colon.

endomorph A person whose body build is characterized by a soft, round physique with a large trunk and thighs, tapering extremities, an accumulation of fat throughout the body, and a predominance of structures derived from the endoderm.

enophthalmos Recession of the globe of the eye within the orbit.

enterocele Herniation of the intestine into the vagina.

entropion Turning inward of the lower lid of the eye.

enuresis Involuntary urination.

epicardium The visceral part of pericardium that closely envelops the heart; also called the visceral pericardium.

epiphora Tearing that results from faulty drainage of the eyes.

episiotomy Surgical procedure in which an incision is made in a woman's perineum to enlarge her vaginal opening for delivery.

epispadias Congenital anomaly in which the urethra opens on the dorsum of the penis.

epistaxis Bleeding or hemorrhage from the nose.

epulis Any tumor or growth on the gingiva.

equilibrium Ongoing process of maintaining the orientation and position of the body in relationship to the ground and in space.

erythema Dilation of capillaries, resulting in redness of the skin.

esophoria Deviation of the visual axis of one eye toward that of the other eye that occurs in the absence of visual stimuli for fusion.

esotropia Strabismus characterized by an inward deviation of one eye relative to the other eye.

essential hypertension Elevated arterial pressure for which no cause can be found and that is often the only significant clinical finding.

ethnic group Group of persons with shared traits, such as common national or regional origin and linguistic, ancestral, and physical characteristics.

ethnocentrism Tendency to view people unconsciously by using one's group and one's own customs as the standard for all judgments.

euphoria False sense of elation or well-being; pathological elevation of mood. This condition is most notable in clients who are experiencing the manic phase of bipolar disorder.

eustachian tube Cartilaginous and bony passage between the nasopharynx and the middle ear that allows equalization of air pressure between the middle ear and the external environment.

evaporation The change of a substance from a solid or liquid state to a gaseous state. The process of evaporation is hastened by an increase in temperature and a decrease in atmospheric pressure.

eversion Turning outward or inside out, as of the eyelid.

exophoria Deviation of the visual axis of one eye away from that of the other eye that occurs in the absence of visual stimuli for fusion.

exophthalmos Abnormal condition characterized by a marked protrusion of the eyeballs.

exostosis Abnormal benign growth on the surface of a bone.

exotropia Strabismus characterized by the outward deviation of one eye relative to the other.

extension Straightening of a limb so that the joint angle is increased.

external rotation Turning of a body part away from the central axis or midline of the body.

extinction Loss of touch perception on one side of the body.

extrapyramidal system Tract of motor nerves from the brain to the anterior horns of the spinal cord, except for the fibers of the pyramidal tract. It controls and coordinates the postural, static, supporting, and locomotor mechanisms and causes contractions of muscle groups in sequence or simultaneously.

extrasystole Cardiac contraction that is abnormal in timing or in origin of impulse; premature contraction of the heart.

facial nerve (CN VII) Cranial nerve that innervates the scalp, forehead, eyelids, muscles of facial expression, cheeks, and jaw.

fasciculation Observable, localized, uncoordinated, uncontrollable twitching movements resulting from contraction of a fasciculus (bundle of muscle fibers) served by one anterior horn cell; usually does not cause movement of a joint.

fever Pyrexia; elevation of the body temperature above normal for a given individual.

fibrillation Fine, continuous twitching caused by irregular, random contraction of a single muscle or group of fibers. Fibrillation of a chamber of the heart results in inefficient random contraction of that chamber and disruption of the normal sinus rhythm of the heart. This condition is usually described by the part that is contracting abnormally (e.g., atrial fibrillation or ventricular fibrillation). Atrial fibrillation is usually benign; ventricular fibrillation can be life-threatening.

fibroadenoma Benign tumor composed of dense epithelial and fibroblastic tissue. A fibroadenoma of the breast is nontender, encapsulated, round, movable, and firm.

fibromyositis Any one of a large number of disorders in which the common element is stiffness and joint or muscle pain accompanied by localized inflammation of the muscle tissues and of the fibrous connective tissues.

field of vision Area simultaneously visible to a motionless eye.

fist percussion Striking the body with the lateral aspect of the hand to elicit pain or tenderness.

flatulence Presence of an excessive amount of gas in the gastrointestinal tract.

flexion Bending of a joint so that the joint angle is decreased.

flight of ideas Nearly continuous flow of rapid speech with abrupt changes from topic to topic. This condition is noted most frequently in organic mental disorders, schizophrenia, and psychotic disorders and as a reaction to stress.

floaters Spots that appear to drift in front of the eye and are caused by a shadow cast on the retina by vitreous debris.

fornix Archlike structure of space.

fourchette Tense band of membranes connecting the posterior angle of the vagina to the posterior ends of the labia minora.

fovea centralis Central spot of color vision on the retina that contains only cones and no rods.

fremitus Palpable vibration.

frenulum Restraining portion or structure. An example is the sublingual frenulum.

friction rub Crackling, grating sound as heard through a stethoscope when two inflamed, roughened surfaces rub together.

fundus The base or deepest part of any organ.

gait Manner of progression in walking. In *ataxic gait* the foot is raised high and the sole strikes down suddenly.

gallop rhythm Heart rate characterized by three sounds.

ganglia Type of nerve cell, chiefly collected in groups outside the central nervous system. Individual cells and very small groups abound in association with alimentary organs.

genogram Diagram that depicts family relationships over at least three generations.

gigantism Excessive growth of the body or its parts; may be a result of hypersecretion of growth hormone in childhood.

gingivitis Inflammation of the papillary and marginal gingiva.

glans Small, rounded mass. *Glans penis:* caplike, conical tip of the penis that covers the end of the corpora cavernosa penis and the corpus spongiosum.

glaucoma Ocular disease in which increased intraocular pressure causes atrophy and excavation of the optic nerve, producing visual field defects.

goiter Increase in size of the thyroid gland.

goniometer Instrument used to measure joint angles.

gout Disease caused by deposition of crystals of monosodium urate; characterized by a disorder in purine metabolism and associated with exacerbations of arthritis of a single joint.

graphesthesia Ability to identify letters or numbers inscribed with a blunt object on the palm of the hand, back, or other areas. Higher cortical integration is required to perform this function.

grasp reflex Normal reflex in young infants elicited by stroking the infant's palms; the examiner's fingers are grasped so firmly that the child can be lifted into the air. (In older individuals the tonic grasp reflex is pathological, occurring in diseases of the premotor cortex.)

Grey Turner's sign Bruising of the flank skin.

gynecomastia Hypertrophy of breast tissue in a male subject.

health history Comprehensive body of information obtained from the client and other select sources. Includes information on the client as a whole, the health/illness status (past and present), the social and physical environment, and past interactions with health care systems.

Heberden's nodes (nodules) Small, hard nodules of the terminal interphalangeal joints, associated with osteoarthritis.

helix Superior and posterior free margin of the ear.

hematemesis Vomiting of blood.

hematopoiesis Relating to the formation and development of blood cells in the bone marrow.

hematuria Presence of blood in the urine.

hemianopsia Defective vision or blindness in one half of the visual field.

hemoptysis Spitting or coughing up of blood from the respiratory tract.

hemorrhoid Dilation of a part of the venous hemorrhoidal plexus in the mucosal membrane of the rectum. A hemorrhoid may occur as a result of increased hydrostatic pressure in the venous system, such as in pregnancy, or from disease that causes portal hypertension and straining at stool. *Internal hemorrhoids:* varicosity of superior or middle hemorrhoidal veins below the anal mucosa; may result in bleeding. *External hemorrhoid:* varicosity of the inferior hemorrhoidal vein under the anal skin; may cause pain and swelling around the anal sphincter and itching and bleeding.

hepatomegaly Abnormal enlargement of the liver, usually a sign of liver disease.

hernia Abnormal protrusion of an organ or tissue through an opening. *Incarcerated hernia:* protrusion of abdominal contents through a weakness in the abdominal wall so that the contents cannot be returned to the abdominal cavity. *Direct inguinal hernia:* protrusion of abdominal contents through a weakness in the abdominal musculature in the region of Hesselbach's triangle. *Indirect inguinal hernia:* protrusion (generally indirect) of abdominal contents into the scrotal sac. *Strangulated hernia:* hernia in which the blood supply to the protruded tissue is obstructed.

herpes zoster Acute infection caused by the varicella-zoster virus, affecting primarily adults and characterized by the development of painful vesicular skin eruptions that follow the underlying route of cranial or spinal nerves inflamed by the virus.

hertz (Hz) Unit of frequency of a periodic process equal to 1 cycle per second.

high-density lipoprotein (HDL) Plasma protein containing about 50% protein with cholesterol and triglycerides. It may serve to stabilize very low-density lipoprotein. Called "good" cholesterol, it is involved in transporting cholesterol and other lipids from the plasma to the tissues.

hirsutism Excessive hairiness, especially in females.

homeostasis Relative constancy in the internal environment of the body, naturally maintained by adaptive responses that promote healthy survival.

homonymous Having the same name.

homonymous hemianopsia Blindness or defective vision in the right or left half of the visual field of both eyes.

hordeolum Inflammation of a sebaceous gland of the eyelid; sty.

horn Projection or protuberance of a body structure. Examples include the gray horns of the spinal cord, horn of the hyoid bone, and iliac horn.

hydrocele Circumscribed collection of fluid, particularly in the scrotum.

hypercholesterolemia Condition in which greater than normal amounts of cholesterol are present in the blood. Higher levels of cholesterol and other lipids may lead to the development of atherosclerosis.

hyperesthesia Abnormally increased sensitivity of one of the body's sense organs, such as pain or touch receptors in the skin.

hyperlipidemia Excess of lipids in the plasma.

hyperopia Farsightedness.

hyperplasia Increase in the number of cells in a body part.

hyperpnea Increased depth of respiration with or without an increase in rate.

hypersomnia (1) Sleep of excessive depth or abnormal duration; (2) extreme drowsiness, often associated with lethargy; (3) a condition characterized by periods of deep, long sleep.

hypertension Common, often asymptomatic disorder characterized by elevated blood pressure that persistently exceeds 140/90 mm Hg.

hyperventilation Increase in rate and depth of respiration.

hyphema Blood in the anterior chamber of the eye.

hypoesthesia Abnormal weakness of sensation in response to stimulation of the sensory nerves.

hypopyon Purulent material in the anterior chamber of the eye.

hyposmia Diminished sense of smell.

hypospadias Developmental anomaly in which the urethra opens on the underside of the penis.

hypotension Abnormal condition in which the blood pressure is not adequate for normal perfusion and oxygenation of the tissues.

hypotonia Decrease in body tonus.

idiopathic Without a known cause.

immediate (direct) percussion Use of the finger or hand to strike the body to evaluate the sound waves produced.

incontinence Failure of control of excretory functions.

incus One of the three ossicles of the inner ear, resembling an anvil. It communicates sound vibrations from the malleus to the stapes.

infarction Obstruction of circulation followed by ischemic necrosis.

inference How one perceives or interprets a cue.

insomnia Chronic inability to sleep or to remain asleep throughout the night; wakefulness; sleeplessness.

inspection Visual evaluation of the body that incorporates the senses of sight, smell, and hearing.

instrumental activities of daily living (IADLs) Life management skills of telephoning, reading, leisure, medication management, money management, transportation, shopping, meal preparation, laundering, housekeeping, home maintenance, etc.

insufficiency Inadequate closure of a heart valve, resulting in backflow of blood into the ventricles or atria.

intensity Loudness of sound.

intercostal space Space between two ribs.

intermittent claudication *Claudication* is a weakness of the legs accompanied by cramplike pains in the calves caused by poor circulation to the leg muscles. *Intermittent claudication* is a form of this disorder that is manifested only at certain times, usually after an extended period of walking, and is relieved by a period of rest.

internal rotation Turning of the body part toward the central axis or midline of the body.

interpersonal distance Distance between two individuals interacting that will vary by the nature of the relationship or cultural practices.

interpretation Sharing the meaning of the facts provided so that the client has an opportunity to confirm, deny, or offer an alternative explanation.

intertrigo (intertriginous) Erythematous irritation in areas where two skin surfaces come together, such as the groin area or the folds between large, pendulous breasts.

intraepithelian Within the epithelium.

introitus Entrance or orifice to a cavity or a hollow tubular structure of the body.

inversion (1) Turning inward. (2) Invagination or depression of the nipple's central portion. Can occur congenitally or as a response to an invasive process.

ipsilateral Pertaining to the same side of the body.

iridescent vision Perception of halos around lights, particularly with corneal edema.

iritis Inflammation of the iris.

ischial spines The two relatively sharp bony projections into the pelvic outlet from the ischial bones that form the lower border of the pelvis.

isolated systolic hypertension Systolic blood pressure greater than 160 mm Hg and normal diastolic blood pressure.

jaundice Accumulation of bilirubin-to-serum concentration greater than 2 mg/dl; produces yellow-green to bronze color of skin and itching.

jugular venous pulse Pulse wave in the jugular veins reflecting cardiac activity on the right side of the heart.

keloid Scar formation caused by a dense overgrowth of fibrous tissue, usually raised and thickened.

keratinization Process by which epithelial cells exposed to the external environment lose their moisture and are replaced by horny tissue.

kinesthetic sensation Feeling facilitated by the proprioceptive receptors in the muscles, tendons, and joints.

Korotkoff sounds Turbulent sounds heard when auscultating the blood pressure.

Kussmaul respiration Rapid and deep respiratory cycles resulting from stimulation of the medullary respiratory center in metabolic acidosis; associated with a pH less than 7.2 in diabetic ketoacidosis.

kyphosis Increased posterior convexity of the spine (humpback).

labile Readily altered, unstable.

labyrinth Intricate communicating passageway, such as the bony and membranous labyrinths of the inner ear.

lacrimation Production of tears, especially in excess.

laminar flow Airflow that is concentrated into a narrow pathway.

lens Transparent biconvex structure located behind the pupil and in front of the vitreous body.

lentigines Flat, tan to brown macules located in sun-exposed surfaces.

leukorrhea White discharge from the vagina.

lichen planus Nonmalignant, chronic, pruritic skin condition characterized by small, flat, purplish papules or plaques. The cause is unknown.

lid lag Condition in which the eyelid margin is above the limbus and some sclera is visible; it may indicate thyroid disease.

limbus Edge of the cornea at the point where it meets the sclera.

linea nigra Pigmentation of the linea alba, the tendinous median line on the anterior abdominal wall, during pregnancy.

lineae albicantes (striae) Atrophic lines or streaks that differ in texture and color from the surrounding skin and are caused by disrupted elastic fibers of the reticular layer of the skin.

lithotomy position Position assumed by the patient lying supine with the hips and the knees flexed and the thighs abducted and rotated externally.

lobes Glandular tissue units in the breast situated in a circular, spokelike fashion.

lobule Small lobe, such as the soft, pendulous lower part of the external ear.

lordosis Anterior concavity of the lumbar spine (swayback, saddleback).

low-density lipoprotein (LDL) Plasma protein containing relatively more cholesterol and triglycerides than protein. Called "bad" cholesterol, it is involved with the formation of atherosclerotic plaques.

lower motor neuron Peripheral neuron with a motor (efferent) function. Its cell body is located in the anterior horns of the spinal cord or brainstem nuclei, and it terminates in skeletal muscles.

lumpectomy Surgical excision of a tumor without removal of large amounts of surrounding tissue or adjacent lymph nodes.

luxation Dislocation.

lymphadenopathy Any disorder of the lymph nodes or lymph vessels.

macula Area of the retina where the receptors for color vision are most concentrated; located temporal to the optic disc.

malaise Feeling of general discomfort or uneasiness.

malleus One of the three ossicles of the middle ear; resembles a hammer; connected to the tympanic membrane.

mammary folds Crescent-shaped ridges of breast tissue found at the inferior portions of very large or pendulous breasts. May be confused with breast masses but are nonpathological.

mammography Radiography of the soft tissues of the breast to allow identification of various benign and malignant neoplastic processes.

mastication Chewing, tearing, or grinding food with the teeth while it becomes mixed with saliva.

mastisis Inflammation of breast tissue.

mastoid process Bony prominence of the posterior portion of the temporal bone, located posterior to the lower part of the auricle, serving as the attachment for various muscles, including the sternocleidomastoid.

McBurney's point Anatomical landmark located approximately 2 inches above the right anterosuperior iliac spine on a line between the umbilicus and the spine.

McMurray's sign Inability to extend the flexed knee may indicate a loose object in the knee (cartilage) due to a torn meniscus.

meatus Passage or opening, especially at the external portion of a canal.

mediastinum Portion of the thoracic cavity in the middle of the thorax, between the pleural sacs that contain the two lungs.

mediate (indirect) percussion Technique in which the middle finger of one hand strikes the middle finger of the other hand to emit a sound of vibration.

meibomian gland One of several sebaceous glands that secrete sebum from the ducts on the posterior margin of each eyelid. The glands are embedded in the tarsal plate of each eyelid.

melanocyte Body cell capable of producing melanin.

menarche First menstruation and commencement of cyclic menstrual function.

menopause Gradual cessation of the menses, usually occurring between 45 and 60 years of age.

menorrhagia Abnormally heavy or long menstrual periods.

mental status examination Record of current findings that includes a description of a client's appearance, behavior, motor activity, speech, alertness, mood, cognition, intelligence, reactions, views, and attitudes.

mesomorph A person whose physique is characterized by a predominance of muscle, bone, and connective tissue, structures that develop from the mesodermal layer of the embryo.

metrorrhagia Irregular and/or dysfunctional uterine bleeding.

microaneurysm Outpouching in the wall of a capillary that appears as a red dot on the retina.

middlescence Term for the years of middle adulthood.

migraine Recurring vascular headache characterized by a prodromal aura, unilateral onset, severe pain, photophobia, and autonomic disturbances during the acute phase, which may last for hours or days.

minority group Any group that receives different and unequal treatment from others in the larger group or society and whose members see themselves as victims of discrimination.

miosis Constriction of the pupil.

mitral regurgitation Backward flow of blood from the left ventricle to the left atrium associated with an incompetent mitral valve.

mitral valve Left atrioventricular valve.

mitral valve stenosis Fibrosis and thickening of the cusps of the mitral valve with narrowing of the aperture between the left atrium and the left ventricle.

mixed hearing loss Combination of conductive and sensorineural loss in the same ear.

mixed sleep apnea Condition marked by signs and symptoms of both central sleep apnea and obstructive sleep apnea.

Montgomery's glands Small sebaceous glands located on the areola.

morning sickness Nausea and vomiting occurring from the fifth or sixth week through the fourteenth to sixteenth week of pregnancy.

Moro reflex Normal mass reflex in a young infant elicited by a sudden loud noise resulting in flexion of the legs, an embracing posture of the arms, and usually a brief cry. Also called startle reflex.

morphology Study of the physical shape and size of a specimen, plant, or animal.

multiparous Having delivered one or more viable infants.

murmur Blowing sound caused by turbulence of blood flow; heard through the stethoscope over the heart; when heard in the great vessels, the sound is called a bruit.

Murphy's sign Sign noted by a maneuver done during deep palpation in the approximate location of the gallbladder. On deep inspiration, the liver descends, bringing the gallbladder in contact with the examiner's hand. Pain is elicited in the presence of cholecystitis.

mycelia Masses of interwoven, branched, threadlike filaments that make up most fungi.

mydriasis Dilation of the pupil.

myelination Development of the myelin sheath around a nerve fiber.

myocardial infarction Occlusion of a coronary artery caused by atherosclerosis or thrombosis, resulting in damage to the myocardium.

myocardium Thick, contractile middle layer of the heart; composed of muscle tissue that forms the bulk of this organ.

myopia Nearsightedness; condition in which parallel rays of light come to focus in front of the retina.

myxedema Hypothyroidism. Hypometabolism is present, and nonpitting edema results from the presence of hydrated mucopolysaccharides in connective tissue.

nabothian cysts Cystlike formations of the mucosa of the uterine cervix resulting from an accumulation of retained secretion in occluded glands.

narcolepsy Syndrome characterized by sudden sleep attacks, cataplexy, sleep paralysis, and visual or auditory hallucination at the onset of sleep.

nasolabial fold Crease in the skin extending from the angle of the nose to the corner of the mouth.

nausea Feeling that vomiting is impending.

neoplasia New and abnormal development of cells that may be benign or malignant.

neuromuscular spindle Any one of a number of small bundles of delicate muscular fibers, enclosed by a capsule, in which sensory nerve fibers terminate. Spindles vary in length from 0.8 to 5 mm, accommodating as many as four large myelinated nerve fibers that piece the capsule and lose their myelin sheaths.

nevus Well-demarcated, pigmented, congenital skin blemish that is usually benign but may become cancerous.

nicking Appearance of indentation of an optic vein where an arteriole crosses it.

night blindness Slow adjustment from bright to dim light.

nocturia Excessive urination at night.

nocturnal enuresis Urinary voiding during sleep.

nodularity Lumpiness.

nuchal Pertaining to the nape of the neck.

nuchal rigidity Pertaining to limited range of motion of the cervical spine, usually associated with pain.

nullipara (nulliparous) Woman who has not given birth to a viable offspring.

nursing diagnosis Statement that describes a client's health state, or response to illness, treatable by a nurse.

nystagmus Involuntary rhythmic motion of the eye; may be horizontal, vertical, rotary, or mixed.

obesity Condition in which the amount of fat in the body is excessive in relation to total body weight; exceeding 20% of ideal body weight.

obstipation Severe constipation.

obstructive sleep apnea Form of sleep apnea involving a physical obstruction of the upper airway.

oligomenorrhea Decreased frequency of menstruation with an interval of 38 to 90 days.

oliguria Abnormally decreased urine secretion (less than 400 ml/24 hr).

opening snap Snapping sound produced by the opening of a diseased mitral or tricuspid valve. It is an early diastolic sound heard soon after the second heart sound.

orchiopexy Operation in which an undescended testis is mobilized, brought into the scrotum, and attached so that it will not retract.

orientation Conscious awareness of person, place, and time.

orifice An opening.

oropharynx One of the three anatomical divisions of the pharynx. It extends behind the mouth from the soft palate (above) to the level of the hyoid bone (below) and contains the palatine tonsils and the lingual tonsils.

orthopnea Dyspnea that begins or increases when the client lies down, and is relieved by sitting upright.

orthostatic (postural) hypotension Lower blood pressure of greater than 30 mm Hg that occurs on rising from a lying or sitting to an erect position.

osteoporosis Disorder characterized by loss of bone density, occurring most frequently in postmenopausal women, in sedentary or immobilized individuals, and in persons on long-term steroid therapy.

ostium Orifice.

otalgia Earache.

palpation Examination technique that involves feeling or touching the object to be evaluated.

palpebra Eyelid.

palpebral fissure Opening between the margins of the upper and lower eyelids when the eye is open.

palpitation Pulsations of the heart and arteries that are perceptable to the client and are associated with normal emotional responses or with certain heart disorders.

papilledema Edema of the optic disc.

paranasal sinus One of the air cavities in various bones around the nose. Examples are the frontal sinus in the frontal bone lying deep to the medial part of the superciliary ridge and the maxillary sinus within the maxilla between the orbit, the nasal cavity, and the upper teeth.

paraphimosis Condition characterized by an inability to replace the foreskin in its normal position after it has been retracted behind the glans penis.

parenchyma Tissue of an organ as distinguished from supporting or connective tissue.

paresis Slight or incomplete paralysis; weakness.

paresthesia Abnormal or perverted sensation; may include burning, itching, pain, or a feeling of electric shock.

Parkinson's disease Progressive disorder of the basal ganglia, characterized by tremor, difficulty in initiating voluntary movements, muscle weakness and rigidity, and a peculiar gait.

paronychia Inflammation and infection of the folds of tissue surrounding a fingernail.

parous Having borne one or more visible offspring.

paroxysmal nocturnal dyspnea Sudden onset of dyspnea after a period of lying down. Sitting upright helps relieve the dyspnea.

pars flaccida Less taut portion of the tympanic membrane.

pars tensa Taut portion of the tympanic membrane.

passive range of motion Joint movement of the client that is produced by the examiner.

peau d'orange Orange-peel appearance of the breast caused by edema of the breast and resultant blocked lymph drainage.

pectus carinatum Structural deformity of the thoracic cage where the sternum is displaced anteriorly, increasing the anteroposterior diameter. The costal cartilages adjacent to the sternum are depressed.

pectus excavatum Structural deformity of the thoracic cage where the lower sternum is depressed. Compression of the heart and great vessels may cause murmurs.

perception Awareness of objects and relations that follows stimulation of the peripheral sense organs.

percussion Examination technique used to evaluate the size, borders, and consistency of certain internal organs and to determine the presence of and evaluate the amount of air and fluid in a body cavity. It involves listening to reverberation of tissue after striking the surface with short, sharp blows.

pericardium Fibrous sac that surrounds the heart and the roots of the great vessels.

periorbital edema Accumulation of fluid in the eyelids and other tissues surrounding the eye.

peritonitis Inflammation of the peritoneum.

petechiae Tiny purple or red spots that appear on the skin as a result of minute hemorrhages within the dermal or submucosal layers.

Peyronie's disease Disease of unknown cause resulting in fibrous induration of the corpora cavernosa of the penis. The chief symptom is painful erection.

phimosis Narrowness of the opening of the prepuce that causes difficulty in retraction of the foreskin of the penis.

phobia Persistent and exaggerated fear of a particular object or situation.

phoria Mild weakness of the extraocular muscle(s); appears as a deviation of the eye when fusion is suspended.

photophobia Abnormal sensitivity to light.

physiologic cup (physiologic depression) Small depression just temporal to the center of the optic disc.

pincer grasp The index finger in apposition to the thumb.

pinguecula Small, yellowish white subconjunctival elevation located between the corneoscleral limbus and the canthus.

pinna Projecting part of the external ear; the auricle.

pitch Quality of a tone or sound that is dependent on the relative rapidity of the vibrations by which it is produced.

pituitary dwarfism Condition of being abnormally small, especially small of stature due to a deficiency of growth hormone.

plantar flexion Bending of the foot toward the floor.

platypnea Respiratory distress that increases when a person is upright.

plethora Pertaining to a red, florid complexion.

pleural effusion Fluid of any kind in the pleural cavity.

pleurisy Pleural inflammation accompanied by pain.

polydipsia Excessive thirst.

polymenorrhea Abnormally frequency menstruation.

polyphagia Excessive ingestion of food.

polysomnography Multicomponent sleep study that monitors arterial oxygen saturation, brain waves (electroencephalogram [EEG]), eye movements (electrooculogram [EOG]), muscle tone and movements (electromyelogram [EMG]), intraesophageal pressure, inspiratory flow, and rib cage and abdominal circumference changes. The length of time slept, the total number of apneic periods, the number of apneic periods per hour, the percentage of apneic time, the mean duration of apneas, and the cumulative SaO_2 are calculated for each individual.

polyuria Excessive urinary excretion.

posterior triangle Landmark on the neck formed by the sternocleidomastoid muscle (laterally), the trapezius muscle (posteriorly), and the clavicle (inferiorly), used to describe the location of physical findings.

Poupart's ligament Inguinal ligament; the fibrous band that runs from the anterosuperior iliac spine to the pubic spine.

precordium Area of the anterior chest wall overlying the heart and the great vessels.

prepuce Foreskin.

presbycusis Age-related hearing loss.

presbyopia Decreased ability of the optic lens to accommodate to near vision with increasing age.

preterm infant Infant born before 37 weeks of gestation.

proctitis Inflammation of the rectal mucosa.

proctoscopy Examination of the rectum with a short cylindrical instrument called a proctoscope.

pronation (1) Assumption of the prone (face down) position; (2) turning the forearm so that the palm is posterior; or (3) eversion and abduction of the foot.

prostatitis Acute or chronic inflammation of the prostate gland, generally in conjunction with cystitis and urethritis. Symptoms include low back and perineal pain, fever, urinary frequency, and dysuria.

pruritus Itching.

pterygium Abnormal triangular thickening of the bulbar conjunctiva on the cornea, with the apex directed toward the pupil.

ptosis Drooping of the upper eyelid, often interfering with vision.

puberty The period of life at which the ability to reproduce begins.

pulmonic valve Heart valve separating the right ventricle from the pulmonary artery.

pulse Palpable, rhythmic expansion of an artery caused by ejection of blood from the left ventricle during systole.

pulse deficit Condition that exists when the periphera; pulse count is less than the ventricular rate taken at the apex of the heart. It indicates a lack of peripheral perfusion for some of the heart contractions.

pulse pressure The difference between the systolic and diastolic blood pressure.

pulsus alternans (alternating pulse) Pulse characterized by a regular alternation of weak and strong beats without changes in the length of the cycle.

pulsus bisferiens Arterial pulse that has two palpable peaks, the second of which is slightly stronger than the first.

pulsus paradoxus (paradoxical pulse) Abnormal decrease in systolic pressure and pulse-wave amplitude during inspiration. The normal fall in pressure is less than 10 mm Hg. An excessive decline may be a sign of precordial tamponade adhesive pericarditis, severe lung disease, advanced heart failure, or other conditions.

puncta Tiny apertures in the margins of each eyelid that open into the lacrimal ducts.

pupil Aperture in the iris that allows for the passage of light.

pyogenic Substance that tends to cause a rise in body temperature.

pyorrhea Purulent inflammation of the gums.

pyramidal tract Pathway composed of groups of nerve fibers in the white matter of the spinal cord through which motor impulses are conducted to the anterior horn cells from the opposite side of the brain. These descending fibers regulate the voluntary and reflex activity of the muscles through the anterior horn cells.

pyrexia Fever; elevation of the body temperature above normal for a given individual.

pyrosis Heartburn.

pyuria Presence of pus in the urine.

race Classification of human beings on the basis of physical characteristics, such as skin pigmentation, head form, or stature, that are transmitted through generations.

radiation Emission of energy, rays, or waves.

Raynaud's phenomenon Intermittent attacks of ischemia of the extremities, especially in fingers, toes, ears, and nose.

rectocele Herniation of the rectum into the posterior vaginal wall.

reflection Repeating a phrase or sentence the client has said. Allow a period of silence lasting at least 5 to 10 seconds to allow the client to think before answering a question or response to a suggestion; after 10 seconds without a response, the interviewer will need to initiate another question or suggestion.

reflex Involuntary functioning or movement of any organ or part of the body in response to a particular stimulus. The function or action occurs immediately, without the involvement of the will or consciousness.

regurgitation Backward flow of blood through a defective heart valve.

REM sleep Rapid eye movement sleep characterized by episodic bursts of rapid eye movements on the electrooculogram and by low-voltage, high-frequency waves on the electroencephalogram.

resonance Low-pitched, hollow sound produced over normal lung tissue when the chest is percussed.

reticular activating system Functional system in the brain that is essential for wakefulness, attention, concentration, and introspection. A network of nerve fibers in the thalamus, hypothalamus, brainstem, and cerebral cortex contribute to the system.

retina Delicate nervous tissue membrane of the eye that is continuous with the optic nerve; receives images of external objects and transmits visual impulses through the optic nerve to the brain.

retinal exudates White or yellow infiltrates that develop on the retina.

retraction (1) Condition of being drawn back. (2) Appears as a depression or pucker on the skin (also called dimpling). It usually is caused by the fibrotic shortening and immobilization of Cooper's ligament by an invasive process.

rhonchus Wheezing or snoring sound produced by airflow across a partially constricted air passage. *Sibilant rhonchus:* high-pitched wheeze produced in a small air passage. *Sonorous rhonchus:* low-pitched wheeze produced in a large air passage.

rigor Common term for shivering accompanying a chill or for muscle rigidity accompanying depletion of adenosine triphosphate, such as in death (rigor mortis).

Rinne test Test comparing air conduction and bone conduction through the use of a tuning fork. In normal hearing, air conduction sounds are heard longer than bone conduction sounds (positive Rinne).

rugated Having ridges or folds.

S_1 First heard sound in the cardiac cycle. It is associated with closure of the mitral and tricuspid valves and is synchronous with the apical pulse. Auscultated at the apex, it is louder, longer, and lower than the second sound (S_2), which follows it.

S_2 Second heart sound in the cardiac cycle. It is associated with closure of the aortic and pulmonary valves immediately before ventricular diastole. Auscultated at the base of the heart, the second sound is louder than the first.

S_3 Third heart sound; related to early ventricular filling. Normally, this sound is audible only in children and physically active young adults. In older people it is an abnormal finding and usually indicates myocardial failure.

S_4 Fourth heart sound; related to late ventricular filling. This sound occurs late in diastole on contraction of the atria. Rarely heard in normal clients, it indicates an abnormally increased resistance to ventricular filling, such as in hypertensive cardiovascular disease, coronary artery disease, myocardiopathy, and aortic stenosis.

salpingitis Inflammation of the fallopian tubes as a result of infection. Leukorrhea, adnexal tenderness, abdominal pain, and fever may be present.

sciatica Pain, weakness, or paresthesias, associated with the course of the sciatic nerve may affect the posterior aspect of the thigh and the posterolateral and anterolateral aspects of the leg into the foot.

sclera Tough, inelastic opaque membrane that covers the posterior five sixths of the eye bulb; maintains the size and form of the bulb and attaches to muscles that move the bulb.

scoliosis Lateral deviation of the spine.

scotoma Islandlike area of blindness in the field of vision.

screening Preliminary procedure, such as a test or examination, to detect the most characteristic sign or signs of a disorder that may require further investigation.

sebaceous Pertaining to or secreting sebum, an oily secretion composed of fat and epithelial debris.

sebaceous cyst Retention of the fatty secretion of the sebaceous gland.

seborrheic keratoses Benign, raised, wartlike skin lesions appearing with increasing age.

self-esteem The degree of worth and competence one attributes to oneself.

semilunar valves Valves with half-moon–shaped cusps located between the ventricles and the great vessels. The left semilunar valve is the aortic valve. The right semilunar valve is the pulmonic valve.

senile purpura Skin bruising caused by leakage of blood through fragile skin capillaries.

sensorineural hearing loss Diminished ability to hear caused by the inability of the acoustic nerve to transmit nervous impulses from the middle ear to the brain. Also called perceptive hearing loss.

sequela Any abnormal condition that follows and results from a disease, treatment, or injury.

sign Objective evidence of disease that is perceptible to the examiner.

sinus Hollow cavity in a bone or other tissue.

skin tags Benign, soft, flesh-colored skin lesions.

sleep State marked by reduced consciousness, diminished activity of the skeletal muscles, and depressed metabolism. People normally experience sleep in patterns that follow four observable, progressive stages.

sleep apnea Periodic cessation of breathing during sleep.

sleep apnea syndrome (SAS) Sleep disorder characterized by multiple episodes of cessation of breathing during sleep.

sleep terror disorder Condition occurring during stage 3 or 4 of nonrapid eye movement (nonREM) sleep that is characterized by repeated episodes of abrupt awakening, usually with a panicky scream, accompanied by intense anxiety, confusion, agitation, disorientation, unresponsiveness, marked motor movements, and amnesia concerning the event.

somnambulism Sleepwalking; a condition occurring during stage 3 or 4 of nonrapid eye movement (nonREM) sleep that is characterized by complex motor activity, usually culminating in leaving the bed and walking about, with no recall of the episode on awakening.

spasm Involuntary sudden contraction of a muscle or group of muscles accompanied by pain and interference with function.

speculum Device made of two narrow blades or a hollow tube, used to assist in opening a body cavity.

spermatogenesis Process of development of spermatozoa, the male germ cells.

spinal accessory nerve (CN XI) Function of this nerve is essential for speech, swallowing, and certain movements of the head and shoulders.

squamocolumnar junction Area of the cervix where the membranes covered by squamous cells of the vaginal portion of the cervix meet the membranes of the columnar portion of the cervix.

standard precautions Constellation of safeguards for handling materials, tissues, and fluids that may contain human pathogens; exposure to blood and body fluids is minimized by using removable and disposable barriers (e.g., latex and vinyl gloves, protective eyewear, mask and gowns, and "sharps" containers).

stapes One of the three ossicles of the middle ear, resembling a tiny stirrup. It transmits sound vibrations from the incus to the internal ear.

steatorrhea Abnormal increase of fat in the feces.

stereognosis Faculty of perceiving and understanding the form and nature of objects by the sense of touch. Higher cortical integration is required to perform this function.

sternocleidomastoid muscles Symmetrical muscles of the neck extending from the upper sternum and proximal portion of the clavicle to the mastoid process of the temporal bone behind the ear.

strabismus Disparity in the anteroposterior axes of the eyes; the optic axes cannot be directed to the same object because of lack of muscular coordination.

stress incontinence Involuntary urination incurred by straining, coughing, or lifting.

stressor Stimulus perceived by the individual or the organism as challenging, threatening, or damaging.

stria (*pl.* striae) (linease albicantes) Atrophic line or streak that differs in texture and color from the surrounding skin because of disrupted elastic fibers of the reticular layer of the cutis.

striae gravidarum Atrophic, pinkish or purplish scarlike lesions observed on the breasts, thighs, abdomen, and buttocks during pregnancy; lesions later become silvery white.

stridor Abnormal, high-pitched respiratory sound caused by an obstruction in the trachea or larynx.

sty Inflammation of a sebaceous gland of the eyelid; also called hordeolum.

subculture Group of persons within a culture with one or more shared traits.

subluxation Partial discoloration.

sulcus Shallow groove, depression, or furrow on the surface of an organ, such as one that separates the convolutions of the cerebral hemisphere.

supination Assumption of the supine (lying down) position.

symmetry Similarly in size, shape, and position to the body part on the opposite side.

symptom Client's subjective perception of an alteration of bodily or mental function from basal conditions; change perceived by the individual.

synapse Joining; point of contact between two neurons or between a neuron and an effector organ, across which nerve impulses are transmitted through the action of a neurotransmitter, such as acetylcholine or norepinephrine.

syncope Fainting; temporary unconsciousness.

systolic (systole) The force of blood against the arterial wall during the ejection phase of the cardiac cycle, or contraction of the heart.

tachycardia Rapid heart rate ($\geq$100 beats per minute). *Atrial flutter:* rapid, regular, uniform atrial contraction caused by AV block; ventricular rhythm varies with the degree of AV block. *Atrial tachycardia:* arrhythmia caused by the atria; rapid, regular beat of the entire heart. *Ventricular tachycardia:* arrhythmia caused by the ventricles; rapid, relatively regular heartbeat.

tachypnea Rapid respiratory rate.

tangential lighting Use of light shining from the side to create shadows over the area being examined; accentuates subtle differences in contour and movement.

taxonomy Framework for classifying and organizing information according to hierarchical categories.

telangiectasias Visible dilated capillaries located in skin.

temporal Of or limited by time.

temporal artery Artery on the head that runs anterior to the ear over the temporal bone and onto the forehead.

temporomandibular joint One of two joints connecting the mandible of the jaw to the temporal bone of the skull.

tenesmus Persistent, ineffectual spasms of the rectum accompanied by the desire to empty the bowel.

term infant Infant born between 37 and 41 weeks of gestation.

therapeutic relationship Relationship in which the focus of exchange is on the client and the client's needs.

therapeutic use of self Communication technique in which the use of personal qualities of the interviewer supports the client's perspective or feelings by finding a common connection. This technique can be especially helpful when the client's ethnicity, race, or socioeconomic status appear to be very different from that of the interviewer.

thrill Fine vibration accompanying rubulent blood flow in the heart or the great vessels. It is palpable when the examiner's fingers are placed over the site of the altered blood flow.

thrombophlebitis Inflammation of a vein, often accompanied by formation of a clot.

thrombus Aggregation of platelets, fibrin, clotting factors, and the cellular elements of the blood attached to the interior wall of a vein or artery that sometimes occludes the lumen of the vessel.

thyroid gland Endocrine gland at the front of the neck, consisting of bilateral lobes connected in the middle by a narrow isthmus. Secretes thyroxine, which is essential for growth and metabolic stability.

timbre The quality of a sound that distinguishes it from other sounds of the same pitch and volume.

tinnitus Sensation of noise in the ear caused by abnormal stimulation of the auditory apparatus or its afferent pathways; may be described as ringing, buzzing, swishing, roaring, blowing, or whistling.

tonic neck reflex Normal response in newborns to extend the arm and the leg on the side of the body to which the head is quickly turned while the infant is supine and to flex the limbs of the opposite side. The reflex prevents the infant from rolling over until adequate neurological and motor development occurs and disappears by 3 to 4 months of age. At this time the reflex is replaced by symmetrical positioning of both sides of the body.

tophi Deposits of monosodium urate, associated with gout.

torticollis Abnormal condition in which the contraction of neck muscles causes the head to be inclined to one side. This condition may be congenital or acquired.

tragus Projection of the cartilage of the auricle at the opening of the external auditory meatus.

transient ischemic attack Occlusion of a central nervous system vessel that results in a focal neurological disturbance.

transillumination Passage of light through a solid or liquid substance.

trapezius muscles Symmetrical, large, flat triangular muscles of the shoulder and upper back. These muscles extend from the occipital bone, the ligamentum nuchae, and the spinous processes of the seventh cervical and all the thoracic vertebrae. They act to rotate the scapula, raise the shoulder, and abduct and flex the arm.

tremor Involuntary, somewhat rhythmic, oscillatory quivering of muscles caused by alternating contraction of opposing groups of muscles. *Cerebellar tremor:* occurs during intentional movement, becoming more pronounced near the end of the movement; associated with lesions of the dentate nucleus. *Coarse tremor:* slow and large-amplitude movements. *Essential (familial) tremor:* usually initially appears around age 50 with fine tremors of the hands; aggravated by intentional movement; commonly affects the head, jaws, lips, or voice. *Fine tremor:* rapid (10 to 20 oscillations/sec) and low-amplitude movements, usually in the fingers and hands. *Moderate tremor:* medium-rate and medium-amplitude movements. *Passive tremor:* present at rest; may improve during intentional movement (e.g., pill-rolling tremor or Parkinson's disease). *Physiological tremor:* experienced by healthy people in fatigue, cold, and stress. *Toxic tremor:* caused by endogenous (thyrotoxicosis, uremia) or exogenous toxins (alcohol, drugs).

tricuspid valve Right atrioventricular valve.

trigeminal nerve (CN V) Cranial nerve that mediates sensation of the face. It has three branches: ophthalmic, maxillary, and mandibular.

trimester Period of 13 weeks.

trochanteric Pertaining to the two bony projections on the proximal end of the femur that serve as the attachment of various muscles.

trophoblast Peripheral cell layer of the blastocysts that attaches the fertilized ovum to the uterine wall and becomes the placenta and the membranes.

tropia Permanent deviation of the axis of an eye; strabismus.

tuberosity Elevation or protuberance, especially of a bone.

two-point discrimination Ability to sense the simultaneous stimulation of two areas of skin. Higher cortical integration is required to perform this function.

tympanic membrane Eardrum; membranous structure separating the external ear from the middle ear.

tympany Resonant sound produced over an air-filled region obtained by percussion.

ulnar deviation Turning the wrist away from the midline of the body.

umbo Landmark on the tympanic membrane created by the attachment of the membrane to the malleus.

upper motor neuron Long neurons with cell bodies in the motor portion of the cerebral cortex and axons that extend down the spinal cord, terminating at segmental levels of the spinal cord. They transmit impulses to lower motor neurons.

uvula Small cone-shaped process, suspended in the mouth from the middle of the posterior border of the soft palate.

valgus Deviation of an extremity outward, away from the midline. *Genu valgum:* condition in which the knees are abnormally close together; knock-knee.

validation Process of making sure the information or data collected is factual or true.

varicocele Distention of the veins of the spermatic cord.

varicose Dilated, distended, or bulging. This term is used particularly to describe a vein.

varus Deviation of an extremity toward the midline. *Genu varum:* condition in which the knees are abnormally separated; bowleg.

ventricle One of two muscular pumping chambers of the heart. The left ventricle pumps blood into the pulmonary artery.

ventricular fibrillation Cardiac arrhythmia marked by rapid, disorganized depolarization of the ventricular myocardium.

ventricular tachycardia Tachycardia that usually originates in the ventricular Purkinje system.

vertigo Illusion of movement, with imagined rotation of one-self (*subjective vertigo*) or one's surrounding (*objective vertigo*).

vestibule Space or cavity that serves as the entrance to a passageway.

vital or cardinal signs Indicators of bodily function such as blood pressure, temperature, pulse, and respiration.

vitreous humor Transparent substance contained in the posterior chamber of the eye.

von Recklinghausen's disease Also known as neurofibromatosis, this congenital condition is characterized by fibrous tumors of the nerve tissue (neurofibromas), café-au-lait spots on the skin, and, in some cases, developmental anomalies of the muscles, bones, and viscera.

Weber test Test of bone conduction through the use of a tuning fork placed on the top of the skull or middle forehead. A normal result occurs when the client reports that the sound is heard equally in both ears. The sound lateralizes when hearing loss is present.

wheeze Form of rhonchus characterized by a high-pitched musical quality. Caused by a high-velocity flow of air through a narrowed airway, it is heard during both inspiration and expiration.

whispered pectoriloquy Increased resonance of the whispered voice as heard through a stethoscope in an area of consolidation.

xanthelasma Soft yellow spot or plaque that usually occurs in groups on the eyelids.

xeromammography Done with a xerographic plate instead of film.

xerostomia Dry mouth, usually caused by medications or radiation therapy.

xiphoid Lowest portion of the sternum; composed of bone and cartilage.

Bibliography

Chapter 1

Alfaro R: *Applying nursing diagnosis and the nursing process: a step-by-step guide,* Philadelphia, 1990, JB Lippincott.

Doenges ME, Moorhouse MF, Geissler AC: *Nursing care plans: guidelines for individualizing patient care,* ed 5, FA Davis, 2000.

Geissler EM: Transcultural nursing and nursing diagnosis, *Nurs Health Care* 12(4):190-123, 1991.

Gordon M: *Nursing diagnosis: process and applications,* ed 4, St Louis, 1999, Mosby.

Maslow A: *Motivation and personality,* New York, 1970, Harper & Row.

Potter PA, Perry AG: *Basic nursing: a critical thinking approach,* ed 4, St Louis, 1999, Mosby.

US Department of Health and Human Services: website: http://www.health.gov/healthypeople. Accessed June 28, 2000.

Yura H, Walsh MB: *The nursing process: assessing, planning, implementing, and evaluating,* ed 5, New York, 1988, Appleton-Century-Crofts.

Chapter 2

Berlin EA, Fowkes WC: A teaching framework for cross-cultural health care, *West J Med* 139:934-938, 1983.

Kleinman A, Eisenberg L, Good B: Culture, illness, and care, *Ann Intern Med* 88:251-258, 1978.

Long L: *Understanding/responding: a communication manual for nurses,* ed 2, Boston, 1992, Jones & Bartlett.

Molde S: Understanding patient agendas, *Image J Nurs Sch* 18:145-147, 1986.

Putsch RW: Cross-cultural communication, *JAMA* 254:3344-3348, 1985.

Stuart GW, Laraia MT: *Principles and practices of psychiatric nursing,* ed 7, St Louis, 2001, Mosby.

Sundeen SJ et al: *Nurse-client interaction: implementing the nursing process,* ed 6, St Louis, 1998, Mosby.

Chapter 3

Anderson KN, Anderson LE, Glanze WD: *Mosby's medical, nursing, and allied health dictionary,* ed 5, St Louis, 1998, Mosby.

Billings JA, Stoeckel JD: *The clinical encounter: a guide to the medical interview and case presentation,* ed 2, St Louis, 1999, Mosby.

Cohen-Cole SA, Bird J: *The medical interview: the three function approach,* ed 2, St Louis, 2000, Mosby.

Davis CM: *Patient practitioner interaction: an experiential manual for developing the art of health care,* ed 3, Thorofare, NJ, 1998, Slack.

Elkin MK, Perry AG, Potter PA, editors: *Nursing interventions and clinical skills,* ed 2, St Louis, 2000, Mosby.

Geyman JP, Deyo RD, Ramsey SD: *Evidence-based clinical practice: concepts and approaches,* Boston, 2000, Butterworth Heinemann.

Giger JN, Davidhizar RE: *Transcultural nursing: assessment and intervention,* ed 3, St Louis, 1999, Mosby.

Gordon M: *Nursing diagnosis: process and application,* ed 3, St Louis, 1994, Mosby.

Kraytman M: *The complete patient history,* ed 2, New York, 1991, McGraw-Hill.

Lipson LG, Dibble SL, Minarik PA, editors: *Culture and nursing care: a pocket guide,* San Francisco, 1996, UCSF Nursing Press.

Mengel MB, Fields SA: *Introduction to clinical skills: a patient-centered approach,* New York, 1997, Plenum Medical Book Publishing.

North American Nursing Diagnosis Association: *Nursing diagnosis: definitions and classification 2001-2002,* Philadelphia, 2001, Nursecom.

Purnell LD, Paulanka BJ: *Transcultural health care: a culturally competent approach,* Philadelphia, 1998, FA Davis.

Smith RC: *The patient's story: integrated patient-doctor interviewing,* Boston, 1996, Little, Brown.

Thibodeau GA, Patton KT: *Anatomy and physiology,* ed 4, St Louis, 1999, Mosby.

Tomlinson J: ABC of sexual health: taking a sexual history, *Br Med J* 317:1573, 1998.

US Department of Health and Human Services Public Health Service: *Healthy people 2010,* Washington, DC, 2000, US Government Printing Office.

US Preventive Services Task Force: *Guide to clinical preventive services: report of the US Preventive Services Task Force,* ed 2, Baltimore, 1996, Williams & Wilkins.

Wasson JH et al: *The common symptom guide: a guide to the evaluation of common adult and pediatric symptoms,* ed 4, New York, 1997, McGraw-Hill.

Wong DL et al: *Whaley and Wong's nursing care of infants and children,* ed 6, St Louis, 1999, Mosby.

Woolf SH, Jonas S, Lawrence, RS: *Health promotion and disease prevention in clinical practice,* Baltimore, 1996, Williams & Wilkins.

Chapter 4

Azjen I: *Attitudes, personality, and behavior,* Chicago, 1988, Dorsey Press.

Ajzen I: The theory of planned behavior, *Org Behav Human Decision Processes* 50:179, 1991.

Ajzen I, Fishbein M: *Understanding additudes and predicting social behavior,* Englewood Cliffs, NJ, 1980, Prentice Hall.

Bandura A: *Social learning theory,* Englewood Cliffs, NJ, 1977, Prentice Hall.

Bandura A: *Social foundations of thought and action: a social cognitive theory,* Englewood Cliffs, NJ, 1986, Prentice Hall.

Connor M, Warren R, Close S: Alcohol consumption and the theory of planned behavior: an examination of the cognitive mediation of past behavior, *J Appl Soc Psychol* 29:1676, 1999.

Davis CM: *Patient practitioner interaction: an experimental manual for developing the art of health care,* ed 3, Thorofare, NJ, 1998, Slack.

Eisen M, Zellman GL, McAlister AL: A Health Belief Model-Social Learning theory approach to adolescents' fertility control: findings from a controlled field trial, *Health Educ Q* 19:249, 1992.

Giger JN, Davidhizar RE: *Transcultural nursing: assessment and intervention,* ed 3, St Louis, 1999, Mosby.

Fishbein M, Ajzen I: *Belief, attitude, intention and behavior: an introduction to theory and research,* Reading, Mass, 1975, Addison-Wesley.

Fisher WA, Fisher JD, Rye BJ: Understanding and promoting AIDS-preventive behavior: insights from the theory of reasoned action, *Health Psychol* 14:255, 1995.

Glanz K, Lewis FM, Rimer BK, editors: *Health behavior and health education: theory and practice,* San Francisco, 1997, Jossey-Bass.

Jemmott LS, Jemmott JB: Applying the theory of reasoned action to AIDS risk behavior condom use among black women, *Nurs Res* 40:228, 1991.

Keller ML, Ward S, Baumann L: Process of self-care: monitoring sensations and symptoms, *Adv Nurs Sci* 12:54, 1989.

Leventhal H, Meyer D, Nerez DR: The common sense representation of illness danger. In Rachman S: *Medical psychology,* vol II, New York, 1980, Pergamon Press.

Leventhal S, Safer MA, Panagis DM: The impact of communications on the self-regulation of health beliefs, decisions, and behavior, *Health Educ Q* 10(1):3, 1983.

McKenzie JF, Smeltzer JL: *Planning, implementing, and evaluating health promotion programs,* ed 3, Boston, 2001, Allyn and Bacon.

Meyer D, Leventhal H, Gutmann M: Commonsense models of illness: the example of hypertension, *Health Psychol* 4:115, 1985.

North American Nursing Diagnosis Association: *Nursing diagnosis: definitions and classification 2001-2002,* Philadelphia, 2001, Nursecom.

Pender NJ: *Health promotion in nursing practice,* ed 3, Stamford, Conn, 1996, Appleton & Lange.

Prochaska JO: *Systems of psychotherapy: a transtheoretical analysis,* Homewood, Ill, 1979, Dorsey Press.

Prochaska JO, Redding CA, Evers KE: The Transtheoretical Model and stages of change. In Glanz K, Lewis FM, Rimer BK, editors: *Health behavior and health education,* San Francisco, 1997, Jossey-Bass.

Prochaska JO et al.: Stages of change and decision balance for 12 problem behaviors, *Health Psychol* 13:39, 1994.

Purnell LD, Paulanka, BJ: *Transcultural health care: a culturally competent approach,* Philadelphia, 1998, FA Davis.

Rosenstock IM: Why people use health services, *Milbank Memorial Fund Q* 44:94, 1966.

Strecher VJ, Rosenstock IM: The Health Belief Model. In Glanz K, Lewis FM, Rimer BK, editors: *Health behavior and health education,* San Francisco, 1997, Jossey-Bass.

US Department of Health and Human Services: *Healthy people 2010,* Washington, DC, 2000, US Government Printing Office.

Woolf SH, Jonas S, Lawrence RS: *Health promotion and disease prevention in clinical practice,* Baltimore, 1996, Williams & Wilkins.

Chapter 5

Ballard J et al: New Ballard Score, expanded to include extremely premature infants, *Pediatrics* 119:417-423, 1991.

Bayley N: *Bayley scales of infant development,* New York, 1993, Psychological Corp.

Berk LE: *Child development,* ed 2, Boston, 1991, Allyn & Bacon.

Blair KA: Aging: physiological aspects and clinical implications, *Nurse Pract* 15(2):14-28, 1990.

Brazelton TB: *The neonatal behavioral scale,* ed 2, *Clinics in developmental medicine,* No. 88, London, 1983, Spastics International Medical Publications; Philadelphia, JB Lippincott.

Carey WB, McDevitt S: Revision of the Infant Temperament Questionnaire, *Pediatrics* 61:735-739, 1978.

Chew AL: *The lollipop test: a diagnostic screening test of school readiness,* Atlanta, 1992, Humanics Ltd.

Coddington RD: The significance of life events as etiologic factors in diseases of children. Part II. A study of a normal population, *J Psychosom Res* 16:205-213, 1972.

Comfort A: *A good old age,* New York, 1976, Crown.

Darling-Fisher C, Leidy NK: Measuring Eriksonian development in the adult: the Modified Erikson Psychosocial Stage Inventory, *Psychol Rep* 62:747-754, 1988.

DeLongis A, Folkman S, Lazarus R: The impact of daily stress on health and mood: psychological and social resources as mediators, *J Pers Soc Psychol* 54(3):486-495, 1988.

Dixon SD, Stein MT: *Encounters with children: pediatric behavior and development,* ed 3, St Louis, 2000, Mosby.

Duvall E, Miller B: *Marriage and family development,* ed 6, New York, 1984, Harper & Row.

Erikson EH: Identity and the lifecycle, *Psychol Iss* 1(monograph 1), 1959.

Erikson EH: *Childhood and society,* ed 2, New York, 1963, WW Norton.

Erikson EH: *Identity: youth and crisis,* New York, 1968, WW Norton.

Erikson EH: *Adulthood,* New York, 1978, WW Norton.

Erikson EH: *The lifecycle completed,* New York, 1982, WW Norton.

Erikson H, Tomlin EM, Swain MA: *Modeling and role modeling: a theory and paradigm for nursing,* Englewood Cliffs, NJ, 1983, Prentice Hall.

Flavell J: *The developmental psychology of Jean Piaget,* Princeton, 1963, Van Nostrand.

Foster RLR et al: *Family-centered nursing care of children,* Philadelphia, 1989, WB Saunders.

Frankenburg WK, Camp BW, editors: *Pediatric screening tests,* Springfield, Ill, 1975, Charles C Thomas.

Frankenburg WK, Dodds JB: The Denver Developmental Screening Test, *J Pediatr* 71:181-191, 1967.

Fung K, Lau S: Denver Developmental Screening Test: cultural variables, *J Pediatr* 106(2):343, 1985.

Gilligan C: *In a different voice, psychological theory and women's development,* Cambridge, Mass, 1982, Harvard University Press.

Havinghurst R: *Human development and education,* St Louis, 1953, Warren H Green.

Hegvik R, McDevitt S, Carey W: The Middle Childhood Temperament Questionnaire, *J Dev Behav Pediatr* 3:197-200, 1982.

Holmes TH, Rahe RH: The social readjustment rating scale, *J Psychosom Res* 11:213-218, 1967.

Kimmel DC: *Adulthood and aging: an interdisciplinary development view,* ed 3, New York, 1989, John Wiley & Sons.

Kane R, Kane RL: *Assessing the elderly,* Lexington, Mass, 1984, Lexington Books.

Kaplowitz PB, Oberfield SE: Reexamination of the age limit of defining when puberty is precocious in girls in the United States: implications for evaluation and treatment, *Pediatrics* 104(4):936-941, 1999.

Kemper DW, Giuffre J, Drabinski G: *Pathways,* Boise, Idaho, 1986, Healthwise.

Kicklighter RH, Richmond BO: *Children's adaptive behavior scale revised and expanded manual,* Atlanta, 1983, Humanics Ltd.

Leidy NK, Darling-Fisher CS: Reliability and validity of the modified Erikson psychosocial stage inventory in diverse samples, *West J Nurs Res* 17(2):168-187, 1995.

Levinson DJ et al: *The seasons of a man's life,* New York, 1979, Ballantine.

Marlow DR, Redding BA: *Textbook of pediatric nursing,* ed 6, Philadelphia, 1988, WB Saunders.

McCubbin HI, Thompson AI, editors: *Family assessment inventories for research and practice,* Madison, Wisc, 1987, The University of Wisconsin-Madison.

McDevitt SC, Carey WB: *The Carey temperament scale,* Scottsdale, Ariz, 1995, Behavioral Developmental Initiatives.

Miller V, Onotera R, Deinard A: Denver Developmental Screening Test: cultural variations in southeast Asian children, *J Pediatr* 104(3):481-482, 1984.

Moos RH, Moos BS: A typology of family social environments, *Fam Process* 15:357-371, 1976.

Murray RB, Zentner JP: *Nursing assessment and health promotion strategies through the life span,* ed 6, Norwalk, Conn, 1997, Appleton & Lange.

Myers I, Briggs-Myers PB: *Gifts differing,* Palo Alto, Calif, 1980, Consulting Psychologists Press.

Olade RA: Evaluation of the Denver Developmental Screening Test as applied to African children, *Nurs Res* 33a94a0:204-207, 1984.

Olson DH: Circumplex model VII: validation studies and FACES III, *Fam Process* 25:337-351, 1986.

Piaget J: *The construction of reality in the child,* New York, 1975, Ballantine.

Psychological Corporation: *Tests and other products for psychological assessment,* San Antonio, 1995, Harcourt Brace.

Rahe RH: Epidemiological studies of life changes and illness, *Int J Psychiatry Med* 6(1-2):133-146, 1975.

Reidy M, Thibaudeau MF: Evaluation of family functioning: development and validation of a scale which measures family competence in measures of health, *Nurs Papers* 16:42-56, 1984.

Robinson RA: The diagnosis and prognosis of dementia. In Anders WF, editor: *Current achievements in geriatrics,* London, 1964, Cassell.

Sarason IG, Johnson JH, Siegel JM: Assessing the impact of life changes: development of the life experiences survey, *J Consult Clin Psychol* 46:932-946, 1978.

Schaefer MT, Olson DH: Assessing intimacy: the pair inventory, *J Marital Fam Ther* 4:47-60, 1981.

Schuster CS, Ashburn SS: *The process of human development: a holistic life span approach,* ed 3, Philadelphia, 1992, JB Lippincott.

Shader RI, Harmatz JS, Salzman C: A new scale for clinical assessment in geriatric populations: Sandoz Clinical Assessment Geriatric (SCAG), *J Am Geriatr Soc* 22:107-113, 1974.

Sheehy G: *The silent passage: menopause,* New York, 1991, Random House.

Sheehy G: *New passages,* New York, 1995, EP Dutton.

Stevenson JS: *Issues and crises during middlescence,* New York, 1977, Appleton-Century-Crofts.

Stokes S, Gordon S: *Development of a tool to measure stress in the older individual,* New York, 1986, Stewart Research Conference, Nursing in the 21st Century, Perspectives and Possibilities.

Wadsworth B: *Piaget's theory of cognitive and affective development,* ed 3, White Plains, NY, 1988, Longman.

Weinberger M, Hiner S, Tierney W: In support of Hassles as a measure of stress in predicting health outcomes, *J Behav Med* 10(1)19-31, 1987.

Welch JB, Instone SL: In Dixon SD, Stein MT: *Encounters with children: pediatric behavior and development,* ed 3, St Louis, 2000, Mosby.

Wong DL et al: *Whaley and Wong's nursing care of infants and children,* ed 6, St Louis, 1999, Mosby.

Wright L, Leahey M: *Nurses and families: a guide to family assessment and intervention,* ed 3, Philadelphia, 2000, FA Davis.

Chapter 6

Abrams B, Altman SL, Pickett KE: Pregnancy weight gain: still controversial, *Am J Clin Nutr* 71(5):1233S-1241S, 2000.

Algert SJ, Brzezinski E, Ellison TH, editors: *Ethnic and regional food practices: Mexican-American food practices, customs, and holidays,* Chicago, 1998, American Dietetic Association.

Allen LH: Anemia and iron deficiency: effects on pregnancy outcome, *Am J Clin Nutr* 71(5(S))(:1280S-1284S, 2000.

American College of Sports Medicine: *ACSM's guidelines for exercise testing and prescription,* Philadelphia, 2000, Lippincott Williams & Wilkins.

American Diabetes Association: Screening for type 2 diabetes, *Diabetes Care* 22(suppl):S20-S23, 1999.

American Diabetes Association: Nutrition recommendations and principles for people with diabetes mellitus, *Diabetes Care* 22(suppl):42S-45S, 1999.

American Heart Association: *Heart and stroke: statistical update,* Dallas, 1999, American Heart Association.

Appel LJ et al: A clinical trial of the effects of dietary patterns on blood pressure: Dash collaborative research group, *N Engl J Med* 336(16): 1117-1124, 1997.

Chumlea WC, Guo SS, Steinbaugh ML: Prediction of stature from knee height for black and white adults and children with application to mobility-impaired or handicapped persons, *J Am Diet Assoc* 94(12):1385-1388, 1994.

Expert Panel on Detection, Evaluation, and Treatment of High Blood Cholesterol in Adults: Summary of the second report of the national cholesterol education program (NCEP) expert panel on detection, evaluation, and treatment of high blood cholesterol in adults (adult treatment panel II), *JAMA* 269(23):3015-3023, 1993.

Flegal KM et al: Overweight and obesity in the United States: prevalence and trends, 1960-1994, *Int J Obes Relat Metabol Disord* 22(1):39-47, 1998.

Haddad EH: Development of a vegetarian food guide, *Am J Clin Nutr* 59(5 suppl):1248S-1254S, 1994.

Haddad EH, Sabate J, Whitten CG: Vegetarian food guide pyramid: a conceptual framework. *Am J Clin Nutr* 70(3 suppl):615S-619S. 1999.

Harris MI et al: Prevalence of diabetes, impaired fasting glucose, and impaired glucose tolerance in US adults: the third national health and nutrition examination survey, 1988-1994, *Diabetes Care* 21(4):518-524, 1998.

Harrison GG et al: Anthropometric standardization reference manual. In Lohman TG, Roche AF, Martorell R, editors: *Skinfold thicknesses and measurement technique,* Champaign, Ill, 1988, Human Kinetics.

Heyward VH: *Advanced fitness assessment exercise prescription,* Champaign, Ill, 1998, Human Kinetics.

Heymsfiels SB, Baumgartner RD, Pan S. In: Shils ME et al, editors: *Nutrition, diet, and hypertension,* ed 9, Baltimore, 1999, William & Wilkins.

Hoffbrand AV, Herbert V: Nutritional anemias, *Semin Hematol* 36(4 suppl 7):13-23, 1999.

Institute of Medicine: *Dietary reference intakes for thiamine, riboflavin, niacin, vitamin B_6, folate, vitamin B_{12}, pantothenic acid, biotin, and choline,* Washington, DC, 1998, National Academy Press.

Institute of Medicine: *Dietary reference intakes for vitamin C, vitamin E, selenium and carotenoids,* Washington, DC, 2000, National Academy Press.

Institute of Medicine: Dietary reference intakes, 2000, Website: www.nap.edu.

Jarvis C: *Physical examination and health assessment,* Philadelphia, 1999, WB Saunders.

Kotchen TA, Kotchen JM: Modern nutrition in health and disease. In Shils ME, Olson JA, Shike M, Ross AC, editors: *Nutrition, diet, and hypertension,* ed 9, Baltimore, 1999, William & Wilkins.

Kraus RM et al: AHA dietary guidelines: revision 2000: a statement for healthcare professionals from the nutrition committee of the American Heart Association, *Circulation* 102(18):2284-2299, 2000.

Lau G, Ma KM, Ng A, editors: *Ethnic and regional food practices: Chinese American food practices, customs, and holidays,* Chicago, 1998, American Dietetic Association.

McGinnis JM, Foege WH: Actual causes of death in the United States, *JAMA* 270(18):2207-2212, 1993.

Morey SS: CDC issues guidelines for prevention, detection and treatment of iron deficiency, *Am Fam Physician* 58(6):1475-1477, 1998.

National Dairy Council: Managing lactose intolerance, *Dairy Council Dig* 65(2):7-12, 1994.

National High Blood Pressure Education Program: *The sixth report of the joint national committee on prevention, detection, evaluation, and treatment of high blood pressure,* Bethesda, Md, 1997, Public Health Service, US Department of Health and Human Services.

NHLBI Obesity Education Initiative: *Clinical guidelines on the identification, evaluation, and treatment of overweight and obesity in adults,* Bethesda, Md, 1998, Public Health Service, US Department of Health and Human Services.

Nicoll D et al: *Pocket guide to diagnostic tests,* ed 2, Stamford, Connecticut, 1997, Appleton & Lange.

Panfilli R: Nursing diagnosis. In Carpenito LJ: *Nutrition, altered: more than body requirements,* ed 7, Philadelphia, 1997, JB Lippincott.

Patterson BH et al: Food choices of whites, blacks, and Hispanics: data from the 1987 national health interview survey, *Nutr Cancer* 23(2):105-119, 1995.

Provan D: Mechanisms and management of iron deficiency anemia, *Br J Haematol* 105(suppl 1):19S-26S, 1999.

Purnell LD, Paulanka BJ: *Transcultural health care,* Philadelphia, 1998, FA Davis.

Recommendations to prevent and control iron deficiency in the United States, Centers for Disease Control and Prevention: *MMWR* 47(RR-3):1-29, 1998.

Schilling B, Brannon E: *Cross-cultural counseling: a guide for nutrition and health counselors,* Bethesda, Md, 1986, USDHHS.

Scholl TO, Johnson WG: Folic acid: influence on the outcome of pregnancy, *Am J Clin Nutr* 71(5 suppl):S1295-S1303, 2000.

Simko MD, Cowell C, Gilbride JA: *Nutrition assessment: a comprehensive guide for planning intervention,* Gaithersburg, Md, 1995, Aspen.

The Expert Committee on the Diagnosis and Classification of Diabetes Mellitus: Report of the expert committee on the diagnosis and classification of diabetes mellitus, *Diabetes Care* 22 (suppl 1):5S-19S 1999.

Underwood LE: Normal adolescent growth and development, *Nutr Today* 26(2):11-16, 1991.

US Department of Health and Human Services: PHS, NHANES III Anthropometric Procedure Video, US Government Printing Office Stock Number 017-022-01355-5, Washington, DC, 1996, US GPO, US Public Health Services.

USDA: The dietary guidelines for Americans, ed 5, 2000, website: http://www.usda.gov/cnpp/dietary_guidelines.htm.

Wardlaw GM: *Perspective in nutrition,* ed 4, New York, 1999, McGraw-Hill.

Weaver CM, Proulx WR, Heaney R: Choices for achieving adequate dietary calcium with a vegetarian diet, *Am J Clin Nutr* 70(3 suppl):543S-548S, 1999.

Willett WC: Modern nutrition in health and disease. In Shils ME et al, editors: *Diet, nutrition, and prevention of cancer,* ed 9, Baltimore, 1999, William & Wilkins.

Willett WC: Convergence of philosophy and science: the third international congress on vegetarian nutrition, *Am J Clin Nutr* 70(3 suppl):434S-438S, 1999.

Woolf N et al, editors: *Ethnic and regional food practices: northern plains Indian food practices, customs, and holidays,* Chicago, 1998, American Dietetic Association.

Worthington-Roberts BS, Williams SR: *Nutrition in pregnancy and lactation,* ed 6, Madison, Wisc, 1997, Brown & Benchmark.

Yip R: Iron deficiency, *Bull WHO* 76(suppl 2)(:121S-123S, 1998.

Zeman FJ, Ney DM: *Applications in medical nutrition therapy,* ed 2, Englewood Cliffs, NJ, 1996, Prentice Hall.

Chapter 7

AAN Expert Panel on Culturally Competent Nursing Care: AAN expert panel report: culturally competent health care, *Nurs Outlook* 40:277-283, 1992.

American Nurses Association: *Cultural diversity in the nursing curriculum: a guide for implementation (ANA No G-171:11),* Kansas City, Mo, 1986, American Nurses Association.

Andrews MM, Bouyle JS: *Transcultural concepts in nursing care,* ed 3, Philadelphia, 1999, JB Lippincott.

Barker JC: Cultural diversity: changing the context of medical practice in cross-cultural medicine: a decade later, *East J Med* 157 (special issue):248-254, 1992.

Buchwald D et al: Caring for patients in a multicultural society, *Patient Care* 28(11):105-120, 1994.

Campinha-Bacote J: Cultural diversity in nursing education: issues and concerns, *J Nurs Educ* 37:3-4, 1998.

Campinha-Bacote J: A model and instrument for addressing cultural competence in health care, *J Nurs Educ* 38(5):203-207 1999.

CDC: www.CDC.gov/growthcharts.

Felice ME: Reflections on caring for Indo-Chinese children and youths, *J Behav Pediatr* 7(2):124-128, 1986.

Fuchs VR, Hahn JS: How does Canada do it? A comparison of expenditures for physicians' services in the United States and Canada, *N Engl J Med* 323:884-890, 1990.

Giger JN, Davidhizar RE: *Transcultural nursing: assessment and intervention,* ed 3, St Louis, 1999, Mosby.

Hanson S, Boyd S: *Family health care nursing,* Philadelphia, 1996, FA Davis.

Hartog J, Hartog EA: Cultural aspects of health and illness behavior in hospitals, *West J Med* 139:911-916, 1983.

Hautman MA: Folk health and illness beliefs, *Nurse Pract* 4:4, 1979.

Health Resources and Service Administration: *Health status of minorities and low income groups,* DHHS Pub No HRS-P-DV 85-1, Washington, DC, 1985, US Government Printing Office.

Helman C: *Culture, health and illness,* ed 2, London, 1990, John Wright & Sons.

Henderson G, Primeaux M: *Transcultural health care,* Menlo Park, Calif, 1981, Addison-Wesley.

Kleinman A, Eisenberg L, Good B: Culture, illness and care: clinical lessons from anthropologic and cross-cultural research, *Ann Intern Med* 88:251-258, 1978.

Kluckhohn F: Dominant and variant value orientations. In Brink PJ, editor: *Transcultural nursing: a book of readings,* Englewood Cliffs, NJ, 1976, Prentice Hall.

Krause N, Goldenhar LM: Acculturation and psychological distress in three groups of elderly Hispanics, *J Gerontol* 47:S279-S288, 1992.

Leininger MM: *Transcultural nursing: concepts, theories and practices,* New York, 1978, John Wiley & Sons.

Lipson JG, Dibble SL, Minarik PA: *Culture and nursing care: a pocket guide,* San Francisco, 1996, USCF Nursing Press.

Martin MM, Henry M: Cultural relativity and poverty, *Public Health Nurs* 6:28-34, 1989.

Morse JM, Young DE, Swartz L: Cree Indian healing practices and Western health care: a comparative analysis, *Soc Sci Med* 32:1361-1366, 1991.

National Center for Health Statistics: *Prevention profile, Health United States,* 1991, Hyattsville, Md, 1992, Public Health Service.

Olness K: Cultural issues in primary pediatric care. In Hoekelman RA et al: *Primary pediatric care,* ed 2, St Louis, 1992, Mosby.

Overfield T: Biological variation: concepts from physical anthropology. In Henderson G, Primeaux M, editors: *Transcultural health care,* Menlo Park, Calif, 1981, Addison-Wesley.

Purnell LD, Paulanka BJ: *Transcultural health care: a culturally competent approach,* Philadelphia, 1998, FA Davis.

Rauh VA, Wasserman GA, Brunelli SA: Determinants of maternal childrearing attitudes, *J Am Acad Child Adolesc Psychiatry* 29:375-381, 1990.

Rogler LH, Cortes DE, Malgady RG: Acculturation and mental health status among Hispanics, *Am Psychol* 46:585-605, 1991.

Shelly J, Fish S: *Spiritual care: the nurse's role,* ed 3, Downer's Grove, Ill, 1988, Intervarsity Press.

Smith LS: Ethnic differences in knowledge of sexually transmitted diseases in North American Black and Mexican-American migrant farmworkers, *Res Nurs Health* 11:51-58, 1988.

Snow LF: Folk medical beliefs and their implications for the care of patients: a review based on studies of black Americans. In Henderson G, Primeaux M, editors: *Transcultural health care,* Menlo Park, Calif, 1981, Addison-Wesley.

Snow LF, Johnson SM: Folklore, food, female reproductive cycle, *Ecol Food Nutr* 7:41-49, 1978.

Spector R: *Cultural diversity in health and illness,* ed 4, Norwalk, Conn, 1996, Appleton & Lange.

Starn JR: Family culture and chronic conditions. In Jackson PL, Vessey JA: *Primary care of the child with a chronic condition,* ed 2, St Louis, 1996, Mosby.

Stulc DM: The family as bearer of culture. In Cookfair JN, editor: *Nursing process and practice in the community,* St Louis, 1991, Mosby.

Syme SL: Social determinants of disease, *Ann Clin Res* 19:44-52, 1987.

Thierderman SB: Ethnocentrism: a barrier to effective health care, *Nurse Pract* 11:53-59, 1986.

Tripp-Reimer T: Cultural assessment. In Bellack J, Edlund B, editors: *Nursing assessment and diagnosis,* Boston, 1992, Jones & Bartlett.

Tripp-Reimer T, Brink PJ, Pinkham C: Culture brokerage. In Bulechek GM, McCloskey JC:: *Nursing interventions: effective treatments,* ed 3, Philadelphia, 1999, WB Saunders.

Tripp-Reimer T, Brink PJ, Saunders JM: Cultural assessment: content and process, *Nurs Outlook* 32:78-82, 1984.

US Bureau of the Census: *Statistical abstract of the United States,* ed 112, Washington, DC, 1992, US Government Printing Office.

US Bureau of the Census: *Current population reports,* Washington, DC, 1997, US Government Printing Office.

US Department of Health and Human Services, Public Health Service: *Healthy people 2010,* Washington, DC, 2000, US Government Printing Office.

Villarruel AM, Ortiz de Montellano B: Culture and pain: a Meso-American perspective, *Adv Nurs Sci* 15:21-32, 1992.

Wong DL et al: *Whaley and Wong's nursing care of infants and children,* ed 6, St Louis, 1999, Mosby.

Zborowski M: Cultural components in response to pain, *Soc Issues* 8:16-30, 1952.

Zborowski M: *People in pain,* San Francisco, 1969, Jossey-Bass.

Zola IK: Culture and symptoms: an analysis of patients presenting complaints, *Am Soc Rev* 31:615-630, 1966.

Chapter 8

Breslow L, Somers AR: The lifetime health monitoring program: a practical approach to preventive medicine, *N Engl J Med* 296:601, 1977.

Gruendemann BJ: Hand hygiene: a manual for health care professionals, Arlington, Tex, 1992, Johnson & Johnson Medical, Inc.

King C: Refining your assessment techniques, *RN* 46:42-47, 1983.

Kozier B, Erb G, Blais K: *Fundamentals of nursing: concepts, process and practice,* ed 5, Menlo Park, Calif, 1995, Addison-Wesley.

Leavell HR, Clark EG: *Preventive medicine for the doctor in his community,* ed 3, New York, 1965, McGraw-Hill.

Potter PA, Perry AG: *Basic nursing: a critical thinking approach,* ed 4, St Louis, 1999, Mosby.

Talbot LA, Marquardt M: *Pocket guide to critical care assessment,* ed 3, St Louis, 1997, Mosby.

US Preventive Services Task Force: *Guide to clinical preventive services,* ed 2, Alexandria, Va, 1996, International Medical Publishing.

Wilson SF, Giddens JF: *Health assessment for nursing practice,* ed 2, St Louis, 2001, Mosby.

Chapter 9

American Heart Association of Wisconsin: *Blood pressure education program instructor's manual,* Milwaukee, 1996, The Association.

Centers for Disease Control and Prevention: Recommendations for prevention of HIV transmission in health-care settings, *MMWR* (suppl 36):SS, August 1987.

Francis CC, Martin AH: *Introduction to human anatomy,* ed 7, St Louis, 1975, Mosby.

Gelfand JA, Dinarello CA, Wolff SM: Alteration in body temperature. In Fauci AS et al, editors: *Harrison's principles of internal medicine,* vol 1, ed 14, New York, 1998, McGraw-Hill.

Gordon M: *Nursing diagnosis: process and applications,* ed 4, St Louis, 1999, Mosby,.

Guyton AC: *Textbook of medical physiology,* ed 10, Philadelphia, 2000, WB Saunders.

Hill MN, Grim CM: How to take a precise blood pressure, *Am J Nurs* 91:38, 1991.

Joint National Committee on Prevention, Detection, Evaluation, and Treatment of High Blood Pressure: The sixth report of the Joint National Committee on Detection, Evaluation, and Treatment of High Blood Pressure, NIH Publication No. 98-4080, 1997.

Magee DJ: *Orthopedic physical assessment,* ed 3, Philadelphia, 1997, WB Saunders.

Mountcastle VB: *Medical physiology,* vol 2, ed 14, St Louis, 1980, Mosby.

National High Blood Pressure Education Program Working Group on Hypertension Control in Children and Adolescents: Update on the 1987 Task Force Report on High Blood Pressure in Children and Adolescents, *Pediatrics* 98(4):649-658, 1996.

Potter PA, Perry AG: *Basic nursing: a critical thinking approach,* ed 4, St Louis, 1999, Mosby.

Summers S: Axillary, tympanic and esophageal temperature measurement: descriptive comparisons in postanesthesia patients, *J Post Anesth Nurs* 6:420, 1991.

Thibodeau GA, Patton KT: *Anatomy and physiology,* ed 4, St Louis, 1999, Mosby.

Timby BK, Lewis LW: *Fundamental skills and concepts in patient care,* ed 6, New York, 1996, JB Lippincott.

Wong DL et al: *Whaley and Wong's nursing care of infants and children,* ed 6, St Louis, 1999, Mosby.

Chapter 10

Archer CB, Robertson SJ: *Black and white skin diseases,* Cambridge, Mass, 1995, Blackwell Science.

Baran R, Dawber RPR, Levene GM: *Color atlas of the hair, scalp, and nails,* London, 1991, Wolfe.

Bates B: *A guide to physical examination and history taking,* ed 6, Philadelphia, 1995, JB Lippincott.

Coheb BA: *Atlas of pediatric dermatology,* St Louis, 1993, Mosby.

Daniel CR et al: Don't overlook skin surveillance, *Patient Care* 30(11):90-107, 1996.

Farrar WE et al: *Infectious diseases,* ed 2, London, 1992, Gower.

Fitzpatrick TB et al: *Dermatology in general medicine,* ed 4, New York, 1993, McGraw-Hill.

Gaskin F: Detection of cyanosis in the person with dark skin, *J Natl Black Nurses Assoc* 1(1):52-60, 1986.

Goldman MP, Fitzpatrick RE: *Cutaneous laser surgery: the art and science of selective photohemolysis,* St Louis, 1994, Mosby.

Gordon M: *Nursing diagnosis: process and application,* ed 3, St Louis, 1994, Mosby.

Habif TP: *Clinical dermatology: a color guide to diagnosis and therapy,* ed 2, St Louis, 1990, Mosby.

Habif TP: *Clinical dermatology: a color guide to diagnosis and therapy,* ed 3, St Louis, 1996, Mosby.

Kopf AW et al: Techniques of cutaneous examination for detection of skin cancer, *Cancer* 75(suppl 2):684-690, 1995.

Lawrence CM, Cox NH: *Physical signs in dermatology,* London, 1993, Mosby-Wolfe.

Marks JG Jr, DeLeo VA: *Contact and occupational dermatology,* St Louis, 1992, Mosby.

The NIH Consensus Development Panel on Melanoma: Diagnosis and treatment of early melanoma, *JAMA* 268:1314-1319, 1992.

Pariser RJ, editor: Diagnostic and therapeutic techniques for evaluation and treatment of skin disorders, *Primary Care* 16(3):823-846, 1989.

Samman PD: *The nails in disease,* ed 4, London, 1986, William Heinemann Medical Books.

Sauer GC: *Manual of skin diseases,* ed 7, Philadelphia, 1996, JB Lippincott.

Sawaya ME, Stough DB: Untangling misconceptions about hair, *Patient Care* 26:193-213, 1992,.

Seidel HM et al: *Mosby's guide to physical examination,* ed 4, St Louis, 1999, Mosby

US Preventive Services Task Force: *Guide to clinical preventive services,* ed 2, Alexandria, Va, 1996, International Medical Publishing.

Weston WL, Lane AT: *Color textbook of pediatric dermatology,* St Louis, 1991, Mosby.

Weston WL, Lane AT: *Color textbook of pediatric dermatology,* ed 2, St Louis, 1996, Mosby.

White GM: *Color atlas of regional dermatology,* St Louis, 1994, Mosby.

Wilson SF, Giddens JF: *Health assessment for nursing practice,* ed 2, St Louis, 2001, Mosby.

Chapter 11

Abrams DI, Foon KA, Gold JWM: Lymphadenopathy: a diagnostic plan, *Patient Care* 4(30):94-112, 1988.

Carpenter DR, Hudacek S: Polymyalgia rheumatica: a comprehensive review of this debilitating disease, *Nurse Pract* 19(6):50-58, 1994.

DeGroot LJ et al: *The thyroid and its diseases,* ed 5, New York, 1984, John Wiley & Sons.

Derman H: Migraine headache: precision in diagnosis and improved therapeutic prospects, *Consultant* 31(5):57-63, 1991.

Diamond ML, Solomon GD, editors: *Diamond and Dalessio's the practicing physician's approach to headache,* ed 4, Baltimore, 1986, Williams & Wilkins.

Giger JN, Davidhizar RE: *Transcultural nursing,* ed 3, St Louis, 1999, Mosby.

Gilbert R, Warfield C: Evaluating and treating the patient with neck pain, *Hosp Pract* 22(8):223-232, 1987.

Gordon M: *Nursing diagnosis: process and applications,* ed 4, St Louis, 1999, Mosby.

Haase GR et al: When facial pain is the problem, *Patient Care* 24(12):119-124, 1990.

Heitman R, Irizarry A: Hypothyroidism: common complaints, perplexing diagnosis, 20(3):54-60, 1995.

Peatfield RC: *Headache,* Berlin, 1986, Springer-Verlag.

Thompson JM et al: *Mosby's clinical nursing,* ed 4, St Louis, 1997, Mosby.

US Preventive Services Task Force: *Guide to clinical preventive services,* ed 2, Alexandria, Va, 1996, International Medical Publishing.

Chapter 12

Apple DJ, Rabb MF: *Ocular pathology: clinical applications and self-assessment,* ed 4, St Louis, 1991, Mosby.

Arffa RC: *Grayson's diseases of the cornea,* ed 4, St Louis, 1997, Mosby.

Boyd-Monk H: Assessing acquired ocular diseases, *Nurs Clin North Am* 25(4):811-822, 1990.

Gordon M: *Manual of nursing diagnosis 1997-1998,* St Louis, 1997, Mosby.

Harrington DO, Drake MV: *The visual fields: text and atlas of clinical perimetry,* ed 6, St Louis, 1990, Mosby.

Hoskins HD, Kass MA: *Becker-Shaffer's diagnosis and therapy of the glaucomas,* ed 6, St Louis, 1989, Mosby.

Jones M, Tippett T: Assessment of the red eye, *Nurse Pract* 5:10-15, Jan-Feb 1980.

Lawlor MC: Common ocular injuries and disorders. 2. Red eye, *J Emerg Nurs* 15(1):36-41, 1989.

Newell FW: *Ophthalmology: principles and concepts,* ed 8, St Louis, 1996, Mosby.

Sapira JD, Schneiderman H: The funduscopic examination: how to make the most of it, *Consultant* 30(6):22-27, 1990.

Small RG: Red eye: five steps toward a differential diagnosis, *Consultant* 31(7):29-32, 1991.

US Preventive Services Task Force: *Guide to clinical preventive services,* ed 2, Alexandria, Va, 1996, International Medical Publishing.

Chapter 13

Gordon M: *Nursing diagnosis: process and applications,* ed 4, St Louis, 1999, Mosby.

Koufman JA: *Core otolaryngology,* Philadelphia, 1990, JB Lippincott.

Lee KJ: *Textbook of otolaryngology and head and neck surgery,* New York, 1989, Elsevier.

Netter FH: *CIBA collection of medical illustrations.* vol 3, Digestive system. Part I, Upper digestive tract, Summit, NJ, 1983, CIBA Medical Education Division.

Potter PA, Perry AG: *Basic nursing: theory and practice,* ed 3, St Louis, 1995, Mosby.

Riley MAK: *Nursing care of the client with ear, nose and throat disorders,* New York, 1987, Springer.

Schuller DE: *DeWeese and Saunders' otolaryngology—head and neck surgery,* ed 8, St Louis, 1994, Mosby.

Seidel HM et al: *Mosby's guide to physical examination,* ed 4, St Louis, 1999, Mosby.

Serra AM: *Ear, nose and throat nursing,* Cambridge, Mass, 1986, Blackwell Science.

Chapter 14

Barth V, Prechtel K, Heywang SH: *Atlas of breast diseases,* Philadelphia, 1991, BC Decker.

Blackwell RE, Grotting JC: *Diagnosis and management of breast disease,* Cambridge, Mass, 1996, Blackwell Science.

Bobak IM, Jenses MD, Zalar MK: *Maternity and gynecologic care: the nurse and the family,* ed 5, St Louis, 1993, Mosby.

Denton S, editor: *Breast cancer nursing,* San Diego, 1995, Singular Publishing.

Donegan WL, Spratt JS, editors: *Cancer of the breast,* ed 4, Philadelphia, 1995, WB Saunders.

Eskin BA, Sucha OA, Jardines L: *Breast disease for primary care physicians,* New York, 1999, Parthenon.

Evans, AJ et al: *Atlas of breast disease management,* London, 1998, WB Saunders.

Gordon M: *Nursing diagnosis: process and application,* ed 3, St Louis, 1994, Mosby.

Giger JN, Davidhizar RE: *Transcultural nursing: assessment and intervention,* ed 3, St Louis, 1999, Mosby.

Hindle WH, editor: *Breast care: a clinical guidebook for women's primary health care providers,* New York, 1999, Springer.

Hughes LE, Mansel RE, Webster DJT: *Benign disorders and diseases of the breast: concepts and clinical management,* ed 2, London, 2000, WB Saunders.

Johnson ET: *Breast cancer, black women,* Montgomery, Ala, 1993, Van Slyke & Bray.

Kline TS, Kline KL, Howell LP: *Breast,* Philadelphia, 1999, Lippincott Williams & Wilkins.

Love SM: *Dr. Susan Love's breast book,* ed 2, Reading, Mass, 1995, Addison-Wesley.

Mansel RE, Bundred NJ: *Color atlas of breast diseases,* London, 1995, Mosby-Wolfe.

Moore-Higgs GJ, editor: *Women and cancer: a gynecologic oncology nursing perspective,* ed 2, Sudbury, Mass, 2000, Jones and Bartlett.

North American Nursing Diagnosis Association: *Nursing diagnosis: definitions and classification 2001-2002,* Philadelphia, 2001, Nursecom.

Pagana KD, Pagana TJ: *Mosby's diagnostic and laboratory test reference,* ed 4, St Louis, 1999, Mosby.

Purnell LD, Paulanka BJ: *Transcultural health care: a culturally competent approach,* Philadelphia, 1998, FA Davis.

Singletary SE, Robb GL: *Advanced therapy of breast disease,* Hamilton, Ont, 2000, BC Decker.

Stoll BA, editor: *Reducing breast cancer risk in women,* Dordrecht, 1995, Kluwer Academic Publishers.

Thibodeau GA, Patton KT: *Anatomy and physiology,* ed 4, St Louis, 1999, Mosby.

US Department of Health and Human Services: *Clinician's handbook of preventive services,* ed 2, Washington, DC, 1998, USDHHS.

US Department of Health and Human Services: *Healthy people 2010,* Washington, DC, 2000, US Government Printing Office.

US Preventive Services Task Force: *Guide to clinical preventive services: report of the US Preventive Services Task Force,* ed 2, Baltimore, 1996, Williams and Wilkins.

Vetto J et al: Accurate and cost-effective evaluation of breast masses in males, *Am J Surg* 175:383, 1998.

Woolf SH, Jonas S, Lawrence RS: *Health promotion and disease prevention in clinical practice,* Baltimore, 1996, Williams & Wilkins.

Chapter 15

Albert RK, Spiro SG, Jett JR, editors: *Comprehensive respiratory medicine,* London, 1999, Mosby.

Anderson KN, Anderson LE, Glanze WD: *Mosby's medical, nursing, and allied health dictionary,* ed 5, St Louis, 1998, Mosby.

Burton GG, Hodgkin JE, Ward JJ, editors: *Respiratory care: a guide to clinical practice,* ed 4, Philadelphia, 1997, JB Lippincott.

Corrin B: *Pathology of the lungs,* London, 2000, Churchill Livingstone.

Cotes JE: *Lung function: assessment and application in medicine,* ed 5, Oxford, 1993, Blackwell Science.

Davis GS, Marcy TW, Seward EA: *Medical management of pulmonary diseases,* New York, 1999, Marcel Dekker.

Ferris BG: Epidemiology Standardization Project (American Thoracic Society), *Am Rev Respir Dis* 118(6 Pt 2):1-120, 1978.

Fink JB, Hunt GE, editors: *Clinical practice in respiratory care,* Philadelphia, 1999, Lippincott Williams & Wilkins.

Giger JN, Davidhizar RE: *Transcultural nursing: assessment and intervention,* ed 3, St Louis, 1999, Mosby.

Gordon M: *Nursing diagnosis: process and application,* ed 3, St Louis, 1994, Mosby.

Hoeman SP, editor: *Rehabilitation nursing: process and application,* ed 2, St Louis, 1995, Mosby.

North American Nursing Diagnosis Association: *Nursing diagnosis: definitions and classification 2001-2002,* Philadelphia, 2001, Nursecom.

Pagana KD, Pagana TJ: *Mosby's diagnostic and laboratory test reference,* ed 4, St Louis, 1999, Mosby.

Providing respiratory care, Springhouse, Pa, 1996, Springhouse.

Purnell LD, Paulanka BJ: *Transcultural health care: a culturally competent approach,* Philadelphia, 1998, FA Davis.

Scanlan RL, Wilkins RL, Stoller JK: *Egan's fundamentals of respiratory care,* ed 7, St Louis, 1999, Mosby.

Seidel HM et al: *Mosby's guide to physical examination,* ed 4, St Louis, 1999, Mosby.

Thibodeau GA, Patton KT: *Anatomy and physiology,* ed 4, St Louis, 1999, Mosby.

US Department of Health and Human Services: *Clinician's handbook of preventive services,* ed 2, Washington, DC, 1998, USDHHS.

US Department of Health and Human Services: *Healthy people 2010,* Washington, DC, 2000, US Government Printing Office.

US Preventive Services Task Force: *Guide to clinical preventive services: report of the US Preventive Services Task Force,* ed 2, Baltimore, 1996, Williams and Wilkins.

West JB: *Respiratory physiology—the essentials,* Philadelphia, 2000, Lippincott Williams & Wilkins.

Wilby ML: *Instant nursing assessment: respiratory,* Albany, NY, 1996, Delmar.

Wilkins RL, Hodgkin JE, Lopez B: *Lung sounds: practical guide,* ed 2, St Louis, 1996, Mosby.

Wilkins RL, Krider SJ, Sheldon RL: *Clinical assessment in respiratory care,* ed 4, St Louis, 2000, Mosby.

Wilson SF, Thompson JM: *Respiratory disorders,* St Louis, 1990. Mosby.

Woolf SH, Jonas S, Lawrence, RS: *Health promotion and disease prevention in clinical practice,* Baltimore, 1996, Williams & Wilkins.

Chapter 16

Adolph RJ: The value of bedside examination in an era of high technology, part 1, *Heart Dis Stroke* 3(3):128-131, 1994.

Baker JD: Assessment of peripheral arterial occlusive disease, *Crit Care Nurs Clin North Am* 3(3):493-498, 1991.

Blank CA, Irwin GH: Peripheral vascular disorders: assessment and intervention, *Nurs Clin North Am* 25(4):777-793, 1990.

Braunwald E, editor: *Heart disease: a textbook of cardiovascular medicine,* ed 5, Philadelphia, 1996, WB Saunders.

Bright LD, Georgi S: Peripheral vascular disease: is it arterial or venous? *Am J Nurs* 92(9):34-43, 1992.

Butman SM et al: Bedside cardiovascular examination in patients with severe chronic heart failure: importance of rest or inducible jugular venous distension, *J Am College Cardiol* 22(4):968-974, 1993.

Davis E: The diagnostic puzzle and management challenge of Raynauds syndrome, *Nurse Pract* 18(3):18-20, 1993.

DeLeon AC: Fine-tuning the examination of the heart, *Consultant* 29(4): 51-61, 1989.

Epstein DE: Changing interpretations of angina pectoris associated with transient myocardial ischemia, *J Cardiovasc Nurs* 7(1):1-13, 1992.

Erickson B: *Heart sounds and murmurs: a practical guide,* ed 3, St Louis, 1997, Mosby.

Fabius DB: Solving the mystery of heart murmurs, *Nursing 94* 24(7):39-44, 1994.

Fabius DB: Uncovering the secrets of snaps, rubs, and clicks, *Nursing 94* 24(7):45-50, 1994.

Fellows E, Jocz AM: Getting the upper hand on lower extremity arterial disease, *Nursing 91* 21(8):34-41, 1991.

Gehring P: Vascular assessment, *RN* 55(1):40-47, 1992.

Gersony WM: Coarctation of the aorta, *Hosp Med* 27(5):53-63, 1991.

Herr KA: Night leg pain in the elderly, *Geriatr Nurs* 13(1):13-16, 1992.

Jessup M et al: CHF in the elderly: is it different? *Patient Care* 26(14): 40-61, 1992.

Meyers DG: Review of cardiac auscultation, (part 1), *Hosp Med* 29(10): 25-52, 1993.

Notowitz LB: Normal venous anatomy and physiology of the lower extremity, *J Vasc Nurs* 11(2):39-42, 1993.

Recognizing valvular heart disease, *Emerg Med* 22(7):56-71, 1990.

Tilkian AG, Conover MB: *Understanding heart sounds and murmurs,* ed 3, Philadelphia, 1993, WB Saunders.

US Preventive Services Task Force: *Guide to clinical preventive services,* ed 2, Alexandria, Va, 1996, International Medical Publishing.

Whitaker L, Kelleher A: Raynaud's syndrome: diagnosis and treatment, *J Vasc Nurs* 12(1):10-13, 1994.

Wilson SF, Giddens JF: *Health assessment for nursing practice,* ed 2, St Louis, 2001, Mosby.

Wong DL et al: *Whaley and Wong's nursing care of infants and children,* ed 5, St Louis, 1995, Mosby.

Yacone-Morton L: Cardiac assessment, *RN* 54(12):28-35, 1991.

Chapter 17

Bowers AC, Thompson JM: *Clinical manual of health assessment,* ed 4, St Louis, 1992, Mosby.

Centers for Disease Control and Prevention: Hepatitis B virus: a comprehensive strategy for eliminating transmission in the United States through universal childhood vaccination: recommendations of the Immunization Practices Advisory Committee (ACIP), *MMWR* vol 40 (No RR-13), 1991.

Christensen J: *Bedside logic in diagnostic gastroenterology,* New York, 1987, Churchill Livingstone.

Gordon M: *Nursing diagnosis: process and application,* ed 3, St Louis, 1994, Mosby.

Johnson LR: *Gastrointestinal physiology,* ed 5, St Louis, 1997, Mosby.

Reece SM: Immunization strategies for the elimination of hepatitis B, *Nurse Pract* 18:42-50, 1993.

Seidel HM et al: *Mosby's guide to physical examination,* ed 3, St Louis, 1995, Mosby.

Thompson JM et al: *Mosby's clinical nursing,* ed 4, St Louis, 1997, Mosby.

US Preventive Services Task Force: *Guide to clinical preventive services,* ed 2, Alexandria, Va, 1996, International Medical Publishing.

Chapter 18

American Academy of Orthopaedic Surgeons: *Joint motion: method of measuring and recording,* Chicago, 1965, The Academy.

Ausenhus MK: Osteoporosis: prevention during the adolescent and young adult years, *Nurse Pract* 13:19-24, 1988.

Beetham W, Polley H: *Rheumatologic interviewing and physical examination of the joints,* ed 2, Philadelphia, 1978, WB Saunders.

Collo MC et al: Evaluating arthritic complaints, *Nurse Pract* 16:9-20, 1991.

Daniels L, Worthingham C: *Muscle testing: techniques of manual examination,* ed 5, Philadelphia, 1986, WB Saunders.

Gordon M: *Nursing diagnosis: process and application,* ed 3, St Louis, 1994, Mosby.

Hoppenfeld S: *Physical examination of the spine and extremities,* New York, 1976, Appleton-Century-Crofts.

Magee DJ: *Orthopedic physical assessment,* ed 3, Philadelphia, 1997, WB Saunders.

Mann RA, editor: *DuVries' surgery of the foot,* ed 5, St Louis, 1986, Mosby.

McCarty DJ, Koopman WJ, editors: *Arthritis and allied conditions,* ed 12, Philadelphia, 1993, Lea & Febiger.

Mendelsohn BA, Paiement GD: Physical examination of the knee, *Primary Care* 23:321-328, 1996.

Mercier LR: *Practical orthopedics,* ed 4, St Louis, 1995, Mosby.

Mourad LA: *Orthopedic disorders,* St Louis, 1991, Mosby.

US Preventive Services Task Force: *Guide to clinical preventive services,* ed 2, Alexandria, Va, 1996, International Medical Publishing.

Chapter 19

Alspach JG: *Core curriculum for critical care nursing,* ed 5, Philadelphia, 1998, WB Saunders.

Bowers AC, Thompson JM: *Clinical manual of health assessment,* ed 4, St Louis, 1992, Mosby.

Chipps EM, Clanin NJ, Campbell VG: *Neurologic disorders,* St Louis, 1992, Mosby.

DeJong RN et al: *Essentials of the neurological examination,* Philadelphia, 1978, SmithKline.

Hickey JV: *The clinical practice of neurological and neurosurgical nursing,* ed 4, Philadelphia, 1997, JB Lippincott.

Jones DA: *Health assessment manual,* New York, 1986, McGraw-Hill.

Lewis SM, Heitkemper MM, Dirksen SR: *Medical-surgical nursing: assessment and management of clinical problems,* ed 5, St Louis, 2000, Mosby.

Matthews P, Carlson CE: *Spinal cord injury: a guide to rehabilitation nursing,* Rockville, Md, 1987, Aspen.

Potter PA: *Pocket guide to health assessment,* ed 4, St Louis, 1998, Mosby.

Rudy EB, Gray VR: *Handbook of health assessment,* ed 3, Norwalk, Conn, 1991, Appleton & Lange.

Scanlon VC, Sanders T: *Essentials of anatomy and physiology,* ed 2, Philadelphia, 1995, FA Davis.

Seidel HM et al: *Mosby's guide to physical examination,* ed 4, St Louis, 1999, Mosby.

Snyder M: *A guide to neurological and neurosurgical nursing,* ed 2, Albany, NY, 1991, Delmar.

Sparks SM, Taylor CM: *Nursing diagnosis reference manual,* ed 5, Springhouse, Pa, 2001, Springhouse.

Stuart GW, Laraia MT: *Principles and practices of psychiatric nursing,* ed 7, St Louis, 2001, Mosby.

Thompson JM et al: *Mosby's clinical nursing,* ed 4, St Louis, 1997, Mosby.

Watson C: *Basic human neuroanatomy: an introductory atlas,* ed 5, Boston, 1995, Little, Brown.

Wilson SF, Giddens JF: *Health assessment for nursing practice,* ed 2, St Louis, 2001, Mosby.

Chapter 20

Betesh S, editor: *Diseases of the urinary tract and male genital organs,* Geneva, 1974, Council for Internal Organizations for Medical Sciences.

Caine KW, Garfinkel P, editors: *The male body: an owner's manual: the ultimate head-to-toe guide to staying healthy and fit for life,* Emmanus, Pa, 1996, Rodale Press.

US Department of Health and Human Services: *Clinician's handbook of preventive services,* ed 2, Washington, DC, 1998, USDHHS.

Devlin HB et al: *Management of abdominal hernias,* ed 2, London, 1998, Chapman & Hall Medical.

Gillenwater JY et al: *Adult and pediatric urology,* ed 3, St Louis, 1996, Mosby.

Giger JN, Davidhizar RE: *Transcultural nursing: assessment and intervention,* ed 3, St Louis, 1999, Mosby.

Gordon M: *Nursing diagnosis: process and application,* ed 3, St Louis, 1994, Mosby.

Lipshultz LI, Kleinman I: *Urology and the primary care practitioner,* London, 1995, Mosby-Wolfe.

Klingman L: Assessing the male genitalia, *Am J Nurs* 99(7):47, 1999.

Maddern GJ, Hiatt JR, Phillips EH: *Hernia repair: open vs. laparoscopic approaches,* New York, 1997, Churchill Livingstone.

Mundy AR et al: *Scientific basis of urology,* Oxford, 1999, Isis Medical Media.

Nieschlag E, Behre HM, editors: *Andrology: male reproductive health and dysfunction,* ed 2, New York, 2001, Springer.

North American Nursing Diagnosis Association: *Nursing diagnosis: definitions and classification 2001-2002,* Philadelphia, 2001, Nursecom.

Nyhus LM, Condon RE: *Hernia,* ed 3, Philadelphia, 1989, JB Lippincott.

Pagana KD, Pagana TJ: *Mosby's diagnostic and laboratory test reference,* ed 4, St Louis, 1999, Mosby.

Presti JC: Prostate cancer: assessment of risk using digital rectal examination, tumor grade, prostate-specific antigen, and systematic biopsy, *Radiol Clin North Am* 38(1):49, 2000.

Purnell LD, Paulanka BJ: *Transcultural health care: a culturally competent approach,* Philadelphia, 1998, FA Davis.

Rous SN: *Urology: a core textbook,* ed 2, Cambridge, Mass, 1996, Blackwell Science.

Seidel HM et al: *Mosby's guide to physical examination,* ed 4, St Louis, 1999, Mosby.

Smith LE, editor: *Practical guide to anorectal testing,* ed 2, New York, 1994, Igaku-Shoin Medical Publishers.

Tanner JM: *Growth at adolescence,* ed 2, Oxford, 1962, Blackwell Scientific Publications.

Thibodeau GA, Patton KT: *Anatomy and physiology,* ed 4, St Louis, 1999, Mosby.

US Department of Health and Human Services: *Clinician's handbook of preventive services,* ed 2, Washington, DC, 1998, USDHHS.

US Department of Health and Human Services: *Healthy people 2010,* Washington, DC, 2000, US Government Printing Office.

US Preventive Services Task Force: *Guide to clinical preventive services: report of the US Preventive Services Task Force,* ed 2, Baltimore, 1996, Williams & Wilkins..

Watson J: *Male bodies: health, culture, and identity,* Buckingham, England, 2000, Open University Press.

Woolf SH, Jonas S, Lawrence RS: *Health promotion and disease prevention in clinical practice,* Baltimore, 1996, Williams & Wilkins.

Chapter 21

Agency of Health Care Policy and Research: Evaluation of cervical cytology, summary, evidence report/technology assessment: No. 5, Rockville, Md, January 1999, Agency for Health Care Policy and Research.

Anderson KN, Anderson LE, Glanze WD: *Mosby's medical, nursing, and allied health dictionary,* ed 5, St Louis, 1998, Mosby.

Beckmann CRB: *Obstetrics and gynecology,* ed 2, Baltimore, 1995, Williams & Wilkins.

Brown K: *Management guidelines for women's health nurse practitioners,* Philadelphia, 2000, FA Davis.

Firth PA, Watanabe SJ: *Instant nursing assessment: women's health,* Albany, NY, 1996, Delmar Publishers.

Giger JN, Davidhizar, RE: *Transcultural nursing: assessment and intervention,* ed 3, St Louis, 1999, Mosby.

Gordon M: *Nursing diagnosis: process and application,* ed 3, St Louis, 1994, Mosby.

Gulanick M, Gradishar D, Puzas MK: *Obstetric and gynecologic nursing,* Albany, NY, 1994, Delmar Publishers.

Hawkins JW, Roberto-Nichols DM, Stanley-Haney JL: *Protocols for nurse practitioners in gynecologic settings,* ed 5, New York, 1995, Tiresias Press.

James M et al: *Obstetrics and gynaecology: a problem-solving approach,* Edinburgh, 1999, WB Saunders.

Klingman L: Assessing the female reproductive system, *Am J Nurs* 99(8): 37, 1999.

Knaus JV, Isaacs JH, editors: *Office gynecology,* New York, 1993, Springer-Verlag.

Moore-Higgs GJ, editor: *Women and cancer: a gynecologic oncology nursing perspective,* ed 2, Sudbury, Mass, 2000, Jones and Bartlett.

National Cancer Institute Workshop: The Bethesda System for reporting cervical/vaginal cytologic diagnoses: revised after the second National Cancer Institute Workshop, *Acta Cytol* 37(2):115, 1991.

North American Nursing Diagnosis Association: *Nursing diagnosis: definitions and classification 2001-2002,* Philadelphia, 2001, Nursecom.

Pagana KD, Pagana TJ: *Mosby's diagnostic and laboratory test reference,* ed 4, St Louis, 1999, Mosby.

Purnell LD, Paulanka BJ: *Transcultural health care: a culturally competent approach,* Philadelphia, 1998, FA Davis.

Ransom SB et al: *Practical strategies in obstetrics and gynecology,* Philadelphia, 2000, WB Saunders.

Ryan KJ et al: *Kistner's gynecology and women's health,* ed 7, St Louis, 1990, Mosby.

Scott JR et al: *Danforth's obstetrics and gynecology,* Philadelphia, 1999, Lippincott Williams & Wilkins.

Secor MC: Skills workshop. Part 1. The challenging pelvic examination, *Patient Care Nurse Pract* 2(7):36, 1999.

Secor MC: Skills workshop. Part 2. The bimanual pelvic examination, *Patient Care Nurse Pract* 2(8):12, 1999.

Seidel HM et al: *Mosby's guide to physical examination,* ed 4, St Louis, 1999, Mosby.

Symonds EM, Macpherson MBA: *Color atlas of obstetrics and gynecology,* London, 1995, Mosby-Wolfe.

Thibodeau GA, Patton KT: *Anatomy and physiology,* ed 4, St Louis, 1999, Mosby.

US Department of Health and Human Services: *Clinician's handbook of preventive services,* ed 2, Washington, DC, 1998, USDHHS.

US Department of Health and Human Services: *Healthy people 2010,* Washington, DC, 2000, US Government Printing Office.

US Preventive Services Task Force: *Guide to clinical preventive services: report of the US Preventive Services Task Force,* ed 2, Baltimore, 1996, Williams & Wilkins.

Woolf SH, Jonas S, Lawrence RS: *Health promotion and disease prevention in clinical practice,* Baltimore, 1996, Williams & Wilkins.

Zitelli BJ, Davis HW: *Atlas of pediatric physical diagnosis,* ed 3, St Louis, 1997, Mosby.

Chapter 22

Bailey HR, Snyder MJ, editors: *Ambulatory anorectal surgery,* New York, 2000, Springer.

Dunphey HR, Botsford TW: *Physical examination of the surgical patient: an introduction to clinical surgery,* ed 4, Philadelphia, 1975, WB Saunders.

Giger JN, Davidhizar RE: *Transcultural nursing: assessment and intervention,* ed 3, St Louis, 1999, Mosby.

Gordon M: *Nursing diagnosis: process and application,* ed 3, St Louis, 1994, Mosby.

Kirsner JB, Shorter RG, editors: *Diseases of the colon, rectum, and anal canal,* Baltimore, 1988, Williams & Wilkins.

Marti MC, Givel JC: *Surgery of anorectal diseases,* Berlin, 1990, Springer-Verlag.

North American Nursing Diagnosis Association: *Nursing diagnosis: definitions and classification 2001-2002,* Philadelphia, 2001, Nursecom.

Pagana KD, Pagana TJ: *Mosby's diagnostic and laboratory test reference,* ed 4, St Louis, 1999, Mosby.

Porrett T, Daniel N: *Essential coloproctology for nurses,* London, 1999, Whurr.

Purnell LD, Paulanka BJ: *Transcultural health care: a culturally competent approach,* Philadelphia, 1998, FA Davis.

Seidel HM et al: *Mosby's guide to physical examination,* ed 4, St Louis, 1999, Mosby.

Smith LE, editor: *Practical guide to anorectal testing,* ed 2, New York, 1994, Igaku-Shoin Medical Publishers.

Thibodeau GA, Patton KT: *Anatomy and physiology,* ed 4, St Louis, 1999, Mosby.

US Department of Health and Human Services: *Clinician's handbook of preventive services,* ed 2, Washington, DC, 1998, USDHHS.

US Department of Health and Human Services: *What you need to know about cancers of the colon and rectum,* Bethesda, Md, 1999, USDHHS.

US Department of Health and Human Services: *Healthy people 2010* (conference edition in two volumes), Washington, DC, 2000, USDHHS.

US Preventive Services Task Force: *Guide to clinical preventive services: report of the US Preventive Services Task Force,* ed 2, Baltimore, 1996, Williams & Wilkins.

Woolf SH, Jonas S, Lawrence RS: *Health promotion and disease prevention in clinical practice,* Baltimore, 1996, Williams & Wilkins.

Chapter 24

Brown SJ: *Knowledge for health care practice: a guide to using research evidence,* Philadelphia, 1999, WB Saunders.

Johnson M, Maas ML, Moorhead S: *Nursing outcomes classification,* ed 2, St Louis, 2000, Mosby.

McCloskey J, Bulechek GM: *Nursing interventions classification,* ed 3, St Louis, 2000, Mosby.

Sackett DL et al: *Evidence-based medicine: how to practice and teach EBM,* ed 2, New York, 2000, Churchill Livingstone.

Chapter 25

American Academy of Pediatrics, American College of Obstetrics and Gynecology: *Guidelines for perinatal care,* ed 4, Elk Grove Village, Ill, 1997, The Academy.

American College of Obstetricians and Gynecologists: *Precis V: an update in obstetrics and gynecology,* Washington, DC, 1998, ACOG.

Anderson KN, Anderson LE, Glanze WD: *Mosby's medical, nursing, and allied health dictionary,* ed 5, St Louis, 1998, Mosby.

Andolsek KM, Kelton GM: Risk assessment, *Prim Care* 27(1):71, 2000.

Barber HRK, Fields DH, Kaufman SA: *Quick reference to OB-GYN procedures,* ed 3, Philadelphia, 1990, JB Lippincott.

Beckmann CRB: *Obstetrics and gynecology,* ed 2, Baltimore, 1995, Williams & Wilkins.

Bennett VR, Brown LK: *Myles textbook for midwives,* ed 3, Edinburgh, 1999, Churchill Livingstone.

Benson MD: *Obstetrical pearls,* ed 3, Philadelphia, 1999, FA Davis.

US Department of Health and Human Services: *Clinician's handbook of preventive services,* ed 2, Washington, DC, 1998, USDHHS.

DeCherney AH, Pernoll ML: *Current obstetric and gynecologic diagnosis and treatment,* ed 8, Norwalk, Conn, 1994, Appleton & Lange.

Firth PA, Watanabe SJ: *Instant nursing assessment: women's health,* Albany, NY, 1996, Delmar Publishers.

Giger JN, Davidhizar RE: *Transcultural nursing: assessment and intervention,* ed 3, St Louis, 1999, Mosby.

Gordon M: *Nursing diagnosis: process and application,* ed 3, St Louis, 1994, Mosby.

Gulanick M, Gradishar D, Puzas MK: *Obstetric and gynecologic nursing,* Albany, NY, 1994, Delmar Publishers.

James M et al: *Obstetrics and gynaecology: a problem-solving approach,* Edinburgh, 1999, WB Saunders.

North American Nursing Diagnosis Association: *Nursing diagnosis: definitions and classification 2001-2002,* Philadelphia, 2001, Nursecom.

Oxorn H: *Oxorn-Foote human labor and birth,* Norwalk, Conn, 1986, Appleton-Century-Crofts.

Pagana KD, Pagana TJ: *Mosby's diagnostic and laboratory test reference,* ed 4, St Louis, 1999, Mosby.

Purnell LD, Paulanka, BJ: *Transcultural health care: a culturally competent approach,* Philadelphia, 1998, FA Davis.

Ransom SB et al: *Practical strategies in obstetrics and gynecology,* Philadelphia, 2000, WB Saunders.

Scott JR: *Danforth's obstetrics and gynecology,* Philadelphia, 1999, Lippincott Williams & Wilkins.

Symonds EM, Macpherson MBA: *Color atlas of obstetrics and gynecology,* London, 1994, Mosby-Wolfe.

Tucker S: *Pocket guide to fetal monitoring,* ed 4, St Louis, 2000, Mosby.

US Department of Health and Human Services: *Clinician's handbook of preventive services,* ed 2, Washington, DC, 1998, USDHHS.

US Department of Health and Human Services: *Healthy people 2010* (conference edition in two volumes), Washington, DC, 2000, USDHHS.

US Preventive Services Task Force: *Guide to clinical preventive services: report of the US Preventive Services Task Force,* ed 2, Baltimore, 1996, Williams & Wilkins.

Woolf SH, Jonas S, Lawrence, RS: *Health promotion and disease prevention in clinical practice,* Baltimore, 1996, Williams & Wilkins.

Chapter 26

American Academy of Pediatrics: *Guidelines for health supervision II,* ed 2, Elk Grove Village, Ill, 1998, The Academy.

American Academy of Pediatrics: Committee on Practice and Ambulatory Medicine Recommendation for Preventive Pediatric Health Care, 2000. website: aap.org/policy.

American Academy of Pediatrics: Committee on Immunization Practice, Recommended childhood vaccination schedule—United States, January through December 2000, *Pediatrics* vol 105, no 1, 2000, http://www.cdc.gov/nip/.

Barlow SE, Dietz WH: Obesity evaluation and treatment: expert committee recommendations, *Pediatrics* 120(3):E291, 1998.

Barness LA: *Handbook of pediatric physical diagnosis,* Philadelphia, 1998, JB Lippincott.

Burns C et al: *Pediatric primary care: a handbook for nurse practitioners,* ed 2, Philadelphia, 2000, WB Saunders.

CDC: www.CDC.gov/growthcharts.

Chess S, Thomas A: *Temperament in clinical practice,* New York, 1986, Guilford Press.

Daniels SR: Primary hypertension in childhood and adolescence, *Pediatr Ann* 21:224-234, 1992.

Dixon SD, Stein MT: *Encounters with children: pediatric behavior and development,* ed 3, St Louis, 2000, Mosby.

Gemberling C: Preparticipation sports evaluation: an overview, *Nurse Pract Forum* 7(3):125-135, 1996.

Goldenring JM, Cohen E: Getting into adolescent heads, *Contemp Pediatr* 5:75-86, 1988.

Hoekelman RA et al: *Primary pediatric care,* ed 3, St Louis, 1997, Mosby.

Levenberg P, Elster A, editors: *Guidelines for adolescent preventive services (GAPS): clinical evaluation and management handbook,* Chicago, 1995, American Medical Association.

Lichtman R, Papera S: *Gynecology: well woman care,* Norwalk, Conn, 1990, Appleton & Lange.

Lowrey GH: *Growth and development of children,* ed 8, St Louis, 1986, Mosby.

National Heart, Lung and Blood Institute: Report of Second Task Force on Blood Pressure Control in Children, 1987, *Pediatrics* 79:1-25, 1987.

National High Blood Pressure Education Program Working Group on Hypertension Control in Children and Adolescents: Update on the 1987 Task Force Report on High Blood Pressure in Children and Adolescents, *Pediatrics* 98(4):649-658, 1996.

Satter E: *Child of mine: feeding with love and good sense,* Palo Alto, Calif, 1991, Bull Publishing.

Schwartz MW et al: *Pediatric primary care: a problem-oriented approach,* ed 3, St Louis, 1996, Mosby.

Seidel HM et al: *Mosby's guide to physical examination,* ed 4, St Louis, 1999, Mosby.

Strassburger V, Brown R: *Adolescent medicine: a practical guide,* Boston, 1991, Little, Brown.

Tanner JM: *Growth at adolescence,* ed 2, Oxford, 1962, Blackwell Scientific Publications.

US Department of Health and Human Services: : *Healthy people 2010,* Washington, DC, 2000, US Government Printing Office.

Wong DL et al: *Whaley and Wong's nursing care of infants and children,* ed 6, St Louis, 1999, Mosby.

Zitelli B, Davis H: *Atlas of pediatric physical diagnosis,* ed 3, New York, 1996, Gower Medical Publishing.

Chapter 27

Abbasi A: Nutrition. In Duthie EH, Katz PR, editors: *Practice of geriatrics,* Philadelphia, 1998, WB Saunders.

Administration on Aging (AoA): 2001 (Online). website: http://www.aoa.dhhs.gov/network.html.

American Psychiatric Association: *Diagnosis and statistical manual of mental disorders,* ed 4, Washington, DC, 1994, The Association.

Cassel CK et al: *Geriatric medicine,* ed 2, New York, 1990, Springer-Verlag.

Dwyer J: *Screening older Americans' nutritional health: current practices and future possibilities,* Washington, DC, 1992, Nutritional Screening Initiative.

Ebersole P, Hess P: *Toward healthy aging,* St Louis, 1998, Mosby

Fantl JA, Newman DK, Colling J et al: Urinary incontinence in adults: acute and chronic management, Clinical Practice Guideline, No 2, 1996 Update. Rockville, Md, March 1996, US Department of Health and Human Services, Public Health Services, Agency for Health Care Policy and Research, AHCPR Publication No. 96-0682.

Fleming KC et al: Practical functional assessment of elderly persons: a primary care approach, *Mayo Clin Proc* 70:890-903, 1995.

Folstein M: Differential diagnosis of dementia: the clinical process, *Psychiatr Clin North Am* 20:45-57, 1997.

Folstein M, Folstein SE, McHugh PR: Mini-mental state: a practical method for grading the cognitive state of patients for the clinician, *J Psychiatr Res* 12:189-198, 1975.

Geriatric assessment methods for clinical decision-making, National Institutes of Health Consensus Development Conference Statement, *J Am Geriatr Soc* 36:342-347, 1988.

Gordon M: *Manual of nursing diagnosis 1997-1998,* St Louis, 1993, Mosby.

Hirsch CH et al: The natural history of functional morbidity in hospitalized older patients, *Am Geriatr Soc* 38:1296-1303, 1990.

Katz S et al: Studies of illness in the aged: the index of ADL: a standard measure of biologic and psychosocial function, *JAMA* 185:914-919, 1963.

Lawton MP, Brody EM: Assessment of older people: self maintaining and instrumental activities of daily living, *Gerontologist* 9:180, 1969.

Lebowitz BD et al: Diagnosis and the treatment of depression in late life. Consensus statement update, *JAMA* 278:1186-1190, 1997.

Levkoff SE et al: Delirium: the occurrence and persistence of symptoms among elderly hospitalized patients, *Arch Intern Med* 152:334-340, 1992.

Lyness JM et al: The importance of subsyndromal depression in older primary care patients: prevalence and associated functional disability, *Am Geriatr Soc* 47:647-652, 1999.

Mahoney Fl, Barthel DW: Functional evaluation: the Barthel Index, *Maryland State Med J* 14:61-65, 1965.

Miller KE, Zylstra RG, Standridge JB: The geriatric patient: a systematic approach to maintaining health, *Am Fam Physician* 61:1089-1104, 2000.

National Osteoporosis Foundation Physician Guide (Online). website: ttp://www.nof.org/physguide.

NIH Consensus Panel on Diagnosis and Treatment of Depression in Late Life, *JAMA* 268:1018-1024, 1992.

Podsiadlo D, Richardson S: The timed "up and go": a test of basic functional mobility for frail elderly persons, *J Am Geriatr Soc* 39:142-148, 1991.

Schor JD et al: Risk factors for delirium in hospitalized elderly, *JAMA* 267:827-831, 1992.

Williams TF: Comprehensive geriatric assessment. In Duthie EH, Katz PR, editors: *Practice of geriatrics,* Philadelphia, 1998, WB Saunders.

Yesavage JA et al: Development and validation of a geriatric depression screening scale: preliminary report, *J Psychiatr Res* 17:37-49, 1983.

Chapter 28

Anderson KN, Anderson LE, Glanze WD: *Mosby's medical, nursing, and allied health dictionary,* ed 5, St Louis, 1998, Mosby.

Brorsson B, Asberg KH: Katz index of independence in ADL: reliability and validity in short-term care, *Scand J Rehabil Med* 16:125-132, 1984.

Buchanan B: Functional assessment: measurement with the Barthel index and PULSES profile, *Home Health Nurse* 4:11-17, 1986.

Curtis KA: Communicating with persons who have disabilities. In Davis CM: *Patient practitioner interaction: an experiential manual for developing the art of health care*, ed 3, Thorofare, NJ, 1998, Slack.

Delisa JA, Gans BM, editors: *Rehabilitation medicine: principles and practice*, Philadelphia, 1998, Lippincott-Raven.

Dittmar SS, Gresham GE, editors: *Functional assessment and outcome measures for the rehabilitation health professional*, Gaithersburg, Md, 1997, Aspen.

Forer SK: *Revised functional status rating instrument*, Glendale, Calif, 1981, Rehabilitation Institute, Glendale Adventist Medical Center.

Fortinsky RH, Granger CV, Seltzer GB: The use of functional assessment in understanding home care needs, *Med Care* 19:489, 1981.

Frattali CM: Perspectives on functional assessment: its use for policy making, *Disabil Rehabil* 15:1, 1993.

Fuhrer MJ, editor: *Rehabilitation outcomes: analysis and measurement*, Baltimore, 1987, Brookes.

Gallo JJ et al: *Handbook of geriatric assessment*, ed 3, Gaithersburg, Md, 2000, Aspen.

Gardent H et al: *Use of the international classification of impairments, disabilities and handicapped (ICIDH) in relation to elderly people*, Strasbourg, 1997, Council of Europe.

Giger JN, Davidhizar RE: *Transcultural nursing: assessment and intervention*, ed 3, St Louis, 1999, Mosby.

Gordon M: *Nursing diagnosis: process and application*, ed 3, St Louis, 1994, Mosby.

Granger CV: Health accounting—functional assessment of the long-term patient. In Kottke FJ, Stillwell GK, Lehmann JF, editors: *Krusen's handbook of physical medicine and rehabilitation*, ed 3, Philadelphia, 1982, WB Saunders.

Granger CV, Albrecht GL, Hamilton BB: Outcome of comprehensive medical rehabilitation: measurement by PULSES profile and the Barthel Index, *Arch Phys Med Rehab* 60:145, 1979.

Granger CV, Seltzer GB, Fishbein CF: *Primary care of the functionally disabled: assesment and management*, Philadelphia, 1987, JB Lippincott.

Hoeman SP: *Rehabilitation nursing*, ed 3, St Louis, 2002, Mosby.

Jette AM: State of the are in functional status assessment. In Rothstein JM: *Measurement in phisical therapy*, New York, 1985, Churchill Livingstone.

Katz S, Akpom CA: Index of ADL, *Med Care* 14:116, 1976.

Katz S et al: Studies of illness in the aged: the index of ADL: a standardized measure of biological and psychosocial function, *JAMA* 185:914, 1963.

Keith RA et al: The functional independence measure: a new tool for rehabilitation. In Eisenberg MG, Grzesiak RC, editors: *Advances in clinical rehabilitation*, New York, 1987, Spring.

Lawton MP, Brody EM: Assessment of older people: self-maintaining and instrumental activities of daily living, *Gerontologist* 9:180, 1969.

Lawton MP: Assessing the competence of older people. In Kent D, Kastenbaum R, Sherwood S, editors: *Research, planning and action for the elderly*, New York, 1972, Behavioral Publications.

Linn MW, Linn BS: The rapid disability rating scale-2, *J Am Geriatr Soc* 30:378-382, 1982.

Mahoney FI, Barthel DW: Functional evaluation: the Barthel index, *Maryland State Med J* 14:61, 1965.

McDowell I, Newell C: *Measuring health: a guide to rating scales questionnaires*, ed 2, New York, 1996, Oxford University Press.

McGinnis GE et al: Program evaluation of physical medicine and rehabilitation departments using self-report Barthel, *Arch Phys Med Rehabil* 67:123-135, 1986.

Moskowitz E: PULSES profile in retrospect, *Arch Phys Med Rehabil* 66:647-648, 1985.

Moskowitz E, McCann CB: Classification of disability in the chronically ill and aging, *J Chron Dis* 5:342-346, 1957.

Nagi S: Disability, concepts and prevalence. Unpublished paper presented at the First Mary Switzer Memorial Seminar, Cleveland, Ohio, May 1975.

Nolan BS: Functional evaluation of the elderly in guardianship proceedings, *Law Med Healthcare* 12(2):10-12, 18, 1984.

North American Nursing Diagnosis Association: *Nursing diagnosis: definitions and classification 2001-2002*, Philadelphia, 2001, Nursecom.

O'Toole DM, Goldberg RT, Ryan B: Functional changes in vascular amputee patients: evaluation by Barthel, PULSES profile and ESCROW scale, *Arch Phys Med Rehabil* 66:508-511, 1985.

Pfeffer RI et al: Index in older adults: reliability, validity, and measurement of change over time, *Am J Epidemiol* 120:922-935, 1984.

Pinholt EM et al: Functional assessment of the elderly: a comparison of standard instruments with clinical judgment, *Arch Intern Med* 147:484-488, 1987.

Purnell LD, Paulanka BJ: *Transcultural health care: a culturally competent approach*, Philadelphia, 1998, FA Davis.

Rothstein JM: *Measurement in physical therapy*, New York, 1985, Churchill Livingstone.

Rubenstein LZ et al: Systematic biases in functional status assessment of elderly adults: effects of different data sources, *J Gerontol* 39:686-691, 1984.

Sheikh K et al: Repeatability and validity of a modified activities of daily living (ADL) index in studies of chronic disability, *Int Rehab Med* 1:51, 1979.

Special issue—Critical issues in functional assessment, *Am J Occup Ther* 47:199-259, 1993.

Spiegel JS, Hirshfield MS, Spiegel TM: Evaluation of self-care activities: comparison of a self-reported questionnaire with an occupational therapist interview, *Br J Rheumatol* 24:357-361, 1985.

Teresi JA, Golden RR, Gurland BJ: Concurrent and predictive validity of indicator scales developed for the comprehensive assessment and referral evaluation interview schedule, *J Gerontol* 39:158-165, 1984.

Teresi JA et al: Construct validity of indicator scales developed from the comprehensive assessment and referral evaluation interview schedule, *J Gerontol* 39:147-157, 1984.

US Department of Health and Human Services: *Healthy people 2010*, Washington, DC, 2000, US Government Printing Office.

Wood P: *Classification of impairments and handicaps*, Geneva, 1975, World Health Organization.

World Health Organization: *International classification of impairments, disabilities, and handicaps*, Geneva, 1980, The Organization.

Woolf SH, Jonas S, Lawrence RS: *Health promotion and disease prevention in clinical practice*, Baltimore, 1996, Williams & Wilkins.

Index

INITIAL ASSESSMENT IN SPANISH

Helpful Hints

- Have an English-Spanish dictionary available.
- If you are not familiar with Spanish, ask questions that require only a "yes" (si), "no" (no), or "I don't know" (yo no se) response.
- Assume you have only a brief time to determine the client's problem and instruct the client in what to do next.
- Use as much body/sign language as possible. This allows the client to do the same.

Some Rules of Pronunciation

- All vowels are pronounced openly (e.g., semana = "seh-**ma**-nah"; duele = "doo-**eh**-lay").
- The letters "ll" are pronounced "y" as in "yellow" (e.g., llama = "**yah**-ma").
- A "u" in front of an "i" or an "e" is silent (e.g., alguien = "al-**gee**-ain"; que = "kay").
- A "g" before a consonant or a "u" (whether the "u" is pronounced or not) is pronounced hard, as in "gate" (e.g., alguien = "al-**gee**-ain").
- A "g" in front of an "i" or an "e" is pronounced as an "h" (e.g., alergia = "ah-lair-**hee**-ha").
- A "j" is pronounced as an "h" (e.g., ojos = "**oh**-hos").
- An "h" is always silent (e.g., hacer = "**ah**-sair").
- An "n" that has a tilde (~) over it is pronounced "nyah" (e.g., Español = "ess-pan-**yole**").
- In Spanish, the second-to-last syllable is accented, except where the accent is written (bold indicates accent).

First, Greet the Client and State Your Name

Buenos días/buenas tardes. Me llamo . . .	Good morning/good afternoon. My name is . . .
Soy enfermera.	I am a nurse.
No hablo español.	I don't speak Spanish.
Le voy a hacer unas preguntas.	I am going to ask you some questions.

Assess the Client

¿Cómo se llama usted?	What is your name?
*¿Está usted enfermo?	Are you ill?
¿Cuál es el problema?	What is the problem?
¿Me puede enseñar donde?	Can you point to it?
¿Por cuántos días/semanas/meses ha tenido este problema?	How many days/weeks/months have you had this problem?
*¿Tiene usted dolor?	Are you in pain?
Enséñeme donde le duele.	Show me where it hurts.
*¿Está tomando algún medicamento?	Are you taking any medicine?
*¿Tien sus medicamentos aquí?	Do you have your medications here?
¿Sabe los nombres de suis medicamentos?	What are they called? (Write down the names the client tells you.)
*¿Es usted alérgico a algo?	Are you allergic to anything?
*¿Tiene usted alguna enfermedad crónica?	Do you have a chronic illness?
*¿Tiene diabetes?	Do you have diabetes?
*¿Tiene la presión alta?	Do you have hypertension?
*¿Ha bajado de peso reciéntemente?	Have you lost weight recently?
*¿Trabaja usted?	Do you work?
*¿Está usted embarazada?	Are you pregnant?
¿Cúantos meses?	How many months?
Por favor acuéstese.	Please lie down.
Por favor siéntese.	Please sit up.
Usted necesita:	You need:
ver a un doctor	to see a doctor.
una radiografiá	an x-ray
una prueba de sangre	blood examined
una prueba de orina	urine examined
Voy a examinar:	I will examine:
sus ojos, oídos, nariz, y garganta	your eyes, ears, nose, and throat
su abdomen	your abdomen
su espalda	your back
*¿Vino usted solo?	Did you come alone?
*¿Conoce usted a alguien que habla ínglés y español?	Do you know someone who speaks English and Spanish?
*¿Puede usted venir el día . . . ?	Can you come on . . . ?
*¿Puede traer una persona que habla inglés y español?	Can you bring someone who speaks English and Spanish?

*Questions requiring only a "yes," "no," or "I don't know" response.

NOTE: This material can be photocopied and used as an initial assessment questionnaire.

Suggested Reeferences

Chase R, Medina de Chase CB: *An introduction to Spanish for health care workers,* New Haven, 1998, Yale.

Kelland B, Jordan L: *CommuniMed: multilingual patient assessment manual,* ed 3, St Louis, 1994, Mosby.

Nasr I, Cordero M: *Medical Spanish,* Philadelphia, 1996, WB Saunders.

NANDA–Approved Nursing Diagnoses (2001-2002)

Activity intolerance
Activity intolerance, risk for
Adjustment, impaired
Airway clearance, ineffective
Allergy response, latex
Allergy response, risk for latex
Anxiety
Anxiety, death
Aspiration, risk for
Attachment, risk for impaired
    parent/infant/child
Autonomic dysreflexia
Autonomic dysreflexia, risk for
Body image, disturbed
Body temperature, risk for imbalanced
Bowel incontinence
Breast-feeding, effective
Breast-feeding, ineffective
Breast-feeding, interrupted
Breathing pattern, ineffective
Cardiac output, decreased
Caregiver role strain
Caregiver role strain, risk for
Communication, impaired verbal
Conflict, decisional
Conflict, parental role
Confusion, acute
Confusion, chronic
Constipation
Constipation, perceived
Constipation, risk for
Coping, ineffective
Coping, ineffective community
Coping, readiness for enhanced community
Coping, defensive
Coping, compromised family
Coping, disabled family
Coping, readiness for enhanced family
Denial, ineffective
Dentition, impaired
Development, risk for delayed
Diarrhea
Disuse syndrome, risk for
Diversional activity, deficient
Energy field, disturbed
Environmental interpretation syndrome,
    impaired
Failure to thrive, adult
Falls, risk for
Family processes, dysfunctional: alcoholism
Family processes, interrupted
Fatigue
Fear
Fluid volume, deficient
Fluid volume, excess

Fluid volume, risk for deficient
Fluid volume, risk for imbalanced
Gas exchange, impaired
Grieving, anticipatory
Grieving, dysfunctional
Growth and development, delayed
Growth, risk for disproportionate
Health maintenance, ineffective
Health-seeking behaviors
Home maintenance, impaired
Hopelessness
Hyperthermia
Hypothermia
Identity, disturbed personal
Incontinence, functional urinary
Incontinence, reflex urinary
Incontinence, stress urinary
Incontinence, total urinary
Incontinence, urge urinary
Incontinence, risk for urge urinary
Infant behavior, disorganized
Infant behavior, risk for disorganized
Infant behavior, readiness for enhanced
    organized
Infant feeding pattern, ineffective
Infection, risk for
Injury, risk for
Injury, risk for perioperative-positioning
Intracranial adaptive capacity, decreased
Knowledge, deficient
Loneliness, risk for
Memory, impaired
Mobility, impaired bed
Mobility, impaired physical
Mobility, impaired wheelchair
Nausea
Neglect, unilateral
Noncompliance
Nutrition, imbalanced: less than body
    requirements
Nutrition, imbalanced: more than body
    requirements
Nutrition, risk for imbalanced: more than
    body requirements
Oral mucous membrane, impaired
Pain, acute
Pain, chronic
Parenting, impaired
Parenting, risk for impaired
Peripheral neurovascular dysfunction,
    risk for
Poisoning, risk for
Post-trauma syndrome
Post-trauma syndrome, risk for
Powerlessness

Powerlessness, risk for
Protection, ineffective
Rape-trauma syndrome
Rape-trauma syndrome: compound reaction
Rape-trauma syndrome: silent reaction
Relocation stress syndrome
Relocation stress syndrome, risk for
Role performance, ineffective
Self-care deficit, bathing/hygiene
Self-care deficit, dressing/grooming
Self-care deficit, feeding
Self-care deficit, toileting
Self-esteem, chronic low
Self-esteem, situational low
Self-esteem, risk for situational low
Self-mutilation
Self-mutilation, risk for
Sensory perception, disturbed
Sexual dysfunction
Sexuality patterns, ineffective
Skin integrity, impaired
Skin integrity, risk for impaired
Sleep deprivation
Sleep pattern, disturbed
Social interaction, impaired
Social isolation
Sorrow, chronic
Spiritual distress
Spiritual distress, risk for
Spiritual well-being, readiness for enhanced
Suffocation, risk for
Suicide, risk for
Surgical recovery, delayed
Swallowing, impaired
Therapeutic regimen management, effective
Therapeutic regimen management,
    ineffective
Therapeutic regimen management,
    ineffective community
Therapeutic regimen management,
    ineffective family
Thermoregulation, ineffective
Thought processes, disturbed
Tissue integrity, impaired
Tissue perfusion, ineffective
Transfer ability, impaired
Trauma, risk for
Urinary elimination, impaired
Urinary retention
Ventilation, impaired spontaneous
Ventilatory weaning response, dysfunctional
Violence, risk for other-directed
Violence, risk for self-directed
Walking, impaired
Wandering

From North American Nursing Diagnosis Association: *Nursing diagnosis: definitions and classification* 2001-2002, Philadelphia, 2001, Nursecom.